P9-EDX-359

Diagnostic
Medical Sonography
A Guide to Clinical Practice
SECOND EDITION

OBSTETRICS AND GYNECOLOGY

Diagnostic Medical Sonography

A Guide to Clinical Practice

SECOND EDITION

SERIES EDITORS

Mimi C. Berman, Ph.D., R.D.M.S.
Professor Emeritus
College of Health Related Professions
State University of New York
Health Science Center at Brooklyn
Brooklyn, New York

Diane M. Kawamura, Ph.D, R.T.(R), R.D.M.S.
Professor, Radiologic Sciences
College of Health Professions
Weber State University
Ogden, Utah

Marveen Craig, R.D.M.S.
Author, Lecturer, Private Consultant
Dallas, Texas

Mark Allen, M.B.A., R.D.C.S., R.D.M.S.
Chief Cardiac Sonographer and Administrator
Echocardiography Laboratory and Mobile Cardiovascular
 Imaging Sciences
University of Rochester
Rochester, New York

OBSTETRICS
AND
GYNECOLOGY

SECOND EDITION

EDITED BY

Mimi C. Berman, Ph.D., R.D.M.S.

Professor Emeritus
College of Health Related Professions
State University of New York
Health Science Center at Brooklyn
Brooklyn, New York

Harris L. Cohen, M.D., F.A.C.R.

Professor of Clinical Radiology
State University of New York
Health Science Center at Brooklyn
Brooklyn, New York

With 59 additional contributors

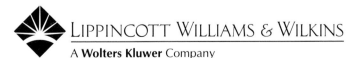

LIPPINCOTT WILLIAMS & WILKINS
A **Wolters Kluwer** Company
Philadelphia • Baltimore • New York • London
Buenos Aires • Hong Kong • Sydney • Tokyo

Acquisitions Editor: Lawrence McGrew
Editorial Assistant: Holly Collins
Senior Production Editor: Virginia Barishek
Production Service: P.M. Gordon Associates, Inc.
Compositor: Tapsco, Inc.

Color Separator: Chroma Graphics
Insert Printer: The Sheridan Press
Printer/Binder: The Maple Press Company
Cover Designer: William T. Donnelly
Cover Printer: Lehigh Press

Second Edition

Copyright © 1997 by Lippincott–Raven Publishers. Copyright © 1991 by J.B. Lippincott Company. All rights reserved. This book is protected by copyright. No part of it may be reproduced, stored in a retrieval system, or transmitted, in any form or by any means—electronic, mechanical, photocopy, recording, or otherwise—without the prior written consent of the publisher, except for brief quotations embodied in critical articles and reviews. Printed in The United States of America. For information write Lippincott Williams & Wilkins 227 East Washington Square, Philadelphia, PA 19106-3780.

Materials appearing in this book prepared by individuals as part of their official duties as U.S. Government employees are not covered by the above-mentioned copyright.

Library of Congress Cataloging-in-Publication Data

Obstetrics and gynecology / edited by Mimi C. Berman and Harris L. Cohen—2nd ed.
     p.   cm.—(Diagnostic medical sonography ; v. 1)
     Includes bibliographical references and index.
    ISBN-13: 978-0-397-55261-0
    ISBN-10: 0-397-55261-0
    1. Ultrasonics in obstetrics.   2. Generative organs, Female—Ultrasonic imaging.
I. Berman, Mimi C.   II. Cohen, Harris L.   III. Series: Diagnostic medical
sonography (2nd ed.) ; v. 1.
    [DNLM: 1. Genital Diseases, Female—ultrasonography.
2. Ultrasonography—in pregnancy.   WB 289 D5355 1997 v. 1 / WB 289
D5355   1997 v. 1]
RC78.8.U4D48   1997 vol. 1
[RG527.5]
616.07′543 s—dc21
[618′.047543]
DNLM/DLC
for Library of Congress   96–39954
                                                                                  CIP

Care has been taken to confirm the accuracy of the information presented and to describe generally accepted practices. However, the authors, editors, and publisher are not responsible for errors or omissions or for any consequences from application of the information in this book and make no warranty, express or implied, with respect to the contents of the publication.

The authors, editors, and publisher have exerted every effort to ensure that drug selection and dosage set forth in this text are in accordance with current recommendations and practice at the time of publication. However, in view of ongoing research, changes in government regulations, and the constant flow of information relating to drug therapy and drug reactions, the reader is urged to check the package insert for each drug for any change in indications and dosage and for added warnings and precautions. This is particularly important when the recommended agent is a new or infrequently employed drug.

Some drugs and medical devices presented in this publication have Food and Drug Administration (FDA) clearance for limited use in restricted research settings. It is the responsibility of the health care provider to ascertain the FDA status of each drug or device planned for use in their clinical practice.

9 8 7

To all the sonographers and physicians who undertook the challenging assignment of updating their chapters or who adopted an equally difficult task—revising chapters initially written by others. Most of the authors are full-time clinicians or educators who were willing to spend precious time and energy documenting their expertise for the benefit of fledgling ultrasound practitioners. Without sonographers and sonologists such as they, our profession would not be as popular as it is today.

To my husband, Marvin, who has cheerfully tolerated and encouraged me during the preparation of this edition. It would have been difficult, if not impossible, to complete it without his warm, accepting attitude. To Bogart, whose furry being was the needed distraction to preserve my equilibrium.

To my father, who has left me with memories of his gentle, wise nature, and to my mother and friend, for giving me love, education, and a home that provided the foundation for everything I have accomplished thus far.

To my colleagues and students whose appreciation of the first edition encouraged me to undertake this second edition.

Mimi C. Berman, PhD, RDMS

To Sandra W. Cohen, MD—my wife, a penultimate internist, ethicist, and mother and the "Grove Avenue Kids": David Mathew, Lauren Elizabeth, and Benjamin Cohen who bear with me as I continue to tilt with academic radiology's windmills now strewn within the uncertain fields of managed care. I owe you a lot.

To Samuel "G" Cohen and in memory of Esther Leah bas Elazar Hertz nee Altman who built new, if not easy, lives along Emma Lazarus' welcoming shores and in an America that has enjoyed great benefits from those who live its dreams and take advantage of its opportunities.

To Phil B. who taught me to weigh and measure my deeds.

To my Chairmen, Drs. Joshua A. Becker, Harry L. Stein, and Irwin Bluth who allowed me to burn the candle at both ends.

To my Ultrasound and Radiology mentors and colleagues, including a fine array of sonographers, diagnostic radiology residents, and imaging fellows, who have reinforced my view that the best imagers combine an inquisitive mind, careful clinical and imaging correlation and judgment, tempered enthusiasm, and a concern for the patient as a human being.

To my Clinical colleagues and mentors in Obstetrics and Gynecology, Pediatric Surgery, Urology, and Pediatric Medicine who have inspired, encouraged, and even provoked me into making those all-important diagnoses on those all-important and very real patients . . . which reminds me. . . .

To my patients and their families—they are what it is all about.

Harris L. Cohen, MD

Contributors

Dunstan Abraham, MPH, PA-C, RDMS
Staff Physician Assistant
Primary Care Clinic
Beth Israel Medical Center
New York, NY
Sonographer
Bronx Lebanon Hospital
Bronx, NY

Tamara Allen, BS, RDMS
Sonographer, Obstetrics and Gynecology
University of Rochester
Strong Memorial Hospital
Perinatal Ultrasound
Rochester, NY

Birgit Bader-Armstrong, BS, RDMS
Adjunct Faculty
Rochester Institute of Technology
Allied Health Department
Diagnostic Medical Sonography Program
Rochester, NY

Frances R. Batzer, MD
Associate Clinical Professor
Obstetrics and Gynecology
Thomas Jefferson University School of Medicine
Attending Physician
Department of Obstetrics and Gynecology
Pennsylvania Hospital, St. Mary's Hospital
Philadelphia, PA

Carol B. Benson, MD
Associate Professor of Radiology
Harvard Medical School
Department of Radiology
Brigham and Women's Hospital
Boston, MA

Mimi C. Berman, PhD, RDMS
Professor Emeritus
College of Health Related Professions
State University of New York
Health Science Center at Brooklyn
Brooklyn, NY

Michael L. Blumenfeld, MD
Associate Clinical Professor
Department of Obstetrics and Gynecology
Director, Division of General Obstetrics and
  Gynecology
The Ohio State University
Columbus, OH

Luis A. Bracero, MD
Director of Maternal-Fetal Medicine/Obstetrics and
  Gynecology
Maimonides Medical Center
Brooklyn, NY

Frank Cervantes, BA, BS, RDMS
Associate Director of Radiography
Supervisor, Division of Ultrasound
State University of New York
Health Science Center at Brooklyn
Brooklyn, NY

Linda M. Chase, BS, RDMS, RDCS
Assistant Professor
Diagnostic Medical Imaging Program
College of Health Related Professions
State University of New York
Health Science Center at Brooklyn
Brooklyn, NY

Frank A. Chervenak, MD
Director of Obstetrics
Director of Maternal-Fetal Medicine
Department of Obstetrics and Gynecology
The New York Hospital-Cornell Medical Center
New York, NY

Harris L. Cohen, MD, FACR
Professor of Clinical Radiology
State University of New York
Health Science Center at Brooklyn
Director
Division of Ultrasound
University and Kings County Hospitals of Brooklyn
Brooklyn, New York

Marveen Craig, RDMS
Author, Lecturer, Private Consultant
Dallas, TX

Dale R. Cyr, BS, RDMS, RDCS
Diagnostic Sonographer
Department of Radiology
Division of Diagnostic Ultrasound
University of Washington Medical Center
Seattle, WA

Marie DeLange, RT(R), BS, RDMS, RDCS
Program Director/Ultrasound Vascular Manager
Loma Linda University Medical Center
Loma Linda, CA

Mark A. Dennis, MD
Radiologist
Radiology Imaging Associates
Englewood, CO

Dail A. De Souza, BA, BS, RDMS
Sonographer
UMDNJ/Robert Wood Johnson Medical School
St. Peters Medical Center
New Brunswick, NJ

Peter M. Doubilet, MD
Associate Professor of Radiology
Harvard Medical School
Co-Director of Ultrasound
Co-Director of High Risk Obstetrical Ultrasound
Department of Radiology
Brigham and Women's Hospital
Boston, MA

Julia A. Drose, BA, RDMS, RDCS
Chief Technologist
Ultrasound Department
Senior Instructor
University of Colorado Health Science Center
Denver, CO

Terry J. DuBose, MS, RDMS, RT(R)
Program Director, Diagnostic Medical Sonography
Assistant Professor
Department of Radiologic Technology
College of Health Related Professions
University of Arkansas for Medical Sciences
Little Rock, AR

Pamela M. Foy, BS, RDMS
Clinical Coordinator of Ultrasound Services
Department of Obstetrics and Gynecology
The Ohio State University
Columbus, OH

Mary Beth Geagan, BS, RT(R), RDMS
Ultrasound Supervisor
Roosevelt Site O
St. Luke's–Roosevelt Hospital Center
New York, NY

Linda W. Graves, RDMS, RVT
Staff Sonographer
Radiology
University Hospital
State University of New York
Health Science Center
Syracuse, NY

William M. Greenhut, BA, RDMS
Supervisor, Department of Ultrasound
Radiology Department
Montefiore Medical Center
Bronx, NY

Gerald L. Grube, MD
Assistant Professor of Radiology
School of Medicine
Loma Linda University
Director of Outpatient Ultrasound
Loma Linda Medical Center
Loma Linda, CA

Warren G. Guntheroth, MD
Professor
Department of Pediatrics (Cardiology)
Attending Pediatric Cardiologist
University of Washington School of Medicine
Seattle, WA

Edith D. Gurewitsch, MD
Division of Maternal-Fetal Medicine
The New York Hospital/Cornell Medical Center
New York, NY

Rebecca Hall, PhD, RDMS
Program Director
Department of Radiology
Medical Imaging Programs
University of New Mexico, School of Medicine
Albuquerque, NM

Jack O. Haller, MD
Professor of Radiology
Director Pediatric Radiology
State University of New York Health Science Center
    at Brooklyn
Brooklyn, New York

Diane M. Kawamura, PhD, RT(R), RDMS
Professor, Radiologic Sciences
College of Health Professions
Weber State University
Ogden, UT

Harry J. Khamis, PhD
Director and Professor, Math and Statistics
Math Department
Statistical Consulting Center
Wright State University
Dayton, OH

Mordecai Koenigsberg, MD
Director of Ultrasound
Unified Department of Radiology
Albert Einstein College of Medicine and Affiliated
    Hospitals
Bronx, NY

Rosalyn Kutcher, MD, FACR
Professor of Radiology
Director of Ultrasound
Montefiore Medical Center, Moses Division
Associate Director of Sonography
Albert Einstein College of Medicine
Bronx, NY

Ji-Bin Liu, MD
Research Assistant, Professor of Radiology
Department of Radiology
Division of Diagnostic Ultrasound
Thomas Jefferson University Hospital
Philadelphia, PA

Laurence B. McCullough, PhD
Professor of Medicine, Community Medicine and
    Medical Ethics
Center for Medical Ethics and Health Policy
Baylor College of Medicine
Houston, TX
Adjunct Professor of Ethics in Obstetrics and
    Gynecology
Cornell University Medical College
New York, NY

Joyce A. Miller, MA, RDMS
Assistant Professor
Diagnostic Medical Imaging Program
State University of New York
Health Science Center at Brooklyn
Brooklyn, New York

Dara Muller, MBA, RDMS
Coordinating Manager
Division of Ultrasound
Kings County Hospital
Brooklyn, NY

Susan E. Nealer, BS, RDMS
Chief Sonographer, Department of Radiology
State University of New York
Health Science Center at Syracuse
Syracuse, NY

Wayne Persutte, BS, RDMS
Instructor and Co-Director
Perinatal Research
Prenatal Diagnostic and Genetics
Department of Obstetrics and Gynecology
University of Colorado Health Science Center
Denver, CO

Lawrence D. Platt, MD
Professor of Obstetrics and Gynecology
UCLA School of Medicine
Chairman, Department of Obstetrics and
    Gynecology
Cedars-Sinai Medical Center
Los Angeles, CA

Joanne C. Rosenberg, BS, RDMS
Parinatal Ultrasound Manager
UMDNJ/Robert Wood Johnson Medical School
St. Peters Medical Center
New Brunswick, NJ

Ruth Rosenblatt, MD, FACR
Professor
Department of Radiology
Albert Einstein College of Medicine
Montefiore Medical Center
Bronx, NY

Shraga Rottem, MD, Dsc
Associate Professor
Department of Obstetrics and Gynecology
State University of New York
Health Science Center at Brooklyn
Brooklyn, NY
International Registry of Fetal Anomalies
    (IRONFAN)

James E. Schneider, MS, RDMS, RT
Lecturer
Department of Cell Biology, Neurobiology, and
    Anatomy
The Ohio State University
Columbus, OH

Judy Schwartz, BS, RDMS
Staff Sonographer
Ultrasound Department
Kings County Hospital
Brooklyn, NY

Karin M. Smith, BS, RDMS
Diagnostic Sonographer
Department of Radiology
Division of Diagnostic Ultrasound
University of Washington Medical Center
Seattle, WA

George I. Solish, MD, PhD
Professor
Department of Obstetrics and Gynecology
State University of New York
Health Science Center at Brooklyn
Brooklyn, NY

Beverly A. Spirt, MD, FACR
Professor of Radiology
Professor of Obstetrics and Gynecology
State University of New York
Health Science Center
Syracuse, NY

Jean Lea Spitz, MPH, RDMS
Professor and Chairman
Department of Radiologic Technology
University of Oklahoma Health Sciences Center
Oklahoma City, OK

Jane Streltzoff, BS, RDMS
Research Associate/Chief Sonographer
Division of Maternal-Fetal Medicine
Department of Obstetrics and Gynecology
Cornell Medical Center/New York Hospital
New York, NY

Maria Sykora, RDMS, RTR
Staff Sonographer
Department of Radiology
State University of New York
Health Science Center at Syracuse
Division of Diagnostic Radiology
Syracuse, NY

Phil-Ann Tan-Sinn, RT, RDMS, RDCS
Diagnostic Ultrasound Specialist
Loma Linda University Medical Center
Loma Linda, CA

Jean M. Torrisi, MD
Assistant Professor
Department of Radiology
State University of New York
Health Science Center at Brooklyn
Brooklyn, NY

Larry Waldroup, BS, RDMS
Technical Manager
Manager of Jefferson Ultrasound Research and
    Education Institute
Division of Diagnostic Ultrasound
Department of Radiology
Thomas Jefferson University Hospital
Philadelphia, PA

Catherine A. Walla, RN, MA, MNA
Coordinator of Clinical Research
Cedars-Sinai Medical Center
Department of Obstetrics and Gynecology
Assistant Clinical Professor
UCLA School of Nursing
Los Angeles, CA

Roger W. Warner, MS, RDMS
Vice President of Physician Services
St. James Hospital and Health Center
Chicago Heights, IL

Yansheng Wei, BS, RDMS, RDCS
Sonographer
Obstetrics and Gynecology
New York Methodist Hospital
Brooklyn, NY

Thomas C. Winter, III, MD
Assistant Professor
Department of Radiology
Director, Diagnostic Ultrasound
University of Washington
Seattle, WA

Paula S. Woletz, BA, RDMS, RDCS
Supervisor, Division of Maternal-Fetal Medicine
Fetal Evaluation Unit
St. Luke's–Roosevelt Hospital Center
New York, NY

Diana Kawai Yankowitz, BS, RDMS, RDCS
Staff Sonographer
Department of Obstetrics and Gynecology
University of Iowa Hospital and Clinics
Iowa City, IA

Daniel L. Zinn, MD
Assistant Professor
Department of Radiology
State University of New York
Health Science Center at Brooklyn
Brooklyn, NY

Preface

When the first edition of *Diagnostic Medical Sonography* was published in 1991, diagnostic ultrasound had begun to be more readily recognized and accepted by the general public—after more than 30 years of clinical use. Now it is a household word, in large part because just about every female member of every American family has had or will have a sonogram during her lifetime. In this manner, for most people, obstetrical/gynecologic ultrasound has been the overture to the many movements of our ever broadening field. The field of ultrasonography is an unfinished symphony which continues to be written by newer technological developments and innovative clinical applications. In obstetrics we may believe we have almost reached the denouement of our ability to visualize two-dimensional details, but our potential to study the physiology of the fetus is accelerating through the use of power Doppler combined with transvaginal ultrasound. And the field of three-dimensional imaging is in its infancy. New developments in gynecologic ultrasound include sonohysterography in combination with saline or contrast agents, continuing investigation of the value of various forms of Doppler in diagnosing malignancies, and ultrasound's ability to observe the uterine and ovarian anatomical changes necessary for successful ovum implantation. These and other new developments have been incorporated into our book's didactic discussions of the major areas of obstetrical and gynecologic diagnostic ultrasound. Our goal has been to provide a comprehensive discussion of each topic including anatomy, pathophysiology, sonographic theory, and sonographic technique along with representative ultrasonographic images. This text is intended to serve as both an introduction to obstetrical/gynecologic ultrasound and as a long-term on-your-shelf reference. Writing this second edition has permitted us to improve on the first by incorporating suggestions you have offered. We hope you find this edition useful and we continue to welcome your comments.

Mimi C. Berman, PhD, RDMS
Harris L. Cohen, MD, FACR
Diane M. Kawamura, PhD, RT(R), RDMS
Marveen Craig, RDMS
Mark N. Allen, MBA, RDCS, RDMS

Contents

xvii

PART III
**Psychosocial, Professional, and
Technical Topics**

List of Tables

Diagnostic Medical Sonography

A Guide to Clinical Practice

SECOND EDITION

OBSTETRICS AND **GYNECOLOGY**

PART I

Gynecologic Sonography

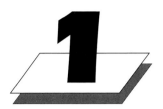

1

Principles of Scanning Technique in Obstetric and Gynecologic Ultrasound

MIMI C. BERMAN and DIANA KAWAI YANKOWITZ

Proper technique is essential to produce an optimally diagnostic gynecologic or obstetric sonogram. Optimizing the examination improves cost effectiveness, reduces exposure to ultrasound energy, and minimizes discomfort for the patient. Some of the art of scanning has disappeared with the retirement of the static scanner, but the importance of a scientific approach to each examination has increased with the advent of real-time, Doppler, and other new technologies as well as with the introduction of transvaginal and other new transducers. Although manipulation of the equipment has become easier, the production of diagnostic images now requires better knowledge of normal and abnormal anatomy, the disease processes being imaged, and the sonographic data that can be obtained. More than ever, it is imperative that sonographers develop a systematic approach in their scanning to ensure obtaining a complete study. Unlike our predecessors, sonographers today have the benefit of a large body of research and experience that provides guidelines on technique and diagnostic criteria.

In this chapter, the basic techniques and protocols of scanning in obstetrics and gynecology are described. A brief discussion of emerging techniques is also included. Routines specific to the topics discussed are explained in greater detail in subsequent chapters.

Patient Preparation

GYNECOLOGIC EXAMINATIONS

A full urinary bladder has become the hallmark of obstetric and gynecologic scanning (Fig. 1-1). Instructions to a patient on how to prepare for an examination should be tailored to the patient, the examination objectives, and the transducer type. A premenopausal woman who is to be examined for a possible ovarian cyst can be instructed to eat normally, void, and then drink four 8-ounce glasses of water 1 hour before the examination and not void again until after the examination. These directions should ensure that she will be properly prepared for the study. A postmenopausal woman in her 60s or 70s who is scheduled because of uterine bleeding may have decreased bladder capacity or may suffer from incontinence.[46] The directions to her could be modified by asking her to drink only three 8-ounce glasses of water. If a patient is scheduled for a transvaginal examination, no urinary blad-

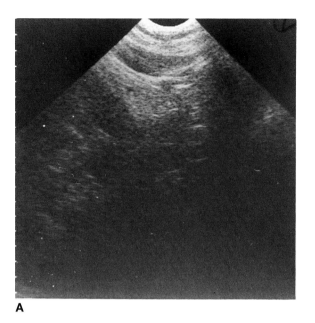

A

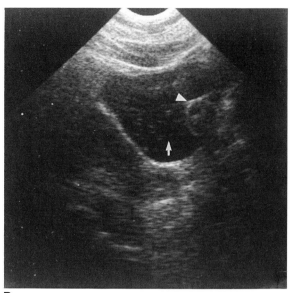

B

C

Figure 1-1. (A) This sagittal transabdominal scan through an empty bladder does not visualize the uterus and adnexa. **(B)** The bladder has been partially filled with saline. Although the uterus is visualized better, the bladder is not filled enough to allow complete evaluation of the fundal region. The balloon (*arrowhead*) from the Foley catheter can be seen, as can echoes (*arrow*) produced by the air that entered the bladder with the fluid. **(C)** With the bladder adequately filled, the fundus (*arrow*) can be evaluated, as can the echogenicity of the myometrium and endometrium (*arrowhead*, balloon from the catheter).

der filling is required unless a transabdominal scan is to be performed before the transvaginal examination.

An adequately filled bladder usually extends slightly beyond the fundus of a nongravid uterus. If the uterus and adnexa are clearly delineated, the bladder is full enough; if not, the patient should be instructed to drink more water or wait for her bladder to fill more. Patient positioning techniques may be particularly helpful with a less than optimally filled bladder. Ask the patient to lie in a left or right posterior oblique position, so that the bladder drapes over the structure of interest, such as the lateral section of the uterus, the adnexa, or a mass.

If the patient's bladder is so distended that it compresses and displaces the pelvic viscera, or the patient cannot tolerate the examination, have her partially empty by giving her a cup and telling her how many cups she may void. Many patients are skeptical of their ability to stop the flow of urine, but most are successful.

In many cases, it is possible to evaluate most of the low-lying pelvic structures with an empty urinary bladder by using a transvaginal transducer. The transabdominal approach is used primarily to rule out pelvic masses that are beyond the imaging range of the transvaginal transducer.

OBSTETRIC EXAMINATIONS

The degree of bladder filling required depends on the stage of gestation. In the first trimester, a full bladder is needed for transabdominal scanning because the air-filled intestines have not been pushed out of the false pelvis by the uterus and therefore obstruct sound beam penetration (Fig. 1-2). Once the second trimester begins, it is usually not necessary for the patient to have a full bladder because the uterus fills the pelvic cavity and displaces the intestines.[43]

A moderately filled bladder enhances visualization of the internal os by providing an unobstructed view of that area.[41] This is useful when assessing competency of the internal os, in determining placental position relative to the os when there is a low-lying placenta, and in displacing a low fetal head upward into a position where the biparietal diameter can be measured. Transvaginal or perineal studies enable the sonographer to evaluate the cervix or presenting fetal part[63] in more detail than may be possible by the transabdominal approach.

Getting Set Up

When the patient arrives for her sonographic examination, the sonographer should introduce him- or herself, confirm the patient's identity, and inform her about the examination procedure. It is a good idea to ask her why she has been sent for the examination, because on occasion, the request form may be incomplete. Tell her approximately how long the study will take, what she may expect to feel, and where and how the transducer will be moved.

All pertinent clinical information should be included on the ultrasound report. This includes patient age, date of the last menstrual period (LMP; also whether it was normal), gravidity, parity, symptoms such as pain or bleeding, history of pelvic procedures, and any other pertinent medical or surgical history. This information should be obtained from the patient if it is not on the examination request. It is desirable to obtain this information

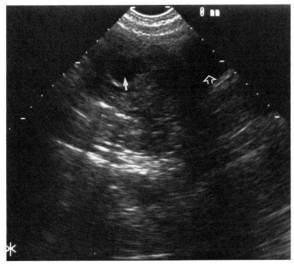
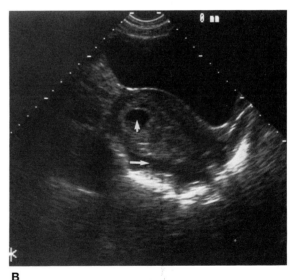

A   B

Figure 1-2. (A) The urinary bladder *(open arrow)* has a small amount of urine in it, but not enough to determine whether the fluid-filled structure *(short arrow)* is a gestational sac and whether it is within or outside the uterus. **(B)** The uterus with the fundal gestational sac *(arrow)* can now be clearly delineated because the bladder is full. A cul-de-sac fluid collection *(long arrow)* is also apparent.

Display 1-1.   Guidelines for the Performance of the Antepartum Obstetrical Ultrasound Examination

GUIDELINES FOR FIRST TRIMESTER SONOGRAPHY

Overall Comment. Scanning in the first trimester may be performed either abdominally, vaginally, or using both methods. If an abdominal examination is performed and fails to provide diagnostic information, a vaginal scan should be done when possible. Similarly, if a vaginal scan is performed and fails to image all areas needed for diagnosis, an abdominal scan should be performed.

1. The uterus and adnexa should be evaluated for the presence of a gestational sac. If a gestational sac is seen, its location should be documented. The presence or absence of an embryo should be noted and the crown–rump length recorded.

Comment. (1) Crown–rump length is a more accurate indicator of gestational age than gestational sac diameter. If the embryo is not identified, the gestational sac should be evaluated for the presence of a yolk sac. The estimate of gestational age should then be based on either the mean diameter of the gestational sac or on the morphology and contents of the gestational sac.
(2) Identification of a yolk sac or an embryo is definitive evidence of a gestational sac. Caution should be used in making a definitive diagnosis of gestational sac prior to the development of such structures. Without these findings an intrauterine fluid collection can sometimes represent a pseudogestational sac associated with an ectopic pregnancy.
(3) During the late first trimester, biparietal diameter and other fetal measurements also may be used to establish fetal age.

2. Presence or absence of cardiac activity should be reported.

Comment. (1) Real-time observation is critical for this diagnosis.
(2) With vaginal scans, cardiac motion should be appreciated by a crown–rump length of 5 mm or greater. If an embryo less than 5 mm in length is seen with no cardiac activity, a follow-up scan may be needed to evaluate for fetal life.

3. Fetal number should be documented.

Comment. Multiple pregnancies should be reported only in those instances where multiple embryos are seen. Occasionally, more than one sac-like structure may be seen early in pregnancy and incorrectly thought to represent multiple gestations, owing to incomplete fusion between the amnion and chorion, or elevation of the chorionic membrane by intrauterine hemorrhage.

4. Evaluation of the uterus, adnexal structures, and cul-de-sac should be performed.

Comment. (1) This will allow recognition of incidental findings of potential clinical significance. The presence, location, and size of myomas and adnexal masses should be recorded. The cul-de-sac should be scanned for presence or absence of fluid. If there is fluid in the cul-de-sac, the flanks and subhepatic space should be scanned for intraabdominal fluid.
(2) Because differentiation of normal pregnancy from abnormal pregnancy and ectopic pregnancy can be difficult, the correlation of serum hormonal levels with ultrasound findings often is helpful.

GUIDELINES FOR SECOND AND THIRD TRIMESTER SONOGRAPHY

1. Fetal life, number, presentation, and activity should be documented.

Comment. (1) Abnormal heart rate and/or rhythm should be reported.
(2) Multiple pregnancies require the documentation of additional information: number of gestational sacs, number of placentas, presence or absence of a dividing membrane, fetal genitalia (if visible), comparison of fetal sizes, and comparison of amniotic fluid volume on each side of the membrane.

2. An estimate of amniotic fluid volume (increased, decreased, normal) should be reported.

Comment. Physiologic variation with stage of pregnancy should be considered in assessing the appropriateness of amniotic fluid volume.

3. The placental location, appearance, and its relationship to the internal cervical os should be recorded. The umbilical cord should be imaged.

(continued)

Display 1-1. (Continued)

Comment. (1) It is recognized that apparent placental position early in pregnancy may not correlate well with its location at the time of delivery.
(2) An overdistended maternal urinary bladder or a lower uterine contraction can give the examiner a false impression of placenta previa.
(3) Abdominal, transperineal, or vaginal views may be helpful in visualizing the internal cervical os and its relationship to the placenta.

4. Assessment of gestational age should be accomplished at the time of the initial scan using a combination of cranial measurement such as the biparietal diameter or head circumference, and limb measurement such as the femur length.

Comment. (1) Third trimester measurements may not accurately reflect gestational age. If one or more previous studies have been performed, the gestational age at the time of the current examination should be based on the earliest examination that permits accurate measurement of crown–rump length, biparietal diameter, head circumference, and/or femur length by the equation: current fetal age = estimated age at time of initial study + number of weeks elapsed since first study.
(2) Measurements of structurally abnormal fetal body parts (such as the head in a fetus with hydrocephalus or the limbs in a fetus with a skeletal dysplasia) should not be used in the calculation of estimated gestational age.

4A. The standard reference level for measurement of the biparietal diameter is an axial image that includes the thalamus.

Comment. If the fetal head is dolichocephalic or brachycephalic, the biparietal diameter measurement may be misleading. Occasionally, computation of the cephalic index, a ratio of the biparietal diameter to fronto-occipital diameter, will be needed to make this determination. In such situations, other measurements of head size, such as the head circumference, may be necessary.

4B. Head circumference is measured at the same level as the biparietal diameter, around the outer perimeter of the calvarium.

4C. Femur length should be routinely measured and recorded after the 14th week of gestation.

Comment. As with head measurements, there is considerable biological variation in normal femur lengths late in pregnancy.

5. Fetal weight should be estimated in the late second and in the third trimesters and requires the measurement of abdominal diameter or circumference.

5A. Abdominal circumference should be determined on a true transverse view, preferably at the level of the junction of the left and right portal veins.

Comment. Abdominal circumference measurement is necessary to estimate fetal weight and may allow detection of growth retardation and macrosomia.

5B. If previous fetal biometric studies have been performed, an estimate of the appropriateness of interval growth should be given.

6. Evaluation of the uterus (including the cervix) and adnexal structures should be performed.

Comment. This will allow recognition of incidental findings of potential clinical significance. The presence, location, and size of myomas and adnexal masses should be recorded. It is frequently not possible to image the maternal ovaries during the second and third trimesters. Vaginal or transperineal scanning may be helpful in evaluating the cervix when the fetal head prevents visualization of the cervix from transabdominal scanning.

(continued)

Display 1-1. (Continued)

7. The study should include, but not necessarily be limited to, assessment of the following fetal anatomy: cerebral ventricles, posterior fossa (including cerebellar hemispheres and cisterna magna), four-chamber view of the heart (including its position within the thorax), spine, stomach, kidneys, urinary bladder, fetal umbilical cord insertion site and intactness of the anterior abdominal wall. While not considered part of the minimum required examination, when fetal position permits, it is desirable to examine all areas of the anatomy.

Comment. (1) It is recognized that not all malformations of the above-mentioned organ systems can be detected using ultrasonography. (2) These recommendations should be considered a minimum guideline for the fetal anatomic survey. Occasionally some of these structures may not be well visualized, as occurs when fetal position, low amniotic volume, or maternal body habitus limit the sonographic examination. When this occurs, the report of the ultrasound examination should include a notation delineating structures that were not well seen. (3) Suspected abnormalities may require a targeted evaluation of the area(s) of concern.

(American Institute of Ultrasound in Medicine. Guidelines for Performance of the Antepartum Obstretical Ultrasound Examination. Laurel, MD: AIUM; 1994.)

before beginning the examination to minimize the chance that the patient will conclude the questions are related to something the sonographer is seeing on the screen.

Knowing the patient's reproductive history gives the sonographer information with which to design and interpret the sonographic examination. Although variations of the obstetric coding system may be used, the following is the most common: *Gravidity* (G) refers to the number of pregnancies the patient has had and includes the current one. A pregnant woman who had a nonviable ectopic pregnancy and later gave birth to twins would be G3. *Parity* (P) refers to the number of pregnancies the patient has carried to term; thus, an ectopic pregnancy would be recorded as PO and a twin gestation would be P1. The numbers used after P refer, in order, to the number of term pregnancies, premature deliveries, abortions (spontaneous or induced), and living children. Thus, G3P1012 would mean the woman has had three pregnancies, one full-term pregnancy, no premature deliveries, one abortion (the ectopic pregnancy in this case), and two full-term births, in this case, a set of twins.[25]

It is generally accepted that the first day of the LMP is used to date pregnancies. The LMP usually occurs about 2 weeks before conception. The LMP is chosen because women can document this date. Still, some 20% to 40% of pregnant women are

uncertain of their LMP, so this date may be unreliable for dating a pregnancy. Ultrasound can narrow the estimated date of delivery, also referred to as estimated date of confinement, to as little as ±2.7 days by using the average of at least three crown–rump length measurements.[27]

After all pertinent clinical information is obtained, the patient should be assisted onto the examination table and made as comfortable as possible. A pillow or two under the patient's knees relieves back strain. For a transabdominal examination, gel should be applied liberally to the lower abdomen to provide an effective medium for sound transmission. The gel should be warmed to body temperature to minimize patient discomfort. If a laboratory is not equipped with a gel warmer, the gel may be warmed carefully (it should not be too hot!) in a microwave oven. If it is anticipated that a transvaginal examination will be necessary, the patient should be given privacy while she takes everything from the waist down off and drapes herself with a sheet.

Every laboratory should develop scanning protocols for each type of examination. These should be printed in a reference manual. Suggested protocols have been developed for obstetric and gynecologic scanning by the American Institute of Ultrasound in Medicine (AIUM; Displays 1-1 and 1-2). The Society of Diagnostic Medical Sonographers'

Display 1-2.   Guidelines for Performance of the Ultrasound Examination of the Female Pelvis

The following guidelines describe the examination to be performed for each organ and anatomic region in the female pelvis. All relevant structures should be identified by the abdominal and/or vaginal approach. If an abdominal examination is performed and fails to provide the necessary diagnostic information, a vaginal scan should be done when possible. Similarly, if a vaginal scan is performed and fails to image all areas needed for diagnosis, an abdominal scan should be performed. In some cases, both an abdominal and a vaginal scan may be needed.

GENERAL PELVIC PREPARATION

For a pelvic sonogram performed from the abdominal wall, the patient's urinary bladder should, in general, be distended adequately to displace the small bowel and its contained gas from the field of view. Occasionally, overdistention of the bladder may compromise evaluation. When this occurs, imaging should be repeated after the patient partially empties the bladder.

For a vaginal sonogram, the urinary bladder is preferably empty. The vaginal transducer may be introduced by the patient, the sonographer, or the physician. A female member of the physician's or hospital's staff should be present, when possible, as a chaperone in the examining room during vaginal sonography.

UTERUS

The vagina and uterus provide anatomic landmarks that can be used as reference points when evaluating the pelvic structures. In evaluating the uterus, the following should be documented: (a) uterine size, shape, and orientation; (b) the endometrium; (c) the myometrium; and (d) the cervix.

Uterine length is evaluated on a long axis view as the distance from the fundus to the cervix. The depth of the uterus (anteroposterior dimension) is measured on the same long axis view from its anterior to posterior walls, perpendicular to its long axis. The width is measured on the axial or coronal view.

Abnormalities of the uterus should be documented. The endometrium should be analyzed for thickness, focal abnormality, and the presence of fluid or mass in the endometrial cavity. Assessment of the endometrium should allow for normal variations in the appearance of the endometrium expected with phases of the menstrual cycle and with hormonal supplementation. The myometrium and cervix should be evaluated for contour changes, echogenicity, and masses.

The endometrial thickness measurement should include both layers, measured anterior to posterior, in the sagittal plane. Any fluid within the endometrial cavity should be excluded from this measurement.

ADNEXA (OVARIES AND FALLOPIAN TUBES)

When evaluating the adnexa, an attempt should be made to identify the ovaries first since they can serve as a major point of reference for assessing the presence of adnexal pathology. Although their location is variable, the ovaries are most often situated anterior to the internal iliac (hypogastric) vessels, lateral to the uterus, and superficial to the obturator internus muscle. The ovaries should be measured and ovarian abnormalities should be documented. Ovarian size can be determined by measuring the ovary in three dimensions (width, length, and depth), on views obtained in two orthogonal planes. It is recognized that the ovaries may not be identifiable in some women. This occurs most frequently after menopause or in patients with a large leiomyomatous uterus.

The normal fallopian tubes are not visualized in most patients. The para-adnexal regions should be surveyed for abnormalities, particularly fluid-filled or distended tubular structures that may represent dilated fallopian tubes.

If an adnexal mass is noted, its relationship to the uterus and ipsilateral ovary should be documented. Its size and echopattern (cystic, solid, or mixed; presence of septations) should be determined. Doppler ultrasound may be useful in select cases to identify the vascular nature of pelvic structures.

(continued)

Display 1-2. (Continued)

CUL-DE-SAC

The cul-de-sac and bowel posterior to the uterus may not be clearly visualized. This area should be evaluated for the presence of free fluid or mass. When free fluid is detected, its echogenicity should be assessed. If a mass is detected, its size, position, shape, echopattern (cystic, solid, or complex), and its relationship to the ovaries and uterus should be documented. Identification of peristalsis can be helpful in distinguishing a loop of bowel from a pelvic mass. In the absence of peristalsis, differentiation of normal or abnormal loops of bowel from a mass may, at times, be difficult. A transvaginal examination may be helpful in distinguishing a suspected mass from fluid and feces within the normal rectosigmoid. An ultrasound water enema study or a repeat examination after a cleansing enema may also help distinguish a suspected mass from bowel.

(American Institute of Ultrasound in Medicine. Guidelines for Performing of the Ultrasound Examination of the Female Pelvis, Laurel, MD: AIUM; 1995.)

(SDMS) Guidelines for Obstetrics and Gynecology Review includes a section on Scanning Techniques.[54] A sonographer developing his or her own protocols should keep in mind that the sonographic examination must clearly demonstrate the normality or abnormality of each anatomic structure through a series of representative images.

Developing an examination protocol ensures that every study is done in a consistent and complete manner, thereby reducing the likelihood of missing pathology. Many recent articles[5,18,24] have discussed the weaknesses of the Routine Antenatal Diagnostic Imaging with Ultrasound Study (RADIUS),[20] which concluded that routine obstetric ultrasound was not cost effective. Of interest to sonographers is that the study illustrated the difference in the rate of fetal anomaly detection between tertiary care centers and nontertiary care centers.[18,24] The rate of detection was 60% lower in nontertiary care centers than in tertiary care centers, which presumably had more experienced sonographers and physicians. This study illustrated the importance of being thorough and optimizing image quality when performing a sonographic study.

Performing the Gynecologic Examination

Regardless of clinical indication, a gynecologic examination should include the following images: sagittal midline of the uterus, including the cervix and vagina, right and left parasagittal views of uterus and both adnexa, and transverse views of the uterine fundus with cornua, the uterine corpus, cervix, vagina, and each ovary. Characteristics of any suspected pathology should be clearly demonstrated and recorded in addition to the standard views. The sonographic record should include several sagittal and transverse views of any suspected abnormality. Documentation should include measurements and a demonstration of the echogenicity and transsonicity of the abnormal structure. Every attempt should be made to delineate clearly the mass and its relationship to surrounding organs and structures. If results of the sonographic examination are negative, the area of interest should be imaged to prove that no pathology was seen.

The sonographer must also be aware of findings that are often associated with particular diseases. For instance, when a solid ovarian mass is seen, the sonographer should also carefully examine the cul-de-sac, Morison's pouch, the liver edge, and the flanks for ascites. The liver, kidneys, and perivascular areas should also be examined for evidence of metastases. Every examination must be performed thoroughly; the additional time required is minimal when using real-time scanners and the findings may be critical to the patient's well-being. Although sonographic images of gynecologic masses often are frustratingly nonspecific, with optimal technique, characteristics related to particular masses can be visualized (Table 1-1). It is also important to understand when Doppler and color Doppler may enhance diagnosis. Specific techniques are described in more detail in following chapters.

A good understanding of the physical principles

TABLE 1-1. GENERAL PRINCIPLES OF GYNECOLOGIC SCANNING TECHNIQUES

Characteristics of Mass	Scanning Technique
Size	Measure three longest dimensions: length, height, width
Mobility	Turn patient, empty bladder, apply transducer pressure
Tissue composition	Change transducer: high to low frequency
	Compare to urine, which is fluid and anechoic
	Raise gain settings to see septations, lower gain to see shadows from calcifications
	Look for edge shadowing and anterior reverberation artifacts in fluid-filled structures
	Check for peristalsis in mass to determine whether it is bowel
Extension	Examine bladder wall, which should appear as clean, echogenic line measuring 3 to 6 mm
	Examine cul-de-sac, flanks, Morison's pouch for ascites
	Examine liver for metastases
	Examine kidneys for hydronephrosis and metastases
	Examine perivascular area for enlarged nodes

of ultrasound enables the sonographer to solve imaging problems. Many excellent textbooks explain these principles.[28,32,35]

Chapter 30 describes artifacts sonographers should be aware of when scanning. Every sonographer should make efforts to minimize them. The following basic scanning principles should be used to achieve the most diagnostic images:

1. The sonographic beam should be perpendicular to the area of interest to use superior axial resolution.
2. The best resolution occurs within the focal zone of the transducer.
3. Higher-frequency transducers provide better resolution.
4. Lower-frequency transducers provide greater depth of penetration.
5. Fluid-filled structures enhance the transmission of sound.
6. Solid structures attenuate sound to varying degrees.

Performing the Obstetric Examination

Scanning a pregnant patient before the 15th week of gestation requires basically the same technique as a gynecologic ultrasound examination. The pro-

tocol detailing the number of examinations and measurements that need to be taken is summarized in Display 1-1 and is described more fully in subsequent chapters.

After about 20 weeks' gestation,[27] some women suffer from caval compression syndrome and cannot lie on their back for long periods. This may begin earlier in cases of multiple gestations. The patient will begin to fidget as she becomes uncomfortable, and may complain that she is hot, nauseous, or feels she is going to faint. At the first sign of these symptoms, the patient should be turned to a side, or have her back elevated. A drink of cold water or a cold, wet washcloth to the forehead will enable her to recover more quickly. Once she has recovered, the examination may resume after putting a pillow under one side of the patient, so that her body is tilted. This provides the patient with relief from her symptoms while providing the sonographer with access to her pelvis. Scanning in the most efficient manner possible minimizes the time the patient lies on the table.

The sonographer should establish an organized routine for scanning; for example, begin the scan at the fetal head and carefully examine each organ and limb while moving toward the lower legs. Representative images should be recorded as they are obtained through this survey. Consistency in performing each scan saves the sonographer from hav-

---

Display 1-3. American Institute of Ultrasound in Medicine Official Statement on Clinical Safety. Approved October 1982; revised and approved March 1988, reaffirmed March 1993.

Diagnostic ultrasound has been in use since the late 1950s. Given its known benefits and recognized efficacy for medical diagnosis, including use during human pregnancy, the AIUM herein addresses the clinical safety of such use:

No confirmed biological effects on patients or instrument operators caused by exposure at intensities typical of present diagnostic ultrasound instruments have ever been reported. Although the possibility exists that such biological effects may be identified in the future, current data indicate that the benefits to patients of the prudent use of diagnostic ultrasound outweigh the risks, if any, that may be present.

American Institute of Ultrasound in Medicine. Bioeffects and Safety of Diagnostic Ultrasound. Laurel, MD: AIUM; 1993.)

---

ing to design a new approach for each patient, makes doing complete examinations habitual, and alerts the sonographer very quickly when something is unusual or abnormal. Having a checklist of fetal anatomy and measurements is also very helpful in ensuring each study is complete.

Safety of Ultrasound

The patient undoubtedly will ask questions about the findings of the examination and the safety to the fetus and herself of exposure to diagnostic ultrasound. The sonographer must answer these questions accurately and clearly. Extensive research has been done on the potential deleterious effects of diagnostic ultrasound. The AIUM, the SDMS, the National Institutes of Health (NIH), and the United States Food and Drug Administration (FDA) carefully monitor results of epidemiologic and biologic studies. In 1984, the NIH and the FDA convened a Consensus Development Conference on Diagnostic Ultrasound Imaging in

Pregnancy. The report generated by the proceedings of that meeting states[40]:

It is the consensus of the panel that ultrasound examination in pregnancy should be performed for a specific medical indication. The data on clinical efficacy and safety do not allow a recommendation for routine screening at this time.

Although the ultrasound community continues to uphold the rationale for this guideline, nearly every pregnant woman now receives at least one sonogram. The AIUM regularly publishes statements and reports informing the ultrasound community of the most recent information regarding safety issues and epidemiologic information.[1–8] The statements presented in Displays 1-3, 1-4, and 1-5 continue to reinforce the NIH's conclusion that no deleterious effects have been demonstrated as resulting from the use of diagnostic ultrasound, but that it should continue to be used prudently.

These conclusions and statements apply equally to the use of Doppler ultrasound, although output from Doppler instruments tends to be higher than for gray-scale imaging.[35] The FDA has established guidelines that restrict the power levels used in Doppler fetal scanning to those used before 1976. Recently, the FDA approved some devices that use higher-output data if power output information is displayed in real-time on the equipment's monitor. The AIUM, FDA, the National Electrical Manufacturers Association, and 38 other professional organizations have developed an output display standard for all ultrasound equipment that requires that mechanical and thermal indices (the mechanisms relating to bioeffects) be visible on the monitor.[2] By knowing the mechanical and thermal indices values, the sonographer can adjust power levels to minimize the patient's exposure to diagnostic ultrasound. It is incumbent on the sonographer to always minimize the patient's exposure to ultrasound energy by efficient scanning and by using the lowest exposure levels possible (as low as reasonably achievable—ALARA).[33,34]

The AIUM's position statement on the use of Doppler ultrasound is as follows:

AIUM feels that there is currently sufficient information to justify clinical use of continuous wave, pulsed and color flow Doppler ultrasound to evaluate blood flow in uterine, umbilical and fetal vessels, the fetal cardiovascular system and to image flow in these structures using color flow imaging technology.[1]

Display 1-4. Conclusions Regarding Epidemiology. Approved October 1995.

Based on epidemiologic evidence to date and on current knowledge of interactive mechanisms, there is insufficient justification to warrant a conclusion that there is a causal relationship between diagnostic ultrasound and adverse effects.

(American Institute of Ultrasound in Medicine. Conclusions Regarding Epidemiology. Laurel, MD: AIUM; 1995.)

Display 1-5. AIUM Statement on Non-Human Mammalian In Vivo Biological Effects. Approved October 1992.

Information from experiments utilizing laboratory mammals has contributed significantly to our understanding of ultrasonically induced biological effects and the mechanisms that are most likely responsible. The following statement summarizes observations relative to specific ultrasound parameters and indices:

In the low megahertz frequency range there have been no independently confirmed adverse biological effects in nonhuman mammalian tissues exposed in vivo under experimental ultrasound conditions, as follows:

a) When a thermal mechanism is involved, these conditions are unfocused-beam intensities[a] below 100mW/cm^2, focused[b]-beam intensities below 1 W/cm^2, or thermal index values less than 2. Furthermore, such effects have not been demonstrated for higher values of thermal index when it is less than

$$6 - \frac{\log_{10} t}{0.6}$$

where t is the exposure time ranging from 1 to 250 minutes, including off-time for pulsed exposure.

b) When a nonthermal mechanism is involved,[c] in tissues that contain well-defined gas bodies, these conditions are *in situ* peak rarefactional pressures below approximately 0.3 MPa or mechanical index values less than approximately 0.3. Furthermore, for other tissues no such effects have been reported.

[a] Free-field spatial peak, temporal average (SPTA) for continuous wave exposures and pulsed exposures.
[b] Quarter-power (6-dB) beam width smaller than 4 wavelengths or 4 mm, whichever is less at the exposure frequency.
[c] For diagnostically relevant ultrasound exposures.

(American Institute of Ultrasound in Medicine. Statement on Non-human Mammalian In-Vivo Biological Effects. Laurel, MD: AIUM; 1992.)

If the patient asks, the sonographer should convey the gist of these statements to allay any immediate fears, but should also indicate that examinations should not be performed indiscriminately.

Sharing the results of the examination with the patient depends on many factors, most of them involving common sense. The physician who ordered the sonographic examination is the best person to explain and discuss the findings with the patient. Whether patients are given immediate reassurance and are allowed to view the images, especially in a normal pregnancy, depends on the philosophy of the ultrasound laboratory. The impact on the patient of seeing the images should be the primary consideration. The bonding that occurs when the mother and father view the sonogram is discussed in Chapter 32. Ethical considerations are discussed in Chapter 34. The sonographer should be aware of all aspects of the ultrasound examination before deciding how much information to share with the patient. A discussion of this and other controversial topics appears in Chapter 31.

Transducer Selection

The choice of transducer should be based on patient habitus, stage of pregnancy, and examination objectives. Each laboratory should have a selection of transducers of varying frequencies with m-mode, Doppler, and color Doppler capabilities. Many transducers are now duplex; a two-dimensional image is seen on the screen with a simultaneous m-mode or Doppler spectral display. Transducers that also show color information are sometimes referred to as triplex. Most transducers are electronically focused, enabling the sonographer to optimally image the structure of interest by changing the depth of the focal point, and, in some cases, the number of focal points. Broadband transducers enable the operator to change imaging frequencies to optimize resolution at different depths.[28]

The small scanning surface or footprint of sector transducers make them easily maneuverable and therefore effective in most gynecologic and early gestation applications. Linear transducers in a variety of sizes and shapes provide various fields of view related to their length and produce more accurate measurements of linear structures (e.g., femur), making them particularly useful in late pregnancy. Curved linear array transducers combine the wider field of view of sector transducers with the greater near-field visualization and more accurate linear measurements of linear transducers.

Patient body habitus affects the choice of transducer frequency. Large patients may require the use of a 2.5-MHz transducer, whereas 5.0 MHz provides excellent resolution on slender women and on children. Infants are often best imaged with 7.5-MHz transducers. In pregnant women, the stage of gestation also influences the choice of frequencies. A 5-MHz transducer may provide optimal images well into the third trimester on a slender patient. In later pregnancy and in heavier women, a 3.5-MHz transducer usually provides better depth penetration. Improvement in image processing has enhanced resolution, thereby allowing patients to be studied with higher-frequency transducers than was previously feasible. To optimize image quality, the sonographer should change transducers depending on the depth of the structure being imaged. For example, if the fetal spine is up, and the kidneys appear suspect, change to a higher-frequency transducer to improve resolution. If a patient is obese, and therefore the fetus is far from the transducer face, change to a lower-frequency transducer.

The utility of the transvaginal transducer, and the superior imaging it provides in most gynecologic and some obstetric applications, make it an essential addition to the transducer arsenal of any laboratory doing gynecologic and obstetric ultrasound. Transvaginal transducers range from 3.0 to more typically 6.0 to 7.5 MHz. Selection of frequency is determined by the distance from the cervix of the structure to be evaluated. Transvaginal transducers produced by different manufacturers vary in size, shape, orientation of the imaging plane in relation to the shaft of the transducer, whether the shaft has an angle to it, and the addition of duplexed m-mode (simultaneous display of m-mode with two-dimensional images), Doppler, and color Doppler capabilities. Some machines and transducers now have the capability of beam steering.[28]

Transvaginal transducers are used primarily for evaluating the nongravid female pelvis[37] and the first trimester fetus. Later in pregnancy, the transvaginal transducer may be useful in the evaluation of presenting fetal parts and the cervix, and to rule out a placenta previa or vasa previa.[61] Transvaginal transducers have also been found to be useful in delineating fetal anatomy in obese pregnant patients when imaging through the maternal umbilicus, where the subcutaneous fat thickness is significantly reduced.[49] When selecting equipment, the laboratory should consider the applications for which various transducers may be used.

Transvaginal Scanning

Transvaginal scans are often performed in conjunction with transabdominal scans. Because the transvaginal transducer depicts anatomy best within a focal range of 2 to 7 cm and cannot be inserted past the area of the vaginal fornices[60,61] (see Fig. 2-7), it is limited to visualizing the uterus and adnexa in the nongravid patient without an enlarged leiomyomatous uterus, and the lower uterine segment in a gravid patient. In most clinical situations, a more extensive view of the pelvis and abdomen is required than can be provided by the transvaginal probe alone (Fig. 1-3). The many applications for transvaginal sonography include evaluation of ectopic pregnancy, uterine, ovarian, and pelvic inflammatory disease,[61] placenta previa[60] or accreta, fetal anatomy and cardiovascular systems, and monitoring ovulation. It may also be used to guide procedures such as ova aspiration, embryo transfer, drainage or aspiration of pelvic fluid, and treatment of ectopic pregnancies. The SDMS publication, *Guidelines for Performing Endovaginal/Transvaginal Procedures*[55] provides a good overview of the technique and, the AIUM's Ultrasound Practice Committee has issued recommendations[11] for cleaning endocavitary transducers.

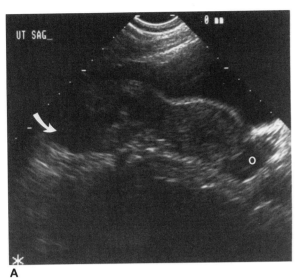
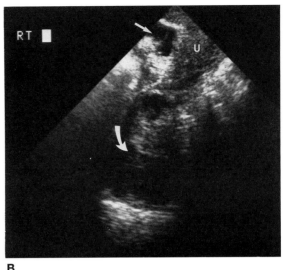

A   **B**

Figure 1-3. (**A**) A transabdominal scan demonstrates a large, complex mass (*curved arrow*) located superior to and to the right of the uterus (O, ovary). The mass was thought to represent a chronic ectopic pregnancy. On a follow-up examination 1 week later, the size of the mass had decreased slightly. (**B**) The endovaginal scan in the area of the right adnexa provided a vague outline of the mass (*curved arrow*) that did not contribute additional diagnostic information (U, uterus; *straight arrow*, bowel).

TECHNIQUE

The procedure should be explained carefully to the patient before beginning the examination procedure.[61] In some institutions, the patient is asked to sign an informed consent form before the examination.[51]

1. Patients are usually scanned with an empty bladder. A distended bladder may distort pelvic anatomy.[59,61] Patients being examined for low-lying placenta should have a half-full bladder to help outline the internal os and anterior portion of the cervix.[60]
2. The lithotomy position is used, or a pillow may be placed under the supine patient's buttocks. The patient's upper body should be positioned higher than the pelvis, to permit pooling of any fluid in the cul-de-sac.
3. The transducer should be covered with a transducer cover designed for this purpose. The cover reduces the patient's risk of infection. If a transducer cover is not available, a condom or a digit of a surgical glove may be substituted. A small amount of gel should be placed on the face of the transducer before covering to provide a fluid contact between the scanning face and the cover. Care should be taken to remove all air bubbles between the transducer face and the cover to optimize image quality.[63]
4. The transducer cover should be lubricated with K-Y jelly to minimize patient discomfort. If the patient is being treated for infertility, no coupling gel should be used because of its spermicidal effect[50]; instead, the probe can be lubricated with saline.
5. Depending on institutional policy, either patient, physician, or sonographer can insert the transducer into the vagina. It is advisable for a female chaperone to be present when an examination is being performed.[51]
6. The sonographer manipulates the transducer to image sagittal, coronal, and transverse sections of the uterus and adnexa. This is done by pushing or pulling the transducer and by tilting or rotating the handle. Advancement of the transducer should be done only while imaging, to avoid advancing the transducer too far.[59,63] As with standard scanning, enlarging the image enhances visualization.
7. Because the orientation of the images differs from transabdominal scans, it is important to indicate the location and directions on each scan. Orientation and labeling have not been standardized[61]; therefore, referencing images by using anatomic landmarks is recommended (e.g., demonstrating the ovaries in relationship to the iliac vessels).

8. At the completion of the examination, the condom should be removed carefully and the transducer disinfected as recommended by the manufacturer of the transducer.[11,63]

Transperineal Scanning

In some cases, transvaginal scanning may be contraindicated. If there is a concern about introducing infection, for example in the case of ruptured membranes, or if the patient refuses a transvaginal scan, the transperineal approach may enable the sonographer to obtain images of the cervix and the lower uterine segment. The patient is positioned as for a transvaginal scan. The study is done by using a conventional ultrasound transducer that has been covered with a transducer cover, as described in the section on transvaginal technique, and scanning between the labia on the perineum.[62] Occasionally the view may be obstructed by bowel gas. To improve visualization, the patient's buttocks may be elevated onto a pillow or towels, shifting the bowel and changing the angle of the ultrasound beam relative to the cervix[29] (Fig. 1-4).

New Developments in Diagnostic Medical Ultrasound

Sonohysterography is a technique in which 25 to 30 ml of sterile saline is infused into the endometrial cavity to enhance visualization by either the trans-

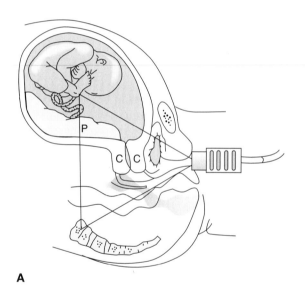

A

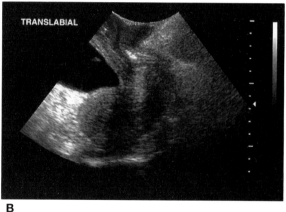

B

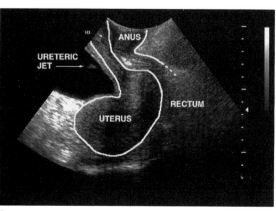

C

Figure 1-4. (**A**) Schematic diagram of transperineal scanning plane. (Hertzberg BS, Bowie JD, Carroll BA, et al. Diagnosis of placenta previa during the third trimester: Role of transperineal sonography. Am J Roentgenol. 1992; 159:83–87). (**B**) Transperineal sonogram of normal uterus, (**C**) with machine-generated outline of structures. (Sonograms courtesy of Susan Schultz, RDMS, Technical Coordinator of Education, The Jefferson Ultrasound Institute, Philadelphia, PA.)

abdominal or transvaginal approach. The saline is infused through a fine, flexible catheter that is placed through the cervix. Patient preparation may include testing for *Chlamydia, Ureaplasma,* and gonorrhea and the use of prophylactic antibiotics. As in transvaginal examinations, the dorsal lithotomy position is assumed. A speculum is inserted into the vagina to expose the cervix, the external os is cleaned with Betadine, and then the catheter is inserted.[19] Patients tolerate the procedure well, reporting little or no pain. The endometrial cavity is delineated by the anechoic saline that often initially appears echogenic because of contained microbubbles of air. Passage of the saline through the fallopian tubes can be demonstrated by imaging fluid in the cul-de-sac.[48] The technique has proven superior to transvaginal sonography alone in characterizing the thickened endometrium for contained polyps, submucous myomas, synechiae, endometrial hyperplasia, and signs of cancerous masses, and in investigating tubal patency.[16,22]

Contrast agents such as Echovist (Schering, Germany) have been used in gynecologic scanning to enhance visualization of the endometrial cavity and fallopian tubes. Echovist injected through the vagina has successfully demonstrated patent and blocked tubes, but sterile saline has proven just as acceptable and certainly is less costly.[12,48,57,58] Some intravenously injected contrast agents have been shown to enhance color and spectral Doppler signals of small blood vessels,[23,57] which holds promise for the investigation of uterine and ovarian blood flow and the study of neovascularity in pelvic tumors. The use of contrast agents, be they saline or other agents, will certainly expand if research continues to prove diagnostic improvement. What role the sonographer will take will depend, as it does today, on the setting in which he or she practices. Usually the sonographer acts as an assistant to the physician instilling the saline or contrast. However, as sonographers begin developing the role of the advanced practitioner, that person might be considered qualified to perform the entire examination.

Three-dimensional ultrasound, an outgrowth of computer technology, is one of the most dynamic new developments in sonographic imaging. Several types of three-dimensional ultrasound are being investigated, such as two-dimensional serial scanning,[28] volume imaging,[14,47] and the use of a defocusing lens.[31] Studies of the efficacy of two-dimensional serial scanning (commonly referred to as three-dimensional imaging) in obstetric scanning, particularly in the evaluation of the fetal face,[45] limbs, and digits, have shown it to add important detail to the study.[15,26] One group of investigators who have been working with the technique since 1989 have reported they found it enhanced their evaluation of fetal anomalies in 62% of the 204 cases studied.[38] Their cases included virtually all categories of defects, with the technique not adding any information to the conventional ultrasound study in 36% of the cases. They found fetal cardiac anomalies could not be evaluated because of movement, although recently Nelson and colleagues successfully overcame this problem and were able to produce diagnostic-quality three-dimensional images of the fetal heart.[40] Other groups have found the technique to be useful in the evaluation of congenital uterine anomalies,[30] estimation of fetal weight,[21] and the study of embryologic development.[14]

Scanning technique does not change appreciably. The volume transducer mechanically obtains sequen-

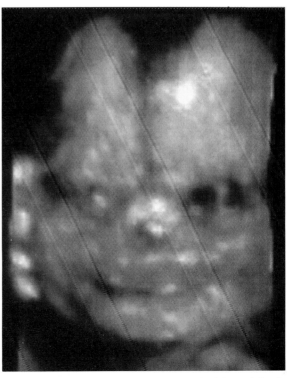

Figure 1-5. Three-dimensional image of a 20-week fetal face.

tial images, which are stored on disc as volume data. At some time after the scan, the data may be recalled and volumetric reconstructions produced that may be rotated approximately 360°. Entire organs, rather than sections, may be evaluated. The technique enables the user to study an infinite variety of orthogonal views through an area of interest at any time after storage of the volume data.

The other form of three-dimensional imaging being investigated involves the use of a defocusing lens. This technique enables the user to view the surface of an object in three dimensions in real time. The image resembles that of a topographic map. The surface to be studied must have a fluid interface. Some of the anomalies that are being detected more easily with this type of evaluation include facial features (Fig. 1-5), ear anomalies, finger and toe numbers and positions, neural tube defects, and limb malformations.[44]

Time domain correlation is a new development that provides an alternative to color Doppler technology. In this technique, velocity is determined by measuring the distance a target has moved during a given time interval.[28] One of the advantages of this technique is that it is not angle dependent. It is hoped that the technique may be useful in evaluating fetal circulation, particularly of small vessels, which are difficult to evaluate by traditional color flow Doppler methods.[36]

Professional Responsibilities of the Sonographer

Although debate as to whether sonographers are regarded as technicians or professionals continues,[13,42] sonographers must strive for professional status by behaving as such and developing their field. It is essential that they be familiar with the Sonographer's Code of Professional Conduct[52] (Table 1-2), Code of Ethics,[56] The Scope of Practice,[54] that they abide by the Patients' Bill of Rights, and that they practice infection control techniques to protect their patients and themselves.

People who choose diagnostic ultrasound as a profession should take the certifying examination given by the American Registry of Diagnostic Medical Sonographers (ARDMS) and should become members of the professional society that represents sonographers, the Society of Diagnostic Medical Sonographers. Although in most hospitals it is not mandatory to be registered, passing the registry examination attests that the sonographer has a practicing level of knowledge in the specialties in which he or she is registered. The registered sonographer can use the designation RDMS (registered diagnostic medical sonographer) after his or her name. To maintain this status, the sonographer must compile 30 hours of continuing education credits every 3 years. In a field as dynamic as diagnostic ultrasound, keeping informed of its innovations is imperative.

The AIUM has instituted a procedure for the accreditation of obstetric and gynecologic ultrasound practices.[10] One of its criteria is the proper education of the sonographers in the practice, which will further encourage sonographers to take the ARDMS examinations.

Membership in the SDMS brings with it the benefits of being part of a professional organization whose mission is to keep its members informed and competent. Among the resources the SDMS provides are educational guidelines, profiles of sonographer characteristics (including salary levels), a peer-reviewed journal (*The Journal of Diagnostic Medical Sonography*), and annual national and regional scientific meetings. It also keeps its membership informed of legislation and current societal trends that can affect the practice of ultrasound.

TABLE 1-2. CODE OF PROFESSIONAL CONDUCT FOR DIAGNOSTIC MEDICAL SONOGRAPHERS

I. Sonographers shall act in the best interests of the patient.
II. Sonographers shall provide sonographic services with compassion, respect for human dignity, honesty, and integrity.
III. Sonographers shall respect the patient's right to privacy, safeguarding confidential information within the constraints of the law.
IV. Sonographers shall maintain competence in their field.
V. Sonographers shall assume responsibility for their actions.

(The Society of Diagnostic Medical Sonographers. Code of Professional Conduct for Diagnostic Medical Sonographers. Dallas: SDMS; 1990.)

REFERENCES

1. American Institute of Ultrasound in Medicine. Position statement on fetal Doppler. AIUM Newsletter. October 1988; 3.
2. American Institute of Ultrasound in Medicine. Standard for Real-Time Display of Thermal and Mechanical Acoustic Output Indices on Diagnostic Ultrasound Equipment. Laurel, MD: AIUM; 1992.
3. American Institute of Ultrasound in Medicine. Statement on Non-human Mammalian In Vivo Biological Effects. Laurel, MD: AIUM; 1992.
4. American Institute of Ultrasound in Medicine. Bioeffects and Safety of Diagnostic Ultrasound. Laurel, MD: AIUM; 1993.
5. American Institute of Ultrasound in Medicine. Bioeffects committee reviews RADIUS study. AIUM Reporter. 1994; 10:2–4.
6. American Institute of Ultrasound in Medicine. Guidelines for Performance of the Antepartum Obstetrical Ultrasound Examination. Laurel, MD: AIUM; 1994.
7. American Institute of Ultrasound in Medicine. Medical Ultrasound Safety. Laurel, MD: AIUM; 1994.
8. American Institute of Ultrasound in Medicine. Conclusions Regarding Epidemiology. Laurel, MD: AIUM; 1995.
9. American Institute of Ultrasound in Medicine. Guidelines for Performance of the Ultrasound Examination of the Female Pelvis. Laurel, MD: AIUM; 1995.
10. American Institute of Ultrasound in Medicine. Ultrasound Practice Accreditation Commission. AIUM Reporter. 1995; 11(9):3.
11. American Institute of Ultrasound in Medicine. Report for cleaning and preparing endocavitary ultrasound transducers between patients. AIUM Reporter. 1995; 11(11):7.
12. Balen FG, Allen CM, Lees WR. Ultrasound contrast agents. Clin Radiol. 1994; 49:77–82.
13. Berman M. Defining the role of the sonographer. J Diagn Med Sonogr. 1984; 8:55–60.
14. Blaas HG, Eik-Nes SH, Kiserud T, et al. Three-dimensional imaging of the brain cavities in human embryos. Ultrasound in Obstetrics and Gynecology. 1995; 5:228–232.
15. Bonilla-Musoles F, Raga F, Osborne NG, et al. Use of three-dimensional ultrasonography for the study of normal and pathologic morphology of the human embryo and fetus: Preliminary report. J Ultrasound Med. 1995; 14:757–765.
16. Bonilla-Musoles F, Simon C, Serra V, et al. An assessment of hysterosalpingosonography (HSSG) as a diagnostic tool for uterine cavity defects and tubal patency. J Clin Ultrasound. 1992; 20:175–181.
17. Devonald KJ, Ellwood DA, Griffiths KA, et al. Volume imaging: Three-dimensional appreciation of the fetal head and face. J Ultrasound Med. 1995; 14:919–925.
18. DeVore GR. The routine antenatal diagnostic imaging with ultrasound study: Another perspective. Obstet Gynecol. 1994; 84:622–626.
19. Dubinsky TJ, Parvey R, Gormaz G, Curtis M, Maklad N. Transvaginal hysterosonography: Comparison with biopsy in the evaluation of postmenopausal bleeding. J Ultrasound Med. 1995; 14:887–893.
20. Ewigman BG, Crane JP, Frigoletto FD, et al. Effect of prenatal ultrasound screening on perinatal outcome. N Engl J Med. 1993; 329:821–827.
21. Favre R, Bader AM, Nisand G. Prospective study on fetal weight estimation using limb circumferences obtained by three-dimensional ultrasound. Ultrasound in Obstetrics and Gynecology. 1995; 6:140–144.
22. Gaucherand P, Piacenza JM, Salle B, Rudigoz R. Sonohysterography of the uterine cavity: Preliminary investigations. J Clin Ultrasound. 1995; 23:339–348.
23. Goldberg BB, Liu JB, Burns PN, Merton DA, Forsberg F. Galactose-based intravenous sonographic contrast agent: Experimental studies. J Ultrasound Med. 1993; 12:463–470.
24. Gomez KJ, Copel JA. Routine ultrasound screening. Curr Opin Obstet Gynecol. 1994; 6:426–429.
25. Hacker NF, Moore JG. Essentials of Obstetrics and Gynecology. Philadelphia: WB Saunders; 1986.
26. Hamper UM, Trapanotto V, Sheth S, et al. Three-dimensional US: Preliminary clinical experience. Radiology. 1994; 191:397–401.
27. Hansman M, Hackeloer BJ, Staudach A. Ultrasound Diagnosis in Obstetrics and Gynecology. Berlin: Springer-Verlag; 1985.
28. Hedrick WR, Hykes DL, Starchman DE. Ultrasound Physics and Instrumentation. 3rd ed. St. Louis: Mosby; 1995.
29. Hertzberg BS, Kliewer MA, Baumeister LA, et al. Optimizing transperineal sonographic imaging of the cervix: The hip elevation technique. J Ultrasound Med. 1994; 13:933–936.
30. Jurkovic D, Geipel A, Gruboeck K, et al. Three-dimensional ultrasound for the assessment of uterine anatomy and detection of congenital anomalies: A comparison with hysterosalpingography and two-dimensional sonography. Ultrasound in Obstetrics and Gynecology. 1995; 5:233–237.
31. Kossoff G, Griffiths KA, Warren PS. Real-time quasi-three-dimensional viewing in sonography, with conventional, gray-scale volume imaging. Ultrasound in Obstetrics and Gynecology. 1994; 4:211–216.
32. Kremkau F. Diagnostic Ultrasound: Principles and Instruments. 4th ed. Philadelphia: WB Saunders; 1993.

33. Kremkau FW. Bioeffects and safety: III. Output indices and bioeffects statement. J Diagn Med Sonogr. 1993; 9:336–338.

34. Kremkau FW. Editorial: Contemporary ultrasound technology. Ultrasound in Obstetrics and Gynecology. 1995; 6:233–236.

35. Kremkau FW. Doppler Ultrasound: Principles and Instruments. 2nd ed. Philadelphia: WB Saunders; 1995.

36. Lee W, Bendick P, Best AM, et al. Time-domain ultrasonography during pregnancy. J Ultrasound Med. 1994; 13:457–463.

37. Leibman AJ, Kruse B, McSweeney MB. Transvaginal sonography: Comparison with transabdominal sonography in the diagnosis of pelvic masses. Am J Roentgenol. 1988; 151:89–92.

38. Merz E, Bahlmann F, Weber G. Volume scanning in the evaluation of fetal malformations: A new dimension in prenatal diagnosis. Ultrasound in Obstetrics and Gynecology. 1995; 5:222–227.

39. National Institute of Child Health & Human Development. Consensus report: Diagnostic ultrasound imaging in pregnancy. U.S. Dept of Health and Human Services, Public Health Service, NIH Publication No. 84-667. Washington, DC: Government Printing Office; 1984.

40. Nelson TR, Pretorius DH, Sklansky M, Hagen-Ansert S. Three-dimensional echocardiographic evaluation of fetal heart anatomy and function: Acquisition, analysis, and display. J Ultrasound Med. 1996; 15:1–9.

41. Parulekar SG, Kiwi R. Dynamic incompetent cervix uteri. J Ultrasound Med. 1988; 7:481–485.

42. Persutte WH. Advanced practice sonography in obstetrics and gynecology. J Diagn Med Sonogr. 1995; 11:147–152.

43. Persutte WH, Lenke RR. Maternal urinary bladder filling for middle- and late-trimester ultrasound: Is it really necessary? J Ultrasound Med. 1988; 7:207–209.

44. Pretorius DH, House M, Nelson RT, Hollenbach KA. Evaluation of normal and abnormal lips in fetuses: Comparison between three- and two-dimensional sonography. Am J Roentgenol. 1995; 165:1233–1237.

45. Pretorius DH, Nelson TR. Fetal face visualization using three-dimensional ultrasonography. J Ultrasound Med. 1995; 14:349–356.

46. Raz S. Female Urology. Philadelphia: WB Saunders; 1983.

47. Riccabona M, Nelson TR, Pretorius DH, Davidson TE. Distance and volume measurement using three-dimensional ultrasonography. J Ultrasound Med. 1995; 14:881–886.

48. Richman RS, Viscomi GN, Cherney A, Polan M, Alcebo LO. Fallopian tube patency assessed by ultrasound following fluid injection. Radiology. 1984; 152:507–510.

49. Rosenberg JC, Guzman ER, Vintzileos AM, Knuppel RA. Transumbilical placement of the vaginal probe in obese pregnant women. Obstet Gynecol. 1995; 85:132–134.

50. Schwimer SR, Rothman CR, Lebovic J, et al. The effect of ultrasound coupling gels on sperm motility in vitro. Fertil Steril. 1984; 42:946.

51. Society of Diagnostic Medical Sonographers. Midwest region conducts survey on endocavitary ultrasound. SDMS Newsletter. 1989; 10(2):1. March/April 1989.

52. Society of Diagnostic Medical Sonographers. Code of Professional Conduct for Diagnostic Medical Sonographers. Dallas: SDMS; 1990.

53. Society of Diagnostic Medical Sonographers. Guidelines for Obstetrics and Gynecology Review. Dallas: SDMS; 1990.

54. Society of Diagnostic Medical Sonographers. The Scope of Practice for the Diagnostic Medical Sonographer. Dallas: SDMS; 1993.

55. Society of Diagnostic Medical Sonographers. Guidelines for Performing Endovaginal/Transvaginal Procedures. Dallas: SDMS; 1995.

56. Society of Diagnostic Medical Sonographers. Code of Ethics for the Profession of Diagnostic Medical Ultrasound. Dallas: SDMS; 1996.

57. Schlief R. Ultrasound contrast agents. Current Opinion in Radiology. 1991; 3:198–207.

58. Stern J, Peters AJ, Coulam CB. Color Doppler ultrasonography assessment of tubal patency: A comparison study with traditional techniques. Fertil Steril. 1992; 58:897–900.

59. Timor-Tritsch IE. How to do vaginal sonography. Presented at the First International Conference on Transvaginal Sonography: Clinical Applications. Columbia University College of Physicians and Surgeons and Sloane Hospital for Women, March 17–18, 1988, New York, New York.

60. Timor-Tritsch IE, Yunis RA. Confirming the safety of transvaginal sonography in patients suspected of placenta previa. Obstet Gynecol. 1993; 81:742–744.

61. Timor-Tritsch IE, Monteagudo A, Brown GM. Transvaginal sonographic evaluation of the obstetric and gynecologic patient. In: Callen PW, ed. Ultrasonography in Obstetrics and Gynecology. 3rd ed. Philadelphia: WB Saunders; 1994:52–62.

62. Weber TM, Hertzberg BS, Bowie JD. Transperineal US: Alternative technique to improve visualization of the presenting fetal part. Radiology. 1991; 179:747–750.

63. Zimmer EZ, Timor-Tritsch IE, Rottem S. The technique of transvaginal sonography. In: Timor-Tritsch IE, Rottem S, eds. Transvaginal Sonography. New York: Elsevier; 1991:61–75.

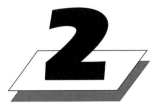

Endovaginal Ultrasound

DAIL A. De SOUZA, YANSHENG WEI, and SHRAGA ROTTEM

Endovaginal (EVS) or transvaginal sonography (TVS) is performed by placing a transducer into the vagina. It can provide excellent images of pelvic anatomy or gestational structures that fall within the transducer's field of view. The limitations of this technique are the relatively small field of view (approximately 6 cm from the transducer)[1] and the confined vaginal space, which restricts lateral movement and anterior and posterior angulation of the transducer. The typical TVS transducer has frequencies between 5.0 to 9 MHz, higher than those generally used in transabdominal scanning (TAS). The higher frequencies result in enhanced near-field resolution but also a smaller field of view due to a lesser depth of penetration.

Transvaginal sonography can be used not only as a diagnostic modality but as a therapeutic modality by assisting invasive procedures. Tables 2-1 and 2-2 summarize various applications of TVS.

Equipment and Procedure

TRANSVAGINAL TRANSDUCERS

The first transvaginal transducers, developed in 1985, were simple adaptations of transabdominal transducers. Since then, TVS transducers have been designed to accomodate the limited anatomic space they are placed in and be more comfortable to the patient and imager.

These transducers should have a smooth and preferably circular shape, measuring not more than two fingers or 1 inch in diameter. They should be long enough to allow for scanning without touching the labia with the fingers of the scanning hand.

Most of the TVS probes produced since 1992 meet these specifications and can be used to perform any of the procedures listed in Tables 2-1 and 2-2. In elderly patients or those with dyspareunia, a transducer with a smaller diameter is preferable. The application of sufficient scanning gel on the condom-covered transducer and insertion by the patient herself often helps the examination in these patients.

FREQUENCY AND RESOLUTION

Given the physical principles of ultrasonography, TVS has several advantages over TAS.

The distance between the TVS transducer and the gynecologic structure being examined is shorter, permitting the use of higher frequencies with the concomitant improved resolution. The distance between the transducer and the ovary using TVS is half of that for TAS.

The lesser amounts of tissue separating the transvaginal transducer and the organ of concern (usually the ovary) do not attenuate sound as much as do the abdominal wall and intrapelvic intestines traversed by a TAS examination. A full urinary bladder used in TAS helps push the intestines and their obscuring intraluminal gas out of the field of view, but the filled bladder adds to the distance between the TAS transducer and the pelvic organs.

TABLE 2-1. DIAGNOSTIC APPLICATIONS OF TRANSVAGINAL ULTRASOUND

Early detection of intrauterine pregnancy
Direct and indirect signs of ectopic pregnancy
Detection of early pregnancy failure and pathology
Detection of embryonal and early fetal anomalies
Location, numeration, and chorionicity in multiple gestations
Early dating by biometry
Diagnosis of placenta previa
Monitoring cervical dynamics to rule out cervical incompetence
Evaluation of the presenting fetal part in patients with oligohydramnios
Scanning of fetal head in cephalic presentations
Diagnosis of uterine disease
Detection of uterine malformations
Detection and scoring of ovarian lesions
Evaluation of posterior cul-de-sac
Monitoring follicular growth
Periovulatory monitoring of endometrial, cervical, and pelvic changes
Evaluation of nongynecologic lesions (i.e., urinary bladder and tract, and bowel)
Evaluation of urodynamics

Small physiologic amounts of free fluid in the pelvis, too deep or beyond the resolution of the TAS, can on occasion enhance the outline of the pelvic organs.

It is recognized that the higher frequency range of transvaginal transducers provides enhanced resolution, but it remains incumbent on the operator to decide which frequency should be used and to know how to manipulate the equipment for the best imaging. Pelvic structures are mobile and may lie at different distances from the vaginal vault. If the pelvis is considered a three-dimensional space and its contained structures (e.g., endometrium, anterior uterine wall, the cervix, the ligaments, and the ovarian parenchyma) as objects in this space, each patient has a slightly different arrangement of these structures possibly requiring the use of different frequencies and, at the very least, different angulations. In most normal uteri, either the 6- or 7.5-MHz frequency is effective, but in patients with enlarged uteri due to fibroids or those with large adnexal masses, a 5-MHz transducer may be needed. Masses beyond the TVS transducer's field of view cannot be imaged.

Changing TVS frequencies has been made eas-

ier with the introduction of newer, multifrequency transducers that have mechanisms for switching insonating frequencies as needed.

Ultrasound units with broad-band technology and transvaginal transducers continuously select frequencies ranging between 5 to 9 MHz. These units can filter the reflecting echo and modulate the image according to the best match of frequency with imaged structure distance and intervening attenuation. The frequency is not selected or controlled by the operator but by the machine. Currently, broad-band technology is relatively expensive.

A TAS provides a more global perspective on pelvic masses. It should be performed when a large pelvic mass is suspected because the field of view of any transvaginal probe, whether multifrequency or broad band, is limited. The scan can be performed with or without filling the urinary bladder. Some sonologists will preface all TVS examinations with a standard TAS examination.

TRANSVAGINAL COLOR FLOW DOPPLER AND THREE-DIMENSIONAL ULTRASONOGRAPHY

Compared with conventional duplex Doppler, color flow Doppler permits faster imaging and spectral analysis to determine the frequency shift of insonated blood vessels. When available, power Doppler further enhances visualization of the vascularity of an organ or area, although with loss of directional information. Moreover, power Doppler is more sensitive to low blood-flow velocities. As a research tool, color Doppler contributed to our knowledge of the physiology of ovulation and early pregnancy vascularization. However, as a clinical tool, color Doppler has not proved to be significantly superior to conventional gray-scale technology and thus may not be warranted in routine scanning. It continues to be of use in tertiary, teaching, and research facilities.

Three-dimensional ultrasound is still in its infancy. Its growth in clinical utility will depend on the development of fast computers and a decrease in the cost of the technology. We believe that three-dimensional technology will probably become a standard option in all equipment and will necessitate the same leap in learning that real-time sonography did in the late 1970s.

TVS-GUIDED PROCEDURES

An important medical principle is to perform, whenever possible, a diagnostic or therapeutic procedure of less invasiveness before proceeding to a more invasive one. In gynecology, the order of least to most invasive diagnostic procedures is sonohysterography, hysterosalpinography, hysteroscopy, dilatation and curettage, laparoscopy, and laparotomy. With TVS guidance, less invasive biopsies, drainage, and other procedures may be performed successfully, eliminating the need for the more aggressive studies (see Table 2-2).

Orientation of Images

Transvaginal sonography images are oriented on the screen slightly differently from conventional transabdominal images because of the location of transducer. Sound waves emitted from the transducer in the vagina first intercept vaginal or cervical tissue, depending on the angling of the transducer.

The structures closest to the transducer are represented at the top of the screen. This results in the anatomically inferior-most structures being depicted uppermost on the screen.

The transvaginal image may be considered a 90-degree counterclockwise rotation of the transabdominal image of the same region (Fig. 2-1). However, this applies only to longitudinal plane TVS scans and is affected by the flexion of the uterus. Depending on the angle at the vaginocervical junction, the uterine fundus can be depicted in the lower right or left of the sector image. In an anteverted uterus, the fundus is directed anteriorly, toward the anterior pelvic wall, and is depicted sonographically toward the lower right of the screen (Fig. 2-2).

Varying degrees of anteflexion cause the fundus to lie more anteriorly, which places it toward the middle to upper right of the screen. In a retroverted uterus, the fundus is directed backward, away from the anterior pelvic wall, and is depicted sonographically toward the lower left of the screen (Fig. 2-3).

TABLE 2-2. PROCEDURES GUIDED WITH TRANSVAGINAL ULTRASOUND (TVS)

TVS-Guided Procedure	Indication	Alternative Procedures	Observations
Puncture of ovarian cyst	Ovum retrieval Histology	Laparoscopy Laparotomy	
Treatment of ectopic pregnancy	Tubal, cornual, ovarian, or cervical ectopic	Laparotomy Laparoscopy	
Reduction of multifetal pregnancy	Super-multifetal pregnancy Twin with major anomaly		Timely reduction compared to transabdominal sonography
Drainage of pelvic content	Pelvic abscess Peritoneal cysts Postoperative collection of blood or lymph	Laparotomy Laparoscopy	
Culdocentesis	Ectopic pregnancy Corpus luteum rupture	Blind culdocentesis	
Early amniocentesis			Rarely performed
Chorionic villus sampling (CVS)	Multiple anterior uterine fibroids	Abdominal CVS Cervical CVS	Rarely performed
Coelocentesis	Early extra amniotic cytogenetics		Rarely performed
Hysterosonography	Pathology of the endometrial cavity	Dilatation and curettage Hysteroscopy	
Salpingosonography Saline Contrast medium Air	Pathology of the fallopian tube	Laparoscopy Hysterosalpingography	

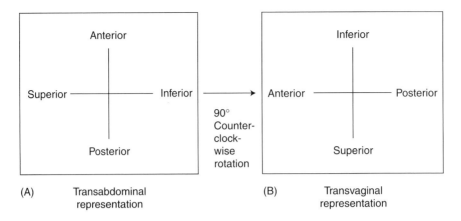

Figure 2-1. Orientation of transabdominal sonographic images (**A**) as compared to transvaginal sonograms (**B**).

Varying degrees of retroflexion cause the fundus to be directed more anteriorly, which places it in the bottom left section of the screen.

Axial images produced by TVS are actually a combination of a transverse and coronal plane. This occurs because the uterus is anteflexed when the bladder is empty. The sound wave intercepts the anteroinferior uterine wall first before intercepting a slightly superior and posterior aspect of the uterus. In transverse TVS imaging, as in the conventional transabdominal orientation, the right side of the patient corresponds to the right of the screen (Fig. 2-4).

Obtaining as nearly a perpendicular plane of an organ as possible is as important in TVS as in TAS, but Rottem et al. have found it easier to use "organ-oriented" scanning rather than trying to locate traditional anatomic planes. This approach entails scanning the target organ, which because of the smaller field of view, often fills the entire image. The organ itself is examined from axial, longitudinal, as well as other planes.[2]

TECHNIQUE

Once the basic concept of image representation is understood, the technique of TVS examination and image interpretation becomes easier to discuss. Trans-

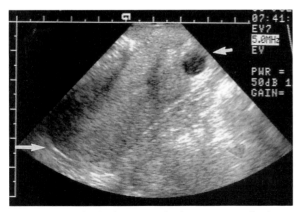

Figure 2-2. Sagittal transvaginal sonogram of uterus. This is an anteverted uterus with the fundus (*long arrow*) oriented toward the lower right corner of the image and the cervix, with a Nabothian cyst (*small arrow*), toward the upper left.

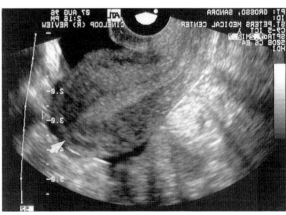

Figure 2-3. Sagittal transvaginal sonogram of a retroverted uterus. The fundus (*arrow*) is oriented toward the lower left corner of the image and the cervix.

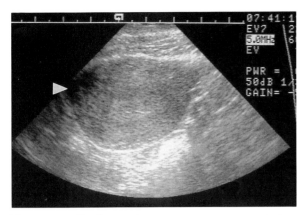

Figure 2-4. Semicoronal/transverse sonogram of the uterus. This is an anteverted uterus with the right side (*arrowhead*) of the uterus oriented on the right of the image.

ducer preparation and infection control techniques are described in Chapter 1. The most frequent transducer/patient manipulations are the following:

1. Anteroposterior angulation
2. Lateral (side-to-side) angulation
3. Depth of penetration (push-pull)

4. Rotation
5. Bimanual maneuvers

Anteroposterior Angulation

In the longitudinal plane, anteroposterior angulation (Fig. 2-5) allows the operator to optimize imaging of the uterus. A slight and gradual downward movement of the scanhead handle angles the transducer upward, allowing better visualization of an anteverted uterus. Conversely, an upward motion of the handle angles the transducer toward the patient's back, allowing better visualization of a retroverted uterus.

Lateral Angulation

Side-to-side manipulation of the transducer (Fig. 2-6) improves visualization of a uterus deviated to the right or left of midline; the cornua of the uterus; and the ipsilateral ovary, fallopian tube, pelvic vas-

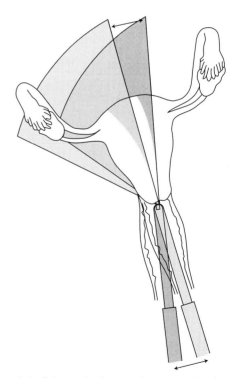

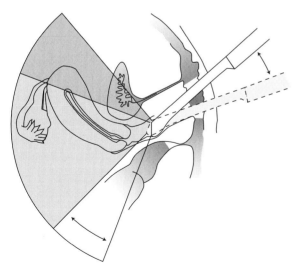

Figure 2-5. Schematic diagram demonstrating the movement of the transducer to produce sagittal views of the uterus in the same plane. The transducer handle is moved anterior and posterior to view all the sections of the uterus in the sagittal plane. (From DuBose TJ. Fetal Sonography. Philadelphia: WB Saunders; 1996:61–64; illustration by Victoria Vescovo Alderman, MA, RDMS.)

Figure 2-6. Schematic diagram demonstrating the movement of the transducer to view sagittal images in different planes. As the transducer is angled from one side to the other, parallel slices of the uterus are imaged. (From DuBose TJ. Fetal Sonography. Philadelphia: WB Saunders; 1996: 61–64; illustration by Victoria Vescovo Alderman, MA, RDMS.)

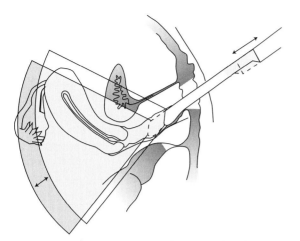

Figure 2-7. *Schematic diagram demonstrating the movement of the transducer to view structures at various distances from the fornix. Pushing the transducer deeper into the fornix brings more distant structures into the field of view, whereas withdrawing the transducer permits visualization of the cervix. (From DuBose TJ. Fetal Sonography. Philadelphia: WB Saunders; 1996:61–64; illustration by Victoria Vescovo Alderman, MA, RDMS.)*

Bimanual Maneuver

Another aid in optimizing vaginal imaging is the bimanual examination. The maneuver is achieved by the operator placing his or her free hand on the patient's pelvic area and gently applying pressure over the site of interest. This maneuver displaces bowel and moves organs or structures located higher in the pelvis into the TVS transducer's field of view. The bimanual maneuver can also help the examiner discriminate between a uterine and non-uterine mass. A uterine mass moves with the rest of the uterus, whereas a nonuterine mass slides past the uterine wall.

The TVS examination of the female pelvis should begin by imaging the cervix, which means the transducer should be pulled out slightly, increasing the distance between it and the cervix. Beginning the examination by imaging the cervix may allow the examiner to avoid image obscuration from air being introduced into the vagina and cervix

culature, ligaments, bowel, and other organs or structures.

Depth of Penetration

Changes in depth of penetration created by a gradual advancement or withdrawal of the vaginal probe (Fig. 2-7) allows the operator to image better an organ or structure by placing it within the field of view of the transducer. Some equipment has a built-in feature that allows the sonographer to vary the field of view by changing the frequency. A lower frequency enlarges the field of view to include structures higher in the pelvis, whereas a higher frequency limits the field of view to structures in the true pelvis. The operator must remember that the resolution of structures further from the transducer deteriorates more rapidly with higher-frequency transducers.

Rotation

A 90-degree counterclockwise rotation of the transducer allows for imaging in the "semicoronal" transverse plane (Fig. 2-8). This rotation, coupled with an anteroposterior angulation, produces views of the superior to inferior regions of the pelvis.

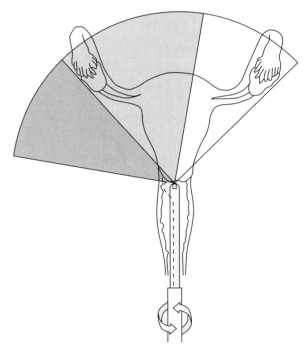

Figure 2-8. *Schematic diagram demonstrating the movement of the transducer to view semicoronal/transverse images of the uterus. Beginning in a sagittal plane, the transducer is rotated 90 degrees counterclockwise to image the uterus in transverse, with the right adnexa appearing on the right side of the screen. (From DuBose TJ. Fetal Sonography. Philadelphia: WB Saunders; 1996:61–64; illustration by Victoria Vescovo Alderman, MA, RDMS.)*

by the TVS examination. The entire uterus should be imaged sagitally by angling the transducer from one side to the other. To view the transverse planes, the transducer is then rotated 90 degrees counterclockwise and angled anteriorly to posteriorly until all sections of the uterus and the cul-de-sac are visualized. The ovaries should be imaged in both planes, using the same landmarks as in TAS. They are often found medial to the iliac vessels, and can be easily identified when they contain follicles. In postmenopausal women who are not on hormone replacement therapy, the lack of follicles may make them more difficult to locate.

As with abdominal scanning, it is advisable for sonographers and sonologists to follow a standard scanning routine. Timor-Tritsch has proposed the following[3]:

1. Scanning the cervix in the sagittal plane and measuring the distance between the internal and external os. The cervix should then be imaged in the coronal or transverse plane. While examining the cervix, the urinary bladder, if it contains any fluid, may be interrogated.
2. The transducer should be advanced to the fornix of the vagina to examine the uterus.
3. The examiner should then proceed to evaluate both adnexa by evaluating each side with longitudinal and transverse scans.
4. Finally, the pelvic cul-de-sac should be examined for fluid, normal anatomic structures such as the ovaries and fallopian tubes, and any pathology.

Patient Considerations

A chaperone should be present when a male sonographer or physician performs the examination. The examination should be well explained to the patient to alleviate any unnecessary anxiety. Comparing the insertion of the transducer to that of a tampon gives the woman an idea of the sensation to expect. Usually the patient is asked to empty her bladder before the examination. However, if the examination is performed to rule out placenta previa, the patient is asked not to empty her bladder totally because a small amount of residual urine in the bladder helps to define the anterior cervical lip.[4]

The patient is placed in the lithotomy position, ideally on a gynecologic examination table. If such

a table is not available, the patient's hips can be elevated with a foam pad or pillow. The patient should be properly draped to have her pelvis and legs covered.

The transducer should be gently inserted into the vagina by the sonographer, the physician, or the patient herself. Extreme angling of the transducer should be avoided because this may cause unnecessary discomfort. When properly performed, the transvaginal examination is well tolerated by nongravid and pregnant patients.

Special Considerations

Transvaginal sonography usually is not performed on patients who are virgins. Its use is not advised in the presence of premature rupture of membranes because of the possibility of introducing infection. In postmenopausal patients, vaginal secretion is reduced, and therefore a generous amount of lubricant should be applied for easier insertion of the transducer. The old belief that TVS can cause bleeding or hemorrhage when placenta previa is present has been found groundless. Rather, TVS is a helpful tool to rule out placenta previa.[5]

Summary

Although the diagnostic ultrasound community in the United States was initially hesitant to embrace the use of TVS, it is now a well established part of the armamentarium of most ultrasound laboratories. TVS is a well accepted part of the scanning protocol for obstetric and gynecologic examinations. Clinical research into improvements in the diagnostic sensitivity of TVS, with or without color Doppler, is ongoing. The enhanced imaging obtained in gynecologic settings and particularly first trimester obstetrics has already been well documented.

There is consensus that the transvaginal examination contributes additional information through its superior near-field resolution. However, there is no consensus among sonographers, radiologists, and obstetricians/gynecologists as to the exact role of TVS. Many radiologists look at TVS as an adjunct to the more panoramic transabdominal imaging of the female pelvis, uterus, and gestation. They report having diagnosed ectopic pregnancies in a cephalad pelvic position on TAS examinations that were not visible on TVS. On the other hand, many obstetricians/gynecologists view the transvaginal examination as the primary diagnostic tool, and may forego a transabdominal examination and its required bladder filling, especially in first trimester patients and with gynecologic studies. In fact, some physicians foresee the time when TVS will be performed in lieu of a bimanual examination. All seem to agree that TAS is necessary for second and third trimester ultrasound examinations and when an ectopic pregnancy is suspected.

Sonographers usually adopt the practice advocated by their particular laboratory—be it in a Radiology or Obstetrics/Gynecology Department or office. Even though the protocol they follow may be that of the particular laboratory, sonographers do not have the same implied status to perform the invasive, transvaginal examinations at will, and must continue to be sensitive to the patients', clinicians', and imagers' concerns about this fact.

REFERENCES

1. Fleischer AC, Kepple DM. Normal pelvic anatomy as depicted with transvaginal sonography. In: Fleischer AC, Manning FA, Jeanty P, Romero R, eds. Sonography in Obstetrics and Gynecology. 5th ed. Stamford, CT: Appleton & Lange; 1996:43–52.
2. Rottem S, Thaler I, Goldstein SR, Timor-Tritsch IE, Brandes JM. Transvaginal sonographic technique: Targeted organ scanning without resorting to "planes." J Clin Ultrasound. 1990;18:243–247.
3. Timor-Tritsch IE. Conducting the gynecologic ultrasound examination. In: Goldstein SR, Timor-Tritsch IE, eds. Ultrasound in Gynecology. New York: Churchill Livingstone; 1995:49–54.
4. Timor-Tritsch IE, Monteagudo A. Diagnosis of placenta previa by transvaginal sonography. Ann Med. 1993;25:279–283.
5. Timor-Tritsch IE, Yunis RA. Confirming the safety of transvaginal sonography in patients suspected of placenta previa. Obstet Gynecol. 1993;81:742–744.

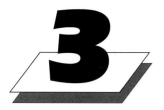

Embryonic Development of the Female Genital System

JOYCE A. MILLER

Knowledge of the embryogenesis of any internal organ is essential to understanding its anatomy. This is especially true in the female pelvis, where developmental anomalies may distort the normal sonographic appearance of the uterus and present diagnostic dilemmas. An understanding of the close developmental relationship between the primitive urinary system and the reproductive system can guide the sonographer to examine both when an anomaly exists in either one. The urogenital system can be demonstrated in utero and in later life, permitting diagnosis of morphologic anomalies when they are large enough for sonographic resolution or when they produce sonographic or clinical symptoms. Sonographers may discover evidence of pelvic anomalies in three different periods of life.

Fetal Period

Most congenital anomalies discovered in fetuses in utero have occurred in the genitourinary system.[12] In a large epidemiologic study of approximately 12,000 pregnant women, the overall prevalence of fetal malformations was found to be 0.5%; urinary tract abnormalities represent about 50% of the total number.[7] These anomalies presented in a wide range, from complete agenesis of the kidney and ureter to partial malformations, duplications, and obstructions with concomitant cyst formation. Prenatal ultrasound may also detect congenital anomalies in the ovaries, uterus, and vagina, especially when they enlarge and produce a pelvic mass. Hydrometrocolpos of the vagina and uterus, which presents as a hypoechoic mass posterior to the bladder, is the most common genital anomaly detected in utero.[4] In some fetuses with this condition, the hydrometrocolpos also compresses the urinary tract and causes hydronephrosis or hydroureter.

Neonatal Period

As in the fetal period, the most common mass lesions in neonates are of renal origin[10]; however, hydrometrocolpos secondary to an atretic vagina is a well known cause of abdominal masses in newborn girls.[3] Sonographic survey of a newborn girl should include identification of normal urinary bladder, uterus, vagina, and (whenever possible) ovaries, to rule out masses and obstructions.

Premenarche Through Adulthood

It is in this age group that the sonographer most frequently finds genital anomalies. Presentation of genital anomalies often occurs at the onset of puberty, when menstrual irregularities are apparent. For example, in the patient with a duplicated uterus with one septated vagina, obstruction to menstrual flow from one side can present as unilateral hematocolpos.[2] Some patients, however, have no symptoms and their congenital anomalies may first be discovered while scanning to rule out other conditions.

A review of the embryonic development of the female genitalia elucidates how such conditions arise.

Expression of Gender in an Embryo

THE PRIMORDIAL GERM CELLS

The gender or sex of an embryo is determined at fertilization. If the male gamete (the spermatozoon) contributes an X chromosome to its union with the female gamete (the ovum), which always contains an X, a female embryo (XX) results. If the male gamete contributes a Y chromosome, a male embryo (XY) results. The *primordial germ cells* that express or produce this femaleness or maleness are first discernible in the embryo about 21 days after conception. They differentiate from cells in the caudal part of the yolk sac, close to the allantois, a small diverticulum of the yolk sac that extends into the connecting stalk (Fig. 3-1*A*). Simultaneously, the *genital* or *gonadal ridges* are formed. They are the precursors to the ovaries in females and to the testes in males. These ridges are located on the anteromedial sides of the wolffian bodies, the embryonic regions where the kidneys develop (see Fig. 3-1*B*).[12] The urinary system and the reproductive system are intimately associated in origin, development, and certain final relations. Both arise from mesoderm that initially takes the form of a common ridge (wolffian body) located on both sides of the median plane. Both systems continue to develop in close proximity; they drain into a common cloaca, and slightly later into a urogenital sinus, which is a subdivision of the cloaca. Some parts of the urogenital system disappear after a transitory existence.[1] For example, by the fifth developmental week, the first-stage kidney (pronephros) has differentiated and has already disappeared.[9] Certain common primordia transform differently in males and females.

INDUCER GERM CELLS

During the fifth week of development, the primordial germ cells migrate by ameboid movement from their origin in the yolk sac along the dorsal mesentery. In the sixth week they invade the gonadal ridges (see Fig. 3-1*B*). If by chance they do not reach the ridges, the gonads cease to develop. Thus these primordial germ cells act as *inducers* of the gonads. Note that at this time in development (the sixth week), the mesonephros, or second-stage kidney, and its wolffian duct have developed lateral to the gonadal ridges.[8,11]

As the primordial cells are invading the ridges, an outer layer of fetal tissue called coelomic epithelium grows into the underlying mesenchymal tissue, or embryonic connective tissue. Active tissue growth here forms a network, or rete, called the primitive sex cords (Fig. 3-2). This rete forms anastomoses with a portion of the wolffian duct, thus establishing the first urogenital connections in the embryo. After the degeneration of the second-stage kidney, the mesonephros, the male embryo appropriates its wolffian duct and converts it into genital canals. This stage of development is often termed the *indifferent gonad stage,* because it is still not possible to distinguish morphologic sex differences.[8,11,12]

In the seventh week, if the embryo is a genetic male, the primitive sex cords continue to proliferate and eventually give rise to the rete testis. If the embryo is a genetic female, the primitive sex cords break up into irregularly shaped cell clusters, which eventually disappear. They are replaced by a vascular stroma, a supporting tissue, that later forms the ovarian medulla.[12]

In a female gonad (the ovary), the outer layer of epithelium continues to proliferate, giving rise to a second group of cords, which eventually occupy the cortex of the ovary. These are the *cortical cords,* or *Pluger's tubules* (Fig. 3-3).[12]

In the fourth month, the cortical cords split into isolated cell clusters, each surrounding one or more primitive germ cells. Now the primitive germ cells differentiate into *oogonia,* which divide repeatedly by mitosis to reach a maximum number of 7 million by the fifth month of prenatal life. Many oogonia subsequently degenerate, so at birth their number is approximately 1 million (Fig. 3-4).[6]

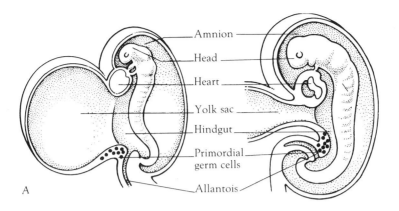

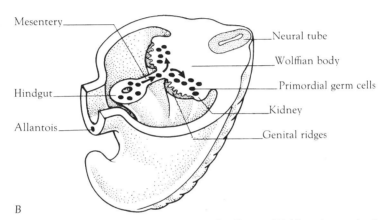

Figure 3-1. (**A**) Primordial germ cells in wall of yolk sac. (**B**) Migration path of primordial germ cells.

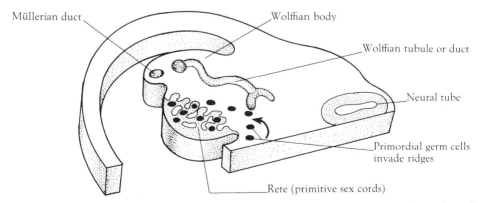

Figure 3-2. Development of embryo on one side. Indifferent gonad stage; formation of primitive sex cords.

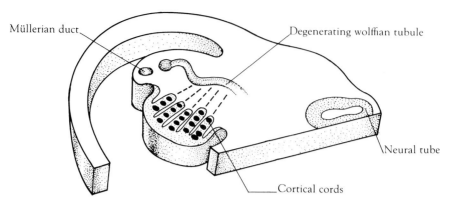

Figure 3-3. Formation of the cortical cords.

The surviving oogonia differentiate into *primary oocytes* during prenatal life and are surrounded by a single layer of granulosa cells derived from the cortical cords. The primary oocyte with its surrounding granulosa cells is called a *primordial follicle.* Many undergo degeneration during childhood and adolescence, so that by puberty approximately 500,000 remain. Between puberty and menopause approximately 300 to 400 fertile ova are produced.[6]

Genital Ducts

It is necessary to backtrack in time to trace the development of the ductal system that occurs simultaneously with the development of the gonads (ovaries or testes). In the indifferent gonad stage (until the seventh week), the genital tracts of both male and female embryos have the same appearance and comprise two pairs of ducts. The wolffian ducts arise from the second-stage kidney, the mesonephros. The müllerian ducts arise from an invagination or pocket of coelomic epithelium lateral to the cranial end of each wolffian duct. Growth progresses caudad, eventually hollowing out to form an open duct.[8] Development of the embryonic ductal system and external genitalia occurs under the influence of circulating hormones in the fetus. In males, fetal testes produce an inducer substance that causes differentiation and growth of the wolffian ducts and inhibition of the müllerian ducts. In females, because the male inducer substance is absent, the wolffian ducts regress while the müllerian ductal system, influenced by maternal and placental estrogens, develops into the fallopian tubes and uterus.[8]

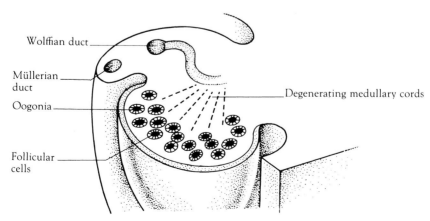

Figure 3-4. Differentiation of primitive germ cells into oogonia in the fourth month.

The müllerian ducts first extend downward parallel to the wolffian ducts, then turn mediad in the lower abdomen, crossing anterior to the wolffian ducts and fusing together in the midline to form a single duct, the *uterovaginal canal* (Fig. 3-5). This fusion begins caudally and progresses up to the site of the future fallopian tubes. In normal development, the midline septum disappears by the end of the third month and the uterine corpus and cervix are formed. They are surrounded by a layer of mesenchyme, which eventually forms the muscular coat of the uterus (the myometrium) and its peritoneal covering (the perimetrium).[8,11]

Formation of the Fallopian Tubes

After the formation of the uterovaginal canal, the segment of each müllerian duct positioned above the junction of the inguinal ligament becomes a fallopian tube. The craniad orifice of the müllerian duct, which stays open to the peritoneal cavity, becomes the fimbriae of the fallopian tube. Initially, the fallopian tube lies in a vertical position. As development proceeds, it moves to the interior of the abdominal cavity to lie horizontally. This causes the ovary, which is attached to the fallopian tube by

the mesovarium, to descend and finally to assume a position dorsal to the fallopian tube (Table 3-1, Fig. 3-6).[6,8,11]

Formation of the Broad Ligament

As the müllerian duct fuses medially and the ovary is successfully located cranial and finally dorsal to the fallopian tubes, the mesenteries follow these positional changes.[11] This movement causes the folds of the peritoneum to be elevated from the posterolateral wall, thus creating a large transverse pelvic fold called the *broad ligament*, which extends from the lateral sides of the fused müllerian ducts toward the wall of the pelvis. The fallopian tube will be located on its superior surface and on its posterior surface, the ovary (see Fig. 3-6). The ovary is suspended by several structures: (1) the *mesovarium* is a double-layered fold of peritoneum that is continuous with the posterosuperior layer of the broad ligament. (2) The *proper ligament of the ovary* is a band of connective tissue that lies between the two layers of the broad ligament and connects the lower pole of the ovary with the lateral uterine wall. (3) The *suspensory ligament* is a triangular fold of peritoneum that actually forms the upper lateral corner of the broad ligament. This ligament sus-

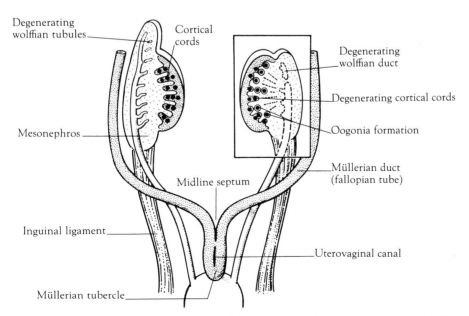

Figure 3-5. Formation of uterovaginal canal, eighth week. Inset: ovary at fourth month, forming the oogonia.

◤◢◤◢ TABLE 3-1. EMBRYONIC DEVELOPMENT CHART FOR FEMALE UROGENITAL SYSTEM

	Urinary System	Gonads	Ducts	Mesenteries
3rd Week	Pronephros differentiates	Primordial cells seen in allantois		
4th Week	Pronephros disappears and mesonephros differentiates	Formation of genital ridges		
5th Week	Metanephros starts to differentiate	Migration of primordial germ cells		
6th Week		Primitive germ cells invade gonadal ridges	Two sets of ducts exist: wolffian (kidney) and müllerian (genital ridge)	
		Formation of primitive sex cords: "indifferent stage"		
7th Week		Primitive sex cords disappear		
		Cortical cords arise		
8th Week	Mesonephros disappears, only its duct (wolffian) remains			
8th Week ↓	Wolffian duct regresses almost completely		Müllerian ducts fuse to form uterovaginal canal and fallopian tubes	
12th Week		Ovary descends	Median septum disappears	
12th Week ↓	Metanephros—3rd– stage kidney	Cortical cords split up and surround primitive germ cells to produce 7,000,000 oogonia		Formation of mesosalpinx, mesovarium, broad ligament, proper ovarian ligament, and suspensory ligament
5th Month				

pends both the ovary and the fallopian tube by its confluence with the parietal peritoneum at the pelvic brim.[5]

Formation of the Vagina

The vagina has a dual origin: its upper region is derived from the mesodermal tissue of the müllerian ducts and its lower region, from the urogenital sinus. The urogenital sinus is the ventral half of the primitive cloaca (hindgut) after it has been divided by the urorectal septum. The upper portion of the urogenital sinus becomes the urinary bladder and the lower portion is divided into two portions—the pars pelvina, involved in formation of the vagina, and the pars phallica, which is related to the primordia (developing organs) of the external genitalia. This can best be understood by following the development of the vagina step by step. First, the distal end of the uterovaginal canal makes contact with the posterior wall of the urogenital sinus (Fig. 3-7A). As these structures fuse, a solid group of cells called the *vaginal plate* is formed (see Fig. 3-7B). From the vaginal plate, two outgrowths (*sinovaginal bulbs*) surround the uterovaginal canal and fuse on opposite sides (see Fig. 3-7C). If the sinovaginal bulbs do not fuse normally, a vagina with two outlets, or a vagina with one normal outlet and one atretic one, may result.[8,11]

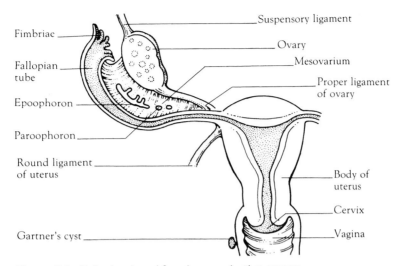

Figure 3-6. Fully developed female reproductive organs.

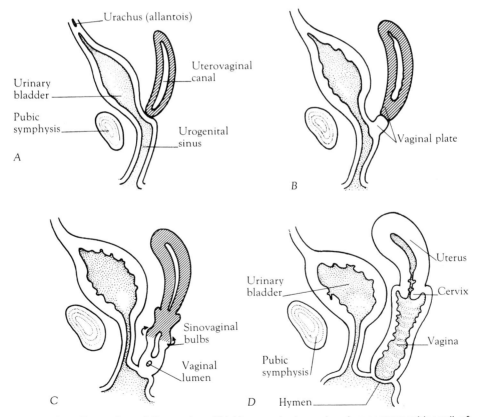

Figure 3-7. Formation of the vagina. (**A**) Uterovaginal canal makes contact with wall of urogenital sinus. (**B**) Formation of vaginal plate. (**C**) Sinovaginal bulbs encircle the vaginal plate and elongate. (**D**) Canalization of vaginal plate to form the vagina; separation of vagina and urogenital sinus by the hymen.

After normal development, the center core of cells hollows out to form a lumen in the vagina. The vagina is now separated from the urogenital sinus only by a thin tissue plate, the *hymen* (see Fig. 3-7*D*). The vaginal fornices, which surround the ends of the uterus (cervix), are thought to be of müllerian duct origin.

In most female fetuses, these developmental steps proceed uneventfully to culminate in normal pelvic viscera, which can be examined with ultrasound. Chapter 5 discusses ultrasound's role in diagnosing congenital abnormalities.

REFERENCES

1. Arey L. Developmental Anatomy. 7th ed. Philadelphia: WB Saunders; 1974.
2. Benson R. Obstetric and Gynecologic Diagnosis and Treatment. 2nd ed. Los Altos, CA: Lange; 1978.
3. Burbige KA, Hensle T. Uterus didelphis and vaginal duplication with unilateral obstruction presenting as a newborn abdominal mass. J Urol. 1984; 132: 1195–1198.
4. Crade M, Gilloley L, Taylor K. Ovarian cystic mass in utero. J Clin Ultrasound. 1980; 8:251–252.
5. Crafts RC, Krieger HP. Gross anatomy of the female reproductive tract, pituitary, and hypothalamus. In: Danforth DN, Scott JR, eds. Obstetrics and Gynecology. 5th ed. Philadelphia: JB Lippincott; 1986.
6. Crowley LV. Introduction to Clinical Embryology. Chicago: Year Book Medical Publishers; 1974.
7. Helin I, Persson P. Prenatal diagnosis of urinary tract abnormalities by ultrasound. Pediatrics. 1986; 78: 879–883.
8. Langeman J. Medical Embryology. 4th ed. Baltimore: Williams & Wilkins; 1981:234–267.
9. Ramsey EM. Embryology and developmental defects of the reproductive tract. In: Danforth DN, ed. Obstetrics and Gynecology. 5th ed. Philadelphia: JB Lippincott; 1986.
10. Schulman CC, Elkhazen N, Picard C. Diagnostic chez le foetus des malformations urinaires par l'echographie. J Urologie. 1981; 87:431.
11. Tuchmann-Duplessis H, Haegel P. Illustrated Human Embryology. Berlin: Springer-Verlag; 1972:2.
12. Zuckerman L, Weir B. The Ovary. 2nd ed. New York: Academic Press; 1977; 1:42–52.

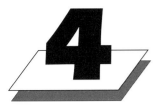

4

Sonographic Anatomy of the Female Pelvis

LARRY WALDROUP and JI-BIN LIU

A thorough knowledge of the gross and cross-sectional anatomy of the female pelvis is essential for the sonographer who must seek pathologic processes in this area. This anatomy can more easily be assimilated and understood by building up a mental picture of the layers of the pelvis, beginning with the bony framework.

The female pelvis serves three principal functions. First, it provides a weight-bearing bridge between the spinal column and the bones of the lower limbs through the sacrum and the innominate bones. Second, it directs the pathway of the fetal head during childbirth (parturition). Third, it protects the organs of reproduction.

The Pelvic Skeleton

In adults, the osseous pelvis is essentially a ring composed of four bones: the *sacrum,* the *coccyx,* and the two large *innominate bones,* which result from fusion of the ilium, ischium, and pubis (Fig. 4-1).[6] The sacrum and coccyx form the posterior wall of the pelvis, and the innominate bones form the lateral and anterior walls (Fig. 4-2). The innominate bones are joined together posteriorly through the sacrum and anteriorly in the midline at the pubic symphysis. The outer surface of the innominate bone forms the acetabulum, the socket for the femoral head (see Fig. 4-2).

The sacrum and coccyx are modified segments of the vertebral column. The sacrum results from fusion of the five sacral vertebrae, and the coccyx (our vestigial tail) consists of four fused coccygeal vertebrae (Fig. 4-3). Between the sacrum and coccyx is an articulation that permits little or no motion.

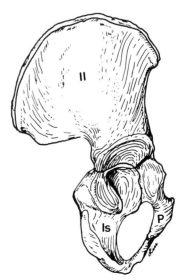

Figure 4-1. Three bones fuse to form the innominate bone. (Il, ilium; Is, ischium; P, pubis.)

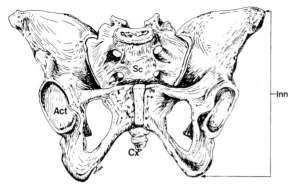

Figure 4-2. The female pelvis viewed from the front. The pelvis has been tilted up to show better the acetabula and pubic rami. See Figure 4-5 for the correct angle of the pelvis in life. (Act, acetabulum; Inn, innominate bone; Sc, sacrum; Cx, coccyx.)

The bones of the pelvis define two distinct spaces, the true pelvis and the false pelvis, which are separated by an imaginary line (the *linea terminalis*) extending from the sacral prominence along the inner surface of the innominate bone down to the symphysis pubis anteriorly (Figs. 4-4 to 4-6).[6] The true pelvis lies below the linea terminalis and has a horizontally oriented inlet but a vertically oriented outlet (Fig. 4-7). The inlet of the true pelvis is entirely walled by bone, but the outlet is only partially so (see Figs. 4-2, 4-5, and 4-6). It is apparent that other structures are needed to fill in the gaps, and these include the membranes, ligaments, and muscles of the pelvic floor.

The Pelvic Muscles

Forming much of the abdominal body wall and lining the osseous framework of the pelvis are muscles that can be demonstrated by ultrasound. Most are paired structures that are bilaterally symmetric. Table 4-1 lists the pelvic muscles by region and pelvic location. The pelvic skeletal muscles, along with the osseous pelvis, define the limits of the space that must be investigated by pelvic sonography. The sonographer should be able to recognize these pelvic muscles to avoid confusing them with a mass. Skeletal muscle appears less echoic than fat or smooth muscle and exhibits linear internal echoes outlining the muscle bundles (see Fig. 4-11). The borders of the muscle are outlined by the echogenic fascia and retroperitoneal fat.

Two of the muscles commonly demonstrated on transverse pelvic scans (rectus abdominis and psoas) are not exclusively pelvic muscles because they also extend through the abdominal region. The *rectus abdominis* muscles form much of the anterior body wall. They extend from the pubic symphysis and pubic crest to the costal cartilages of the fifth, sixth, and seventh ribs and the xiphoid process (Fig. 4-8).[5] On cross section, each rectus muscle is ovoid or lens shaped (lenticular), most strikingly so in the lower abdomen.

The *psoas major* muscle originates from the lower thoracic and the lumbar vertebrae.[5] This cylindrical muscle then courses laterad and ante-

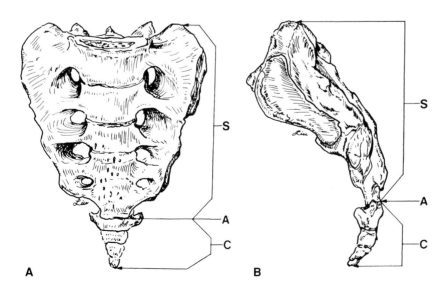

A   **B**

Figure 4-3. (**A**) Ventral and (**B**) lateral surfaces of the adult sacrum (S) and coccyx (C). Note the five fused vertebral bodies forming the sacrum, the four fused bodies that form the coccyx, and the shallow **S**-shaped curve that these bones establish in the posterior wall of the pelvis. (A, articulation between sacrum and coccyx.)

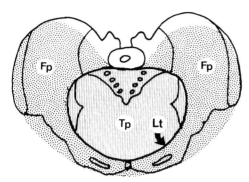

Figure 4-4. The true and false pelvic cavities. The wide but shallow false pelvis (Fp) surrounds the deep central true pelvis (Tp.) The dividing line between the two spaces is the linea terminalis (Lt).

rior as it descends through the lower abdomen (Fig. 4-9). Above the level of the fourth lumbar vertebra (L4), the psoas is closely attached to the lateral margins of the vertebral column. At about L5, it separates from the spine and begins

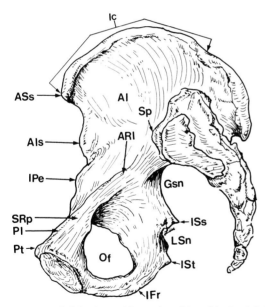

Figure 4-5. Pelvis viewed from the side with the left innominate bone removed. The linea terminalis (innominate line) is made up of the pectineal line and the arcuate line. (Sp, sacral prominence; Al, ala [wing] of the ilium bone forming iliac fossa; Ic, iliac crest; ASs, anterior superior iliac spine; Als, anterior inferior iliac spine; Pt, pubic tubercle; ISt, ischial tuberosity; ISs, ischial spine; Gsn, greater sciatic notch; LSn, lesser sciatic notch; IFr, inferior ramus of pubis; Of, obturator foramen; SRp, superior ramis of pubis; IPe, iliopubic eminence; Pl, pectineal line; ARI, arcuate line.)

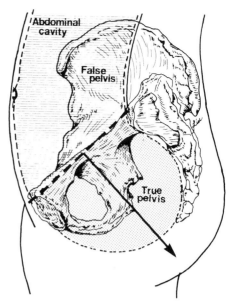

Figure 4-6. Relationship of the abdominal cavity to the true and false pelvic cavities. The false pelvis forms the walls of the most inferior part of the abdominal cavity. The true pelvis extends farther posterior than the false pelvis. When viewed from the side, the axis of the true pelvic cavity is directed posterior and inferior at about 45 degrees. The inlet is steeply tilted (about 60 degrees from horizontal) whereas the outlet is almost horizontal. The curve of the sacrum provides the transition between these two angles, and serves to direct the fetal head downward and then forward during parturition.

to move more laterad, creating a gutter or trough-like space between the psoas and spine. The common iliac vessels run through this space. Below the level of the iliac crest, fibers of the psoas major lie adjacent to or begin to interdigitate with fibers from the medial aspect of the *iliacus muscle*, thus creating the *iliopsoas*. This

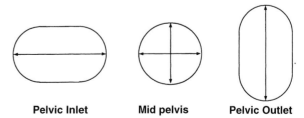

Figure 4-7. Shape of the true pelvis at its inlet, mid-pelvis, and outlet. Although the inlet and outlet are similar in shape, their axes differ by 90 degrees. Consider how these shapes affect the orientation of the fetal head during parturition.

▰▰▰ TABLE 4-1. THE PELVIC MUSCLES		
Region	**Muscle**	**Location**
Abdominopelvic	Rectus abdominis	Anterior wall
	Psoas major	Posterior wall
False pelvis	Iliacus	Iliac fossa
True pelvis	Obturator internus	Lateral wall
	Piriformis	Posterior wall
	Coccygeus	Posterior floor
	Levator ani	Middle and anterior floor

composite muscle continues its lateral and anterior course through the false pelvis, passing over the pelvic brim to insert on the lesser trochanter of the femur.

Through most of the false pelvis, the cross-sectional shape of the psoas–iliopsoas is that of an oddly shaped hook with a bulbous medial limb (Fig. 4-10, section 4). On sagittal ultrasound scans, these muscles appear as a long, dark strip whose posterior margin courses upward toward the anterior body wall as the muscle complex descends through the pelvis (Fig. 4-11). The iliopsoas never enters the true pelvis. In the false pelvis, its medial margin coincides with the linea terminalis and thus marks the border between the true and false pelvis (Fig. 4-12).

Within the true pelvic space is the *obturator internus* (Fig. 4-13). This triangular sheet of muscle originates as bands of fibers anchored along the brim of the true pelvis and from the inner surface of the obturator membrane, which closes the obturator foramen.[5] The muscle extends posteriorly and medial along the sidewall of the true pelvis, passing beneath the levator ani muscles to exit from the pelvic space through the lesser sciatic foramen. Because it lies parallel and adjacent to the lateral pelvic wall, the obturator internus is difficult to identify on a sagittal ultrasound image. At normal gain levels it is often obscured on transverse scans as well; however, when it is visible, the obturator appears as a thin, hypoechoic, vertical strip lining the wall of the pelvis (Fig. 4-14).

Deeply posterior in the true pelvis is another roughly triangular muscle, the *piriformis,* which takes origin from the sacrum and then courses laterally through the greater sciatic foramen to insert on the greater trochanter of the femur (Fig. 4-15).[5] Unless the urinary bladder is very full, the piriformis is usually obscured by overlying bowel gas in the sigmoid colon.

The floor of the true pelvis is made up of a complex group of similar muscles that collectively form a two-layered pelvic diaphragm. The outermost layer is composed of the muscles of the *perineum,* which are rarely identifiable in transabdominal ultrasound images. In contrast, the innermost layer of the pelvic diaphragm is commonly visualized in transverse ultrasound scans. The named muscles of the innermost group include (from posterior to anterior) the coccygeus,

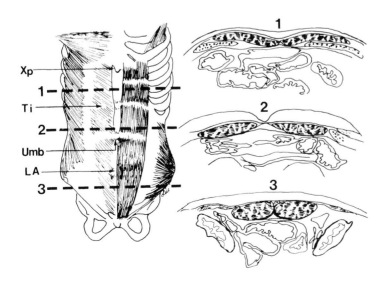

Figure 4-8. The rectus abdominis muscles seen from the front with representative cross sections (*dashed lines*). The left and right columns of muscle are separated by the midline linea alba (LA) and are interrupted by transverse tendinous intersections (Ti) at the level of the umbilicus, between the umbilicus (Umb) and the xiphoid, and at the xiphoid process (Xp).

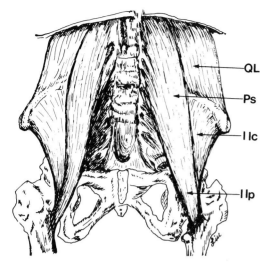

Figure 4-9. *Muscles of the posterior body wall and the false pelvis, viewed from the front. (Ps, psoas major; QL, quadratus lumborum; Ilc, iliacus; Ilp, iliopsoas.)*

ties include the coccygeus as part of the levator ani, but some do not because it functions only to support the sacrum.

The levator ani is like a hammock stretched between the pubis and the coccyx. Its lateral margins attach to a thickened band of the fascia that covers the obturator internus muscle, thus anchoring the levator ani to the lateral pelvic walls.[5] In the midline, fibers from the levator ani insert on the walls of the rectum, vagina, and urethra as they pass through the pelvic diaphragm.

The levator ani functions to resist increased intraabdominal pressure (as from coughing or straining) and to resist gravity, holding the pelvic organs in place (Fig. 4-17).[5] If these muscles fail to function properly, one of the results is "prolapse" of the pelvic organs through the pelvic diaphragm.

the iliococcygeus, and the pubococcygeus (part of which is classified as the puborectalis; Figs. 4-15 and 4-16).[5] The iliococcygeus, pubococcygeus, and puborectalis are more correctly described as the *levator ani* muscles. Most authori-

The Pelvic Organs

The pelvic organs include three hollow muscular viscera and one pair of parenchymatous organs. These are (1) the urinary bladder and urethra; (2)

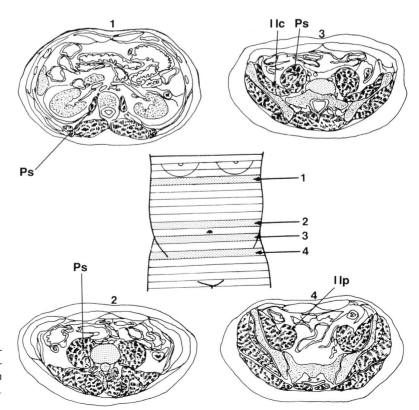

Figure 4-10. *Shape of the psoas-iliacus-iliopsoas muscles on cross section at various levels in the abdomen and pelvis. (Ps, psoas; Ilc, Iliacus; Ilp, iliopsoas.)*

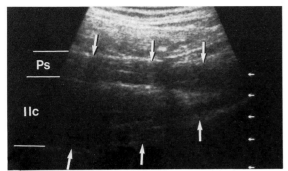

Figure 4-11. Sagittal scan of the psoas major (Ps) and iliac muscles (Ilc) in the false pelvis. Faint lines within the muscle arise from the fiber bundles and fascial planes. Note the upward slant of the posterior wall of the muscle group and how the image ends at the bone of the ilium.

provides a relatively rigid framework that supports a layer of fascia composed of loose connective tissue, through which runs the plumbing (arteries, veins, and lymphatics) and the electrical and communication lines (nerves). Almost everywhere in the pelvis, the membranous fascia is covered by a layer of insulation (the retroperitoneal fat, which lies between the peritoneum and the endopelvic fascia). The "wallpaper" over the surface of the walls is the peritoneum. Inside the "room" defined by these walls are found the organs. The analogy breaks down a bit here, because most of the organs of the female pelvis (urinary bladder, uterus, rectum) technically are not inside the room but push into it from the walls or floor without ever breaking through the wallpaper (peritoneum). From a practical stand-

the uterus, fallopian tubes, and vagina; (3) the pelvic colon and rectum; (4) and the ovaries.

Before beginning a detailed examination of the organs of the female pelvis, the reader should take a moment to conceptualize the various layers of the pelvic walls formed by the bones, muscles, and tendons. Like the walls of a house, this organic wall

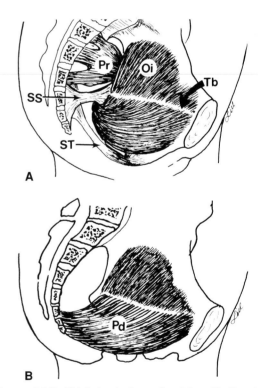

Figure 4-13. (**A**) Lateral view of pelvis with the deep pelvic sidewall muscles shown. The piriformis muscle (Pr) exits the true pelvic space through the greater sciatic foramen; the obturator internus (Oi) exits the true pelvis through the lesser sciatic foramen. These foramina are defined by the sacrospinous (SS) and the sacrotuberous (ST) ligaments. (Tb, tendinous band.) (**B**) The obturator internus muscle exhibits a tendinous band (Tb) that runs anterior to posterior across the muscle. This band is the point of attachment for the pelvic diaphragm (Pd), which is in part suspended from the surface of the obturator internus muscle.

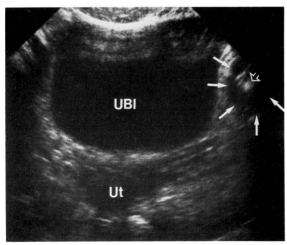

Figure 4-12. Transverse scan of the mid-pelvis. The iliopsoas muscle complex is almost always seen on transverse pelvic scans. The bright echo (*open arrow*) within the muscle arises from the femoral nerve, the iliopsoas tendon, and fat filling in a groove formed by the line of fusion between the two contributor muscles. Although the anatomic location of this bright echo complex is not actually central to the iliopsoas composite muscle, it usually appears central on the sonogram because the lateral region of the iliacus is rarely seen well owing to overlying bowel gas. (UBI, urinary bladder; Ut, uterus.)

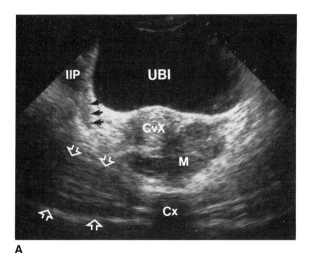
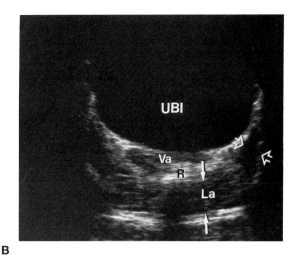

A   B

Figure 4-14. (**A**) Transverse scan of the pelvis demonstrates the obturator internus muscle as a thin, hypoechoic strip (*black arrows*) adjacent to the lateral pelvic wall. The upper margin of the muscle is just below the brim of the pelvis. The levator ani muscle group is also well seen (*open arrows*). (UBI, urinary bladder; CvX, cervix; Cx, coccyx; M, mass adjacent to cervix; Ilp, iliopsoas muscle.) (**B**) Forming the floor of the true pelvic space is the levator ani muscle group (*arrows*), which attaches to the medial surface of the obturator internus muscle (*open arrows*). (UBI, urinary bladder; La, levator ani muscle; R, rectum; Va, vagina.)

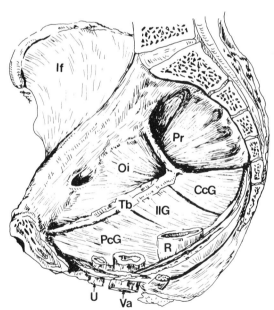

Figure 4-15. A more detailed view of the pelvic muscles with the pelvic diaphragm in place. The ragged edges along the tendinous band of the obturator internus are the cut edges of the fascial membrane that covers these muscles. The major orifices that pass through the pelvic diaphragm are also shown. (Oi, obturator internus muscle; Pr, piriformis muscle; Tb, tendinous band; CcG, coccygeus muscle; IIG, iliococcygeus; PcG, pubococcygeus; U, urethra; Va, vagina; R, rectum; If, iliac fossa.)

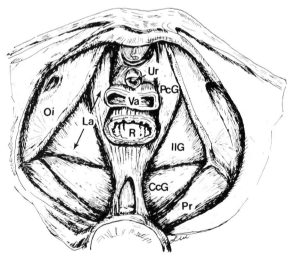

Figure 4-16. A view from above and posterior looking down into the true pelvis. Relate the position of the muscles in this view to the view shown in Figure 4-15. (Oi, obturator internus muscle; Pr, piriformis muscle; CcG, coccygeus muscle; IIG, iliococcygeus; PcG, pubococcygeus; La, levator ani muscle group; R, rectum; Ur, urethra; Va, vagina.)

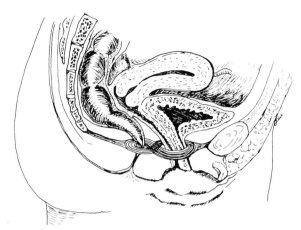

Figure 4-17. Relationship of the pubococcygeus muscle of the levator ani to the orifices that pass through the pelvic diaphragm.

point, however, the pelvic organs should be conceptualized as being inside the "room" defined by the pelvic walls. These organs constantly change dimensions. The urinary bladder and the rectum must expand and contract over relatively brief periods of time. Over a longer time frame, the uterus must expand during pregnancy and contract after expulsion of the fetus.

The arrangement of the organs within the pelvic space (Fig. 4-18) facilitates dimensional changes, but it also means that the position and contour of each organ varies in response to the degree of filling of the other organs that share the same space. These variations dramatically affect the ultrasound image, as is seen later in this chapter.

URINARY BLADDER AND URETHRA

The *urinary bladder* is a thick-walled, highly distensible muscular sac that lies between the symphysis pubis and the vagina. When empty, its shape on a sagittal section is an inverted triangle whose apex is formed by the orifice of the urethra.

The anterior surface of the bladder is loosely anchored to the pubic arch by fibrous connective tissue (the pubovesical ligament) but is separated from the symphysis pubis by an interposed pad of extraperitoneal fat in the space of Retzius, or retropubic space.[12] The posterior wall is composed largely of the *trigone* region, which is defined by the orifices of the two ureters and the urethra (Fig. 4-19). The trigone region is thicker and more rigid than the rest of the bladder wall and is separated from the anterior vaginal wall only by a thin layer of fat and loose connective tissue. The superior wall (the *dome* of the bladder) is covered by the coe-

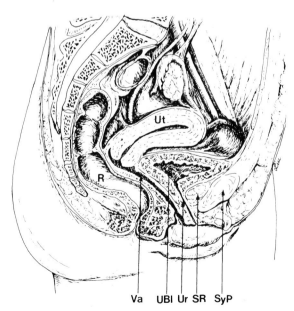

Figure 4-18. Organs of the pelvis. (Ut, uterus; R, rectum; Va, vagina; UBl, urinary bladder; Ur, urethra.) Also noted are certain nonorgan structures, including the space of Retzius (SR) and the symphysis pubis (SyP).

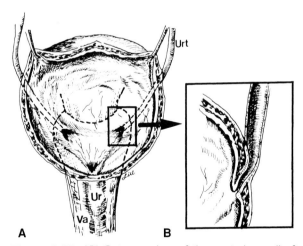

Figure 4-19. (**A**) Cutaway view of the posterior wall of the urinary bladder. Deeper structures, including the cervix and the upper region of the vagina, are indicated by dotted lines. (**B**) The ureters enter the bladder at the level of the cervix and on the posterior and inferior wall of the bladder. Their passage through the bladder wall is oblique, forming a passive valve system that resists urine reflux. (Ur, urethra; Va, vagina; Urt, ureter.)

lomic peritoneum and usually is in contact with the anterior wall of the uterus, which folds forward to rest on the dome of the bladder (see Fig. 4-18).

The walls of the urinary bladder are composed of three layers, but only two are visible on sonography. The thick middle layer (the muscularis or detrusor muscle) is composed predominantly of smooth muscle fibers, which give the bladder its contractility. The outer epithelial layer is not visible in ultrasound scans because it is thin and in intimate contact with adjacent layers of fascia and fatty tissues that cover most of the anterior and posterior walls. The inner layer of the bladder is the mucosa, which is very echogenic. Sonographic demonstration of the muscularis and mucosa depends on the degree of bladder filling. When the urinary bladder is empty, the bladder mucosa is quite thick and easily demonstrated (Fig. 4-20*A*). When the bladder is distended, the stretched mucosa becomes so thin that it can no longer be recognized as a discrete layer of the bladder wall.

Extending from the urinary bladder are three tubular structures: the two *ureters,* which carry urine from the kidneys to the bladder, and the *urethra,* which conducts urine from the bladder to the urethral orifice, which lies between the labia minora of the external female genitalia. At its exit from the bladder the urethra is surrounded by a thickened region of bladder wall known as the internal sphincter. This thickening may be observed on the sagittal sonogram, marking the urethral exit (see Fig. 4-20*B*).

Urine is transported through the ureters by peristaltic contraction of the walls. As the contraction reaches the bladder, back-pressure from the bladder must be overcome; the ureteral valve pops open and a bolus of urine enters the bladder in a brief jet (Fig. 4-21). Urine jets can be observed routinely on sonography with high gain in gray-scale imaging or with color Doppler, but the jet is transient and the echoes disappear quickly. The cause of these echoes is the subject of debate, but it is probable that the pressure differential between the jet and the surrounding urine is sufficient explanation. Urine in the renal pelvis, ureters, and urinary bladder is normally sterile and completely anechoic.

The contour of the urinary bladder does not change uniformly as it expands with filling. The dome is the most distensible region of the bladder, so it might be expected to expand uniformly upward in the pelvis, but two factors dictate nonuniform expansion of the bladder walls. First, the trigone is thicker and more rigid; second, the bladder must accommodate the space requirements of the other organs in the pelvis, chiefly the uterus. Be-

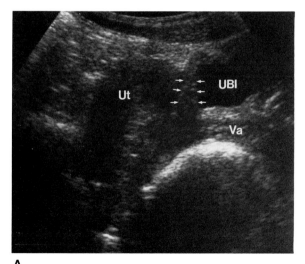
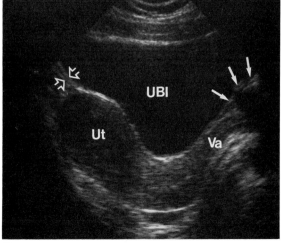

A   **B**

Figure 4-20. (**A**) *Sagittal scan in midline. When the urinary bladder contains only a small amount of urine, the bladder walls (arrows) are thick and easily demonstrated. (Ut, uterus; UBl, urinary bladder; Va, vagina.) (**B**) Sagittal scan in midline. When fully distended, the bladder walls (open arrows) nearly disappear from the image. The "urethral hump" formed by the internal sphincter is clearly visible in this scan (solid arrows). (UBl, urinary bladder; Ut, uterus; Va, vagina.)*

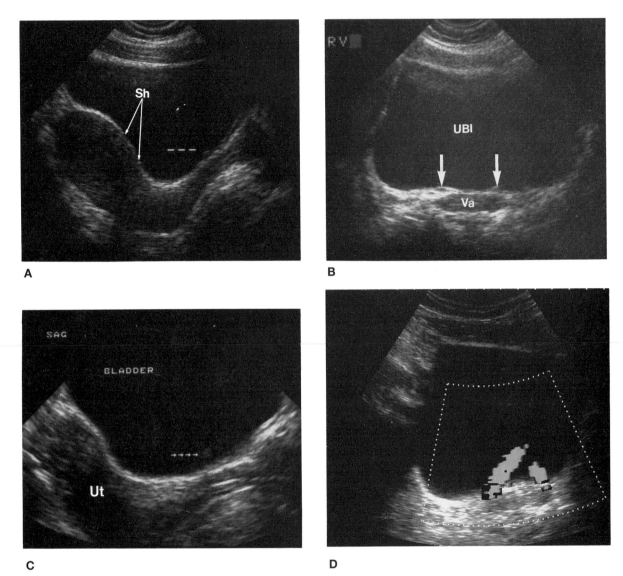

Figure 4-21. (**A**) Sagittal scan slightly to the left of midline. The ureteric valve is visible occasionally as a small projection (*dashed line*). When the valve structure is normal, this projection appears only briefly as the valve pops open. If persistent, it may represent a ureterocele. This image is also a good example of the typical reflection shadow (Sh), which occurs as a result of the relationship between the curve of the anterior uterine wall and the angle of incidence of the acoustic beam. This shadow is artifactual but normal. (**B**) A slightly oblique transverse scan shows the right ureter (*left arrow*) anterior to the vagina (Va) and just beneath the urinary bladder (UBl) wall. The left ureteric valve (*right arrow*) is in the process of opening. (**C**) A ureteric jet (*arrows*). This echo pattern lasts only a second or two (Ut, uterus). (**D**) Color Doppler of the region of the ureteric orifices often shows dramatic plumes of color when the jets enter the urinary bladder. (See also Color Plate 1.)

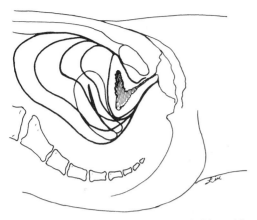

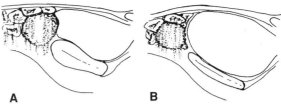

A   B

Figure 4-24. The cephalad margin of the urinary bladder can provide an important clue to the presence of a mass superior to the urinary bladder and uterine fundus (**A**). If the bladder is only moderately distended, it can respond to the weight of a mass by forming a gentle curve around the mass (**B**). As the bladder becomes tense with overdistention, the weight of a cephalad mass may be insufficient to alter the bladder contour. Because masses cephalad to the urinary bladder and uterine fundus may be surrounded by loops of small bowel, the bladder contour may be the only indication of the presence of the mass.

Figure 4-22. Contours of the urinary bladder with progressive filling. The uterus is shown in its initial position, folded forward over the dome of the empty urinary bladder. For clarity, the corresponding positions of the uterus are not shown, although the indentation of the posterior bladder wall by the uterus is indicated for each stage of filling.

cause the uterus normally folds forward to rest on the posterior and mid-regions of the dome, the part of the bladder wall that experiences least resistance to expansion is the extreme anterior portion. This region needs displace only highly mobile loops of small bowel, which normally fill any unoccupied space in the true pelvis. So the anterior part of the urinary bladder expands upward most easily, resulting in the typical asymmetric shape of the distended bladder on sagittal section (Fig. 4-22).

Because the bladder contour molds to or "reflects" structures with which it is in contact, the examiner should look carefully at the urinary bladder before trying to determine the identity and relationship of other structures in the pelvis. The urinary bladder contours provide a "reverse map" of the pelvis (Figs. 4-23 and 4-24). In addition, urine in the bladder provides both a window and a reference standard. Like water, urine attenuates ultrasound frequencies only slightly, permitting transmission deep into the pelvis with minimal energy loss. If there are echoes in the urine (with the exception of the normal anterior wall artifact seen on transabdominal sonography), then either the gain setting is too high or the urine is abnormal.

Cell casts from the renal tubules and uric acid crystals can cause punctate echoes in the urine, but sonographers encounter these only rarely. More often, echoes in the urine represent "noise" associated with a gain or output level that is too high. If such false echoes are appearing in the urine, they will also appear in soft tissues, where they may not be recognized as false. The most common technical error in gynecologic sonography is excessive gain obscuring subtle details within the soft tissues. A good rule of thumb is to use the minimum output and gain level consistent with adequate demonstration of tissue echo patterns. The second way in which urine serves as a reference standard is for comparison with other echo patterns in pelvic structures. If the gain is set so that no echoes appear in the normally anechoic urine, then no echoes should appear within cysts (such as follicles), which are wider than the ultrasound beam and which contain homogeneous fluid (Fig. 4-25).

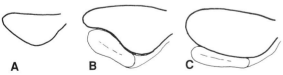

A   B   C

Figure 4-23. The urinary bladder contour is directly influenced by the presence of the uterus within the fixed space of the pelvis. When the uterus has been surgically removed or is congenitally absent, the bladder contour is distinctly deltoid (**A**). The normal anteflexed uterus creates a gentle indentation of the moderately distended bladder (**B**). The degree of indentation is influenced by the size of the uterus and the degree of bladder filling. If overdistended, the bladder can compress the uterus excessively, altering the uterine shape and echo pattern (**C**). The ideal degree of filling results in extension of the bladder 1 to 2 cm above the fundus of the uterus, while preserving the normal uterine contour.

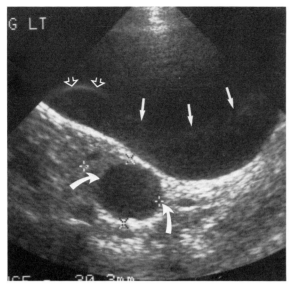

Figure 4-25. Excessive gain is evidenced by false echoes (*straight arrows*) in the bladder. These false echoes also appear in the follicular cyst in the ovary (*curved arrows*). Also noted on this scan is a typical "thumbnail" artifact within the bladder (*open arrows*) caused by rough handling of the film used to record the scan.

By comparing the echogenicity of the urine with the echogenicity of the unknown structure at various gain levels, the sonographer can qualitatively assess the structural similarity or dissimilarity of the two. A word of caution is in order here: too often, the assumption is made that anechoic content always represents fluid; this is not so. Echogenicity alone cannot be used as a definitive criterion for the presence of fluid. Homogeneous solids (e.g., myoma) can be anechoic at normal gain levels and fluids (e.g., blood, pus) can be echogenic. Both echogenicity and through-transmission must be used as criteria for distinguishing fluids from solids.

THE VAGINA

The *vagina* is a relatively thin-walled, 7- to 10-cm-long muscular tube that extends from the cervix of the uterus to the vestibule of the external genitalia and lies between the urinary bladder and the rectum.[7] Its wall is composed of smooth muscle and elastic connective tissue and is lined with stratified squamous epithelium, very similar to skin (hence its name; the vagina is essentially an invagination of the skin). The outer surface of the vagina (the adventitial coat) is a thin, fibrous layer that is continuous with the sur-

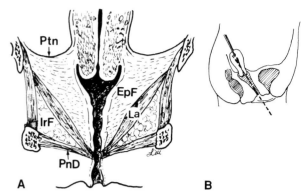

Figure 4-26. (**A**) Oblique section through lower uterus and vagina. The plane of section is indicated in (**B**). The uterus has been elevated to stretch the vagina and align it with the plane of section. Note the relationship between the perineal diaphragm and the levator ani muscle group. (PnD, perineal diaphragm; La, levator ani; EpF, endopelvic fascia; Ptn, peritoneum; IrF, ischiorectal fossa.)

rounding endopelvic fascia (Fig. 4-26). Normally, the vaginal canal is a potential space, because the anterior and posterior walls are in apposition. When collapsed, the vagina assumes a rounded "H" shape on cross section, and the inner mucosal surface of the wall wrinkles up to form transverse ridges (rugae), which largely disappear when the vaginal wall is stretched (Fig. 4-27).

The posterior wall of the vagina is longer than the anterior wall. The upper end of the vagina attaches to the cervix of the uterus along an oblique line about halfway up the length of the cervix.[12] This form of attachment creates a ring-shaped, blind pocket (the *fornix*) between the outer wall of the cervix and the inner surface of the vaginal wall. By convention, this continuous ring-shaped space is

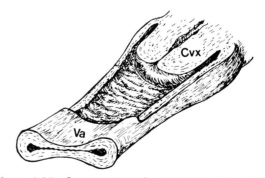

Figure 4-27. Cutaway view of vagina. Note cross section when collapsed and relationship of uterine cervix (Cvx) to vaginal (Va) walls.

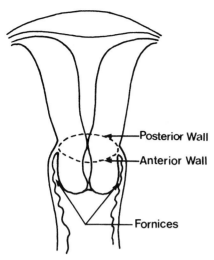

Figure 4-28. Relationship between uterus and vagina. The posterior vaginal wall attaches higher on the cervix than the anterior wall. The fornices are the blind pockets formed by the inner surface of the vaginal walls and the outer surface of the cervix. These spaces are normally collapsed or contain only a small amount of mucus.

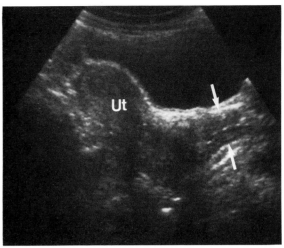

Figure 4-29. Median sagittal scan with the bladder only moderately filled. Note the thickness (*arrows*) and cephalocaudad length of the vaginal walls. The vaginal canal is indicated by the interrupted bright line separating the anterior and posterior walls. (Ut, uterus.)

divided into anterior, lateral, and posterior fornices (Fig. 4-28). Because of the oblique attachment of the vagina to the cervix, the posterior fornix is deeper than the anterior, and its posterior location causes it to be the site of pooling of urine, pus, blood, or other fluid that originates in the vagina or escapes into it.

The length and wall thickness of the vagina vary in response to filling of the urinary bladder. The vagina is attached to the uterus, which is displaced upward and backward by bladder filling, thus stretching and reducing the thickness of the vaginal wall as the bladder expands. The combined thickness of the normal anterior and posterior vaginal walls should not exceed 1 cm[17] when measured from a transvesical scan made with the urinary bladder distended.

On sonograms, the muscular walls of the vagina produce a moderately hypoechoic pattern typical of smooth muscle (Fig. 4-29). The mucosa of the vagina is highly echogenic, but it may be difficult to visualize when the vaginal walls are stretched by a distended bladder (Fig. 4-30). Although the vagina can move laterally in response to pressure from a distended rectum, it is most commonly found at or near the sagittal midline of the pelvis. Its anteroposterior position, however, varies substantially in response to the degree of filling of the urinary blad-

der and the rectum. In addition, the upper part of the vagina follows the cervix if the uterus is displaced laterally by a pelvic mass or a distended rectum or sigmoid colon.

The introduction of transvaginal ultrasound imaging has placed new emphasis on the importance of a complete understanding of the anatomy of the vagina and its relationship to the surrounding organs.

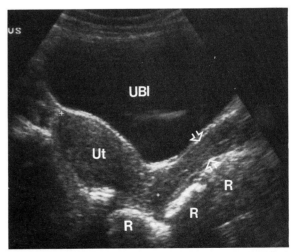

Figure 4-30. Echo pattern of the vagina when the bladder is fully distended. The vaginal walls can be identified readily (*open arrows*). The linear echo in the bladder is an artifact. (Ut, uterus; UBl, urinary bladder; R, rectum.)

The typical transvaginal scan is performed with the urinary bladder empty or containing only a little urine (Fig. 4-31). A specially designed transducer is inserted into the vagina so that the active face of the transducer is positioned at the tip of the cervix or in the fornix. The ultrasound beam may then be directed anteriorly and cephalad to image the uterus, fallopian tubes, and ovaries, or the transducer can be rotated to view the lateral pelvic walls.[19] The higher frequency used by transvaginal probes and the ability to place the transducer close to the structure of interest results in markedly improved detail resolution of the ultrasound image (see Fig. 4-31B,C) at the sacrifice of depth of penetration and, hence, depth of field of view.

Although the remarkable flexibility of the vagina affords substantial latitude in positioning the ultrasound probe, the shape of the pelvic cavity imposes some limitations. In addition, the probe must be manipulated judiciously. The patient may have

limited tolerance for probe movement, particularly in the case of pelvic inflammation or adhesions. The examiner also must be aware of the differences in anatomic position and mobility of the pelvic organs when the urinary bladder is empty. For example, the uterus is much lower and more anterior in the pelvic cavity when the bladder is empty, and the ovaries are usually in the posterolateral region of the pelvis and may lie at some distance from the uterus. This is in contrast with transabdominal pelvic scans, on which the ovaries are usually deeper in the true pelvic space and are pressed against the lateral or superior margins of the uterus.

THE UTERUS

In nulliparous women the *uterus* is a small, pear-shaped muscular viscus suspended in the mid-pelvis. In one sense, the uterus is only a prominent bulge in

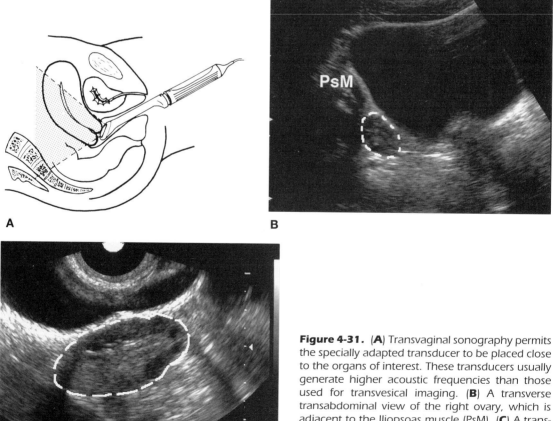

A

B

C

Figure 4-31. (**A**) Transvaginal sonography permits the specially adapted transducer to be placed close to the organs of interest. These transducers usually generate higher acoustic frequencies than those used for transvesical imaging. (**B**) A transverse transabdominal view of the right ovary, which is adjacent to the Iliopsoas muscle (PsM). (**C**) A transvaginal image of the same ovary. Note the improved visualization of the internal structure of the ovary.

the middle section of a continuous muscular canal that begins with the fallopian tubes and ends with the external orifice of the vagina (Fig. 4-32), but, because its structure and size differentiate it so dramatically from the fallopian tubes and the vagina, the uterus is usually considered as a separate organ. Its sole function is reproductive—that is, to receive the fertilized egg, to nourish the developing conceptus, and ultimately to expel the fetus.

Regions of the Uterus

The uterus is described as having four parts or regions—fundus, corpus, isthmus, and cervix. The regions are arbitrarily defined on the basis of the uterine contour and structure (Fig. 4-33).

FUNDUS. The uppermost region of the uterus is the fundus ("bottom"), which begins at the point where the fallopian tubes arise from the uterine walls. (The "bottom" of the uterus is its uppermost region because the uterine regions are named for the Greek wine bottle, the amphora, which it resembles. In this case, the wine bottle is upside down with its neck pushed into the vaginal canal.) The fundus is the least distinctive region of the uterus.

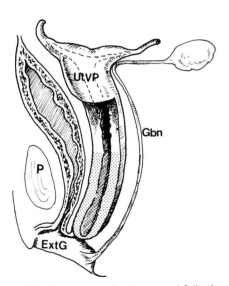

Figure 4-32. *The embryonic uterus and fallopian tubes arise from the paired paramesonephric ducts. The upper (cranial) regions of these ducts remain separate and form the fallopian tubes. The caudal regions fuse to form the uterovaginal primordium, which later differentiates into the uterus and the vagina. The shaded area on the figure indicates the area that will differentiate into the vagina. (P, pubis; Gbn, gubernaculum; UtVP, uterovaginal primordium; ExtG, external genitalia.)*

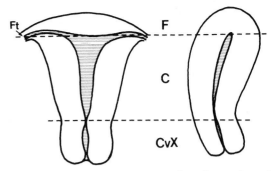

Figure 4-33. *Schematic diagram of uterine regions. (F, fundus; C, corpus; CvX, cervix; Ft, fallopian tube.)*

It is a rounded or dome-shaped area characterized only by its location above the level of the uterine cavity. It narrows at its outer and lateral margins to form the cornu (horn) of the uterus,[13] through which passes the interstitial portion of the fallopian tube (see Fig. 4-33).

CORPUS AND ISTHMUS. The corpus (body) is the largest uterine region and houses the uterine cavity. On cross section, the corpus appears rounded or ovoid (Fig. 4-34). In both sagittal and coronal sections, the corpus usually appears cylindrical or slightly tapered, narrowing as it approaches the isthmus, or waist, of the uterus. The isthmus marks the transition from the corpus to the cervix, or neck. The isthmus is important in that it is the point at which the uterus is most flexible. With the urinary bladder empty, the uterus folds or bends at the isthmus, so that the axis of the corpus and the axis of the cervix form a shallow angle.

CERVIX. The cervix is the cylindrical neck of the uterus (Fig. 4-35). It is different from the rest of the uterine tissue in being more fibrous and less muscular, and by having a distinctive endothelium. It may be described as a barrel-shaped cylinder, slightly wider in the middle and 2 to 3 cm long in nulliparous women.[13] It is penetrated by the spindle-shaped endocervical canal, which extends from the internal to the external os (small opening). The canal is lined with a mucosa whose anterior and posterior surfaces are characterized by oblique ridges or palmate folds that slant downward toward the external os.[13] The endocervical mucosa is richly supplied with mucous glands (Fig. 4-36*A,B*). The mucus serves to impede upward migration of bacteria from vagina to uterus. In pregnancy, the mucosa of the endocervical canal undergoes hypertrophy and the glands produce a dense, sticky mucous plug (the

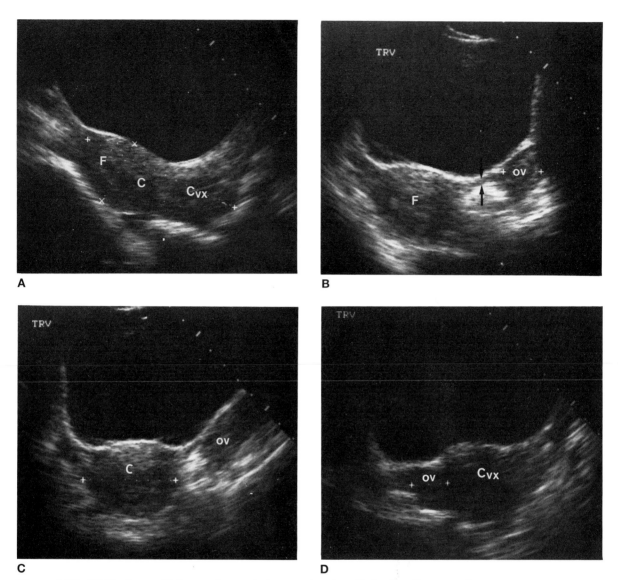

Figure 4-34. (**A**) Median sagittal scan of normal uterus and vagina. (F, fundus; C, corpus; Cvx, cervix). (**B**) Transverse scan at the level of the fundus. The left ovary (OV) is demonstrated. The broad ligament and/or fallopian tube (*arrows*) bridges the space between the uterine fundus and the ovary. (**C**) Transverse scan at the level of the corpus. (**D**) Transverse scan at the level of the cervix. The right ovary (OV) is seen adjacent to the cervix. In this position, it occupies most of the posterior cul-de-sac.

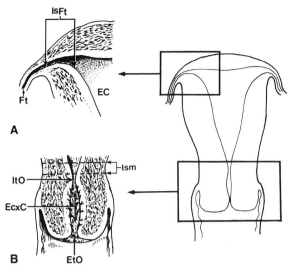

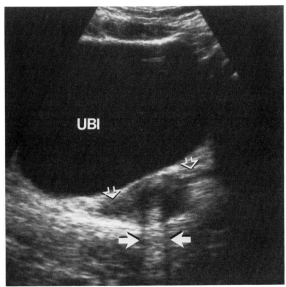

Figure 4-35. Structure of the cornual (**A**) and cervical (**B**) regions of the uterus. (EC, endometrial cavity; Ft, fallopian tube; ItO, internal os; EtO, external os; EcxC, endocervical canal; IsFt, interstitial portion of the fallopian tube; Ism, isthmus.)

mucous plug of pregnancy) that effectively seals the uterus.

The Uterine Cavity

The uterine cavity is shaped like an inverted triangle with its basal angles defined by the ostia of the fallopian tubes and its apex defined by the internal os of the cervix. The cavity is widest at the fundus and narrowest at the isthmus and is flattened front to back, so that the anterior and posterior endometrial surfaces are normally separated only by a thin layer of mucus.

Layers of the Uterus

The walls of the uterus are composed of three tissue layers (Fig. 4-37). The outermost layer is the serosa, which is quite thin and not visible on sonography. The serosa is continuous with the pelvic fascia. The thick middle layer (the myometrium) is composed of smooth muscle cells and interspersed connective tissue fibers. Lining the inner surface of the uterus is a mucosa known as the endometrium, which forms the walls of the uterine cavity.

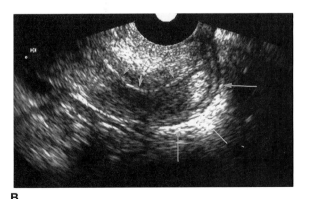

Figure 4-36. (**A**) Transverse scan of a cervix that is shifted to the left side of the pelvic cavity. Note the lateral extensions of the cervical echo pattern (*open arrows*). These ill-defined "wings" are the transverse cervical ligaments. Also note the edge shadows (*solid arrows*), which bracket a central zone of enhanced echoes. This pattern is characteristic of the cervix. (UBl, urinary bladder.) (**B**) Endovaginal sagittal image of the cervix. Note the posterior vaginal wall (*long arrows*), which extends around the cervical tip to insert on the posterior wall. The prominent endocervical canal (*short arrows*) is readily visible throughout the length of the cervix.

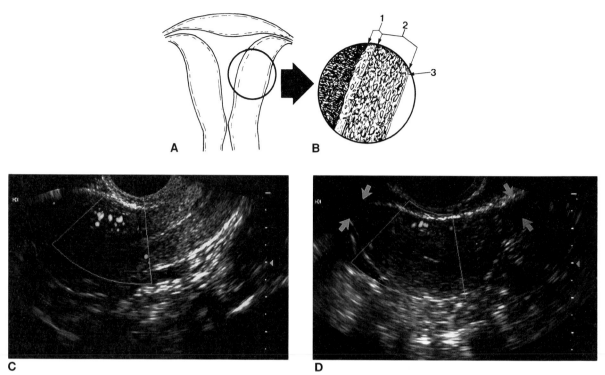

Figure 4-37. (**A**) Frontal plane schematic of the uterus. (**B**) Enlarged view of tissues that form the uterine wall. (1, endometrium; 2, myometrium; 3, serosa.) (**C**) An endovaginal sagittal of the uterus with a power-Doppler sample box placed over the mid-corpus region. Power Doppler is not sensitive to direction of blood flow, but is more sensitive to the presence of flow. Note the rich vascularization of the middle layer of the myometrium, indicated by the bright spots of color where blood flow was detected. (**D**) An endovaginal transverse scan of the same uterus, again illustrating the vascularization of the middle layer of the myometrium. These vessels are normally not visible on gray scale imaging alone. Also note the conical "ears" (*arrows*) which extend from the lateral margins of the uterus. These represent the cornua or "horns" of the uterus, where the fallopian tubes, the round ligaments and the ovarian ligaments are attached to the uterus. (See also Color Plate 2.)

MYOMETRIUM. The thick, muscular middle layer of the uterus (the myometrium) forms most of the bulk of the uterine body. Within this layer, the major muscle fibers are arranged in a complex spiral pattern (Fig. 4-38). The myometrium may be further subdivided into three rather indistinct layers: an outer layer characterized by longitudinal muscle fibers, a thick middle layer that is richly vascular (see Fig. 4-37C,D), and a denser inner layer whose muscle fibers are arranged both longitudinally and obliquely.[13] Throughout the reproductive years, the muscular tissues of the uterus participate in low-amplitude contractile activity, which serves to maintain the muscle tone of the uterus. Just before and during the menstrual flow, this contractile activity becomes more focused and results in slow, subsensate, ripple-like contractions, which originate in the fundus and sweep down the length of the uterus to the internal os. These contractions are of very low amplitude and quite slow, requiring several seconds to progress from fundus to isthmus. They can be recognized during transvaginal imaging of the uterus as a progressive focal rippling distortion of the endometrial echo pattern. In contrast to these menstrual contractions, one group of investigators[15] has described contractions that sweep upward from the internal os to the fundus. These contractions were observed during transvaginal sonography and were found to be most frequent at the time of ovulation. The investigators speculate that these contractions assist migration of sperm upward through the uterus to the fallopian tubes.[15]

ENDOMETRIUM. The endometrium is a specialized mucosa that varies in thickness and composition

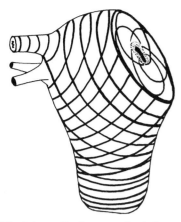

Figure 4-38. *Schematic diagram of spiral smooth muscle fibers of the uterus. Contraction of these fibers tends to increase pressure in the uterine lumen.*

through the menstrual cycle. Covering the surface are ciliated cells interrupted at intervals by the orifices of mucous glands.[14] The hair-like cilia flex in synchronized waves that tend to force surface mucus toward the cervix. This steady downward flow of a sticky tide of mucus impedes bacteria from migrating upward into the uterine cavity. Although the vagina is richly colonized by bacteria, the endometrium and the endocervical canal are normally free of foreign organisms. The amount of mucus present at any given time is highly variable, but typically is greatest just before the menstrual flow begins or at the onset of pregnancy.

After menstruation, the thickness of a single layer of endometrium is about 0.5 to 1 mm[12]; it increases to a maximum 5 to 7 mm at the onset of the next menstrual flow. Sonographic measurements of the endometrium are usually made across the long axis of the uterus, including layers of endometrium on the anterior and posterior walls. When measured this way, endometrial thickness ranges from approximately 1 mm immediately after menstruation to about 14 mm immediately before menstruation (Fig. 4-39*A*). When measuring the endometrium, the outermost, hypoechoic layer should be excluded, because it is myometrial in origin. Within the endometrium proper, two or even three layers may be identified (see Fig. 4-39*A*). Their exact clinical significance is a matter of debate, but Hackeloer[9] and others[3] have noted that a thin hypoechoic layer can sometimes be seen lining the innermost surface of the endometrial cavity at the time of ovulation or immediately afterward (see

Fig. 4-39). This "inner ring" sign may be useful as a confirmation of ovulation, but it has not been identified consistently in studies by other investigators.[3] (See also Chap. 28.)

Attempts have been made to correlate precisely the echo pattern or thickness of the endometrium with the stage of the menstrual cycle. Although the variations during the menstrual cycle for an individual are relatively consistent from cycle to cycle, the range of variation from individual to individual is great, and only generalizations may safely be made. The average menstrual cycle of 28 days may be regarded as having four phases associated with histomorphologic changes in the endometrium. These phases, their duration, endometrial thickness, and echo pattern are shown in Table 4-2.

Although transvaginal scanning has greatly improved our ability to delineate the endometrium with ultrasound (see Fig. 4-39*C,D*), it is doubtful that endometrial thickness or echo pattern will prove to be reliable clinical indicators, except when either is grossly abnormal.

Uterine Size and Shape

The size and shape of the uterus vary markedly with age and obstetric history (Fig. 4-40*A*). In the fetus, the uterus grows at a rate consistent with the rest of the body until early in the third trimester. For the remainder of the gestational period, growth of the uterine corpus is accelerated because of the high level of maternal estrogen produced as term approaches. As a result, the uterus is larger and has a more "adult" contour in newborns than in children.[11] Immediately after birth, withdrawal of the influence of maternal estrogen causes the uterine corpus to shrink, and significant growth does not occur again until the ovaries begin to produce hormones as a prelude to puberty. In infants, the uterus rides high in the pelvis, is cylindrical, and lies along the same axis as the vagina. In young girls, the uterus remains nearly cylindrical (see Fig. 4-40*B*), but the body (corpus and fundus) of the uterus becomes more globular as it matures. By puberty, the uterus has assumed the characteristic inverted pear shape. With each pregnancy the corpus and fundus grow thicker, increasing the globularity of the multiparous uterus (Fig. 4-40*C*). After menopause the corpus and fundus shrink and regress to the prepubertal state (Fig. 4-40*D*), and in elderly women, they may appear as little more than a cap above the cervix. Throughout life, changes in uter-

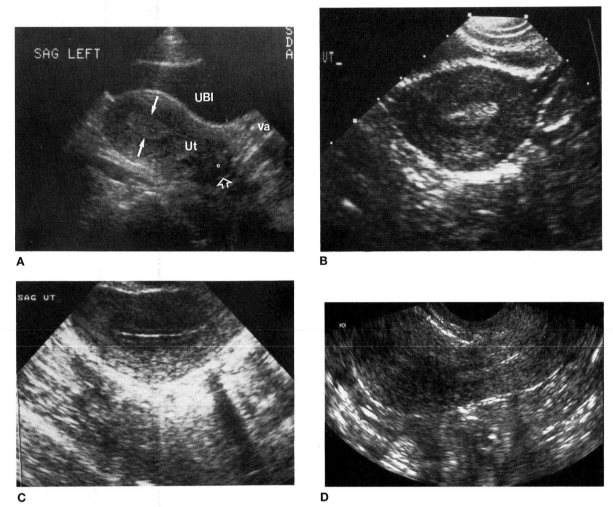

Figure 4-39. (**A**) Sagittal scan of uterus (Ut) and vagina (Va). This immediately premenstrual (day 27) endometrium (*arrows*) is producing abundant mucus, which has outlined the uterine cavity. Four distinct echo layers can be identified. The outermost dark layer is myometrium and should not be included in measurement of the endometrium. This layer abuts on the thick, echogenic glandular layer that forms the bulk of the endometrium. A hypoechoic inner layer separates the echogenic glandular layer from a thin, highly echogenic line formed by mucus and the surfaces of the endometrium. Mucus has also outlined the posterior fornix (*open arrow*). (UBl, urinary bladder.) (**B**) In this transverse transvesical scan of a midsecretory-phase endometrium, the layers are more difficult to identify precisely, and the echo pattern in the glandular layer is patchy. (**C**) The distinct layers are more easily appreciated in this transvaginal sagittal scan of the uterine corpus during the late proliferative stage. (**D**) Transvaginal sagittal scan of the uterus immediately postmenstruation. The endometrium is not visible through most of the uterus.

▰▰▰ TABLE 4-2. THE ENDOMETRIUM

Phase	Days of Cycle	Thickness (mm)	Endometrial Echo Pattern
Menstrual	1–5	<0.5	Thin echogenic line
Postmenstrual	6–9	1–2	Mostly anechoic
Proliferative	10–13	2–4	Slightly echogenic
Secretory	14–28	5–7	Highly echogenic

ine size are mostly the result of changes in the muscularis layer, predominantly in the corpus. Because of its smaller proportion of muscle to connective tissue, the cervix varies least in size and is least flexible of all the uterine regions.

A CAVEAT ABOUT UTERINE DIMENSIONS. The range of individual variation in organ size increases steadily from the fetal period through adulthood. In addition, the linear dimensions of the uterus are influenced by many factors, including pressure from surrounding organs, stage of the menstrual cycle, and obstetric history. Normal dimensions given for the uterus must be regarded only as arbitrarily defined points on the continuum of uterine development, growth, and regression (see Fig. 4-40). The uterus of a child typically is 2.5 cm long and has an anteroposterior diameter of about 1 cm.[18] The length of the adult nulliparous uterus typically is 8 cm or less, the width 5.5 cm, and the anteriorposterior dimension 3 cm.[11] The sonographer should use a consistent method to measure the uterus. One such method is shown in Figure 4-41. Small variations of uterine size are not clinically significant.

The Uterine Ligaments

Unlike the urinary bladder and rectum, which are relatively closely attached to the walls of the pelvic space, the uterus is loosely suspended in the center of the pelvic cavity.

The *cardinal ligaments* (also called transverse cervical ligaments) consist of ill-defined, wide bands of condensed fibromuscular tissue that originate from the lateral region of the cervix and along the lateral margin of the uterine corpus. These bands insert over a broad region of the lateral pelvic wall and extend posteriorly to the margins of the sacrum.[12] The posterior edge of the cardinal ligaments is more condensed than other regions and is identified as the uterosacral ligaments (Fig. 4-42). These extend from the posteriolateral margin of the cervix to the sacrum. Together, the cardinal and uterosacral ligaments anchor the cervix and orient its axis so that it is roughly parallel to the central axis of the body.

The *round ligaments* (see Fig. 4-42) are fibromuscular bands originating from the uterine cornua and extending across the pelvic space from posterior to anterior. They cross over the pelvic brim, pass through the inguinal ring, and then disperse as fibers anchored in the labia majora of the external genitalia.[12] They serve to loosely tether the uterine fundus and tilt it forward in the pelvis, aiding in the normal anteflexion of the uterus at the isthmus.

Of all the ligaments of the pelvis, the *broad ligament* is the most difficult to describe because it is not a true ligament but simply a double fold of *peritoneum*. The peritoneum is a thin, glistening serous membrane that forms a sac that lines the abdominopelvic cavity. Its function is to permit organs to slide over each other with minimal friction, and this is aided by a thin layer of serous fluid produced by the peritoneum.

To understand the relationship of the peritoneum to the organs in the pelvis, the reader might imagine a container that represents the abdominopelvic cavity. Put into it a pear to represent the uterus. Now, stuff a sac into the container so that it covers the pear, folding back on itself, and extending down in front and back. At the sides of the pear, the sac forms a double layer, which is analogous to the broad ligament. The broad ligament is simply the double layer of peritoneum, with fat, vessels, and nerves between the two layers. This arrangement probably has only minimal function in suspension of the uterus, but the broad ligament is important because it incompletely divides the true pelvis into anterior and posterior pelvic compartments. The ovaries are attached to the posterior surface of the broad ligament, thus constraining their movements to the posterior pelvic compartment.

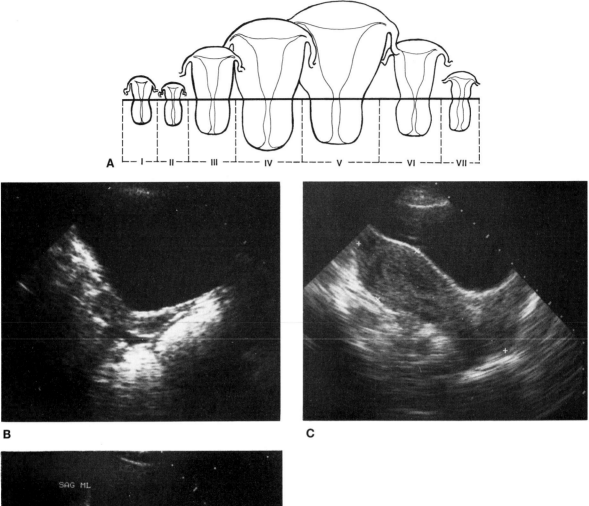

Figure 4-40. (**A**) Relationship between cervical length and the length of the combined corpus and fundus at various stages of a woman's life. In childhood, the cervix may constitute two thirds and the corpus and fundus one third of the total uterine length. By puberty, the ratio has become 1 to 1 and continues to shift steadily until the adult nulliparous ratio is two-thirds corpus and fundus to one-third cervix. (I, birth; II, childhood; III, at puberty; IV, adult nuliparous; V, adult parous; VI, at menopause; VII, elderly.) (**B**) Sagittal scan of the uterus in a child, aged 8 years. The uterus is mostly cylindrical with only slight rounding of the corpus and fundus. (**C**) Sagittal scan of the uterus of a multiparous woman. (**D**) Sagittal scan of the uterus of a postmenopausal, 58-year-old woman.

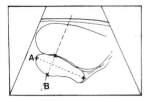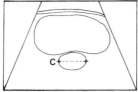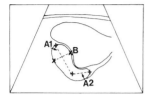

Figure 4-41. Measurement technique for the uterus. The long axis of the uterus should be measured from the fundus to the tip of the cervix (line A). When making this measurement, carefully identify the true long axis of the uterus, because it is seldom parallel to the pelvic midline. Gain and scan plane are then adjusted to demonstrate optimally the tip of the cervix. The posterior wall of the vagina serves as a guide; its curve can be followed around the posterior lip of the cervix to identify more precisely where the cervix ends and the vaginal wall begins. On the same image, the greatest anteroposterior diameter of the uterus should be measured along a line perpendicular to line A at a point where the uterus appears widest in the anteroposterior plane. Then the midpoint of the field of view is centered on the same line used to measure the anteroposterior diameter, and the transducer is rotated 90 degrees, maintaining a constant tilt. This ensures that the transverse diameter (line C) is measured in the same plane as the anteroposterior diameter (line B), which results in more consistent and accurate measurements of the uterus. If the uterus is strongly anteflexed, two measurements of the long axis (lines A1 and A2) should be made and added together to obtain the true length.

Spaces Adjacent to the Uterus

In addition to its anatomic function of isolating and lubricating the surfaces of organs, the peritoneum is also responsible for formation of certain spaces in relationship to the uterus and other organs of the pelvis (see Fig. 4-42; Fig. 4-43). The peritoneum reflects, or folds back, from the anterior wall of the pelvic cavity to cover the dome of the bladder, and then folds more sharply to cover the anterior surface of the uterus. This fold forms the relatively shallow *anterior cul-de-sac* (vesicouterine pouch), which lies between the anterior wall of the uterus and the urinary bladder.[12] This space virtually disappears as the urinary bladder fills; normally it is not significant to the sonographer. In contrast, the similar pocket formed by reflection of the peritoneum from the posterior wall of the pelvis (covering the rectum)

to the posterior wall of the uterus is very important. The *posterior cul-de-sac* (pouch of Douglas or recto-uterine pouch) is the most posterior and dependent portion of the peritoneal sac lining the abdominopelvic cavity.[8] Fluid originating anywhere in the peritoneal sac tends to drain into the posterior cul-de-sac. This space is relatively complex in its configuration. Its most inferior extent consists of a deep, narrow pocket that extends down between the rectum and the cervix and is defined at its upper margins by the uterosacral ligaments. Above these ligaments, the cul-de-sac widens out and is continuous with the broad, shallow spaces to the side of the uterus. These shallow *adnexal* spaces are lined by the peritoneum, forming the broad ligament.

Variants of Uterine Position

In some women, the uterus does not maintain the anteflexed position, instead bending backward so that the fundus of the uterus comes to rest in the posterior cul-de-sac (Fig. 4-44).[14] This retroflexion of the uterus is relatively common, rarely has clinical significance, and may be transient or persistent in a specific individual.

Retroflexion of the uterus is responsible for significant alterations in the echo pattern of the uterus when demonstrated by transabdominal scanning.

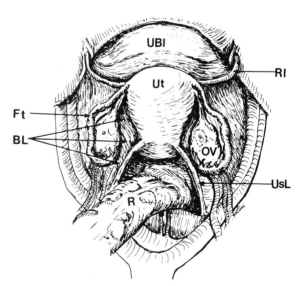

Figure 4-42. View looking down into the pelvic cavity from behind, with the organs in place: Ut, uterus; OV, ovary; Ft, fallopian tube; Rl, round ligament; UsL, uterosacral ligament; R, rectum; UBl, urinary bladder; Bl, broad ligament.

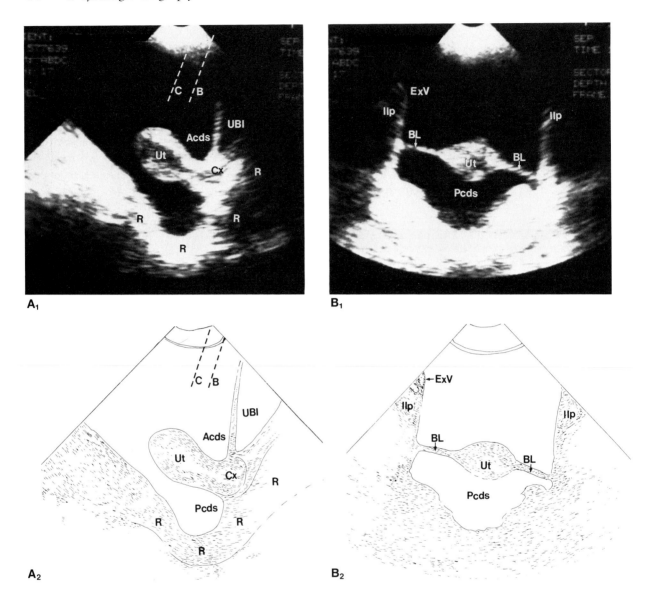

Figure 4-43. (**A₁**) Sagittal scan of the pelvis of a patient with massive ascites. Fluid fills the pelvic cavity, outlining the uterus. Note how the shape of the posterior cul-de-sac compares with the shape of the anterior cul-de-sac. The dashed lines indicate the plane of scan for images **B** and **C**. (**A₂**) UBl, urinary bladder; Acds, anterior cul-de-sac; Ut, uterus; Cx, cervix; Pcds, posterior cul-de-sac; R, rectum. (**B₁**) Transverse scan at the level of the uterine isthmus demonstrates the broad ligaments and posterior cul-de-sac. (**B₂**) ExV, external iliac artery and vein; Ilp, iliopsoas muscle; BL, broad ligament; Ut, uterus; Pcds, posterior cul-de-sac. (**C₁**) Transverse scan at the level of the uterine fundus demonstrates the uterus, ovaries, fallopian tubes, and rectum. (**C₂**) Ilp, iliopsoas muscle; Ft, fallopian tube; Ut, uterus; OV, ovary; Pcds, posterior cul-de-sac; R, rectum. (**D**) Typical pattern of a moderate amount of fluid in the posterior cul-de-sac (*curved arrow*). Compare with image **A₁** to appreciate the shape of the posterior cul-de-sac with varying amounts of fluid in it.

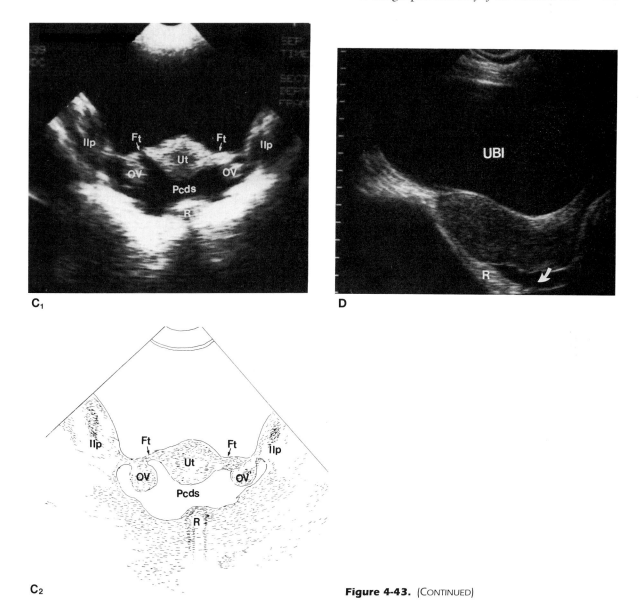

C₁

C₂

D

Figure 4-43. (Continued)

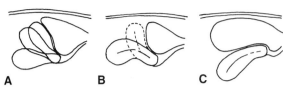

Figure 4-44. Variants of uterine position within the pelvis. (**A**) Normal physiologic retroversion of the uterus by filling of the urinary bladder. (**B**) Retroflexion of the uterus. The cervix maintains a normal position but the corpus and fundus flex backward into the posterior pelvic compartment. Note that the point of flexion is at the isthmus. (**C**) Retroflexion and retroversion. All regions of the uterus are abnormal in position. Positions **B** and **C** are commonly lumped together in the category of "retroversion."

Normally, the uterus lies in a plane roughly perpendicular to an ultrasound beam entering through the full urinary bladder. Most of the uterus lies at a relatively constant depth from the transducer, so the echo pattern is uniform throughout the myometrium. In contrast, the corpus and fundus of a retroflexed uterus are tilted back into the posterior pelvic cavity, and the acoustic beam must traverse the muscle tissue of the corpus to reach the fundus. As a result, the fundus of a retroflexed uterus often appears echo poor compared with the corpus (Fig. 4-45).[11] This difference is due to absorption of the

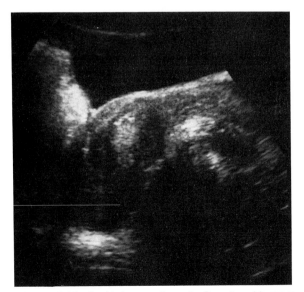

Figure 4-45. Sagittal scan of a retroflexed multiparous uterus. The ill-defined fundus mimics a mass in the posterior cul-de-sac. Note the abnormal contour of the posterior wall of the urinary bladder.

ultrasound beam by the muscle of the corpus. In extreme cases, the hypoechoic fundus may be mis-identified as a mass in the cul-de-sac.

THE FALLOPIAN TUBES

The *fallopian tubes* (*oviducts* or *salpinges* [singular: *salpinx*]) are paired musculomembranous tubes that extend from the fundus of the uterus to the ovary and lateral pelvic wall. Most of the length of the fallopian tube lies within the free edge of the fold of peritoneum that forms the broad ligament. Like the uterine wall, the wall of the fallopian tube consists of three layers: an outer serosal coat (which is continuous with the overlying peritoneum over the isthmic portion of the tube), a middle muscular layer, and an inner mucosa. By convention, the tube is divided into the intramural, isthmic, and ampullary portions (Fig. 4-46). The total tubal length in an adult (7 to 14 cm)[12] is usually greater than the distance from the uterus to the lateral pelvic wall, so in its normal state the tube is more tortuous than its wall structure alone would impose. The tubal lumen widens as it moves away from the uterus. The intramural portion is the narrowest (~1 mm), and the third portion or ampulla is the widest (~6 mm).[13] The ampullary portion terminates in the trumpet-shaped infundibulum, which is open to the inside of the peritoneal sac that lines the abdominopelvic cavity. This trumpet-shaped opening is about 1 cm wide and is fringed by delicate, finger-like projections called fimbriae. Usually one of these, the *fimbria ovarica*, is attached to the ovary and serves to maintain a close relationship between the opening of the tube and the ovarian surface.[12]

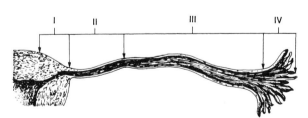

Figure 4-46 Regions of the fallopian tube. For this illustration, the tube has been stretched horizontally. The intramural (interstitial) portion (I) is relatively straight and is located within the uterine wall. The isthmic portion (II) is longer and slightly wavy in its course. The ampullary portion (III) is the longest section of the tube and is quite tortuous in vivo. It terminates in the trumpet-shaped infundibulum (IV), which is fringed with finger-like projections, the fimbriae.

Because the echo pattern of the fallopian tube is similar to that of the surrounding structures, it is commonly demonstrated but rarely recognized in transabdominal ultrasound images, except when distended with fluid. Occasionally, a typical pattern is seen at the lateral pole of the ovary where the infundibulum is usually located (Fig. 4-47*A*). Because of the relative thinness of its wall, the characteristic echo pattern of the fallopian tube is that of a thin layer of hypoechoic muscle tissue lined by the hyperechoic mucosa surrounding a crescentic or cylindrical lumen. The fallopian tube is more easily demonstrated during endovaginal scanning, where it appears as a tubular extension of the myometrium, often with high-amplitude echoes representing the tubal mucosa (see Fig. 4-47*B,C*). The fallopian tube is the final element of a channel that connects the interior of the peritoneal cavity with the exterior of the female body. This channel is composed of the external genitalia, the vagina, the uterus and the fallopian tubes. No equivalent tract exists in the male.

THE OVARIES

The *ovary* is unlike the other organs of the female pelvis in many respects. It is a solid (parenchymatous) structure; it secretes hormones; it is not covered by peritoneum; and it is the only organ that is entirely "inside" the peritoneal sac.

In a term infant, the ovary is an elongated structure shaped like a round-edged prism and located in the posterior segment of the false pelvis, directly adjacent to the posterior uterine surface. Its size is approximately 25 × 15 × 5 mm.[10] By menarche, the ovary has moved into the true pelvic space and has assumed its almond-shaped adult contour and location.

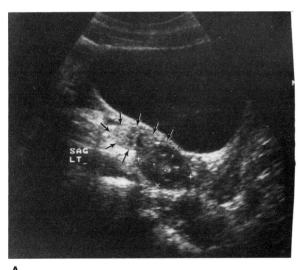

A

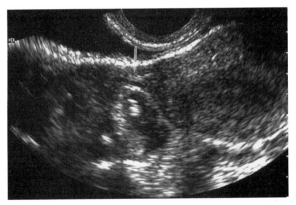

B

Figure 4-47. (**A**) Sagittal scan of the left ovary (outlined by the measurement markers). The fallopian tube (*small arrows*) is seen over the upper pole of the ovary in this transvesical scan. Without the small amount of fluid that defines the crescentic lumen, it would not be possible positively to identify these echoes as representing the tube. (**B,C**) Transvaginal scan of the uterus at the cornua shows the fallopian tube extending from the uterine body to the ovary. Beneath the tube are two loops of small bowel. Differentiation of these structures is more easily performed in real-time imaging because the small bowel is actively peristaltic. Note that a short section of tubal lumen is seen as a linear high-amplitude echo pattern (*arrow*) within the isthmic portion. (OV, ovary; B, bowel; FT, fallopian tube.)

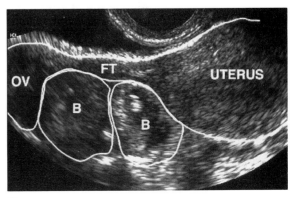

C

The normal dimensions for the adult ovary are length, 2.5 to 5.0 cm; width, 1.5 to 3.0 cm; and anteroposterior thickness, 0.6 to 2.2 cm.[10] Individual variation for a single linear dimension of the ovary is greater than either the average of the three linear dimensions or the volume. In other words, short ovaries tend to be thicker, and thin ovaries tend to be longer. For this reason, a single linear dimension of the ovary should not be used to assess normality of size. Instead, a volume calculation should be used (length × width × height/2 = volume in cm³). With this approach, the upper normal value for the prepubertal ovary is 1 cm³. During the reproductive years, ovarian volumes average 6–9 cc.[2a]

The anterior margin of the ovary is relatively thin and is attached to the posterior surface of the broad ligament by the mesovarium (Fig. 4-48). The posterior or free edge of the ovary is thicker and bows outward, giving the ovary its characteristic asymmetric almond shape.

The ovary is suspended in the pelvic space by three anchoring structures (Fig. 4-49). The *ovarian ligament* is a flattened fibromuscular band extending from the uterine cornu, where the fallopian tube exits the uterine wall, to the inferior (medial or uterine) pole of the ovary. The *infundibulopelvic ligament* consists of fibromuscular strands intertwined with the ovarian vessels and lymphatics as they pass from the brim of the pelvis to the lateral pole of the ovary. These vessels and their supporting

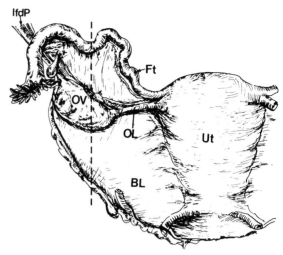

Figure 4-49. *The ovary and its suspensory structures. This view of the posterior surface of the broad ligament shows the relationship of the ovary to the broad ligament, fallopian tube, infundibulopelvic ligament, and ovarian ligament. The fallopian tube has been lifted up to expose the ovary and its ligaments. (Ft, fallopian tube; OL, ovarian ligament; IfdP, infundibulopelvic ligament; OV, ovary; Ut, uterus; BL, broad ligament.)*

fibers form a ridge in the overlying peritoneum, which is thicker in this region and contributes to the suspensory effect. The infundibulopelvic ligament suspends the superior (lateral or pelvic brim) pole of the ovary from the posteriolateral pelvic wall at the brim of the true pelvic space. The *mesovarium* is a short double layer of peritoneum extending from the posterior surface of the broad ligament. The mesovarium provides only a minimal suspensory effect in comparison with the fibromuscular ovarian ligament, but it does provide the primary route of access for vessels traveling into and out of the ovarian hilus.

The outer layer of the ovary is composed of so-called *germinal epithelium*, which is neither germinal nor a true epithelium. (The early anatomists made some incorrect assumptions.) It is actually a modified form of the peritoneum but sufficiently different to result in the ovary's being considered "nude," that is, not covered by the coelomic peritoneum.[12] Immediately beneath the germinal epithelium is a thin layer of fibrous tissue, which forms the *tunica albuginea* (*white coat*), or capsule, of the ovary.

The bulk of the ovarian substance consists of a thick layer of ovarian parenchyma (the cortex)

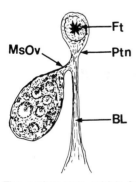

Figure 4-48. *The peritoneum, which forms the broad ligament, covers the fallopian tube and forms a short suspensory ligament, the mesovarium, which supports and anchors the ovary to the posterior surface of the broad ligament. The plane of this figure is shown on Figure 4-49 as a dotted line. (Ft, fallopian tube; Ptn, peritoneum; MsOv, mesovarium; BL, broad ligament.)*

containing a large number of primordial follicles (Fig. 4-50*A*). In the center of the ovary is the medulla, which contains blood vessels (Fig. 4-50*B,C*) and connective tissue but no follicles.[12] Along the margins of the ovarian hilus, the ovarian germinal epithelium is continuous with the peritoneum that forms the broad ligament. Occasionally the hilus also contains vestigial remnants of the primitive mesonephros, which persist in the adult ovary as a cluster of tubules known as the epoöphoron.[12] These are of some interest to the sonographer because they occasionally give rise to benign simple cysts (parovarian cysts), which, when very large, can be mistaken for the urinary bladder.

Each ovary of a newborn infant contains about a million or more primordial follicles, but this number is substantially reduced through spontaneous follicular regression as the infant matures. Only 300 to 400 of the many thousands of follicles that persist into adult life will actually progress through development and ovulation over the 30 or more reproductive years.[10] It is interesting to contemplate that

ovulation occurring when a woman is 40 years old will release an egg that is approximately 40 years and 8 months old, containing DNA-encoded patterns that extend back through time to the primordial organism with which life began on this planet.

Follicular Development

The stages of follicular development (see Fig. 4-50) have been of particular interest to sonographers since the advent of fertility therapy using ultrasound monitoring of follicular growth. These stages are controlled by a complex cycle of chemical interchanges between the brain, the anterior hypophysis of the pituitary gland, and the ovary. (For more information on follicular development, see Chaps. 12 and 28.) The early developing follicle is a solid mass consisting of granulosa cells surrounding the central ovum. External to the granulosa layer are two thinner layers of theca cells, the theca interna, which is richly vascularized, and the theca externa, which is primarily connective tissue. With further development, a fluid-filled cres-

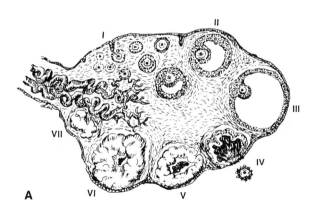

A

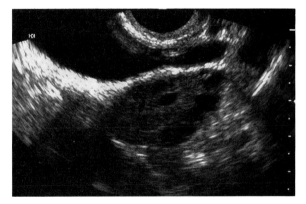

B

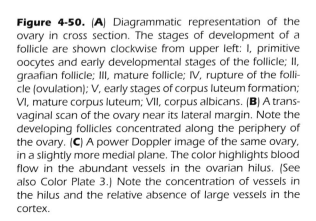

C

Figure 4-50. (A) Diagrammatic representation of the ovary in cross section. The stages of development of a follicle are shown clockwise from upper left: I, primitive oocytes and early developmental stages of the follicle; II, graafian follicle; III, mature follicle; IV, rupture of the follicle (ovulation); V, early stages of corpus luteum formation; VI, mature corpus luteum; VII, corpus albicans. **(B)** A transvaginal scan of the ovary near its lateral margin. Note the developing follicles concentrated along the periphery of the ovary. **(C)** A power Doppler image of the same ovary, in a slightly more medial plane. The color highlights blood flow in the abundant vessels in the ovarian hilus. (See also Color Plate 3.) Note the concentration of vessels in the hilus and the relative absence of large vessels in the cortex.

centic cavity forms eccentrically within the granulosa layer. As this cavity (the antrum) enlarges, the ovum contained within a surrounding mound of granulosa cells projects into the cavity, forming a structure known as the cumulus oöphorus (also called discus proligerus).[10] As the follicle continues to develop, it enlarges and becomes a follicular cyst, eventually impinging on the tunica albuginea of the ovarian surface. Typically, a mature follicle reaches 20 mm in size before rupturing.

The ripening follicle is referred to as a graafian follicle. Each month during the reproductive years, five to seven or more of these follicles in each ovary are triggered into rapid growth by follicle-stimulating hormone produced by the pituitary gland (Fig. 4-51A). In a normal ovulatory cycle, only one of these follicles becomes dominant and ruptures through the tunica albuginea, releasing its contained egg; this is known as ovulation (see Fig. 4-51B). The other follicles undergo atresia,[10] rapidly shrinking eventually to become an amorphous mass of hyalin scar tissue known as the corpus albicans. Artificial stimulation of follicular development (i.e., fertility therapy) can result in simultaneous development of multiple follicles (see Fig. 4-51C).

At ovulation, the combination of the discharged liquor folliculi and hemorrhage associated with follicular rupture results in accumulation of 5 to 10 ml of fluid in the posterior cul-de-sac, where it can be observed as a crescentic anechoic collection behind the cervix (see Fig. 4-51D).[1] The process of ovulation may be associated with mid-cycle pain (mittelschmerz). The stigma (the opening through which the egg was discharged) is sealed by a blood clot, thus reestablishing a closed cystic structure filled with clotted blood. The theca interna layer of the ruptured follicle undergoes rapid proliferation and luteinization through deposit within the cells of golden or reddish brown pigment and fat.[10] The follicle thus becomes the corpus luteum (yellow or golden body). In the normal development of the corpus luteum, the blood clot is gradually resorbed, sometimes forming strands of fibrin within the liquefied center of the corpus luteum.[19]

If the discharged egg is fertilized, the corpus luteum is maintained and enlarges to become the corpus luteum cyst of pregnancy. This cystic structure can become quite large (5 to 6 cm is not unusual) and persists through the early stages of pregnancy. If fertilization does not occur, the corpus luteum undergoes regression, involuting to become the corpus albicans.

The surface of the ovary where rupture of the follicle occurred becomes puckered inward as a scar forms, giving the aging ovary a quilted or cobbled surface. At menopause, the remaining follicles undergo atresia over the subsequent 4 or 5 years, although occasionally a postmenopausal follicle may undergo development, ovulation, and corpus luteum formation.[10] This, however, is rare, and any persistent cyst in the postmenopausal ovary must be regarded with suspicion. After menopause the ovary shrinks steadily until it is less than one third of its mature size.[10] Occasionally, dilated veins can mimic follicles in postmenopausal women, and the sonographer may misinterpret the persistent fluid-filled structure as a persistent follicle. Doppler ultrasound can be used to differentiate a true cyst from a dilated vessel.

Ultrasound measurements of the follicle are most often performed using an average of the follicular diameter in three planes, but when precise measurements are required, the follicle can be measured in the same manner as the ovary. A volume can be calculated using (length × width × height)/2 = volume in cm^3. If only two diameters are available, the formula is (diameter A × diameter B × diameter B)/2.

Location and Acoustic Patterns of the Ovary

When the bladder is empty, the ovary rests in the ovarian fossa, a shallow depression on the posteriolateral pelvic wall just beneath the brim of the pelvis and formed by the external iliac vessels and the ureter. In this position, with the uterine fundus in its normal position resting on the dome of the urinary bladder, the ovary is substantially superior and posterior to the fundus of the uterus. As the bladder fills, the uterus is physiologically retroverted and pushed upward toward the sacral prominence. As filling progresses, the ovaries tend to remain stationary in their ovarian fossae and come to lie at the sides of the uterine fundus. (The uterus moves upward while the ovaries stay in place; Fig. 4-52.) With further filling of the bladder, the ovaries are subjected to increasing pressure from the bladder and are usually forced downward in the adnexal space. Frequently one of them slips farther down into the posterior cul-de-sac. With excessive filling of the bladder, the ovaries are often forced out of the lower regions of the posterior pelvic compartment and come to rest above (cephalad to) the fundus of the uterus in what is often called the axial position.

The ovary may be found in any of three regions

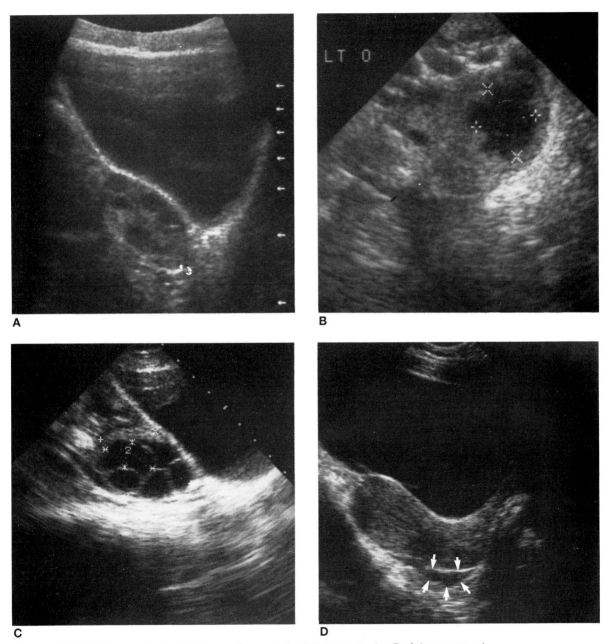

Figure 4-51. (**A**) Transvesical sagittal scan of a normal adult ovary on day 7 of the menstrual cycle. Several small follicles are seen within the ovarian substance. (**B**) Transvaginal sagittal scan of a dominant follicle immediately after its rupture at ovulation. Note the partially collapsed walls resulting from loss of most of the liquor folliculi. (**C**) Transvesical scan of an ovary that has been artificially stimulated during fertility therapy. Five follicles are seen in this scan plane. (**D**) Transvesical sagittal scan of the uterus immediately after ovulation, showing a small amount of echogenic fluid in the posterior cul-de-sac (*arrows*). This fluid most likely represents blood and serous fluid from the follicle.

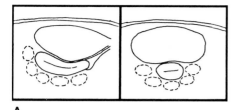

A

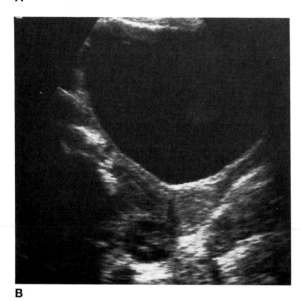

B

Figure 4-52. (**A**) Positions of the ovary. Because of its attachment to the posterior surface of the broad ligament, the ovary may be found in the posterior pelvic compartment or above the fundus of the uterus, in the adnexal spaces or in the posterior cul-de-sac, but not in the anterior cul-de-sac or between the urinary bladder and the uterus. (**B**) Parasagittal scan slightly to the right of midline shows a normal ovary located in the posterior cul-de-sac. Part of the fundus of the uterus is not visualized in this plane of scan. Note the excellent acoustic penetration deep to the ovary.

of the posterior pelvic compartment: the posterior cul-de-sac, the adnexal space to the side of the uterus, or above (cephalad to) or behind the fundus of the uterus. The normal ovary is not found anterior to the broad ligament (in front of the uterus, between the uterus and the urinary bladder, or in the anterior cul-de-sac) because of its attachment by the mesovarium to the posterior surface of the broad ligament (see Fig. 4-49).

Movements of the ovaries are governed by the complex relationship of the configuration of the true pelvic space, the degree of filling of the rectum, ovarian and uterine size, and the degree of filling of the urinary bladder. When meticulous scanning

with gain variations does not reveal the ovary, the sonographer should consider having the patient void partially, especially if the bladder is highly distended. This usually causes the ovaries to assume a new position, most commonly adjacent to the uterine fundus, where they may be more easily visualized.

Transvaginal ultrasound imaging is the method of choice when the primary interest is detailed visualization of the ovaries; however, the advantages of

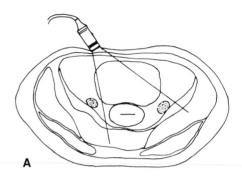

A

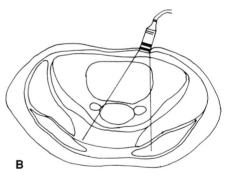

B

Figure 4-53. (**A**) The ovary can be differentiated from the obturator internus muscle by scanning in a transverse plane and angling the beam in from the side of the pelvis opposite the ovary to be demonstrated. This steep angle brings the ultrasound beam more perpendicular to the surface of the obturator internus muscle and usually demonstrates the thin layer of fat overlying the muscle, thus separating the dark echo pattern of the ovary from the similar dark pattern of the muscle. (**B**) A more difficult task is to separate the ovary from the myometrium when the two are in opposition. Scanning in a transverse plane with the transducer positioned on the same side of the pelvis as the ovary of interest and angled slightly back toward the midline often permits demonstration of a thin line between the ovary and the uterus, which confirms that the structure is an ovary and not a small subserosal fibroid. Careful attention to matching ovarian position with the focal zone of the ultrasound beam also helps. Placing the patient in a decubitus position may make it easier to obtain certain steeply angled scan planes.

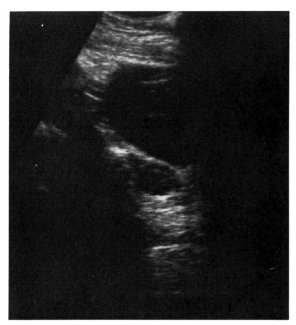

Figure 4-54. *Sagittal scan of the right ovary at very low gain setting. Note the burst of bright echoes that "marks" the position of the overlying ovary.*

transvaginal imaging must be balanced against the limitations of less depth of penetration of the ultrasound beam and a limited range of transducer positions. For the initial evaluation of the pelvic organs, especially when a pelvic mass is suspected, transabdominal imaging is the method of choice. This examination may then be supplemented by transvaginal imaging to obtain more detailed images of specific structures as needed. Transvaginal imaging alone can be used for follow-up examinations and in cases in which only the ovaries are to be evaluated (e.g., in fertility therapy), and for the few cases in which the patient is unable to maintain a distended urinary bladder.

The normal echo pattern of the adult ovary consists of a background of low-amplitude echoes (compared to the uterine myometrium) through which is scattered a coarse pattern of punctate bright reflectors and the distinctive anechoic spaces of the developing follicles. The bright reflections are most likely caused by corpora albicantia in the ovarian cortex and small vessels in the ovarian medulla. On both transvesical and transvaginal ultrasound, the ovary can be identified by its characteristic "Swiss cheese" pattern of anechoic follicles against the low-amplitude gray of the ovarian cortex.

Infants' ovaries may be difficult or impossible to locate, and in postmenopausal women the ovaries become increasingly difficult to detect as they become isoechoic with the surrounding parametrial ("around the ovary") tissues. With transabdominal scanning of patients in the reproductive years of life, the ovary may be difficult to separate from the adjacent myometrium or obturator internus muscle (Fig. 4-53). Because the echo patterns of the uterus and the ovary are subtly different, placing the focal zone at a level where both structures intersect permits optimal differentiation. Many instruments today permit selective positioning of the focal zone, greatly facilitating demonstration of the ovary as separate from the adjacent uterus.

In especially difficult cases, an acoustic property of the ovary may provide the only clue to its location. The ovary exhibits nearly as much acoustic transmission as a serous cyst of the same size. To locate a difficult ovary, the examiner should reduce gain levels so that most of the echoes from the uterus and the parametrium disappear. The ovary will be revealed by the burst of acoustic enhancement (increased through-transmission) seen beneath it as a column of brighter echoes (Fig. 4-54).

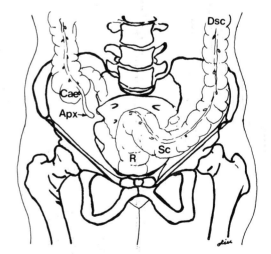

Figure 4-55. *Schematic diagram of the large bowel and its relationship to the false pelvis. The false pelvis is usually filled with loops of small bowel. The cecum and appendix are found on the right side of the false pelvis, and the pelvic portion of the descending colon and the proximal (upper) part of the sigmoid colon are found on the left. The location of the appendix is highly variable, and it may be found virtually anywhere in the right false pelvis, or even in the true pelvis. (Cae, cecum; Apx, appendix; Dsc, descending colon; Sc, sigmoid colon; R, rectum.)*

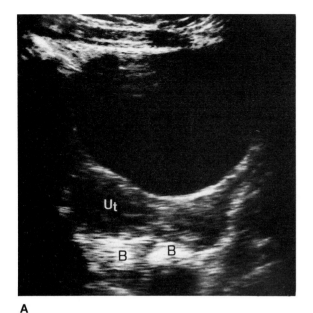

A

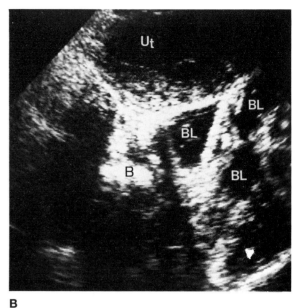

B

C

Figure 4-56. (**A**) Parasagittal scan of the pelvis demonstrating boluses of fecal material (B) with typical "dirty" shadows (*arrows*). (Ut, uterus.) (**B**) Transvaginal scan of the uterus. Fluid-filled loops of bowel (BL) are seen posterior to the uterus. (**C**) Sagittal view of the pelvis. The space between the posterior uterine wall and the curve of the sacrum is occupied by the rectum (*arrows*). In this person, the fecal material contains little gas, permitting good visualization of the curve of the sacrum, as indicated by the abrupt cutoff of the ultrasound image.

TABLE 4-3. ECHO PATTERN OF BOWEL

	Echo Pattern	**Shadows**
Small bowel	Variably echogenic content with thin, anechoic ring representing the muscular wall	Shifts with movement of bowel and content
Cecum	Variably echogenic content with thin, anechoic ring representing the muscular wall	Constant except when peristalsis occurs
Sigmoid	Echogenic content with thin, anechoic ring representing the muscular wall	Constant except when peristalsis occurs
Rectum	Echogenic content with thin, anechoic ring representing the muscular wall	Constant and nearly complete; only top surface of fecal boluses can be seen

The Pelvic Bowel

Sonographers often fail to recognize bowel when it is evident in the image, and so fail fully to appreciate its influence on other organs in the pelvis. To a large extent, the position of the uterus and ovaries is influenced by the degree of filling of the rectum, and bowel may be easily mistaken for a pelvic mass, especially when peristalsis is not readily evident in the real-time image. The *descending colon* becomes the *sigmoid colon* and enters the pelvic space through the left iliac fossa. The sigmoid typically forms one or more S-curves, which loop back and forth along the curve of the sacrum (Fig. 4-55).

Whereas the descending colon is partially buried in the retroperitoneal fat of the colic gutter, the sigmoid emerges to become completely covered by peritoneum, which forms a short suspensory membrane known as the *mesocolon*. It is the flexibility of this mesocolon that permits the sigmoid colon to move about over a relatively wide area of the posterior pelvic compartment. When the urinary bladder is empty, the sigmoid (along with loops of small bowel) occupies the posterior cul-de-sac. This location of the sigmoid can create some difficulty during transvaginal sonography. If the transducer is placed in the posterior fornix, curves of the sigmoid colon may lie between the transducer and the ovaries. In such cases, transfer of the probe to the lateral fornix may permit better visualization. This is not a problem in transvesical scanning because the distended urinary bladder forces the sigmoid and loops of small bowel upward so that they move above and behind the fundus of the uterus.

When filled with fecal material, the sigmoid colon usually can be followed from its entry at the left posterolateral brim of the pelvis, down into the cul-de-sac. At about the midpoint of the sacral curve, the sigmoid moves posterior to the peritoneum and, like the descending colon, becomes partially buried, so that only its anterior surface and part of its lateral surfaces are covered by peritoneum. From this point to its terminus at the anus, the large bowel is the *rectum,* which is characterized by thicker and more muscular walls.

In the ultrasound image, the rectum is commonly recognized by deduction. That is, the rectum walls usually are not visible, but the content of the rectum is easily demonstrated. Boluses of fecal material in the rectum cause irregular ("dirty") shadows and produce a pattern of very

dense, bright echoes typical of material containing many small bubbles of gas (Fig. 4-56A). Fluid in the rectum or fecal material containing little gas permits visualization of the anterior surface of the sacrum lying deep to the rectum (see Fig. 4-56C). On real-time observation, the upper parts of the pelvic bowel and any intruding loops of small bowel are actively peristaltic and can be easily differentiated as bowel, particularly if filled with fluid (see Fig. 4-56B). In contrast, rectal peristalsis is infrequent and the rectum must be identified by location and echo pattern rather than by its motion.

The *cecum* and *appendix* can usually be identified in the right iliac fossa. The appendix is one of the most variable structures in the human body, and although technically it is an abdominal structure, it may be found in the pelvis.[2]

Bowel is relatively easy to differentiate from other pelvic organs and from muscle in most cases. If there appears to be a mass in the posterior cul-

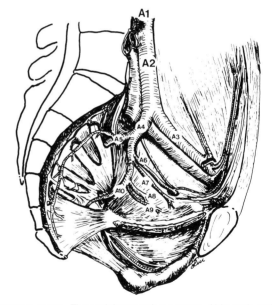

Figure 4-57. The pelvic vascular system. Although only the arteries are shown in detail, the veins follow the same pattern but lie posterior to the arteries. The one exception to the pattern of naming the vessels is the hypogastric artery, whose companion vein is named the internal iliac vein rather than the hypogastric. Note the triangular space defined by the vessels at the bifurcation of the common iliac vessels. This open-based triangle is the ovarian fossa (Waldeyer's fossa). (A1, aorta; A2, common iliac artery; A3, external iliac artery; A4, hypogastric artery; A5, superior gluteal artery; A6, obturator artery; A7, umbilical artery; A8, uterine artery; A9, superior vesical artery; A10, internal pudendal and inferior gluteal arteries.)

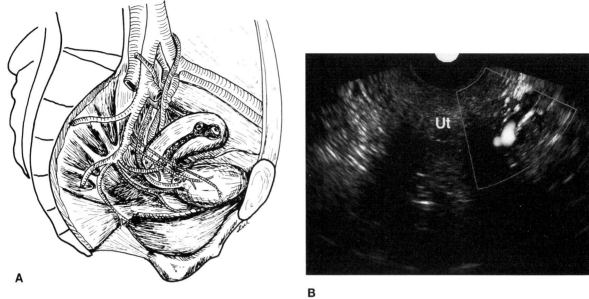

A

B

Figure 4-58. (**A**) Arterial supply to the uterus. The broad ligament has been removed to expose the uterine artery as it courses upward from the level of the cervix to the cornu of the uterus, where it makes a sharp turn to run along the underside of the fallopian tube. The uterine artery forms an anastomosis with the ovarian artery beneath the fallopian tube. Thus, although the uterine artery is the principal supplier of blood to the uterus, it is not the sole supplier. Anastomotic connections are not limited to the uterine–ovarian arteries. They are found throughout the pelvis, providing an elaborate fail-safe network of alternate channels to each of the organs. (**B**) This transverse endovaginal scan of the region of the uterine isthmus (Ut) uses power Doppler imaging to demonstrate the abundant vessels which lie along the lateral cervical margins. Blood flow is indicated by the presence of color, with the volume of flow indicated by brighter shades of color. Power Doppler is not directional, so we cannot determine if flow in any specific vessel is toward or away from the transducer. (See also Color Plate 4.)

de-sac but it is not possible to determine whether it is bowel, a water enema may be administered while the suspect area is simultaneously observed with real-time ultrasound imaging. Movement of water through the rectum and sigmoid should permit positive identification of these structures. Table 4-3 lists some of the salient features of the echo pattern and shadowing for each of the pelvic bowel segments.

The Pelvic Vascular System

Until the early 1990s, information about the pelvic vascular system had little direct value for sonographers. Occasionally, they encountered dilated pelvic veins mimicking a complex mass, but these were rare. Today, Doppler examination of the pelvic vessels is becoming an increasingly important tool in obstetric ultrasound, and it shows promise of having applications in gynecologic sonography as well.

The pelvic vascular system consists of three distinct components: the arteries, the veins, and the lymphatics. The lymphatic channels usually have no significance in pelvic sonography.

The spatial relationship of the great vessels (aorta and vena cava) changes as they descend through the abdomen. In the upper abdomen, the vena cava is more anterior than the aorta. Just above the level of the umbilicus, these two vessels come to lie side by side, and then at their bifurcation the veins come to lie posterior to the arteries.[16] From the bifurcation through the pelvic region, the arteries are more anterior than the veins. A simple way to remember this is with the phrase "*a*rteries before *v*eins."

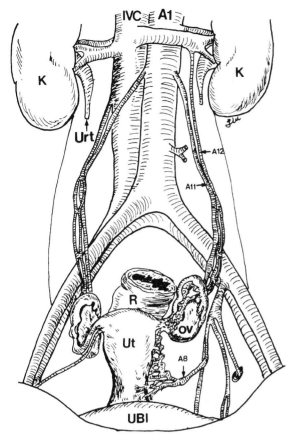

Figure 4-59. The blood supply of the ovaries (OV). The uterine artery (A8) and the ovarian artery (A11) form anastomoses in the region of the ovarian hilus. Note the difference in the pattern of ovarian artery origin versus ovarian vein (A12) termination. Because lymphatics follow the gonadal (ovarian) vessels, tumor spread from the pelvis to the paraaortic nodes at the level of the renal pelvis is common. (Urt, ureter; K, kidney; Ut, uterus; UBl, urinary bladder; IVC, inferior vena cava; R, rectum.)

ARTERIAL SYSTEM OF THE PELVIS

The *aorta* usually bifurcates at a point slightly higher than the inferior vena cava, giving rise to the *common iliac arteries,* which are quite short, extending only for a few centimeters until they branch into the large *external iliac artery* and the smaller *internal iliac (hypogastric) artery* (Fig. 4-57). The external iliac artery runs along the medial border of the iliopsoas muscle at the brim of the true pelvic space. When it reaches the lower margin of the pelvis, the external iliac artery passes beneath the inguinal ligament to enter the thigh.

The hypogastric or internal iliac artery is smaller than the external iliac artery, and it courses from the bifurcation at the upper and posterior margin of the true pelvic space down into the pelvic cavity along the lateral wall for a distance of only 1 or 2 cm. It then gives rise to the relatively large and posteriorly directed *superior gluteal artery.* The hypogastric artery continues downward along the pelvic wall, giving rise to four small branches that course anterior along the pelvic wall: the *obturator artery,* the *umbilical artery,* the *uterine-vaginal artery,* and the *superior vesical artery.* Finally, the hypogastric terminates in two posteriorly directed branches: the *internal pudendal* and the *inferior gluteal arteries.* Except for these last two posteriorly directed branches, the branches of the hypogastric artery and their many subdivisions fan out along the lateral wall of the pelvis, descending to the pelvic floor to pass over the pelvic diaphragm to reach their target organs or muscles.[16] The hypogastric artery is the primary blood supply for the uterus, vagina, urinary bladder, and most of the muscles of the pelvic floor. It should be kept in mind that branching patterns of blood vessels are highly variable.

Most of the smaller branches of the hypogastric artery are not individually identifiable in the ultrasound image, but one branch, the uterine artery, is important to sonographers. The uterine artery extends across the pelvic floor to reach the uterus at approximately the level of the tip of the cervix (Fig. 4-58A). At this point, it bifurcates into a uterine branch and a descending vaginal branch. Its uterine component turns upward to run along the lateral margin of the uterus (see Fig. 4-58B) to the fallopian tube, where it again makes a sharp turn to run along the length of the fallopian tube. Just past the cervical "right-angle" turn, the uterine artery is relatively straight as it ascends alongside the cervix. It is at this point that the artery is most accessible for Doppler evaluation with a transvaginal probe. As it courses upward along the lateral border of the uterus, the uterine artery becomes very tortuous.

On the basis of the description thus far, it might reasonably be concluded that the uterine artery is the exclusive supplier of arterial blood to the uterus; however, the organs of reproduction, like the brain, are provided with an elaborate fail-safe blood supply. In addition to terminating in capillaries embedded in the target organ, the

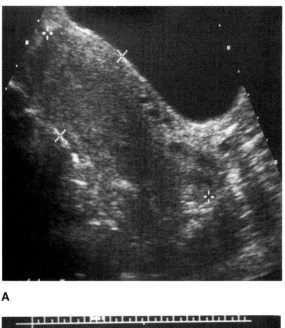

A

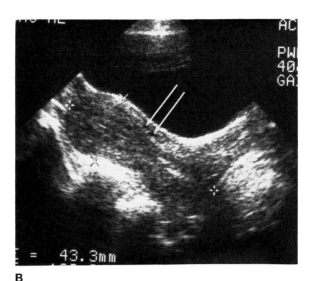

B

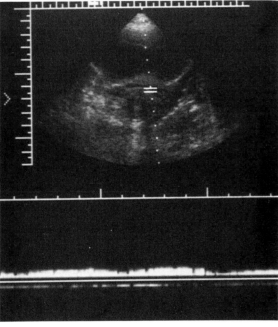

C

Figure 4-60. (**A**) *Parasagittal along the left margin of the uterus (outlined by measurement cursors). Note the prominent veins along the anterior margin of the lower corpus and cervix.* (**B**) *More typical vascular channels (arrows) in the uterine myometrium. These appear as small, often irregular or serpiginous anechoic spaces within the myometrium. They are most commonly seen within the superficial layers.* (**C**) *Doppler can be used to determine whether flow is present in the suspected vascular channel. Because the dilated vessels are veins, the Doppler signal typically is low in amplitude and the flow nearly constant.*

internal pudendal artery, vaginal artery, and uterine artery all have anastomotic branches that form a complex network of interconnected channels around the vagina and most of the uterus. This anastomotic network ensures that compromised flow through any one of these arteries does not result in tissue damage in the target organ. Other feeder vessels of the network provide an immedi-

ate compensatory flow, thus preserving tissue function. An even more elaborate system exists to supply the ovary.

The embryonic ovaries originate in the abdominal region from a common mesenchymal tissue, which also gives rise to the adrenal glands. This explains why tumors in the region of the adrenal may produce sex hormones and why tumors that

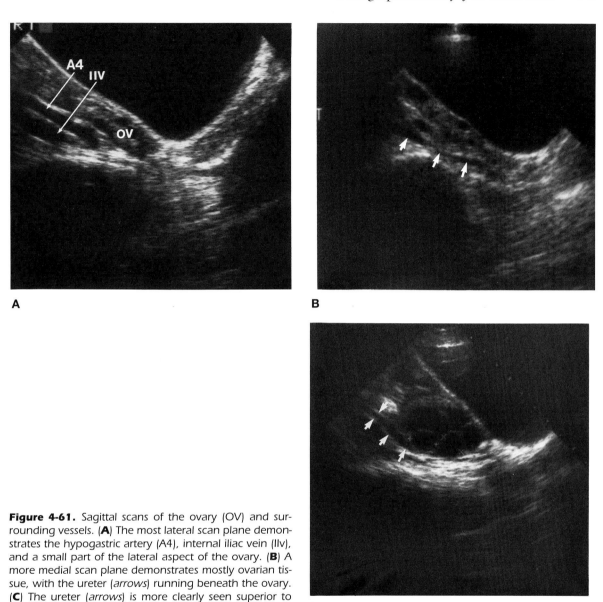

Figure 4-61. Sagittal scans of the ovary (OV) and surrounding vessels. (**A**) The most lateral scan plane demonstrates the hypogastric artery (A4), internal iliac vein (IIv), and a small part of the lateral aspect of the ovary. (**B**) A more medial scan plane demonstrates mostly ovarian tissue, with the ureter (*arrows*) running beneath the ovary. (**C**) The ureter (*arrows*) is more clearly seen superior to and deep to a hormonally stimulated ovary.

have adrenal characteristics may be found in the pelvis. In the later stages of embryonic life, the ovaries descend into the pelvis, guided by a ligamentous band called the *gubernaculum*. As the embryonic ovaries descend, they bring with them their original blood supply derived from the aorta and draining into the vena cava. These vessels persist in adult life as the *ovarian artery* and *vein*. The ovarian arteries originate as lateral branches of the aorta at about the level of the lower margin of the renal

pelvis (Fig. 4-59). These arteries course downward over the psoas muscles and along the same path followed by the ureters, crossing over the common iliac artery just superior to its bifurcation into the external and internal iliac arteries. The ovarian artery then bridges across from the upper margin of the pelvis to the ovary through the infundibulopelvic ligament. From the infundibulopelvic ligament it passes through the mesovarium to reach the ovarian hilus, where it supplies the ovarian parenchyma.

In addition, the ovarian artery forms anastomoses with the ovarian branches of the uterine artery, thus providing a closed-loop or fail-safe blood supply originating from two widely divergent points in the arterial system.

VENOUS SYSTEM OF THE PELVIS

The venous system of the pelvis follows a pattern virtually identical to that of the arterial system. The *inferior vena cava* bifurcates slightly below the level of the aortic bifurcation, giving rise to the *common iliac veins,* which run beneath the *common iliac arteries.* These short vessels in turn give rise to the large *external iliac veins,* which drain the legs, and the smaller *internal iliac veins,* which drain the pelvic organs and muscles. The ovarian veins follow the same course as the ovarian arteries until they reach the mid-abdomen, where the *right ovarian vein* drains directly into the vena cava and the *left ovarian vein* drains into the left renal vein.

Because the veins are thin walled, they are highly distensible and vary in size with certain conditions, most notably pregnancy. After parturition, the venous channels usually shrink, but rarely to the prepregnant state, and they may remain prominent and easily visible. If venous congestion occurs, the veins may form pelvic varices, which are readily identifiable in the ultrasound image. In some women, particularly after parturition, the venous channels in the outer regions of the myometrium may appear to separate the muscle layer into two regions (Fig. 4-60).

The Ureter

The *ureter* is commonly observed as it courses along the lateral pelvic wall posterior to the ovary. These musculomembranous tubes move urine by peristalsis, and enter the pelvis at a point just caudad to the bifurcation of the common iliac vessels. This results in the ureter being the most anterior and lateral of the three tubular structures seen deep to the ovary in its most common position lateral to the uterus (Fig. 4-61). As the ureter descends into the pelvic space, it moves mediad, to reach the trigone of the urinary bladder, and therefore oblique scan planes are usually required to demonstrate long segments of the ureter in the pelvis. Ureteral contractions are readily observed with real-time ultrasound, and the ureter can be identified most clearly with vaginal scanning.

REFERENCES

1. Athey PA. Sonographic appearance of the normal female pelvis. In: Athey PA, Hadlock FP, eds. Ultrasound in Obstetrics and Gynecology. St. Louis: CV Mosby; 1981.
2. Blount RF. The digestive system. In: Schaeffer JP, ed. Morris' Human Anatomy. 11th ed. New York: McGraw-Hill; 1953.
2a. Cohen HL, Tice H, Mandel F. Ovarian volumes measured by US: Bigger than we think. Radiology 1990; 177:189–192.
3. Fleischer AC, Kalemeris GC, Entman SS. Sonographic depiction of the endometrium during normal cycles. Ultrasound Med Biol 1986; 12:271–277.
4. Fleischer AC, Kalemeris GC, Machin JE, et al. Sonographic depiction of normal and abnormal endometrium with histopathologic correlation. J Ultrasound Med. 1986; 5:445–452.
5. Grant JCB, Smith CG. The musculature. In: Schaeffer JP, ed. Morris' Human Anatomy. 11th ed. New York: McGraw-Hill; 1953.
6. Gray H. Osteology. In: Goss CM, ed. Gray's Anatomy. 28th ed. Philadelphia: Lea & Febiger; 1966.
7. Gray H. The urogenital system. In: Goss CM, ed. Gray's Anatomy. 28th ed. Philadelphia: Lea & Febiger; 1966.
8. Green JH, Silver PHS. An Introduction to Human Anatomy. New York: Oxford University Press; 1981.
9. Hackeloer B. The role of ultrasound in female infertility management. Ultrasound Med Biol. 1984; 10:44.
10. Kistner RW. Gynecology: Principles and Practice. 3rd ed. Chicago: Year Book Medical Publishers; 1980.
11. Kurtz AB, Rifkin MD. Normal anatomy of the female pelvis. In: Sanders RC, James AE, eds. The Principles and Practice of Ultrasonography in Obstetrics and Gynecology. 3rd ed. New York: Appleton-Century-Crofts; 1985.
12. Markee JE. The urogenital system. In: Schaeffer JP, ed. Morris' Human Anatomy. 11th ed. New York: McGraw-Hill; 1953.
13. Muckle CW. Clinical anatomy of the uterus, fallopian tubes, and ovaries. In: Droegemueller W, Sciarra J, eds. Gynecology and Obstetrics. Philadelphia: JB Lippincott; 1988.
14. Netter FH, Oppenheimer E, eds. The CIBA Collection of Medical Illustrations: Reproductive System. West Caldwell, NJ: Ciba Pharmaceutical Company; 1965.

15. Oike K, Obata S, Takagi K, et al. Observation of endometrial movement with transvaginal ultrasonography (Abstract). J Ultrasound Med. 1988; 7:S99.
16. Patten BM. The cardiovascular system. In: Schaeffer JP, ed. Morris' Human Anatomy. 11th ed. New York: McGraw-Hill; 1953.
17. Sample WF. Gray scale ultrasonography of the normal female pelvis. In: Sanders RC, James AE, eds. The Principles and Practice of Ultrasonography in Obstetrics and Gynecology. 2nd ed. New York: Appleton-Century-Crofts; 1980.
18. Sample WF, Lippe BM, Gyepes MT. Gray-scale ultrasonography of the normal female pelvis. Radiology 1977; 125:477–483.
19. Timor-Tritsch IE, Rottem S, Elgali S. How transvaginal sonography is done. In: Timor-Tritsch IE, Rottem S, eds. Transvaginal Sonography. New York: Elsevier; 1988.

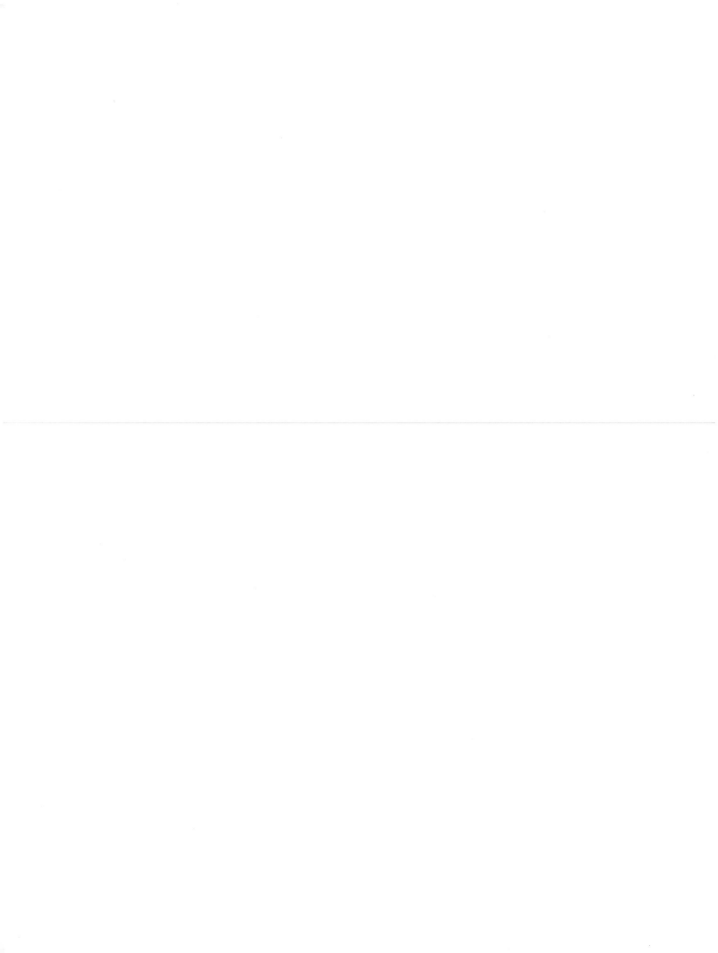

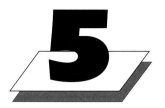

Congenital Anomalies of the Female Genital System

MIMI C. BERMAN and **JOYCE A. MILLER**

Congenital anomalies of the female reproductive tract are uncommon. The reported incidence is between 0.1% and 0.5%, with an occasionally reported figure as high as 12%.[1,2,20,35] When they do occur, most prevalent congenital anomalies are septate, bicornuate, and didelphic uteri.[33]

Congenital malformations usually present with no clinical symptoms.[21] They can, however, mimic other pelvic lesions, such as leiomyoma, adnexal mass, ectopic pregnancy, and twin gestation, making it important for practitioners to be familiar with the appearance of the different anomalies. Usually patients are sent for a sonogram to investigate the cause of infertility or reproductive problems or, during a pregnancy, when suspicion arises that there may be some irregularity in the configuration of the uterus. Also, because uterine anomalies occur in at least 50%[22,29] of patients with developmental urinary tract disorders, such as renal agenesis or ectopic kidney, sonographers should make it a practice to examine both systems whenever an anomaly is found in either one.

In 1979, Buttram and Gibbons proposed a classification system that took into account the configuration of the anomaly, its clinical symptoms, treatment options, and prognosis.[1,10] This system, which has been adapted by the American Fertility Society, provides a useful reference system when discussing congential anomalies (Table 5-1).

Anatomy of Congenital Anomalies

The vagina and uterus are formed by the müllerian ducts fusing together in the midline to form a single duct, the *uterovaginal canal*. At first, there is a midline septum in this canal that normally disappears by the end of the third month of prenatal development (see Fig. 3-5). Most types of malformations in this region may be attributed to total or partial atresia of the müllerian ducts, failure of the müllerian ducts to fuse properly, or failure of the uterovaginal septum to be resorbed.

VAGINA

The vagina, which is the connection between the interior and exterior portions of the genitalia, is a frequent site of maldevelopment of the müllerian system. The lumen of the vagina is separated from the urogenital sinus by a thin tissue plate, the *hymen*. This tissue usually ruptures during prenatal life; however, if it does not, an *imperforate hymen* results (see Fig. 3-7). This diagnosis is usually made at menarche, when a physician observes a tense, bulging membrane. Sonography can image hema-

▨▨▨ **TABLE 5-1. CLASSIFICATION SYSTEM OF MÜLLERIAN DUCT ANOMALIES**

Class I
  Hypoplasia or agenesis of :
    A. Vagina
    B. Cervix
    C. Fundus
    D. Tubal
    E. Combined
Class II
  Unicornuate:
    A1a. Communicating
    A1b. Noncommunicating
    A2. No cavity
    B.   No horn
Class III
  Uterus didelphys
Class IV
  Bicornuate:
    A. Complete
    B. Partial
    C. Arcuate
Class V
  Septate uterus:
    A. Complete
    B. Partial
Class VI
  DES- and drug-related anomalies, or arcuate

(From Buttram VC, Gibbons WE. Müllerian anomalies: A proposed classification [an analysis of 144 cases]. Fertil Steril. 1979; 32:40–46.)

tometrocolpos, a combination of menstrual blood, fluid, and secretions in a distended vagina (hematocolpos) and in a distended uterus (hematometra).[17]

Vaginal Agenesis or Atresia

Vaginal agenesis or atresia may occur if the sinovaginal bulbs do not develop or develop improperly. Transverse septa, or partitions, can also form during embryonic development of the vagina; when they do, they are usually located in the upper third of the vagina. These septa, like an imperforate hymen, may close off the vagina to the exterior and result in similar clinical and sonographic findings.[17]

UTERUS

Fusion Failure

Vaginal abnormalities are often associated with concomitant cervical and uterine anomalies, because virtually all are caused by failure of some stage of devel-opment in the müllerian duct system.[32] Partial or total failure of fusion of the müllerian ducts may cause any degree of duplication of the system, from the minor anomaly seen in uterus arcuatus, which has a slightly indented fundus, to a completely duplicated uterus, *uterus didelphys,* including duplicate cervix and vagina (Fig. 5-1).[27] One of the most common anomalies encountered in the uterus is *uterus bicornis,* either *bicervical* or *unicervical* (see Fig. 5-1D, 5-1F), which has two horns entering a common vagina.[44]

Müllerian Duct Atresia

Another cause of uterine and cervical anomalies occurs when there is partial or complete atresia of one of the müllerian ducts. *Aplasia* or *hypoplasia* of the entire uterus or cervix may occur, or only one side may be atretic and may not communicate with the vagina. A rudimentary or hypoplastic uterus usually is not functional, but if menstrual bleeding does occur in a horn that has no communication with the vagina, hydrometra can result (see Fig. 5-1H).[44]

Failure of the Urogenital Septum to Disappear

The septum can persist to variable degrees, causing any degree of separation of the uterine corpus from slight (see Fig. 5-1D,F) to complete.[44] In *uterus subseptus,* the septum is only partially resorbed (see Fig. 5-1C).

Diethylstilbestrol Syndrome

From the late 1940s to the early 1970s, many women were exposed in utero to diethylstilbestrol (DES) administered to their mothers primarily for the treatment of threatened abortion. Women exposed to DES in utero are able to conceive, but many have poor pregnancy outcomes. Thirty-five percent of them have been found to have vaginal epithelial changes (adenosis), and 42% have an abnormally shaped uterine cavity. The most significant DES stigmata are a T-shaped uterus, constricting bands in the uterus, and intrauterine wall defects.[17,42]

FALLOPIAN TUBES

Very rarely, both fallopian tubes are absent. Unilateral absence is associated with absence of the uterus on that side. Rare doubling of the tube can also occur on one side. The most common problem encountered here is *atresia* of a portion of a tube,

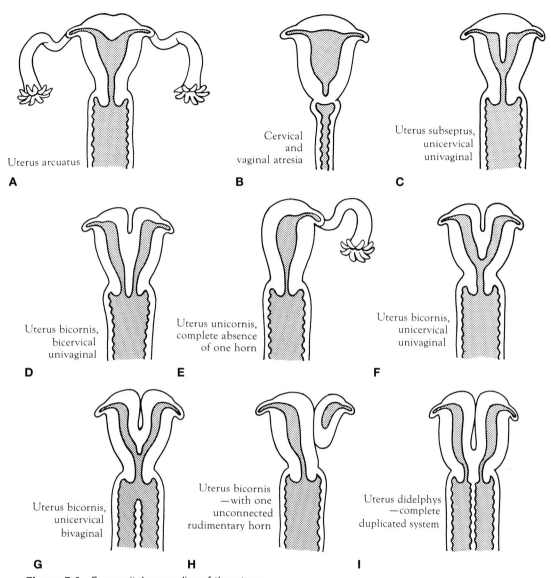

Figure 5-1. Congenital anomalies of the uterus.

which may cause infertility or tubal pregnancy.[17] Patency of fallopian tubes are usually imaged with hysterosalpingography. Although routine sonographic techniques do not visualize nondilated fallopian tubes, sonohysterography using saline or contrast agents has made their imaging feasible.[4]

OVARIES

Congenital agenesis or atresia of the ovaries is very rare.[17] When it does occur, the fallopian tubes usually are also absent (see Fig. 5-1E). It has also been re-

ported that the ovaries are more frequently malpositioned above the iliac vessels in patients with congenital uterine anomalies, particularly in women without uteri or unicornuate uteri.[16] *Supernumerary* (extra) ovaries are found occasionally at a site remote from the normal ovary. They probably result from development of separate primordia in an ectopic portion of the gonadal ridge. Benign teratomas and dermoid cysts of these supernumerary ovaries have been found in the omentum and in the retroperitoneum.[17]

Occasionally, an ovary may be split into separate portions. *Accessory ovarian tissue,* usually less than 1 cm in diameter, can be found in the broad ligament near the normal ovary or near the cornua of the uterus.[17] Ectopic ovarian tissue may also be found near the kidney or in the retroperitoneal space.

Parovarian cysts arising from the Rosenmüller's organ, a vestigial portion of the wolffian duct system, may be found. The outer extremity of this "duct" can become dilated and form a cystic, pedunculated structure known as the *hydatid cyst of Morgagni.* These may become infarcted and cause pain when they twist on their pedicles. Gartner's duct, a remnant of the wolffian duct in the broad ligament, has a propensity to cystic dilatation and infection.[17,36]

Clinical Manifestations of Congential Anomalies

In nonpregnant patients, congenital anomalies are suspected when at or after puberty a mass is palpated in the pelvis. An anomaly may also be considered as part of the differential diagnosis when a patient experiences amenorrhea, dysmenorrhea, dyspareunia, or pelvic pain. These symptoms are often caused by obstruction at some level of the uterus, cervix, or vagina, resulting in an accumulation of mucus or menstrual blood. Obstruction can be caused by an intact hymen or by congenital absence or stenosis of the vagina. Ultrasound can contribute essential information when no vagina is found on physical examination and when a mass is palpated.

After menarche, patients present with reproduction related problems such as infertility, habitual abortion, unsuccessful dilation and curettage (because only one uterus was treated), cervical incompetence, and failure of an intrauterine device. Many uterine anomalies allow zygote implantation, but they are associated with increased rates of abortion and premature delivery, possibly owing to the weakness of the cervical muscles, the diminished uterine space, or the decreased vascularity in some implantation sites, such as the septum.[1,18,19] In septate uteri, the conceptus may implant on the septum, often resulting in an early abortion.[18,38] An 8% to 12% incidence of congenital anomalies has

been reported in women who experience habitual abortion and infertility.[35]

Once the patient becomes pregnant, it is important to be aware of any unusual configurations that could interfere with a normal pregnancy. Higher incidences of premature deliveries, abnormal fetal presentations, premature labor, prolonged labor, low birth weight, and fetal malformations have been reported.[19,24,35] A sonogram is the first imaging modality to use to examine pregnant patients for structural anomalies.

Sonographic Scanning Technique and Appearance

VAGINAL ANOMALIES

Most vaginal anomalies, such as transverse and longitudinal septa and duplicated vagina, cannot be imaged by transabdominal or transvaginal ultrasound.[30] An intact hymen can be imaged using a transverse perineal approach, but with standard sonographic techniques, only the sequelae, such as accumulations of mucus or blood in the vagina (colpos) or endometrial canal (metra), are seen[12] (Fig. 5-2). As in all ultrasound imaging, gross changes in the normal appearance of the vagina can be seen. Thus, a Gartner's duct cyst appears as a small anechoic mass in the anterolateral portion of the vagina (Fig. 5-3). Complete absence of the vagina is apparent by the missing normal central coapted vaginal echoes (Fig. 5-4). This condition occurs in about 1 in 5000 patients[6] and may affect part of the vagina. When there is agenesis of a small inferior section, ultrasound can be useful in identifying the atretic area[40] by mapping out the section where no normal echoes are visualized.

The importance of ultrasound in detecting the cause of pelvic masses in women with asymmetric duplication of the uterus resulting in one imperforate vagina has been reported.[8,25,31] Although the shape of the masses varied because each duplication above the vagina was somewhat different, the basic sonographic appearance was of a mass adjacent to a uterus and filled with either clear fluid (anechoic) or with low-level echoes (hypoechoic) from blood or mucus. The ultrasound findings spared several of these patients from having hysterectomies or exploratory surgery. Subsequently they had corrective

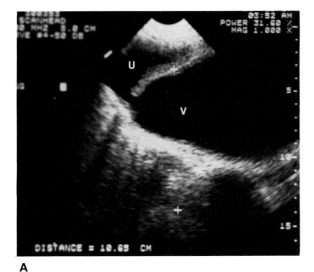

A

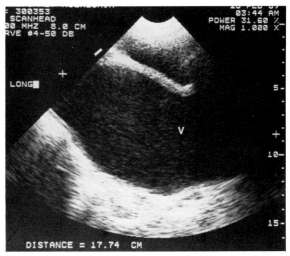

B

Figure 5-2. (A) A 12-year-old girl with hematometro-colpos. Sagittal sonogram demonstrates the fluid-filled dilated vagina (V). Superior to the vagina is a smaller blood-filled structure representing the dilated uterus (U). **(B)** This sagittal section of the hematometrocolpos has the characteristic low-level echoes representing clotted blood. The lack of convergence of the inferior borders of the dilated vagina is characteristic of hematocolpos. **(C)** Hematometro-colpos, transverse perineal view. A transducer placed on an intact hymen (H) shows a vagina (V) distended by menstrual debris. This technique allowed presurgical measurement of the hymen of this 13-year-old child who presented with fever of unknown etiology and was cured by hymenectomy. (Cohen HL, Bober SE, Bow SN. Imaging the pediatric pelvis: The normal and abnormal genital tract and simulators of its diseases. Urologic Radiology. 1992; 14:273–283.)

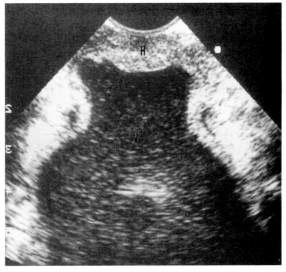

C

surgery that involved incision and drainage of the fluid followed by reconstruction of a vagina or excision of a septum if it was causing the obstruction.[13] The kidney on the side of the asymmetric duplication is almost always absent.[43]

Technique

In a longitudinal plane, using transabdominal scanning, the vaginal canal with the surrounding vaginal muscles should appear continuous with the cervix. Absence of this continuity could indicate atresia and can be further documented with transverse scans.

The transvaginal approach should be performed cautiously if there is suspicion of an atretic or absent vagina. If duplication is suspected, water vaginography using transabdominal technique may help elucidate the configuration by demonstrating one intact vagina, a connection between two vaginas, or a vagina with a contiguous obstructed one.[39] Transperineal scanning can also be attempted to visualize the area of the obstruction or if absence of the vagina is suspected.

In cases of hydrocolpos or hematocolpos, no vagina is visible separate from the fluid-filled

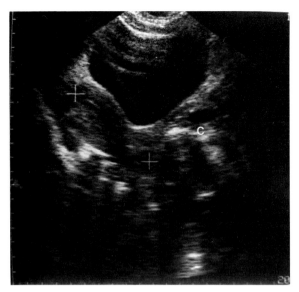

Figure 5-3. A cyst (C) in the vagina, a Gartner's duct cyst.

mass. The typical appearances of vaginal anomalies are summarized in Table 5-2.

UTERINE ANOMALIES

Because uterine anomalies run the gamut from absence of uterus and vagina (Mayer-Rokitansky-Kuster-Hauser syndrome) to complete duplication of uterus, cervix, and vagina (uterus didelphys), there is a wide variety of sonographic appearances (Table 5-3).[7] In the nonpregnant patient without symptoms, unless the anomaly manifests itself with gross changes to the morphology of the uterus (see Figs. 5-4 through 5-7), transabdominal pelvic ultrasound may be of limited value in making a diagnosis. However, directed transabdominal ultrasound, transvaginal ultrasound, sonohysterography with sterile saline or ultrasound contrast agents, as well as recently reported three-dimensional ultrasound imaging, have shown improved sensitivity[4,26,28,34] (Fig. 5-5).

Distinguishing between bicornuate and septate uteri is critical for planning surgery, particularly because the repair of a bicornuate uterus requires transabdominal surgery, whereas a septate uterus often can be treated on an outpatient basis by excising the septum hysteroscopically.[34,45]

When examining a patient for a uterine anomaly, the sonographer must keep in mind the various combinations of uterine, cervical, and vaginal malformations. Transverse images best visualize duplications of the cervix and uterus. The transverse scan through a duplicated cervix shows two echogenic connected or contiguous cervices (Figs. 5-6 and 5-7). Duplications of the endometrium or separation of the endometrial cavity by a septum are imaged as two endometrial echoes. For optimal visualization of the endometrial echoes, it is best to perform the examination during the late secretory phase when the endometrium is at its thickest and most echogenic. Careful sonographic examination of the fundal region provides anatomic information that can help differentiate between bicornuate and septated uteri (Fig. 5-8).

A uterus widened on transverse plane that contains two endometrial echoes is characteristic of duplication. One study found that women with septated uteri typically had fundi measuring between 6.5 to 9 cm in breadth, which is wider than normal.[41] Although both didelphic and bicornuate uteri have widened and divided fundi representing the two uterine bodies, a didelphic uterus can be diagnosed by noting duplication of endometria and

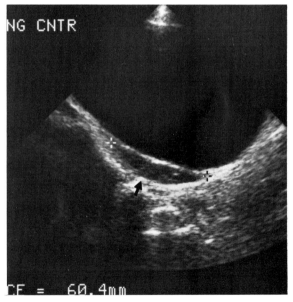

Figure 5-4. Sagittal scan through the rudimentary uterus (arrow) of a 16-year-old girl with primary amenorrhea. Reconstructive surgery was performed to create a vagina. (Courtesy Dr. Ruth Rosenblatt, Montefiore Hospital, Bronx, NY.)

▰▰▰ **TABLE 5-2. SONOGRAPHIC APPEARANCE OF CONGENITAL VAGINAL ANOMALIES**

Anomaly	Sonographic Appearance
Hydrocolpos or hematocolpos	Anechoic to hypoechoic pear-shaped mass with no normal vaginal echoes located adjacent and posterior to the bladder (see Fig. 5-2)
Vaginal septa	Normal vaginal echoes
Double vagina	Either no significant change in appearance of normal vagina or enlarged vagina; transvaginal scanning may demonstrate second vagina
Absent vagina	Absence of normal vaginal echoes (see Fig. 5-4)
Duplicated uterus with unilateral imperforate vagina	Vagina appears normal; lateral to normal uterus, an anechoic or echo-filled mass might be seen. Kidney ipsilateral to mass is usually absent.
Intact hymen	In postmenarchal symptomatic patient, hematocolpos or hematometrocolpos might be found (see Fig. 5-2)
Gartner's duct cyst	Anechoic small mass in anterolateral vagina (see Fig. 5-3)

endocervical echoes, whereas a bicornuate uterus demonstrates separation of endometrial echoes only to the area of the cervix. The real diagnostic challenge is sonographically differentiating between duplication representing a bicornuate uterus from that of a septate uterus, because the septum can divide the uterine cavity to the same level as imaged in bicornuate uteri. By scanning transabdominally with a nearly empty bladder to permit the uterus to lie in its normal anteverted position, or coronally through the fundus with transvaginal technique, the clinician can improve the chances of making this diagnosis sonographically.[18,37] The completely separate fundi of a bicornuate uterus may be differentiated from a septated uterus (flat or slightly indented intact fundus—see Fig. 5-8) by identifying a fundal notch 10 mm or greater[18,34] or a 75° or greater separation between the endometrial cavities. Differentiating between these entities has become easier with the endometrial analysis allowed by sonohysterography.[4,15] Three-dimensional scanning has likewise proven effective.[26]

Because aplasia and hypoplasia of the uterus are possible anomalies, the size of the uterus relative to the patient's age and parity should be accounted for. If the uterus is absent or small, it is particularly important to examine for a vagina, because it is frequently absent in these cases of Mayer-Rokitansky-Kuster-Hauser syndrome (see Fig. 5-4).[2]

The T-shaped uterine cavity, characteristic of some women exposed to DES in utero, is most easily seen on hysterosalpingogarphy but ultrasound can visualize a thin endometrial cavity in the uterine corpus which widens in the region of the cornua to represent the cross-bar in the "T" (Fig. 5-9; see also Fig. 28-14).

Potential Pitfalls

Pedunculated and subserosal myomas located in the cervical or fundal areas can present as enlargements of these structures simulating their duplication (Fig. 5-10).[5] Myomas do not have endocervical echoes and usually do not have the same degree of echogenicity as endometrial tissue. Most important, on sagittal scans masses due to myoma are not continuous with the rest of the uterus.

UTERINE ANOMALIES IN PREGNANT PATIENTS

After 22 weeks' gestation, the enlargement of the pregnant uterus obliterates some subtle findings suggestive of anatomic variants. If there is clinical suspicion of an anomaly, the patient should be ex-

▰▰▰ **TABLE 5-3.** Sᴏɴᴏɢʀᴀᴘʜɪᴄ Aᴘᴘᴇᴀʀᴀɴᴄᴇ ᴏғ Uᴛᴇʀɪɴᴇ Aɴᴏᴍᴀʟɪᴇs

	Sonographic Appearance	
Anomaly	**Nonpregnant Uterus**	**Pregnant Uterus***
Cervical atresia	No cervical echoes but corpus of uterus appears as echogenic mass[29]	
Uterine agenesis	Absence of echoes in area of uterus or small remnant of apparently fibrous tissue[29]	
Unicornuate uterus	Normal to slightly asymmetric uterus,[9] loss of pear shape,[29] lateral displacement	In advanced pregnancy, no abnormalities
Didelphic uterus	Double cervix, uterine corpora, enlarged uterus, two endometrial canal echoes visualized (see Figs. 5-6 and 5-7)	Pregnancy in one uterus; decidual reaction and enlarged other
Bicornuate uterus	Dependent on degree of cleft between horns: broad uterine fundus, two distinct cornua, with a cleft between them of over 1 cm and angle between horns of over 75°, two endometrial cavity echoes or normal-looking uterus[18,34]	Eccentric implantation of gestational sac (see Figs. 5-11 and 5-12)
Subseptate uterus	Depends on extent of septum (partial or complete). Undivided and widened fundus, convex or flat in contour[18,34]. Two endometrial echoes might be seen until fusion of endometrium (see Fig. 5-8).	Thick septum might be seen in early pregnancy. Sac might extend across septum (see Fig. 12-31) Differentials include large ovarian cyst, degenerated cystic fibroid, ectopic gestation

* After 22 weeks' gestation, most anomalies cannot be visualized.

amined before this juncture. It is important for the physician to know whether an anomaly exists, because uterine anomalies tend to be associated with unusual fetal presentation, premature delivery, low birth weights, and complicated delivery, often requiring cesarean section.[19]

Pregnancy can occur in one or both duplicated uteri and in arcuate (see Fig. 5-1A), unicornuate, and septate uteri; therefore, the sonographic appearance varies with the individual anomaly and pregnancy. Pregnant women with a second uterine corpus not connected to the vagina may present with a pelvic mass representing the nonpregnant uterus that is enlarged in response to hormonal stimulation or that is filled with blood or mucus. Early in pregnancy the gravid uterus is located off midline, and the nongravid uterus often demonstrates a decidual reaction and enlargement (Figs. 5-11 and 5-12). The decidual reaction may look

like a gestational sac but has neither an embryo nor the double sac sign of a true pregnancy on either initial or follow-up examinations. Transvaginal scanning can clearly differentiate between a true gestation and the endometrial reaction.

The septum in a septate uterus can be seen when it is surrounded by amniotic fluid. A subseptate uterus can also be imaged and the septum appears as a broad uterine linear echogenicity. The septum often causes the fetus to lie in an abnormal position.

Potential Pitfalls

Sonographic findings of pregnancy can simulate one of the many variations of uterine anomalies. A gestational sac in a fallopian tube may look like a pregnancy in a uterine horn. A cornual uterine fibroid may look like a nonpregnant horn (see Fig. 5-10). The decidual reaction in the nonpregnant

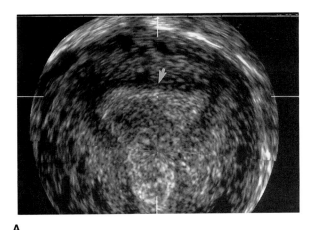

A

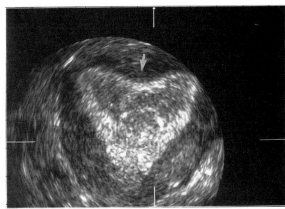

B

Figure 5-5. Planar reformatted sections producing 3D images of uteri. (**A**) Normal uterus with a convex fundus and endometrial cavity (arrow). (**B**) Arcuate uterus with a concave endometrial cavity (arrow). (**C**) Subseptate uterus with a septum (arrow) separating half of the uterine cavity. (Courtesy of Davor Jurkovic, MRCOG, PhD, King's College School of Medicine and Dentistry, London, England. Jurkovic D, Geipel A, Gruboeck K, Jauniaux E, Natucci M, Campbell S. Three-dimensional ultrasound for the assessment of uterine anatomy and detection of congenital anomalies: A comparison with hysterosalphingography and two-dimensional sonography. Ultrasound in Obstetrics and Gynecology. 1995; 5:233–237.)

C

uterus may suggest a twin gestation. Being alert to the patient's symptoms and the sonographic characteristics of each entity helps to differentiate among these.[3]

Treatment

Modern surgical techniques and more potent antibiotics have allowed improvements in treatment, surgery, and reconstruction of the anomalous gynecologic tract.[14]

Metroplasty, the joining of two uteri by excising the adjacent walls and connecting the fundi, can be performed to try to improve pregnancy potential. Septa are removed hysteroscopically to create one uterine cavity.[38] The success of this procedure has been judged by the fetal survival rate. Fedele and colleagues re-

ported a slight improvement in pregnancy outcome, whereas Ayhan and coworkers reported that fetal survival rates improved from 0% to 31% to 50% to 90% after metroplasty.[3,19] Vaginal surgery may range from simple hymenectomy to removal of septa to significant construction and reconstruction.

Other Imaging Modalities

Until the advent of magnetic resonance imaging, hysterosalpingography was the standard diagnostic modality for identifying congenital anomalies of the gynecologic tract. It is limited in that it delineates the morphology only of the internal uterine cavity. This limits its ability to differentiate between a separation of the endometrium due to a septum from

(Text continues on page 92)

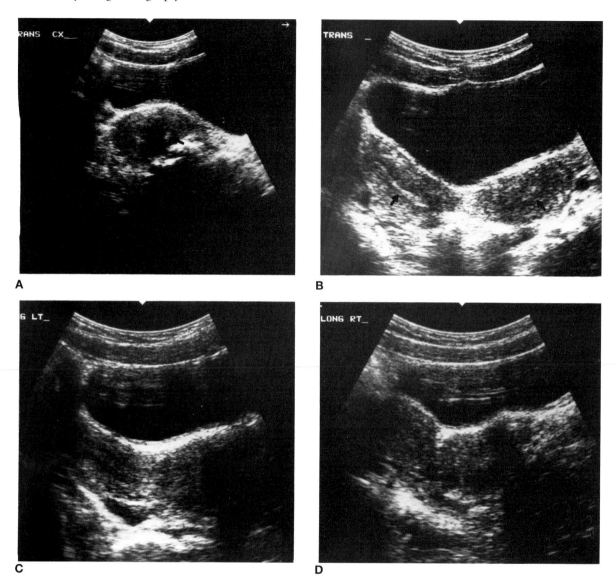

Figure 5-6. (**A**) Transverse scan through the cervix of a patient with uterus didelphys. Two separate endocervical echoes (*arrows*). (**B**) Transverse scan through a more superior section of the uterus demonstrates separate uterine bodies with their endometrial canal echoes (*arrows*). (**C,D**) Sagittal scans through the left (**C**) and right (**D**) uteri. With anomalous uteri, it may be difficult to outline clearly each individual uterus. (Courtesy Birgit Bader-Armstrong, University of Rochester Medical Center, Rochester, NY.)

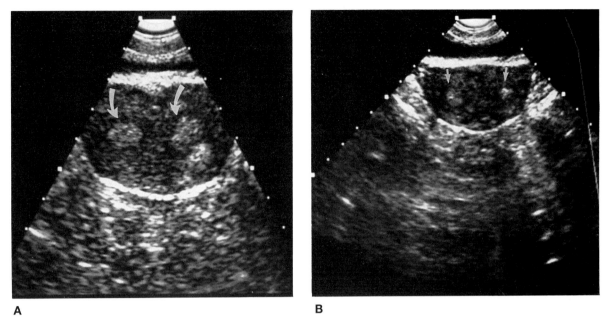

A   **B**

Figure 5-7. (**A**) Transvaginal coronal view of uterine fundus didelphys showing two endometrial echoes (*curved arrows*). (**B**) More caudad coronal transvaginal view of uterus at level of cervix again shows two groups of echoes (*arrows*) continuous with the duplicated endometria. (Mendelson EB, Bohm-Velez M, Neiman HL, Russo J. Transvaginal sonography in gynecologic imaging. Ultrasound CR MR. 1988; 9:102–121.)

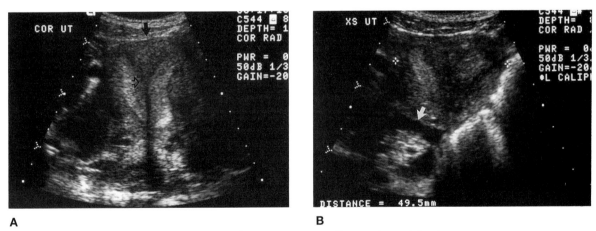

A   **B**

Figure 5-8. (**A**) Transvaginal coronal view of a septate uterus. Two endometrial echoes are separated by a hypoechoic septation (*open arrow*). Note the smooth, intact fundal contour (*black arrow*) characteristic of this anomaly. (**B**) Transvaginal axial view of the same uterus. Note the presence of a benign cystic teratoma in the right adnexal region (*white arrow*). (Courtesy Catherine Carr-Hoefer, Corvallis Radiology, Corvallis, OR).

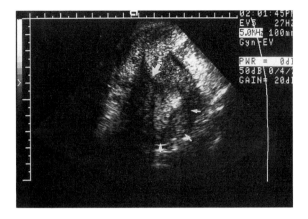

Figure 5-9. T-shaped uterus in a patient exposed to DES in utero. Uterus is retroverted and demonstrates a very thin endometrial cavity echo (*large arrow*), which expands at the cornua to form the characteristic T shape. Small arrows point to retroverted fundus. (Courtesy Jane Streltzoff, BS, RDMS, New York Hospital, New York, NY.)

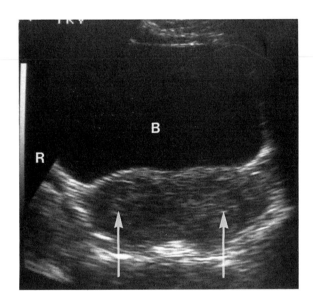

Figure 5-10. Transverse sonogram of a young woman with a history of several first-trimester miscarriages who was thought to have a bicornuate uterus. Uterus has a symmetric bilobed appearance. Echoes from two apparent canals (*arrows*) are seen, although entire right side is slightly more hypoechoic. Hysterosalpingography revealed a normal central cavity and outlined a mass consistent with a fibroid on the right side (R), confirmed on a follow-up sonogram. (B, bladder) (Baltarowich OH, Kurtz AB, Pennell RG, et al. Pitfalls in the sonographic diagnosis of uterine fibroids. Am J Roentgenol. 1988; 151:725–728.)

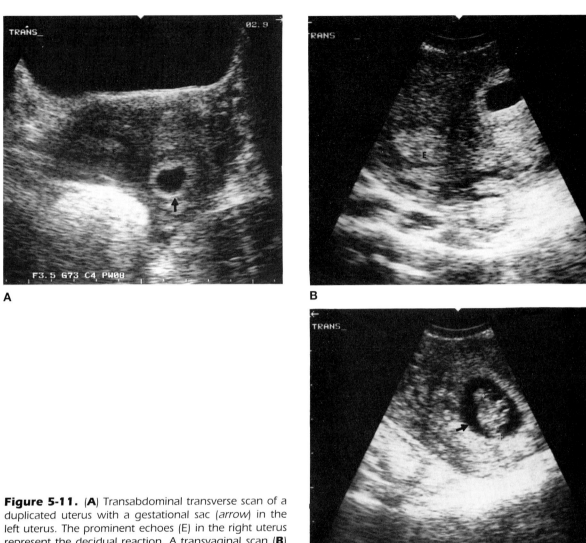

Figure 5-11. (**A**) Transabdominal transverse scan of a duplicated uterus with a gestational sac (*arrow*) in the left uterus. The prominent echoes (E) in the right uterus represent the decidual reaction. A transvaginal scan (**B**) more clearly defines the decidual reaction (E) in the right uterus and (**C**) the embryo (*arrow*) in the left uterus. (Courtesy Birgit Bader-Armstrong, University of Rochester Medical Center, Rochester, NY.)

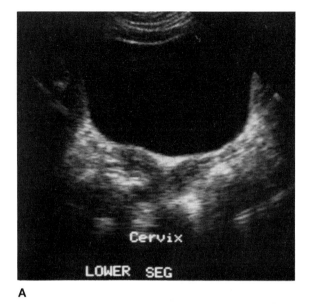

A

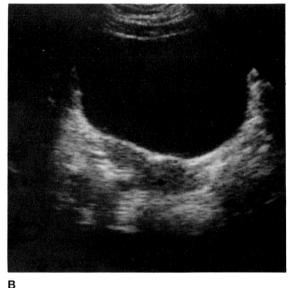

B

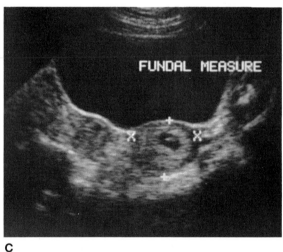

C

Figure 5-12. Example of clearly separated fundi in a pregnant patient with uterus didelphys. (**A**) Sonogram through the cervices, which are joined. (**B**) More cephalad section through the uterine bodies demonstrates that they are still joined, but the left (pregnant) uterus (*arrow*) is enlarged. (**C**) A sonogram through the fundal area shows two separate fundi with a gestational sac in the uterus. (Courtesy Ultrasound Lab, Raritan Bay Medical Center, Raritan, NJ.)

separation due to separate uterine walls, as in bicornuate or didelphic uteri.

Laparoscopy does permit observation of the external structure of the uterus, but it is an invasive, costly surgical procedure.

Magnetic resonance imaging has been shown to be highly sensitive and specific in identifying congenital anomalies and particularly in distinguishing between septated and bicornuate uteri by characterizing the dividing tissue as being fibrous, representing a septum, or muscular, representing the myometrial medial walls of the bicornuate uteri. When proper

techniques are used, ultrasound has shown almost comparable accuracy in identifying anomalies. With sonohysterography and three-dimensional techniques, ultrasound is becoming increasingly reliable. If the cost of ultrasound remains low, and its diagnostic accuracy improves, it will continue to gain acceptance as the diagnostic modality of choice in identifying causes of infertility and pregnancy wastage. It certainly remains the first examination to be used to evaluate the gynecologic tract.[26,28,34] With a good knowledge of the characteristics of congenital anomalies and the use of transvaginal scanning, the sonographer's ability to identify these developmental variations should improve dramatically.

REFERENCES

1. Akhtar AZ. Congenital abnormalities of genital tract-uterine malformation. J Pak Med Assoc. 1986; 36:261–266.
2. Alper MM, Garner PR, Spence JEH. Coexistence of gonadal dysgenesis and uterine aplasia. J Reprod Med. 1985; 30:232–234.
3. Ayhan A, Yucel I, Tuncer ZS, Kisnisci HA. Reproductive performance after conventional metroplasty: an evaluation of 102 cases. Fertil Steril. 1992; 57:1194–1196.
4. Balen FG, Allen CM, Lees WR. Ultrasound contrast agents. Clin Radiol. 1994; 49:77–82.
5. Baltarowich OH, Kurtz AB, Pennell RG, et al. Pitfalls in the sonographic diagnosis of uterine fibroids. Am J Roentgenol. 1988; 151:725–728.
6. Barach B, Falces E, Benzian SR. Magnetic resonance imaging for diagnosis and preoperative planning in agenesis of the distal vagina. Ann Plast Surg. 1987; 19:192–194.
7. Baramki TA. Treatment of congenital anomalies in girls and women. J Reprod Med. 1984; 29:376–384.
8. Berman L, Stringer DA, St Onge O, et al. Case report: Unilateral haematocolpos in uterine duplication associated with renal agenesis. Clin Radiol. 1987; 38:545–547.
9. Bowie JD. Sonography of the uterus. In: Sabbagha RE, ed. Diagnostic Ultrasound. Philadelphia: JB Lippincott; 1987.
10. Buttram VC. Mullerian anomalies and their management. Fertil Steril. 1983; 40:159–163.
11. Buttram VC, Gibbons WE. Müllerian anomalies: A proposed classification (an analysis of 144 cases). Fertil Steril. 1979; 32:40–46.
12. Cohen HL, Bober SE, Bow SN. Imaging the pediatric pelvis: The normal and abnormal genital tract and simulators of its diseases. Urologic Radiology. 1992; 14:273–283.
13. Cohen RC, Davey RB, LeQuesne GW. Ultrasonography in the diagnosis and management of unilateral hematometracolpos and associated renal agenesis. Australian Paediatric Journal. 1982; 18:287–290.
14. Cukier J, Batzofin JH, Conner JS, et al. Genital tract reconstruction in a patient with congenital absence of the vagina and hypoplasia of the cervix. Obstet Gynecol. 1986; 68:32S–36S.
15. Cullinan JA, Fleischer AC, Kepple DM, Arnold AL. Sonohysterography: A technique for endometrial evaluation. Radiographics. 1995; 15:501–514.
16. Dabirashrafi H, Mohammad K, Moghadami-Tabrizi N. Ovarian malposition in women with uterine anomalies. Obstet Gynecol. 1994; 83:293–294.
17. Durfee RB. Congenital anomalies in female genital tract. In: Benson R, ed. Current Obstetrics and Gynecology: Diagnosis and Treatment. 2nd ed. Los Altos, CA: Lange; 1978:147–156.
18. Fedele L, Dorta M, Brioschi D, et al. Pregnancies in septate uteri: Outcome in relation to site of uterine implantation as determined by sonography. Am J Roentgenol. 1989; 52:781–784.
19. Fedele L, Zamberletti D, d'Alberton A, et al. Gestational aspects of uterus didelphys. J Reprod Med. 1988; 33:353–355.
20. Ferrazzi E, Fedele L, Dorta M, Candiani GB. Uterine malformations. In Chervenak FA, Isaacson GC, Campbell S, eds. Ultrasound in Obstetrics and Gynecology. Vol. 1. Boston: Little, Brown & Co. 1993:1655–1663.
21. Fliegner JRH. Uncommon problems of the double uterus. Med J Aust. 1986; 145:510–512.
22. Hacker NF, Moore JG. Essentials of Obstetrics and Gynecology. Philadelphia: WB Saunders; 1986.
23. Hansmann M, Hackeloer B-J, Staudach A. Ultrasound Diagnosis in Obstetrics and Gynecology. Berlin: Springer-Verlag; 1985.
24. Hochner-Celnikier D, Hurwitz A, Beller U, et al. Ultrasound diagnosis in the case of an adnexal mass as a presenting symptom in early pregnancy. Eur J Obstet Gynecol Reprod Biol. 1984; 16:339–342.
25. Johnson J, Hillman BJ. Uterine duplication, unilateral imperforate vagina and normal kidneys. Am J Roentgenol. 1986; 147:1197–1198.
26. Jurkovic D, Geipel A, Gruboeck K, Jauniaux E, Natucci M, Campbell S. Three-dimensional ultrasound for the assessment of uterine anatomy and detection of congenital anomalies: A comparison with hysterosalpingography and two-dimensional sonography. Ultrasound in Obstetrics and Gynecology. 1995; 5:233–237.
27. Langman J. Medical Embryology. 4th ed. Baltimore: Williams & Wilkins; 1981.
28. Letterie GS, Haggerty M, Lindee G. A comparison of pelvic ultrasound and magnetic resonance imaging as diagnostic studies for mullerien tract abnormalities. Int J Fertil. 1995; 40:34–38.
29. Malini S, Valdes C, Malinak R. Sonographic diagnosis and classification of anomalies of the female genital tract. J Ultrasound Med. 1984; 3:397–404.
30. Mendelson EB, Bohm-Velez M, Neiman HL, et al. Transvaginal sonography in gynecologic im-

aging. Semin Ultrasound CT MR. 1988; 9:102–121.

31. Miyazaki Y, Ebisuno S, Uekado Y, et al. Uterus didelphys with unilateral imperforate vagina and ipsilateral renal agenesis. J Urol. 1986; 135:107–109.

32. Novak ER, Jones GS, Jones HW. Novak's Textbook of Gynecology. 8th ed. Baltimore: Williams & Wilkins; 1970:131–140.

33. Patton PE. Anatomic uterine defects. Clin Obstet Gynecol. 1994; 37:705–721.

34. Pellerito JS, McCarthy SM, Doyle MB, Glickman MG, DeCherney AH. Diagnosis of uterine anomalies: Relative accuracy of MR imaging, endovaginal sonography, and hysterosalpingography. Radiology 1992; 183:795–800.

35. Pennes DR, Bowerman RA, Silver TM. Congenital uterine anomalies and associated pregnancies. J Ultrasound Med. 1985; 4:531–538.

36. Ramsey D. Embryology and developmental defects of the female reproductive tract. In: Danforth DN, Scott JR, eds. Obstetrics and Gynecology. 5th ed. Philadelphia: JB Lippincott; 1986:106–119.

37. Reuter KL, Daly DC, Cohen SM. Septate versus bicornuate uteri: Errors in imaging diagnosis. Radiology 1989; 172:749–752.

38. Rock JA, Zacur HA. The clinical management of repeated early pregnancy wastage. Fertil Steril. 1983; 39:123–140.

39. Rosenberg HK, Sherman NH, Tarry WF, Duckett JW, Snyder HM. Mayer-Rokitansky-Kuster-Hauser syndrome: US aid to diagnosis. Radiology 1986; 161:815–819.

40. Rulin MC, Yoder DA, Hayashi TT. Congenital atresia of the lower vagina with regular menses through a fistula: A therapeutic approach. Obstet Gynecol. 1985; 65:88S–90S.

41. Sheth SS. Broad uterine fundus: A sign to suspect intrauterine septum. Int J Gynaecol Obstet. 1993; 40:65–66.

42. Sharp H. Reproductive tract disorders. In: Danforth DN, Scott JR, eds. Obstetrics and Gynecology. 5th ed. Philadelphia: JB Lippincott; 1986: 561–568.

43. Stassart JP, Nagel TC, Prem KA, Phipps WR. Uterus didelphys, obstructed hemivagina, and ipsilateral renal agenesis: The University of Minnesota experience. Fertil Steril. 1992; 57:756–761.

44. Tuchman-Duplessis H, Haegel P. Organogenesis. Illustrated Human Embryology. Vol. 2. New York: Springer-Verlag; 1972:88–99.

45. Valle RF, Sciarra JJ. Hysteroscopic treatment of the septate uterus. Obstet Gynecol. 1986; 67(2):253–257.

Pediatric Gynecologic Ultrasound

MARY BETH GEAGAN, JACK O. HALLER, and HARRIS L. COHEN

Major indications for gynecologic ultrasound examination of young girls include vaginal bleeding or discharge, ambiguous genitalia, and abdominal mass. Although pregnancy is often found to be the cause of an abdominal mass in older adolescents, because this chapter deals with premenarchal patients, pregnancy is not discussed here.

Because internal pelvic examination of young girls is not generally desirable or possible, ultrasound assumes a role of great importance as a relatively simple and painless method of viewing the internal anatomy. Transvaginal ultrasound, helpful in the older patient, is not used in the virginal patient or child.[4,8,17,58] Transperineal imaging has occasionally proven useful by providing imaging close to the uterus without transducer insertion.[50] Ultrasonography has opened new horizons in the field of pediatric gynecologic imaging. Much information about the nature and extent of the abnormality can be collected with little trauma to the child. More invasive procedures, such as examination under anesthesia, diagnostic laparoscopy, or exploratory laparotomy, may be avoided or postponed.

In recent years, spectral, color flow, and duplex Doppler have added to our ability to examine the child sonographically.

Anatomy and Physiology

The uterus is approximately 3.5 cm long for the first 6 to 8 weeks of life and, owing to maternal hormonal stimulation, it has the adult configuration. After the immediate postnatal period, the uterus gradually decreases in length to 2.5 cm and regresses to premenarchal shape, in which the cervix predominates (Fig. 6-1). The ratio of cervix to corpus length in premenarchal girls is 2:1.[32] Hansmann and coworkers report the prepubertal length to be 1.5 to 3 cm and the corpus width, 0.5 to 1 cm; the cervix width is 1.5 to 3 cm.[33] The size of the uterus increases gradually between 3 to 8 years of age. At this point, it begins to increase in size, with a proportionally greater increase in the corpus than in the cervix.[49] The mean total uterine length increases from 2.5 cm at 7 years, to 3.5 cm at 10 years, to 6.2 cm at 13 years of age (Fig. 6-2).[33]

At birth, the ovaries usually have descended to their normal position in the pelvis. As in adults, the adnexae may be found in the posterior cul-de-sac, at the lateral pelvic wall, or, rarely, above the pelvic brim. Identifying the iliac vessels and pelvic musculature may aid in locating the ovaries. The ovaries' shape may vary, but usually they are elongated and symmetric, as in adults. The pediatric ovary measures 15 mm long, 2.5 mm thick, and 3 mm wide and grows gradually until the onset of puberty, when it has adult proportions—24 to 41 mm long, 8.5 to 19.4 mm thick, and 15 to 24 mm wide.[30] Ovarian mean volumes increase from 1 cm^3 in the first year of life to the reported adult value of 9.8 cm^3.[16] Studies by Cohen and colleagues[14-16] have shown that mean ovarian volumes in patients younger than 2

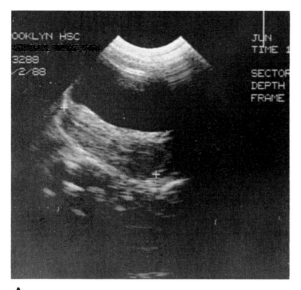
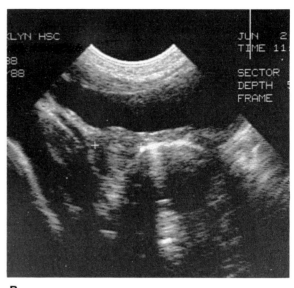

A   B

Figure 6-1. Normal infantile uterus. A 5-day-old infant had vaginal bleeding; no hematocolpos was found. Enlargement is caused by maternal hormonal situation. (**A**) Sagittal scan through the uterus. (**B**) Transverse scan through uterine fundus.

years of age are slightly greater than 1.00 cm³ for the first year of life, and may be as high as 3.6 cm³ in girls 1 day to 3 months of age, and as great as 2.7 cm³ in girls 4 to 12 months of age. In the second year of life, the mean volume was 0.67 cm³, with values as great as 1.7 cm³. It appears that values that may previously have been worrisome fall within the 95% confidence interval of normal.

A cyst in a child's ovary is usually no cause for concern. Many follicles in all stages of development are present constantly in girls' ovaries, and a greater portion of these follicles are in earlier stages of development than those in women.[31]

Usually, follicular regression in fetal or postnatal life begins before the follicle attains any appreciable size, but follicles can measure several millimeters. These may occur at any time before menarche, and they differ from true follicles in that they contain no ova.[32] Although the work of Salardi and colleagues[49] and Orsini and associates[46] suggested that cysts were uncommon in patients younger than 6 years of age and that macrocysts (cysts >9 mm) were uncommon in patients younger than 11 years of age, Cohen and colleagues have shown cysts in 68% of the adequately visualized ovaries of 101 children 2 to 12 years of age.[14] In addition, cysts, in-

cluding macrocysts, were noted in 84% of 98 patients 1 day to 24 months of age,[15] which disputes the findings of Stanhope and colleagues, who found that a maximum follicular diameter of 7 mm was normal in early childhood.[60]

The presence of these multiple cysts leads to a more typically heterogeneous, rather than homogeneous, sonographic appearance of the ovary in the normal child (Fig. 6-3).

Vascularization increases slowly in infants and young children to approximately the adult level by age 6 or 8 years, at which time the medullary zone of the ovary becomes identifiable histologically. By age 11 or 12 years, primordial follicles are seen in the cortical zone. Under normal conditions, these primordial follicles regress as follicles containing ova develop.[30]

Sonographic Examination Technique and Protocols

Before beginning a sonographic examination of a pediatric patient, it is wise to spend a few minutes explaining "the test" and the equipment, at least to older girls. The explanation and demonstration should be tailored to the age of the patient. For

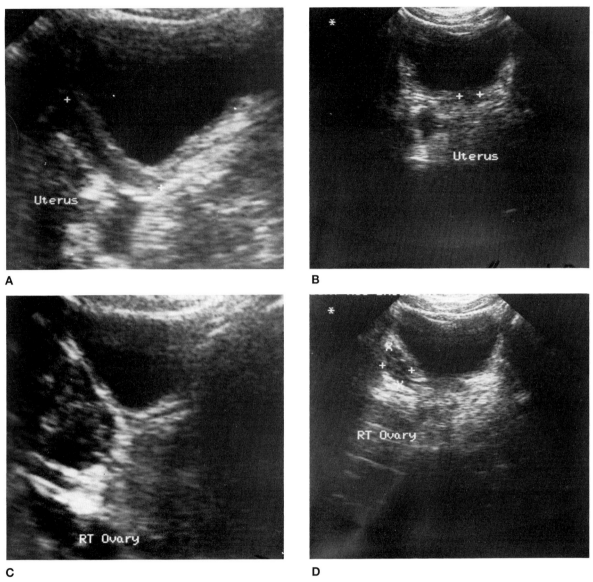

Figure 6-2. Normal prepubertal uterus and ovaries of 10-year-old. Sagittal (**A**) and transverse (**B**) scans of uterus. (**C,D**) Sagittal and transverse scans of ovary.

example, the child should be allowed to touch the transducer, feel the "jelly," and locate the "TV" where she will "see her belly." Allowing one or both parents to stay with the child during the examination may reduce the anxiety level of all concerned. A bottle, pacifier, and a key ring for an infant and perhaps a favorite toy for an older child may also alleviate the patient's anxiety. Nursery rhymes, songs, and riddles can also be used to dis-

tract the child's attention from "the test." Often a child will cry at the start of the examination despite the examiner's explanations and endeavors; invariably she will stop once she realizes the examination is not painful and that her parents are not going to leave her. At the termination of the ultrasound procedure, the examiner might give the patient a "happy face" or some similar sticker as a reward.

As for adults, pelvic sonography of a pediatric

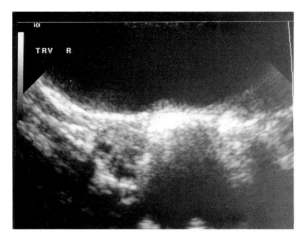

Figure 6-3. *Normal ovary in an 18-month-old girl. Transverse image shows a 1.3 cm right ovary with several small cysts up to 6 mm.*

patient requires a full urinary bladder. The older child should drink 24 ounces of noncarbonated fluid 45 minutes to 1 hour before the study and can usually maintain a full bladder for the time required to complete the examination. A bottle 30 minutes before the study may provide adequate bladder filling in a patient who is not toilet trained, but catheterization may be necessary to ensure proper filling for optimal pelvic evaluation. An 8-French feeding tube is usually an adequate catheter substitute for an infant; age and size determine the catheter of choice for older children. Sedation is rarely necessary, but it may be indicated when repeated attempts fail to calm the child enough to permit a diagnostically adequate examination. Speed and accuracy are of prime importance in scanning pediatric patients because bladder control is limited and the patient, especially a very young child, may void at any time.

The scanning planes used and the images obtained are the same as for adults. Considerable patience and fortitude may be required to obtain these views, however, if the child presents a squirming, moving target. The cineloop feature of today's newer equipment allows the recall of images and makes the sonographer's job somewhat easier in this respect. Transducer frequency usually ranges from 5 to 7.5 MHz; the higher-frequency transducer is preferred for younger children. The prepubertal uterus and ovaries are usually small in com-

parison to the filled urinary bladder. Therefore, the gain must be set low enough to allow these structures to be distinguished from surrounding muscle and bowel.

Transperineal imaging may be helpful, particularly for evaluating cases of suspected vaginal or uterine obstruction.

Schaarschmidt and Willital have described the use of high-frequency, small-diameter radial endoscopic scanners for intraanal scanning in children. Excellent detail, particularly of retrorectal structures, has been reported. In their series of 200 children, the technique was also helpful in evaluating pelvic floor structures and the sphincter mechanism in cases of incontinence.[51]

The "water enema" technique is occasionally used in children. Fluid, instilled by means of a syringe through a Foley catheter in the rectum, can be followed to differentiate between a true mass anterior to the colon and posterior to the uterus, and a pseudomass formed by air and stool within the bowel.[3,12,13]

As in adults, if an abnormality is found in the pelvis, the appropriate upper abdominal organs should be examined to preclude related findings, such as hydronephrosis or metastatic lesions in the lymph nodes or liver.

Pathology

Genital tumors are quite rare in children and young adolescents, but approximately 50% of those found are malignant or potentially malignant.[4] Almost every tumor that occurs in an adult has also been described in a child.[25] Here, we emphasize the more common pathologic lesions of children, which are grouped into benign and malignant categories.

VAGINA, UTERUS, AND FALLOPIAN TUBES

Primary tumors are rare in children. Malignant tumors are more common, and the vagina is involved more often than the uterus.[52] The most common reason for vaginal bleeding in the child is a foreign body, often toilet paper. Other causes are less common. The workup of vaginal bleeding may include measurement of blood estradiol levels, gonadotropin-releasing hormone stimulation test, pelvic sonography and possibly computed tomography (CT) or magnetic resonance imaging (MRI) to rule out adrenal or gonadal tumors, and a head CT to rule out central nervous system lesions,[4] particularly in the evaluation of precocious puberty.

Benign Lesions

Gartner's duct cysts and pelvic inflammatory disease occur most often. Gartner's duct cysts are the most common cystic lesions of the vagina. These benign mesonephric duct remnants are rare in children and are found as single or multiple lesions along the anteromedial aspect of the vaginal wall[19,36] (see Fig. 5-3). If large enough, a Gartner's duct cyst may block the vagina, simulating an imperforate hymen.[4,26]

It is possible for hydrosalpinx or pyosalpinx to occur, often in a sexually abused child. Inflammatory debris may be present, which together with the fusiform shape and thickened tubal walls, help differentiate this entity from an ovarian cyst. Tuboovarian abscess occurs when the infection extends to involve the ovary.[7]

Malignant Lesions

Sarcoma botryoides is the most common malignant vaginal and uterine lesion of young girls. It is a polypoid form of embryonal rhabdomyosarcoma, which usually originates in the vagina and spreads to the uterus, although the reverse may occur. The mass is soft and may fill the entire abdomen without being palpable. Symptoms include a bloody vaginal discharge and a grape-like mass in the vagina or protruding from it.[4,23,24,29,52]

On sonography, a large, poorly circumscribed mass with a mixed echogenic pattern and areas of cystic degeneration is usually demonstrated. Invasion of the bladder and surrounding pelvic structures often makes it impossible to determine the organ of origin.[29] Radiation and chemotherapy are used to shrink the mass to a size suitable for conservative excision. Ultrasound, MRI, and CT may be used for serial follow-up examinations.

Primary adenocarcinoma of the uterus and vagina has been reported, some in daughters of mothers exposed to diethylstilbestrol (DES). Approximately one third occur in children younger than 1 year of age. Almost all cases occur before age 11 years.[29] It presents with vaginal bleeding and a rap-

idly growing tumor not associated with sexual precocity. Sonography usually reveals a solid tumor with no distinguishing characteristics.

Endodermal sinus tumor, a soft, often cystic and highly malignant tumor of the vagina and cervix, usually occurs by age 3 years and simulates sarcoma botryoides clinically.[25]

OVARY

Aside from simple follicular cysts, ovarian cysts and tumors are infrequent in childhood, with an estimated incidence of 2.6 to 2.7 per 100,000 population.[44] The ovary is the most common site of tumors in the female genital tract in childhood, and in the premenarchal girl, one third of these are malignant.[4] Ovarian tumors often present with pain, abdominal swelling, or a palpable abdominal mass. Ultrasound is often useful in determining the organ of origin, narrowing the possible differential diagnoses, and directing further diagnostic work-up.

Benign Masses

Single or multiple cysts, usually nonneoplastic, account for more than 70% of ovarian masses and are the most common pelvic tumors of childhood and adolescence. These are usually follicular retention cysts, corpus luteum cysts, or hemorrhagic cysts. Hormone secretion by the lining cells of some cysts may lead to precocious puberty. Fetal ovarian cysts have been reported, which may cause dystocia if they are large. They are thought to be related to excessive stimulation of maternal placental chorionic gonadotropin.[45] In utero torsion may occur, leading to a mass in the fetal and neonatal abdomen on sonography (Fig. 6-4). Parovarian cysts, located in the mesosalpinx between the tube and ovary, are usually indistinguishable from simple ovarian cysts.[30] With the exception of hemorrhagic cysts, which may contain internal debris, these masses are usually purely cystic and often asymptomatic. Polycystic ovaries may have a sonographic appearance identical to that of multiple primordial follicles. The cysts may be too small to distinguish and simply appear as enlarged ovaries. All of these masses are subject to torsion when they attain sufficient size.[52]

The management of neonatal ovarian cysts has evolved. Because many cysts regress in the first few months of life once high newborn gonadotropin

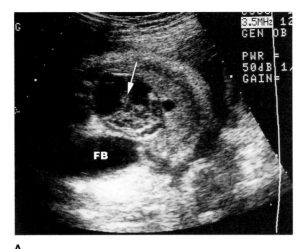
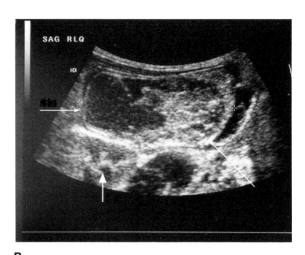

A   **B**

Figure 6-4. In utero ovarian torsion. (**A**) Transverse scan through the lower fetal abdomen at 37.5 weeks of gestation shows a complex mass to the right of the fetal bladder with a "beak" at its inferomedial aspect. (FB, fetal bladder; arrow points to mass). (**B**) Sagittal scan through the right lower quadrant of the infant on the day of delivery. A 4.2-cm complex mass representing the torsed, necrotic ovary is seen anteroinferior to the lower pole of the kidney (*small arrows,* mass; *large arrow,* kidney).

levels decrease, conservative management with serial ultrasound monitoring has replaced routine excision of the cyst or oophorectomy for simple cysts.[20,65]

Some continue to advocate removal for those cysts larger than 5 cm, hemorrhagic cysts that may be caused by torsion or infarction, and even small cysts if they persist longer than 4 months, enlarge, or become symptomatic.[1,65] It is thought that surgery may avoid the potential morbidity of ovarian autoamputation due to torsion, peritonitis caused by cyst rupture, or intestinal obstruction due to cyst size. The presence of ascites in association with a neonatal ovarian cyst raises the possibility of a potentially lethal cyst rupture, or peritonitis from cyst torsion with infarction, or bowel obstruction.[45]

The use of color Doppler ultrasound does not increase specificity in the diagnosis of cystic ovarian lesions in the child. Its principal role is to demonstrate the presence of flow, which may be of help in excluding the diagnosis of torsion. A cyst should demonstrate flow in the adjacent parenchyma and absence of central flow within the cyst itself, whether cystic or hemorrhagic.[47]

The benign cystic teratoma (BCT, dermoid cyst)

is the most common tumor during the reproductive years, but it is relatively uncommon before puberty. It occurs more often on the right side and often presents with abdominal pain secondary to torsion, which may easily be confused with appendicitis.[7] In children, the mass is predominantly cystic, with small foci of fat, hair, and calcification, the latter being less than in adults.[25] Sisler and Siegel found that ovarian teratomas in prepubertal girls contained sonographically visible mural nodules in only 38%, and exhibited posterior acoustic shadowing in only 13% of patients, compared with a 70% incidence of mural nodules and shadowing in postpubertal girls.[59] This is probably a result of the known evolution of the contents of ovarian teratomas over time. The appearance of a cyst-within-a-cyst has been described by Haller and colleagues. Fifteen to 20% of BCTs are reported to be bilateral.[30]

There have been reports of serous and mucinous cystadenomas in prepubertal girls. These tumors of epithelial origin are almost exclusively unilateral in children, and although rare, they are more common than their malignant counterparts.[25] The diagnosis can be suspected by demonstrating septa, a frequent finding in these masses. Ovarian fibroma, which may be associated with Meigs' syndrome, is a rare benign solid connective tissue tumor occasionally found in children. It also is subject to torsion.[22,42]

Malignant Masses

As a group, germ cell tumors are the most common malignant tumors involving the pediatric genital tract. Dysgerminoma is the most common pediatric ovarian mass and is thought to be the counterpart of the testicular seminoma. Fortunately, this tumor has low-grade malignancy and is very radiosensitive, so it is potentially curable. The sonogram usually demonstrates a solid mass ranging in size from a small nodule to one of pelvoabdominal proportions. The mass may be multilobulated with areas of hemorrhagic necrosis and fibrovascular septa.[37] Ascites, retroperitoneal adenopathy, and hepatic metastases may be seen in advanced cases.[30]

Kim and Kang describe three cases, including a 7-year-old girl, in which color Doppler ultrasound demonstrated prominent arterial flow within the fibrovascular septa of dysgerminoma. The RI (0.44 to 0.70, mean 0.59) and PI (0.60 to 1.32, mean 0.98) differed from the reported normal values of resistance index (RI) less than 0.4 and pulsatility index (PI) less than 1.0 for spectral Doppler determination of malignant versus benign lesions. The septa were hypointense or isointense on T2-weighted images and showed marked enhancement on both contrast-enhanced CT and contrast enhanced T1-weighted MRI, a finding also described by Tanaka and coworkers.[37,62]

Dysgerminoma is bilateral in 10% to 15% of cases and may contain foci of calcification. Levels of human chorionic gonadotropin (HCG), lactic dehydrogenase (LDH), and α_1-fetoprotein (AFP) may all be elevated.[25] The image is nonspecific and the differential diagnosis requires appropriate clinical and laboratory correlation. Ovarian torsion and appendiceal abscess have a similar sonographic appearance and must be ruled out.

Treatment is somewhat controversial. When the tumor is localized to one ovary, some advocate unilateral oophorectomy, with or without postoperative radiation; others recommend total abdominal hysterectomy with postoperative radiation. The more aggressive surgery is always indicated if the tumor is bilateral or locally extensive or if ascites or adenopathy is present.[49]

The other germ cell tumors are endodermal sinus tumor, malignant teratoma, primary choriocarcinoma of the ovary, and embryonal carcinoma. Endodermal sinus tumor, the second most common of the germ cell tumors, grows rapidly and is unilateral.[25] Malignant teratoma may be indistinguishable from BCT, but usually contains more solid components. The peak incidence is at age 3 years, and 60% of teratomas show calcification on radiographic examination.[40] Embryonal carcinoma is highly malignant, unilateral, and may lead to precocious puberty. Nongestational choriocarcinoma, although rarer, likewise may lead to precocious puberty.[25] The appearance of these tumors ranges from almost purely cystic to purely solid and highly echogenic. Cul-de-sac fluid is found in 50% of these patients. Nodal metastases, abdominal ascites, and liver metastases are not uncommon.[52]

Tumors of gonadal (sex cord) origin such as the granulosa-theca cell and arrhenoblastoma (Sertoli-Leydig cell) are usually less malignant and exert hormonal influences. Granulosa-theca cell tumors are feminizing tumors that lead to precocious puberty. Approximately 5% occur prepubertally, and less than 5% are bilateral. They are prone to late recurrence, which requires lifelong postoperative follow-up of the patient. Arrhenoblastomas are masculinizing tumors. When they recur in children it is usually during the first 3 years after operation.[25]

Serous and mucinous cystadenocarcinomas are malignant tumors of epithelial origin. In children, they are even rarer than their benign counterparts. The serous type is twice as common as the mucinous type. These tumors are often multilocular with thick septa and solid elements.[25,40]

The ovary may be involved by tumor metastases. Neuroblastoma, rhabdomyosarcoma, Krukenberg's tumor, lymphoma, and leukemia have all been reported to involve the ovary.[21,28,30] The genital involvement of acute lymphocytic leukemia at autopsy is 11.5% to 80% in females. The sonographic appearance has been described as solid, hypoechoic ovarian masses. Gonadal involvement often coincides with marrow remission.[9] Tumor recurrence is likely if the sequestered tumor is not treated adequately.[24]

Genital Anomalies, Gonadal Dysgenesis, Ambiguous Genitalia

Congenital uterine anomalies are difficult to detect in infants and young children. Often the sonogram is obtained as a precaution in the presence of other anomalies such as absence of the vagina, imperforate anus, or urinary tract anomalies. Sonographic demonstration of a smaller than normal uterus or one with partial obstruction suggests a congenital anomaly of the uterus, whereas a uterus with a distended endometrial cavity and distended vagina suggests an anomaly of the vagina or an imperforate hymen. If there is dysgenesis involving the müllerian systems, the uterus or vagina may be absent, as in patients with Mayer-Rokitansky-Kuster-Hauser syndrome, who have normal karyotypes and develop normal secondary sexual characteristics but have coexistent renal (50%) and skeletal (12%) anomalies.[12,48] In DES-exposed infant girls, a T-shaped uterus (one that is relatively short and wide) has been described (see Fig. 5-9). Ultrasound may be of some use in identifying this anomaly,[24] although it is usually diagnosed after menarche. Vaginal anomalies are even more difficult to detect than uterine ones, and often it is possible to establish only that a vagina is indeed present. Occasionally, an increased anteroposterior vaginal diameter may suggest an abnormality when compared to a child of the same age. In the case of vaginal atresia, stenosis, or hypoplasia, sonography can provide useful information on the presence or absence of the upper one third of the vagina, the uterus, and the ovaries before corrective surgery.[29]

Ovarian agenesis is extremely rare and is thought to be an acquired condition secondary to torsion and necrosis in utero. Hypoplasia is often associated with endocrine disorders, intersex disorders, and gonadal dysgenesis.[29]

Gonadal dysgenesis is marked by rudimentary gonads. In the most familiar type, Turner's syndrome, the ovaries are deficient. They may reach varying stages of development, ranging from absent to infantile to adult. Turner's patients have a 45,XO karyotype (chromosome pattern). Anomalies include dwarfism, webbed neck, shield-shaped chest, infantile sexual development, and amenorrhea. The ovary has no primordial follicles and is often represented only as a fibrous streak.[60] Sonographic study

of these patients before the commencement of hormonal therapy rarely demonstrates the ovaries (volume less than 1 cm^3) and reveals a uterus with a prepubertal size and configuration, even in older adolescents. Ultrasound is useful to follow and document the changes in size and shape that occur in response to hormone therapy.[30]

In androgen insensitivity (testicular feminization) the karyotype is 46,XY and the patient often has uterine or vaginal defects, normal breast development, little or no pubic or axillary hair, and abdominal or inguinal testes. The testosterone level is close to normal, but the end organs are insensitive.[32] Patients with gonadal dysgenesis may have "streak" gonads. These resemble ovaries but contain no germ cells or follicular apparatus. The presence of a Y chromosome in such a child is cause for concern because the child's risk for development of a tumor such as a dysgerminoma or a gonadoblastoma is greater than 30%. Gonadectomy is recommended for these patients.[5,11]

Ambiguous genitalia is one of the main indications for sonography of neonates. Early diagnosis is important to avoid serious psychological disturbances. The presence of vaginal atresia, fused labia, clitorimegaly, or cryptorchidism should prompt an effort to define the internal anatomy with sonography and to locate a uterus, vagina, ovaries, or testes. Images of the adrenal glands and kidneys should be obtained to exclude congenital adrenal hyperplasia and renal anomalies.[32] The sonogram can easily be obtained while awaiting results of hormonal and chromosomal studies and may afford the parents some peace of mind.

Approximately 1 in 5000 babies is born with ambiguous genitalia.[39] Intersex occurs as an isolated entity in 1 birth in 1000 and is more common in association with other anomalies.[29] By defining the internal anatomy, ultrasound helps speed diagnosis and sex assignment of such infants.[29,52] A true hermaphrodite has both ovarian and testicular tissue. The structures may be joined, as an ovitestis, or separate ovaries and testes may be seen on each side of the pelvis. A uterus may or may not be present. A female pseudohermaphrodite is a chromosomal female (46,XX) with ovaries but with masculinized external genitalia, including an enlarged clitoris and prominent fused labia. This condition may be caused by congenital adrenal hyperplasia, in which case a uterus is always present, or by increased androgen production due to a virilizing maternal condition, in which case a uterus may not be present.

A male pseudohermaphrodite is a chromosomal male (46,XY) with feminized external genitalia due to decreased androgens, poor target organs, or an enzyme defect. Sonography is difficult and usually fails to locate undescended testicles unless they lie in the inguinal canal or high in the scrotum, but it can exclude the presence of a uterus and ovaries. These patients may have two testes or one testicle and one streak gonad. MRI may be of use in locating the undescended testicles, particularly in areas above the inguinal crease.

Precocious Puberty

True isosexual precocious puberty is idiopathic in most cases, secondary to activation of the hypothalamic–pituitary–gonadal axis. It can be defined as the onset of the normal physiologic and endocrine processes of puberty in girls before age 8 years. There is pubertal luteinizing hormone and follicle-stimulating hormone response to gonadotropin-releasing hormone (G_nRH), elevated levels of gonadal sex steroids, and advanced bone age.[2] It usually follows the developmental sequence seen in normal children, that is, breast development followed by pubic and axillary hair development, followed by the onset of menstruation. The ovaries reach postpubertal size and volume and the uterus assumes the adult configuration, with a corpus-to-cervix ratio of 1:1.[32] True precocious puberty may occasionally be related to a central nervous system lesion that affects the hypothalamus.[24] Isolated premature development of the breasts (thelarche) or pubic hair (adrenarche) is not considered true precocious puberty.

Pseudoprecocious or incomplete precocious puberty is independent of the action of pituitary gonadotropins and results from adrenal or ovarian dysfunction.[38] The accompanying clinical signs may be identical to those of the true type, although the menses are usually more irregular. Granulosa-theca cell tumors account for 60% of the cases with an ovarian cause.[52] Rarely, dysgerminoma, choriocarcinoma, arrhenoblastoma, follicular retention cysts, and autonomous function of an ovarian cyst have been demonstrated as the cause of pseudoprecocious puberty.[6] Adrenal causes include congenital hyperplasia, adenoma, and carci-

noma. Hypothyroidism has occasionally been reported as a cause of breast development but has not produced menses.[24,52]

McCune-Albright syndrome, characterized by fibrous dysplasia of bone associated with café-au-lait skin pigmentation and possible endocrine hyperfunction has also been associated with precocious puberty. These patients tend to have the largest ovarian cysts and the largest size discrepancy between the two ovaries.[53]

Before the development of ultrasound, surgical exploration was required to search for ovarian or adrenal masses in patients with precocious puberty. Sonography has virtually eliminated this. The size of the uterus and ovaries can be assessed accurately. Findings of a large uterus and symmetric ovarian enlargement lead to a diagnosis of pituitary axis stimulation (true precocious puberty; Fig. 6-5). Unilateral ovarian enlargement and a prepubertal-sized uterus suggest ovarian tumor; however, primordial cysts may be a normal cause of ovarian enlargement. In a study by King and colleagues that looked at ovarian cysts in patients with precocious puberty, the presence of small (<9 mm) cysts alone could not separate those patients with precocious puberty from normal girls. In their study, the best predictor of true precocious puberty was bilateral ovarian enlargement, whereas unilateral enlargement associated with macrocysts (>9 mm) was suggestive of pseudoprecocious puberty.[38] An infantile uterus and ovaries suggest premature thelarche or adrenarche rather than true precocious puberty (Fig. 6-6).[21] Therefore, careful study of the adrenal and hypothalamic regions must also be undertaken before precocious puberty can be attributed to an ovarian cyst.[30] Both areas are better studied by CT or MRI than by sonography.

When true precocious puberty is treated by hormone replacement therapy (luteinizing hormone-releasing factor analog therapy to decrease the pituitary response to G_nRH), sonography is part of the protocol, to monitor the size and volume changes of the uterus and ovaries.[27,57] G_nRH-a (G_nRH agonist) medications are aimed at suppression of the pituitary–gonadal axis and down regulation of pituitary gonadotropin secretion, leading to a return to hypogonadal status as soon as possible.[2,43] Serial sonograms document regression in response to therapy.

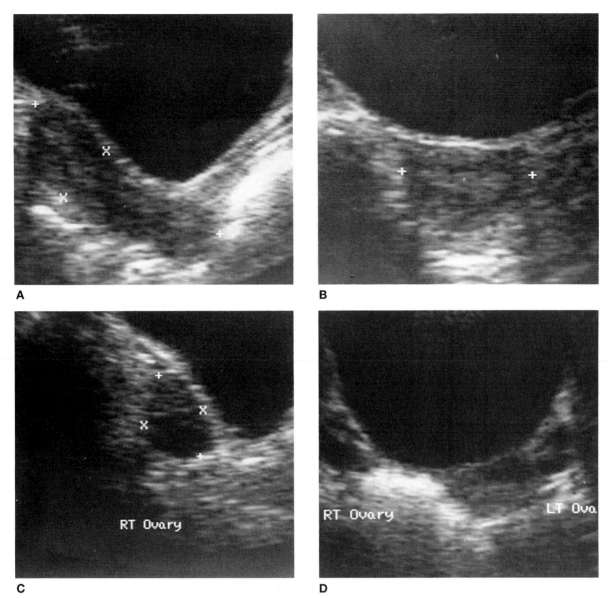

Figure 6-5. Precocious puberty. Note adult size and configuration of the uterus and ovaries of an 8-year-old girl with true precocious puberty. (**A**) Sagittal scan through uterus. (**B**) Transverse scan through uterine fundus. (**C**) On sagittal scan of right ovary, note follicles. (**D**) Transverse scan of ovaries and uterus.

In a study by Ambrosino and coworkers, ovarian volume was the most sensitive indicator of neuroaxis stimulation or suppression. A trend toward decreasing ovarian volume and uterine length was indicative of suppression despite the fact that the values may still be above normal threshold values. They found that although the presence of ovarian cysts alone is not a reliable indicator of stimulation, the absence of visible cysts is a good indicator of suppression.[2]

Hydrocolpos

Fluid or blood may accumulate in the vagina (hydrocolpos, hematocolpos), the uterus (hydrometra, hematometra), or both (hydrometrocolpos, hema-

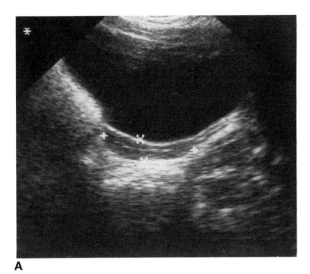
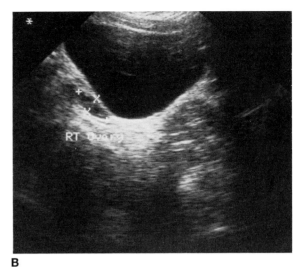

A   B

Figure 6-6. Premature thelarche. Normal prepubertal uterus and ovaries in a 7.5-year-old with precocious breast development (thelarche). (**A**) Sagittal scan through uterus. (**B**) Sagittal scan through right ovary; note small follicles.

tometrocolpos). The cause is most often related to imperforate hymen, vaginal septum, duplication anomaly with unilateral obstruction, or acquired obstructing lesion.[7,23,24,29,40,52] In addition, distention of the cervix with blood may also occur, usually secondary to atresia or stenosis, and may be associated with vaginal atresia.[55] Although these conditions often go undetected until menarche, they may present in a neonate as an abdominal mass or bulging hymen. Indeed, they account for 15% of abdominal masses in newborn girls; the incidence is slightly greater than that of ovarian cysts.[32] Maternal hormones prompt increased uterine secretions in newborns. This leads to distention of the uterus or vagina proximal to the point of obstruction (Fig. 6-7).

Sonography reveals a hypoechoic, transonic, pear-shaped mass in the midline arising from the pelvis between the bladder and rectum (Fig. 6-8). Because they both may present (see Fig. 5-2) with internal echoes resulting from cellular debris or blood, pyometria and hematometria may not be differentiated.[67] A normal uterus and vagina cannot be identified.[7,52] It is important for the urinary bladder to be distended to prove that this mass is not the bladder.

Scanlan and associates recommend transperineal sonography, placement of the transducer on the perineum (with or without a standoff pad), to visualize adequately the entire length of the vagina.

Sagittal and coronal scans allow visualization of low-lying obstruction and evaluation of the thickness of an obstructing vaginal septum, and may be helpful in planning vaginal reconstruction.[50]

Severe distention can lead to hydronephrosis

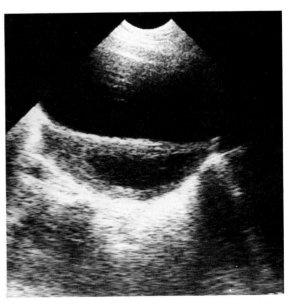

Figure 6-7. Hydrocolpos. Sagittal scan through an infant uterus. Note hypoechoic material distending the cervix and vagina.

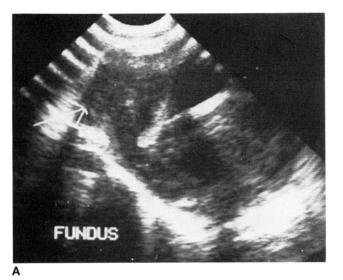

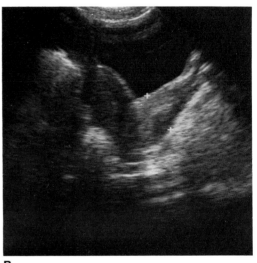

A   **B**

Figure 6-8. Hematometrocolpos. Abdominal mass in a 13-year-old. (**A**) Sagittal scan shows distended vagina and uterus; arrow indicates fundus. (**B**) Postoperative scan after surgery for vaginal web shows normal uterus.

and obstruction of the venous and lymphatic channels of the lower extremity.[54] If the condition presents in utero, urinary tract obstruction associated with fetal anuria, oligohydramnios, and pulmonary hypoplasia may result.[40]

Except for pure imperforate hymen, hydrocolpos is often accompanied by other severe congenital malformations, such as imperforate anus and urinary tract anomalies as well as genital, cardiac, and skeletal anomalies. Therefore, an attempt should be made to identify associated anomalies such as unilateral renal agenesis or hypoplasia. Uterine anomalies occur in only 0.1% to 0.5% of all females, but the incidence is 48% to 70% in females with renal abnormalities. Accordingly, discovery of a major renal anomaly should prompt evaluation of the uterus for potential anomalies.[10] In the case of a double uterus with an obstructed hemivagina, the septum must be resected surgically to avoid the possibility of pyocolpos due to spontaneous closure after drainage. Early diagnosis can lead to conservative treatment, thus preserving the maximum reproductive capability of these patients.[56] In cases in which corrective surgery is performed, serial sonograms may be obtained to follow the postoperative course.

Ovarian Torsion

Torsion of a normal or an abnormal ovary is an infrequent but important cause of abdominal pain. There is rotation of the ovary or adnexa about the ovarian pedicle, causing lymphatic followed by venous and then arterial obstruction.[34] There is an unexplained right-sided predominance ratio of 3:2.[61] Torsion of the normal adnexa usually occurs in the first decade of life and is less common than torsion of an ovary containing a mass (i.e., BCT or dysgerminoma). It is thought to be related to the particular mobility of the pediatric adnexa, which allows twisting at the mesosalpinx as a result of changes in intraabdominal pressure or in body position. The torsion may involve the tube, the ovary, or both. If the ovary is to be salvaged, surgical treatment must be carried out promptly.[30]

Clinical symptoms include lower abdominal pain, usually of more than 48 hours' duration, fever, anorexia, nausea, and vomiting. The pain is often acute in onset, sharp, and radiates to the groin or flank. The presence of fever and leukocytosis usually indicates that necrosis or abscess formation has begun. Fifty percent of patients have a history of pain with spontaneous recovery.[19,64] Diagnostic confusion may result, especially in the case of pediatric patients, whose symptoms are often attributed to such entities as appendicitis, gastroenteritis, pyelonephritis, intussusception, or Meckel's diverticulitis.[30]

Sonographic signs are often nonspecific and include a markedly enlarged ovary (mean volume may be 28 times normal), cul-de-sac fluid, peripheral structures most likely representing follicles, and other adnexal lesions such as a cyst or tumor.[26,64] Sonographically noted cul-de-sac fluid, when caused by the torsion itself, is usually a late manifestation and associated with hemorrhagic, nonviable ovarian tissue.[18,66] Vascular congestion in the mass leads to good sound transmission and numerous internal echoes. Incomplete torsion, with its associated abnormal venous and lymphatic drainage, can lead to marked ovarian enlargement over several days and the appearance of a solid mass. Massive ovarian edema, a tumor-like condition caused by an accumulation of edema fluid in the ovarian stroma with normal follicular structures, is generally thought to be the result of partial or intermittent torsion leading to obstruction of ovarian venous and lymphatic drainage. However, it is unclear whether the torsion is the primary event or the result of the enlarged size of the ovary. This condition has also occurred in an ovary previously fixed to the pelvic sidewall (oophoropexy), where torsion would not be the etiology. The sonographic appearance varies from solid to multicystic to complex.[35] When torsion is associated with an intraovarian mass, a complex pelvoabdominal mass is usually identified.[24]

Duplex and color flow Doppler may aid in the diagnosis of ovarian torsion.[18,58] Transducers that are highly sensitive to slowly flowing blood are necessary when trying to establish this diagnosis in young children. The normal ovary should be imaged first, to establish the proper technical factors. Then, the abnormal side is examined for the presence or absence of flow.[63] Even with proper technique, however, many normal ovaries do not show definitive flow on color Doppler.

The sonographic differential diagnosis includes ovarian neoplasm, ectopic pregnancy, hemorrhagic cyst, pelvic inflammatory disease, and periappendiceal abscess. A proper index of suspicion in the face of a clinical history that is atypical for these entities

may lead to early diagnosis of torsion and salvage of the ovary.[19]

Subsequent asynchronous torsion of the remaining normal ovary in a girl with a previous oophorectomy for torsion is a catastrophic event from both the reproductive and emotional perspective. Some authors, therefore, advocate the consideration of oophorepexy, tacking the ovary to the broad ligament or pelvic sidewall to prevent subsequent torsion on the noninvolved side.[18]

Diagnostic Criteria

The diagnostic criteria are essentially the same for pediatric as for adult gynecologic disorders. Masses can be described as cystic, solid, or complex. Examination techniques such as gain studies should be used to ensure that hypoechoic, homogeneously solid masses, such as lymphoma, are not mistaken for cystic masses. The presence of ascites, irregular borders, or papillary projections with thickened septa in a mass favors, but is not diagnostic of, malignancy. Identification of the abnormality in relation to normal landmarks often reveals the organ of origin even in confusing cases.

Sonography is a method to describe and characterize, not make a specific diagnosis. The final diagnosis in most cases requires clinical, radiographic, and laboratory input to narrow the differential possibilities and arrive at the diagnosis. Sonography is of prime importance in directing further workup.

Differential Diagnosis

The differential diagnosis of a pediatric gynecologic disorder is extensive and varied. Cystic masses may be of gynecologic origin (ovarian cyst, hydrosalpinx, hydrocolpos) or of urinary tract origin (bladder diverticulum, hydroureter). In addition, mesenteric cyst, gastrointestinal duplication cyst, pseudocyst, and presacral meningocele must be considered.

Complex masses may be secondary to abscesses, including appendiceal abscess, hematoma (depends on stage of clot), torsion of a mass, or ectopic pregnancy.

▰▰▰ **TABLE 6-1.** **DIFFERENTIAL DIAGNOSES OF THE COMPLEX PEDIATRIC OVARIAN MASS**

Mass	History	Physical Findings	Laboratory Studies	Sonographic Findings
Hemorrhagic ovarian cyst	Lower abdominal pain, occasional nausea	None, or palpable mass; fever with torsion	↑ WBC if torsion	Variable: thick-walled cyst; septated cyst; homogeneous low-level echoes with poor sound attenuation; cyst containing solid components, may have fluid in cul-de-sac; change in appearance in follow-up study
Benign cystic teratoma	Lower abdominal pain, nausea, vomiting; pain increase with torsion	Lower abdominal or pelvic mass; torsion in 25% cases, with associated fever and acute abdomen	↑ WBC if torsion	Complex mass with hyperechoic zones with acoustic shadowing; "tip-of-the-iceberg sign"; solid mass with cystic components with or without scattered internal echoes; fat-fluid level; pelvic radiograph shows calcification in 47% to 54%
Torsion of normal uterine adnexa	Acute abdominal pain; 50% have had similar episodes with spontaneous recovery in past; nausea, vomiting	Small, tender adnexal mass or lower abdominal mass, possible rebound tenderness, fever	↑ WBC	Predominantly solid ovarian mass with good through-transmission; may have fluid in cul-de-sac; solid mass (enlarged ovary) with peripheral cysts; infarction may mimic hemorrhagic cyst
Appendiceal abscess	Right lower quadrant pain, nausea, fever, vomiting	Tender right, lower abdominal mass; may have rebound tenderness; fever	↑ WBC	Nonspecific complex adnexal mass; fecalith with or without shadowing; fluid in cul-de-sac
Tuboovarian abscess	Lower abdominal pain, vaginal discharge, history of pelvic inflammatory disease	Tender lower abdominal or adnexal mass; fever; purulent cervical drainage	↑ WBC	Nonspecific complex mass; may simulate hemorrhagic cyst in enlarged adnexa; fluid in cul-de-sac
Malignant neoplasm	May have lower abdominal pain that is acute, subacute, or chronic; nausea, vomiting	Lower abodominal mass; fever with torsion; ascites, lymphadenopathy, metastases	↑ WBC if torsion	Nonspecific complex ovarian mass; central cystic area of necrosis; may be cystic with multiple septations; uterus may not be identifiable; fluid in cul-de-sac in 50%; ascites, liver and peritoneal metastases, lymphadenopathy may occur

WBC, white blood cell count.
(Adapted from Haller JO, Bass IS, Friedman AP. Pelvic masses in girls: An 8-year retrospective analysis stressing ultrasound as the prime imaging modality. Pediatr Radiol 1984;14:367.)

TABLE 6-2. DIFFERENTIAL DIAGNOSES OF CYSTIC AND SOLID GYNECOLOGIC MASSES OR THEIR SIMULATORS IN CHILDREN

Cystic	Solid
Anterior meningocele	Chordoma
Neurenteric cysts	Neuroblastoma
Retrorectal cysts	Ganglioneuroma
Ectopic kidney (hydronephrotic)	Neurofibroma
Massive hydroureter	Sacral bone tumors
Bladder diverticulum	Retroperitoneal sarcomas
Hydrosalpinx	Lymphosarcoma
Ovarian cyst	Rhabdomyosarcoma
Hydrometrocolpos	Yolk sac carcinoma
	Intussusception

Solid masses may represent torsiverted tumors, gynecologic tumors, presacral neural tumors, intussusception, lymph nodes, and sarcomas of bone origin. Tables 6-1 and 6-2 describe some of the pediatric gynecologic masses and their differential diagnoses.

The sonographic information, clinical history, laboratory values, and hormone assays must all be used in conjunction to narrow the possibilities and arrive at the most likely diagnosis.

REFERENCES

1. Alrabeeah A, Galliani CA, Giacomantonio M, et al. Neonatal ovarian torsion: Report of three cases and review of the literature. Pediatr Pathol. 1988; 8:143–149.
2. Ambrosino MM, Hernanz-Schulman M, Genieser NB, et al. Monitoring of girls undergoing medical therapy for isosexual precocious puberty. J Ultrasound Med. 1994; 13:501–508.
3. Athey P. Introduction to gynecologic ultrasound. In: Athey P, Hadlock F, eds. Ultrasound in Obstetrics and Gynecology. 2nd ed. St. Louis, MO: CV Mosby; 1985:134.
4. Baldwin DD, Landa HM. Common problems in pediatric gynecology. Urol Clin North Am. 1985; 22:161–176.
5. Baramki TA. Treatment of congenital anomalies in girls and women. J Reprod Med. 1984; 29:376–384.
6. Baran GW, Alkema RC, Barkett GK, et al. Autonomous ovarian cyst in isosexual precocious pseudopuberty. J Clin Ultrasound. 1988; 16:58–60.
7. Bass IS, Haller JO, Friedman A, et al. Sonography of cystic masses of the pelvis in children: Part 2. Masses originating in female genitalia. Appl Radiol. 1984; 13:144–149.
8. Bellah RD, Rosenberg HK. Transvaginal ultrasound in a children's hospital: Is it worthwhile? Pediatr Radiol. 1991; 21:570–574.
9. Bicker GH, Siebert JJ, Anderson JC, et al. Sonography of ovarian involvement in childhood acute lymphocytic leukemia. Am J Roentgenol. 1981; 137:399–401.
10. Bowie JD. Sonography of the uterus. In: Sabbagha RE, ed. Diagnostic Ultrasound Applied to Obstetrics and Gynecology. 2nd ed. (Ch. 39). Philadelphia: JB Lippincott; 1987.
11. Cabrol S, Haseltine FP, Taylor KJ, et al. Ultrasound examination of pubertal girls and of patients with gonadal dysgenesis. Journal of Adolescent Health Care 1981; 1:185–192.
12. Cohen HL. The female pelvis. In: Siebert J, ed. Syllabus: Current Concepts: A Categorical Course in Pediatric Radiology. Chicago: RSNA Publications; 1994:65–72.
13. Cohen HL. Sonography of the pediatric pelvis: Imaging in gynecologic health and disease. In: Mendelson E, Seeds J, eds. Ultrasound and Women's Health Course Syllabus. Laurel, MD: American Institute of Ultrasound in Medicine; 1994.
14. Cohen HL, Eisenberg P, Mandel F, et al. Ovarian cysts are common in premenarchal girls: A sonographic study of 101 children 2–12 years old. Am J Roentgenol. 1992; 159:89–91.
15. Cohen HL, Shapiro MA, Mandel FS, et al. Normal ovaries in neonates and infants: A sonographic study of 77 patients 1 day to 24 months old. Am J Roentgenol. 1993; 160:583–586.
16. Cohen HL, Tice HM, Mandel FS. Ovarian volumes measured by US: Bigger than we think. Radiology 1990; 177:189–192.
17. Coleman BG. Transvaginal sonography of adnexal masses. Radiol Clin North Am. 1992; 30:677–691.
18. Davis AJ, Feins NR. Subsequent asynchronous torsion of normal adnexa in children. J Pediatr Surg. 1990; 25:687–689.
19. Farrell TP, Boal DK, Teele RL, et al. Acute torsion of normal uterine adnexa in children: Sonographic demonstration. Am J Roentgenol. 1982; 139:1223–1225.
20. Fernbach SK, Feinstein KA. Selected topics in pediatric ultrasonography—1992. Radiol Clin North Am. 1995; 30:1011–1131.
21. Fleischer AC, Entmann SS. Sonographic evaluation of the ovary and related disorders. In: Sabbagha RE,

ed. Diagnostic Ultrasound Applied to Obstetrics and Gynecology. 2nd ed. (Ch. 40). Philadelphia: JB Lippincott; 1987.

22. Fleischer AC, Entmann SS, Burnett LS, et al. Principles of differential diagnosis of pelvic masses by sonography. In: Sanders RC, James AE, eds. The Principles and Practice of Ultrasonography in Obstetrics and Gynecology. 3rd ed. (Ch. 35). Norwalk, CT: Appleton-Century-Crofts; 1985.

23. Fleischer AC, Entmann SS, Porrath SA, et al. Sonographic evaluation of uterine malformations and disorders. In: Sanders RC, James AE, eds. The Principles and Practice of Ultrasonography in Obstetrics and Gynecology. 3rd ed. (Ch. 38). Norwalk, CT: Appleton-Century-Crofts; 1985.

24. Fleischer AC, Shawker TH. The role of sonography in pediatric gynecology. Clin Obstet Gynecol. 1987; 30:735–746.

25. Foster CM, Feuillan R, Padmanabhan V, et al. Ovarian function in girls with McCune-Albright syndrome. Pediatr Res. 1986; 20:859–863.

26. Gallup D, Talledo OE. Benign and malignant tumors. Clin Obstet Gynecol. 1987; 30:662–670.

27. Graif M, Shaler J, Strauss S, et al. Torsion of the ovary: Sonographic features. Am J Radiol. 1984; 143:1331.

28. Hall DA, Crowley WF, Wierman ME, et al. Sonographic monitoring of LHRH analogue therapy in idiopathic precocious puberty in young girls. J Clin Ultrasound. 1986; 14:331–338.

29. Haller JO, Bass IS, Friedman AP. Pelvic masses in girls: An 8-year retrospective analysis stressing ultrasound as the prime imaging modality. Pediatr Radiol. 1984; 14:363–368.

30. Haller JO, Fellows RA. The pelvis. In: Haller JO, Shkolnik A, eds. Ultrasound in Pediatrics (Clinics in Diagnostic Ultrasound, Vol. 8). New York: Churchill Livingstone; 1981.

31. Haller JO, Friedman AP, Schaffer R, et al. The normal and abnormal ovary in childhood and adolescence. Semin Ultrasound. 1983; 4:206–225.

32. Haller JO, Schneider M. The reproductive system. In: Haller JO, Schneider M, eds. Pediatric Ultrasound. Chicago: Year Book Medical Publishers; 1980.

33. Hansmann M, Hackeloer B-J, Staudach A. Examination of the female pelvis. In: Hansmann M, Hackeloer B-J, Staudach A, eds. Ultrasound Diagnosis in Obstetrics and Gynecology. Berlin: Springer-Verlag; 1985.

34. Helvie MA, Silver TM. Ovarian torsion: Sonographic evaluation. J Clin Ultrasound. 1989; 17: 327–332.

35. Hill LM, Pelekanos M, Kanbour A. Massive edema of an ovary previously fixed to the pelvic sidewall. J Ultrasound Med. 1993; 12:629–632.

36. Ivarsson SA, Nilsson KO, Persson PH. Ultrasonography of the pelvic organs in prepubertal and postpubertal girls. Arch Dis Child. 1983; 58:352–354.

37. Kim SH, Kang SB. Ovarian dysgerminoma: Color Doppler ultrasonographic findings and comparison with CT and MR imaging findings. J Ultrasound Med. 1995; 14:843–848.

38. King LR, Siegel MJ, Solomon AL. Usefulness of ovarian volume and cysts in female isosexual precocious puberty. J Ultrasound Med. 1993; 12:577–581.

39. Kutteh WH, Santos-Ramos R, Ermel LD. Accuracy of ultrasonic detection of the uterus in normal newborn infants: Implications for infants with ambiguous genitalia. Ultrasound in Obstetrics and Gynecology. 1995; 5:109–113.

40. McCarthy S, Taylor KJW. Sonography of vaginal masses. Am J Radiol. 1983; 140:1005.

41. Merten DF, Kirks DR. Diagnostic imaging of pediatric abdominal masses. Pediatr Clin North Am. 1985; 32:1397–1425.

42. Morely P, Barnett E. The ovarian mass. In: Sanders RC, James AE, eds. The Principles and Practice of Ultrasonography in Obstetrics and Gynecology. 3rd ed. (Ch. 36). Norwalk, CT: Appleton-Century-Crofts; 1985.

43. Navot D, Rosenwaks Z, Anderson F, et al. Gonadotropin-releasing hormone agonist-induced ovarian hyperstimulation: Low-dose side effects in women and monkeys. Fertil Steril. 1991; 55:1069–1075.

44. Nour S, MacKinnon AE, Dickson JAS. Ovarian cysts and tumors in childhood. J R Coll Surg Edinb. 1992; 37:39–41.

45. Nussbaum AR, Sanders RC, Hartman DS, et al. Neonatal ovarian cysts: Sonographic–pathologic correlation. Pediatr Radiol. 1988; 168:817–821.

46. Orsini L, Salardi S, Pilu G, et al. Pelvic organs in premenarchal girls: Real-time ultrasonography. Radiology. 1984; 153:113–116.

47. Quillen SP, Siegel MJ. Color Doppler US of children with acute lower abdominal pain. Radiographics. 1993; 13:1281–1293.

48. Rosenberg H, Sherman N, Tarry W, et al. Mayer-Rokitansky-Kuster-Hauser syndrome: US aid to diagnosis. Radiology. 1986; 161:815–819.

49. Salardi S, Orsini LF, Cacciari E, et al. Pelvic ultrasonography in premenarchal girls: Relation to puberty and sex hormone concentrations. Arch Dis Child. 1985; 60:120–125.

50. Scanlan KA, Pozniak MA, Fagerholm M, et al. Value

of transperineal sonography in the assessment of vaginal atresia. Am J Roentgenol. 1990; 154:545–548.

51. Schaarschmidt K, Willital GH. Intraanal ultrasound: A new aid in the diagnosis of pelvic processes and their relation to the sphincter complex. J Pediatr Surg. 1992; 27:604–608.

52. Schaffer RM, Haller JO, Friedman AP, et al. Sonographic diagnosis of ovarian dysgerminoma in children. Medical Ultrasound. 1982; 6:118–119.

53. Schneider M, Grossman H. Sonography of the female child's reproductive system. Pediatr Ann. 1980; 9:180–186.

54. Shawker T, Comite F, Rieth KG, et al. Ultrasound evaluation of female isosexual precocious puberty. J Ultrasound Med. 1984; 3:309.

55. Sherer DM, Beyth Y. Ultrasonographic diagnosis and assisted surgical management of hematotrachelos and hematoma due to cervical atresia with associated vaginal agenesis. J Ultrasound Med. 1989; 8:321–323.

56. Sherer DM, Rib DM, Nowell RM, et al. Sonographic-guided drainage of unilateral hematometrocolpos due to uterus didelphys and obstructed hemivagina associated with ipsilateral renal agenesis. J Clin Ultrasound. 1994; 22:454–456.

57. Shkolnik A. Applications of ultrasound in the neonatal abdomen. Radiol Clin North Am. 1985; 23:361–365.

58. Siegel MJ. Female pelvis. In: Siegel MJ, ed. Pediatric Sonography. 2nd ed. New York: Raven Press; 1995: 437–477.

59. Sisler CL, Siegel MJ. Ovarian teratomas: A comparison of the sonographic appearance in prepubertal and postpubertal girls. Am J Roentgenol. 1990; 154:139–141.

60. Stanhope R, Adams J, Jacobs HS, et al. Ovarian ultrasound assessment in normal children, idiopathic precocious puberty, and during low-dose pulsatile gonadotrophin-releasing hormone treatment of hypogonadotrophic hypogonadism. Arch Dis Child. 1985; 60:116–119.

61. Stedman TL. Stedman's Medical Dictionary Illustrated. 23rd ed. Baltimore: Williams & Wilkins; 1976:1391.

62. Tanaka YO, Kurosaka Y, Nishida M, et al. Ovarian dysgerminoma: MR and CT appearance. J Comput Assist Tomogr. 1994; 18:443–448.

63. Teele RL, Share JC. Ultrasonography of the female pelvis in childhood and adolescence. Radiol Clin North Am. 1992; 30:743–758.

64. Warner M, Fleischer A, et al. Torsion of the adnexa: Sonographic findings. Radiology. 1985; 154:773.

65. Widdowson DJ, Pilling DW, Cook RCM. Neonatal ovarian cysts: Therapeutic dilemma. Arch Dis Child. 1988; 63:737–742.

66. Worthington-Kirsch RL, Raptopoulos V, Cohen IT. Sequential bilateral torsion of normal ovaries in a child. J Ultrasound Med. 1986; 5:663–664.

67. Yaghoobian J, Yankelevitz DF, Pinck RL, et al. Pyometrium in a three-year-old girl: Sonographic findings. J Ultrasound Med. 1984; 3:87–88.

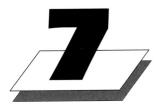

Benign Disease
of the Female Pelvis

PAMELA M. FOY, JAMES E. SCHNEIDER, FRANCES R. BATZER,
and MICHAEL L. BLUMENFELD

For many years, diagnostic ultrasound has been the modality of choice for evaluating the female pelvis. Although ultrasound is of limited use for making definitive histologic diagnoses, a reliable clinical diagnosis can usually be made through correlation with clinical and laboratory information. In this chapter, we focus on benign diseases of the female pelvic viscera, which include the uterus, ovaries, and fallopian tubes. Leiomyomas and adenomyosis are common benign conditions seen within the uterus. The ovaries can be involved in a variety of benign processes, including ovarian cyst development (physiologic, functional, miscellaneous), inflammatory disease (tuboovarian abscesses), and neoplasms (germ cell tumor, epithelial tumor, stromal tumor). Neoplasms are new tissue growths or tumors.[83] They may image as solid, cystic, or a combination of the two, and they may be histologically benign or malignant. This chapter discusses only benign conditions.

Sonographic Technique

In the evaluation of the pelvis, the ultrasound practitioner must pay careful attention to the patient's history. An adequate history should include the pa-

tient's age, menstrual history, surgical history, complaints and symptoms (e.g., pain, fever, bleeding), use of contraceptive devices, potential pregnancy state, history of previous pregnancies, and history of use of medications, including oral contraceptives. Knowledge of history and significant findings on physical examination are important in helping to formulate an ultrasound diagnosis.

The uterus and adnexa should be thoroughly examined sonographically and the findings documented. Documentation should include the location, size, and sonographic appearance of normal structures as well as any masses. Whenever possible, anatomic landmarks such as a urinary bladder, uterus, ovaries, or pelvic vessels should be included with the images of an unknown mass to verify its location. Labeling all images on "hard copy" should also be done. Documentation should identify a mass's origin, when possible. A mass should be measured in three dimensions: length, width, and height. Characteristics such as mass contour, mass echo texture, degree of sound transmission, the presence of fluid–fluid or fluid–solid levels, septa, nodularity, and mobility should be documented.

The question always arises as to which technique should be used to evaluate the pelvis of the female patient, the transvaginal approach or the transabdominal approach. We believe that most of the sonographic information will be obtained with

The authors thank J. Bruce Nestleroth, PhD for his technical assistance in digitizing many of the ultrasound images for inclusion in this chapter.

the transvaginal approach. Because of probe proximity to the organ of interest and higher insonating frequency transducers (5.0 to 6.5 MHz), resolution is dramatically improved. A study by Fleischer and colleagues has shown that transvaginal sonography (TVS) adds diagnostically specific information to transabdominal sonography (TAS) in over three fourths of women studied.[24] However, the goal of the examination is complete evaluation of the pelvis, and frequently the sonographer may need to evaluate for hydronephrosis, ascites, or pleural effusions. This can be accomplished only with a transabdominal approach. In many radiology-based ultrasound laboratories, TVS is used only as an adjunct to TAS in cases of inadequate bladder distention, incomplete evaluation of the pelvis, and equivocal findings that require improved visualization for diagnosis.[16] Although different schools of thought on the position of vaginal sonography exist, the sonographic technique used to evaluate the female pelvis should include the full array of sonographic approaches so that pelvic pathology will not be missed.

TRANSVAGINAL SONOGRAPHY

The introduction of TVS has produced renewed interest in the evaluation of the female pelvis.[79] The technique of TVS does not require a full bladder and has high patient acceptance. Problems previously encountered during TAS, such as obesity, bowel gas, and a retroverted uterus, no longer preclude accurate diagnosis.[27] When evaluating the uterus or bladder, the probe should be placed in the anterior fornix. The probe should be moved laterally into the lateral fornix when evaluating the adnexa. This technique permits transducer placement closer to the structures in the adnexa. In women who are having pelvic pain, the probe can be touched against the ovary to see if that organ is causing the patient pain. The push–pull motion that can be obtained with the vaginal probe, plus use of the free hand abdominally, allows assessment of organ motion, organ fixation, and fluid loculation. The sonographer's free hand should also be used for organ palpation (uterus and ovaries), to position the pelvic structures better within the transducer's field of view, and to displace overlying bowel gas from an organ of interest such as the ovaries. In many ways, the vaginal probe can be

looked on as an extension of the hand, as if performing a bimanual examination.

Transvaginal sonography is certainly not without its drawbacks. A narrow or stenotic introitus, either in a virginal or postmenopausal woman, can prohibit insertion of the vaginal probe. Infrequently, obesity may cause difficulty even with the vaginal sonogram, if there is a significant amount of adipose tissue in the pelvis. A pelvic mass greater than 10 cm may be missed or not completely imaged by the higher-frequency probes because of the limited field of view and limited penetration.

TRANSABDOMINAL SONOGRAPHY

The transabdominal approach (3.5 to 5.0-MHz transducers) permits an overall panoramic view of the pelvic structures. The technique uses a full bladder, which creates an acoustic window permitting visualization of the uterus and adnexa. Mechanical and phased-array transducers allow the greatest degree of manipulation, and are therefore ideally suited for angling around pelvic bones and through the urinary bladder to obtain as much sonographic information as possible.

Adnexal structures may be difficult to visualize, so repositioning the patient from the supine position can be helpful. Patient position may be changed to right side up or left side up, or the pelvis may be tilted anteriorly (supported on a pillow). Different positions change the relationship of the bladder to the other pelvic organs, creating a new acoustic window. The transducer may then be angled obliquely from one side of the pelvis to the other through the newly positioned urinary bladder. This technique can create perpendicularity for the structure, improving its imaging. If bowel is adjacent to and visually obscuring a pelvic organ, having the patient perform a Valsalva maneuver may move the structure into the transducer's field of view.

Tampons as well as the vaginal contraceptive device, the sponge, can be visualized within the vaginal canal when scanning with a transabdominal technique, and should not be mistaken for an abnormality. A tampon within the vaginal canal can be easily identified sonographically as an irregularly shaped echogenic focus[60] (Fig. 7-1). As the tampon absorbs menstrual blood, it enlarges to fill the vaginal cavity and may appear to distort the vaginal wall. Vaginal contraceptive sponges produce a curvilinear

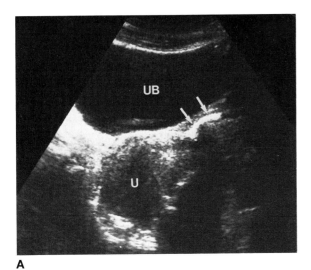

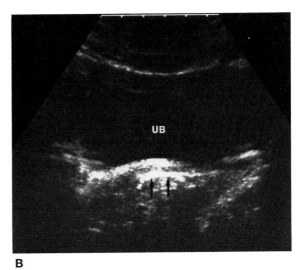

A
B

Figure 7-1. A curvilinear, brightly echogenic structure (*arrows*) is present in the vagina in longitudinal (**A**) and transverse (**B**) views. This represents a tampon (U, uterus; UB, urinary bladder).

echo that casts an acoustic shadow when visualized within the vaginal canal.[60]

Often, a loop of fluid-filled sigmoid or rectum can mimic a cystic or complex adnexal mass. In such cases, especially when peristalsis cannot be demonstrated, it may be necessary to reevaluate the "mass" on another day or during or after a cleansing enema. A warm tap water enema may also be used to identify the rectum, sigmoid colon, and cecum and to delineate the posterior cul-de-sac.[67] The urinary bladder should be emptied before the procedure is begun for patient comfort as well as optimal visualization of pelvic structures.

Complementary Imaging Modalities

Although computed tomography (CT) and magnetic resonance imaging (MRI) are more expensive, they may provide information ultrasound cannot. MRI may be contraindicated in patients with metallic objects of any type.[71] Pelvic CT, which may require a contrast medium, is rarely used primarily to evaluate the adnexa because of its delivery of radiation to the gonads.[71] CT is often used to demonstrate the extent of complicated pelvic disease, such as pelvic inflammatory disease, endometriosis, or malignancy.[53] CT is also a useful modality when diagnosing metastatic peritoneal implants.[71] CT is the most reliable modality in identifying fat and

calcifications and, if necessary, can improve a diagnosis of cystic teratoma.[71] The multiple anatomic planes provided by MRI are reportedly helpful in delineating the origins of pelvic masses by demonstrating connection to the ovary or uterus when ultrasound is inconclusive. Hemorrhagic fluid may be differentiated more reliably from protein-free fluid, fat, and solid lesions by MRI than by ultrasound. Next to ultrasound, MRI is particularly useful in evaluating adnexal masses in pregnant women because it does not use ionizing radiation.[85] This imaging technique is helpful later in pregnancy, when diagnostic ultrasound may be limited not only by the large, gravid uterus but by the displacement of the adnexa out of the true pelvis.[69] Both CT and MRI are useful for evaluating pelvic disease in patients whose ultrasound examination results are suboptimal because of obesity or bowel gas.[53]

The Uterus

THE CERVIX

Anomalies of uterine development are relatively frequent. They can be divided into those caused by abnormal uterine fusion (see Chap. 5), those caused by abnormal cervical function (incompetent cervix), and those produced by maternal exposure to diethylstilbestrol (DES). Benign conditions that may produce an enlarged cervix include cervical myoma, nabothian cysts, and cervical polyps (Table 7-1).

TABLE 7-1. BENIGN LESIONS OF THE VAGINA, CERVIX, AND UTERUS

Lesion	Ages Affected	Sonographic Characteristics
Gartner's duct cyst	Reproductive years	Anechoic fluid-filled mass with well defined margins and good through-transmission. Located in the anterolateral wall of the vagina.
Nabothian cyst	Usually seen after pregnancy	Fluid-filled mass located in the cervical canal, often with refractive edge shadowing.
Polyps	Perimenopausal and postmenopausal	Appear increased in echogenicity when compared to the surrounding endometrium. May be focal or diffuse.
Adenomyosis/adenomyoma	Later reproductive years	Nonspecific; enlarged uterus with normal contours and intact endometrial lining. Multiple small cysts may be found in myometrium.
Leiomyoma ("fibroids")	Reproductive years	May be increased, decreased, or same echogenicity as myometrium. Hyaline degeneration; anechoic mass with poor sound transmission. Cystic degeneration: anechoic mass with good sound transmission. Calcific degeneration: echogenic focal areas with distal acoustic shadowing.

Nabothian Cysts/Inclusion Cysts

Nabothian cysts or inclusion cysts are formed in the cervix when the opening of a nabothian duct, located within the cervix, is covered by epithelial cells and the fluid is "retained."[26] These cysts are found so commonly they are considered to be a normal feature of the adult cervix. Nabothian cysts are often noted after pregnancy[3]; they are usually asymptomatic and require no treatment.

Sonography, particularly TVS, is helpful in detecting cysts within the cervix. They may be multiple and range in size from 3 mm to 3 cm. Sonographically, these cysts are seen as fluid-filled masses with smooth borders and enhanced transmission, and may demonstrate refractive edge shadowing (Fig. 7-2). Care must be taken not to confuse these cysts with developing ovarian follicles; with proper scanning techniques, this mistake can be avoided.

Polyps

Cervical polyps are the most common benign neoplasms of the cervix. Found in at least 4% of women, they most often occur in multigravidas in the perimenopausal and postmenopausal years. Cervical polyps are usually found incidentally and are almost always asymptomatic, although less commonly they may be a cause for profuse bleeding or discharge.[3] Polyps are usually attached to the cervical wall by a pedicle and may reach a size of several centimeters.[20,58] Although it is easier to identify small polyps with the transvaginal approach than transabdominally,[78] they may be difficult to identify sonographically because of their size.

Myomas

Cervical myomas are similar histologically to myomas of the uterine corpus. Three to 8% of myomas are classified as cervical, and most are small and cause no symptoms. If symptoms do occur, they

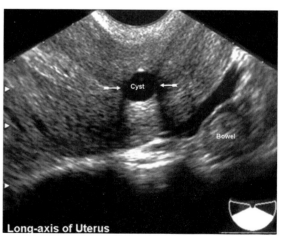

Figure 7-2. Long-axis view transvaginally of the cervix in an anteverted uterus. A rounded, fluid-filled mass (*arrows*, with refractive edge shadows distally) is consistent with a nabothian cyst.

may include dyspareunia, dysuria, urgency, genito-urinary obstruction, cervical obstruction, prolapse, bleeding, and obstructed labor. Symptomatic lesions may be resected, or a hysterectomy may be indicated, depending on the age and reproductive plans of the patient.[20,36] Sonographically, cervical myomas may distort the cervix. The sonographic pattern may be similar to that of corpus myomas. Like corpus myomas, asymptomatic tumors are observed for growth.

Incompetent Cervix

The uterine cervix has a unique role in pregnancy. It must remain closed, retaining the fetus within the uterus until maturity, and then dilate to allow delivery. The anatomic and physiologic changes in the cervix that allow delivery are known as cervical competence. Cervical incompetence can result from congenital Müllerian duct abnormalities, DES exposure, or surgical trauma from conization or procedures involving dilatation of the canal.[66] Dilation of the cervix at any gestational age is preceded by progressive shortening of the cervical canal. TVS aids in identifying women with cervical changes suggestive of cervical incompetence[42] by providing measurements of the length of the cervix.[3] Because TAS requires a distended bladder, which can cause variations in cervical length, it is not as accurate as the transvaginal approach.[66] With the transvaginal probe placed in the anterior fornix, the length of the cervix is measured in the sagittal plane from the external to the internal os. Shorter-than-normal measurements are suggestive of cervical incompetence. Because the pregnant cervix is a dynamic structure that varies in size and opening, at least three measurements should be taken over a minimum of 3 minutes. The shortest measurement is considered the most accurate.[43] If the cervix is incompetent, a funnel-shaped anechoic mass may be seen effacing the cervix. This represents the membranes and amniotic fluid bulging into the cervix[43] (Fig. 7-3).

Diethylstilbestrol (DES)

DES-exposed women are at increased risk for pregnancy complications such as ectopic pregnancy, first trimester abortion, and premature labor.[49,74] Premature labor may be caused in part by an incompetent cervix,[51,52] another side effect of DES exposure. Serial sonography has been recommended to

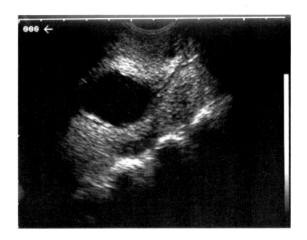

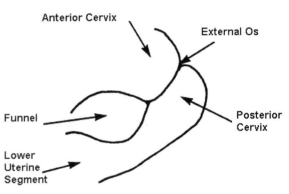

Figure 7-3. *Transvaginal long-axis view of the cervix demonstrating a dynamic lower uterine segment. Funneling membranes can be seen invaginating into the cervix.*

assess the cervix for incompetency during pregnancy.[51,52] Documented uterine anomalies include a small uterus and T-shaped uterus.[59,63,81] The T-shaped uterus, although hard to document sonographically, is best demonstrated in a transverse view.[63,68] Uterine tissue resembling a "T" may be seen in the fundal area. Careful technique and attention to detail are necessary because the uterus may be smaller than normal. Hysteroscopy and hysterosalpingography are better diagnostic examinations than ultrasound for confirmation of an abnormal uterine configuration (see Figs. 5-9 and 28-14).

THE ENDOMETRIUM

Polyps

Endometrial polyps are a common lesion. The peak age of occurrence is during the perimenopausal years, from 40 to 49 years of age.[3] Although the

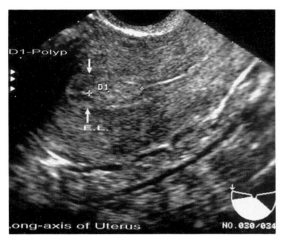

Figure 7-4. Transvaginal long-axis view shows a focal area of increased echogenicity (between the plus signs) that proved to be an endometrial polyp.

etiology is unknown, they originate as local growths of endometrial tissue covered by epithelium containing a variable amount of glands, stroma, and blood vessels.[3] Endometrial polyps are usually solitary and most frequently originate at the fundus in the cornual region. They are often asymptomatic, but the most common presenting symptom is bleeding, either intermenstrual or excessive (menorrhagia).[3] Larger polyps are frequently associated with bleeding.

Sonographically, focal polyps are increased in echogenicity compared to the surrounding normal endometrium (Fig. 7-4). The sonographer should evaluate the endometrial lining in short axis, looking for contour irregularities during the proliferative phase of the menstrual cycle. Polyps (which are echogenic) may be missed if the ultrasound examination is performed during the secretory phase of the cycle. The recently described technique of sonohysterography may be used to confirm the location of endometrial polyps[17,62,76] (Fig. 7-5). They can be differentiated from submucous myomas by their greater echogenicity.[76]

Tamoxifen

Tamoxifen, a nonsteroidal antiestrogen hormonal drug, has been used effectively in the treatment of postmenopausal women with breast cancer. Results of pharmacologic studies have shown that the drug acts predominantly as an estrogen antagonist within the uterus, and it has been shown to stimulate the endometrium.[15]

As a result, it has been suggested there may be a relationship between tamoxifen therapy and the development of endometrial cancer, polyps (Fig. 7-6), increased growth of leiomyomas, and uterine enlargement.[14] An article by Goldstein showed a heterogenous, bizarre ultrasonographic appearance of the endometrium in five women by TVS.[29] None of the

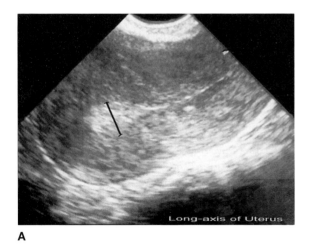

A

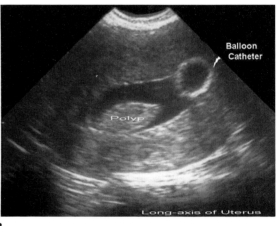

B

Figure 7-5. (**A**) Conventional transvaginal sonography reveals a thickened fundal endometrial lining (*black line*). No distinct mass was seen. (**B**) Sonohysterogram of same patient demonstrates a distinct polyp (balloon catheter is seen in the lower uterine segment). (Courtesy of Nancy Spangler, Ultrasound Specialist, Reproductive Specialty Center, Milwaukee, WI.)

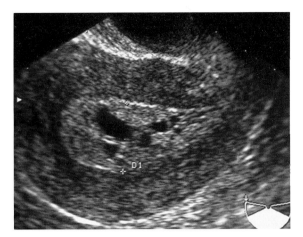

Figure 7-6. A 62-year-old woman undergoing tamoxifen therapy with postmenopausal bleeding. Transvaginal long-axis view of the uterus reveals a thickened endometrial lining (19 mm) with cystic changes. A polyp was confirmed.

patients was bleeding clinically. Sonohysterography of the same patients revealed a normal-appearing endometrial lining with small subendometrial sonolucencies in the proximal myometrium.[29] It was believed that the sonolucent areas represented abnormal adenomyomatous-like changes in the proximal myometrium.[29]

SONOGRAPHIC TECHNIQUE. When a patient presents who is undergoing tamoxifen therapy, careful attention should be payed to the endometrial lining as well as the rest of the uterus. Goldstein and colleagues have developed a plan of management for tamoxifen-treated patients using endometrial screening with TVS and sonohysterography.[30] If the endometrium measured no more than 5 mm, serial monitoring with ultrasound was conducted. For patients with an endometrial lining thicker than 5 mm, sonohysterography was performed. If the results of the sonohysterogram demonstrated a thickened endometrium, hysteroscopy, a dilation and curettage, or endometrial biopsy was performed.[30]

THE MYOMETRIUM

Leiomyoma

Leiomyomas are the most common tumor of the female pelvis. They have been estimated to occur in 20% to 25% of women of reproductive age. The rate of occurrence is markedly greater in African

Americans than whites. The cause of leiomyoma is unknown; however, they typically arise after menarche and regress after menopause, implicating estrogen as a promotor of growth.[2]

Uterine leiomyomas are benign tumors of smooth muscle cells and fibrous connective tissue arising from uterine smooth muscle. Other frequently used descriptive terms include myoma, fibroid, and fibromyoma. They may be single or multiple, may range in size from 1 mm to 20 cm in diameter,[2] and are surrounded by a pseudocapsule of compressed muscle fibers. Myomas are described by their relation to the uterine cavity. Those located within the myometrium are termed intramural (Fig. 7-7). The submucous forms lie beneath the endometrium and often protrude into the endometrial cavity (Fig. 7-8). Those located at the serosal surface of uterus are called subserosal. Five to 10% of myomas are submucosal, and these are the most symptomatic.[3] Subserosal myomas may become pedunculated at times, and are the most difficult to assess sonographically (Fig. 7-9). The term "parasitic myomas" is used when the blood supply of a myoma is from other organs. These myomas may be attached to omentum or intestine or may grow laterally into the broad ligament.[3] Because treatment approaches may differ, exact location of a myoma is important.

DEGENERATIVE CHANGES. When myomas outgrow their blood supply, degeneration can occur. The extent of degeneration depends on the severity of the

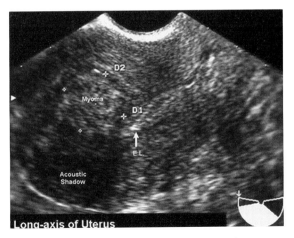

Figure 7-7. Transvaginal long-axis view of an anteverted uterus reveals an anterior myoma approximately 18 × 17 mm with distal acoustic shadowing. This myoma is deviating the endometrial lining (E.L.) posteriorly.

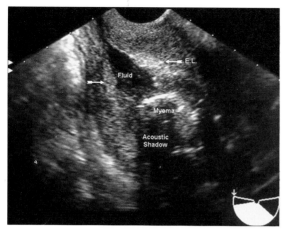

Figure 7-8. Transvaginal long-axis view of a retroverted uterus reveals a solid mass (myoma) with a distal acoustic shadow within the endometrial lining. Fluid is also seen within the endometrial cavity. This proved to be a submucous myoma.

discrepancy between the myoma's growth and its blood supply.[31] Two thirds of all myomas show some form of degeneration. The signs and symptoms of degeneration depend on the size and location of the myoma. Various types of degeneration can occur, including hyaline, myxomatous, cystic, calcific, fatty, red degeneration, and necrosis.[2] Pain may indicate some

form of a degenerative process, or may be the result of torsion of a pedunculated myoma or large tumors pressing on pelvic nerve roots.

In hyaline degeneration, smooth muscle cells are replaced by fibrous tissue. In cystic degeneration (4%), degeneration of hyaline tissue occurs, which leads to liquefaction necrosis. Calcific degeneration occurs most often after menopause[58] and is easily recognized sonographically. Red degeneration is an acute form resulting from muscle infarction, and occurs more commonly during pregnancy.[48] This may cause acute pain requiring surgical treatment. If laparotomy or myomectomy is necessary in the pregnant patient, there is usually a favorable maternal and fetal outcome.[2]

SIGNS AND SYMPTOMS. The size and location of myomas determine the symptomatology; however, many women with myomas have no symptoms. Submucous (see Fig. 7-8) and intramural myomas that distort or deviate the endometrial cavity (Fig. 7-10) often result in abnormal bleeding that presents clinically as menorrhagia, but intermenstrual spotting and irregular periods may also occur. A very large myomatous tumor may result in increasing abdominal girth without associated pain.[3] A myoma pressing on the bladder anteriorly often produces urinary frequency and urgency exaggerated perimenstrually. A posterior myoma may

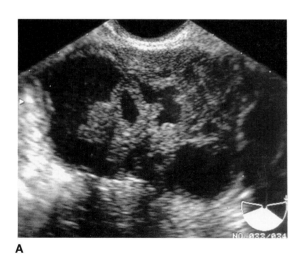

A

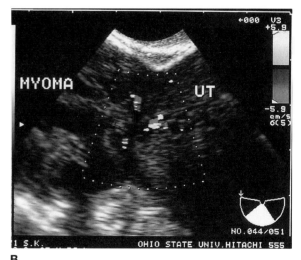

B

Figure 7-9. (**A**) This large, complex mass, with cystic degeneration, anterior to the uterus proved to be a degenerating pedunculated myoma. (**B**) In this long-axis view, color flow Doppler shows vessels at the attachment site of the pedunculated myoma to the uterus. (See also Color Plate 5.)

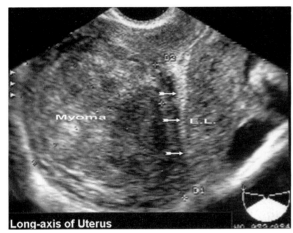

Figure 7-10. A large fundal intramural myoma, 72 × 57 mm, can be seen deviating the echogenic endometrial lining posteriorly.

produce rectal pressure, causing constipation or lower back and leg discomfort.[3]

SONOGRAPHIC FINDINGS. Routine sonography for imaging of myomas allows for accurate assessment of dimensions, number, and location of tumors.[2] Measurements should be obtained of all the tumors in three dimensions: length, width, and height. Frequently, the sonographer may need to use the lowest-frequency transducer possible or increase the overall gain because myomas tend to attenuate the sound beam, which in turn makes it difficult to define the posterior wall of the tumor. Serial examinations may also be performed to document interval growth. Physical assessment of the adnexa may be compromised by an enlarged uterus. In these instances, sonography is an excellent modality to evaluate the ovaries. Frequently, with a large myomatous uterus, the ovaries are low in the pelvis, best evaluated with the transvaginal approach, or extremely high in the pelvis, best evaluated with a transabdominal approach. When the uterus is enlarged, an evaluation of the patient's kidneys should be performed sonographically to inspect for hydronephrosis, because ureteral obstruction can result from a large myoma filling the pelvis.

A wide range of sonographic findings is associated with myomas.[10,34] The sonographic appearance of myomas depends on their size, location, and whether degeneration exists. Small myomas appear as subtle changes in myometrial echogenicity and may displace the endometrial cavity echo. Degeneration may present

and can range from hypoechoic to echogenic. Cystic degeneration can cause hypoechoic areas within the myoma. A whorled internal architecture may be seen when bundles of smooth muscle and fibrous tissue are arranged concentrically within a myoma. Calcific degeneration is commonly seen and sonographically is recognized as clusters of bright reflectors that are associated with a distal acoustic shadow (Fig. 7-11). A whorled, calcific myoma can even resemble a fetal head. Red degeneration can present as medium echoes with good through-transmission.[48]

Large myomas can disrupt uterine contour more than smaller ones. Multiple large subserosal myomas may result in an enlarged uterus with a lobulated contour; large intramural and submucous myomas can distend the uterine cavity and distort the endometrial lining (Fig. 7-12). Large myomas in the anterior and posterior uterine musculature can cause extrinsic compression of the urinary bladder and rectum that appears sonographically to indent the usually smooth uterus–bladder (Fig. 7-13) and rectum interface. It is important to indicate the location of myomas, whether subserosal, intramural, and/or submucosal, and whether distortion of the endometrial lining is present. Different surgical approaches may be used depending on the position and size of the myomas.

Because leiomyomas can enlarge the uterus considerably and may present outside the uterus in a pedunculated form (see Fig. 7-9), care must be taken to demonstrate the entire pelvic area to docu-

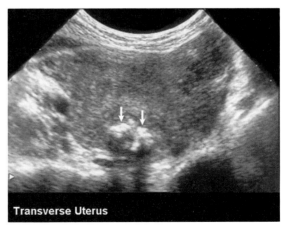

Figure 7-11. Transabdominal transverse view of uterus reveals an intramural myoma with calcific degeneration. Calcifications (arrows) are seen as punctate echogenic foci with distal acoustic shadowing.

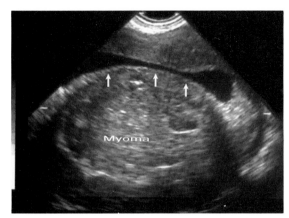

Figure 7-12. Sonohysterography reveals a large intramural myoma disrupting and thinning the endometrial lining (*arrows*). (Courtesy of Nancy Spangler, Ultrasound Specialist, Reproductive Specialty Center, Milwaukee, WI.)

ment both uterine and extrauterine myomas. A pedunculated fibroid can be mistaken for a number of conditions, including bicornuate uterus, blind uterine horn, ovarian mass, hydatidiform mole, and ectopic pregnancy.[10] A push–pull technique (sliding the scanning hand back and forth so that the probe is in the proximal and distal portion of the vagina) with the vaginal probe can often help identify the stalk of the myoma and its movement.

Studies indicate that MRI may in some in-stances visualize leiomyomas better than ultrasound.[21,84] MRI evaluation may be recommended to locate myomas before surgery,[21] but this diagnostic examination is much more expensive than an ultrasound examination.

Adenomyosis

Adenomyosis is defined as the presence of endometrial glands and stroma within the myometrium. Frequently seen in women older than 50 years of age, the common symptoms are abnormal bleeding, secondary dysmenorrhea, and an enlarged, tender uterus. Because these symptoms are nonspecific, it is not surprising that adenomyosis is seldom correctly diagnosed clinically. The cause of adenomyosis is not clear, but it is usually associated with multiparity and often endometriosis. Adenomyosis is frequently a diffuse process involving the entire uterine musculature and resulting in uterine enlargement. Up to 80% of adenomyotic uteri are associated with such conditions as leiomyomata, endometrial hyperplasia, peritoneal endometriosis, and uterine cancer.[3] It occurs in association with leiomyomata in up to 57% of the time.[3] Although adenomyosis is considered distinct from endometriosis, the two are associated in 13% of women.[82] A focal form of adenomyosis, the adenomyoma, ca occur with discrete nodules presenting in the myometrium (Fig. 7-14)[20,36,58] or cervix.

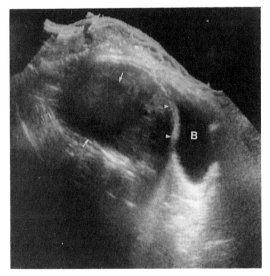

Figure 7-13. Longitudinal static image shows an enlarged uterus with a large hypoechoic fundal myoma (*arrows*). There is extrinsic compression (*arrowheads*) on the urinary bladder.

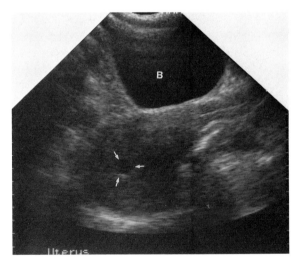

Figure 7-14. Longitudinal sonogram of the uterus shows 1-cm cystic mass (*arrows*) in the myometrium of a retroverted uterus. Although the lesion appeared similar to cystic degeneration of a small leiomyoma, it was found to be a focal adenomyoma (B, urinary bladder).

Sonographic findings for adenomyosis are non-specific, including an enlarged uterus with normal contours and an intact endometrial lining.[13,72] Uterine echogenicity may range from normal[72] to slightly hypoechoic,[13] and multiple small cysts may be found in the myometrium. Areas of decreased echogenicity and inhomogeneity within the myometrium may represent menstrual engorgement of the endometrial glands.[82]

Sonographers must pay careful attention to technique to accurately assess uterine size, contour, and texture in the presence of adenomyosis. Measurements of the uterus, in three dimensions, should be obtained transabdominally. Careful attention should be paid to the fundus because generalized adenomyosis results in focal widening of this region.[13] If proper bladder distention is not possible or the uterus is too large, the transducer should be placed at the pubis and angled sharply cephalad. This may help identify the fundal area by enlarging the bladder window. MRI has proved useful in diagnosing adenomyosis in difficult cases.[80]

THE VAGINA

Gartner's Duct Cyst

Gartner's duct cysts are usually asymptomatic and are most commonly discovered on routine pelvic examinations.[3] These cysts may be single or multiple, and are a common lesion of the vagina. They are a remnant of the mesonephric duct, an embryonic urogenital structure. They rarely cause symptoms, but if large, they may cause pressure symptoms and dyspareunia. When symptomatic, they often originate high in the vagina adjacent to the cervix and extend into the labia at the vaginal opening. Sonography is helpful in delineating the location of the cyst in the anterolateral vaginal wall. The lesion appears as an anechoic mass, with well defined margins and good sound transmission (see Fig. 5-3).

The Fallopian Tubes

The normal fallopian tubes are narrow and are not routinely seen with the transabdominal approach, unless surrounded by fluid (see Fig. 4-43). Transvaginally, a combination of the fallopian tube and the suspensory ligament may be seen in a short-axis view, and frequently may assist in locating the ovary. This normal structure is easier to see with TVS when surrounded by fluid. Benign disease of the fallopian tubes is restricted to pelvic inflammatory processes.

INFLAMMATORY PROCESSES

Inflammatory processes in the pelvis include pelvic inflammatory disease (PID; pyosalpinx and tubo-ovarian abscess) and nongynecologic abscesses. PID is associated primarily with gynecologic infections and also with intrauterine contraceptive devices. A complete discussion of PID is presented in Chapter 10. Patients with pelvic abscesses present with fever, pain, and elevated white blood cell count.

A variety of sonographic patterns can be displayed by pelvic abscesses. Such collections usually demonstrate good through-transmission and may have irregular borders, internal septa, debris levels, and air. Gas within an abscess produces bright echoes and may shadow.

Pyosalpinx may appear sonographically similar to hydrosalpinx, but usually there are low-level internal echoes representing pus. If the ovary can be visualized at one wall of the abscess, the diagnosis of tuboovarian abscess (Fig. 7-15) may be entertained.[23]

The differential diagnosis for a pelvic abscess should include hematoma, endometrioma, ectopic pregnancy, necrotic gynecologic tumor, and abscess of nongynecologic origin (e.g., diverticular abscess, periappendiceal abscess, Crohn's disease, psoas abscess, postsurgical abscess). Because many of these entities have similar sonographic patterns, a complete patient history is critical for distinguishing which disease process has most likely been demonstrated.

HYDROSALPINX

Hydrosalpinx is a fluid collection in a scarred or blocked fallopian tube. Usually secondary to pyosalpinx, it evolves when the purulent material is replaced by serous fluid.[11] This appearance suggests a chronic or old infection. Frequently patients have no acute symptoms and the hydrosalpinx is discovered transvaginally as an incidental finding.

Sonographically, hydrosalpinx appears as a tubular, tortuous, fluid-filled mass with smooth, well de-

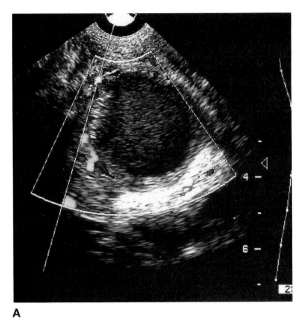

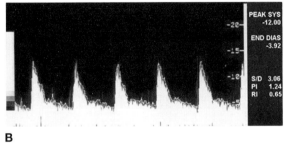

A

B

Figure 7-15. (**A**) This solid-appearing adnexal mass displaying good through-transmission distally has multiple vessels peripherally displayed with color Doppler. (See also Color Plate 6.) (**B**) The pulsed Doppler revealed an RI of 0.65 and a slight notch in early diastole. A tuboovarian abscess was found surgically.

fined walls (Fig. 7-16). Hydrosalpinx can be unilateral or bilateral, and the tube may become quite large. The distinguishing sonographic characteristic of a hydrosalpinx is that the proximal end of the fusiform fluid-filled structure tapers as the tube enters the cornual region of the uterus.[23] This fluid collection may mimic sonographically an adnexal cyst or surrounding bowel. However, the lack of peristalsis should help to differentiate this entity from bowel. Bladder diverticulum, urachal cyst, and mesenteric cyst are some of the nongynecologic entities that can also appear as fluid-filled pelvic masses.

The Ovaries

BENIGN CYSTS

Most fluid-filled pelvic masses are ovarian in origin.[22] The sonographic criteria for simple cysts are (1) smooth, well defined borders, (2) absence of internal echoes, and (3) increased posterior acoustic enhancement (Fig. 7-17). Thick, irregular walls or thick septations (>3 mm) may be associated with inflammation, endometriosis, or malignancy.[41,50] Adnexal masses containing extremely echogenic foci may be benign cystic teratomas. Adnexal masses that are of homogeneously increased echogenicity tend to be solid masses,[55,56] hemorrhage, or endometriomas.[22] A list of benign cystic masses of the adnexa is presented in Table 7-2.

Ovarian cysts may be visualized sonographically in women of all reproductive stages, including preg-

Figure 7-16. Anechoic tubular structure displays good through-transmission, representing a hydrosalpinx.

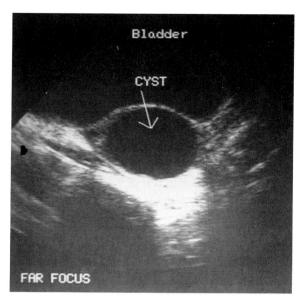

Figure 7-17. *This cyst demonstrates the criteria for a simple cyst of the ovary: smooth walls and good acoustic transmission with posterior acoustic enhancement and no internal echoes.*

nancy. Cysts measuring less than 3 cm in greatest diameter usually regress spontaneously and represent follicles and physiologically normal functioning of the ovary. Sonographic follow-up is recommended for cysts between 3 and 5 cm; most regress spontaneously, but some continue to enlarge. The best time to reevaluate the ovary is 6 to 8 weeks later, immediately after menses or after several menstrual cycles. Careful sonographic evaluation to detect septa or solid components is recommended for any ovarian cyst, especially those measuring more than 5 cm in greatest dimension.[64] Up to 60% of cysts with thin septa and no solid components have been reported to regress spontaneously, usually within 3 months.[64] Even cysts that appear simple by sonographic criteria rarely resolve if they measure more than 10 cm in greatest diameter. Cysts of this size have a greater potential to be malignant or invasive, and thus are usually removed.[64] Cysts detected during pregnancy that measure more than 5 to 8 cm in diameter traditionally have been removed during the second trimester because they may complicate the pregnancy or delivery and may represent a malignancy. However, Thornton and Wells have suggested that, unless complications have occurred or are likely at delivery, simple cysts measuring between 5 and 10 cm in diameter should

be treated conservatively until the postpartum period, because most of these cysts are benign.[77]

Traditionally, ovarian cysts of any size found in postmenopausal women have been excised. Hall and McCarthy reported that only 1 of 13 simple cysts excised from postmenopausal women in their facility was found to be malignant on histopathologic evaluation. Although the high incidence of ovarian cancer in postmenopausal women necessitates further investigation of any adnexal cyst, they suggested that their findings may reduce the anxiety experienced by postmenopausal women in whom adnexal cysts are discovered.[39] More recently, Goldstein and others have reported that postmenopausal, unilocular, ovarian cysts measuring less than 5 cm in largest dimension are usually benign (in the absence of ascites). They suggest that these cysts may be safely monitored with serial sonograms, particularly because TVS is now available and provides superior resolution.[28,61,70]

FUNCTIONAL CYSTS

Functional or physiologic cysts of the ovary include ovarian follicles, follicular cysts, corpus luteum cysts, and theca lutein cysts. Ovarian follicles are visualized as anechoic structures in the ovary. Follicles as small as 5 mm may be appreciated sonographically. Approximately 10 days before ovulation, the ovaries contain many small follicles. Not all of the follicles mature to the point of ovulation. A single follicle usually becomes dominant, measuring 2.0 to 2.5 cm in greatest dimension. One to 3 days before ovulation, the domi-

TABLE 7-2. BENIGN CYSTIC MASSES OF THE ADNEXA

PHYSIOLOGIC OR FUNCTIONAL
Ovarian follicles
Follicular cysts
Corpus luteum cysts
Theca lutein cysts

MISCELLANEOUS
Paraovarian cysts
Peritoneal inclusion cysts
Hemorrhagic cysts
Endometriomas
Hydrosalpinx
Paratubal cysts
Polycystic ovary
Inflammatory processes

nant follicle may appear sonographically as a "cloudy cone," with its wide end leading out to the periphery of the ovary.[44] During the mid-portion of the menstrual cycle, a release of luteinizing hormone leads to ovulation with follicular rupture and conversion into a corpus luteum. If conception occurs, the corpus luteum continues to produce progesterone until approximately the 11th or 12th week of pregnancy, when the placenta takes over production of progesterone. If conception does not occur, the corpus luteum usually regresses within 2 weeks of ovulation.

Follicular Cysts

Follicular cysts result from either nonrupture of the dominant mature follicle[3,22] or failure of an immature follicle to undergo the normal process of atresia, with absence of follicular fluid reabsorption.[3] They may be multiple but are usually unilateral. They range in diameter from 1 to 10 cm,[55] averaging 2 cm.[3] Solitary follicular cysts are common and may occur from fetal life to menopause.[3] Most patients with physiologic cysts experience no symptoms because these cysts usually regress spontaneously. Sonographically, follicular cysts meet the criteria for a simple cyst, as described earlier. In general, any simple ovarian cyst measuring less than 5 cm in greatest dimension in an ovulating woman should be reevaluated sonographically, 6 to 8 weeks later. A change in the size or appearance or complete resolution of the cyst usually is seen. In some cases, patients with follicular cysts present with mild to severe pelvic pain.[44] The cyst may become symptomatic, with the occurrence of hemorrhage, torsion, or rupture into the peritoneal cavity.[55] Sonographically, hemorrhage within the cyst will appear variable in its echo pattern. In the case of a ruptured cyst, changes in the appearance of the cyst may be associated with free fluid in the cul-de-sac.

Corpus Luteum Cysts

Corpus luteum cysts are less prevalent than follicular cysts.[3] The corpora lutea forms from the graafian follicle within hours of ovulation. As the dominant follicle ruptures, the corpora lutea develops. The corpora lutea measures 1.5 to 2.5 cm and may appear hypoechoic and possess irregular or thick borders around a central anechoic area.[46] Because of their variable appearance, these cysts have been called "the great pretender." These cysts are routinely visualized with the transvagi-

nal approach but frequently are not seen with the transabdominal approach. Corpora lutea are not considered to be corpus luteum cysts unless their size is at least 3 cm in diameter.[3] This cyst results from intracystic hemorrhage.[3] Low-level echoes or a fluid–debris level are seen when hemorrhage has occurred (Fig. 7-18). Most patients present with acute pain of less than 24 hours' duration, although one fourth of patients have pain for a duration of 1 to 7 days.[3] Corpus luteum cysts usually are unilocular and unilateral and measure 6 to 8 cm,[12] with an average diameter of 4 cm.[3] Unless torsion occurs, no treatment is required,[45] and regression occurs after two to three menstrual cycles.[12] Rupture results in fluid in the cul-de-sac and elsewhere in the abdomen. Hemorrhage and rupture frequently cause increased symptoms.

Should fertilization take place, a corpus luteum cyst of pregnancy may result.[37] In Figure 7-19, a corpus luteum cyst of pregnancy and a gravid uterus are demonstrated on a single sonographic image. During pregnancy, corpus luteum cysts typically reach a maximum size of 3 cm, but can enlarge up to 5 to 10 cm.[23] They usually resolve by 16 weeks' gestation.[5] At any point during this time, hemorrhage or rupture can occur, causing pelvic pain and posing a threat to both mother and fetus.[37]

Theca Lutein Cysts

Theca lutein cysts are the largest of the functional cysts and may range in size from 3 to 20 cm. Theca lutein cysts represent an exaggerated corpus luteum

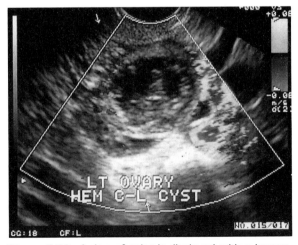

Figure 7-18. A ring of color is displayed with a hemorragic corpus luteum cyst. This hemorrhagic corpus luteum cyst is complex in appearance. (See also Color Plate 7.)

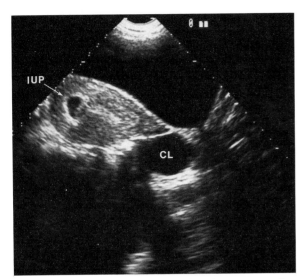

Figure 7-19. Corpus luteum cyst (CL) of pregnancy visualized posterior and inferior to a uterus containing an intrauterine pregnancy (IUP).

response in patients with high levels of human chorionic gonadotropin,[23] the hormone produced by a pregnancy. In 14% to 30% of cases, theca lutein cysts are associated with gestational trophoblastic diseases such as hydatidiform mole, chorioadenoma destruens, and choriocarcinoma. Montz and colleagues have observed an increased incidence of postmolar trophoblastic disease in hydatidiform mole patients who also had theca lutein cysts, particularly if the cysts became complicated or were bilateral.[54] Theca lutein cysts may also be seen with ovarian hyperstimulation syndrome, a complication of infertility drug therapy.[38,44] In rare instances, theca lutein cysts are seen with a normal singleton or multiple gestations.[38,44,54]

Sonographically, theca lutein cysts are multilocular, thin-walled, large, bilateral, fluid-filled masses (Fig. 7-20).[37] Bilateral development is thought to be a response to hormonal stimulation. Because of their association with gestational trophoblastic disease, it is important to evaluate the uterus carefully when theca lutein cysts are seen. A good patient history also is helpful in evaluating the cause of theca lutein cysts.[57]

Theca lutein cysts are usually treated conservatively because they involute when the source of gonadotropin is removed, although they may persist for several months after trophoblastic evacuation. In some patients, the cysts persist long after the

human chorionic gonadotropin levels are no longer detectable.[54] On occasion, theca lutein cysts, like other functional cysts, may undergo hemorrhage, torsion, or rupture, causing the patient pain. Surgery may be necessary if they become very large or in the event of intraperitoneal rupture or hemorrhage.

HEMORRHAGIC CYSTS

Any adnexal cyst or mass may twist, causing pain of sudden onset. The acute pain is caused by the vascular occlusion that results from the twisting of the base of the cyst or mass. When a pelvic ultrasound examination is requested for a nonpregnant patient with acute onset of pelvic pain (regardless of whether an adnexal mass is appreciated on physical examination), hemorrhage and torsion should be entertained as the primary diagnoses.

Hemorrhagic cysts usually display good through-transmission with variable sonographic features.[9,65] Sonographically fresh blood appears anechoic, progresses subacutely to a mixed echogenicity, and finally becomes anechoic again.[9] Any pattern or combination of these patterns may be seen. Debris may be seen in the posterior portion of a hemorrhagic cyst. In some cases, septa (Fig. 7-21) may be present. Frequently, free fluid is seen in the cul-de-sac. The onset of pain and these sonographic features seen vaginally are specific but may be encountered with other adnexal masses. A follow-up ultrasound examination can prove helpful in diagnosis in cases in which clot lysis has taken place.

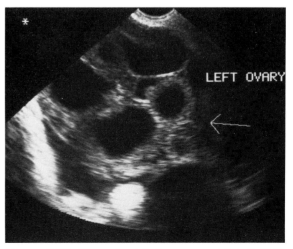

Figure 7-20. Hyperstimulated ovary contains multiple theca lutein cysts of varying sizes.

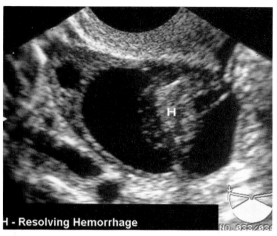

Figure 7-21. Transvaginal complex ovarian mass that is solid and cystic in appearance. This represents a resolving hemorrhage.

Torsion

The ovary's pedicle may also twist. Although torsion may occur with normal ovaries, most reported cases have involved children with ovarian masses or in women younger than 30 years of age. The fallopian tube is often involved as well. An increased incidence has been noted in pregnant patients. The clinical presentation is recurrent or acute onset of localized pain and tenderness. If the torsion is incomplete and intermittent, the ovary may enlarge with edema. Areas of decreased and increased echogenicity in the ovary may be appreciated.[33] These areas represent hemorrhage or infarct. Multifollicular enlargement is thought to result from fluid transudation into follicles due to the ovarian congestion caused by circulatory impairment.[33] Intraperitoneal fluid may be present secondary to obstruction of venous and lymphatic return, resulting in a transudate from the capsule of the ovary.[23] Doppler evaluation may be useful in determining whether the ovary is receiving blood,[32] because torsion initially involves the ovarian vein but may progress to involve the ovarian artery as well. Fleischer and associates published data on 13 patients with surgically proven adnexal torsion. In 10 cases, the ovaries were considered nonviable because they lacked venous flow centrally.[25] In contrast, the viable ovaries demonstrated venous flow centrally.[25]

POLYCYSTIC OVARY DISEASE

Polycystic ovary disease (Stein-Leventhal syndrome) is an endocrine disorder associated with obesity, amenorrhea, anovulation, hirsutism, and infertility. Anovulation is thought to result from the unusually thick capsule surrounding the ovaries and the associated endocrine abnormalities in these patients. The clinical presentation varies greatly with the degree and duration of the hormone imbalance. Because certain adrenal tumors can also cause oligomenorrhea or amenorrhea and infertility, adrenal tumor should be considered in the clinical differential diagnosis of these patients.

The sonographic appearance of the ovaries in patients with polycystic ovary disease varies widely. In classic cases, the ovaries are enlarged bilaterally and contain multiple, tiny peripheral cysts (Fig. 7-22). The cysts may range in diameter from 2 to 6 mm.[75] Because they can be quite small, often only the echogenic linear wall may be visualized. The cysts may be subcapsular or randomly distributed throughout the parenchyma of the ovary. Up to

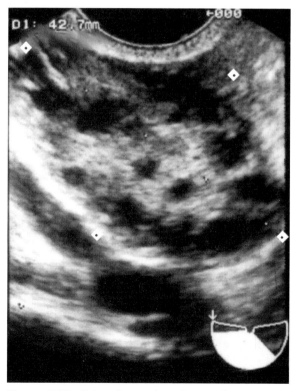

Figure 7-22. Polycystic ovarian disease shows an enlarged ovary with multiple small cysts.

TABLE 7-3. BENIGN OVARIAN NEOPLASMS

Lesions	Ages Affected	Laterality	Sonographic Characteristics
GERM CELL TUMORS			
Benign teratoma	Any age; usually reproductive or younger	15% Bilateral	Varied; may be cystic, complex with calcifications, fat–fluid levels, diffusely echogenic, predominantly solid with echogenic foci.
EPITHELIAL TUMORS			
Serous cystadenoma	40s and 50s	25% Bilateral	Typically unilocular; may have thin septations; may have papillary projections.
Mucinous cystadenoma	40s and 50s	5% Bilateral	Usually multilocular; may reach 30 cm diameter; may contain debris.
Brenner tumor	Any age, usually around 50 y	6.5% Bilateral	Solid; hypoechoic, may exhibit acoustic enhancement; ranges in size from microscopic to 8 cm in diameter.
STROMAL TUMORS			
Fibroma	50s and 60s	Usually unilateral, but multiple in 10% of cases	Hypoechoic; attenuates sound, which can produce distal acoustic shadow; measures 5–16 cm in diameter.
Thecoma	Common among postmenopausal women, but age distribution ranges from 15 to 86 y	Usually unilateral	Hypoechoic; attenuates sound, which can produce distal acoustic shadow; can measure up to 30 cm in diameter.
Sertoli-Leydig cell tumor	Usually younger than 30 y	Unilateral	Echogenic mass

25% of pelvic sonograms performed on patients with the clinical findings of polycystic ovary syndrome reveal sonographically normal ovaries.[40,75]

Women with true polycystic ovary disease may have no clinical manifestations; however, the cysts are always bilateral. The sonographic appearance of polycystic ovaries may also be seen in women being treated with follicle-stimulating hormones or in newborn girls whose ovaries are responding to maternal hormones.[40] If patients are under ovulation induction, the sonographic presence of polycystic ovaries at the beginning of a menstrual cycle should be recorded.

BENIGN NEOPLASMS

Eighty percent of all ovarian tumors are benign. Benign ovarian neoplasms may be categorized as germ cell tumors, epithelial tumors, or stromal tumors, depending on the ovarian tissue elements and derivation of these tumors. The most common benign adnexal neoplasms are benign cystic teratomas (germ cell tumor) and cystadenomas (epithelial tumors). Stromal tumors include fibroma and the-

coma.[44] Benign neoplasms are summarized in Table 7-3.

Koonings and associates performed a retrospective study spanning 10 years (encompassing real-time sonography) evaluating 861 surgically confirmed cases of ovarian neoplasm.[45] In their series, cystic teratoma was the most prevalent neoplasm, accounting for 44% of all ovarian tumors (Table 7-4). Twenty-eight percent of the neoplasms measured less than 6 cm, 53% ranged from 6 to 11 cm,

TABLE 7-4. INCIDENCE OF BENIGN OVARIAN NEOPLASMS

Type	Occurrence
Cystic teratoma	58%
Serous cystadenoma	25%
Mucinous cystadenoma	12%
Benign stromal	4%
Brenner tumor	1%

(Modified from Koonings PP, Campbell K, Mishell DR, Grimes DA. Relative frequency of primary ovarian neoplasms: A 10-year review. Obstet Gynecol. 1989; 74:921. Reprinted with permission from The American College of Obstetricians and Gynecologists.)

whereas 19% were larger than 11 cm. In premenopausal women, 75% of the tumors were benign, whereas 25% were benign in postmenopausal women (Table 7-5).

Benign Cystic Teratoma

Benign cystic teratomas are the most common germ cell tumor. They are also the most frequently seen ovarian tumor in women younger than age 20 years. Although teratomas may occur in any age group, they are most often seen during the second and third decades. The terms "dermoid tumor" and "teratoma" are often used interchangeably, although teratomas contain tissue of all three germ layers (ectoderm, mesoderm, endoderm), whereas dermoids are composed of ectodermal tissue only.[38] Pathology specimens of teratomas include teeth, hair, and glandular tissues (sweat, apocrine, sebaceous). Neural and thyroid tissue have also been seen on histopathologic examination. The malignant potential of a teratoma is related inversely to its tissue maturity, but malignant change rarely occurs (<1%) in benign cystic teratomas.

Although patients with teratomas usually have no symptoms, they may present with pain or a palpable mass. Teratoma pedicles may twist, but they rarely rupture, because of their thick capsules. Teratomas are often first detected with a bimanual pelvic examination. Teratomas containing high fat content may cause the ovary to be located superior to the uterine fundus.[23] They are bilateral in approximately 10% to 15% of patients.

There is a wide spectrum of sonographic appearances to teratomas, including a predominantly cystic mass, a complex mass with calcifications, fat–fluid level within a complex mass, and a diffusely

echogenic mass without shadowing. Most commonly, teratomas appear sonographically as complex masses that are predominantly solid, containing echogenic foci that represent calcium or fat with or without acoustic shadowing.[22] This type of teratoma is the most difficult to detect because the sonographic appearance mimics that of bowel gas. Occasionally, the "tip of the iceberg" sign is demonstrated; this refers to a very echogenic anterior component with a posterior shadow, which prevents visualization of the more posterior aspect of the mass (Fig. 7-23*A*).[35] When a fat–fluid level is identified, the fluid component is seen in the more dependent position, whereas the echodense fat floats on top of the fluid (see Fig. 7-23*B*). The sonographic appearance of a teratoma varies according to its elemental components—skin, hair, teeth, bone, fat. Strands of hair may be seen floating in fluid (see Fig. 7-23*C*). With the presence of significant bone and teeth components, echogenic foci with distal shadowing should be demonstrated on ultrasound examination.

TRANSABDOMINAL TECHNIQUE. Decubitus positioning while scanning may aid in demonstrating fat–fluid or fluid–debris levels, because shifting should occur when different parts of the mass are dependent. Palpating the mass with the free hand may also produce movement at the fat–fluid interface. Water enemas may help differentiate a teratoma from bowel. The microbubbles in the tap water provide sonographic contrast that helps to distinguish rectum from pelvic masses.

OTHER IMAGING MODALITIES. A pelvic radiograph may show fat, teeth, or bony components of teratomas. CT and MRI also display some characteristic findings of benign cystic teratoma. Fat has a characteristic appearance on CT, and CT can demonstrate fat–fluid or fluid–debris levels in these tumors. Benign cystic teratomas with high fat content have been demonstrated with MRI: the fat component in the tumors gives very high signal intensity on T1-weighted images.[38]

TREATMENT. Surgical removal of benign cystic teratomas is usually indicated. When patients are young, it is particularly important that ovarian function be preserved. It usually is possible to resect the teratoma without removing the entire ovary.

◤◤◤ **TABLE 7-5. Ovarian Neoplasms (861 Cases)**

Type	Occurrence
Premenopausal	75% (13% malignant)
Postmenopausal	25% (45% malignant)
Benign	75%
Malignant	21%
Low malignant potential	4%

(Modified from Koonings PP, Campbell K, Mishell DR, Grimes DA. Relative frequency of primary ovarian neoplasms: A 10-year review. Obstet Gynecol 1989; 74:921. Reprinted with permission from The American College of Obstetricians and Gynecologists.)

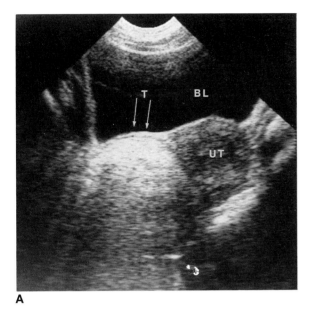

A

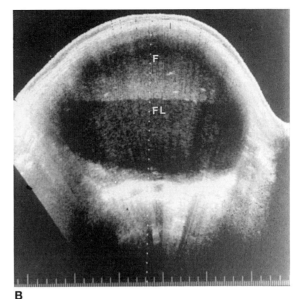

B

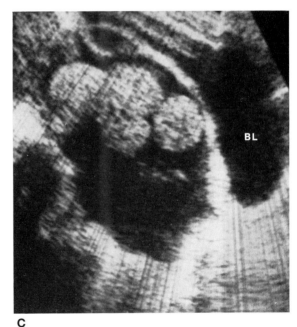

C

Figure 7-23. (**A**) Teratoma (T) located posterior to the urinary bladder (BL) and to the right of the uterus (UT) on a transverse transabdominal scan. The teratoma appears brightly echogenic anteriorly and simulates bowel gas. (**B**) Teratoma with a fat–fluid level is demonstrated on a static scan. The fatty component (F) is floating on the dependently located fluid (FL). (**C**) Teratoma located posterior to the urinary bladder on longitudinal scan. Echogenic "balls" of hair appear to float on fluid located in the dependent portion of the teratoma.

Epithelial Tumors

Epithelial tumors arise from the ovarian epithelium. The benign epithelial tumors include serous cystadenoma and mucinous cystadenoma. Their malignant counterparts are serous cystadenocarcinoma and mucinous cystadenocarcinoma. Less common benign epithelial tumors include Brenner tumors and mixed epithelial tumors.

CYSTADENOMAS. The most common type of cystic ovarian tumor is a cystadenoma. In general, cystadenomas may grow very large and are seen in postmenopausal women, although they are occasionally encountered in women of childbearing ages. As their names suggest, serous cystadenomas contain thin, serous fluid and mucinous cystadenomas contain thicker mucin. Serous cystadenomas are more common than

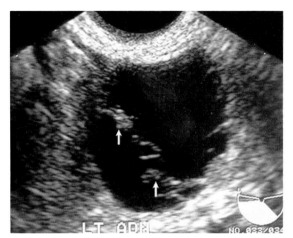

Figure 7-24. Transvaginal scan in a postmenopausal woman reveals a large, fluid-filled mass containing a septation (*arrows*). Surgically, this proved to be a serous cystadenoma.

mucinous cystadenomas and more frequently malignant. They are usually unilocular and may be bilateral in 25% of cases. Serous cystadenomas may contain very thin septations (Fig. 7-24), and, on occasion, papillary projections.[57] Mucinous cystadenomas, the largest of the ovarian cysts, are bilateral less than 5% of the time and can grow extremely large (15 to 30 cm) with multiple prominent septations and debris.[4,38] It may be possible to differentiate serous from mucinous cystadenomas based on the echogenicity of fluid. It is difficult to differentiate sonographically between benign and malignant forms of cystadenoma, so it is important to look for secondary signs of malignancy, such as ascites or fixation of the mass. Histopathologic analysis is required for a definitive diagnosis.

BRENNER TUMORS. Brenner tumors are solid ovarian tumors arising from the ovarian surface epithelium.[8] They account for 1.7% of all ovarian neoplasms.[18] Brenner tumors can be seen in any age group but usually are found in women in the fifth and sixth decades of life who present with abnormal uterine bleeding. The tumors are bilateral in 6.5% of cases and range in size from microscopic to about 8 cm in diameter.[18] The usual sonographic presentation is an echogenic mass that may contain small cystic spaces[5,85] (Fig. 7-25). Brenner tumors often are diagnosed histopathologically as incidental findings in specimens removed for associated pelvic disease. Malignant changes in Brenner tumors are

rare. Malignant forms of this tumor usually are large, fluid-filled masses.[18]

Stromal Tumors

Benign stromal tumors include fibromas, thecomas, and Sertoli-Leydig cell tumors (also referred to as androblastomas and arrhenoblastomas).[57] Fibromas, thecomas, and Sertoli-Leydig cell tumors are all sonographically hypoechoic or echogenic adnexal masses and cannot be distinguished from one another or from other solid benign or malignant tumors of the ovary.[7,57] The differential diagnosis between these ovarian tumors and uterine fibroids may be made by establishing, if possible, the ovarian origin of the mass.[57,87]

OVARIAN FIBROMAS. Fibromas constitute about 5% of ovarian tumors and usually are found in women in the fifth or sixth decades of life. Ranging in size from 5 to 16 cm, they are multiple in 10% of cases.[57] Fibromas may be calcified, but in less than 10% of cases.[88] Bilateral, calcified, multinodular fibromas are atypical and usually are associated with basal cell nevus syndrome, a hereditary disorder. Very small fibromas are relatively common and often are associated with other ovarian neoplasms.[88] Sonographically, fibromas appear homogeneously hypoechoic

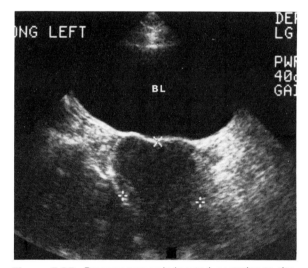

Figure 7-25. Brenner tumor is located posterior to the urinary bladder (BL) on a longitudinal scan. Borders of the solid tumor are marked by the mechanical measuring device. The posterior border is not well delineated. An acoustic shadow may be appreciated posterior to the mass.

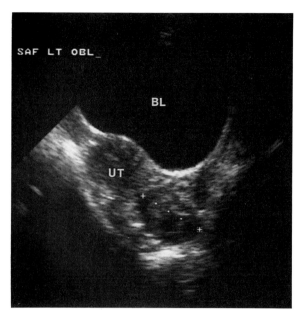

Figure 7-26. *Thecoma located posterior to the cervix on a longitudinal scan. Diameter of solid tumor measured by mechanical measuring device (BL, urinary bladder; UT, uterus).*

and attenuate the sound beam, producing an acoustic shadow posterior to the mass. Ascites and right-sided pleural effusion may be associated with fibromas in 1% to 3% of cases; this triad makes up Meigs' syndrome.[57] Fibromas larger than 10 cm in diameter have been imaged with ascites but without pleural effusion in 10% to 15% of cases.[88]

THECOMAS. Thecomas are estrogen-producing, solid ovarian masses that account for 1% to 2% of ovarian tumors. Estrogen production is responsible for the presenting complaint of abnormal uterine bleeding.[19] Thecomas are usually unilateral[85] and may measure up to 30 cm in diameter. They occur most frequently in postmenopausal women and in young girls. The characteristic sonographic appearance of a thecoma is that of a pelvic mass that casts a large acoustic shadow corresponding to the entire mass. Figure 7-26 is a sonographic image of a small thecoma confirmed by histopathogic examination. Although they are not considered malignant, they may become invasive. Increased estrogen production may place the patient at greater risk for endometrial cancer.[57,87]

SERTOLI-LEYDIG CELL TUMORS. These tumors are unilateral neoplasms. They account for less than 0.5% of all ovarian neoplasms. Patients often present with pain or abdominal swelling, and one third suffer masculinization effects from elevated testosterone levels, because Sertoli-Leydig cell tumors primarily secrete androgens. Seventy-five percent of cases occur in women younger than 30 years of age.[88] Sertoli-Leydig cell tumors appear sonographically as echogenic masses and may not be distinguished from other solid ovarian tumors. Up to 20% are malignant[57] (see Fig. 9-7).

OVARIAN REMNANT SYNDROME

A complication of prior bilateral salpingo-oophorectomy is the ovarian remnant syndrome. In this syndrome, postoperative remnants of ovarian tissue become functional.[3] Women can present with pain, a mass, or both. Sonographically, solid tissue similar in echogenicity to ovarian tissue can be visualized (Fig. 7-27). This occurs most frequently in patients who have undergone pelvic exploration because of severe endometriosis. Ovarian remnant syndrome can also develop in patients who had severe adhesions where dissection of the ovary may have been difficult.

Miscellaneous

PARAOVARIAN AND PARATUBAL CYSTS

Paraovarian or paratubal cysts develop from vestigial wolffian duct structures or arise from the tubal epithelium. The paraovarium is located in the mesosalpinx,

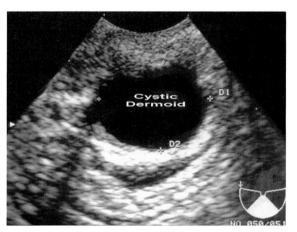

Figure 7-27. *A 32-year-old woman status post total abdominal hysterectomy and bilateral salpingo-oophorectomy presented with pain. Transvaginal examination revealed an adnexal fluid-filled mass consistent with ovarian remnant syndrome. Surgery confirmed a cystic dermoid.*

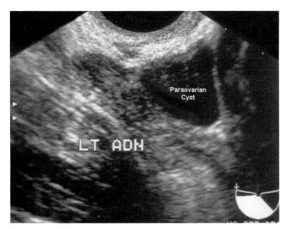

Figure 7-28. Transvaginal ultrasound reveals a unilocular, fluid-filled mass separate from the adjacent ovary, consistent with a paraovarian cyst.

the portion of broad ligament between the fallopian tube and the hilum of the ovary. These cysts represent 10% of all adnexal masses and occur over a wide range of ages.[6] They are seen most commonly in the third and fourth decades of life and range in size from 1.5 to 19 cm.[4] Paraovarian cysts are difficult to distinguish from other ovarian lesions by physical or ultrasound examination. Most symptomatic patients present with menstrual irregularities, increased lower abdominal girth, and pain if the cyst is large. Some small cysts remain asymptomatic and are found incidentally on ultrasound examination or at surgery.

Sonographically, paraovarian cysts appear thin walled, unilocular, and free of internal echoes. They arise from the adnexa and not the ovary, but this may not be a simple ultrasound diagnosis. Because they do not respond to cyclic changes, their size does not change in relation to the menstrual cycle. On occasion, a paraovarian cyst may be recognized when a cyst is noted to be separate from an intact ovary and the fallopian tube is draped or stretched over the cyst (Fig. 7-28). With the transvaginal technique, the sonographer may be able more easily to establish the separation of the paratubal mass from the ovary. As with other cystic masses, hemorrhage, torsion, and rupture alter the sonographic appearance.

PERITONEAL INCLUSION CYSTS

Fluid-filled masses resulting from accumulations of serous fluid between adhesions or layers of peritoneum may be seen sonographically, usually in patients with a history of pelvic adhesions or surgery. These collections are referred to as peritoneal inclusion cysts. Noted almost exclusively in premenopausal women, affected patients present with pelvic pain or mass. The patient histories includes previous surgery (frequently multiple operations), endometriosis, or a history of pelvic inflammatory disease.[73]

Peritoneal inclusion cysts are usually contiguous with the adnexa and may distort the appearance of the ovaries by displacing them (Fig. 7-29). TVS often reveals multiple septations within fluid surrounding an intact ovary, reminiscent of "a spider in a web."[73] When large, these inclusion cysts may be better evaluated with the transabdominal approach. Sohaey and colleagues used color Doppler and pulsed Doppler to reveal relatively low resistive flow in the septations of peritoneal inclusion cysts.[73]

Differential Diagnosis

In the proper clinical setting, it is imperative that ectopic pregnancy and endometriosis be included in the differential diagnosis of the pelvic mass. The sonographic presentation of ectopic pregnancy and endometriosis ranges from predominantly cystic to complex pelvic masses. These entities are discussed in detail in Chapters 9 and 10.

The differential diagnoses for benign cystic and solid ovarian masses are presented in Table 7-6. Fluid-filled bowel or abnormal bowel may mimic

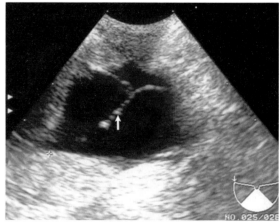

Figure 7-29. A 35-year-old woman status post hysterectomy presented with pelvic pain. A fluid-filled mass with strands (*arrows*) was adjacent to the right ovary. This was consistent with a peritoneal inclusion cyst.

TABLE 7-6. DIFFERENTIAL DIAGNOSIS FOR BENIGN ADNEXAL MASSES

CYSTIC ADNEXAL MASSES
Follicular cyst
Corpus luteum cyst
Paraovarian cyst
Peritoneal inclusion cyst
Hemorrhagic cyst
Hydrosalpinx
Endometrioma
Benign cystic teratoma

PREDOMINANTLY CYSTIC ADNEXAL MASS WITH SEPTATIONS OR DEBRIS
Theca lutein cyst
Hemorrhagic cyst
Cystadenoma
Tuboovarian abscess
Ectopic pregnancy
Cystic adnexal mass

SOLID ADNEXAL MASS
Endometrioma
Hemorrhagic cyst
Brenner tumor
Thecoma
Fibroma

cystic, complex, or solid adnexal masses. Sonography cannot differentiate between benign and malignant masses, but it can identify tissue characteristics suggestive of benignity or malignancy.[41,56] Solid adnexal tumors tend to be more malignant, as do cysts with multiple septations or solid mural nodules.[39,47] Associated ascites, peritoneal implants, or visceral metastases also favor malignancy.

Ultrasound continues as the primary imaging modality in the evaluation of the female pelvis. A sonographic examination by a skilled ultrasound practitioner in conjunction with the appropriate clinical findings should generate a working diagnosis or differential for any pelvic mass.

REFERENCES

1. ACOG. ACOG Technical Bulletin: Gynecologic Ultrasonography. Number 215. Washington, DC: American College of Obstetrics and Gynecology, November, 1995.
2. ACOG. ACOG Technical Bulletin: Uterine Leiomyomata. Number 192. American College of Obstetrics and Gynecology, May, 1994.
3. Adelson MD, Adelson KL. Miscellaneous benign disorders of the upper genital tract. In: Copeland L, ed. Textbook of Gynecology. Philadelphia: WB Saunders; 1993:857–870.
4. Alpern MB, Sandler MA, Madrazo BL. Sonographic features of parovarian cysts and their complications. Am J Roentgenol. 1984; 143:157–160.
5. Athey PA. Adnexa: Nonneoplastic cysts. In: Athey PA, Hadlock FP, eds. Ultrasound in Obstetrics and Gynecology. 2nd ed. St. Louis: CV Mosby; 1985: 206–221.
6. Athey PA, Cooper NB. Sonographic features of parovarian cysts. Am J Roentgenol. 1985; 144:83–86.
7. Athey PA, Malone RS. Sonography of ovarian fibromas/thecomas. J Ultrasound Med. 1987; 6:431–436.
8. Athey PA, Siegel MF. Sonographic features of Brenner tumor of the ovary. J Ultrasound Med. 1987; 6:367–372.
9. Baltarowich OH, Kurtz AB, Pasto ME, et al. The spectrum of sonographic findings in hemorrhagic ovarian cysts. Am J Roentgenol. 1987; 148:901–905.
10. Baltarowich OH, Kurtz AB, Pennell RG, et al. Pitfalls in the sonographic diagnosis of uterine fibroids. Am J Roentgenol. 1988; 151:725–728.
11. Berland LL, et al. Ultrasound evaluation of pelvic infections. Radiol Clin North Am. 1982; 20:367.
12. Blumenfeld M, Zuspan FP. Benign pelvic masses. In: Iams JD, Zuspan FP, eds. Zuspan & Quilligan's Manual of Obstetrics and Gynecology. 2nd ed. St. Louis: CV Mosby, 1990.
13. Bohlman ME, Ensor RE, Sanders RC. Sonographic findings in adenomyosis of the uterus. Am J Roentgenol. 1987; 148:765–766.
14. Bornstein J, Auslender R, Pascal B, et al. Diagnostic pitfalls of ultrasonographic uterine screening in women treated with tamoxifen. J Reprod Med. 1994; 39:674–678.
15. Bourne TH, Lawton F, Leather A, et al. Use of intracavity saline instillation and transvaginal ultrasonography to detect tamoxifen-associated endometrial polyps. Ultrasound in Obstetrics and Gynecology. 1994; 4:73–75.
16. Coleman BG. Transvaginal sonography of adnexal masses. Radiol Clin North Am. 1992; 30:677–691.
17. Cullinan JA, Fleischer AC, Kepple DM, et al. Sonohysterography: A technique for endometrial evaluation. Radiographics. 1995; 15:510–514.
18. Czernobilsky B. Common epithelial tumors of the ovary. In: Kurman RJ, ed. Blaustein's Pathology of the Female Genital Tract. 3rd ed. New York: Springer-Verlag; 1987:560–606.
19. Diakoumakis E, Vieux U, Seife B. Sonographic demonstration of thecoma: Report of two cases. Am J Obstet Gynecol. 1984; 150:787–788.

20. Droegemueller W, Herbst AL, Mishell DR, et al. Comprehensive Gynecology. St. Louis: CV Mosby; 1987.

21. Dudiak CM, Turner DA, Patel SK, et al. Uterine leiomyomas in the infertile patient: Preoperative localization with MR imaging versus US and hysterosalpingography. Radiology. 1988; 176:627–630.

22. Fleischer AC. Gynecologic sonography. In: Fleischer AC, James AE, eds. Diagnostic Sonography: Principles and Clinical Applications. Philadelphia: WB Saunders; 1989:221–340.

23. Fleischer AC, Shah DM, Entman SS. Sonographic evaluation of maternal disorders during pregnancy. In: Fleischer AC, Romero R, Manning FA, Jeanty P, James AE, eds. The Principles and Practice of Ultrasonography in Obstetrics and Gynecology. Norwalk, CT: Appleton & Lange; 1991:521–528.

24. Fleischer AC, Entman S, Gordon A. Transvaginal and transabdominal ultrasound of pelvic masses. J Ultrasound Med Biol. 1989; 15:529–533.

25. Fleischer AC, Stein SM, Cullinan JA, et al. Color Doppler sonography of adnexal torsion. J Ultrasound Med. 1995; 14:523–528.

26. Fogel SR, Slaskey BS. Sonography of nabothian cysts. Am J Roentgenol. 1982; 138:927.

27. Freimanis MG, Jones AF. Transvaginal ultrasonography. Radiol Clin North Am. 1992; 30:955–976.

28. Goldstein SR, Subramanyam B, Snyder JR, et al. The postmenopausal cystic adnexal mass: The potential role of ultrasound in conservative management. Obstet Gynecol. 1989; 73:8–10.

29. Goldstein SR. Unusual ultrasonographic appearance of the uterus in patients receiving tamoxifen. Am J Obstet Gynecol. 1994; 170:447–451.

30. Goldstein SR, Schwartz L, Snyder JR, et al. Screening and monitoring endometrial response to tamoxifen therapy for breast cancer. J Ultrasound Med. 1996; 15:S1–S117.

31. Gompel C, Silverberg SG. Pathology in Gynecology and Obstetrics. 3rd ed. Philadelphia: JB Lippincott; 1985.

32. Graif M, Itzchak Y. Sonographic evaluation of ovarian torsion in childhood and adolescence. Am J Roentgenol. 1988; 150:647–649.

33. Graif M, Shalev J, Strauss S, et al. Torsion of the ovary: Sonographic features. Am J Roentgenol. 1984; 143:1331–1334.

34. Gross BH, Siver TM, Jaffe MH. Sonographic features of uterine leiomyomas: Analysis of 41 proven cases. J Ultrasound Med. 1983; 2:401–406.

35. Gutman PH Jr. In search of the elusive benign cystic ovarian teratoma: Application of the ultrasound "tip of the iceberg" sign. J Clin Ultrasound. 1977; 5:403–406.

36. Hale RW, Krieger J, eds. Gynecology: A Concise Textbook. Garden City, NY: Medical Examination Publishing Co; 1983.

37. Hall DA. Sonographic appearance of the normal ovary, of polycystic ovary disease and of functional ovarian cysts. Semin Ultrasound. 1983; 4:149–165.

38. Hall DA, Hann LE. Gynecologic radiology: Benign disorders. In: Taveras JM, Ferrucci JT, eds. Radiology: Diagnosis–Imaging–Intervention (vol. 4). Philadelphia: JB Lippincott; 1988:1–9.

39. Hall DA, McCarthy KA. The significance of the postmenopausal simple adnexal cyst. J Ultrasound Med. 1986; 5:503–505.

40. Hann LE, Hall DA, McArdle CR, et al. Polycystic ovarian disease: Sonographic spectrum. Radiology. 1984; 150:531–534.

41. Herrmann UJ, Locher GW, Goldhirsch A. Sonographic patterns of ovarian tumors: Prediction of malignancy. Obstet Gynecol. 1987; 69:777–781.

42. Iams JD, Johnson FF, Sonek J, et al. Cervical competence as a continuum: A study of ultrasonographic cervical length and obstetric performance. Am J Obstet Gynecol. 1995; 172:1097–1106.

43. Iams JD, Goldenberg RL, Meis PJ, et al. The length of the cervix and the risk of spontaneous premature delivery. N Engl J Med. 1996; 334:567–572.

44. Jones HW, Jones GS. Novak's Textbook of Gynecology. Baltimore: Williams & Wilkins; 1981.

45. Koonings PP, Campbell K, Mishell DR, Grimes DA. Relative frequency of primary ovarian neoplasms: A 10 year review. Obstet Gynecol. 1989; 74:921.

46. Lenz S. Ultrasonic study of follicular maturation, ovulation and development of corpus luteum during normal menstrual cycles. Acta Obstet Gynecol Scand. 1985; 64:15–19.

47. Leopold GR. Pelvic ultrasonography. In: Sarti DA, ed. Diagnostic Ultrasound: Text and Cases. Chicago: Year Book Medical Publishers; 1987:692–695.

48. Lev-Toaff AS, Coleman BG, Arger PH, et al. Leiomyomas in pregnancy: Sonographic study. Radiology. 1987; 164:375–380.

49. Mangan CE, Borrow L, Burtnett-Rubin MM, et al. Pregnancy outcome in 98 women exposed to diethylstilbestrol in utero, their mothers, and unexposed siblings. Obstet Gynecol. 1982; 59:315–319.

50. Meire HB, Farrant P, Guha T. Distinction of benign from malignant ovarian cysts by ultrasound. Br J Obstet Gynaecol. 1978; 85:893–899.

51. Michaels WH, Montgomery C, Karo J, et al. Ultrasound differentiation of the competent from the incompetent cervix: Prevention of preterm delivery. Am J Obstet Gynecol. 1986; 154:537–546.

52. Michaels WH, Thompson HO, Schreiber FR, et al. Ultrasound surveillance of the cervix during pregnancy in diethylstilbestrol-exposed offspring. Obstet Gynecol. 1989; 79:230–238.

53. Mitchell DG, Mintz MC, Spritzer CE, et al. Adnexal

masses: MR imaging observations at 1.5 T, with US and CT correlation. Radiology. 1987; 162:319–324.

54. Montz FJ, Schlaerth B, Morrow CP. The natural history of theca lutein cysts. Obstet Gynecol. 1988; 72:247–251.

55. Morley P, Barnett E. The ovarian mass. In: Sanders RC, James AE, eds. The Principles and Practice of Ultrasonography in Obstetrics and Gynecology. 2nd ed. Norwalk, CT: Appleton-Century-Crofts; 1980:357.

56. Moyle JW, Rochester D, Sider L, et al. Sonography of ovarian tumors: Predictability of tumor type. Am J Roentgenol. 1983; 14:985–991.

57. Neiman HL, Mendelson EB. Ultrasound evaluation of the ovary. In: Callen PW, ed. Ultrasonography in Obstetrics and Gynecology. 2nd ed. Philadelphia: WB Saunders; 1988:423–447.

58. Novak ER, Woodruff JD, eds. Novak's Gynecologic and Obstetric Pathology. 8th ed. Philadelphia: WB Saunders; 1979.

59. Nunley WC, Pope TL. Upper reproductive tract radiography findings. Am J Roentgenol. 1984; 142: 337–339.

60. Odwin C. Sonographic appearance of a vaginal contraceptive sponge. J Diagn Med Sonogr. 1985; 1:65–67.

61. Parker WH, Berek JS. Management of selected cystic adnexal masses in postmenopausal women by operative laparoscopy: A pilot study. Am J Obstet Gynecol. 1990; 163:1574.

62. Parsons AK, Lense JJ. Sonohysterography for endometrial abnormalities: Preliminary results. J. Clin Ultrasound. 1993; 21:87–95.

63. Peckham B, Shapiro S. Signs and Symptoms in Gynecology. Philadelphia: JB Lippincott; 1983.

64. Pinotti JA, Marussi EF, Zeferino LC. Evolution of cystic and adnexal tumors identified by echography. Int J Gynaecol Obstet. 1988; 26:109–114.

65. Reynolds T, Hill MC, Glassman LM. Sonography of hemorrhagic ovarian cysts. J Clin Ultrasound. 1986; 14:449–453.

66. Romero R, Mazor M, Gomez R, et al. Cervix, incompetence and premature labor. The Fetus. 1993; 3(1):1–10.

67. Rubin C, Kurtz AB, Goldberg BB. A new ultrasound technique in defining pelvic anatomy. J Clin Ultrasound. 1978; 6:28–33.

68. Sabbagha R, ed. Diagnostic Ultrasound Applied to Obstetrics and Gynecology. 2nd ed. Philadelphia: JB Lippincott; 1987:480–482.

69. Sanders R, James AE, eds. Principles and Practice of Ultrasonography in Obstetrics and Gynecology. 3rd ed. New York: Appleton-Century-Crofts. 1985.

70. Schoenfeld A, Levavi H, Hirsch M, et al. Transvaginal sonography in postmenopausal women. J Clin Ultrasound. 1990; 18:350.

71. Schwartz LB, Seifer DB. Diagnostic imaging of adnexal masses: A review. J Reprod Med. 1992; 37:63–71.

72. Siedler D, Laing FC, Jeffrey RB Jr, Wing VW. Uterine adenomyosis: A difficult sonographic diagnosis. J Ultrasound Med. 1987; 6:345–349.

73. Sohaey R, Gardner TL, Woodward PJ, et al. Sonographic diagnosis of peritoneal inclusion cysts. J Ultrasound Med. 1995; 14:913–917.

74. Stillman RJ. In utero exposure to diethylstilbestrol: Adverse effects on the reproductive tract and reproductive performance in male and female offspring. Am J Obstet Gynecol. 1988; 142:905–920.

75. Swanson M, Sauerbrei EE, Cooperberg PL. Medical implications of ultrasonically detected polycystic ovaries. J Clin Ultrasound. 1981; 9:219–222.

76. Syrop CH, Sahakian V. Transvaginal sonographic detection of endometrial polyps with fluid contrast augmentation. Obstet Gynecol. 1992; 79:1041–1043.

77. Thornton JG, Wells M. Ovarian cysts in pregnancy: Does ultrasound make traditional management inappropriate? Obstet Gynecol. 1987; 69:717–721.

78. Timor-Tritsch IE, Rottem S. Transvaginal Sonography. New York: Elsevier; 1988.

79. Timor-Tritsch IE, Rottem S, Thaler I. Review of transvaginal ultrasonography: A description with clinical application. Ultrasound Quarterly. 1988; 6:1–34.

80. Togashi K, Ozasa H, Konishi I, et al. Enlarged uterus: Differentiation between adenomyosis and leiomyoma with MR imaging. Radiology. 1989; 171:531–534.

81. Viscomi GN, Gonzalez R, Taylor KJW. Ultrasound detection of uterine anomalies. Radiology. 1980; 136:733.

82. Walsh JW, Taylor KJW, Rosenfield AT. Gray scale ultrasonography in the diagnosis of endometriosis and adenomyosis. Am J Roentgenol. 1979; 132:87–90.

83. Webster's New Collegiate Dictionary. Springfield, MA: G & C Merriam; 1976.

84. Weinreb JC, Brown CE, Lowe TW, et al. Pelvic masses in pregnant patients: MR and US imaging. Radiology. 1986; 159:717–724.

85. Williams CO. Radiologic seminars CL XXXIV: Brenner tumor of the ovary—ultrasound findings. J Miss State Med Assoc. 1978; 19:168.

86. Woodburne RT, Buricel WE. Essentials of Human Anatomy. New York: Oxford; 1994.

87. Yaghoobian J, Pinck RL. Ultrasound findings in thecoma of the ovary. J Clin Ultrasound. 1983; 11:91–93.

88. Young RH, Scully RE. Sex cord-stromal, steroid cell, and other ovarian tumors with endocrine, paraendocrine and paraneoplastic manifestations. In: Kurman RJ, ed. Blaustein's Pathology of the Female Genital Tract. 3rd ed. New York: Springer-Verlag; 1987:607–658.

Malignant Diseases of the Uterus and Cervix

RUTH ROSENBLATT and ROSALYN KUTCHER

The uterus is the most common site of pelvic malignancy, accounting for 8% of cancers diagnosed in women.[2] A number of pathologically and clinically distinct lesions are encountered. Three of these are discussed here: endometrial carcinoma, carcinoma of the cervix, and gestational trophoblastic neoplasia.

A reversal in the incidence of carcinoma of the endometrium and cervix has been observed in the past several decades. Carcinoma of the endometrium has become statistically more significant, being twice as common now as carcinoma of the cervix. This is due in part to better control of carcinoma of the cervix as a result of early diagnosis by means of the Papanicolaou (Pap) smear. Furthermore, endometrial carcinoma occurs later in life than carcinoma of the cervix, and the increase in normal life spans undoubtedly has a bearing on the increasing incidence of endometrial carcinoma.

Mortality from carcinoma of the endometrium is also currently equal to that of carcinoma of the cervix.[2] This reflects the general aging of our population, patterns of postmenopausal estrogen use, and the widespread use and effectiveness of Pap smear screening.

The role of ultrasound in the diagnosis and management of carcinoma of the uterus and cervix has been expanding. Morphologic changes produced by endometrial carcinoma may be observed with ultrasound. Intracavitary transducers (trans-vaginal and endorectal) may further improve visualization of the regional anatomy, providing information that can aid in staging of endometrial and cervical malignancies. A sonohysterogram, the instillation of sterile saline into the endometrial cavity monitored with transvaginal sonography, can often elucidate the etiology of endometrial thickening.[11] Color and pulsed Doppler evaluation of uterine endometrial and myometrial blood flow is also a helpful adjunct to routine gynecologic ultrasonography.[1]

Endometrial Carcinoma

CLINICAL INFORMATION

Epidemiology and Risk Factors

In the United States, endometrial carcinoma is the most commonly encountered malignancy of the female genital tract. About three quarters of the patients are diagnosed and treated at a relatively early stage, and an overall 5-year cure rate of close to 85% in the white and 56% in the African-American population may be attained.[2] Carcinoma of the endometrium is seen frequently in the clinical setting of obesity, hypertension, diabetes, and, it is claimed, short stature. It is also more common among Jewish women, suggesting some genetic predisposition.[26]

There is evidence to suggest a relationship between elevated estrogen levels in perimenopausal and postmenopausal patients and the development of endometrial carcinoma.[22] Estrogen has a proliferative effect on the endometrium. A number of premenopausal conditions, probably related to estrogen imbalance, place some women at higher risk for development of carcinoma of the endometrium at a later time. These include dysfunctional uterine bleeding with failure of ovulation, adenomatous hyperplasia of the endometrium, and polycystic ovaries (Stein-Leventhal syndrome). In the perimenopausal and postmenopausal age group, the presence of a functioning theca-granulosa cell tumor of the ovary (usually estrogen-producing) is associated with an increased incidence of endometrial carcinoma.[33] Prolonged intake of therapeutic estrogen after menopause, which some women take to alleviate postmenopausal symptoms, including osteoporosis, has been implicated as a risk factor.[22] Tamoxifen, a nonsteroidal antiestrogen, is currently the most widely prescribed antineoplastic agent in the United States for the treatment of breast cancer, especially those cases that are estrogen receptor positive. It has, however, an estrogen agonist effect on the endometrium, and therefore a small but definite risk for carcinoma development exists, requiring careful interval monitoring.[14]

Pathophysiology

On gross examination, endometrial carcinoma may be exophytic and polypoid, sometimes filling the uterine cavity. Growth toward the myometrium is superficial at first, but deep myometrial infiltration may develop. Uterine enlargement is often, but not always, present. Myometrial infiltration is more apt to occur with poorly differentiated tumors and is associated with an increased incidence of lymph node metastases and a poorer prognosis. Spread to the cervix is an important criterion for tumor staging. In late stages, transmural spread of tumor to the adnexa occurs. Another route for pelvic extension is retrograde, toward the fallopian tubes and ovaries. Distant metastases occur through the pelvic lymphatics, eventually involving retroperitoneal lymph nodes. Histologically, endometrial carcinoma is classified into grades 1 through 3, depending on the degree of tumor differentiation. This histologic classification is distinct from the staging of the disease, which is based on extent of tumor spread. Current International Federation of Gynecologists and Obstetricians (FIGO) staging for endometrial

carcinoma is based on both surgical and pathologic findings (Table 8-1). Both tumor grade and stage influence treatment.[9,10]

Clinical Diagnosis

Carcinoma of the endometrium is usually diagnosed in the sixth or seventh decade and the principal presenting symptom is abnormal bleeding or discharge. Pain may also occur because of uterine distention resulting from intracavity bleeding associated with cervical blockage. Symptoms of postmenopausal pelvic inflammatory disease may occur secondary to tumor necrosis and superinfection. Dilation and curettage and endometrial biopsy provide the tissue necessary to confirm the diagnosis of endometrial carcinoma. Important diagnostic features in staging the disease include depth of myometrial invasion; involvement of the cervix; spread to the tubes, ovaries, or pelvic lymph nodes; and distant metastases (see Table 8-1).

Treatment

Carcinoma of the endometrium is treated by total abdominal hysterectomy and bilateral salpingo-oophorectomy. Depending on tumor grade and

 TABLE 8-1. SURGICAL–PATHOLOGIC STAGING OF ENDOMETRIAL CARCINOMA[10]

Stage I*
  A: Tumor limited to endometrium
  B: Invasion to $< \frac{1}{2}$ myometrium
  C: Invasion to $> \frac{1}{2}$ myometrium
Stage II*
  A: Endocervical glandular involvement only
  B: Cervical stromal invasion
Stage III*
  A: Tumor invades serosa or adnexa, or positive peritoneal cytology
  B: Vaginal metastases
  C: Metastases to pelvic or paraaortic lymph nodes
Stage IV*
  A: Tumor invades bladder or bowel mucosa
  B: Distant metastases, including intraabdominal or inguinal lymphatics

---

*Pathologic stages
  G1: Highly differentiated adenomatous carcinomas
  G2: Differentiated adenomatous carcinomas with partly solid areas
  G3: Predominantly solid or entirely undifferentiated carcinomas
(Adapted from the International Federation of Gynecologists and Obstetricians [FIGO] Cancer Committee Report, Rio de Janeiro, Brazil, October, 1989.)

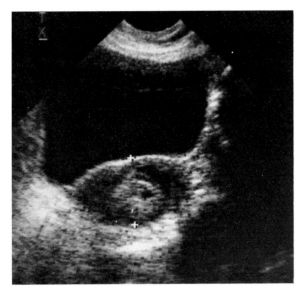

Figure 8-1. Stage I endometrial carcinoma. The 60-year-old patient experienced postmenopausal bleeding. A transverse view of the enlarged uterus demonstrates irregular thickening of the endometrium and fluid collections in the endometrial cavity representing blood and tissue necrosis.

stage, selective pelvic and paraaortic lymphadenectomy is performed. Radiation therapy is frequently added before or after surgery. In more advanced cases, preoperative intrauterine radium therapy is sometimes used.[33] Treatment of stage IV disease is individualized and may include hormonal therapy or chemotherapy. The 5-year survival statistics range from 10% to 75%, depending on the stage of disease at the time of diagnosis.[9,10] Both incidence and mortality rates are higher among African Americans than among whites.[2]

SONOGRAPHIC IMAGING

Diagnostic Features

For patients with abnormal uterine bleeding, pelvic ultrasound is often the initial study. The uterus may appear entirely normal sonographically in the early stage of endometrial carcinoma.[30] In most cases, however, some change in the size, shape, and acoustic texture of the uterus is observed. A common finding is increased uterine size, either in length or anteroposterior diameter. In the absence of fibroids, a postmenopausal uterus should not exceed 7 cm in length and 2 cm in anteroposterior

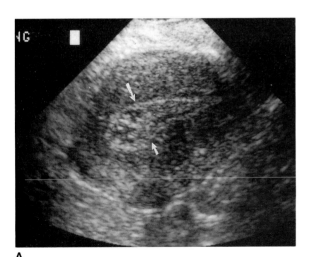

A

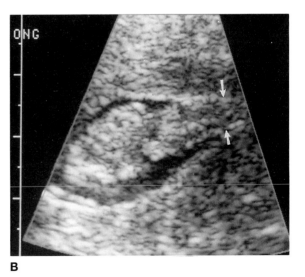

B

Figure 8-2. A 60-year-old patient, 17 years postmenopausal, with onset of bleeding. (**A**) Transvaginal sonogram shows thickened endometrium (*arrows*). (**B**) Sonohysterogram demonstrates large polyp with narrow stalk (*arrows*) projecting from anterior endometrium; surrounding endometrium is thin.

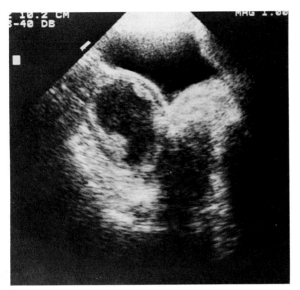

Figure 8-3. Stage I endometrial carcinoma with cervical stenosis. The 91-year-old patient had abdominal pain. The sagittal scan of the pelvis shows hematometra. Note the echogenic fluid and nodular endometrial surface. (Courtesy of Janet Hoffman and Flora Mincer, Albert Einstein College of Medicine, Bronx, NY.)

dimension. A bulbous or lobulated uterine contour may also be present.[8,30] When seen in a postmenopausal woman, a more suspect finding is thickening of the endometrial lining (exceeding 5 to 6 mm; Fig. 8-1). Patterns of endometrial thickening are used to differentiate endometrial hyperplasia, polyps, and carcinoma, the latter demonstrating a more heterogeneous appearance.[20] The instillation of sterile saline into the endometrial cavity resulting in a sonohysterogram may further differentiate a polyp extending into and filling the endometrial cavity from smooth or irregular endometrial thickening. A submucosal leiomyoma may also be differentiated from an endometrial lesion such as a polyp[11] (Fig. 8-2). Fluid distention of the cavity may occur naturally with endocervical occlusion by tumor or stenosis (Fig. 8-3).

Sonographic imaging is of use in staging endometrial carcinoma and determining myometrial extension after the diagnosis has been made histologically. Accurate staging is an important guide to successful management of the disease. For example, if an imaging test suggests myometrial extension (which increases the likelihood of lymphatic involvement), the patient may receive preoperative radiation therapy.

Detailed analysis of the endometrial lining and the subendometrial hypoechoic halo (which corresponds in location to the compact vascular inner myometrial segment) may provide a clue to the presence or extent of myometrial invasion (Fig. 8-4). In a study of 20 cases of endometrial carcinoma, sonographic analysis of the degree of myometrial involvement was accurate within 10% in 14 of 20 cases.[15] It has been suggested that preservation of the subendometrial halo in the presence of endometrial carcinoma would imply superficial involvement only. In many cases, transvaginal scanning facilitates the detailed study of endometrial and myometrial texture (Fig. 8-5). In addition, color and pulsed Doppler sonography can be used to evaluate blood flow to the endometrium and myometrium. In a transvaginal study, patients with endometrial carcinoma were found to have greater myometrial vascularity and higher diastolic flow, leading to lower resistive (RI) and pulsatility indices (PI) when these vessels were visualized and a Doppler spectral pattern obtained. However, other studies suggest overlap of RI and PI in endometrial carcinoma with those obtained in benign disease. Doppler findings are therefore not considered statistically reliable.[1,31] Intrauterine radial scanning has also been advocated as an accurate means of de-

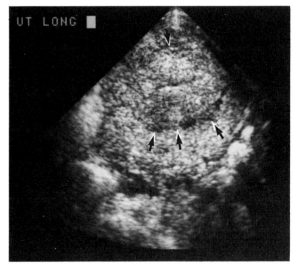

Figure 8-4. Stage I endometrial carcinoma. The 80-year-old patient reported vaginal bleeding. The longitudinal view of the uterus using the transvaginal probe shows marked thickening of endometrium (to 50% of the total uterine thickness). Note the partially visualized sonolucent subendometrial halo (*arrows*).

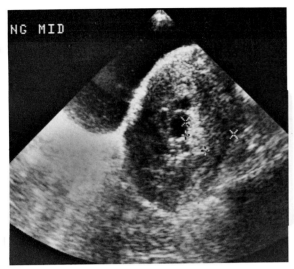

Figure 8-5. *Stage I endometrial carcinoma with myometrial invasion. A 79-year-old woman had vaginal bleeding and a history of breast carcinoma. The sagittal transvaginal view of the uterus demonstrated an irregularly thickened endometrial reflection measuring 11 mm (between cursors), suggesting myometrial extension of tumor.*

termining extent of myometrial invasion by tumor.[25] This procedure, which requires dilation of the cervix and insertion of a high-frequency sterile transducer into the uterus is, of course, more invasive, requiring anesthesia, and it is not likely to be used routinely. Myometrial tumor invasion may be hypoechoic or hyperechoic. The increased echogenicity may be related to a more differentiated, mucin-producing lesion, whereas the hypoechoic areas may indicate zones of necrosis or evidence of an anaplastic lesion that does not form glandular elements.[15]

Ultrasound has a useful role in helping to distinguish carcinoma confined to the uterus (stage I or II) from carcinoma extending beyond the uterus (stage III or IV). Presence of a mass adjacent to the uterus may represent direct extension, metastases to the ovary, lymph node enlargement, or a coincidental ovarian mass. Attention to the uterine cervix, especially to expansion greater than 2 or 3 cm in diameter, and a heterogeneous sonographic pattern may also separate stage I from stage II disease (see Table 8-1). If the urinary bladder is involved with tumor, ureteral obstruction is likely to be present. The kidneys should be scanned for evidence of hydronephrosis.

A potential but not universally used role of ul-

trasound in treatment planning is the delineation and assessment of endometrial length.[17] When intracavitary radiation therapy is contemplated, this information is valuable in facilitating the selection of an appropriate applicator (Fig. 8-6). Proper placement of the applicator can be monitored with ultrasound, and the scan also provides spatial relationships that allow calculation of the radiation dose to the surrounding tissue and bladder wall (see Fig. 8-6).

Although pelvic ultrasound may be used to monitor treated patients for recurrent disease, computed tomography (CT) is more commonly used because it affords better definition of pelvic sidewalls and retroperitoneal anatomy.

Technique and Protocol

A systematic sonographic examination of the pelvis with special attention to the uterus should include a number of key points. The uterus should be depicted in its long axis (which is not necessarily parallel to the long axis of the patient). The dimension from the fundus to and including the cervix should be measured. Insertion of a tampon or Foley cathe-

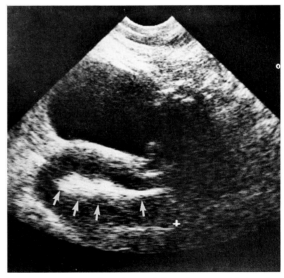

Figure 8-6. *Stage II endometrial carcinoma with involvement of the cervix. The 61-year-old patient presented with bleeding. Patient had preoperative radiation therapy with intracavitary tandem. Sagittal scan of the uterus demonstrates a high-amplitude reflection from the endometrium representing the tandem and the endometrial thickening (arrows). Study was done to monitor position of the tandem before insertion of radioactive sources.*

ter (with balloon inflated) into the vagina before scanning helps to identify the cervix. The sonographer should observe the cervix for changes in size and echogenicity if endometrial carcinoma is suspected. Overall thickness of the uterus is measured in the anteroposterior axis.

It is important to identify the endometrial lining, which represents the endometrial canal. Endometrial thickening, if present, may be expressed as a percentage of total myometrial thickness by dividing the thickness of the thickest portion of the endometrium (from the lumen to the margin) by the myometrial wall thickness and multiplying by 100 (see Fig. 8-4). This represents the half-layer endometrial thickness. Endometrial full thickness can also be measured as an absolute value, referring to current measurement guidelines depending on patient age and menopausal status. Endometrial lining thickness should be obtained on the midline longitudinal image of the uterus. The sonographer should note whether the myometrial echoes are homogeneous or heterogeneous. The pattern of endometrial and myometrial vascularity should be observed with color Doppler. Spectral analysis of arcuate branches of the uterine arteries and any abnormal vascularity should be documented, and RIs and PIs obtained.

Attention should then be focused on the adnexal region, to identify the ovaries and any adnexal masses. The presence of pelvic or abdominal ascites should be noted.

Whenever sonographic findings in the pelvis suggest a neoplasm, the examination should be extended to the liver and other abdominal viscera to search for possible metastases. In addition, the para-aortic and paracaval areas should be scanned to search for adenopathy. Finally, the kidneys should be imaged to document the presence or absence of hydronephrosis.

OTHER IMAGING MODALITIES

Computed tomography is most useful for determining the extent of tumor inside and outside the pelvis of patients who have stage III or IV disease. Enlarged retroperitoneal lymph nodes, urinary tract obstruction, and liver metastases are readily visualized.[5]

The advantages of magnetic resonance imaging (MRI) of the pelvis lie in the ability to provide sagittal, coronal, and transverse images and to display intrinsic tissue contrast of fat, bowel gas, bone, and blood vessels. These factors contribute to good anatomic resolution of the pelvis and its contents. Furthermore, obesity is not an impediment to MRI. (Patients with endometrial carcinoma frequently are obese.) The origin of a mass can be assigned to the appropriate organ with reasonable accuracy. The ability of MRI to resolve different layers of the uterus (e.g., endometrium and myometrium separated by the junctional zone) has made it a valuable tool for assessing the presence and degree of myometrial invasion by tumor.[19] In a study of 40 patients, contrast-enhanced MRI was found to be significantly more accurate than transvaginal sonography in assessing the depth of myometrial invasion.[37] The reported accuracy of MRI in detecting cervical invasion is 85% to 90%.[26]

DIFFERENTIAL DIAGNOSIS

Prominence and thickening of the endometrial layer seen on ultrasound are not specific signs of endometrial carcinoma. The differential diagnosis includes endometrial hyperplasia, which may be a precursor to carcinoma in some cases. Endometrial polyps may also increase echogenicity, as may secretions or blood in the endometrial cavity. In postmenopausal women, all of these conditions are likely to be accompanied by abnormal bleeding and would, in most cases, call for curettage. The most common cause of uterine enlargement is leiomyoma (fibroid); therefore, an enlarged, bulbous or lobulated uterus associated with abnormal bleeding does not necessarily imply endometrial carcinoma but could be due to fibroids, either alone or associated with endometrial carcinoma. Fibroids can also distort the endometrial lining, making it difficult to appreciate any endometrial thickening. The recent advances in sonographic endometrial analysis and the use of the sonohysterogram have improved the sonographer's ability to differentiate these pathologic conditions (see Fig. 8-3). Hematometra and pyometra may also be secondary to cervical carcinoma or cervical stenosis. When endometrial carcinoma extends to the cervix, it may resemble primary cervical carcinoma sonographically.

LEIOMYOSARCOMA

Leiomyosarcoma is a rare malignancy, accounting for only 3% of uterine tumors. This lesion is derived from smooth muscle in the wall of the uterus. It is believed to arise from preexisting leiomyoma. The diagnosis of leiomyosarcoma may be suspected when a fibroid undergoes a growth spurt (rather than regression) in a perimenopausal or postmenopausal patient. The lesion is rarely diagnosed before surgery. Sonographically, leiomyosarcoma may be indistinguishable from the leiomyoma, especially when cystic degeneration is present.

Carcinoma of the Cervix

CLINICAL INFORMATION

Epidemiology and Risk Factors

Carcinoma of the cervix accounts for 6% of malignancies of women. Its incidence is about half that of carcinoma of the endometrium. In the past few decades, a decrease in the incidence of invasive carcinoma of the cervix has been observed. This trend is due largely to the increased availability of the Pap test. Unlike the ovary, which by virtue of its location deep in the pelvis often is not amenable to early clinical diagnosis of malignancy, the cervix is easily accessible to visual inspection and palpation in the course of a gynecologic examination. As a result, there has been an increase in the diagnosis of early carcinoma (carcinoma in situ). The availability of cytologic screening has led to a reduction in mortality.

Epidemiologic studies suggest a number of individual risk factors for carcinoma of the cervix, of which the most consistent are early sexual activity, multiple sex partners, and human papillomavirus infection.[3] Cancer of the cervix develops at an earlier age in India, where early marriage has been customary. Conversely, the disease is virtually unknown among celibate women. In the United States, the disease is more prevalent among the Puerto Rican and African-American populations and least common among Jewish women. This ethnic variation has led some authors to speculate on the possible significance of coitus with uncircumcised men. It has been suggested that secretions contained in the smegma of uncircumcised men constitute an irritant to the cervical mucosa and promote cancer in susceptible women.[22]

The incidence of adenocarcinoma of the cervix and vagina is increased among women who were exposed to diethylstilbestrol in utero. This drug was used during the 1940s and 1950s to support pregnancy for habitual aborters.

Pathophysiology

Two types of cells form the lining of the cervix. The mucosal covering of the lower cervix is squamous epithelium, which gives rise to squamous carcinoma and accounts for 90% to 95% of lesions. The cervical canal (endocervix) is lined with columnar epithelium, which may give rise to adenocarcinoma. The junction between the two types of epithelium, the squamocolumnar junction, is the site of active mitotic activity, or squamous metaplasia. Cervical cancer invariably arises at this junction, initially as carcinoma in situ. The concept that has been proposed is that this site of physiologic mitotic activity is subject to transformation into neoplastic growth by exposure to external carcinogens.

Initially, the carcinoma is confined to the cervix and may form a superficial ulcerating mass with bulky expansion of the cervix. The lesion spreads locally to involve the vagina, upper cervix, and parametria, and may spread to neighboring structures such as bladder and rectum. A clinical staging system proposed by FIGO provides criteria for staging of the disease (Table 8-2).[6] Stage of disease determines the type of therapy. The cervix has a rich plexus of lymphatics that drain to the hypogastric

 TABLE 8-2. SUMMARY OF INTERNATIONAL FEDERATION OF GYNECOLOGISTS AND OBSTETRICIANS (FIGO) CERVICAL CANCER STAGING/CLINICAL FINDINGS*

Stage 0	Carcinoma in situ
Stage I	Confined to cervix
	A: <5 mm invasion depth
	B: All other stage I
Stage II	Extends beyond cervix: upper two thirds of vagina or parametrial tissue
	A: No parametrial involvement
	B: Parametrial involvement
Stage III	Extends to pelvic wall or lower third of vagina or causes ureteral obstruction
	A: No pelvic wall involvement
	B: Pelvic wall involvement or ureteral obstruction
Stage IV	Extends beyond true pelvis or involves bladder or rectal mucosa
	A: Spread to adjacent organs
	B: Spread outside pelvis

* Examination under anesthesia.
(From Burghardt E. Pathology of early invasive squamous and glandular carcinoma of cervix [FIGO stage Ia]. In: Coppelson M, ed. Gynecologic Oncology. 2nd ed. New York: Churchill Livingstone; 1992: 614.)

and presacral area. Lymph node metastases occur early; nodes are involved in 15% of women with stage I disease, 28% with stage II, and 47% with stage III disease.[29]

Five-year survival has remained relatively stable over the past 20 years, averaging 80% to 90% for stage I, 75% for stage II, 35% for stage III, and 10% to 15% for stage IV.[26]

Clinical Diagnosis

Cervical cancer occurs at a younger age than carcinoma of the endometrium (mean age, 45 years). Carcinoma in situ is often diagnosed between ages 25 and 40 years.[22] The incidence of in situ carcinoma is greater than that of invasive carcinoma by 4:1.[26] Abnormal vaginal discharge and bleeding, especially after intercourse, are typical presenting symptoms. Delay in seeking medical attention after the onset of symptoms is common. In more advanced stages, symptoms of bladder irritability, low back pain from lumbosacral root involvement, and parametrial involvement may be seen. Unilateral or bilateral ureteral obstruction is invariably present in advanced disease, and the resultant uremia has been the most common cause of death from carcinoma of the cervix. The diagnosis is often suspected from the Pap smear and can be established with cervical biopsy. Colposcopy has considerable value. Physical examination helps determine the initial clinical stage. Additional methods used for staging include cystoscopy, intravenous pyelography, barium enema, lymphangiography, and chest examination. Since the mid-1980s, CT, ultrasound, and MRI have been added to the diagnostic workup.

Treatment

The type of treatment, whether primarily surgery or radiation therapy, is determined by the stage of disease. Limited surgery—excision of a cone of tissue around the cervical os—is sometimes performed in early cancers when fertility preservation is desired. A radical hysterectomy is usually performed when parametria are free of tumor (stage II or earlier).

Radiation therapy is given to patients whose disease involves the parametria and when nodal extension is likely. Intracavitary radiation therapy consists of placing radioactive sources in the uterus and the vaginal fornices, usually for 24 to 48 hours, to deliver high-intensity local radiation. Knowledge of the distance from the radiation source to sensitive adjacent organs such as bladder is crucial. Radiation dose is calculated on the basis of these distances. A metal tandem (a hollow tube) is placed into the uterine cavity while the patient is in the operating room and anesthetized. Later, the radioactive material is loaded into the tube. A sonographic survey of the uterus with the intracavitary tandem in place may be helpful in demonstrating the spatial relationship of the radioactive material to the urinary bladder and to the lesion (see Fig. 8-6).[13]

SONOGRAPHIC IMAGING

In stage I and II carcinoma of the cervix, ultrasound offers little diagnostic information because the cervix is usually of normal size and echogenicity. Occasionally, expansion of the cervix is observed (Fig. 8-7). Changes in the echogenicity of an enlarged cervix may also be observed with carcinoma. In the presence of cervical stenosis, hematometra may be noted.

Sonographic identification of the cervix may be difficult. Some authors have suggested that placing a fluid-soaked tampon in the vagina facilitates visualization of the cervix.[16] Placing an inflated Foley catheter balloon in the upper vagina is another method that has been used to aid in the identification of the cervix.[4] It is likely that a few milliliters

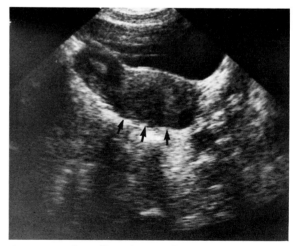

Figure 8-7. *Stage II carcinoma of the cervix with a mass extending to the upper third of the vagina. The 28-year-old patient's Pap smear was abnormal. A sagittal scan of the pelvis shows marked expansion of the cervix (arrows).*

of sterile saline placed vaginally will serve the same purpose and may help define the vaginal fornices.

Involvement of the bladder in stage IV disease may be readily appreciated with ultrasound because of the natural contrast provided by fluid in the bladder (Fig. 8-8*A,B*). Rectal involvement and parametrial infiltration are more difficult to demonstrate unless a bulky adnexal mass is present. Obstruction and dilatation of the distal ureter may, on occasion, mimic an ovarian cyst, but the identification of ipsilateral hydronephrosis usually clarifies this. The kidneys should be scanned routinely to exclude obstructive hydronephrosis, which would indicate stage III disease. Survey of the retroperitoneal nodal areas may disclose adenopathy (see Fig. 8-8*C*), and, as with any pelvic malignancy, the liver should be surveyed for possible metastases.

Reports on the use of transrectal and transvaginal sonography in staging of cervical cancer have suggested that this type of examination may facilitate staging of early lesions and be adjunctive in noting parametrial involvement.[4,21] With transrectal

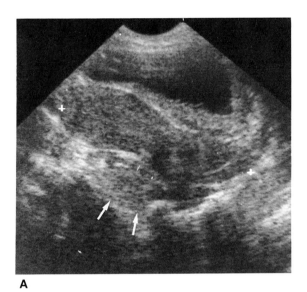

A

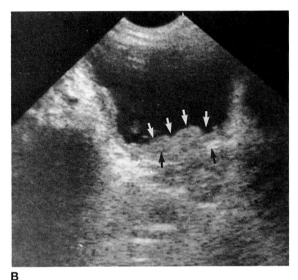

B

Figure 8-8. *Stage IV carcinoma of the cervix. The 32-year-old patient presented with intermenstrual bleeding.* (**A**) *Sagittal scan of the pelvis demonstrates enlargement of the cervix and an ill-defined mass in the cul-de-sac* (arrows). (**B**) *Transverse view shows nodularity and thickening of the posterior wall of the bladder* (arrows). (**C**) *Transverse view of the upper abdomen at the level of the splenic vein demonstrates retroperitoneal adenopathy* (arrows).

C

endosonography, high-frequency transducers scanning at close range, some through a balloon water path, provide sufficient anatomic resolution to distinguish between stage I and stage II disease and to determine depth of tumor infiltration. Although it is not possible to differentiate between a malignant and a benign mass, ultrasound can be used to guide an accurate biopsy. Transrectal and transabdominal pelvic scanning have also been reported to have benefits in treatment planning during intracavitary irradiation and in the diagnosis of recurrence.[4,21]

Conventional real-time ultrasound is used as a guide to interventional procedures in the management of patients with pelvic malignancy. For example, in the presence of bilateral ureteral obstruction, percutaneous nephrostomy is often performed using ultrasound guidance.

OTHER IMAGING MODALITIES
Computed Tomography

Because lymph node involvement is an important parameter in establishing the extent of disease, CT has become the standard imaging modality for staging cervical carcinoma, replacing lymphangiography.[23] Current CT units that provide high-resolution images of thinner sections and improved intravenous contrast techniques may improve staging accuracy. Parametrial extension is manifested by a mass or nodules extending laterally from the cervix, obliteration of fat planes, and loss of periureteral fat. CT has been shown to be more accurate in the diagnosis and staging of lesions beyond stage III, but is less accurate in differentiating stage I from stage II disease.[23] There is also an overall low accuracy rate (30% to 58%) in CT assessment of parametrial tumor invasion.[26,35] MRI with endorectal surface coils is becoming the procedure of choice in these early lesions.

Computed tomographic detection of pelvic lymph node enlargement equal to or greater than 1.5 to 2.0 cm is considered equivalent to pelvic sidewall tumor invasion, and evidence of enlarged paraaortic or inguinal lymph nodes is considered evidence of extrapelvic tumor extension. Size criteria alone, however, are not sufficiently specific or sensitive. CT has remained valuable in assessing recurrence.[35]

Magnetic Resonance Imaging

Cervical carcinomatous masses are consistently well demonstrated on MRI and appear as tumors of high signal intensity.

Parametrial invasion with tumor may be visualized as well, but significant advantages of MRI over CT in this regard are not yet clear.[24] MRI has achieved high staging accuracy rates of 76% to 83%. Invasion into paracervical tissues can be excluded with 100% specificity if a low–signal-intensity rim of cervical stroma surrounds the tumor. Parametrial spread is diagnosed by venous plexus invasion. Invasion along the sacrouterine or cardinal ligaments can also be visualized. The role of various MRI sequencing techniques and the value of gadolinium-diethylenetriamine pentaacetic acid-enhanced images in staging is still evolving.[34,36]

DIFFERENTIAL DIAGNOSIS

The main consideration in the differential diagnosis when a bulky cervix is present on ultrasound is a leiomyoma involving the lower uterine segment. Benign endometrial polyps may prolapse into the cervical canal, causing expansion of the cervix and changes in its acoustic texture. Occasionally cancer of the endometrium may involve the cervix, causing bulky expansion.

Gestational Trophoblastic Neoplasia
CLINICAL INFORMATION
Epidemiology

Gestational trophoblastic disease is a group of rare neoplasms of the uterus that occur as a complication of pregnancy or conception. These lesions include benign hydatidiform mole, invasive (but not metastasizing) mole, and choriocarcinoma, a highly malignant lesion. The reader is referred to Chapter 25 for a complete discussion of the spectrum of gestational trophoblastic disease. The present discussion focuses on invasive mole and choriocarcinoma. In approximately 20% of cases, hydatidiform mole may develop into an invasive mole. Rarely (in 3% to 5% of patients), choriocarcinoma may result, and metastases develop in 5% of these patients.[27] The highest incidence of invasive mole and choriocarcinoma is seen in Southeast Asia and the tropics, where hydatidiform mole is more common.[28]

Pathophysiology of Invasive Mole and Choriocarcinoma

The *invasive mole* is characterized by extensive proliferation of trophoblastic tissue and swollen chorionic villi. These tissue components invade the myometrium, forming hemorrhagic masses. In the case of hydatidiform mole, they distend the endometrial cavity. The focal invasion of myometrium and blood vessels may cause uterine rupture and intraperitoneal hemorrhage. Because the growth is primarily into the myometrium, diagnostic curettage may not yield tumor tissue, yet significant abnormalities may be present on ultrasound and MRI.[18]

Choriocarcinoma is also characterized by extensive proliferation of trophoblastic tissue, but, in contrast to invasive mole, no villi are present. It is possible that the absence of villi is due to their rapid destruction by the malignant tissue. Choriocarcinoma is more aggressive than invasive mole, and extension to the cervix and vagina sometimes occurs. A typical feature of the malignant behavior of choriocarcinoma is invasion of blood vessels and embolization of trophoblastic tissue to the lungs, where the tissue may obstruct the pulmonary venous circulation, causing right-sided heart failure or spread of tumor into the pulmonary arterial system. Embolization to the systemic circulation is not uncommon, accounting for tumor implants in brain, liver, and soft tissues.

Theca-lutein cysts involving one or both ovaries are frequently observed with gestational trophoblastic disease (Fig. 8-9B; see Fig. 25-2). It has been suggested that these cysts may be the result of the high levels of the β subunit of human chorionic gonadotropin (β-hCG), a hormone similar to luteinizing hormone produced by the pituitary.[22] Theca-lutein cysts may be seen in 25% of cases of trophoblastic disease. When they are present, they constitute an additional risk factor for the presence or development of postmolar trophoblastic disease.[24]

Clinical Diagnosis

Invasive mole is usually diagnosed in the setting of previous evacuation of a hydatidiform mole and persistent bleeding as well as elevation of β-hCG titers. Choriocarcinoma may be preceded by a hydatidiform mole in 50% of cases, by a normal pregnancy in 30%, and by a spontaneous abortion in 20%.[22]

Abnormal vaginal bleeding in conjunction with a pregnancy is a common presenting symptom. Often incomplete or impending abortion is suspected. Should intrauterine hemorrhage or perforation occur, the patient is likely to present in shock. The presenting symptoms (cough, hemoptysis, or neurologic disturbances) may be related to metastatic disease.

Malignant trophoblastic disease is divided into two groups: nonmetastatic and metastatic. The nonmetastatic form includes invasive mole or choriocarcinoma that is confined to the uterus. Patients with metastatic disease are classified into low-, intermediate-, or high-risk categories, depending on the duration of disease, the β-hCG titer, and the sites of the metastases.

SONOGRAPHIC IMAGING

Ultrasound appearance of invasive mole or choriocarcinoma may be indistinguishable from that of benign hydatidiform mole. The uterus is usually enlarged in both conditions. When the invasive mole is focal, echogenic masses may be noted within the myometrium (see Fig. 8-9A). Hypoechoic areas may be seen within these masses, representing hemorrhage or vascular lakes with arteriovenous shunting (see Fig. 8-9B; Fig. 8-10).[32]

Endovaginal scanning with color and spectral Doppler analysis has provided additional data, demonstrating the significant increase of tissue perfusion that is associated in many cases with gestational trophoblastic disease.[12,31] Doppler interrogation of the uterine wall and ovarian artery has demonstrated high-amplitude systolic and diastolic frequency shifts, indicating increased perfusion with low impedance to blood flow. Such increase in blood flow is also seen in normal pregnancy during the late second and early third trimester, but not in the first trimester, during which period the diagnosis of trophoblastic disease is usually made. A study reporting the use of color Doppler in the investigation of invasive trophoblastic mole has also confirmed that the vessels with high systolic and diastolic flow may be noted in the endometrial tumor and the myometrial regions of tumor invasion. The Doppler studies were repeated after treatment, and resolution of the hypervascularity usually paralleled the positive response to chemotherapy.[32] Flow abnormalities appear to correlate with the titer of the β-hCG.[7]

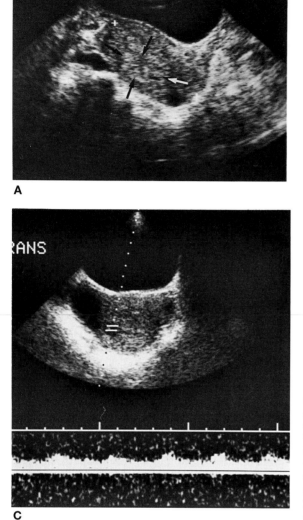

A

B

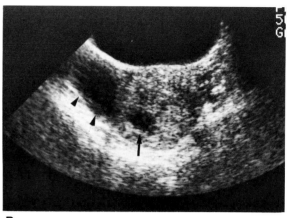

C

Figure 8-9. Choriocarcinoma in a 21-year-old woman with persistent elevation of β-hCG titer after an abortion. (**A**) Sagittal view of the pelvis shows a slightly enlarged uterus with an eccentrically situated echogenic mass (*arrows*) representing tumor tissue in the myometrium. (**B**) Transverse view of the pelvis shows a fluid collection within the uterine outline (*arrows*) and a right-sided adnexal corpus luteum cyst (*arrowheads*). (**C**) A Doppler tracing of the sonolucent zone within the uterus demonstrates pulsatile flow, suggesting the presence of arteriovenous lakes.

Associated adnexal multicystic masses representing theca-lutein cysts may be unilateral or bilateral and range in size from 4 to 10 cm (see Figs. 8-9*B* and 25-2). These cysts occur in association with the classic mole, invasive mole, and choriocarcinoma. The liver is a common site of metastases in choriocarcinoma, and it should be included in the sonographic evaluation.

OTHER IMAGING MODALITIES

Chest radiography is an important part of the evaluation and follow-up of patients diagnosed with choriocarcinoma (Fig. 8-11). CT of the chest may be necessary to find small pulmonary lesions. CT of the brain can help determine the presence of cerebral metastases.

The excellent resolution of MRI of the central nervous system as well as the pelvis and the sensitivity of MRI in detecting hemorrhage suggest that it may also become the modality of choice in evaluating the brain and the uterus.[18]

DIFFERENTIAL DIAGNOSIS

An early failed pregnancy with incomplete abortion and hydropic degeneration of the placenta may be confused with trophoblastic disease and therefore

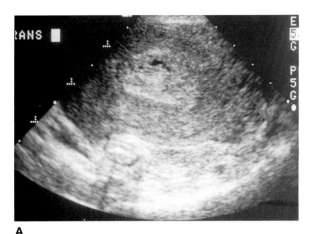

A

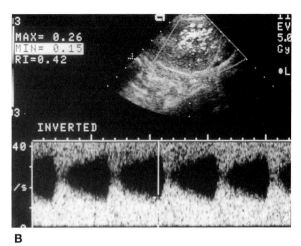

B

Figure 8-10. A 25-year-old patient, 12 weeks pregnant, presented with persistent vaginal bleeding 3 weeks after a dilatation and curettage procedure. (**A**) Transvaginal sonogram shows thickened endometrium with tiny cystic spaces. (**B**) Spectral Doppler shows increased vascularity with high diastolic flow. The patient was diagnosed as having choriocarcinoma.

should be included in the differential diagnosis. However, in this condition, the β-hCG titer is likely to be low because not only is there an absence of trophoblastic proliferation, but function of this tissue is decreased or diminished. Doppler analysis may also confirm the increased systolic and diastolic flow in this functioning tissue. Retained products of conception or a degenerating uterine fibroid with areas of hemorrhage may also produce an appear-ance of numerous small cysts within an expanded uterine outline. Intramural fibroids may resemble invasive molar tissue, especially when they are un-dergoing degeneration. Some ovarian tumors such as cystic papillary adenoma or dermoids may have a morphologic similarity to molar tissue. This source of confusion can be minimized if every at-tempt is made to search for and identify the uterus. In this regard, one of the strengths of transvaginal scanning is its ability to separate uterine from ad-nexal structures, thereby enhancing the value of the ultrasound examination.

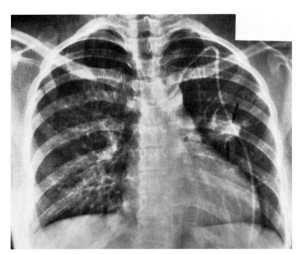

Figure 8-11. Choriocarcinoma in a 16-year-old girl with a history of previous evaluation for hydatidiform mole who presented with hemoptysis. Frontal view of the chest shows a metastatic lung mass (*arrows*).

REFERENCES

1. Aleem F, Predanic M, Calame R, et al. Transvaginal color and pulsed Doppler sonography of the endo-metrium: A possible role in reducing the number of dilatation and curettage procedures. J Ultrasound Med. 1995; 14:139–145.
2. American Cancer Society. Cancer statistics 1996. CA Cancer J Clin. 1996; 46:5–29.
3. Armstrong BK, Munoz N, Bosch FX. Epidemiology of cancer of the cervix. In: Coppleson M, ed. Gyne-cologic Oncology. 2nd ed. New York: Churchill Liv-ingstone; 1992:11–29.
4. Bernaschek G, Dertinger J, Bartl W, et al. Endo-sonographic staging of carcinoma of the uterine cer-vix. Arch Gynecol. 1986; 239:21–36.
5. Boronow RC, Morrow CP, Creasmon WT, et al.

Surgical staging in endometrial CA: Clinicopathologic findings of a prospective study. Obstet Gynecol. 1984; 63:825–832.

6. Burghardt E. Pathology of early invasive squamous and glandular carcinoma of cervix (FIGO stage Ia). In: Coppleson M, ed. Gynecologic Oncology. 2nd ed. New York: Churchill Livingstone; 1992:609–629.

7. Carter J, Fowler J, Carlson J, et al. Transvaginal color flow Doppler sonography in the assessment of gestational trophoblastic disease. J Ultrasound Med. 1993; 12:595–599.

8. Chambers CB, Unis JS. Ultrasonographic evidence of uterine malignancy in the postmenopausal uterus. Am J Obstet Gynecol. 1986; 154:1194–1199.

9. Cohen CJ. Advanced (FIGO III and IV) and recurrent carcinoma of the endometrium. In: Coppleson M, ed. Gynecologic Oncology. 2nd ed. New York: Churchill Livingstone; 1992:791–800.

10. Creasman WT, Weed JC Jr. Carcinoma of endometrium (FIGO Stages I and II): Clinical features and management. In: Coppleson M, ed. Gynecologic Oncology. 2nd ed. New York: Churchill Livingstone; 1992:775–789.

11. Cullinan JA, Fleischer AC, Kepple DM, Arnold AL. Sonohysterography: A technique for endometrial evaluation. Radiographics. 1995; 15:501–514.

12. Desai RK, Desberg AL. Diagnosis of gestational trophoblastic disease: Value of endovaginal color flow Doppler sonography. Case report. Am J Roentgenol. 1991; 157:787–788.

13. De Wit JJ, Smit BJ. The role of ultrasound in the management of cervical carcinoma: A preliminary report. S Afr Med J. 1983; 64:381–383.

14. Fisher B, Constantino C, Redmond CK, et al. Endometrial cancer in tamoxifen treated breast cancer patients: Findings from the National Surgical Adjuvant Breast and Bowel Project (NASBP) B-14. J Natl Cancer Inst. 1994; 86:527–537.

15. Fleischer AC, Dudley BS, Entmann SS, et al. Myometrial invasion by endometrial carcinoma: Sonographic assessment. Radiology. 1987; 162:307–310.

16. Fleischer AC, Entman SS. Sonographic evaluation of the uterus and related disorders. In: Fleischer AC, Manning FA, Jeanty P, Romero R, eds. Sonography in Obstetrics and Gynecology—Priniples and Practice, 5th ed. Stamford, CT: Appleton & Lange; 1996:829–850.

17. Girinski T, Leclere J, Pejovic MH, et al. Prospective comparison of US and CT in evaluation of the size of the uterus: Can these methods be used for intra-cavitary treatment planning of cancer of the uterus. Int J Radiat Oncol Biol Phys. 1987; 13:789–793.

18. Hricak H, Demas BE, Braga CA, et al. Gestational trophoblastic neoplasm of the uterus: MR assessment. Radiology. 1986; 161:11–16.

19. Hricak H, Stern JL, Fisher MR, et al. Endometrial cancer staging by MR imaging. Radiology. 1987; 162:297–307.

20. Hulka CA, Hall DA, McCarthy K, et al. Endometrial polyps, hyperplasia and carcinoma in postmenopausal women: Differentiation with endovaginal sonography. Radiology. 1994; 191:755–758.

21. Innocenti P, Pulli F, Savino F, et al. Staging of cervical cancer: Reliability of transrectal US. Radiology. 1992; 185:201–205.

22. Jones HW, Jones GS. Novak's Textbook of Gynecology. 11th ed. Baltimore: Williams & Wilkins; 1988.

23. Lewis E. The use and abuse of imaging in gynecologic cancer. Cancer. 1987; 60:1993–2009.

24. Montz FJ, Schlaerth JB, Morrow CP. The natural history of theca lutein cysts. Obstet Gynecol. 1988; 72:247–251.

25. Obata A, Akamatsu N, Sekiba K. Ultrasound estimation of myometrial invasion of endometrial cancer by intrauterine radiologic scanning. J Clin Ultrasound. 1985; 13:397–404.

26. Outwater E, Kressel HY. Evaluation of gynecologic malignancy by magnetic resonance imaging. Radiol Clin North Am. 1992; 30:789–806.

27. Park WN. Pathology and classification of trophoblastic tumors. In: Coppleson M, ed. Gynecologic Oncology. New York: Churchill Livingstone; 1981: 745–756.

28. Perez C, Knapp RC, DiSaia PJ, et al. Gynecologic tumors. In: De Vita VT, Hellman S, Rosenberg SA, eds. Cancer: Principles and Practice of Oncology. Philadelphia: JB Lippincott; 1982:872–874.

29. Plentyl A, Friedman E. Lymphatic System of the Female Genitalia. Philadelphia: WB Saunders; 1971.

30. Requard K, Wicks JD, Mettler FA. Ultrasonography in the staging of endometrial adenocarcinoma. Radiology. 1981; 140:781–785.

31. Shimamato K, Sakuma S, Ishigaki T, et al. Intramural blood flow: Evaluation with color Doppler echography. Radiology. 1987; 165:683–685.

32. Taylor KJW, Schwartz PE, Kohorn EI. Gestational trophoblastic neoplasia: Diagnosis with Doppler ultrasound. Radiology. 1987; 165:445–448.

33. Thigpen JT. Approaches to the evaluation and management of endometrial carcinoma. In: Forastiere AA, ed. Gynecologic Cancer. New York: Churchill Livingstone; 1984:215–247.

34. Waggenspack GA, Amparo EG, Hannigan EV, et al. MRI of cervical carcinoma. Semin Ultrasound CT MR. 1988; 9:158–166.

35. Walsh JW. Computed tomography of gynecologic neoplasms. Radiol Clin North Am. 1992; 30:817–830.

36. Yamashita Y, Takhashi M, Sawada T, et al. Carcinoma of the cervix: Dynamic MR imaging. Radiology. 1992; 182:643–648.

37. Yamashita Y, Mizutani H, Torashima M, et al. Assessment of myometrial invasion by endometrial carcinoma: Transvaginal sonography vs contrast enhanced MR imaging. Am J Roentgenol. 1993; 161:595–599.

9

Malignant Diseases of the Ovary

RUTH ROSENBLATT and ROSALYN KUTCHER

Ultrasound has maintained an important role in the imaging of ovarian malignancy. It permits the accurate evaluation of the patient with a suspected pelvic mass. In a patient with the diagnosis of ovarian carcinoma, it helps determine the presence of recurrent or persistent disease after surgery and chemotherapy. Ultrasound as a routine screening modality for the diagnosis of ovarian cancer in the general population has not been successful or cost effective. The combination of ultrasound screening in patients with an elevated tumor marker (CA 125) or in patients with a hereditary propensity for ovarian carcinoma is under active investigation and is proving to be of value.[43,51]

Incidence and Prognosis

Ovarian malignancy is a disease of low prevalence, accounting for only 4% of all cancers in women.[1] However, it causes more deaths than any other cancer of the female reproductive system and is the fourth leading cause of cancer deaths among women, trailing behind cancer of the lung, breast, and colon. The relatively high mortality of ovarian malignancy is a reflection of its low cure rate. The American Cancer Society estimates that approximately 26,700 new cases are diagnosed each year in the United States and that 1 of every 70 newborn girls without genetic predisposition will have ovarian cancer during her lifetime.[1] Although mortality rates from other gynecologic malignancies are declining, there is evidence to suggest that both the incidence and mortality rate of

ovarian cancer are increasing.[2,14,19,20,24,52] There are global variations in the incidence of ovarian cancer. It is much more common in the Scandinavian countries and the United States compared to India and Japan, where it is rare.[29]

The poor prognosis of ovarian malignancy is in great measure related to the fact that the disease is often diagnosed at a late stage. In such cases, the overall 5-year survival rate is about 15% to 20%. Ovarian malignancy is, unfortunately, found late because early in its course the disease is usually silent. When symptoms do appear, they are often vague. On the other hand, if the disease happens to be detected and treated in its early phase, the 5-year survival rate may reach 80% to 90%.[1] Factors that determine the prognosis are: 1) its stage (the extent of the disease when it is first diagnosed); 2) the tumor grade (the histopathologic classification or the degree of cellular differentiation); 3) the extent of residual disease after initial surgical excision; and 4) the tumor response to types of treatment given.

Early detection of ovarian malignancy offers the most effective means of reducing the current high mortality rate. Research in a number of medical disciplines, including epidemiology, gynecologic oncology, and radiologic imaging, has been directed toward this goal. Extensive epidemiologic studies have helped to define the population at risk.[1,49] It is possible that such data will help direct screening so as to make it economically more feasible in light of its low prevalence. Biochemical research has tried to develop immunologic studies to detect even a small population of malignant cells by means of tumor markers such as CA 125.[4,28,49,52] Finally, the ongoing improvement in imaging techniques has enabled the visualization of even minimal ovarian enlargement.

Epidemiology and Risk Factors

Several studies in the epidemiology of ovarian cancer have shed some light on risk factors for this disease. Age is the major risk factor for the most common ovarian malignancies. The peak incidence of occurrence is between 55 and 59 years.

A direct relationship has been observed between the number of years of ovulatory activity and the risk for development of epithelial ovarian cancer, the most common type. A woman whose ovulatory activity extends for more than 40 years is considered at high risk.[49] An interesting theory regarding the relationship of ovulation and the development of ovarian cancer has been postulated. Ovulation involves minor but repeated trauma to the surface epithelium of the ovary, with exposure to estrogen-rich follicular fluid and the formation of inclusion cysts as a reparative process in follicular rupture. This incessant ovulation may predispose to carcinogenesis.[10] Conversely, there appears to be a protective influence against development of ovarian cancer when ovulatory activity is reduced. For example, pregnancy, lactation, oral contraceptives, and a shorter reproductive span due to late menarche or early menopause are all factors that decrease the number of years of ovulatory activity.[29] Current studies suggest bilateral tubal ligation may be as effective as oophorectomy in risk reduction.[25]

As with breast cancer, a strong family history of ovarian cancer (maternal or sibling) places a woman at higher risk, and makes this genetic fact a criterion for screening studies.[21,51,52] Several chromosomal deletions have been identified in patients with ovarian malignancy, in particular an abnormality in chromosome 17q (the *BRCA1* gene). There are several hereditary family cancer syndromes that involve ovarian neoplasms (Table 9-1). Unaffected family members with hereditary breast/ovarian cancer syndrome have a risk factor of 82% by 70 years of age. Fortunately, only 0.5% of the population has a familial syndrome.

Certain environmental factors have been linked to ovarian cancer risk. A three- to five-fold higher incidence of ovarian cancer and mortality has been observed in industrialized countries compared to developing nations.[49] A notable exception is Japan, an industrialized country with a low incidence of ovarian cancer. Countries with the highest incidence of ovarian cancer are Sweden, Norway, and the United States. Global variations have led epidemiologists to postulate that carcinogens in the air, water, or diet of industrialized communities play a role in the higher incidence of this disease.[24]

Talcum powder used for perineal hygiene has also been implicated as a possible causal factor. It has been postulated that insoluble, finely divided powder particles may migrate to the peritoneal cavity through the vagina, uterus, and tubes and act as irritants, promoting cancer growth.[24]

Pathology

HISTOLOGIC CLASSIFICATION

The pathology and pathophysiology of ovarian malignancy are extremely complex. The ovary has both endocrine and reproductive functions and is com-

TABLE 9-1. Ovarian Neoplastic Syndromes

Syndrome	Associated Neoplasms
Gonadal dysgenesis	Gonadoblastoma, dysgerminoma
Multiple nevoid basal cell carcinoma	Ovarian fibroma
Peutz-Jeghers	Granulosa–theca cell tumor
Hereditary site-specific ovarian cancer	Epithelial ovarian cancer
Hereditary breast/ovarian cancer	Breast and epithelial ovarian cancer
Lynch II (hereditary nonpolyposis colorectal cancer)	Colorectal, endometrial, breast, and epithelial ovarian cancer

(From Teneriello MG, Park RC. Early detection of ovarian cancer. CA Cancer J Clin. 1995; 45:71–87.)

TABLE 9-2. MOST COMMON MALIGNANT OVARIAN NEOPLASMS: CORRELATION OF CLINICAL AND SONOGRAPHIC FINDINGS*

Pathology (Frequency)	Clinical Features	Sonographic Findings
EPITHELIAL (90%–95%)		
Cystadenocarcinoma, serous (more common) or mucinous	Peri- and postmenopausal; abdominal pain; distention; gastrointestinal symptoms	Large (10- to 30-cm), complex cysts with clear or echogenic fluid; thick septa and papillations; 25%–60% are bilateral
Undifferentiated adenocarcinoma		Fixation; ascites common; echogenic ascites suggests pseudomyxoma peritonei
Endometrioid	May be associated with benign endometriosis and endometrial cancer	Mixed cystic and solid pattern; 30% are bilateral; may be seen associated with endometrial echo abnormality
SEX CORD NEOPLASMS (2%)		
Granulosa–theca cell tumor	Wide age range; associated with hyperestrinism; vaginal bleeding due to endometrial hyperplasia or carcinoma	Predominantly solid; unilateral; homogenous; may see endometrial thickening
Androblastoma (Sertoli-Leydig cell tumor)	Common in adolescence; may have masculinizing effect	Usually solid and unilateral
GERM CELL NEOPLASMS (1%)		
Dysgerminoma	Often seen in adolescence; radiosensitive; may be cause of primary amenorrhea	Usually solid; variable in size; 10%–20% are bilateral
Choriocarcinoma	May cause precocious puberty; associated with high levels of human chorionic gonadotropin; aggressive growth	Variable consistency
Teratocarcinoma	Rare tumor; often seen in young adulthood	Variable appearance with cystic and highly echogenic areas with acoustic shadow
Endodermal sinus tumor	May be seen in association with teratoma; highly malignant; young adulthood	Predominantly solid, with areas of necrosis
METASTASES TO OVARY (4%–8%)		
Krukenberg tumor (primary in gastrointestinal tract) or from other sites: breast, lung, pancreas, lymphoma	Peri- and postmenopausal; may be first manifestation of extraovarian malignant disease; search for gastrointestinal primary	Large masses; usually complex texture and bilateral; more common on right if unilateral; often indistinguishable from ovarian primary malignancy

* For a complete World Health Organization classification of ovarian tumors, the reader is referred to Jones H, Jones G, eds. Novak's Textbook of Gynecology. 11th ed. Baltimore: Williams & Wilkins; 1988:507.

posed of at least four different cell populations, each of which may undergo malignant transformation. A classification of ovarian tumors has been proposed by the World Health Organization.[23] There are nine broad categories of tumors based on the cell of origin. Each of these categories of neoplasms is further divided into histologically distinguishable lesions that may be benign, borderline malignant, or frankly malignant. Varying degrees of histologic differentiation can be found in different sections of one lesion. Whereas the most differentiated area of

the lesion determines the cell type, the least differentiated portion determines its malignant potential. The degree of cellular differentiation is used for tumor grading and represents an important criterion in assessing the severity of the disease, and therefore its prognosis. Poorly differentiated cancers have a higher likelihood of aggressive growth, and occult metastases may be present even when the primary lesion is small.

Tumors originating from the epithelium covering the ovaries, the serous and mucinous cystade-

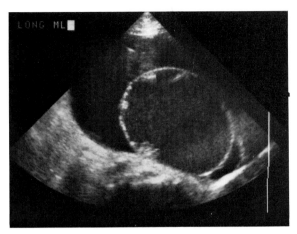

Figure 9-1. Papillary serous cystadenoma of low-grade malignancy, stage Ia, in an 80-year-old woman with abdominal discomfort. Midline sagittal scan demonstrated a cyst within a cyst. Note the palpillations on the inner cyst wall and the echogenic fluid, which contained fine particulate debris and residua of previous bleeding. The entire lesion measured 21 × 17 × 11 cm, unilateral, and confined to the ovary.

nocarcinomas, account for greater than 80% of ovarian malignancies. A much less common group of lesions are the gonadal stromal, or *sex cord,* neoplasms, some of which may be endocrinologically active and therefore may be diagnosed when smaller in size. The least common group are the germ cell lesions. Metastases to the ovary account for about 4% to 8% of ovarian malignancies. Although the sonographic specificity for a particular histologic type of ovarian malignancy is poor, correlation of the clinical features and the sonographic appearance of the ovarian masses may lead to a more accurate diagnosis. Table 9-2 summarizes the pathologic, clinical, and sonographic features of the most common ovarian malignancies.

PATHOPHYSIOLOGY

A characteristic feature of most epithelial cancers is the tendency to form cystic masses with multiple septa. The masses can be enormous, reaching 30 to 40 cm in diameter and weighing 10 to 15 kg and, of course, extending into the abdomen. The cysts contain serous or mucinous fluid. Nodular or papillary growths may project into the cystic fluid and may also be present on the external surface of the cyst (Fig. 9-1). The tissue is friable, and thin-walled blood vessels of the

lesion predispose to intracystic bleeding. Doppler analysis may show prominent blood flow in the septations or solid tissue components with elevated diastolic flow (Fig. 9-2). Areas of the lesion devoid of adequate blood supply may undergo necrosis. Bleeding and necrosis add to the fluid content of the lesion and may increase the echogenicity of the fluid on ultrasound (Fig. 9-3). Dystrophic calcification often occurs within areas of cellular degeneration. These microcrystals, or psammoma bodies, may be seen radiographically. The epithelial tumors that do not secrete fluid are usually smaller but may still have irregular fluid collections within them secondary to hemorrhage and necrosis.

Ascites is often associated with ovarian malignancy. At postmortem examination it is found in 60% to 70% of cases. Typically, the fluid has a high protein content. Protein-rich fluid exudes from the tumor-bearing surfaces of the peritoneum, because tumor vessels are more permeable to protein.[12] Fluid accumulates first in the dependent portion of the peritoneal cavity, such as the pelvic cul-de-sac. Subsequently, the fluid ascends into both paracolic gutters but predominantly on the right side because this space is broader and forms a better communication between the right upper quadrant and the pelvis (Fig. 9-4A).

When spontaneous leakage or rupture of a mucinous cystadenocarcinoma occurs, the peritoneal cavity is contaminated with sticky, gelatinous fluid, leading to massive abdominal distention, a condition known as pseudomyxoma peritonei (Fig. 9-5). Rupture of a mucinous neoplasm of the appendix (most often malignant) is also a cause of this condition.

**Spread and Staging
of Ovarian Malignancy**

The major patterns of spread of ovarian malignancy are direct extension to involve contiguous organs in the pelvis, peritoneal seeding, and lymphatic spread. Ovarian cancer is the most common tumor responsible for peritoneal malignancy in women. Intraperitoneal dissemination occurs when tumor cells are shed from the lesion and establish growth on peritoneal surfaces within the abdomen, particularly the diaphragmatic leaflets, liver capsule, bowel serosa, and omentum. This occurs relatively early in the disease and is often, but not always, associated with ascites. There are several

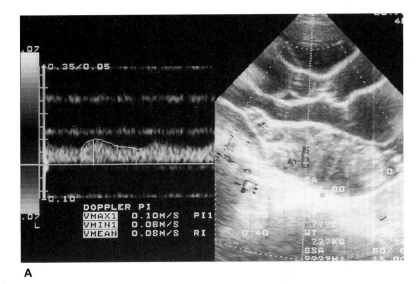

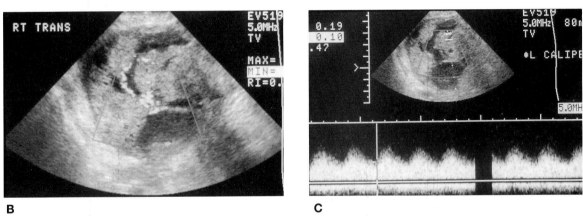

Figure 9-2. (**A**) Borderline epithelial ovarian tumor in a 26-year-old woman presenting with a large pelvic mass. A multiseptated cystic mass in the right adnexa has high diastolic flow with a resistive index of 0.4 and a pulsatility index of 0.5. The mass was confined to the ovary at surgery. (**B,C**) Stage IV poorly differentiated ovarian carcinoma in a 74-year-old woman with abdominal distention and unexplained drainage from the umbilicus. (**B**) Transvaginal sonogram shows large right complex adnexal mass with prominent vascularity. (**C**) Spectral Doppler image shows high diastolic flow.

pathways for the lymphatic spread of tumor cells: peritoneal lymphatics draining toward the diaphragm and pelvic lymphatics draining to the retroperitoneum. The pattern of spread of ovarian tumor is not predictable. Because the diaphragmatic lymphatics are the major pathways of peritoneal fluid drainage, blockage of this pathway by tumor may also produce ascites. The diaphragmatic lymphatics that drain to the retrosternal and mediastinal nodes constitute a major avenue for spread of the disease to the chest.

In advanced cases of ovarian malignancy, ante-grade spread or distal migration of tumor cells to the uterus may be manifested by positive vaginal cytology. Not infrequently, distant metastases occur in the liver. Sonographically, these lesions may have a complex cystic appearance, reflecting the presence of fluid and mucin within them.

The extent of tumor spread or stage of disease at time of diagnosis is an important parameter in determining the patient's clinical course. A staging scheme proposed by the International Federation of Gynecologists and Obstetricians is a widely ac-

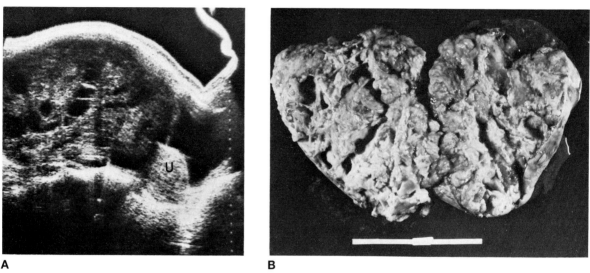

Figure 9-3. Endometrioid carcinoma, stage III, in a 59-year-old woman with increased abdominal girth, weight loss, and mild abdominal discomfort. (**A**) Sagittal view of pelvis and abdomen with minimal bladder distention. The large mass, predominantly solid, contains numerous cystic spaces (U, uterus). (**B**) Cut surface of an 11 × 10 cm tumor, predominantly solid, with areas of necrosis. At surgery, metastatic nodules were found on the mesentery and omentum.

cepted classification (Table 9-3). The stage of disease is determined at the time of laparotomy. Imaging techniques such as computed tomography (CT), magnetic resonance imaging (MRI), and ultrasound add further information to increase the accuracy of staging.[13,31,34,42,45,54]

Clinical Considerations

SYMPTOMS

Ovarian carcinoma is mainly a disease of perimenopausal and postmenopausal women; mean age at diagnosis is 52 years. The often insidious or vague

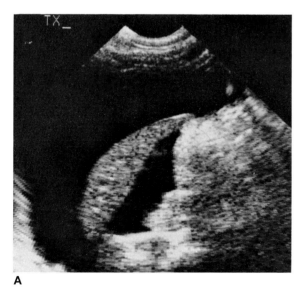
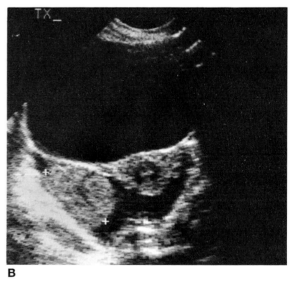

Figure 9-4. Granulosa–theca cell tumor in an 18-year-old woman with abdominal distention. (**A**) Transverse view of the right upper quadrant demonstrating a large amount of ascites, predominantly on the right and surrounding the liver. (**B**) Transverse view of the pelvis showing a right adnexal solid mass, 8 × 7 × 6 cm, homogeneous in texture.

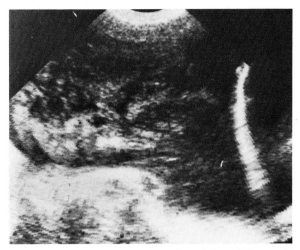

Figure 9-5. *Pseudomyxoma peritonei in a 62-year-old woman with increasing abdominal girth. Midline sagittal scan above the bladder. Echogenic fluid was noted floating between loops of bowel.*

symptoms of ovarian cancer contribute to delays in diagnosis. When symptoms do appear, they are related to pressure from an enlarging pelvic mass or from accumulation of ascites. Less frequently, manifestation of hormone activity (feminizing or masculinizing symptoms) provides clues to the presence of a lesion. Rarely, the diagnosis is made only when the tumor undergoes torsion and the patient presents with an acute abdomen, requiring surgical intervention.

An analysis of 10 clinical studies from the literature, comprising over 2000 patients, disclosed that 50% of ovarian cancer patients presented with pain.[38] An almost equally common complaint was abdominal distention (49%). Gastrointestinal symptoms such as indigestion or bloating were present in 21% of cases. Such complaints are often treated symptomatically, diverting attention from the pelvis and delaying diagnosis. It has been emphasized that undiagnosed, persistent gastrointestinal symptoms in women older than 40 years of age should prompt a search for an ovarian lesion. The pressure from mass and ascites accounts for the urinary symptoms of urgency and frequency seen in 17% of patients. The mass may produce backache, pelvic pressure, or simply a vague feeling of pelvic discomfort. Despite increases in abdominal girth, 17% of patients may experience true weight loss.

A significant number of patients with ovarian malignancy present with or develop vaginal bleeding (17%). Bleeding may be secondary to estrogen secretion by the lesion (see later), concurrent endometrial and ovarian carcinoma, or, rarely, direct spread of the lesion to the endometrium (Fig. 9-6). Not infrequently, the cause of bleeding is undetermined.

Symptoms of abnormal endocrine activity are sometimes a clue to the presence of an ovarian malignancy that is hormonally active or stimulates the normal ovarian tissue to increased hormone production. Feminizing effects due to overproduction

 TABLE 9-3. INTERNATIONAL FEDERATION OF GYNECOLOGISTS AND OBSTETRICIANS STAGING SYSTEM FOR OVARIAN CANCER

Stage I   Growth limited to the ovaries
   A: Only one ovary involved, capsule intact and free of tumor, no ascites
   B: Growth limited to both ovaries, capsule intact and free of tumor, no ascites
   C: Growth limited to ovaries, capsule surface tumor or ruptured, ascites, positive peritoneal cytology
Stage II   Growth beyond ovaries but limited to the pelvis
   A: Extension or metastases to uterus/tubes
   B: Extension to other pelvic structures, including uterus
   C: Extension within pelvis, ovarian capsule surface tumor or rupture, ascites, positive peritoneal cytology
Stage III   Growth beyond the pelvis; retroperitoneal or inguinal nodes or intraperitoneal omental implants; superficial liver metastases
   A: Negative nodes, histologically confirmed microscopic seeding of abdominal peritoneal surfaces
   B: Abdominal peritoneal implants <2 cm diameter, negative nodes
   C: Abdominal peritoneal implants >2 cm diameter or positive retroperitoneal or inguinal nodes
Stage IV   Distant metastases or pleural involvement; liver parenchymal metastases

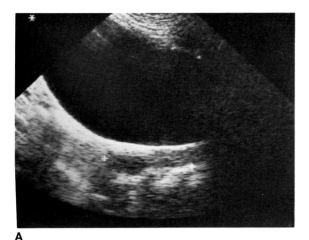
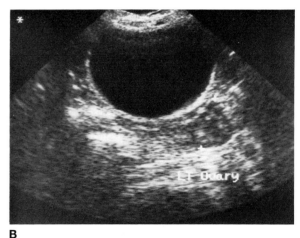

A   **B**

Figure 9-6. Serous papillary carcinoma in a 79-year-old woman. Results of abdominal Pap smear and findings at dilation and curettage were compatible with adenocarcinoma. No mass was palpated on pelvic examination. (**A**) Sagittal view of the uterus demonstrates a normal-sized uterus for patient's age. Despite this, findings at dilation and curettage were positive for papillary carcinoma. (**B**) Transverse view of pelvis shows a 4.4-cm, solid left adnexal mass with good sound transmission. This proved to be an ovarian serous papillary carcinoma.

of estrogen by a granulosa cell tumor are often associated with vaginal bleeding in the postmenopausal patient. In young girls, the rare primary ovarian choriocarcinoma may be a cause of precocious puberty (see Chap. 6). Conversely, a rare cause of primary amenorrhea in adolescents is dysgerminoma, which is the counterpart of, and histopathologically resembles, the seminoma of the testis. A lesion that often produces defeminizing or masculinizing effects is the arrhenoblastoma or Sertoli-Leydig cell tumor. This lesion is more commonly seen in adolescents or young women and is often solid (Fig. 9-7). Other endocrine-like effects, such as Cushing's syndrome, hypoglycemia, hypercalcemia, and hyperthroidism, may be seen in association with ovarian malignancy. One consequence of hormonal activity by the ovarian lesion is the possibility of earlier diagnosis. Inappropriate hormonal activity is not diagnostic of ovarian malignancy, however. A variety of benign ovarian neoplasms as well as ovarian or adrenal hyperplasia may also manifest such abnormalities.

Any mass may undergo sudden compromise of its blood supply due to torsion or incarceration. Such an event is likely to produce acute abdominal symptoms that may mimic inflammatory disease. In the pediatric age group, ovarian malignancy is likely to present as a pelvic or abdominal mass, with or without torsion. Torsion of any ovarian mass is also more likely to occur in the second or third trimester

of pregnancy because of uterine enlargement and the change in position of the ovarian pedicle.[49]

TREATMENT

Treatment options include surgery, radiation therapy, and chemotherapy.[38] Surgery plays a crucial role in the diagnosis, staging, and treatment of ovarian cancer. Surgical planning and management is decisive in the prognosis of ovarian malignancy, and maximum information regarding staging before initial oncologic surgery is important. Surgical excision provides the specimen for histologic confirmation. An attempt is made to remove the bulk of the tumor, to minimize residual disease and enhance the effectiveness of radiation and chemotherapy. Initial inspection at surgery also provides information for staging the disease. Surgical treatment usually includes bilateral salpingo-oophorectomy, total hysterectomy, and omentectomy. In young women with stage I disease, only the involved ovary may be removed. After surgery, a cyclic course of chemotherapy, and in some cases radiation therapy, may be given, especially for stage II through stage IV disease. Promising results have been obtained with newer chemotherapeutic drugs such as paclitaxel in combination with cisplatin.[43] A repeat laparotomy (second-look operation) is sometimes performed after a course of chemotherapy, to determine the presence or absence of residual disease and to plan possible further treatment.

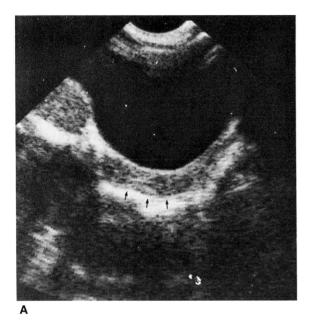
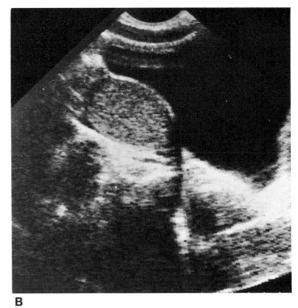

A   **B**

Figure 9-7. *Androblastoma (Sertoli-Leydig cell tumor). A 17-year-old girl with clinical signs of virilization and primary amenorrhea. (***A***) Sagittal view of the small uterus (*arrows*), which is infantile in shape. (***B***) Sagittal view of the right adnexa showing a unilateral solid lesion measuring 7 × 3 cm. Note good sound transmission through the mass.*

LABORATORY TESTS

Much work has been done on laboratory detection of malignancies, including ovarian carcinoma.[49] The work is based on the principle of finding telltale substances in the serum or plasma of patients who harbor a malignancy. Such substances, which may be proteins, hormones, or enzymes, are produced by cancer cells, or by the sensitized nonmalignant tissue of the patient's immune system in response to the presence of cancer cells. These substances have been termed "tumor markers."

Although significant elevations in certain tumor markers have been described in ovarian carcinoma patients, none is unique to the ovary or has been sensitive enough to be used as a screening test. However, in a patient with a known pelvic mass, certain laboratory tests may be helpful in the diagnosis. For example, a serum radioimmunoassay has been developed for an antibody called CA 125. CA 125 is a cell surface glycoprotein present in 80% of ovarian epithelial cancers. In combination with two other newly identified markers—TAG 72 and CA15-3—a malignancy diagnosis specificity of 99.9% has been reported.[28,49]

There is also a new CA 125 II assay in use, and a risk algorithm has been developed by comparing changes in a patient's assay level over time. This method is said to improve the positive predictive value of the assay from 2% to 16%.[25]

Cytologic examination of ascitic fluid is often helpful in the diagnosis of ovarian malignancy. When ascites is only minimal, ultrasound may be used to guide fluid aspiration.

Imaging Diagnosis

CONVENTIONAL RADIOLOGY

Important information is often gained from a plain radiograph of the abdomen and a barium enema study.

The principal value of the *radiograph* of the abdomen, the simplest and least expensive radiographic examination, is that it detects calcifications and abnormal soft tissue masses in patients with abdominal distention. The most common ovarian lesion, serous cystadenoma, and its malignant counterpart, cystoadenocarcinoma, may contain fine, granular calcifications termed psammoma bodies, which may coalesce to form cloudlike aggregates. The calcifications occur in approximately 12% of ovarian cystadenomas and cystadenocarcinomas and may be found in the primary lesion or its metastatic deposits. Coarse, sometimes curvilinear calcifications are seen more often with mucinous cystadenocarcinoma and in pseudomyxoma peritonei. A wide range of plain film densities, sometimes quite specific, may be present in cystic teratomas, including their far less common malignant counterpart, the teratocarcinoma. These include teeth, bone, and fat. Malignant teratomas, which are typically seen in adolescents or very elderly patients, may contain areas of coarse calcification.

The barium enema has a significant role in patients with suspected ovarian malignancy. It may demonstrate extrinsic displacement or encasement of the colon or abnormalities of contour that raise the suspicion of serosal involvement. In addition, the barium enema may demonstrate a primary colonic malignancy, which may be coincidental to the ovarian primary or the source from which metastases to the ovary have spread.

COMPUTED TOMOGRAPHY

Specific strengths of the CT examination include the demonstration of pelvic sidewall masses, nodal enlargement in the retroperitoneum, liver metastases, and calcifications.[36]

When intravenous and oral contrast are given, the CT examination provides accurate anatomic information about the urinary tract, the opacified portions of the gastrointestinal tract, and the presence of ascites, in addition to demonstrating the actual mass. Deep and subcapsular liver metastases that may be difficult or impossible to detect at surgery are readily visualized. Therefore, CT together with the ultrasound examination are complementary to laparotomy as means of staging the disease. CT may also be useful in determining initial operability.[40,46]

After surgery, CT is used to assess residual disease. After chemotherapy, CT is frequently used to assess the response to treatment. In evaluating recurrent disease, the CT scan may show extensive unresectable tumor, thereby obviating unnecessary surgery.[27]

The main limitation of CT is the difficulty in detecting small foci of disease, in particular, bowel surface, mesenteric, or peritoneal implants, and lymph nodes smaller than 2 cm. Current high-resolution CT scanners, however, can detect 50% of peritoneal implants as small as 5 mm.[54]

MAGNETIC RESONANCE IMAGING

Magnetic resonance imaging of adnexal masses offers some refinements in tissue characterization over CT and ultrasound.[37,42] Using various parameters, signal intensities can be noted suggesting fat or blood, but tissue specificity is not sufficient to distinguish ovarian malignancy from benign or inflammatory lesions. Histologic types of ovarian neoplasms also cannot be differentiated. The addition of intravenous gadolinium-DTPA to enhance areas of pathology may improve accuracy. Current opinion is that the accuracy rates of CT and MRI are similar, and therefore routine MRI is not cost effective for ovarian cancer staging.[54] MRI may also fail to demonstrate calcified peritoneal implants.[5] On the other hand, like ultrasound, MRI has the capability of multiplanar imaging, and this feature, together with the good spatial resolution of pelvic anatomy, makes MRI a good tool for determining the origin of a pelvic mass. MRI may therefore be used when ultrasound or CT findings are suboptimal or indeterminate.[16]

POSITRON EMISSION TOMOGRAPHY

Positron emission tomography is a new tagged radionuclide study used primarily to detect occult or recurrent ovarian malignancy. Because an on-site cyclotron is required for tagging, cost currently precludes its routine use. Early results have been promising, suggesting it is more sensitive than either CA 125 assay or CT scan in diagnosing recurrence.[11]

ULTRASOUND

Screening for Ovarian Malignancy

Normally, significant regression in ovarian size as well as changes in texture and surface characteristics occur in the perimenopausal period. Ovarian dimensions change from approximately $3.5 \times 2 \times 1.5$ cm to $2 \times 1 \times 0.5$ cm, making the ovary impalpable in 70% of women.[34] Diminished blood supply and absence of folliculogenesis produce a wrinkled surface and a change in texture. Absence of this normal regression 3 to 5 years after menopause is considered pathologic and has been termed the postmenopausal palpable ovary syndrome, which requires prompt investigation.[3] Early detection of an adnexal mass in perimenopausal and postmenopausal patients is considered the most promising means of favorably influencing the prognosis of patients with ovarian cancer. The yield of detecting asymptomatic ovarian carcinoma in women by means of physical examination is only 1 per 10,000 examinations.[3] Some limitations to a reliable physical examination include obesity, vaginal atrophy, and muscle tension.

Ultrasound screening of the normal population of postmenopausal women for ovarian carcinoma has not developed into a successful or cost effective undertaking, even though the ultrasound examination is a more sensitive tool than the physical examination in measuring ovarian volume and size.[21] In a genetically high-risk population, a multimodality approach that combines tumor markers (i.e., CA 125) with pelvic ultrasound (transabdominal and transvaginal), color flow Doppler analysis, and the physical examination is being investigated in numerous studies to see if it improves detection of early malignancy.[12,13,26,27,28,30,48]

When screening patients for ovarian malignancy, size as well as sonographic texture are important features to note. To date, ultrasound studies of ovarian volume in postmenopausal women have suggested a range of 2.5 to 3.7 cm^3 as the upper limit of normal.[19,22] Significant size inequality when comparing both ovaries is another criterion for ovarian enlargement. It has been suggested that one ovary should not be more than twice the size of the contralateral one,[8] but in postmenopausal women less dramatic size discrepancies should raise suspicion. Transabdominal sonography has a sensitivity of 83% in detecting postmenopausal ovaries, an improvement over the 67% sensitivity of palpation.[34] Transabdominal sonography depicts a more global view of the pelvic viscera, permits inspection of the abdomen and retroperitoneum, and can readily demonstrate ascites. A predominantly solid or complex mass is more suspect than a purely cystic mass (see Fig. 9-4). Benign inclusion cysts are not rare in postmenopausal women. Transvaginal ultrasound allows distinctions in tissue texture to be made with greater confidence and provides further refinements in the assessment of ovarian size. The addition of color flow Doppler and spectral analysis permits added information regarding regional blood flow. To date, the best approach to ultrasound imaging of the postmenopausal ovary combines information from both transabdominal and transvaginal studies.[19]

A significant limitation in the ultrasound study of postmenopausal patients is the difficulty in identifying normal postmenopausal ovaries, which are devoid of follicles, a characteristic feature that aids ovarian identification in premenopausal women. It is important to recognize that when ovaries are not visualized sonographically, they cannot be classified as normal.[15,27] Greater experience, careful scanning technique, and transvaginal scanning will overcome some of the difficulty. In addition, when ovarian enlargement is due to a neoplasm, it is likely that a portion of the mass will be composed of cystic elements containing septa, thereby aiding in its recognition.

Sonographic Diagnosis

Ultrasound is often the initial imaging study for patients with ovarian malignancy. The object of the ultrasound examination is to characterize the mass, define its contours, and measure it. The ovarian origin of the mass can usually be suspected, particularly if a normal uterus is identified. The gross anatomy of the most common form of ovarian malignancy, cystadenocarcinoma, lends itself well to ultrasound depiction because of the propensity of the lesion to form cystic masses with internal septa and soft tissue protrusions (see Fig. 9-1). Diffuse, low-amplitude signals within the cystic mass or a portion thereof suggest the presence of mucin, as is seen in mucinous cystadenoma and cystadenocarcinoma. However, this finding is not specific for mucin, because it may be seen with fresh blood or purulent material. High-amplitude reflections associated with acoustic shadowing are often a clue to the presence of calcifications within the mass.

The ultrasound examination does not have the specificity to distinguish between benign and malignant disease, but a number of sonographic features, if present, favor the diagnosis of ovarian malignancy. As the proportion of solid components of the lesion increases, so does the likelihood of its being malignant. Solid portions of the lesion consist of irregular septations, 2 mm thick or greater, and papillary growths.[39] Using transvaginal sonography, a morphologic scoring system has been devised, based on ovarian volume, cyst wall thickness, and the presence of septations or papillary growths. This will help to quantify findings and assign a risk of malignancy.[47] Not infrequently, an ovarian malignancy has a predominantly or completely solid texture (see Figs. 9-4 and 9-7). Good to excellent sound transmission may be observed in such cases. This is undoubtedly a result of the friable necrotic tissue and high fluid content in the lesion. Nodularity and poor definition of the outer margin of the mass favor malignancy. Immobility or noncompressibility imply fixation of a mass and suggest malignancy. In addition, bilateral disease also favors malignancy. This finding is often difficult to ascertain. If the bilateral lesions are large, they may coalesce in the cul-de-sac to form one large mass (Fig. 9-8). Although ascites can be a feature of a benign ovarian lesion, notably the ovarian fibroma, presence of ascites together with a cystic pelvic mass raises the suspicion of malignancy.[44] In some cases, ascites is the only clue to the presence of ovarian malignancy and the ovarian lesion itself may not be visualized. In such cases, use of a transvaginal probe may help identify the ovarian mass and be of diagnostic value (Figs. 9-9 and 9-10). The ultrasound appearance of the ascitic fluid in pseudomyxoma peritonei is usually echogenic as a result of the thick globular consistency of the fluid (see Fig. 9-5).

Several studies suggest both color flow Doppler and spectral analysis may have value in differentiating benign from malignant ovarian neoplasms. The distribution of vascularity is typically peripheral and orderly in benign lesions, but central and haphazard in malignancy.[6,7,17,33,34,50,53] An overall elevated peak systolic velocity due to neovascularity and arteriovenous shunting has been noted by some authors. A decrease in vascular impedence due to lack of intimal smooth muscle in tumor vessel walls has

been described in several series. A resistive index of less than 0.4 and a pulsatility index less than 1.0 have been used as measurements denoting malignancy (see Fig. 9-2). Initial enthusiasm for these Doppler methods has waned somewhat because of overlap of malignant measurements with those of benign conditions, leading to an unacceptably high false-positive rate. In a series of 167 patients evaluated with both gray-scale and color Doppler, the gray-scale findings alone were sufficient to make a diagnosis in 93% of patients, whereas color flow Doppler added useful information in only 30%. When only the Doppler information was used, it was specific but lacked sensitivity and predictive value.[9] Current practice therefore is to use the Doppler information as an adjunct to the transabdominal and transvaginal imaging evaluation. An important caveat for the Doppler evaluation of ovarian masses in the premenopausal patient in the secretory (premenstrual) phase of the cycle is that a benign periovulatory follicle or persistent corpus luteum cyst can have low impedence similar to that reported in malignant neoplasms. Evaluations should therefore be performed in the proliferative (postmenstrual) phase of the cycle. As previously noted, there may also be overlap of flow characteristics in benign conditions such as leiomyomas, adenomyomatosis, and endometriosis. Conversely, there is an occasional malignancy that is avascular.

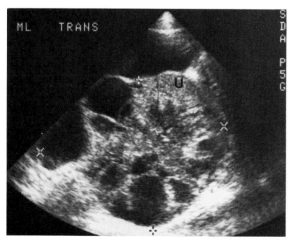

A

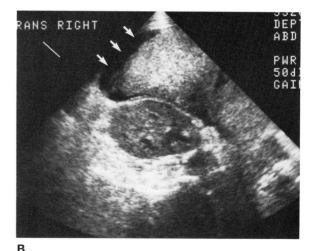

B

Figure 9-8. Metastatic disease to both ovaries in a 42-year-old woman who presented with weight loss and hepatomegaly. (**A**) Complex, multicystic mass distending the cul-de-sac, adherent to posterior surface of the uterus (U), which is compressed. (**B**) Transverse scan of the right upper quadrant demonstrates ascites and nodularity on the liver capsule, representing serosal metastases (*arrows*).

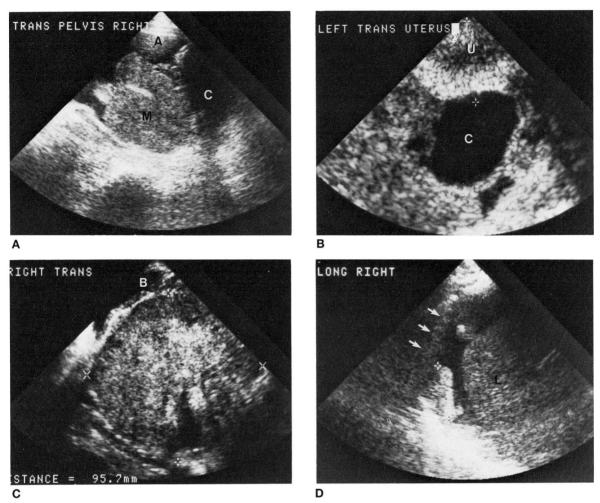

Figure 9-9. Undifferentiated adenocarcinoma, stage IV, in a 68-year-old woman with progressive abdominal distention. (**A**) Transverse view of the pelvis shows a lobulated mass on the right (M) with a cystic component on the left (C). Ascites (A) is seen anteriorly. The patient could not maintain a filled bladder. (**B**) Transvaginal view in the transverse plane shows a partial view of the uterus (between cursors). The cystic component of the mass (C) is seen posterior to the uterus (U). In this case, the transvaginal scan was able to resolve the uterus and adnexal mass as separate structures. (**C**) Transvaginal transverse view of the right adnexa shows a 9- to 10-cm, predominantly solid mass representing the right ovarian carcinoma (B, portion of the bladder). (**D**) Longitudinal view of the right subphrenic area (*arrows* on portions of diaphragm) shows a metastatic nodule on the inferior surface of the right hemidiaphragm (between cursors).

Ultrasound imaging has its limitations in that there is the difficulty in detecting small-volume disease involving retroperitoneal nodes, peritoneal surfaces, and omentum.[31,32] Lesions situated high in the pelvis are partially or entirely outside the field of view of the transvaginal probe. Despite these limitations, ultrasound provides reasonably accurate information for initial staging as well as evaluation for recurrent disease, with a reported accuracy of 90%.[32,45] Ultrasound-guided transvaginal biopsy has been advocated to obtain tissue diagnosis of pelvic masses, but is not currently accepted practice.[18]

Sonographic Monitoring

Ultrasound is often used to monitor patients for persistent or recurrent disease after surgery and during treatment (Fig. 9-11). A scan shortly after surgery may serve as a baseline study. In scanning the patient after total hysterectomy, it is important to

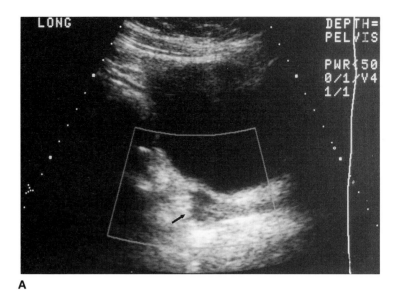

A

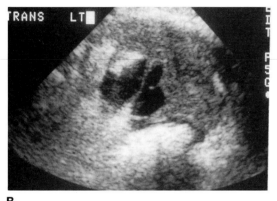

B

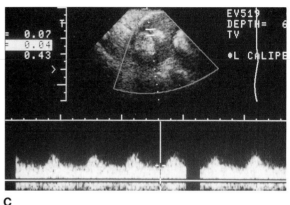

C

Figure 9-10. Recurrent, poorly differentiated papillary serous adenocarcinoma of the vaginal cuff in a 53-year-old woman. (**A**) Transabdominal sonogram shows some irregularity of the proximal vaginal cuff (*arrow*), thought to be caused by bowel. (**B**) Transvaginal image clearly demonstrates a complex mass. (**C**) Diastolic flow is prominent, with a resistive index of 0.43.

adjust the gain settings so that the increased sound transmission through the urinary bladder does not obscure a small pelvic mass. Transvaginal scanning may clarify any question with regard to the presence of a mass in the true pelvis or involving the vaginal cuff. Survey of the liver and retroperitoneal areas should be part of the postoperative examination as well. If pelvic masses, peritoneal nodules, or loculated areas of ascites are observed, ultrasound may be used to guide needle aspiration.

Ultrasound Scanning Protocol

The examination consists of a systematic survey of the pelvis in the sagittal and transverse planes with identification of the bladder, uterus, and adnexal and cul-de-sac areas (Table 9-4). In studying a pelvic mass, depth gain curve, focal zone, and depth of view need to be adjusted to optimize the image and to demonstrate degree of sound transmission through the mass.

Often it is not possible to perform the ideal pelvic sonographic examination in the presence of a large pelvic mass because it is difficult for the patient to maintain a full bladder. It is important, however, to have enough fluid in the bladder so that it can be identified and used as a landmark, and not mistaken for the cystic mass (see Fig. 9-11). In some cases, instillation into the bladder of 300 to 500 ml of normal saline with a Foley catheter may be required. A transvaginal scan is

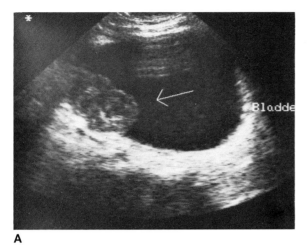
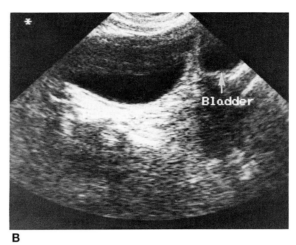

A   B

Figure 9-11. Recurrent cystadenocarcinoma in a 69-year-old woman who underwent total abdominal hysterectomy and bilateral salpingo-oophorectomy for adenocarcinoma of the ovary. (**A**) Sagittal view of the pelvis with nondistended bladder shows a cystic mass, which was initially mistaken for the urinary bladder. Note reverberation artifact anteriorly and nodularity (arrow) in the superior aspect of the cyst. (**B**) Repeat scan with minimal bladder distention confirmed the supravesicular location of the cystic mass, which proved to be a recurrent cancer.

an important adjunct to the examination, especially when an adequate transabdominal scan is not possible; it may provide additional diagnostic information in 70% of patients with pelvic masses. Usually, transvaginal sonography improves delineation of the adnexal mass and better defines the uterus (see

◢◢◢◢ TABLE 9-4. SUMMARY OF ULTRASOUND PROTOCOL FOR OVARIAN MALIGNANCY

Purpose	Sonography Checklist
Screening	Note any ovarian enlargement. In peri- and postmenopausal women, ovarian linear dimension should not exceed 3 cm in length and 1.5 cm in thickness. Note significant asymmetry in ovarian size.
Diagnosis	Observe texture, contour, size, and sound transmission of mass. Determine whether it is unilateral or bilateral. Note uterine contours and endometrial reflection. Check for ascites. Identify liver, retroperitoneal, or omental masses. Check kidneys for hydronephrosis.
Monitor	Compare to baseline study to exclude new masses. Check for ascites, retroperitoneal nodes, and liver masses. Survey pelvis, abdomen, and retroperitoneum before second-look operation.

Fig. 9-9B). It is important to identify uterine texture and contour. Abnormalities of the endometrial lining, usually thickening, suggest hyperplasia or associated endometrial carcinoma (see Table 9-2). Familiarity with Doppler techniques using color flow and spectral analysis is essential for obtaining additional information regarding blood flow to the lesion.

When ovarian malignancy is suspected based on the sonographic appearance of the mass, a complete pelvic and abdominal study should be done to provide information for staging (see Table 9-3). Search for ascites is directed to the cul-de-sac, paracolic gutters, especially on the right, and around the liver edge (Fig. 9-12). The inferior surfaces of the diaphragmatic leaflets may be visualized in the presence of moderate ascites. This enables the sonographer to demonstrate nodules on the liver capsule or on the diaphragmatic surface, which suggest stage IV disease (see Fig. 9-9D). Attention should be directed to the peritoneal surfaces to detect tumor implants (see Figs. 9-8B and 9-9D). Observation of peristalsis is of course an important aspect of real-time scanning and may avoid confusion between tumor nodules and loops of bowel. The sonographer also has the opportunity to perform a "hands-on" maneuver by exerting gentle pressure on the cystic mass (if it is superficially located) to assess it for compressibility, which is a

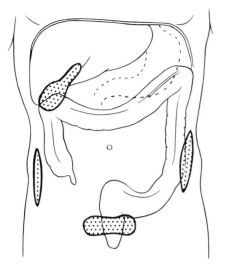

Figure 9-12. *Diagrammatic view of the peritoneal cavity. Dotted areas represent the most common sites of ascites fluid collection.*

feature of bowel and is usually not found with cystic malignant lesions. Evaluation of liver parenchyma is an integral part of the ultrasound study in the search for metastases. The costophrenic angles are also evaluated for the presence of pleural effusion. Both kidneys should be studied to assess the presence or absence of hydronephrosis. In the presence of massive ascites, it may be difficult to image the paraaortic area to demonstrate retroperitoneal adenopathy. In such cases, oblique and coronal scanning should be attempted.

Differential Diagnosis

The differential diagnosis of ovarian malignancies includes a variety of benign ovarian neoplasms. No imaging modality has yet been able to provide the tissue specificity necessary to distinguish between benign and malignant lesions. Most ovarian neoplasms are benign, and their gross pathologic appearance is often indistinguishable from that of their malignant counterparts. In the menstruating woman, nonneoplastic cystic lesions of the ovaries such as large follicular cysts, corpus luteum, and theca-lutein cysts should also be considered in the differential diagnosis. These lesions have a mixed echogenic pattern, particularly when intracystic hemorrhage occurs. Inclusion or paraovarian cysts are nonneoplastic cystic masses of the ovary that, when found in the postmenopausal age group, may resemble neoplasms.

A pedunculated leiomyoma may mimic an ovarian neoplasm, particularly when degeneration due to vascular compromise results in the formation of cystic spaces.[41]

Neoplasms of the fallopian tube are exceedingly rare and often malignant. These lesions are usually mistaken for ovarian malignancies.

Tumor-like conditions that are morphologically similar to ovarian neoplasms include endometriosis and pelvic inflammatory disease. Ectopic pregnancy should always be considered as a potential cause for a mass in menstruating women. Gastrointestinal diseases such as diverticulitis and colitis often produce inflammatory masses and fluid collections in the pelvis and should be considered, particularly in postmenopausal patients.

Distended, fluid- and stool-filled loops of bowel imaged in the pelvis may appear tumor-like. Although the observation of peristalsis identifies them as bowel, absence of peristalsis need not exclude this possibility. Ischemic disease of the bowel may be associated with adynamic ileus, and a small amount of ascites may also be observed.

The examiner faces a number of diagnostic challenges in the presence of a pelvic mass. The first is to determine the origin of the mass: is it ovarian, uterine, or nongynecologic? The second is to identify characteristics that are consistent with benign or malignant neoplasms. Awareness of differential diagnostic possibilities is important because of the morphologic similarity among many masses and disorders in the pelvic area.

REFERENCES

1. American Cancer Society. Cancer statistics 1996. CA Cancer J Clin. 1996; 46:5–29.
2. Andolf E, Svalenius E, Astedt B. Ultrasonography for early detection of ovarian carcinoma. Br J Obstet Gynaecol. 1986; 19:1286–1289.
3. Barber HRK, Graber EA. The PMPO syndrome (postmenopausal palpable ovary syndrome). Obstet Gynecol. 1971; 38:921–923.
4. Bast RC Jr, Klug TL, St. John E, et al. A radioimmunoassay using a monoclonal antibody to monitor the course of epithelial ovarian cancer. N Engl J Med. 1983; 309:883–887.
5. Bies JR, Ellis JH, Kopecky KK, et al. Assessment of primary gynecologic malignancies: Comparison of 0.15T resistine MRI with CT. Am J Roentgenol. 1984; 143:1249–1257.
6. Bourne TH, Campbell S, Reynolds KM, et al.

Screening for early familial ovarian cancer with transvaginal ultrasonography and colour blood flow imaging. Br Med J. 1993; 306:1025–1029.

7. Bromley B, Goodman H, Benacerraf BR. Comparison between sonographic morphology and doppler waveform for the diagnosis of ovarian malignancy. Obstet Gynecol. 1994; 83:331–338.

8. Campbell S, Goswamy R, Goessen L. Real-time ultrasonography for determination of ovarian morphology and volume. Lancet. 1982; 1:425–426.

9. Carter J, Saltzman A, Hartenbach E, et al. Flow characteristics in benign and malignant gynecologic tumors using transvaginal color flow doppler. Obstet Gynecol. 1994; 83:125–130.

10. Casagrande JT, Pike MC, Ross RK, et al. "Incessant ovulation" and ovarian cancer. Lancet. 1979; 2:170–173.

11. Casey MJ, Gupta NC, Muths CK. Experience with positron emission tomography (PET) scans in patients with ovarian cancer. Gynecol Oncol. 1994; 53:331–338.

12. Coates G, Bush RS, Aspin N. A study of ascites using lymphoscintigraphy with ^{99m}Tc sufur colloid. Radiology. 1973; 107:577–583.

13. Cohen CJ, Jennings TS. Screening for ovarian cancer: The role of noninvasive imaging techniques. Am J Obstet Gynecol. 1994; 170:1088–1094.

14. Creasman WT, DiSaia PJ. Screening in ovarian cancer. Am J Obstet Gynecol. 1991; 165:7–10.

15. DiSantis DJ, Scatarige JC, Kemp G, et al. A prosective evaluation of transvaginal sonography for detection of ovarian disease. Am J Roentgenol. 1993; 161:91–94.

16. Dooms GC, Hricack H, Tschalakoff D. Adnexal structures: MR imaging. Radiology. 1986; 158:639–646.

17. Fleischer AC, Rogers WH, Rao BK, et al. Transvaginal color Doppler sonography of ovarian masses with pathological correlation. Ultrasound in Obstetrics and Gynecology. 1991; 1:275–278.

18. Fornage BD, O'Keefe F. Ultrasound-guided transvaginal biopsy of malignant cystic pelvic mass. J Ultrasound Med. 1990; 9:53–55.

19. Goswamy RK, Campbell S, Whitehead ML. Screening of ovarian cancer. Clinics in Obstetrics and Gynecology. 1983; 10:621–643.

20. Granberg S, Wikland M. Comparison between endovaginal and transabdominal transducers for measuring ovarian volume. J Ultrasound Med. 1987; 6:649–653.

21. Granberg S, Wikland M. A comparison between US and gynecologic examination for detection of enlarged ovaries in a group of women at risk for ovarian cancer. J Ultrasound Med. 1988; 7:59–64.

22. Hall DA, McCarthy KA, Kopans DB. Sonographic visualization of the normal postmenopausal ovary. J Ultrasound Med. 1986; 5:9–11.

23. Hart WR. Pathology of malignant and borderline epithelial tumors of the ovary. In: Coppleson M, ed. Gynecologic Oncology: Fundamental Principles and Clinical Practice (Vol. 2.). New York: Churchill Livingstone; 1981:633–654.

24. Heintz APM, Hacker NF, Lagasse LD. Epidemiology and etiology of ovarian cancer: A review. Obstet Gynecol. 1985; 66:127–135.

25. Highlights of the American Cancer Society National Conference on Gynecologic Cancers. CA Cancer J Clin. 1995; 45:254–255.

26. Jacobs I, Bridges J, Reynolds C, et al. Multimodal approach to screening for ovarian cancer. Lancet. 1988; 1:268–271.

27. Jacobs I, Davies AP, Bridges J, et al. Prevalence screening for ovarian cancer in postmenopausal women by CA 125 measurement and ultrasonography. Br Med J. 1993; 306:1030–1034.

28. Jacobs IJ, Oram DH, Bast RC Jr. Strategies for improving the specificity of screening for cancer with tumor-associated antigens CA 125, CA 15-3, and TAG 72.3. Obstet Gynecol. 1992; 80:396–399.

29. Jones HW, Jones GS. Novak's Textbook of Gynecology. 11th ed. Baltimore: Williams & Wilkins; 1988:507–558.

30. Karlan BY, Raffel LJ, Crvenkovic G, et al. A multidisciplinary approach to the early detection of ovarian carcinoma: Rationale, protocol design and early results. Am J Obstet Gynecol. 1993; 169:494–501.

31. Khan O, Cosgrove DO, Fried AM, et al. Ovarian carcinoma follow-up: US versus laparotomy. Radiology. 1986; 159:111–113.

32. Khan O, Wiltshaw E, McGready VR, et al. Role of US in the management of ovarian carcinoma. J Royal Soc Med. 1983; 76:821–827.

33. Kurjak A, Zabed I, Tuckover D, et al. Transvaginal color Doppler for the assessment of pelvic circulation. Acta Obstet Gynaecol Scand. 1989; 68:131–135.

34. Mendelson EB, Bohm-Velez M. Transvaginal ultrasonography of pelvic neoplasms. Radiol Clin North Am. 1992; 30:703–734.

35. Meyer JI, Kennedy AW, Friedman R, et al. Ovarian carcinoma: Value of CT in predicting success of debulking surgery. Am J Roentgenol. 1995; 165:875–878.

36. Mitchell DG, Hill MC, Hill S, et al. Serous carcinoma of the ovary: CT identification of metastatic calcified implants. Radiology. 1986; 158:649–652.

37. Mitchell DG, Mintz MC, Spritzer CE, et al. Adnexal masses: MR imaging observations at 1.5T with US and CT correlation. Radiology. 1987; 162:319–324.

38. Morrow CP. Malignant and borderline epithelial tumors of ovary: Clinical features staging diagnosis. Intraoperative assessment and review of management. In: Coppleson M, ed. Gynecologic Oncology: Fundamental Principles and Clinical Practice (Vol. 2). New York: Churchill Livingstone. 1981:655–679.

39. Moyle JW, Rochester D, Sider L, et al. Sonography of ovarian tumors: Predictability of tumor type. Am J Roentgenol. 1983; 241:985–991.

40. Nelson BE, Rosenfield AT, Schwartz PE. Preoperative abdominopelvic computed tomographic prediction of optimal cytoreduction in epithelial ovarian carcinoma. J Clin Oncol. 1993; 11:166–172.

41. Nocera RM, Fagan CJ, Hernandez JC. Cystic parametrial fibroid mimicking ovarian cystadenoma. J Ultrasound Med. 1984; 3:183–187.

42. Outwater E, Dressel HY. Evaluation of gynecologic malignancy by magnetic resonance imaging. Radiol Clin North Am. 1992; 30:789–803.

43. Qazi F, McGuire WP. The treatment of epithelial ovarian cancer. CA Cancer J Clin. 1995; 45:88–101.

44. Requard CK, Mettler FA Jr, Wicks JD. Preoperative sonography of malignant ovarian neoplasms. Am J Roentgenol. 1981; 137:79–82.

45. Sanders RC, McNeil BJ, Finberg HJ, et al. A prospective study of CT and US in the detection and staging of pelvic masses. Radiology. 1983; 146:439–442.

46. Silverman PM, Osborne M, Dunnick NR, et al. CT prior to second-look operation in ovarian cancer. Am J Roentgenol. 1988; 150:829–832.

47. Sassone AM, Timor-Tritsch IE, Artner A, et al. Transvaginal sonographic characterization of ovarian disease: Evaluation of a new scoring system to predict ovarian malignancy. Obstet Gynecol. 1991; 78:70–76.

48. Schneider VL, Schneider A, Reed KL, et al. Comparison of Doppler with two-dimensional sonography and CA 125 for prediction of malignancy of pelvic masses. Obstet Gynecol. 1993; 81:983–988.

49. Smith LH, Ol RH. Detection of malignant ovarian neoplasms: A review of the literature. Obstet Gynecol Surv. 1984; 39:313–360.

50. Taylor KJW, Morse SS. Doppler detects vascularity of some malignant tumors. Diagnostic Imaging 1988; 10:132–136.

51. Teneriello MG, Hall KL, Lemon S, et al. Genetic alterations in gynecologic cancers. In: Srivastava S, Lippman SM, Hong WK, Mulshine JL, eds. Early Detection of Cancer: Molecular Markers. Armonk, NY: Futura; 1994:96–120.

52. Teneriello MG, Park RC. Early detection of ovarian cancer. CA Cancer J Clin. 1995; 45:71–87.

53. Timor-Tritsch IE, Lerner JP, Monteagudo A, et al. Transvaginal ultrasonographic characterization of ovarian masses by means of color flow directed Doppler measurements and a morphologic scoring system. Am J Obstet Gynecol. 1993; 168:909–913.

54. Walsh JW. Computed tomography of gynecologic neoplasms. Radiol Clin North Am. 1992; 30:817–831.

10

Pelvic Inflammatory Disease and Endometriosis

REBECCA HALL

Endometriosis and pelvic inflammatory disease (PID) are diffuse disease processes of the female pelvis that cause morphologic and vascular changes. As progressive diseases, they display a varied pattern of tissue involvement and clinical presentation. Clinical presentation in the early stages of both diseases is frequently nonspecific. Endometriosis may mimic functional bowel disease, and PID may mimic ectopic pregnancy, or appendicitis. Furthermore, these very different entities may have similar sonographic findings. Sonography of PID and endometriosis, therefore, are discussed together, although their causes, clinical presentations, and progression may be quite different. Close correlation of patient history, clinical findings, and sonographic findings should enable the clinician to distinguish between PID and endometriosis. In this chapter, endometriosis and PID are considered separately in terms of etiology, clinical findings, and sonographic findings. Table 10-1 summarizes the differences and similarities of the two.

Pelvic Inflammatory Disease

Pelvic inflammatory disease is a nonspecific term that refers to all pelvic infections. More commonly, it is related to inflammation caused by infection in the upper genital tract. Locations affected by PID include the endometrium (endometritis), the uterine wall (myometritis), the uterine serosa and broad ligaments (parametritis), and the ovary (oophoritis). The most common location of infection is the oviducts, or fallopian tubes (salpingitis).

Salpingitis is a disease with major economic and health consequences. Approximately 1 million cases of salpingitis are diagnosed each year in the United States, at an estimated cost of care in excess of $3 billion. It is expected that the incidence of PID will increase directly with the current rise in the number of sexually active people.[28] Twenty percent of patients who have had salpingitis subsequently become infertile, and those who do conceive have a 6 to 10 times greater risk of ectopic pregnancy. In addition, chronic pain and tuboovarian abscess (TOA) are common sequelae of salpingitis. The percentage of patients hospitalized with salpingitis progressing to TOA varies.[19,45]

ETIOLOGY

The cause of PID is almost invariably (99%) polymicrobial, and begins with bacterial invasion ascending from the mixed flora of the vagina and cervix. The most common bacteria that cause PID are (in descending order) *Chlamydia trachomatis* and *Neisseria gonorrhoeae* (gonococcus). Endogenous anaerobic bacteria (*Bacteroides, Peptostreptococcus,* and *Peptococcus* species) and aerobic bacteria (*Streptococcus, Escherichia coli,* and *Staphylococcus* organisms) have also been implicated.

TABLE 10-1. CHARACTERISTICS OF PELVIC INFLAMMATORY DISEASE (PID) AND ENDOMETRIOSIS COMPARED

	PID	Endometriosis

Etiology	Variable:
	Bacterial infection
	Neisseria gonorrhoeae
	
	Chlamydia species
	Anaerobic bacteria
	  Bacteriodes
	  Peptostreptococcus
	  Peptococcus
	Aerobic bacteria
	  Streptococcus
	  Escherichia coli
	  Staphylococcus
		Presence of endometrial tissue in abnormal locations outside uterus
		Most commonly held mechanism is retrograde menstruation
		Can be diffuse or focal (endometrium)

Clinical findings	**Stage 1,** early PID or endometriosis 50% to 80% asymptomatic
	Gonococcus culture may still be positive.
	History of venereal disease, intrauterine device, or pelvic surgery
	Pelvic tenderness
	Vaginal discharge
	Urethral burning
	Stage 2, Salpingitis (with or without formation of pyosalpinx and resolution to hydrosalpinx)
	  Fever
	  Chills
	  Acute abdominal complaints
	  Abnormal vaginal bleeding
	Stage 3, tuboovarian abscess or pelvic peritonitis with or without pelvic abscess
	  Fever with shaking chills
	  Acute abdominal pain
	  Significantly increased white blood cell count
	  Fitz-Hugh–Curtis syndrome
		May be asymptomatic. Symptom characteristics:
		  Involuntary infertility
		  Cyclic dysmenorrhea
		  Pelvic pain
		  Dyspareunia
		  Radiating back, leg, or groin pain

Sonographic characteristics	**Stage 1**, early PID
	Nonspecific findings:
	  Thickened, hyperechoic endometrium surrounded by hypoechoic fluid
	  May see fluid within endometrial cavity
	  May see highly reflective interface within endometrial cavity representing gas with "dirty" acoustic shadow
	  May see cul-de-sac fluid (anechoic or complex)
	
	Stage 2, Salpingitis
	  Serpiginous swollen tubes appear as tubular or beaded adnexal masses
	  Pointed beak (tapered end of swollen tube) at the proximal end of the tube
	  Distended section of swollen tube at the distal fimbriated end of the tube
		Variable appearance:
		May see nonspecific contour changes of pelvic structures or indistinct normal tissue planes
		  Diffuse endometriosis can appear as solid, homogeneous adnexal mass or complex
		  Focal endometriosis appears as a cystic or complex, primarily cystic, spherical structure with discrete, thick, irregular walls; commonly exhibits uniform dispersion of low-level internal echoes; enhanced through-transmission

(continued)

▰▰▰ **TABLE 10-1.** (Continued)

PID		Endometriosis
	Pyosalpinx appears hypoechoic or complex, eventually becoming anechoic as resorption occurs and as hydrosalpinx develops Hydrosalpinx appears as sausage-shaped or ovoid adnexal structure with distinct borders and enhanced through-transmission; tail points toward uterus; ampullary segment is expanded portion of cyst	
Differential diagnoses by ultrasound	Endometriosis Hemorrhagic ovarian cyst Ectopic pregnancy Neoplasm	PID Ectopic pregnancy Hemorrhagic ovarian cyst Neoplasm

In the past, *N. gonorrhoeae* was considered "the major pathogen" in salpingitis. However, current thought is that gonococci and chlamydiae may initially penetrate the endocervical barrier and cause mucopurulent endocervicitis that damages the endocervical canal, thus affording other organisms access to the upper genital tract. The initial gonorrheal or chlamydial infection may then be replaced by competing anaerobic or aerobic infective processes.[28]

Although most (85%) patients with PID become infected through sexual transmission, there are other routes of infection. For example, women who use an IUD (intrauterine contraceptive device) have a greater risk of contracting nongonococcal PID than women who use oral or barrier forms of contraception. It has been postulated that the IUD string protruding from the uterus through the cervix into the vagina provides a route of infection. The pathogen causing PID may also be introduced into the upper genital tract through dilation and curettage, postpartum conditions, hysteroscopy, hysterosalpingography, endometrial biopsy, intrauterine artificial insemination, or by other intraabdominal infections. Less than 1% of all cases of PID, however, result from hematogenous or lymphatic spread or from transperitoneal spread as a result of perforated appendix or intraabdominal abscess.[14]

The predominant organisms isolated from TOA aspirates are *E. coli*, *Bacteroides fragilis* and other *Bacteroides* species, aerobic streptococci, peptococci, and peptostreptococci. It has been suggested that PID patients with no history of infectious gonorrhea, chlamydia, or IUD placement who have vaginitis with high concentrations of anaerobic bacteria, may have alterations in the physiologic or immunologic defense system. This in turn promotes invasion of the upper genital tract by normal vaginal and cervical flora.[28] In addition, changes in cervical mucus throughout the menstrual cycle—specifically, thinning occurring as a function of increasing estrogen during the early follicular phase, and thickening occurring as a function of increasing progesterone during the secretory phase respectively—are thought to enhance (thin mucus) and prevent (thick mucus) penetration of bacteria toward the uterine cavity.[21,37]

PROGRESSION

Pelvic inflammatory disease is a progressive disease whose stages are determined by the upward migration of surface-invading bacteria from cervix to endometrium to oviducts to pelvic peritoneum. The initial spread of infection past the cervical barrier results in endometritis, or an intermediate stage of PID. Although the endometrial surface is infected with the pathogen, the uterus itself is usually immune to the inflammatory impact of the infection.[34] The endometrial cavity, however, is a conduit by which microorganisms reach the fallopian tubes. Varying degrees of salpingitis and ovarian and peritoneal involvement resulting from the spread of infection characterize the later stages of PID.[34]

The next stage of pelvic inflammatory disease is characterized by acute or subacute salpingitis in which the tube becomes inflamed and swollen or edematous. With acute gonococcal salpingitis, a purulent exudate may develop within the lumen of the tube, causing it to distend. With pyogenic salpingitis, the tube walls may become grossly edematous and thickened, causing a much greater enlargement of the tube.[34] If the lumen of the tube becomes blocked at the fimbriated orifice, purulent material may build up within the lumen, producing pyosalpinx (pus-filled tube). The obstruction of the tube may occur during the processes of inflammation and tissue repair. Pyosalpinx is usually associated with a chronic tubal infection or reinfection of a previously scarred tube.[34,39]

Hydrosalpinx may be a sequela of salpingitis and pyosalpinx. With the resolution of the acute infection, the purulent exudate is resorbed and a clear, watery fluid remains.[34] The walls of the tube remain distended and stretched, resulting in a thin-walled structure.

Extension of the inflammatory exudate from the salpinges may involve the broad ligaments (parametritis) and the ovaries (oophoritis). Ovaries affected by past or current PID may be adherent to the uterus. They may be enlarged, usually because of acute oophoritis. If the purulent material formed in the tube oozes from the fimbriated opening and over the ovary (perioophoritis), an abscess involving both the tubes and the ovary may form. This is referred to as a tuboovarian complex, although it is really a salpingo-oophoritis complex. If pus escapes from the tube into the peritoneal cavity, a pelvic peritonitis may develop and give rise to a diffuse pelvic abscess.[34] As the inflammatory exudate becomes organized, it glues adjacent surfaces to one another, forming adhesions between uterus, bladder, adnexa, and bowel.[20,28]

As healing occurs, scarring of the tube with adhesion formation usually develops.[34] The course and extent of the disease seem to be related to the type and virulence of the infecting organism, individual response to the infection, and a history of previous infection.[34]

CLINICAL FINDINGS

The patient with pelvic infection is often a young, sexually active woman with a wide range of nonspecific complaints. The clinical presentation ranges from minor complaints to acute, life-threatening illness.[14,17] The most frequent symptoms are lower abdominal pain and cervical motion tenderness. Adnexal tenderness, usually diffuse and bilateral, and constant dull pain, usually described as accentuated by movement or sexual activity, are also reported. Onset of symptoms may be rapid (associated more often with *N. gonorrhoeae*) or insidious (associated more often with *C. trachomatis*). In fact, most chlamydial infections are subclinical, even while the infection is widespread enough to partially obstruct the tube.[11,14] Physical examination may reveal cervical motion tenderness, adnexal tenderness, abdominal tenderness with or without guarding, and adnexal masses.[11,14,17] Seventy-five percent of patients with PID have associated endocervical infection with coexisting purulent vaginal discharge on physical examination.[14,17] About one third of women with acute salpingitis report abnormal vaginal bleeding, 20% report dysuria, and only 30% have fever.[34] This spectrum of clinical findings contributes to the high rate of misdiagnoses when diagnosis is based on clinical criteria alone.

Laboratory findings play only a minor role in the diagnosis of PID. Although 50% of PID patients have leukocytosis, an elevated erythrocyte sedimentation rate is variable (20% to 75%) with the etiology and severity of the infection, so this finding is nonspecific. Many patients, even with advanced abscess formation, may have no fever or elevated white blood cell count.[14,28,34]

Some patients may present with pelvic and right-sided upper quadrant pain. Fitz-Hugh–Curtis syndrome is a constellation of clinical findings that includes right-sided pleuritic pain and right-sided upper quadrant pain and tenderness on palpation. Fitz-Hugh–Curtis syndrome is experienced by 5% to 10% of patients with PID and is caused by perihepatic inflammation from peritonitis, as the infected fluid tracks into the subhepatic space from the lower pelvic peritoneal compartments. Often, ultrasound of these patients shows no definitive abnormality.

Although laboratory findings usually are of little help in establishing the diagnosis of PID, the detection of human chorionic gonadotropin (hCG) has major diagnostic implications.[14,28] A small number (3% to 4%) of patients who present with symptoms of pelvic infection test positive for hCG, indicating pregnancy. Because there is a strong association of PID and ectopic pregnancy, particularly in patients who have a history of PID and TOA, patients suspected of having PID who test positive for hCG should have an ultrasound examination to determine the location of the gestation and the extent of possible pelvic infection.[5]

The gold standard for accurate diagnosis of PID has been direct visualization of pelvic structures by laparoscopic examination, but this varies from country to country. In Swedish studies, laparoscopy was performed on all patients with pelvic infections. In the United States, the most common method of diagnosis is the clinical history and physical examination in conjunction with sonographic findings. Usually, only equivocal cases and patients who do not respond to antibiotic treatment are examined by laparoscopy, although there is considerable variation in its use.[14,29]

TREATMENT

Empiric antimicrobial therapy options initially include doxycycline, azithromycin (for *Chlamydia trachomatis*), and ceftriaxone, cefixime, ciprofloxacin, or ofloxacin (for *N. gonorrhea*).[6,9,11,22] For patients who do not respond to radical drug therapy, ultrasound-guided percutaneous, or surgical drainage of the unruptured abscess or removal of the affected tubes or ovaries may be recommended.[8]

ULTRASOUND IN THE MANAGEMENT OF PELVIC INFLAMMATORY DISEASE

Most PID patients are young women with many years of reproductive life ahead. The scarring of the fallopian tubes, which may be a result of pelvic infection, puts them at increased risk for sterility. Of even more clinical importance is a greater risk for ectopic pregnancy.[11] Ultrasound examination is useful for determining the location of an early gestation in such patients (see Chap. 11).

The sonographic presentation of PID varies with the extent of the infection. Findings may be dynamic, changing rapidly over a short time.[43] This discussion considers the sonographic appearance of the various stages of infection and their sequelae.

Early pelvic inflammatory disease, particularly salpingitis, has no specific ultrasound findings. The images of patients with salpingitis alone are often negative. However, the progression to salpingitis, tuboovarian complex, and pelvic abscess can be detected by ultrasound imaging with a higher degree of specificity and sensitivity. Computed tomography (CT) may provide a more global perspective of pelvic involvement.

Early and Intermediate Pelvic Inflammatory Disease

Early sonographic findings are too nonspecific to provide a definitive diagnosis of PID. A constellation of sonographic findings, however, may be present. Because the infection affects the endometrium, early findings include changes associated with endometritis or myometritis (Fig. 10-1*A*). The endometrium may appear prominent and hyperechoic. It may be surrounded by a hypoechoic ring, or it may contain a fluid collection with or without echogenic foci. A subtle hypoechogenicity of the uterus may signal early uterine infection.[28,42,43] Laparoscopic correlation with sonographic findings has, in fact, shown that 75% of patients with proven endometritis do not demonstrate any sonographic abnormalities.[36] Endometritis as a result of postpartum retained products of conception, IUD perforation, or ascending microorganisms from the vagina such as *E. coli* and *Clostridium perfringens (welchii)* can result in a gas-containing abscess in the endometrial cavity. A typical "dirty acoustic shadow" appearance behind high-level reflectors within the endometrial cavity are characteristic of air and gas.[20,42,43]

Other early findings are indistinct borders of the pelvic structures[4,42] and posterior cul-de-sac fluid. The amount of fluid, whether transudate or exudate, is greater than that often found midcycle in normal subjects, which is known to be 4 to 6 ml.[20,42] The fluid may appear complex if it contains blood or pus. A distended bladder can displace cul-de-sac fluid, resulting in some underestimation of pelvic fluid volume. The presence of cul-de-sac fluid cannot be correlated well with the severity of disease.[5] As the infection ascends the genital tract, acute salpingitis results. Tubal infection has a destructive effect on the tubal mucosa that can result in the formation of purulent exudate.

Severe Pelvic Inflammatory Disease With Tuboovarian Complex

Tuboovarian complex results from the escape of purulent exudate beyond the tube to include a perioophoritis. With salpingo-oophoritis, ovar-

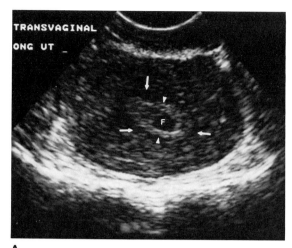

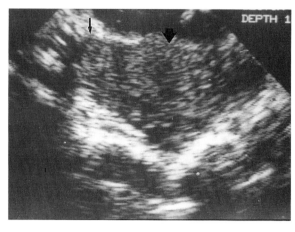

A **B**

Figure 10-1. (**A**) Transvaginal sonogram demonstrates changes in the endometrium as a result of endometritis. Note echogenic endometrium (*arrowheads*) enveloping a definite fluid collection (F). This prominent endometrium is surrounded by hypoechoic ring (*arrows*). (**B**) Transverse image of a 16-year-old with abdominal pain and mild fever with known acute salpingo-oophoritis. *Chlamydia trachomatis* cultured. Long arrow points to right prominent adherent ovary; short arrow points to uterus.

ian enlargement and adherence to adnexal structures makes the pelvic tissue planes ill defined (see Fig. 10-1*B*). A true TOA occurs once the ovarian parenchyma is affected.[20] TOA is usually a bilateral process of varying size and echogenicity. Bilateral TOAs may completely fill the pelvis, obscuring the uterine borders. TOA should be suspected when cystic adnexal masses with indistinct, thick walls, internal septations, or complex internal echoes are imaged (Figs. 10-2 and 10-3). The sonographic characteristics of these masses vary according to the stage of abscess formation. TOA may appear as an indistinct, complex mass (Fig. 10-4), whereas a resorbing mass results in a more cystic appearance. As treatment leads to healing, pelvic structures begin to regain their normal appearances. Color flow and Doppler waveform patterns are variable. TOAs are usually well perfused owing to increased vascularization, and demonstrate low to moderate impedance (PI < 1.0 and RI < 0.50).[16,27]

Pyosalpinx

Pyosalpinx (pus-filled fallopian tubes) may develop and distend the oviducts. These appear as tubular adnexal masses or as a string of beadlike adnexal masses (Fig. 10-5). This appearance results from the blockage of the tubal lumen at the fimbriated end or at various points along the tube with resultant retention of the purulent exudate.[33] These masses are primarily tubular in shape, but their sonographic echogenicity ranges from anechoic, simple cystic appearance to complex, primarily cystic structures with relatively smooth borders due to edema from the inflammatory process (Fig. 10-6).

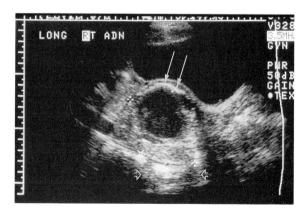

Figure 10-2. Sagittal image of large right adnexal tubo-ovarian abscess on a 24-year-old woman with severe diffuse pelvic pain and leukocytosis. Note the indistinct, thick walls (*closed arrows*) and posterior acoustic enhancement of this complex mass (*open arrows*). Findings were bilateral.

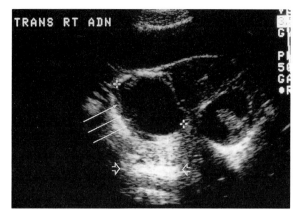

Figure 10-3. Transverse image of large right adnexal tuboovarian mass on a 24-year-old woman with severe diffuse pelvic pain and leukocytosis. Note the indistinct, thick walls (closed arrows) and posterior acoustic enhancement of this complex mass (open arrows). Findings were bilateral.

The stage of active pus formation with varied presence and degree of debris and fluid determine the sonographic characteristics along that spectrum. Usually the walls of the pyosalpinx are relatively smooth, but they may appear shaggy and the lumen may show hyperchoic protrusions caused by endosalpingeal folds.[5,42,45] Pyosalpinx is usually a unilateral process, but it may be bilateral.[20,42]

Peritonitis

The TOA may further involve the bladder, ureter, bowel, and contralateral adnexa.[37] As diffuse infectious involvement of the pelvis occurs, the borders of all the pelvic structures, including the ovaries and tubes, become indistinct owing to parametrial inflammation (Fig. 10-7). This is caused by the development of multiple abscesses forming septa. Some of the bacteria implicated in PID cause gas-forming abscesses, which further obscure tissue planes,[42] including the posterior cul-de-sac. In addition, the gas-forming organisms may create a complex, reflective, echogenic appearance.[17] With abscess formation and the development of peritonitis, loculated fluid collections appear in the pelvis. These loculations may displace adjacent organs or compartments. Some of the infected fluid may not be loculated but may flow freely in the pelvis, paracolic gutters, and mesenteric reflections, shifting with changes in the patient's position. If it flows to the perihepatic space, the patient might experience Fitz-Hugh–Curtis syndrome (Fig. 10-8). Once fluid is discovered, the sonographer should note changes in appearance of the free fluid by moving the patient from supine to right posterior oblique and left posterior oblique positions. Pelvic peritoni-

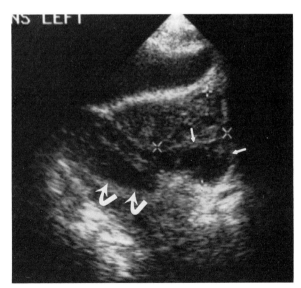

A

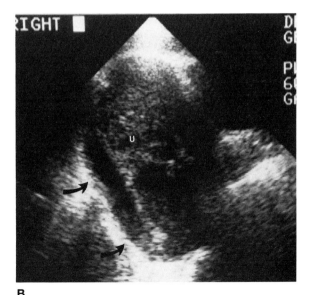

B

Figure 10-4. (A) Severe pelvic inflammatory disease with posterior fluid collection (*curved arrows*). Transverse scan demonstrates indistinct, complex mass in left adnexa (*straight arrows*). **(B)** Midline sagittal section, after partial voiding. Heterogenous appearance of uterus (U) indicates myometritis.

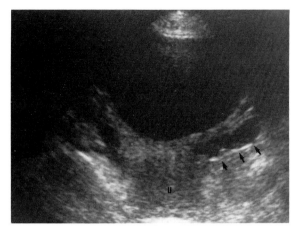

Figure 10-5. Transverse sonogram demonstrates left-sided pyosalpinx (*arrows*). Note the indistinct uterine (u) borders.

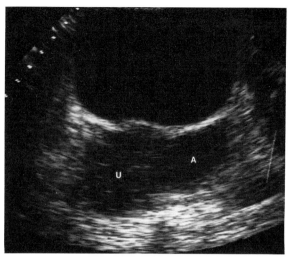

Figure 10-7. Severe pelvic inflammatory disease in transverse section in which the uterus (U) can barely be distinguished from enlarged left adnexa (A).

tis may lead to ileus, which further complicates the sonographic findings by distending the bowel air. Again, CT may provide a more global view of the pelvis and abdomen.

Chronic Pelvic Inflammatory Disease

Chronic PID refers to both the residue of acute infection or the subacute recurrence of a previous inflammation. Clinically, these patients present for infertility problems even without overt PID symptoms. Several studies have concluded that the pathophysiology of these chronic disease conditions is immunologically mediated.[11] Hydrosalpinx, sterile fluid in a scarred, obstructed fallopian tube, can accumulate as a result of long-standing PID. It appears as a sausage-shaped or ovoid, anechoic ad-

nexal structure with enhanced acoustic transmission (Fig. 10-9). It has distinct borders and thin walls, owing to long-standing enlargement. In hydrosalpinx there is typically a tail-shaped structure pointing toward the uterus because the ampullary portion of the tube expands more than the proximal portion (Fig. 10-10).[42] Hydrosalpinx may be difficult to differentiate from an ovarian cyst or small cystadenoma.[43] Like ovarian cysts, hydrosalpinges occasionally undergo torsion.[34]

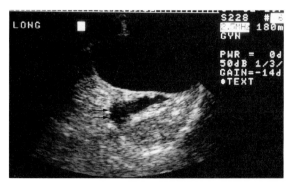

Figure 10-6. Transverse sonogram of pyosalpinx on a 34-year-old woman scanned to rule out abscess. The arrow points to the fimbriated end of the tube.

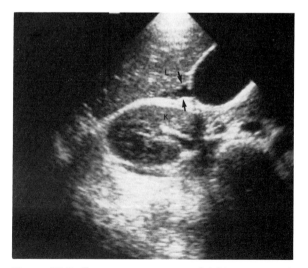

Figure 10-8. Transverse sonogram of right upper quadrant demonstrates subhepatic fluid collection (*arrows*) between liver and right kidney. The presence of this fluid is associated with Fitz-Hugh–Curtis syndrome.

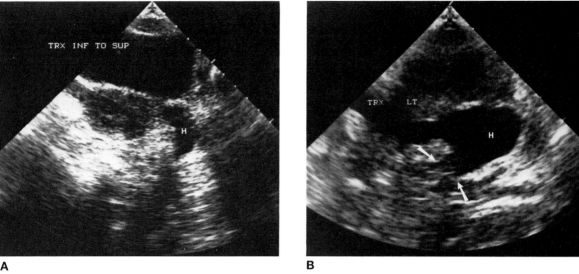

Figure 10-9. Left hydrosalpinx (H) demonstrated in (**A**) transabdominal and (**B**) transvaginal sonogram. Note dilation of fimbriated end of the tube (*arrows*).

When adhesions have developed as the result of long-standing, severe PID, the borders of pelvic structures may become obliterated or ill defined because of fixation of organs by widespread fibrosis.[42] As in all pelvic examinations, it is important to distinguish bowel from possible PID, because bowel may mimic pelvic masses. If peristalsis is not evident, and the patient cannot tolerate an endovaginal ultrasound examination, bowel may be differentiated from a "mass" by using the water enema technique.

After treatment, serial ultrasonographic examinations demonstrate resolution of pelvic infection

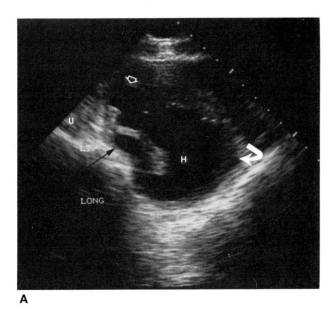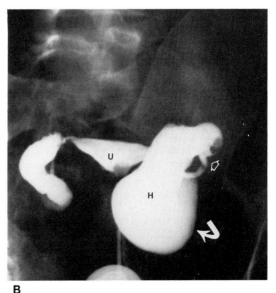

Figure 10-10. Left hydrosalpinx by sonography (**A**) and hysterosalpingography (**B**). Uterus (U), hydrosalpinx (H). The proximal end of the fallopian tube is obscured because of the folding over of the ampullary portion (*curved arrow*) on this view. The fimbriated end of the tube is represented by the open arrow.

by documenting changes in size and appearance of pelvic structures. This may be as simple as documenting the reduction in the size of masses or the amount of free fluid, or as complex as judging the changes in the appearance of pelvic structures as they return to normal.[44] If the disease does not respond to conservative therapy, the ultrasound examination provides valuable information on the size and location of abscesses for surgical drainage with or without sonographic guidance.[26,42] With appropriate treatment, the end result may be return to a completely normal pelvis or one scarred and functionally impaired.[39] Sonographic evidence of resolution should be seen within 6 to 8 weeks after antibiotic therapy begins.[5]

OTHER IMAGING MODALITIES

Although ultrasound is the standard diagnostic imaging procedure in the evaluation of PID, other noninvasive imaging techniques used to differentiate TOA from other masses include CT, magnetic resonance imaging (MRI), and radionuclide scanning.[28,32,37] Mitchell and coworkers recommend MRI or CT as a useful, larger–field-of-view supplement to ultrasound if clearer documentation of the presence or absence of blood, fluid, fat, or protein components in the adnexal masses will increase the physician's confidence in his or her diagnosis of PID.[33] It is the opinion of some investigators that gallium-67 imaging in conjunction with sonographic examination or CT can lead to early diagnosis and treatment of occult infections.[32] Sonography is the primary diagnostic imaging modality, however, because it is inexpensive, readily available, does not expose the patient to ionizing radiation, and lends itself to serial scanning to follow treatment efficacy.[28]

Endometriosis

Endometriosis is defined as heterotopic growth of the glands and stroma of the uterine lining (endometrium) that continues to respond to the hormonal influence of the ovulatory cycle.[13,14] Although the disease is usually regarded as a benign process, cellular activity and progression may lead to adhesion formation and interruption of normal reproduction. Chronic progression can produce a wide range of clinical consequences, including severe cyclic pain and infertility.[46]

ETIOLOGY

The etiology of endometriosis is uncertain, but several theories have been advanced. The dissemination of endometrial tissue fragments throughout the pelvis because of retrograde menstruation is the most popular theory, wherein flow of sloughed endometrial cells during menses is refluxed toward the tubes instead of the cervix. Retrograde menstrual bleeding has been found in most menstruating women.[21] Other theories postulate metaplasia caused by the stimulation of menstrual debris by estrogen and progesterone, vascular or lymphatic spread, genetic predisposition, immunologic defects, and contributing environmental factors.[14,48] Epidemiologic and clinical data suggest that parity is inversely associated with endometriosis risk.[18]

Endometriosis and its symptoms are directly related to the cyclic hormonal stimulation of the reproductive years. Natural menopause gradually brings relief of symptoms. Patients who have had transabdominal hysterectomy with bilateral oophorectomy experience prompt and complete regression of the ectopically located endometrial tissue and, with it, relief of symptoms, although scar tissue may persist. It is assumed that intrapelvic bleeding and the development of adhesions cease when hormonal stimulation of ectopic endometrium ceases.[14,25]

Endometriosis can be diffuse or focal; 66% of implants are located in the pelvis. Focal implants are called endometriomas. The term "chocolate cyst" is used to describe the characteristic appearance of an endometrioma filled with old blood from repeated episodes of hormonally stimulated endometrial sloughing within the implant. Endometriomas are usually small, measuring 2 to 6 cm.[42] The most common site for endometrial implantation is the ovary. Involvement is usually bilateral. Other commonly involved locations include the anterior and posterior cul-de-sac, the broad ligaments, pelvic lymph nodes, the cervix, vagina, vulva, and the fallopian tubes (Fig. 10-11).[14,40,48] Rarely, implantation occurs in areas of previous surgery, the umbilicus, bladder, kidney, extremities, and urinary tract. Pleural endometriosis that has spread from the pelvis through diaphragmatic defects has been documented.[14,24]

The color, shape, size, degree of inflammation, and associated fibrosis of the endometrial implants vary. The differences are associated with cyclic hormonal changes and length of time the implant has been active. New lesions are small (<1 cm in diameter), blood filled, and raised above the surface of surrounding tissue. Lesions within the ovaries may range from these small, 1-mm, "new" implants to larger chocolate cysts, which may be 8 to 14 cm in diameter.[14,40,42]

CLINICAL FINDINGS

The presenting symptoms of patients with endometriosis are common to several conditions, including chronic PID, ovarian malignancy, degeneration of uterine myoma, adenomyosis, primary dysmenorrhea, and functional bowel disease, making the clinical diagnosis difficult.[14,30] It is estimated that 30% to 40% of infertility patients have endometriosis. Five to 10% of female laparotomy patients of childbearing age have been found incidentally to have endometriosis. As many as 30% of all women may have no symptoms despite evidence of endometriosis.

Even with a complex clinical presentation, there are some common features. The typical endometriosis patient is nulliparous and in her thirties. The variety of symptoms is wide, including asymptomatic involuntary infertility, dysmenorrhea, incapacitating pelvic pain, and dyspareunia.[13,14,30,42,47] Endometriosis is rare in women younger than 20 years of age.[30]

One of the most common presenting symptoms is pelvic pain, but there is no direct relationship between the degree of pain and extent of the disease. A minimal amount of tissue implantation may result in excruciating pain if it causes peritoneal stretching, whereas extensive endometrial implants in less sensitive locations may create no symptoms. In fact, pain may be unrelated to the extent of disease. Patients with pelvic pain present with secondary dysmenorrhea (because of successive periods of swelling and extravasation of blood and menstrual debris into the surrounding tissue) and dyspareunia (either because of direct pressure of implants on the uterosacral ligaments or in the cul-de-sac, or as a result of the immobilization of adherent structures).[13,14,40]

Pelvic pain usually begins 24 to 48 hours before menstruation and lasts for several days, or it may be chronic, worsening during menses.[14,43] Descriptions of the pain range from a dull ache to severe unilateral or bilateral pain, which may radiate to the lower back, legs, or groin. Patients also report "pelvic heaviness," describing a feeling of swelling or congestion in the pelvic region. Fifteen to 20% of patients with endometriosis also have menorrhagia or abnormal premenstrual spotting.[14,40]

Endometriosis is a chronic and progressive disease of the childbearing years. Although the degree of pelvic involvement may not necessarily advance with age, depth of infiltration and size of implants may increase.[15]

TREATMENT

Treatment of endometriosis may take several forms: the implant site may be excised or the hormonal stimulation that causes the cyclic growth and swelling may be ablated. More conservatively, the patient may be observed and managed only with analgesics. Treatments for endometriosis include the following:

1. Continuous therapy with oral contraceptives or progestins alone to promote a pseudopregnant state (anovulatory–acyclic hormonal environment), causing ectopic endometrial tissue to atrophy.
2. Use of the synthetic steroid danazol to inhibit ovulation by suppressing luteinizing hormone and follicle-stimulating hormone midcycle surges causes amenorrhea, producing atrophic changes in both the endometrium and the ectopic endometrial implants. Unfortu-

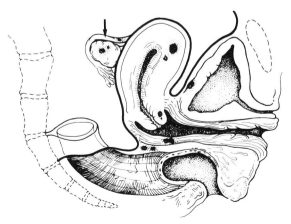

Figure 10-11. *Schematic diagram of the female pelvis showing sites for focal implants of ectopic endometrial tissue. The most common site of implantation is the ovary (arrow).*

▟▟▟▟ **TABLE 10-2.** Ultrasound Examination for Endometriosis or Pelvic Inflammatory Disease

Examination	
Uterus	*Size* is measured and documented on midline sagittal and anteroposterior mid-uterus and transverse.
	Echogenicity is noted; echo patterns are compared to normal homogeneous appearance, especially when performing serial exams.
	Architecture and border definition are noted.
Endometrium	Changes of normal echogenic patterns throughout the ovulatory cycle must be understood by the sonographer (see Chap. 4). For example, a 6-mm echogenic endometrium surrounding a small amount of sonolucent endometrial cavity fluid is the normal premenses appearance of the late secretory phase but is abnormal for the first-week proliferative phase.
Adnexa	Delineation and measurement of ovaries in two planes must be consistently documented.

If Abnormalities Are Found:

If "masses" are seen, the following parameters are characterized in two planes:

Size is marked by caliper measurements.

Shape of "mass(es)." Spherical, ovoid, sausage-shaped? Where is it in relation to the ovaries? Could it be tubal? If you suspect it is tubal, is it dilated? Can you follow tube to the fimbriated end?

Internal definition. It is sonolucent, hypoechoic, complex? Are there septa?

Adjacent structures. Is there indentation or displacement of normal adjacent structures, such as uterus or bladder?

Wall thickness. If the wall is thick, document with measurements. Is there fluid surrounding the border?

Posterior cul-de-sac. Is there free fluid? Is it sonolucent or is there debris in it? If fluid is present, is there also free fluid in Morison's pouch in the right-side upper quadrant? If so, document it.

Patient position. How does the appearance of such "mass(es)" change when the patient is moved to oblique positions, or after partial voiding and complete voiding? If the patient can tolerate transvaginal scanning, how do the "masses" appear in comparison? Do the findings confirm or clarify the transabdominal finding?

Pre- and postprocessing. Proper use of pre- and postprocessing capabilities should help. For example, changing the postprocessing curve on a poorly defined mass may accentuate the borders more effectively.

Remember: The key to a successful serial scanning technique is consistent documentation of all of the above.

---

nately, danazol has significant side effects. These include weight gain, increased muscle mass, acne, deepening of voice, and altered libido, all results of the androgenicity of the drug. Gonadotropin-releasing hormone agonists such as leuprolide acetate and nafarelin acetate have been found to be as effective as danazol, with fewer side effects.[9]

3. Surgical intervention to excise large endometriomas or relieve ureteral obstruction, compromised bowel function, or adnexal masses.

4. Complete hysterectomy with oophorectomy is an option for patients who have completed childbearing.[1,3,13,14,40,42]

5. The combination of drug therapy (as described previously) to reduce endometrioma size, followed by laser therapy by laparoscope to vaporize implants, attempts eradication of endometrial implants while preserving function of adjacent tissue.[10] Use of laser treatment varies by institution, but it is becoming a central tool in endometriosis treatment, especially with the increasing number of laparoscopic procedures being performed.

The main aim of treatment is to keep recurrence to a minimum. Surgery is the only permanent cure. Treatment results may be monitored by second-look laparoscopy.

Studies suggest that the natural history of endometriosis is varied. It may progress to deeper infiltration or new implantation, or it may improve or disappear. Current data indicate potentially progressive disease in 50% of affected patients.[15,41]

Role of Ultrasound

The goal of ultrasound in the management of endometriosis is to add as much detail as possible to the clinical picture, such as location and extent of disease. Ultrasound findings are most useful in the clinical management of advanced stages of the disease, although diffuse endometriosis is more difficult to image than individual endometriomas.

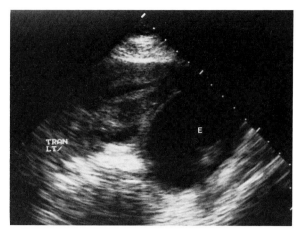

Figure 10-12. Endometrioma (E) with characteristic complex, primarily cystic, appearance.

As in all scanning protocols for gynecologic sonography, the ideal examination should include examination of the uterus and all its borders, the ovaries, pelvic vasculature, bladder, and ureters, all in at least two planes. The careful delineation of structures is particularly important when attempting to diagnose diffuse processes, which may produce subtle sonographic changes. In addition, the blurring of tissue planes associated with progressive PID or endometriosis necessitates more careful scanning to distinguish the mass from neighboring structures (Table 10-2).[42]

A negative ultrasound examination in the presence of clinical findings suggestive of endometriosis does not exclude an active, developing process.[7] Some authors assert that ultrasound plays only a minor role in the diagnosis of endometriosis because it is neither sensitive nor specific.[48]

ULTRASOUND FINDINGS

The sonographic findings in endometriosis are variable.[14,42] The uterus appears normal. Endometrial implants may exhibit sonographic patterns ranging from cystic to solid to complex. In general, there must be a large volume of abnormal endometrial tissue if it is to be detected by ultrasound. Solid echo patterns representing organized blood or fibrin deposits may appear as uniform homogeneous masses, but differentiation from other adnexal disease processes such as PID, neoplasms, hemorrhagic corpus luteum cysts, or chronic ectopic pregnancy is difficult because of image similarities.[20,30,41]

The ultrasound diagnosis of focal endometriosis is made by documentation of heterogeneous structures representing chocolate cysts or endometriomas (Fig. 10-12). These appear as discrete, thick-walled, spherical pelvic masses (Fig. 10-13). Most commonly they exhibit uniform dispersion of low-level internal echoes (Fig. 10-14). In a few patients, they may be totally anechoic or septated with enhanced through-transmission (Fig. 10-15).[20,30,43] The walls of endometrial cysts are irregular, unlike the smooth walls of simple ovarian cysts. They may displace normal structures, such as the bladder, by mass effect.[13,30,40,42]

Transvaginal sonography may aid in the imaging of chocolate cysts, noting with more clarity their uniformly echogenic appearance (Fig. 10-16; see also Fig. 28-6B). When the endometriomas are larger, they may be difficult to visualize because of the limited field of view of transvaginal sonography. Sonographic findings are nonspecific. Their echo pattern may resemble that of sebaceous dermoid cysts and hemorrhagic corpus luteum cysts, which appear as complex structures with variable degrees of solid components.[25,47]

Color Doppler demonstrates flow around and not within these masses, similar to that noted with

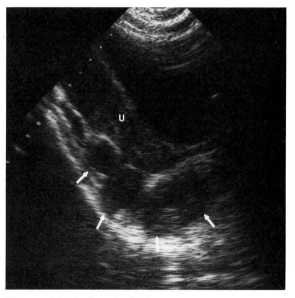

Figure 10-13. Longitudinal sonogram demonstrates multiple endometriomas (*arrows*) posterior to uterus (U). Note the irregular thick walls of these spherical masses and the different levels of echogenicity due to their various stages of aging.

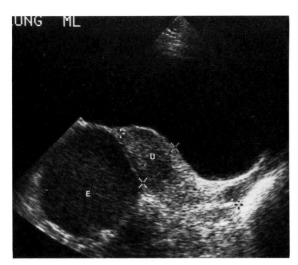

Figure 10-14. Longitudinal sonogram shows the classic low-level echoes within this endometrioma (E) located superior to the uterus (U).

a simple cyst.[2,27] Doppler flow may demonstrate high to low resistance depending on phase of menstrual cycle, with lower impedance in the menstrual phase, and the absorption of degraded blood products and higher resistance in the same patient in the late follicular phase (Fig. 10-17).[16,27] As with all pelvic scans, it is especially important to distinguish bowel from areas of possible pathology when examining a patient whose clinical presentation suggests endometriosis. If peristalsis is not evident in a suspect area, bowel should be differentiated from mass by use of a water enema. Bowel involvement may also produce changes on barium studies.[12,13]

Diagnosis and treatment of endometriosis is based primarily on clinical findings. Other common diseases that involve the pelvic organs, however, must be included in the differential diagnosis because of overlapping patterns of clinical presentation. These include PID, ectopic pregnancy, abscess, neoplasm, hemorrhagic corpus luteum cyst, leiomyoma, ovarian cyst, and cystadenoma.[13,43]

Adenomyosis

DEFINITION

Adenomyosis is a uterine condition in which growth of endometrial glands and stroma occurs within the uterine myometrium at a depth of at least 2.5 mm from the basalis layer of the endome-

trium, usually with more prominent involvement of the posterior wall (Fig. 10-18; see also Fig. 28-13).[14,38,43,48] This may be followed by envelopment of hypertrophied myometrial smooth muscle around it.[50] The aberrant growth of endometrial tissue within the uterine wall, either diffuse or focal, differs from endometriosis in that it remains continuous with the endometrium, yet does not undergo the cyclic changes resulting from ovarian hormone production. The cul-de-sac and ovaries are not involved.

CLINICAL FINDINGS

Patients with adenomyosis are older than those with endometriosis, are usually multiparous, and have a history of hypermenorrhea and progressive dysmenorrhea. When symptomatic, the most common clinical manifestations of adenomyosis are pelvic pain, hypermenorrhea, and intermenstrual spotting.[35] Pain associated with adenomyosis is noticed immediately before or during menstruation. On physical examination, the uterus is found to be normal or enlarged, globular in contour, boggy, and somewhat tender. When enlarged it may often be two or three times normal size. The clinical presentation and physical findings may mimic those of leiomyoma.[35] The usefulness of hysterosalpingography is limited; it may show an enlarged uterus, or results may be normal.[49]

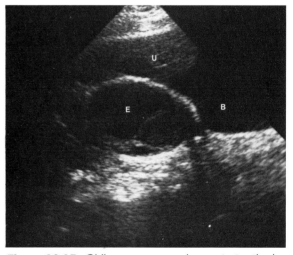

Figure 10-15. Oblique sonogram demonstrates the less common sonographic appearance of endometriomas (E) adjacent to bladder (B) and uterus (U). Note the septae and enhanced through-transmission.

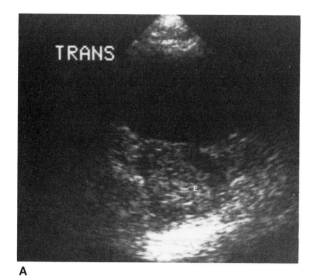

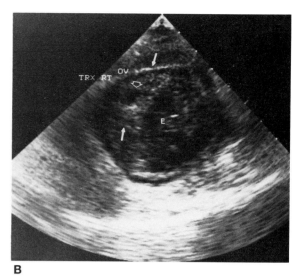

A   **B**

Figure 10-16. Comparison of transabdominal (**A**) and transvaginal sonogram (**B**) of the same endometrioma (E). Note the improved distinction of the endometrioma from the ovary (*closed arrows*) on the transvaginal sonogram. A small follicle is noted in the ovary (*open arrows*).

TREATMENT

Adenomyosis is treated surgically by total hysterectomy with or without removal of the ovaries. Hormonal treatment used for endometriosis has been uniformly unsuccessful.[25] This is because the tissue is composed largely of basal endometrium, which is not fully responsive to endometrial cyclic hormonal changes.[50]

ULTRASOUND FINDINGS

The primary ultrasound finding in adenomyosis is a symmetrically enlarged uterus due to endometrial hyperplasia and hypertrophy of the uterine muscle.[4,5,7,43] The sonographic texture of the uterus is uniform; echogenicity of the lesion is normal, increased, or slightly decreased with poor, if any, border delineation. The endometrial cavity may be displaced, most typically from posterior to anterior, by the thickened myometrium.[7,50] This thickened area may have a heterogeneous appearance previously described as "swiss cheese" or "honeycomb" appearance.[7,13,42]

These findings are also consistent with uterine myomas and endometrial carcinoma. Care must be taken to evaluate further the disease process by us-

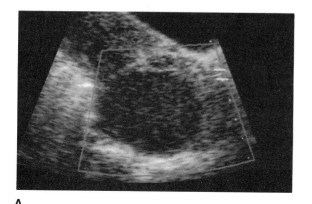

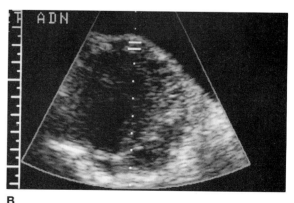

A   **B**

Figure 10-17. (**A**) Sagittal image of a patient with recurring endometrioma on her right ovary. Peripheral flow Doppler waveform reveals a normal resistive index (RI) of 0.75. (**B**) Sagittal image of a patient with a hemorrhagic ovarian cyst. Peripheral flow Doppler waveform reveals a normal RI of 0.85.

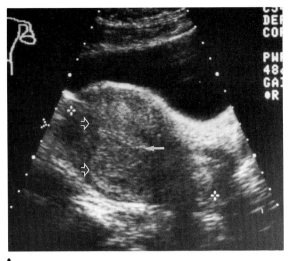
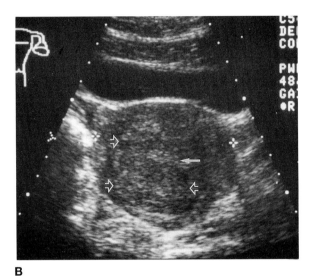

A   **B**

Figure 10-18. (**A,B**) A 43-year-old woman with a history of painful menstrual periods. Sagittal and transverse images demonstrate uterus with global enlargement and increased echogenicity of surgically confirmed adenomyosis (*open arrows*). Endometrium is only mildly displaced anteriorly (*closed arrows*). (Courtesy of Catherine Carr-Hoefer, Corvallis Radiology, Corvallis, OR.)

ing signal-processing capabilities, such as preprocessing and postprocessing, to distinguish better contour and border differentiation of the abnormal uterus. Transvaginal color Doppler studies have proven to be helpful in differentiating uterine pathology. One study reporting color flow patterns of uterine masses noted that myomas typically demonstrate feeding arteries (91%), sarcomas always demonstrate feeding arteries (100%), and adenomyosis rarely demonstrates feeding arteries (9%) around the mass.[23]

Although expensive, MRI is highly accurate in helping to distinguish adenomyosis from leiomyoma. MRI researchers believe that the difference in signal intensities between the two entities as well as the comparison of border definition and effect on surrounding structures may hold a key to this diagnostic problem. The differentiation is important for patients who wish to preserve their reproductive capacity. Presurgical diagnosis of leiomyoma may permit myomectomy instead of hysterectomy. Diagnosis must be confirmed histologically.[31,49]

REFERENCES

1. Adamson GD, Kwei L, Egrea RA. Pain of endometriosis: Effects of navefelin and danazol therapy. Int J Fertil Menopausal Stud. 1994; 39:215–217.

2. Applebaum M. The menstrual cycle, menopause, ovulation induction, and in vitro fertilization. In: Copel JA, Reed KL, eds. Doppler Ultrasound in Obstetrics and Gynecology. New York: Raven Press; 1995:78.

3. Balasch J, Martinez-Román S, Carreras J, Vanrell JA. Acute pancreatitis associated with danazol treatment for endometriosis. Hum Reprod. 1994; 9:1163–1165.

4. Berland L, Lawson T, Foley W, Albarelli JN. Ultrasound evaluation of pelvic infections. Radiol Clin North Am. 1982; 20(2):367–368.

5. Bernstine R, Kennedy W, Waldron J. Acute pelvic inflammatory disease: Clinical follow-up. Int J Fertil. 1987; 32:229–332.

6. Blanchard TJ, Mabey DCW. Chlamydial infections. Br J Clin Pract. 1994; 48:201–205.

7. Bohlman M, Ensor R, Sanders R. Sonographic findings in adenomyosis of the uterus. Am J Roentgenol. 1987; 148:765–766.

8. Casola G, van Sonnenberg E, Varney RR, et al. Percutaneous drainage of tubo-ovarian abscesses. Presented at the 74th Scientific Assembly and Annual Meeting of the Radiologic Society of North America, Chicago, Illinois, November 27–December 2, 1988.

9. Centers for Disease Control and Prevention. Recommendations for the prevention and management of chlamydia trachomatis infections. WMMR 1993; 42(RR-12):1–39.

10. Cohen SM. CO_2 laser microsurgery for pelvic disease

and infertility. In: Fisher W, ed. Laser Surgery in Gynecology: A Clinical Guide. Philadelphia: WB Saunders; 1993:214–215.

11. Czerwenka K, Heuss F, Hosmann J, Manavi M, Jelincic D, Kubista E. Salpingitis caused by *Chlamydia trachomatis* and its significance for infertility. Acta Obstet Gynaecol Scand. 1994; 73:711–715.

12. Dallenbach-Hellweg G. Histopathology of the Endometrium. New York: Springer-Verlag; 1987.

13. Deutsch A, Gosink B. Nonneoplastic gynecologic disorders. Semin Roentgenol. 1982; 17:269–283.

14. Droegemueller W, Herbst A, Michell D, et al. Comprehensive Gynecology. St. Louis: CV Mosby; 1987.

15. Fedele L, Bianchi S, Dinola G, Candiani M, Busacea M, Vignali M. The recurrence of endometriosis. Ann NY Acad Sci. 1994; 734:358–364.

16. Fleischer AC, Rogers WH. Ovarian masses. In: Fleischer AC, Emerson DS, eds. Color Doppler Sonography in Obstetrics and Gynecology. New York: Churchill Livingstone; 1993:60–69.

17. Galask R, Larsen B. Infectious Diseases in the Female Patient. New York: Springer-Verlag; 1986.

18. Gruppo Italiano per lo Studio. Prevalence and anatomical distribution of endometriosis in women with selected gynaecological conditions: Results from a multicentric study. Hum Reprod. 1994; 9:1158–1162.

19. Hager W. Follow-up of patients with tuboovarian abscess(es) in association with salpingitis. Obstet Gynecol. 1983; 61:680.

20. Hagen-Ansert S. Textbook of Diagnostic Ultrasonography. 4th ed. St. Louis: CV Mosby; 1995.

21. Halme J, Hammond MG, Hulka J, et al. Retrograde menstruation in healthy women and in patients with endometriosis. Obstet Gynecol. 1984; 64:151–154.

22. Hemsell D, Santos-Ramos R, Cunningham G, et al. Cefotaxime treatment for women with community-acquired pelvic abscesses. Am J Obstet Gynecol. 1985; 151:771–777.

23. Hirai M, Sagai H, Sekiya S. Transvaginal pulsed and color Doppler sonography for the evaluation of adenomyosis. J Ultrasound Med. 1995; 14:529–532.

24. Kang H, Choi B, Park J, et al. Endometriosis: CT and sonographic findings. Am J Roentgenol. 1987; 148:523–524.

25. Kistner R. Gynecology Principles and Practice. 4th ed. Chicago: Year Book Medical Publishers; 1986.

26. Kuligowska E, Keller E, Ferrucci JT. Treatment of pelvic abscesses: Value of one-step sonographically-guided transrectal needle aspiration and lavage. Am J Roentgenol. 1995; 164:201–206.

27. Kurjak A, Predonic M, Kupesic S, Zalud I. Adnexal masses—malignant ovarian tumors. In: Kurjak A, ed. The Encyclopedia of Visual Medicine Series: An Atlas of Transvaginal Color Doppler—The Current State of the Art. London: The Parthenon Publishing Group; 1994:216–217.

28. Landers D, Sweet R. Current trends in the diagnosis and treatment of tuboovarian abscess. Am J Obstet Gynecol. 1985; 151:1098–1110.

29. Ledger W. Infection in the Female. 2nd ed. Philadelphia: Lea & Febiger; 1986.

30. Manor WF, Zwiebel WJ, Hanning RV Jr, et al. Ectopic pregnancy and other causes of acute pelvic pain. Semin Ultrasound CT MR. 1985; 6:181–184.

31. Mark A, Hricak H, Heinrichs L, et al. Adenomyosis and leiomyoma: Differential diagnosis with MR imaging. Radiology. 1987; 163:527–529.

32. Mettler FA, Guiberteau M. Essentials of Nuclear Medicine Imaging. 3rd ed. Orlando, FL: Grune & Stratton; 1986.

33. Mitchell D, Mintz M, Spritzer C, et al. Adnexal masses: MR imaging observations at 1.5T, with US and CT correlations. Radiology. 1987; 162:319–324.

34. Novak E. Novak's Textbook of Gynecology. 11th ed. Baltimore: Williams & Wilkins; 1988.

35. Nyberg D, Laing F, Jeffrey B. Sonographic detection of subtle pelvic fluid collections. Am J Roentgenol. 1984; 143:261–263.

36. Patten RM, Vincent LM, Wolner-Hanssen P, Thorpe E Jr. Pelvic inflammatory disease: Endovaginal sonography with laparoscopic correlation. J Ultrasound Med. 1990; 9:681–689.

37. Radecki PD, Lev-Toaff AS, Hilpert PL, Horrow MM. Inflammatory diseases. In: Friedman A, Radecki PD, Lev-Toaff AS, Hilpert PL, eds. Clinical Pelvic Imaging, CT, Ultrasound, and MRI. St. Louis: CV Mosby; 1990:107–109.

38. Radecki PD, McKrisky PJ. Female pelvis: Neoplastic and nonneoplastic masses. In: Friedman AC, Radecki PD, Lev-Toaff AS, Hilpert PL, eds. Clinical Pelvic Imaging, CT, Ultrasound, and MRI. St. Louis: CV Mosby; 1990:219–220.

39. Rice PA, Weström LV. Pathogenesis and inflammatory response. In: Burger GS, Weström LV, eds. Pelvic Inflammatory Disease. New York: Raven Press; 1992:35–42.

40. Rosenwaks Z, Benjamin F, Stone M. Gynecology: Principles and Practice. New York: Macmillan; 1987.

41. Ryan K, Barkowitz RS, Barbieri RL. Kistner's Gynecology Principles and Practice. 6th ed. St. Louis: CV Mosby; 1995.

42. Sanders R, James E. The Principles and Practice of Ultrasonography in Obstetrics and Gynecology. 3rd ed. Norwalk, CT: Appleton-Century-Crofts; 1985.

43. Sarti D. Diagnostic Ultrasound: Text and Cases. 2nd ed. Chicago: Year Book Medical Publishers; 1987.

44. Spirtos N, Bernstine R, Crawford W, et al. Sonography in acute pelvic inflammatory disease. J Reprod Med. 1982; 27:312–320.

45. Swayne L, Love M, Karasick S. Pelvic inflammatory disease: Sonographic–pathologic correlation. Radiology. 1984; 151:751–755.

46. Thomas EJ, Cooke ID. Impact of gestrinone on the course of asymptomatic endometriosis. Br Med J. 1987; 294:272–274.

47. Timor-Tritsch I, Rottem S. Transvaginal Sonography. New York: Elsevier; 1988.

48. Wilson E. Endometriosis. New York: Alan R. Liss; 1987.

49. Winfield AC, Wentz AC. The Uterine Cavity in Diagnostic Imaging in Infertility. Baltimore: Williams & Wilkins; 1992.

50. Wynn RM. Obstetrics and Gynecology: The Clinical Core. Philadelphia: Lea and Febiger; 1992.

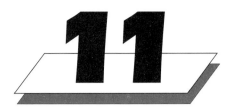

Sonographic Assessment of Ectopic Pregnancy

TAMARA ALLEN and FRANK CERVANTES

An ectopic pregnancy is one in which the fertilized ovum implants in any area outside the endometrial cavity. It accounts for 1% of all pregnancies.[2] Before the advent of modern diagnostic techniques, patients died from hemorrhage secondary to rupture because the diagnosis was not made in time for surgical intervention. The maternal mortality rate from ectopic pregnancy declined markedly starting in 1970, from 3.5 deaths per thousand, and more gradually in recent years, with an overall sevenfold decrease to 0.5 deaths per thousand in 1983. This decline may, in part, be accounted for by greater clinical awareness, improved laboratory methods for earlier diagnosis of pregnancy, and both transabdominal and transvaginal ultrasound. Ectopic pregnancy still, however, continues to be a cause of morbidity and mortality among young women. Currently, 40 to 50 women die each year in the United States as a result of ectopic pregnancy.[10] The incidence of extrauterine pregnancy has been reported to be 1.4 ectopic pregnancies for every 70 reported pregnancies.[23]

The clinical diagnosis of ectopic pregnancy is made by physical examination in conjunction with diagnostic ultrasound and human chorionic gonadotropin (hCG) radioimmunoassay. The anatomic images provided by ultrasound of an extrauterine gestational sac or mass are important in making the diagnosis. A thorough understanding of sono-graphic features, implantation sites, scanning technique, and differential diagnoses is necessary for the practitioner to perform a proper sonographic evaluation of a patient at risk for ectopic pregnancy. A knowledge of the physiology of conception and gestation, along with an awareness of the meaning of pertinent laboratory values, clinical symptoms, and clinical histories that predispose to ectopic pregnancy, supplement the information provided by the sonographic images.

Sites of Ectopic Pregnancy

Normal gestational implantation occurs in the upper corpus or fundal region of the uterine cavity.[3] Those that do not are ectopic in location. Approximately 97% of ectopic gestations occur in the fallopian tubes (93% ampullary; 4% isthmic); 2.5% of ectopic pregnancies are interstitial within the uterine cornua (Fig. 11-1). Other ectopic implantation sites are nontubal and may uncommonly occur in the ovaries (0.5%), the cervix (0.12%), and the abdomen (0.03%).[23] The narrow tubular structure of the fallopian tubes and their unique location in the true pelvis with an opening into the peritoneal cavity account for the occurrence of abdominal pregnancies.

191

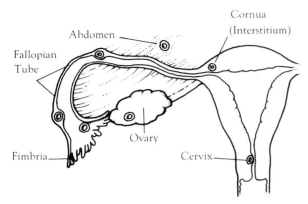

Figure 11-1. Sites of implantation of the fertilized ovum in an ectopic pregnancy.

ETIOLOGY

Each fallopian tube is derived from the müllerian duct system. It is the only connection between the peritoneal cavity and the endometrial cavity. As the ovum is expelled from the dominant follicle and is swept up by the fimbriae into the oviduct, certain conditions may impede its normal course and cause it to implant in the fallopian tube.

Mechanical obstruction and abnormalities in the movement of the embryo through the tube may result in ectopic implantation. Alteration of the tubal transport mechanism and intrinsic embryonic abnormalities cause most ectopic pregnancies to be located in the fallopian tube. Mechanical obstruction may be the result of developmental anomalies, infectious damage, or tubal surgery. Proposed theories regarding the etiology of ectopic pregnancy in normal tubes include transmigration of an ovum, intrinsic embryonic abnormalities (chromosomally abnormal blastocysts), hormonal imbalance, the presence of pelvic masses, the use of an intrauterine contraceptive device (IUD), in vitro fetilization procedures, follicle-stimulating hormone therapy, and reduced tubal motility secondary to pelvic inflammatory disease.[23,52] Processes responsible to a lesser extent for ectopic pregnancy are induced abortion, tubal surgery for infertility or sterilization, conservative management of ectopic pregnancy, delayed childbearing, and douching.[5]

A history of previous ectopic pregnancy increases the likelihood of an extrauterine pregnancy (Table 11-1). Among women who have had an ectopic pregnancy, the subsequent overall conception rate is approximately 60%. Depending on the surgical procedure used to treat the ectopic pregnancy, 10% to 16% have repeat ectopic gestations.[7] Tubal scarring from the first ectopic pregnancy probably accounts for the second ectopic pregnancy or contributes to infertility.

One of the most prevalent contributors to mechanical obstruction is pelvic inflammatory disease (PID) and associated salpingitis. Antibiotic therapy is used to treat the patient, but in so doing may preserve the tube from complete obstruction, with a resulting patent tube with scarring of epithelial tissue and reduced intratubal motility, perhaps from ciliary damage.[41] Congenital abnormalities of the fallopian tube and tubal surgery may also be responsible for causing delayed ovum passage in the oviduct.

Transmigration of the fertilized ovum is another process that can culminate in a tubal pregnancy. Internal transmigration occurs when the ovum is fertilized in one tube and migrates across the uterus to enter the opposite tube and implant there.[51] External transmigration occurs when fertilization occurs in the cul-de-sac and progresses to the blastocyst disc stage; the conceptus is then picked up by the fimbriae and implants in the contralateral tube. Demonstration of a contralateral corpus luteum cyst supports this transmigration theory. Iffy's theory is that cases occur when an ovum is fertilized but the pregnancy is unable to suppress menstruation, which occurs and flushes the fertilized oocyte from the uterus back onto the fallopian tube.[25]

An embryo may implant ectopically if the propulsive mechanism of the tube is inhibited or ren-

TABLE 11-1. RISK FACTORS ASSOCIATED WITH INCREASED INCIDENCE OF ECTOPIC PREGNANCY
History of
Pelvic inflammatory disease
Tubal surgery
Previous ectopic pregnancy
Induced abortion
Intrauterine contraceptive device
Advanced maternal age
Infertility
Infertility treatments
In vitro fertilization
Gamete intrafallopian transfer
Uterine and adnexal masses

dered ineffective. Fetuses with grossly abnormal chromosome patterns have been noted in a number of ectopic pregnancies. Blighted ova are found more frequently in tubal ectopics than in intrauterine pregnancies. This may be the result of an unfavorable location for implantation or indicate that the embryo is too abnormal to generate the proper hormonal signals for intrauterine implantation.[12]

Uterine and adnexal masses can interfere with the normal function of the tube. Myomas, endometriomas, adnexal masses, and pelvic adhesions can result in kinking of the tube or narrowing of the lumen.

Where an ectopic gestation is implanted depends on various mechanisms and particular sequences of events. Myoelectrical activity, more so than the ciliary action within the tube, helps propel the fertilized ovum through the tube. The high concentration of estrogen that develops after ovulation increases the muscular tone in the isthmus, which subsequently retains the fertilized ovum in the ampulla. In normal implantation, the increasing progesterone levels that develop in the luteal phase of the menstrual cycle cause a decrease in myoelectrical activity that relaxes the ampullary wall, allowing the fertilized ovum to enter the uterus. When an estrogen or progesterone imbalance occurs, the risk of an ectopic pregnancy increases.[35]

Although most ectopics implant in the ampulla, those that occur in the interstitium of the tube (cornual pregnancy) often result in the direst consequences. Cornual pregnancies may go undetected for a longer period of time because they are surrounded by myometrium, which allows for greater growth than the thinner and less vascular wall of the oviduct. The fact that maternal veins lie adjacent to the cornua may account for the massive hemoperitoneum that may result from late rupture of this form of ectopic pregnancy.

After implantation of an ectopic pregnancy within the tubal mucosa, there is invasion by the villous trophoblast into the endosalpinx and subsequent layers of the oviduct. Bleeding may occur and may be seen in the cul-de-sac and other dependent areas, such as Morison's pouch, where free fluid collects. Diagnostic ultrasound, even if unable to image an ectopic gestational sac, may readily note the cul-de-sac and other free fluid collections so as to alert the clinician when other clinical and laboratory findings are suggestive.

OTHER IMPLANTATION SITES

Cervical Implantation

Cervical pregnancy—when a fertilized ovum implants below the level of the internal os—is rare, with a reported incidence ranging from 1:1000 to 1:50,000[49] (Fig. 11-2). It is postulated that any factor that alters the entire endometrium or a portion of it, making it unsuitable for uterine implantation, may increase the risk of cervical pregnancy. Endometritis, Ascherman's syndrome, an intrauterine device, previous cesarean section, and leiomyomas are such factors.[3] Another theory suggests that the cervical ectopic pregnancy is due to an abnormally rapid transit of the fertilized ovum through the uterine cavity, placing the ovum in the cervical canal when implantation occurs.[47] Some authors consider the rise in induced abortions to be a factor in the increased numbers of cervical ectopics.[24]

The clinician must first consider an impending abortion in progress, because of similarities in gestational sac location and subsequent sonographic appearance. An abortion in progress would usually demonstrate a more complex sonographic appearance than implantation of the blastocyst below the internal os. Ectopic implantation is diagnosed histologically if cervical glands are found opposite the placental attachment site, and no fetal elements are present in the corpus of the uterus.[29] These patients have a softened and disproportionately enlarged cervix, said to be at least the size of the uterine body.[23] Approximately 50% of cervical ectopic pregnancies have been reported to require hysterectomies because of uncontrollable hemorrhage.[49]

Abdominal Implantation

An abdominal pregnancy is defined as primary or secondary. In the primary sort, both tubes and ovaries are normal, with no evidence of recent or remote injury; there is no evidence of uteroperitoneal fistulas; and the pregnancy is adherent to the peritoneal surface without evidence of secondary implantation after primary implantation in the tube (Fig. 11-3). As of 1988, approximately 300 cases had been reported, including implantations in the spleen (Fig. 11-4), liver, the lesser sac, diaphragm, and on the ovaries.[13,27,30,33,36,48]

Most secondary abdominal pregnancies result from tubal abortion or rupture with extension and implantation of a viable placenta onto the peritoneal

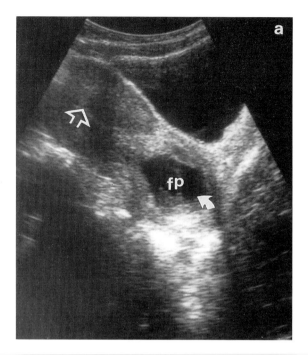

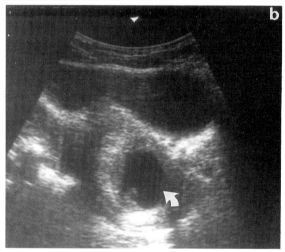

Figure 11-2. (**A**) A longitudinal transabdominal image of a cervical ectopic pregnancy shows the fundal endometrial echo (*open arrow*). The fetal pole (fp) is seen in the ectopic gestational sac (*curved arrow*). (**B**) A transverse transabdominal image shows the ectopic gestational sac and fetal pole.

surfaces.[43] Early diagnosis of abdominal pregnancy is of the utmost importance in light of the possibility of massive hemorrhage secondary to separation of the placenta from its attachment to bowel or other peritoneal viscera.[3] The risk of dying as a result of an abdominal pregnancy is approximately 8 times greater than the risk for a tubal pregnancy, and 90 times greater than when there is an intrauterine pregnancy.[46] Most fetuses of abdominal pregnancies die, and when undiagnosed and untreated result in a calcified mass (lithopedian). The remaining abdominal pregnancies who are delivered live may have complications of growth delay, pulmonary hypoplasia, and pressure deformities of their limbs and face.[19]

Certain signs and symptoms suggest abdominal pregnancy: abdominal pain, nausea or vomiting late in pregnancy, pain on fetal movements, sudden cessation of fetal movement, and fetal movement high in the mother's abdomen.[3]

Ovarian Implantation

Ovarian pregnancy is a rare (less than 0.52%) type of ectopic pregnancy with certain established identifying features. The tube and the fimbriae on the affected side must be intact. The gestational sac must occupy the normal position of the ovary. The

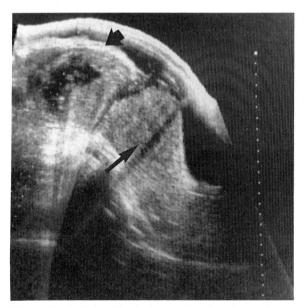

Figure 11-3. A longitudinal scan showing the endometrium in the uterus (*long arrow*). The abdominal pregnancy is visible superior to the fundus (*short arrow*). (Courtesy of Charles Odwin, Brooklyn, NY.)

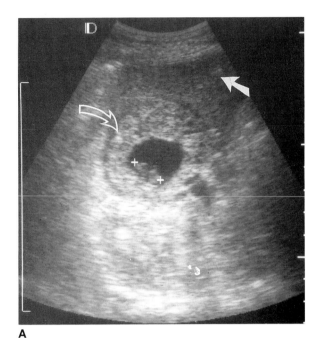

A

B

Figure 11-4. (**A**) A coronal image of the maternal spleen (*solid arrow*) is seen with an 8-week ectopic pregnancy within the parenchyma (*open arrow*). The embryonic pole is between the calipers. (**B**) The embryo within the removed spleen. (See also Color Plate 8.) (*A courtesy Bethany Bentley, RDMS, Jacquelyn C. Howitt, MD, Westfall OB/GYN, Rochester, NY; B courtesy Cynthia Hoeflinger, MD, PhD.*)

gestational sac must be connected to the uterus by the uteroovarian ligament, and ovarian tissue must be identified histologically in the wall of the sac.[44] An ovarian pregnancy is classified as primary or secondary. The primary, or interfollicular, type presumably results from failure of the ovum to be ex-

truded from the follicle; fertilization subsequently occurs within the early corpus luteum. The secondary type probably results from an early tubal abortion that implants on the ovarian surface.[3]

Clinical Information

Symptoms of acute ectopic pregnancy include vaginal spotting or bleeding, abdominal pain, amenorrhea, adnexal tenderness or palpable adnexal mass, and a positive pregnancy test. Tubal rupture results in intraperitoneal hemorrhage, which often causes abdominal pain and referred shoulder pain due to peritoneal blood irritating the diaphragm.[11,15] Less acute pelvic discomfort suggests a chronic ectopic pregnancy. Symptoms may include recurrent, intermittent, low-grade fever along with the clinical evidence of a palpable solid mass.[18] Patients with chronic ectopic pregnancies have higher lactate dehydrogenase levels than patients with acute ectopic symptoms.[4]

Laboratory tests are based on the production of hCG, which is a glycoprotein produced by the syncytiotrophoblast at approximately 7 days postconception.[46] The hCG level in normal pregnancy should double every 2 days and peak at 6 weeks at 100 IU/ml.

Research reports include information on the serum levels of β-hCG that have been determined quantitatively using either the First International Reference Preparation (IRP) or the Second International Standard (2nd IS). It is important to know which method your laboratory uses. Both are based on serum hCG levels quantified as milliInternational units/milliliter (mIU/ml). A common rule of thumb is that 2nd IS values are half their equivalent in IRP. For example, an hCG level of 2000 mIU/ml IRP is equivalent to 1000 mIU/ml 2nd IS.[14]

Kadar and colleagues report that in women with hCG levels exceeding 6500 mIU/ml, IRP sonography should demonstrate a gestational sac; its absence is evidence for an ectopic pregnancy.[26] A gestational sac should be imaged on transvaginal sonography when hCG levels exceed 1000 mIU/mL IRP, and again, its absence is evidence of an ectopic pregnancy.[5,23] Ectopic pregnancies are associated with lower hCG levels than normal pregnancies. Decreasing hCG concentrations indicate a nonviable intrauterine pregnancy or can be evidence of a spontaneous abortion or a nonviable ectopic pregnancy.[34]

The newer urine pregnancy tests (enzyme-linked immunosorbent assay [ELISA]) based on the presence of hCG are very sensitive and can detect hCG concentrations in the range of 15 to 25 mIU/ml. The ELISA test can detect hCG 14 days postconception and has a sensitivity of 90% for ectopic pregnancy. The estimation of serum levels of hCG is clinically superior to the measurement of any other pregnancy protein or biochemical parameter.[23] With intrauterine pregnancy, hCG normally becomes detectable in the bloodstream 7 to 10 days after ovulation, and serum concentration increases exponentially, paralleling the early proliferation of the trophoblast. An abnormally rapid increase may indicate the presence of hydatidiform mole; decreasing concentrations indicate a nonviable pregnancy, such as a spontaneous abortion or ectopic implantation.[34]

Increased serum amylase has been reported in association with ruptured tubal pregnancy, owing to release of tubal amylase when rupture occurs. When an ectopic gestation ruptures, tubal amylase may be released into the peritoneal cavity.[21]

Alternate Diagnostic Modalities

Other diagnostic modalities for evaluating ectopic pregnancy may be used when sonographic findings are equivocal. Although criteria for differentiating between the echogenic decidual reaction and a true intrauterine gestation have been used, when a gestational sac cannot be conclusively identified sonographically, other diagnostic procedures are necessary. If the pregnancy is unwanted, a uterine curettage may be diagnostic because recovery of chorionic villi confirms intrauterine pregnancy, whereas recovery of decidual tissue alone suggests the presence of an extrauterine pregnancy.[31] Simultaneous intrauterine and extrauterine implantation, although unusual, can occur, and its incidence is increasing. In 1948, the incidence of heterotopic pregnancy was calculated to be 1:30,000.[9] It is now considered more common, particularly among patients treated by assisted reproductive technologies (ART), such as in vitro fertilization or gamete intrafallopian transfer. The incidence of heterotopic pregnancies among infertility patients may be as high as 1:100[23,37] (Fig. 11-5). Currently, the incidence among nonassisted reproductive technology patients has been estimated at as great as 1:4000.[6] The increase has been due to the increased incidence of PID in the general population.

Culdocentesis is used widely to diagnose hemoperitoneum in patients with suspected ectopic pregnancy.[38] This procedure has value only for diagnosing *ruptured* tubal pregnancy. It may be guided by transabdominal or transvaginal ultrasound. There is also the possibility of a false-positive result, because culdocentesis cannot predict the site of hemorrhage. Clinical findings with ruptured, but not actively bleeding, corpus luteum cyst may closely resemble those of ectopic pregnancy and can yield a positive result on culdocentesis.[52]

Laparoscopy has replaced laparotomy for diagnosis of ectopic pregnancy. Early unruptured ectopic pregnancy without hemoperitoneum can be diagnosed by laparoscopy or laparotomy.[20] Laparoscopy may be used when sonographic findings are inconclusive (Fig. 11-6).

Sonographic Technical Protocol

Optimal visualization of the uterus and adnexa is crucial in the sonographic evaluation of a suspected ectopic pregnancy. The examiner must be familiar with the patient's medical and surgical history and clinical presentation to correlate the sonographic findings and

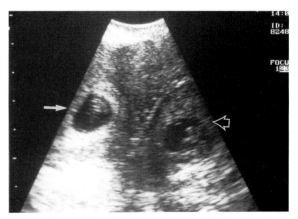

Figure 11-5. Heterotopic pregnancy after in vitro fertilization that was documented only on transvaginal sonography. The uterine pregnancy (*solid arrow*) has a good decidual reaction around the sac. In contrast, the cul-de-sac tubal ectopic pregnancy (*open arrow*) does not.

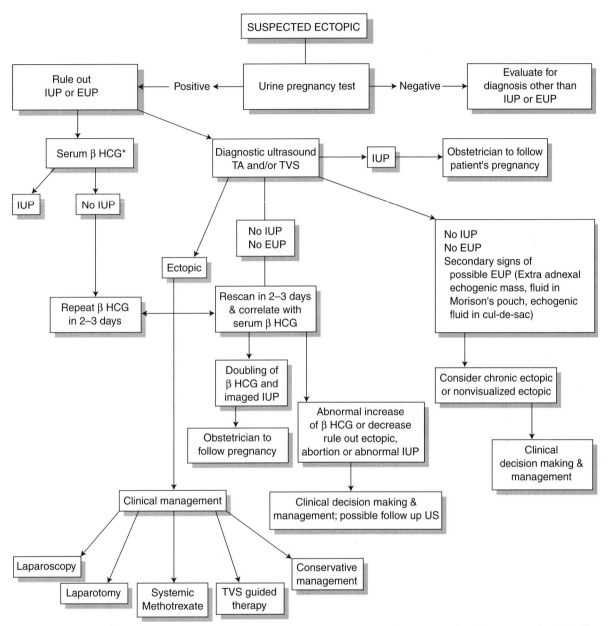

* Intrauterine gestational sac should be seen on TVS with β HCG ≥ 1000 mIU/mL (2nd IS); on TA with β HCG ≥ 3600 mIU/mL (2nd IS).
Values of 1000 mIU/mL and 3600 mIU/mL represent the upper limits of the discriminatory zones.

EUP   = Extra Uterine Pregnancy
IUP   = Intrauterine Pregnancy
TA   = Transabdominal Ultrasound
TVS   = Transvaginal Ultrasound
2nd IS = Second International Standard
US   = Ultrasound

Figure 11-6. *Management of stable patients with suspected ectopic pregnancy. HCG, human chorionic gonadotropin; LMP, last menstrual period; D&C, dilatation and curettage.*

formulate the differential diagnosis. The single most important function of ultrasound in the evaluation of ectopic pregnancy is to establish the presence of a viable intrauterine pregnancy. A sac is usually noted 4 to 5 weeks after the last menstrual period (LMP) with transabdominal scanning, and 3 to 4 weeks after LMP with transvaginal technique; sonographic appearance may suggest an intrauterine pregnancy, but if no yolk sac or embryonic pole is imaged, an ectopic pregnancy with an intrauterine decidual reaction cannot be excluded. The decidual reaction (Fig. 11-7), which takes place with both extrauterine and intrauterine pregnancy, may resemble a sac. Demonstration of a fetal pole with cardiac activity definitively locates the gestation.

Transvaginal scanning has been shown to be almost essential in examinations for possible ectopic pregnancy[32]; however, transabdominal scans usually are performed first by many sonologists/sonographers, to obtain more complete views of the adnexa, fundal region, flanks, and abdomen.[17] To optimize visualization, appropriate bladder filling and transducer selection are important technical aspects. The urinary bladder should be filled enough to cover the uterine fundus. Certain conditions, such as an enlarged leiomyomatous uterus, may prohibit tolerable bladder distention, and the sonographer should use other means, such as patient positioning. Placing the patient in an oblique position shifts the bladder to visualize better the right and left lower quadrants. Placing the patient in the Trendelenburg position may afford a better view of the uterine fundus, facilitated by bladder displace-

ment. An overly distended bladder and submucosal fibroids may both contribute to the eccentric location of an early gestational sac. To differentiate, the patient should be scanned again after voiding partially.

The practitioner must systematically evaluate all potential sites of implantation and must look for other sonographic diagnostic criteria. Evaluation of the endometrial cavity begins by imaging the central endometrial echo and noting its size and contents. If an intrauterine gestational sac cannot be found, this may be due to several factors. It may be too early to demonstrate a sac, or a complete abortion may have occurred. All other areas of the uterus must be evaluated for potential implantation sites. Both adnexa and adnexal regions should be scrutinized. Special attention needs to be given to any suspect masses. They should be demonstrated from a variety of scanning planes, and every technique available, such as looking for peristalsis, should be used to make sure the mass is not a segment of normal bowel. Any complex adnexal mass that has a pole with cardiac activity outside the endometrial cavity is definitely an ectopic pregnancy. A complex mass can represent an ectopic gestation at one of its stages of growth or rupture. When there is clinical suspicion of an ectopic pregnancy, all adnexal findings should be noted, characterized, and treated as potential ectopic pregnancy until proven otherwise.

Sonographic evaluation also includes the hepatorenal space (Morison's pouch) and paracolic gutters (flank areas) to check for the extent of free fluid, such as blood from ruptured ectopic implantation or peritoneal fluid from a ruptured ovarian

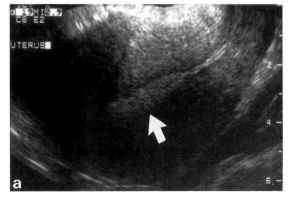
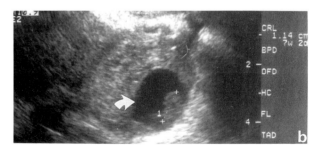

Figure 11-7. (**A**) The uterus is visualized on transvaginal ultrasound with a prominent endometrial echo (*solid arrow*) and no evidence of an intrauterine gestation. (**B**) A tubal ectopic gestation (*curved arrow*) is seen adjacent to the uterus.

TABLE 11-2. SCANNING PROTOCOL FOR ECTOPIC PREGNANCY USING TRANSABDOMINAL OR TRANSVAGINAL TRANSDUCERS

1. Be acquainted with clinical history, pregnancy test results, and last menstrual period.
2. Use bladder distention (transabdominal scanning) and appropriate transducer (3.5 MHz).
3. Examine endometrial cavity in sagittal and transverse planes for signs of ectopia:
   - Decidual cast versus double sac sign
   - Absence of gestational sac
   - Gestational sac located in cervical area
   - Gestational sac located in cornual region
   - Gestational sac in asymmetric location
   - Fluid in endometrial cavity
4. Examine adnexa in sagittal and transverse planes for signs of ectopia:
   - No rupture: look for fetal cardiac motion in adnexal mass
   - Acute rupture: variable complex adnexal mass with free fluid
   - Chronic rupture: echogenic complex mass that may gravitate to cul-de-sac region
5. Examine cul-de-sac for the presence of fluid, blood, or embryonic tissue from ruptured sac or tube.
6. Examine hepatorenal space for free fluid.
7. Describe sonographic findings and establish a preliminary impression.

cyst. Certain cul-de-sac masses may also be bowel related and can usually be differentiated from those that are gynecologic in origin with transvaginal ultrasound or by administering a fluid enema and observing for peristalsis with real-time ultrasonography. The examiner may be faced with a patient who exhibits severe abdominal discomfort, which is a further complication to an already difficult and sensitive examination. This stressful environment should not be allowed to compromise a comprehensive evaluation (Table 11-2).

Sonographic Characteristics

UTERINE

The demonstration of a viable intrauterine pregnancy occupying a high fundal position within the endometrium is usually the conclusive sonographic information that rules out an ectopic pregnancy. A viable intrauterine gestation may be visualized transabdominally from 5 to 6 weeks after LMP,

depending on the mother's body habitus. Vaginal transducers detect gestational sacs and cardiac activity about 10 days earlier than transabdominal ones. Suggestive transvaginal sonographic findings of an intrauterine pregnancy, such as visualization of a double sac sign, a yolk sac, or a gestational sac, eliminate the likelihood of an ectopic implantation.

The normal prominence of the endometrial echo during the secretory phase of the endometrial cycle may appear similar to the decidual reaction of the endometrial lining as it prepares for implantation in response to both intrauterine and extrauterine pregnancies (see Figs. 4-39 and 11-7). Therefore, this finding in itself is not a diagnostic criterion. The appearance of a sac-like structure with a perimeter of high-amplitude echoes, which is due to trophoblastic reaction, can be somewhat suggestive of an early intrauterine pregnancy.

Demonstration of the double sac sign is a stronger and more reliable indicator of an early intrauterine pregnancy. The double sac, which consists of two concentric rings (Fig. 11-8) surrounding a portion of the gestational sac, is thought to represent the decidua parietalis (decidua vera)

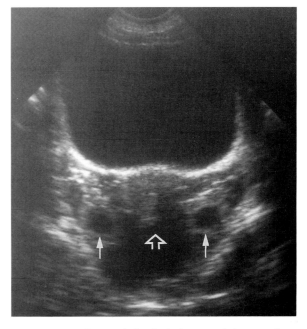

Figure 11-8. A transabdominal ultrasound shows echogenic rings (*solid arrows*) in both fallopian tubes, with the empty uterus (*open arrow*) between. Subsequent transvaginal ultrasound revealed an ectopic pregnancy in each fallopian tube.

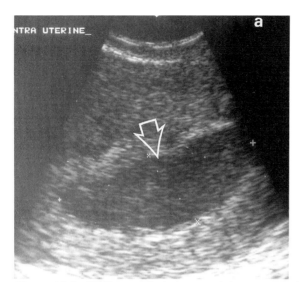
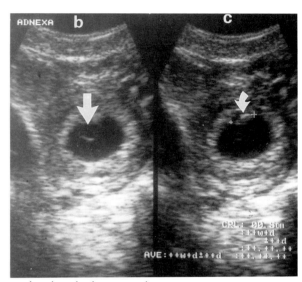

Figure 11-9. (**A**) Transvaginal ultrasound shows a pseudogestational sac in the uterus that on magnification revealed particles within representing blood (*open arrow*). (**B**) Adjacent to the uterus is an ectopic gestation containing a yolk sac (*solid arrow*) and (**C**) embryo (*curved arrow*).

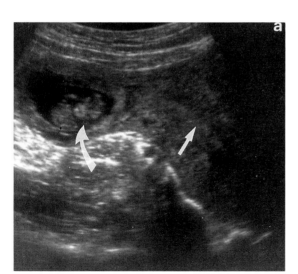
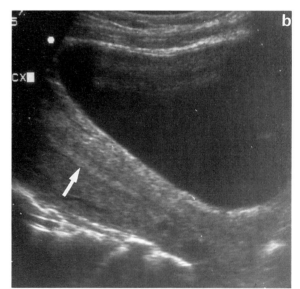

Figure 11-10. (**A**) Adjacent to the fundus is an interstitial ectopic pregnancy containing a fetal pole (*curved arrow*). (**B**) Transabdominal ultrasound shows a normal endometrial echo within the uterus (*straight arrow*).

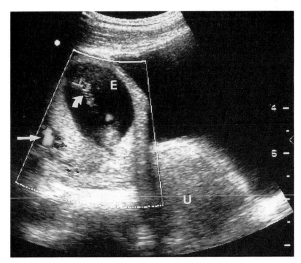

Figure 11-11. *An ultrasound ordered because of a palpable adnexal mass reveals a viable 13-week tubal ectopic pregnancy (E). Color Doppler shows flow in the umbilical cord (curved arrow) and placental vessels (straight arrow). (See also Color Plate 9.)*

sonographer should keep in mind that a pregnant bicornuate uterus may present a confusing picture, with a decidual reaction in the nongravid horn and the gestational sac in the other, resembling an extra-uterine gestational sac (see Fig. 5-11).

ADNEXAL

Unruptured Tubal Pregnancy

An adnexal mass is palpated in a significant number of patients with an ectopic pregnancy (Fig. 11-11). Abnormal sonographic findings of the adnexa are, predictably, more common in patients with an unruptured ectopic pregnancy than in patients with an intrauterine pregnancy.[39] The sonographic appearance of these masses is highly variable, and a number of other lesions mimic them sonographically. Ultrasound may provide definitive diagnosis of an ectopic pregnancy only if an ectopic gestational sac is visible outside the

adjacent to the decidua capsularis.[14] In contradistinction, the pseudogestational sac of an ectopic pregnancy is composed of a single decidual layer surrounding an intraendometrial fluid collection, and thus demonstrates a single echogenic ring[15] (Fig. 11-9). A pseudosac develops when the hormones of pregnancy act on the endometrium, causing it to thicken. Decreases in hormone levels cause decidual degeneration and bleeding into the endometrial cavity. A decidual cast may bleed, simulating a fetal pole and causing the diagnosis of an ectopic pregnancy to be delayed. Intrauterine gestations are clearly distinguished by their asymmetric sonographic pattern, as opposed to the circular decidual sac that is associated with an ectopic pregnancy and postovulation.[22] Lacunar structures also may be visualized, which are the beginning of the placental site. Color Doppler may aid in this respect because a pseudogestational sac does not exhibit the typical significant blood flow seen around a normal gestational sac.[40]

An interstitial pregnancy demonstrates a gestational sac peripherally adjacent to the uterine cornua and never completely surrounded by myometrium (Fig. 11-10). A cervical ectopic pregnancy demonstrates a gestational sac below the level of the internal os. The rarity of the cervical ectopic pregnancy makes the imaging of a sac below the os more often the result of an inevitable abortion. The

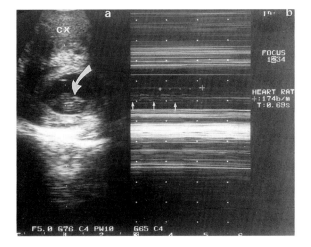

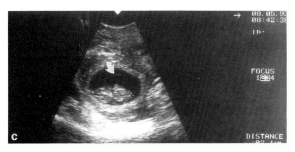

Figure 11-12. *(A) Transvaginal ultrasound shows a tubal ectopic pregnancy containing an embryo (curved arrow) located in the cul-de-sac posterior to the cervix (cx). (B) Viability is noted (arrows). (C) A thin amnion is noted within the sac (curved arrow).*

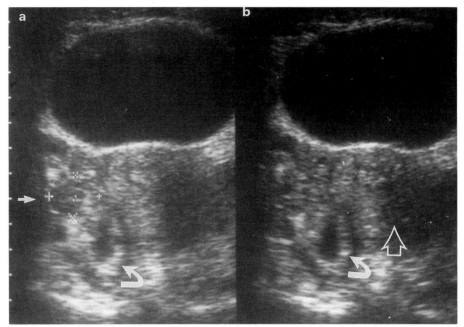

Figure 11-13. (**A**) Transverse transabdominal ultrasound shows the right ovary between calipers (*arrow*) with an echogenic ring (*curved arrow*) around the sonolucent central portion. (**B**) The uterus (*open arrow*) is seen with an empty endometrium.

uterus and fetal heart movements are demonstrable within it (Fig. 11-12). Certain sonographic findings may suggest an unruptured ectopic pregnancy. An echogenic ring is usually noted (due to trophoblastic reaction) with a sonolucent center (Fig. 11-13). This sac-like structure may be located adjacent to or distant from either ovary. Because location may be influenced by bladder filling or bowel arrangement, all areas of the pelvis should be evaluated for suspect extrauterine masses (Fig. 11-14). A corpus luteum cyst may be found in either adnexa, on the side of the ectopic gestation or on the contralateral side. The image of a hemorrhagic corpus luteum cyst may be confused with the image of an ectopic pregnancy, but presence in an ovary make an ectopic pregnancy very unlikely. An extrauterine sac may also apear as a complex mass with both solid and cystic areas that, before rupture, can mimic other pelvic masses. A pelvic hematocele, corpus luteum cysts with internal bleeding, tuboovarian abscess, or PID collections are some of the more common conditions that can sonographically simulate ectopic pregnancy. Other masses that can give the appearance of ectopic pregnancy are small serous and mucinous cystadenomas, cystic teratomas, and single endometriomas. Echoes may be seen within these neoplasms, making them difficult to differentiate from ectopic implantation. Any of these masses can coexist with an ectopic pregnancy. Fluid-filled bowel loops should be differentiated from an ectopic pregnancy by looking for peristalsis.

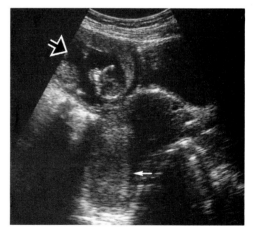

Figure 11-14. A severely retroverted uterus (*solid arrow*) is seen on sagittal transabdominal sonography, with a gestational sac superior to the uterus corresponding to a 13-week viable tubal ectopic gestation (*open arrow*).

Because they look similar on sonographic examination, ovarian ectopic pregnancies are often indistinguishable from more common tubal ectopic pregnancies. This makes a true ovarian pregnancy difficult to identify.[17]

Ruptured Tubal Pregnancy

Acute rupture of a tubal pregnancy initiates formation of a complex mass, which shows further changes as it proceeds to the chronic stage. When there is a partial or complete rupture of the tubal pregnancy, the variety of sonographic appearances that may be imaged expand the differential diagnosis. When rupture occurs, blood and gestational contents add to the complex nature of the adnexal mass (Fig. 11-15). The image of a hemoperitoneum evolves over time. It may simulate a tuboovarian abscess or other complex mass. Typically, however, free fluid with or without hemorrhage conforms to the shape of the space it is contained in. The contained debris may gravitate to the most dependent area of the cul-de-sac.

The presence of free fluid in the cul-de-sac and around the uterus and adnexa, subphrenic spaces, and paracolic gutters is part of the sonographic evaluation of the patient with acute rupture of an ectopic pregnancy. The volume and sonographic appearance of free intraperitoneal fluid are valuable signs in the diagnosis of ectopic

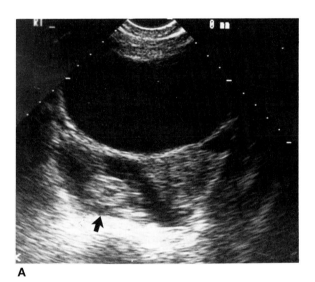

A

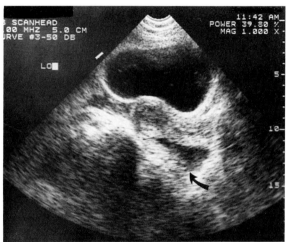

B

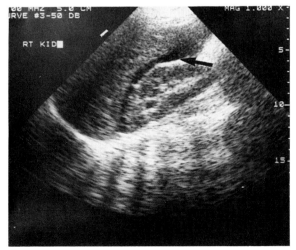

C

Figure 11-15. (**A**) A complex right adnexal mass (*arrow*) represents a gestational sac surrounded by fluid and blood resulting from the tubal rupture. (**B**) In this sagittal scan of the same patient, free fluid is seen in the cul-de-sac (*curved arrow*). (**C**) Fluid in the hepatorenal space of the patient (*arrow*).

pregnancy. Fluid in the cul-de-sac may be exudate, in the presence of PID, or blood, in patients with an ectopic pregnancy or rupture of other abdominal viscera.[8] Acquaintance with a patient's menstrual history may also suggest that cul-de-sac fluid is the result of her ovulatory phase. Aside from identifying cardiac activity in the extragestational sac, adnexal findings tend to be nonspecific, and a differential diagnosis is proposed in conjunction with the clinical and laboratory findings. The sonographer must also consider the concurrent presence of other neoplasms or lesions that further complicate the sonographic presentation.

Chronic ectopic pregnancy is a form of tubal pregnancy in which growth of trophoblastic tissue early in gestation causes gradual disintegration of the tubal wall and slow or repeated episodes of hemorrhage. The presence of blood, trophoblastic tissue, and disrupted tubal tissue in the peritoneal cavity incites an inflammatory response, which seals off the area, creating a pelvic hematocele.[4] The echogenicity of the mass may be similar to that of the uterus, obscuring its borders and creating the "indefinite uterus" sign. Sonographically, a complex extrauterine mass may be seen in the region of the adnexa and cul-de-sac that conforms to the spaces that it occupies. Echogenic foci and sonolucent areas may contribute to a highly complex and variable appearance, depending on the degree of clot and mass organization. The sonographic appearances of endometriosis and chronic PID are similar to those of chronic ectopic pregnancy.

ABDOMINAL PREGNANCY

Most abdominal pregnancies are diagnosed sonographically at a later gestational age than tubal pregnancy. A first trimester abdominal pregnancy may be difficult to distinguish by sonographic criteria from an unruptured tubal pregnancy. Rupture of a tubal ectopic gestation usually occurs between 6 and 12 weeks, although there have been reported cases of unruptured tubal ectopic pregnancies as late as 14 weeks.[42] Certain clinical signs and symptoms suggest the presence of an abdominal pregnancy.[1] Sonographically, a number of specific findings are associated with an abdominal pregnancy. The most frequent and reliable one is an empty uterus separate

from the fetus.[45] Extragestational findings in abdominal pregnancy are listed in Table 11-3.

The sonographer must also be aware of the variability in the appearance of a dead fetus. Signs of intrauterine and extrauterine fetal demise are similar; however, documentation becomes more difficult in abdominal pregnancies, owing to the lack of amniotic fluid and to maceration of fetal parts. This further complicates interpretation, because the fetus may simulate other conditions such as calcific changes in the leiomyomatous uterus. Additional diagnostic imaging modalities such as radiography and hysterosalpingography can be used to confirm sonographic findings. Unfortunately, the diagnosis of abdominal pregnancy is missed in a significant percentage of patients. The sonographer must carefully document criteria that firmly establish an intrauterine pregnancy (placental–myometrial interface), especially when other abnormal features are seen on the sonogram (Table 11-4).

Transvaginal Scanning

Transvaginal sonography has become an integral part of evaluating women who are suspected of having an ectopic pregnancy when conventional transabdominal sonography fails to show a living intrauterine or extrauterine embryo.[32] Although transvaginal sonography is considered by some to be sufficient in early pregnancy evaluation, structures that are superior to the uterus and outside the field of view of the transvaginal transducer cannot be delineated.[16]

The presence of free fluid can be reliably detected by transvaginal examination only in the

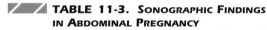

TABLE 11-3. SONOGRAPHIC FINDINGS IN ABDOMINAL PREGNANCY

Oligohydramnios
No placenta–myometrium interface
Poor definition of placenta
    May be seen attached to maternal intestine
    Lack of chorionic plate
Close location of fetal parts to maternal abdominal wall
Unusual fetal presentation
Maternal bowel gas anterior or intermingled with fetal
  parts
Pseudoprevia created by empty uterus superior to
  maternal bladder and free fluid

Ectopic Location	Differential Diagnosis
Tubal	Corpus luteum cyst/adnexal mass Adhesed bowel Salpingitis Acute appendicitis
Ovarian	Tubal ectopic Bowel (mass-like) Hemorrhagic corpus luteum cyst
Abdominal	Severely retroflexed uterus Bicornuate uterus
Cervical	Impending or incomplete abortion Degenerating cervical myoma
Chronic ectopic	Pelvic inflammatory disease Degenerating myoma Endometriomas
Interstitial	Myoma Bicornuate uterus with pregnancy in horn

pouch of Douglas; other collection sites can be out of the field of view of the transducer. For these reasons, many clinical sonologists combine a transabdominal and transvaginal approach in the analysis of ectopic pregnancy.

Color Doppler

Color Doppler has been used to characterize the nature of adnexal and paraadnexal masses seen on ultrasound by determining if blood flow is present (Fig. 11-16). Ectopic pregnancy may be suggested by significant color flow surrounding the periphery of an adnexal mass separate from the ovary and corpus luteum. The typical resistive index of an ectopic pregnancy is low-resistance in type (i.e., high systolic and diastolic flow) and has been reported as below 0.40. The low impedance is thought to be due to the trophoblastic tissue eroding the surrounding area, with resultant bleeding into the intervillous space. The lack of muscle layers could also explain the low-resistance flow. However, low-resistance flow is also noted in the corpus luteum of a normal pregnancy. In one color Doppler study of 103 known ectopic pregnancies, color flow with a resistive index of 0.40 or less was detected in 92 patients. A positive predictive value of 96.8% was

reported in this group of patients.[28] Other authors have not found color Doppler useful and continue to rely on the gray-scale image. However, the combined use of color Doppler and two-dimensional ultrasound may help to differentiate between a pseudogestational sac, which has high-resistance flow, and a true intrauterine pregnancy, which exhibits low-resistance arterial flow.[14]

Treatment of Ectopic Pregnancy

The treatment of ectopic pregnancy may be surgical or nonsurgical intervention. Surgical treatments include laparoscopy or laparotomy. If the patient is

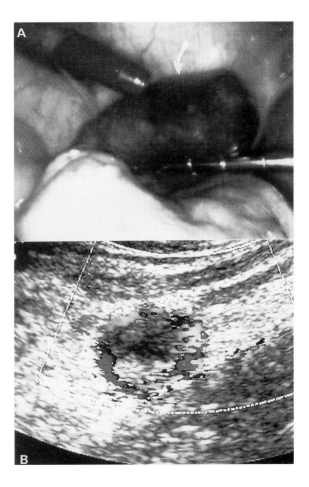

Figure 11-16. (**A**) a laparoscopy confirmed a tubal ectopic pregnancy (*curved arrow*) found on ultrasound and a salingostomy was performed. (**B**) The suspect area was scanned with Doppler showing the typical color pattern exhibited by trophoblastic tissue. (See also Color Plate 10.)

in hemodynamic shock from a ruptured ectopic, or an interstitial or abdominal ectopic is suspected, a laparotomy is indicated. One operation is total salpingectomy; however, when the tube has not ruptured—and sometimes when it has—salpingostomy with removal of the pregnancy and conservation of the tube is feasible. Ruptured contents, such as old blood, clots, and conceptus debris (chronic pregnancy), are removed from the peritoneal cavity during surgery. A hysterectomy may be necessary in cases of ruptured interstitial pregnancy, because the cornua may be so damaged that repair is time consuming, unsatisfactory, and accompanied by considerable blood loss. Wedge resections may be performed to remove the interstitial ectopic.[11,53]

Methotrexate, administered systemically or locally, has proven to be a successful, nontraumatic way of resolving early tubal ectopic pregnancy. Embryonic cardiac activity, however, is a contraindication to systemic therapy.[46] When methotrexate is administered locally, transvaginal ultrasound may be used to direct the injection. Methotrexate is effective in inducing tubal abortion and reabsorption of ectopic pregnancy. The procedure may be performed on an outpatient basis, side effects are relatively few, and the failure rate is at an acceptable level.[46]

Expectant (a "wait-and-see" approach) management of ectopic pregnancies is attempted when five criteria are met. These include decreasing serum hCG, no evidence of an intrauterine pregnancy on transvaginal sonography, an ectopic pregnancy less than 4 cm, no fetal heartbeat, and no sign of bleeding or tubal rupture. The major benefit of expectant management is the avoidance of an invasive procedure, giving future pregnancies a better chance. Expectant management should, however, be done with great care, and the patient should be informed to contact the emergency unit if symptoms worsen.[50]

Regardless of gestational age or fetal condition, the clinical management of abdominal pregnancy is surgical. The maternal mortality rate for abdominal pregnancy is in the range of 4% to 18%. The fetal mortality rate is 90%, and the prevalence of fetal deformity ranges from 1% to 100%. Because removal of the placenta, especially in more advanced pregnancies, can result in acute hemorrhage, it is preferable to leave it in place and allow it to reab-

sorb. It may take several months for complete absorption to occur.[44]

Conclusion

Unfortunately, despite new techniques such as transvaginal scanning, ultrasound cannot always produce a definitive diagnosis of ectopic pregnancy. The combination of clinical findings, hCG values, patient history, and other diagnostic tests increases the degree of certainty when ectopic pregnancy is suspected. A methodical evaluation of pelvic organs, adnexal regions, and dependent body areas for free fluid provides a routine for the sonographer that can contribute diagnostic information. When sonographic results are equivocal and the patient is stable, serial β-hCG assays and repeat scans may provide conclusive evidence of an intrauterine pregnancy. Steadily increasing hCG values and an intrauterine pregnancy, which is sonographically visible in follow-up scans because it grows at the rate of 1.2 mm/day, help rule out an ectopic pregnancy.

REFERENCES

1. Athey PA. Ectopic pregnancy. In: Athey PA, Hadlock FP, eds. Ultrasound in Obstetrics and Gynecology. 2nd ed. Moody; 1985.
2. Atri M, Bret P, Tugandi T. Spontaneous resolution of ectopic pregnancy: Initial appearance and evolution at transvaginal US. Radiology. 1993; 186:83–86.
3. Bayless RB. Nontubal ectopic pregnancy. Clin Obstet Gynecol. 1987; 30:191–199.
4. Bedi D, Fagan C, Nocera R. Chronic ectopic pregnancy. J Ultrasound Med. 1981; 3:347–352.
5. Bree RL, Edwards M, Bohm VM, et al. Transvaginal sonography in the evaluation of normal early pregnancy: Correlation with hCG level. Am J Roentgenol. 1989; 153:75–79.
6. Bright DA, Gaupp FB. Heterotopic pregnancy: A reevaluation. J Am Board Fam Pract. 1990; 3:125.
7. Buster J. Reproductive performance following treatment. In: Stovall T, Ling F, eds. Extrauterine Pregnancy: Clinical Diagnosis and Management. New York: McGraw-Hill; 1993:279–284.
8. deCrespigny LC. The value of ultrasound in ectopic pregnancy. Clin Obstet Gynecol. 1987; 30:136–147.
9. DeVoe RW, Pratt JH. Simultaneous intrauterine and extrauterine pregnancy. Am J Obstet Gynecol. 1948; 56:1119–1126.

10. Dorfman SF. Epidemiology of ectopic pregnancy. Am J Obstet Gynecol. 1987; 30:176.

11. Droegemueller W. Ectopic pregnancy. In: Danforth D, ed. Obstetrics and Gynecology. 4th ed. New York: Harper & Row; 1982.

12. Elias S, LeBeau M, Simpson JL, et al. Chromosome analysis of ectopic human conceptuses. Am J Obstet Gynecol. 1981; 141:698–703.

13. Elzey N. Primary abdominal pregnancy in the lesser peritoneal cavity. Western Journal of Surgery. 1948; 56:410–413.

14. Emerson D, Altieri L, Cartier M. Transabdominal and endovaginal ultrasound. In: Stovall T, Ling F, eds. Extrauterine Pregnancy: Clinical Diagnosis and Management. New York: McGraw-Hill Inc; 1993:146, 149–150, 171.

15. Filly RA. Ectopic pregnancy: The role of sonography. Radiology. 1987; 162:661–668.

16. Fleischer A. Sonography in early intrauterine pregnancy emphasizing transvaginal scanning. Presented at the 12th Annual Spring Weekend Symposium in Diagnostic Ultrasound, SUNY Health Science Center at Brooklyn, Brooklyn, New York, 1988.

17. Fleischer A, Boehr F, James A. Sonographic evaluation of ectopic pregnancy. In: Sanders RC, James AE Jr, eds. The Principles and Practice of Ultrasonography in Obstetrics and Gynecology. 2nd ed. Norwalk, CT: Appleton-Century-Crofts; 1980.

18. Fleischer A, Cartwright P, Pennell R, et al. Sonography of ectopic pregnancy. In: Sanders RC, James AE Jr, eds. The Principles and Practice of Ultrasonography in Obstetrics and Gynecology. 4th ed. Norwalk, CT: Appleton-Century-Crofts; 1991:59.

19. Hallatt J, Grove J. Abdominal pregnancy: A study of twenty-one consecutive cases. Am J Obstet Gynecol. 1985; 152:444–449.

20. Hallatt J. Tubal conservation in ectopic pregnancy: A study of 200 cases. Am J Obstet Gynecol. 1986; 154:1216–1221.

21. Hannon Z, Guzick D. Tubal pregnancy: The significance of serum and peritoneal fluid amylase. Obstet Gynecol. 1985; 66:396.

22. Hansmann M, Hackeloer B, Staudach A. Ultrasound in Obstetrics and Gynecology. 1985; 60.

23. Hill GA, Herbert CM. Ectopic pregnancy. In: Copeland LJ, ed. Textbook of Gynecology. Philadelphia: WB Saunders; 1993:242.

24. Hofmann H, Urdl W, Hofler H, Tamussino K. Cervical pregnancy: Case reports and current concepts in diagnosis and treatment. Arch Gynecol Obstet. 1987; 241:63–69.

25. Iffy L. Embryologic studies of time of conception in ectopic pregnancy and first-trimester abortion. Obstet Gynecol. 1965; 26:490–498.

26. Kadar N, DeVore G, Romero R. Discriminatory hCG zone: Its use in the sonographic evaluation for ectopic pregnancy. Obstet Gynecol. 1981; 58:156.

27. Kirby N. Primary hepatic pregnancy. Br Med J. 1969; 1:296.

28. Kurjak A, Zalud I. Ultrasound assessment of ectopic pregnancy. In: Jaffe R, Warsof S, eds. Color Doppler Imaging. New York: McGraw-Hill; 1992:92–96.

29. Laughlin CL, Lee TG, Richards RC. Ultrasonographic diagnosis of cervical ectopic pregnancy. J Ultrasound Med. 1983; 2:137–138.

30. Norenberg D, Gundersen J, Janis J, et al. Early pregnancy on the diaphragm with endometriosis. Obstet Gynecol. 1977; 49:620–622.

31. Nyberg D, Filly R, Laing F, et al. Ectopic pregnancy diagnosis by sonography correlated with quantitative hCG levels. J Ultrasound Med. 1987; 6:145–150.

32. Nyberg D, Mack LA, Jeffrey RB Jr, et al. Endovaginal sonographic evaluation of ectopic pregnancy: A prospective study. Am J Roentgenol. 1987; 149: 1181–1186.

33. Panda J. Primary ovarian twin pregnancy: Case report. Br J Obstet Gynaecol. 1990; 97:540–541.

34. Pittway D. BHCG dynamics in ectopic pregnancy. Clin Obstet Gynecol. 1987; 30:130–132.

35. Pulkkinen MO, Talo A. Tubal physiologic consideration in ectopic pregnancy. Clin Obstet Gynecol. 1987; 30:164.

36. Raziel A, Golan A, Pansky M, et al. Ovarian pregnancy: A report of twenty cases in one institution. Am J Obstet Gynecol. 1990; 163:1182–1185.

37. Rizk B, Tan SL, Morcos S, et al. Heterotopic pregnancies after in vitro fertilization and embryo transfer. Am J Obstet Gynecol. 1991; 164:161–164.

38. Romero R, Copel J, Kadar N, et al. Value of culdocentesis in the diagnosis of ectopic pregnancy. Obstet Gynecol. 1985; 65:519–522.

39. Romero R, Kadar N, Castro D, et al. The value of adnexal sonographic findings in the diagnosis of ectopic pregnancy. Am J Obstet Gynecol. 1988; 158:52–54.

40. Rottem S, Timor-Tritsch I. Think ectopic. In: Timor-Tritsch I, Rottem S, eds. Transvaginal Sonography. 2nd ed. New York: Elsevier Science Publishing; 1991:377.

41. Russell JB. The etiology of ectopic pregnancy. Clin Obstet Gynecol. 1987; 30:183–184.

42. Sherer D, Smith S, Allen T. Sonographic diagnosis of a viable ampullary tubal pregnancy at 14 weeks gestation. J Diagn Med Sonogr. 1991; 7:12–14.

43. Spanta R, Roffman L, Grissan T, et al. Abdominal pregnancy: Magnetic resonance identification with ultrasonographic follow-up of placental involution. Am J Obstet Gynecol. 1987; 157:887–889.

44. Spiegelberg O. Zur Casuistik der Ovarialschwangerschaft. Arch Gynaekol. 1878; 13:73.

45. Stanley JH, Horger EO III, Fagan CJ, et al. Sonographic findings in abdominal pregnancy. Am J Roentgenol. 1986; 147:1043–1046.

46. Stovall T. Medical management. In: Stovall T, Ling F, eds. Extrauterine Pregnancy: Clinical Diagnosis and Management. New York: McGraw-Hill; 1993: 50, 119, 249–266.

47. Studdiford WE. Cervical pregnancy: A partial review of the literature and a report of two probable cases. Am J Obstet Gynecol. 1945; 49:169–185.

48. Yackel D, Panton O, Martin D, Lee D. Splenic pregnancy: Case report. Obstet Gynecol. 1988; 71:471–473.

49. Yankowitz J, Leake J, Huggins G, et al. Cervical ectopic pregnancy: Review of the literature and report of a case treated by single-dose methotrexate therapy. Obstet Gynecol Surv. 1990; 45:405–414.

50. Ylostalo P, Cacciatore B, Sjoberg J, et al. Expectant management of ectopic pregnancy. Obstet Gynecol. 1992; 80:345–348.

51. Walters MD, Eddy C, Pauerstein CJ. The contralateral corpus luteum and tubal pregnancy. Obstet Gynecol. 1987; 70:823–826.

52. Weckstein LN, Boucher AR, Tucker H, et al. Accurate diagnosis of early ectopic pregnancy. Obstet Gynecol. 1985; 65:393–397.

53. Whitworth C, Hill G. Laparotomy for ectopic pregnancy: Operative procedures. In: Stovall T, Ling F, eds. Extrauterine Pregnancy: Clinical Diagnosis and Management. New York: McGraw-Hill; 1993:205–208, 243–244.

PART II

Obstetric Sonography

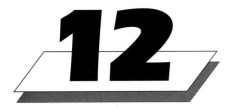

The Use of Ultrasound in the First Trimester

PAULA S. WOLETZ

The use of ultrasound in the first trimester has undergone a rapid change in emphasis in recent years. As technology advanced, first with the introduction of high-resolution, real-time transducers and continuing with the development and acceptance of higher-frequency transvaginal ultrasound, our diagnostic capabilities and expectations have grown. The potential availability of three-dimensional ultrasound imaging in the near future may affect these capabilities and expectations even further.

Our most pressing concern in evaluating the early pregnancy remains the determination of where implantation has occurred and whether the pregnancy is viable. But more and more, we are now being called on to determine whether the pregnancy is normal in appearance or whether the embryo is at risk for structural or chromosomal abnormalities. To that end, the practitioner must have an understanding of the processes that occur from ovulation through the beginning of fetal development.

Ovulation, Fertilization, and Implantation

Ovulation, the release of a mature ovum from a follicle within the ovary, is initiated and controlled by the secretion of hormones from the anterior pituitary gland. Follicle-stimulating hormone causes numerous follicles within an ovary to grow. The follicles produce estrogen, which in turn stimulates the pituitary to release luteinizing hormone. One of the follicles reaches maturity, its final growth influenced by the luteinizing hormone. The rest of the follicles undergo atrophy and are replaced by connective tissue. On day 14 of a 28-day cycle, the mature follicle ruptures, releasing a single ovum. (See Fig. 28-2.)

The ovum is picked up by the fimbriated ends of the fallopian tube and begins its course through the tube. Within the ovary, the ruptured follicle becomes a corpus luteum (yellow body) and produces progesterone. Nearby cells within the ovary continue to secrete estrogen. These hormones cause the endometrium of the uterus to grow, as the glands of the endometrium proliferate. If fertilization does not occur, the estrogen and progesterone levels drop, the endometrium is shed (menstruation), and the cycle begins anew. When fertilization does occur, the corpus luteum continues to produce its hormones and the endometrium continues to grow. The resultant histologic changes seen in the late secretory phase of menses or in early pregnancy cause the endometrium to become decidualized and the uterus is thus prepared to receive the fertilized egg.

Fertilization usually occurs in the ampullary

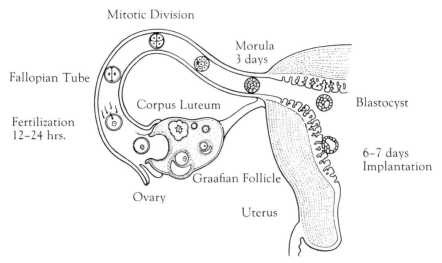

Figure 12-1. *The stages from fertilization of the ovum to implantation of the blasto-cyst. (Courtesy of the Department of Biomedical Communications, State University of New York, Health Science Center at Brooklyn.)*

portion of the tube, 24 to 36 hours after ovulation, when the outer layer of the ovum (the zona pellucida) is penetrated but not destroyed by the sperm. On entering the nucleus of the ovum, the sperm loses its tail and merges its genetic contents with that of the ovum to form a single cell, the zygote. Initial cell division (mitosis) begins 24 to 30 hours after fertilization while the developing zygote moves through the fallopian tube. Cells continue to divide, forming a solid cluster of cells still surrounded and protected by the zona pellucida. This ball of cells, the morula, continues its passage through the fallopian tube, and reaches the uterine cavity about 3 days after fertilization (Fig. 12-1).[50]

As the morula takes on an organized form, it becomes known as a blastocyst. An outer layer of cells, the trophoblast, surrounds a fluid-filled cavity (the blastocele) and an inner cell mass. Within the uterus, the zona pellucida disappears and the blastocyst receives its nutrients from the secretions of the endometrial glands. Implantation has not yet occurred.

The trophoblast differentiates into two layers, an inner single layer of cytotrophoblast and an outer, multicelled layer of syncytiotrophoblast. An important role of the trophoblast is the production of human chorionic gonadotropin (hCG), a hormone that extends the life of the corpus luteum.

Continued secretion of progesterone by the corpus luteum ensures that the uterus does not shed its endometrial lining, and with it the rapidly developing products of conception.

Implantation, made possible by the disappearance of the zona pellucida, begins when the tropho-

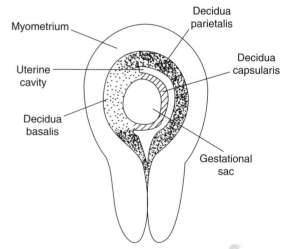

Figure 12-2. *Implantation of an early embryo. The common sonographic term "gestational sac" actually describes the fluid-filled chorionic cavity surrounded by primary villi during a trophoblastic–decidual reaction. A gestational sac can be imaged before the fusion of the decidua capsularis and decidua parietalis.*

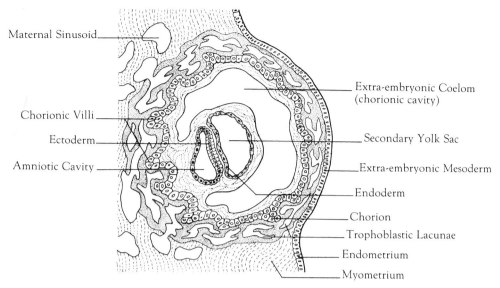

Maternal Sinusoid

Chorionic Villi

Ectoderm

Amniotic Cavity

Extra-embryonic Coelom (chorionic cavity)

Secondary Yolk Sac

Extra-embryonic Mesoderm

Endoderm

Chorion

Trophoblastic Lacunae

Endometrium

Myometrium

Figure 12-3. The bilaminar embryonic disc with its associated structures. (Courtesy of the Department of Biomedical Communications, State University of New York, Health Science Center at Brooklyn.)

blastic cells over the region of the inner cell mass begin to penetrate into the endometrium about 7 days after fertilization. The blastocyst burrows beneath the endometrial surface, and the opening it created is sealed by a blood clot. Decidualized endometrium can be seen to have three distinct layers defined by their relationship to the blastocyst. The decidua capsularis closes over and surrounds the blastocyst. The decidua parietalis, or decidua vera, is the decidua that lines the remainder of the endometrial cavity. The decidua basalis develops at the point of attachment by the blastocyst and

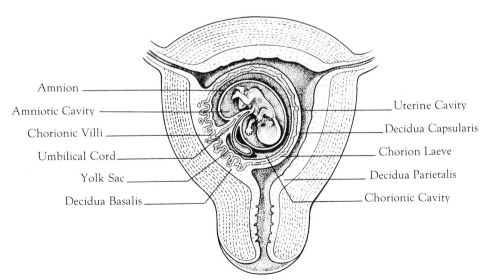

Amnion

Amniotic Cavity

Chorionic Villi

Umbilical Cord

Yolk Sac

Decidua Basalis

Uterine Cavity

Decidua Capsularis

Chorion Laeve

Decidua Parietalis

Chorionic Cavity

Figure 12-4. The membranes and cavities surrounding the embryo. (Courtesy of the Department of Biomedical Communications, State University of New York, Health Science Center at Brooklyn.)

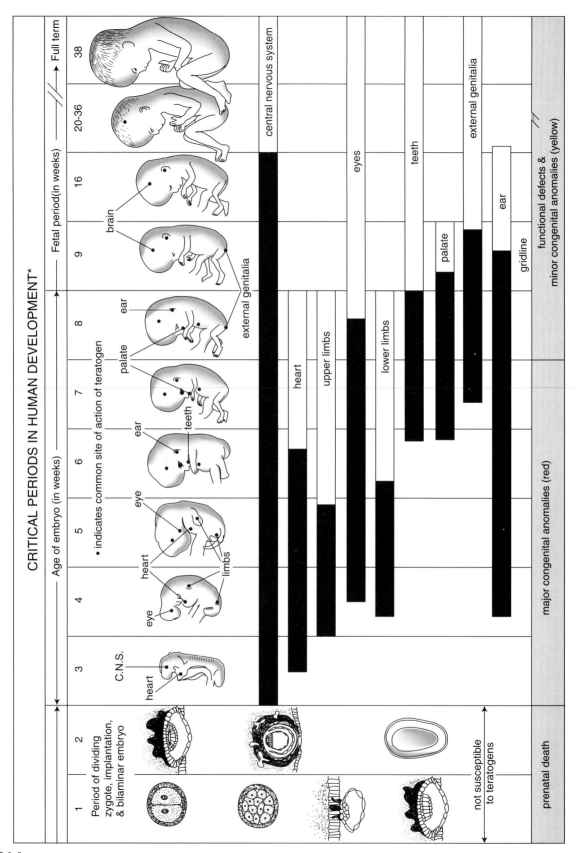

CRITICAL PERIODS IN HUMAN DEVELOPMENT*

contributes the maternal portion of the placenta (Fig. 12-2).

Development of the Conceptus

The inner cell mass, or embryonic pole, differentiates into two layers: the endoderm, which faces the blastocele, and the ectoderm, which lies adjacent to the trophoblast. Within the ectoderm the amniotic cavity begins to form as a small fluid collection. Another fluid-filled structure forms adjacent to the endoderm. This cavity is the primary or primitive yolk sac. Eventually a portion of the primitive yolk sac is pinched off and disappears; the remainder is the secondary yolk sac.

The chorionic cavity, or extraembryonic coelom, is filled with a gel called magma reticulare, and occupies most of the blastocyst. While the inner cell mass is differentiating, a loose network of cells, the extraembryonic mesoderm, develops, lining the cavity, the yolk sac, and the bilaminar embryonic disc with its small amniotic cavity (Fig. 12-3). It also forms a stalk connecting the embryonic disc to the trophoblast.

The trophoblast and the lining of mesoderm are now called chorion. Chorionic villi project outward from the walls of the blastocyst into the decidua. As the gestational sac grows, the decidua parietalis is stretched thin and the chorionic villi that do not proliferate into chorion frondosum disappear, leaving smooth chorion laeve. At the point where implantation into the uterus occured, however, villi continue to grow and proliferate, forming the chorion frondosum. This will become the conceptus' contribution to the formation of the placenta.

Within the embryonic ectoderm, a line of cells thickens to form a primitive streak, which migrates to the area between the ectoderm and endoderm. A third layer of cells, the embryonic mesoderm, arises from the primitive streak. The embryonic disc contains the three germ cell layers from which all future tissue is derived. Development of the trilaminar disc (at the end of the third week after fertilization) marks the transition from the preembryonic period to the embryonic stage.

During the embryonic period, the once-flat embryonic disc folds and further differentiates, and the amniotic cavity expands at the expense of the chorionic cavity. Eventually the amniotic cavity completely fills the gestational sac. The cells lining the amniotic cavity (amnion) fuse with the chorion, but this fusion is not complete until 12 to 17 weeks after the last menstrual period (Fig. 12-4).

The embryonic endoderm, mesoderm, and ectoderm continue to differentiate, and by the end of the eighth week after conception (10 menstrual weeks), the embryo has developed the rudimentary forms of all of its organs and structures. The embryonic period is now complete, and the fetal stage, with its rapid growth and maturation of organ systems, commences (Fig. 12-5).

Sonographic Identification of the Early Intrauterine Pregnancy

The earliest stages of preembryonic and embryonic development take place on a microscopic level, and are impossible to image even with current high-frequency transvaginal probes. An early indication of pregnancy may be seen with the development of prominent arcuate vessels in the periphery of the myometrium and a thick, lush echogenic endometrial echo (Fig. 12-6).

The first definitive evidence of an intrauterine pregnancy as detected by ultrasound is the presence of a gestational sac, which represents a fluid-filled chorionic cavity surrounded by the primary chorionic villi invading the maternal decidua (Fig. 12-7). The inner cell mass, early amniotic cavity, and primitive yolk sac are too small to be resolved at this time. The trophoblastic–decidual reaction

Figure 12-5. *Graph of the critical periods of the development of the embryo/fetus (organogenesis) in weeks from the date of conception. A physical or chemical insult (teratogen) has its most devastating effects when it occurs during the critical period of the susceptible organ or system. During the 2 weeks from conception to the development of the trilaminar embryo, teratogens tend to have an all-or-nothing effect; that is, the most severe insults cause pregnancy loss, whereas other agents are unlikely to affect the undifferentiated cells of the zygote or bilaminar embryo. (Moore K, Persaud TVN. The Developing Human: Clinically Oriented Embryology. 5th ed. Philadelphia: WB Saunders; 1993:473).*

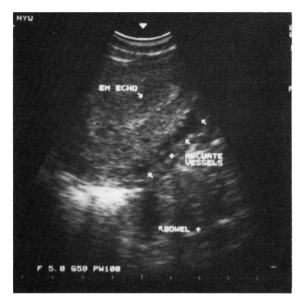

Figure 12-6. A long-axis view of the uterus (vaginal scan) in very early pregnancy. Before the appearance of a true gestational sac, it is possible to visualize the extremely prominent arcuate vessels (*arrows*). The endometrial cavity appears lush and echogenic. These findings are compatible with, although in no way diagnostic of, early pregnancy. Bowel can be seen posterior to the uterus.

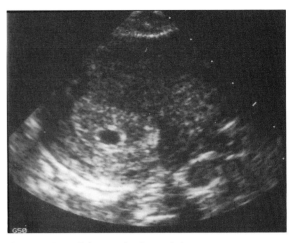

Figure 12-8. A long-axis view of the uterus revealing a very early gestational sac. The thick echogenic rind (trophoblastic–decidual reaction) surrounds an anechoic center (chorionic cavity).

appears as a very thick echogenic rind surrounding an anechoic center (Fig. 12-8).

Transabdominally, it was difficult to distinguish between an early intrauterine gestational sac (before the visualization of structures within the sac) and the decidual reaction associated with ectopic pregnancies. This confusion was significantly reduced by the recognition of the "double decidual sac"

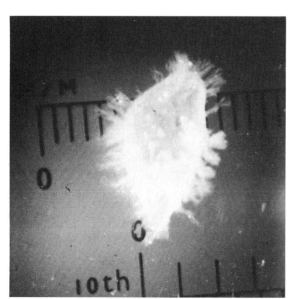

Figure 12-7. An entire gestation (of 5.5 weeks LMP) viewed with low-power microscope magnification. Note the chorion with primary villi projecting from it. This is the anatomic basis for the sonographic appearance that we know as the gestational sac.

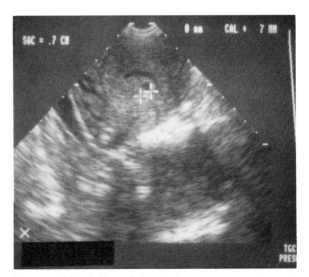

Figure 12-9. A 7-mm intrauterine pregnancy. The calipers have been moved so as not to obscure the landmarks of the gestational sac. The crescent-shaped sonolucency adjacent to it represents decidua capsularis not yet fused to decidua parietalis.

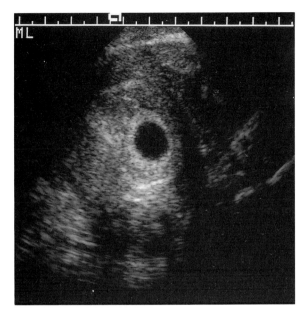

Figure 12-10. A 15-mm intrauterine pregnancy. Even without fluid in the endometrial cavity, as seen in Figure 12-9, recognition of the double decidual sign of an early pregnancy helps the ultrasound practitioner exclude the possibility of a decidual cast associated with an ectopic pregnancy.

sign, which represented the decidua capsularis and the decidua parietalis before they fused (Fig. 12-9).[55] In the absence of an intrauterine pregnancy, the fluid seen with a decidual reaction lies within the endometrial cavity, whereas an early in-

trauterine pregnancy is surrounded in most planes by the two layers of decidua. Although higher-frequency transvaginal probes have made the distinction simpler (Fig. 12-10), it is still a useful marker for the identification of an intrauterine pregnancy before the visualization of structures within the gestational sac.

As mentioned earlier, the embryonic disc, early amniotic cavity, and primary yolk sac are initially too small to be identified sonographically. The first structure within the gestational sac that can be seen using ultrasound is the secondary yolk sac (Fig. 12-11A). This appears as a round, anechoic structure measuring approximately 4 mm in diameter, surrounded by a highly reflective echogenic ring. It is seen transvaginally about 5 weeks after the last menstrual period (LMP), and transabdominally by 6 to 7 weeks post LMP.[57] The "double-bleb sign," which was first identified transabdominally, represents the complex of the early sonolucent amniotic sac and the yolk sac, with the developing embryo between them (Fig. 12-12).[81] The yolk sac remains fairly constant in size and appearance until about 11 weeks' menstrual age. Meanwhile, the embryo and the amniotic sac that encloses it are growing at the expense of the chorionic cavity (Fig. 12-13). Eventually, the chorionic cavity is completely filled by the amniotic cavity, and the amnion and chorion fuse.

The embryonic heart begins pulsating by 21

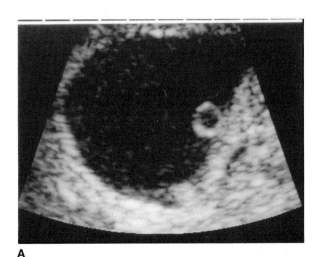

A

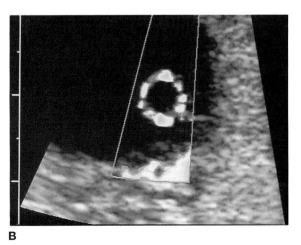

B

Figure 12-11. **(A)** The yolk sac appears as a round, anechoic structure surrounded by a highly reflective echogenic ring located within the chorionic cavity. **(B)** Low-velocity flow detected in the walls of the secondary yolk sac. The yolk sac plays a role in the transport of nutrients to the embryo and is the first site of blood cell formation. (See also Color Plate 11.)

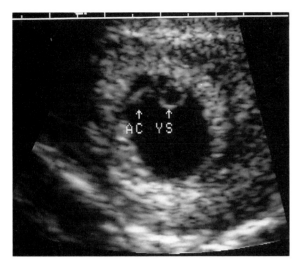

Figure 12-12. The "double-bleb" describes the appearance of the yolk sac (YS) adjacent to the early amniotic cavity (AC). The collection of echoes along a wall of the amniotic cavity represents the embryonic pole, in which cardiac pulsations were identified.

days after conception; however, a very early embryonic pole may initially be too small to identify cardiac pulsations within it.[67] Failure to visualize cardiac activity in embryos measuring 4 mm or less may be a normal finding, and warrants a follow-up examination to establish viability.[45] Cardiac pulsations should be identified in all normal embryos measuring 5 mm or larger, and can be documented using M-mode or Doppler.

Perhaps one of the most exciting results of enhanced ultrasound resolution has been the ability to observe milestones of embryonic development.[5,7,12,25,35,73,74] Although a full discussion of "sonoembryology" is beyond the scope of this chapter, certain highlights should be mentioned. The embryo grows at a rate of about 1 to 2 mm per day. By 8 weeks' menstrual age, it begins to unfold. At this time, the head accounts for approximately one half its size (Fig. 12-14). Limb buds begin to develop (Fig. 12-15). Around 8 weeks post LMP, the embryonic gut herniates out of the abdominal cavity into the base of the cord (Fig. 12-16). It then goes through a process of rotation and eventually recedes back into the abdominal cavity. This physiologic herniation is a normal process, and should not be mistaken for an omphalocele.[21,68]

The development of the hindbrain has been well described.[6,7] The cavity of the rhombencephalon, the future fourth ventricle, can be seen by the seventh week as a posterior lucency initially lying superiorly in the embryonic head (Fig. 12-17). By the eighth week, the cerebellum can be distinguished. The echogenic choroid plexus within the lateral ventricles can be seen by the 10th week (Fig. 12-18). The fetal spine can be identified, although

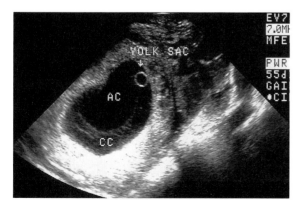

Figure 12-13. The yolk sac is seen outside the amniotic cavity (AC), but within the chorionic cavity (CC) in this image taken in a plane that does not include the embryo. The embryo and the amniotic cavity in which it develops grow at a faster rate than that of the chorionic cavity. Eventually the chorionic cavity is completely filled by the amniotic cavity and the membranes, the amnion and the chorion, fuse.

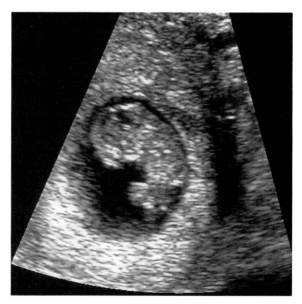

Figure 12-14. By 8 weeks LMP, the embryo is seen beginning to unfold. The head is about half the size of the embryo.

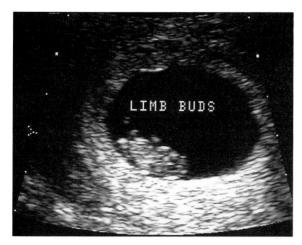

Figure 12-15. Limb buds may be seen before 9 weeks after LMP.

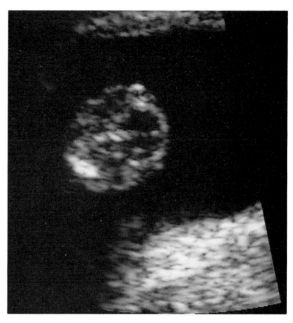

Figure 12-17. The sonolucent structure seen in the posterior portion of the brain in this axial view of the head at 10 weeks, 2 days after LMP, represents the cavity of the rhombencephalon. This structure gives rise to the fourth ventricle.

it is not yet sufficiently ossified to cause acoustic shadowing (Fig. 12-19). By 11 weeks, the umbilical cord and its normal insertion can be seen. By all definitions, the developing organism ceases to be an embryo and becomes a fetus by 10 weeks post LMP.

Pregnancy Detection

The use of higher-frequency transvaginal ultrasound has modified expectations of *when* we should be able to see evidence of an intrauterine pregnancy.[32] In 1981, Kadar and colleagues proposed

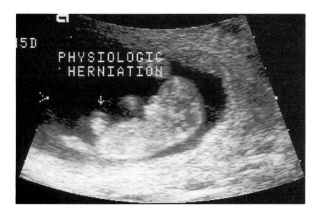

Figure 12-16. This 10-week, 5-day fetus demonstrates the normal physiologic herniation of midgut into the base of the umbilical cord. The bowel will undergo a 270-degree rotation before returning to the abdominal cavity. This should not be mistaken for an abdominal wall defect.

a "discriminatory zone" of hCG.[42] Using a transabdominal sonographic approach, they concluded that when the β-subunit level of serum hCG reached 6000 to 6500 mIU/ml (International Reference Preparation), a normal intrauterine pregnancy should be sonographically visualized. Its absence at those levels would indicate either an ectopic or abnormal intrauterine pregnancy. Several years later, the discriminatory zone was further refined to 1800 mIU/ml (Second International Standard).[53] It should be noted that the values of the Second International Standard are approximately one-half those of the International Reference Preparation. Today, using higher-frequency transvaginal probes, the discriminatory β-hCG zone is in the range of 1025 mIU/ml (IRP)[34,61] or 300 to 700 mIU/ml (2nd IS).[5,34] Failure to visualize an intrauterine gestation in a patient whose serum hCG has exceeded these levels may be a strong indication of an ectopic pregnancy.

Most normal intrauterine gestational sacs can be visualized at 4 weeks plus 1 to 4 days from the LMP.[7] Transabdominally, they should be detectable by 6 weeks' menstrual age.[25] Maternal obesity or significant scarring from previous lower abdomi-

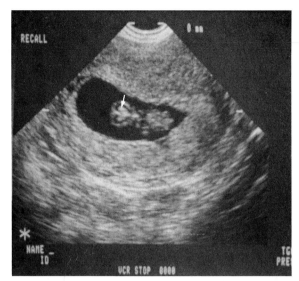

Figure 12-18. *The echogenic choroid plexus is distinctly seen within the head of this embryo at 9.5 weeks after LMP.*

nal or pelvic surgery may make visualization difficult with this approach. Once an intrauterine gestation is sonographically identified, correlation with the hCG titer may provide a clue as to whether the pregnancy is progressing normally.

Establishing Gestational Age in the Very Early Pregnancy

Before detecting a measurable embryonic pole, the pregnancy can be dated by measuring the gestational sac. To obtain a mean sac diameter (MSD),

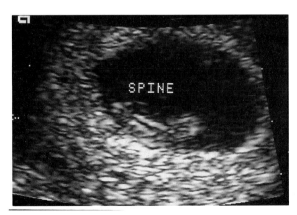

Figure 12-19. *The embryonic spine, as seen at 8 weeks, 4 days after LMP, is insufficiently ossified to cause acoustic shadowing.*

the height, width, and depth of the fluid portion of the sac taken at the fluid–chorionic tissue interface is measured by scanning in two planes at right angles to one another and calculating an average of the three measurements. Other authors have used the maximal sac diameter, which requires only a single measurement. Gestational sacs as small as 4 mm, corresponding to a menstrual age of 4.5 weeks, have been identified. The smallest sacs are usually uniformly spherical, so a single diameter would yield virtually the same results as a mean of the three diameters.

The developing and enlarging embryonic pole can routinely be visualized by the 7th week. By measuring the embryo along its longest axis, taking care to exclude the yolk sac, a crown–rump length (CRL) can be obtained (Fig. 12-20).[22] This is the single, most accurate method of establishing an estimated date of delivery, although using multiple parameters early in the second trimester approaches the accuracy of the CRL.

Nomograms are available to establish gestational age based on these measurements. See Chapter 19 for a complete discussion of pregnancy dating techniques.

Expanding the Role of First Trimester Ultrasound

In the second and third trimesters of pregnancy, diagnostic ultrasound is used to determine gestational age, identify multiple gestations, evaluate fe-

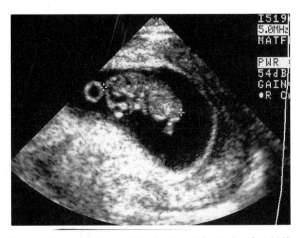

Figure 12-20. *A transvaginal scan at 9 weeks after LMP demonstrates the landmarks (crosses) for measuring the crown–rump length. Caution must be exercised not to include the yolk sac, the fetal limbs, or a portion of the uterine wall. The transvaginal approach is preferable because it more clearly delineates these structures.*

tal anatomic structures to identify anomalies, and assess fetal well-being. Until recently, ultrasound examination in the first trimester was indicated only to establish the presence of an intrauterine pregnancy (or verify an ectopic pregnancy) and predict its viability. Its role is now being greatly expanded.

Routine first trimester ultrasound is not included in the accepted standard of care in the United States at this time.[75] In part, this reflects a cautious approach to avoid potential bioeffects of ultrasound. The first trimester, with its rapid cell growth and differentiation, is the period of greatest susceptibility to physical and chemical insults. Resultant abnormalities may not be manifested immediately. Therefore, caution must be exercised when introducing any unnecessary influences to the intrauterine environment. Although no significant bioeffects have been documented at the current diagnostic levels of ultrasound, prudence demands a conservative approach to a modality that is still under investigation.

When a patient reports a problem during the first trimester of pregnancy, or when the clinician perceives an unusual or discrepant finding, ultrasound is often the method of choice to confirm or rule out the clinician's suspicions. Additionally, groundbreaking research in the identification of markers for chromosomal abnormalities and the early identification of structural malformations have shifted the risk-benefit ratio of very early ultrasound towards a greater acceptance. The following discussion will focus first on the most commonly presenting clinical symptoms in the first trimester. This will be followed by the expanded criteria to predict pregnancy viability, new findings that raise the suspicion of chrommosomal abnormalities, and the early detection of structural anomalies.

Vaginal Bleeding

Clinically, pregnancy is confirmed after a woman has missed a menstrual period and has had a positive urine or serum pregnancy test. A surprisingly large number of undetected pregnancies are aborted spontaneously before a woman has missed her menstrual period, and thus neither she nor her obstetrician is aware of the pregnancy and its loss. Of those pregnancies that progress to the point of detection, approximately one quarter are complicated by some degree of first trimester vaginal bleeding.[27] When vaginal bleeding occurs with a closed cervical os in

a pregnancy of less than 20 weeks, the diagnosis is that of a threatened abortion. Although other factors not related to the pregnancy (such as cervical polyps) may be the source of the bleeding, first consideration goes to establishing the viability of the pregnancy.

Traditionally, it has been said that half of all women with threatened abortion eventually abort, and half proceed to a normal outcome. Although various attempts to influence these results have been investigated, none holds much promise for increasing the proportion of successful pregnancies. It is thought that many spontaneous abortions are due to chromosomal abnormalities that are not compatible with life. The value of ultrasound in threatened abortion lies not in any endeavor to alter the outcome of the pregnancy, but in the ability to predict which pregnancies will continue successfully to term. At the same time, the possibility of ectopic pregnancy can be ruled out, as discussed in Chapter 11.

Examination of the uterus and its contents enables the sonographer to determine whether the patient's condition is an early viable pregnancy or an abnormal development.[77] The rate of early pregnancy loss decreases as gestational age increases. Goldstein reports that if an intrauterine gestational sac develops, subsequent loss of viability occurs in 11.5% of first trimester pregnancies. Spontaneous loss occurs in 8.5% of intrauterine gestational sacs in which a yolk sac is identified. Embryos with a CRL up to 5 mm have a 7.2% loss rate, which decreased to 3.3% in embryos between 6 to 10 mm, and to 0.5% in embryos larger than 10 mm.[30,31]

A mean or maximal sac diameter can be used not only to date a very early pregnancy, but to establish whether development is proceeding normally. Using a transabdominal scanning technique, an embryo should be apparent in all normal gestational sacs with an MSD of 25 mm or larger.[56] Transvaginally, the embryo should be detected in a gestational sac 16 mm or larger.[44] Using these limits as a standard, the absence of an embryo at this time is indication of an abnormal condition commonly referred to as a blighted ovum, or anembryonic pregnancy. Blighted ova may occur when the embryo has died and been resorbed, or development ceased before the formation of a discrete embryo (Fig. 12-21). The sac of a blighted ovum appears too large to be devoid of internal structures. It

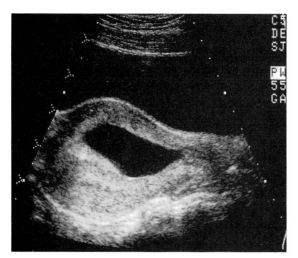

Figure 12-21. *Large, irregular sac without evidence of embryonic development, compatible with the diagnosis of a blighted ovum. In some cases, this may actually represent embryonic resorption rather than lack of embryonic development.*

typically looses its smooth, round, or ovoid shape, becoming irregular in form.

In examining gestational sacs of even earlier pregnancies, the sonographer should attempt to find a yolk sac. The yolk sac can be identified before the embryo can be visualized and should be evident by transabdominal technique in all normal gestational sacs with an MSD of 20 mm or greater,[57] whereas transvaginally the yolk sac should be seen in all normal gestational sacs greater than or equal to 8 mm in MSD.[44] Its absence in a gestational sac of this size is sonographic proof of a nonviable pregnancy.

Once the yolk sac has been identified, an embryo within a small amniotic cavity should be identified. Between 6.5 to 10 weeks' gestation, the length of the amniotic cavity is very close to the length of the embryonic pole. It has been reported that an empty amniotic cavity, even in the presence of a yolk sac, is another indicator of early pregnancy failure.[48]

In clearly identifiable embryos with a CRL of 4 mm or greater, the absence of cardiac activity is diagnostic of embryo demise (Fig. 12-22). It is advisable for the sonographer to scan the embryo for a full 3 minutes before assuming embryo demise, and the findings should be confirmed by another observer, usually the radiologist or obstetrician. If there is any doubt, especially in studies that

are technically limited, follow-up scans are warranted after an appropriate interval, usually 7 to 10 days. A dead embryo that has not been expelled from the uterus is termed a missed abortion.[66]

The presence of a sonographically identifiable intrauterine embryo with an obviously pulsating heart is the best predictor of a favorable outcome. Among patients diagnosed with threatened abortion, those who sonographically demonstrate a living embryo have an 84% to 98% chance of successfully carrying to term.[16,70,78]

The range in estimates is due largely to the patient populations from which the data were collected. Only three fourths of pregnancies in women with a history of recurrent pregnancy loss (defined as three or more pregnancy losses) have a live embryo at the first trimester sonogram. In this subset of patients, demonstration of a living fetus results in a viable live birth 83% of the time. Therefore, the rate of spontaneous abortion or fetal death among these women is higher than in a normal obstetric population.[76]

In addition, advanced maternal age was associated with higher spontaneous loss rates.[78] Finally, as might be expected, the highest success rates were obtained from exclusively private patients who are presumably more affluent, better nourished, and more likely to receive prenatal and preconception care, whereas the lower rates reflected a large clinic population from a lower socioeconomic stratum.[70]

Occasionally, a normal-looking gestational sac may be partially surrounded by a crescent-shaped sonolucent collection (Fig. 12-23). This is evidence of a

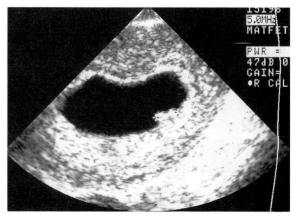

Figure 12-22. *Embryo demise (missed abortion) in a patient who reported vaginal bleeding at 9 weeks after LMP. A small-for-dates embryonic pole without cardiac pulsations is seen within the uterus.*

subchorionic hemorrhage (bleeding between the endometrium and the gestational sac). Coexistence of a subchorionic hemorrhage with embryonic heart activity leads to a slightly reduced continuation rate, but most of these pregnancies progress to term.[33] Detection of subchorionic bleeding as documented by Doppler flow as well as static collections was thought to have little significance unless clinical vaginal bleeding occurred.[23] A recent study, however, indicates that there is not only a statistically increased risk of miscarriage in patients with subchorionic hemorrhage, but that the incidence of stillbirth, abruptio placentae, and preterm labor rises as well.[3]

When a patient is noted to have profuse bleeding and the cervical os has begun to dilate, abortion is said to be inevitable and imminent. A sonogram may be requested to inform the obstetrician of the progress or completion of the evacuation of the uterine contents. Sonographically, a gestational sac may be seen in the cervix or vagina as it is expelled (Fig. 12-24). If the uterus appears empty and has moderate to bright endometrial echoes, the patient has had a complete abortion. A complex collection of echoes within the endometrial cavity indicates an incomplete abortion (Fig. 12-25). These ultrasound findings may determine whether the patient requires dilatation and curettage.

Size–Dates Discrepancy

When a patient is unsure of her LMP, or if a clinical examination of the uterus does not agree with the patient's reported LMP, her clinician may request

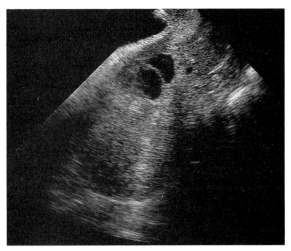

Figure 12-24. The two sacs of an early twin gestation are seen approaching the cervix of a patient who went on to abort spontaneously.

a sonogram to date the pregnancy. Although this is usually requested early in the second trimester, several factors, such as the presence of uterine fibroids, maternal obesity, surgical scars, or multiple gestation, may make it difficult for the obstetrician to estimate the size of the uterus, from which the gestational age is estimated. Because other aspects of pregnancy management (e.g., methods of termination, interpretation of α-fetoprotein levels, timing of chorionic villi sampling or amniocentesis) hinge on the correct assessment of the duration of

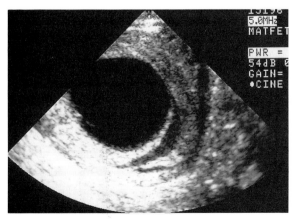

Figure 12-23. A patient at 9 weeks after LMP, scanned for vaginal bleeding. The crescent-shaped anechoic area outside the gestational sac represents subchorionic hemorrhage. An embryo with cardiac activity was identified in another plane within the gestational sac.

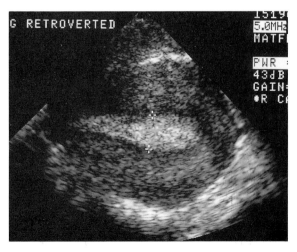

Figure 12-25. Irregular, heterogeneous, dense endometrial echo (*arrows*) compatible with a diagnosis of incomplete abortion.

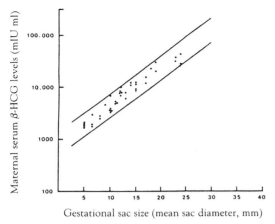

Figure 12-26. Correlation of mean sac diameter with simultaneous serum human chorionic gonadotropin level for 39 normal gestations. Solid lines represent 95% confidence limits. (From Nyberg D, Laing FC, Filly RA, et al. Threatened abortion: Sonographic distinction of normal and abnormal gestational sacs. Radiology. 1986; 158:395.)

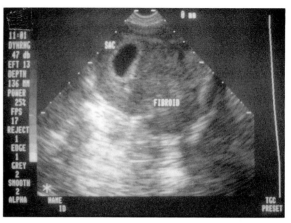

Figure 12-28. Sonogram of a patient who presented at 7 weeks dates with a 14-week–sized uterus reveals a 7-week intrauterine gestation within a large myomatous uterus.

pregnancy, the patient may be sent for ultrasound evaluation in the first trimester.

A mean sac diameter of 5 mm can be obtained by the fifth week after LMP using a transvaginal transducer, but other fluid collections in the endometrial cavity can have a similar appearance. It

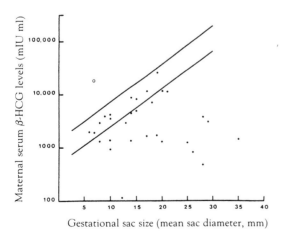

Figure 12-27. Mean sac diameter compared with serum human chorionic gonadotropin (hCG) levels for 31 abnormal gestations. In 20 cases (65%), the hCG level was disproportionately low. Only one woman (with a molar pregnancy) had an elevated hCG determination (○). (From Nyberg D, Laing FC, Filly RA, et al. Threatened abortion: Sonographic distinction of normal and abnormal gestational sacs. Radiology. 1986; 158:395.)

is therefore helpful to correlate the MSD to the level of hCG.[15,53,54,61] A 5-mm MSD should correspond to an hCG level of 1800 mU/ml (2nd IS). The MSD and serum levels should continue to rise proportionally in normal pregnancies (Figs. 12-26 and 12-27). By the eighth week after LMP, hCG levels start to plateau, but by this time the embryo should be seen clearly on ultrasound, and its CRL measured. Normal embryos are consistently identified by the time they reach a CRL of 5 mm or more.

When the obstetrician reports that the patient is large for her dates, the gestational age should be estimated from either the MSD or CRL. The pregnancy may simply be more advanced than was anticipated. The uterus should be surveyed carefully to rule out the presence of leiomyomas (Fig. 12-28). If fibroids are found, the sonographer should be able to demonstrate their number, size, and location for future follow-up. Care must be taken not to mistake a focal myometrial contraction for a fibroid. These contractions are transient thickenings of a portion of the myometrium (Fig. 12-29). They tend to indent the gestational sac or endometrial cavity, whereas fibroids more often distort the outer contours of the uterus.[80] The sonographer should begin the examination with a survey of the uterus. Focal thickenings seen at the beginning of the examination often have disappeared by the end, and this change can be noted to make the diagnosis. When the thickening persists, the patient can be asked to empty

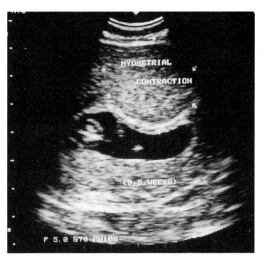

Figure 12-29. Sonographic appearance of a focal myometrial contraction (arrows). Note how the gestational sac is indented. This should not be confused with a fibroid uterus. This is extremely important when performing chorionic villus sampling. The patient with a focal myometrial contraction may be allowed to walk about for 15 to 20 minutes before the scan is repeated.

her bladder or walk around for a half hour, and then be rescanned.

A large-for-dates uterus accompanied by hyperemesis and elevated serum hCG levels may be an indication of hydatiform mole (see Chap. 25). Another cause of an enlarged uterus is a multiple gestation (Fig. 12-30). The uterus must be scanned carefully in several planes to establish the number of sacs and embryos and to rule out uterine anomalies, such as a septate uterus, that may distort a gestational sac and in some planes make a singleton appear to be twins (Fig. 12-31). It is also important to keep in mind the large number of early pregnancies that fail to develop. Although some of them are shed and the woman experiences vaginal bleeding, others are simply resorbed. As with a singleton pregnancy, this process can occur with one or more of a multiple gestation, and is known as the "vanishing twin" (Fig. 12-32). In as many as 70% of cases, when twins are identified at or before 10 weeks' gestational age, only a singleton is born.[28]

When the uterus is smaller than expected, careful measurements are again taken to establish the gestational age. If the development of the gestational sac and its contents is indeed less advanced than the patient's dates would indicate, again, cor-

relation with the hCG levels is in order. Once spontaneous abortion and blighted ovum have been ruled out, serial sonograms should be performed to establish a normal rate of growth. Although most cases of intrauterine growth restriction are due to uteroplacental insufficiency and therefore occur in the third trimester (or, in severe cases, in the second), congenital anomalies, particularly those associated with chromosomal abnormalities and certain congenital viral infections, cause disturbed growth patterns as well.[4,66]

Advances in Predicting Viability

Documenting cardiac activity on real-time, M-mode, or Doppler in the first trimester was at one time thought to be an unequivocally favorable sign of viability. Once heart motion has been detected, the heart rate can be measured using either Doppler or M-mode. It is now known that the heart rate has great significance in predicting outcome. Bradycardia is associated with a high likelihood of first trimester demise. Age-specific norms for heart rates in the first trimester have been established. The lower limit of normal is now thought to be 100 bpm before 6.2 weeks' gestational age, and 120 bpm between 6.3 and 7 weeks.[26] Embryos with lower heart rates are much less likely to survive the first trimester.

The size of the gestational sac has added sig-

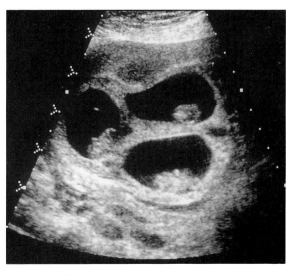

Figure 12-30. Transvaginal sonogram reveals a triplet pregnancy with three distinct gestational sacs. Multiple gestation is a common source of size–dates discrepancy.

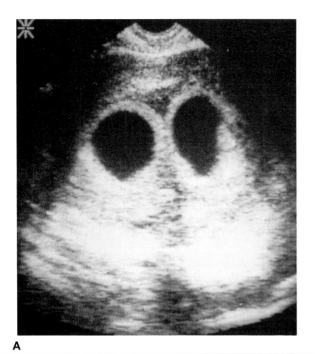

A

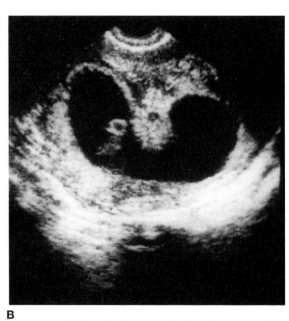

B

Figure 12-31. (**A**) Sonogram reveals an apparent twin gestation. (**B**) Sonogram of the same patient taken at a slightly different scan angle reveals a septate uterus containing a single intrauterine pregnancy. Careful scanning helps avoid misdiagnosing a twin gestation.

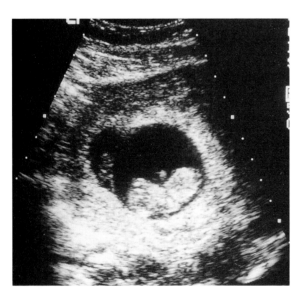

Figure 12-32. A normal embryo is seen within a gestational sac. In the much smaller, adjacent sac, an embryonic pole without cardiac activity is identified. If the dead twin becomes completely resorbed, it will be said to have "vanished." This process occurs much more commonly than was thought before the widespread use of detailed first trimester endovaginal sonography.

nificance when viewed in relation to the size of the embryo. A small sac size is another predictor of a poor outcome. When the CRL (in millimeters) is subtracted from the MSD, the difference should measure 5 mm or greater. In pregnancies in which the difference was less than 5 mm, as many as 94% had spontaneous abortions, even after demonstrating normal cardiac activity.[10,29]

The yolk sac should also be examined. Abnormally large, abnormally small, and abnormally shaped yolk sacs are all associated with a poor outcome (Fig. 12-33).[43,46,63] A yolk sac of more than 5.6 mm in a pregnancy of less than 10 weeks' menstrual age is a particularly strong indicator of an abnormal outcome. An additional, serendipitous advantage of investigating yolk sacs in multiple pregnancies is the ability to determine amnionicity in monochorionic pregnancies. Monochorionic pregnancies in the first trimester present as a single gestational sac. In monochorionic–diamniotic pregnancies, two yolk sacs are identified (Fig. 12-34) within a gestational sac. In monochorionic–monoamniotic pregnancies, only one yolk sac can be seen at 9 weeks despite the identification of two embryos.[9]

The Nuchal Lucency

In 1990, a letter appeared in *Lancet* describing an unusual finding that was discovered by scanning the embryos of patients who had undergone chorionic villus sampling. An accumulation of subcutaneous fluid in the nuchal region was seen in 7 of 7 embryos with trisomy 21, whereas only 1 of 105 chromosomally normal embryos was found to have a similar appearance.[71] Concurrently, an article in *Prenatal Diagnosis* described the significance of "cystic hygroma" in the first trimester, noting that embryos with this finding had a 50% chance of having chromosomal abnormalities, including trisomy 21.[19] These communications, which were confirmed by other researchers,[11,17,18,40,51,58,59,60,69,79] heralded a new era in first trimester ultrasound, leading many to propose ultrasound performed between 9 to 12 weeks' gestational age as a screening tool to rule out aneuploidies.[8,9,13,37,39,52,72]

The nuchal lucency, also described as nuchal edema or a simple (as opposed to septated) cystic hygroma, is seen as a sonolucent area enclosed by a membrane that extends from the posterior aspect of the embryo's head to a variable point along the spine (Fig. 12-35). The upper limits of normal vary according to

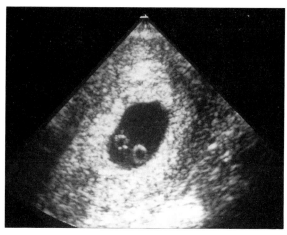

Figure 12-34. Two yolk sacs are seen within a single gestational sac, indicating monochorionic–diamniotic twins. Monochorionic–monoamniotic twins would have a single yolk sac, although two embryos would develop within a single gestational sac. Dichorionic–diamniotic twins present as two distinct gestational sacs.

authors, with anything from less than or equal to 3 to 6 mm (in an anterior-to-posterior plane) being offered as a cutoff point. If the embryo is in a "face up" position during the scan, care must be taken not to mistake the amnion on which the embryo is lying for the nuchal membrane (Fig. 12-36). If in doubt, wait for the embryo to move and see if the membrane moves with it, or have the patient turn to her side. The embryo will usually float away from the membrane

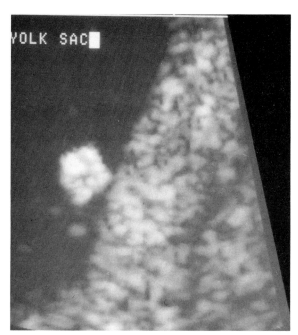

Figure 12-33. A thickened, collapsed, unusually echogenic yolk sac that was associated with an embryo demise.

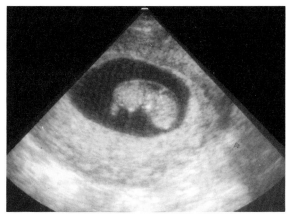

Figure 12-35. The nuchal translucency, a sonolucent area enclosed by a membrane along the posterior aspect of the embryonic head and body, is seen in an embryo subsequently diagnosed as having Turner syndrome (45XO).

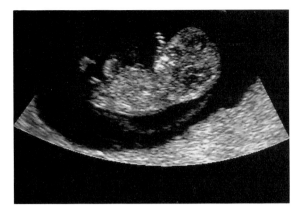

Figure 12-36. An apparent example of an embryo with a nuchal lucency is created by displaying a normal embryo lying against the amnion. In real-time scanning, the embryo could be seen moving away from the membrane.

if it is truly the amnion. Confusion can be caused as well by the presence of nuchal blebs, which are small fluid collections seen in the occipital region in 40% of embryos before 10 weeks' gestation and are considered to be normal variants that have no lasting significance.[36] Confirming the diagnosis of a nuchal lucency may best be made after 10 weeks to avoid this problem. Once the presence of a nuchal lucency is confirmed, the patient should be offered appropriate counseling and karyotyping.[41]

Structural Abnormalities Detected in the First Trimester

In 1993, the International Society of Ultrasound in Obstetrics and Gynecology formally established the International Registry of the Onset of Fetal Anomalies (IRONFAN), which is a database of the early detection of structural abnormalities. From this information, it is hoped that ultrasound professionals and those who rely on their expertise will learn not only the earliest time an abnormality *can* be detected, but, equally important, the earliest time it *should* be detected.

The list of anomalies detected in the first trimester is ever-growing.[37,49,65] However, when normal development can mimic an abnormality, careful follow-up is required to avoid unnecessarily alarming the patient and perhaps resulting in termination of a desired pregnancy in the mistaken belief that something is wrong. For example, correct diagnosis of omphalocele has been made (distinct from

the normal physiologic herniation) by noting that the herniated mass had the appearance of homogeneous tissue compatible with liver rather than the more heterogeneous bowel.[20] Some of the other anomalies detected in the first trimester include du-

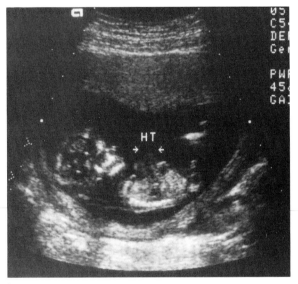

A

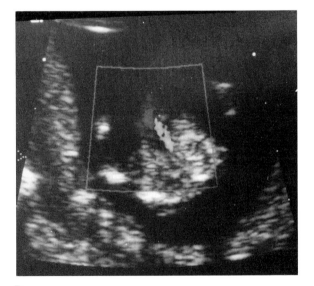

B

Figure 12-37. (**A**) First trimester diagnosis of ectopic cordis. The heart (HT) is seen outside the fetal thorax. (**B**) First trimester diagnosis of ectopic cordis. (See also Color Plate 12.) (*A* and *B* courtesy of Patricia Mayberry, RT, RDMS, RVT; St. Luke's Roosevelt Hospital Center, New York, NY.)

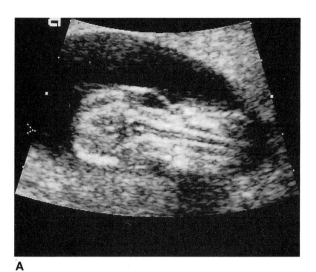
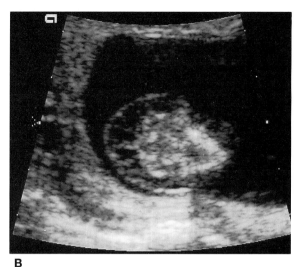

A   **B**

Figure 12-38. (**A**) *A sonolucent area is seen on the lateral aspect of the neck of an 11-week gestation.* (**B**) *An axial view demonstrates the septations characteristic of cystic hygroma. Although the fetus had a normal karyotype, the patient elected to terminate the pregnancy.*

odenal atresia,[62] hydrolethalus syndrome,[2] ocular defects,[14] and cardiac defects (Fig. 12-37).[1,24,38] Septated cystic hygromas have been identified (Fig. 12-38).[64] The bifid appearance of an embryo has led to the correct diagnosis of conjoined twins.[47]

Unfortunately, normal appearance in the first trimester does not necessarily ensure a normal fetus by the second trimester. In one example, visualizing a normal amount of cortical tissue at 10 weeks' gestational age could not preclude abnormal structure and vascularization and resultant degeneration that gave rise to anencephaly, as seen at 16 weeks.[36] It is therefore unwise either to confirm or exclude a diagnosis prematurely.

Conclusion

The clinical value of ultrasound in the first trimester is growing rapidly. It has gained wider acceptance in the areas of predicting viability, ruling out abnormally developing pregnancies, and identifying chromosomally and structurally abnormal embryos. Competent ultrasound practitioners must therefore have detailed knowledge of developmental processes and be aware of the most current sonographic research to play a role in the management of early pregnancy.

REFERENCES

1. Achiron R, Rotstein Z, Lipitz S, et al. First-trimester diagnosis of fetal congenital heart disease by transvaginal ultrasonography. Obstet Gynecol. 1994; 84:69–72.

2. Ammala P, Salonen R. First trimester diagnosis of hydrolethalus syndrome. Ultrasound in Obstetrics and Gynecology. 1995; 5:60–62.

3. Ball RH, Ade CM, Schoenborn JA, et al. The clinical significance of ultrasonigraphically detected subchorionic hemorrhages. Am J Obstet Gynecol. 1996; 174:996–1002.

4. Benacerraf BR. Intrauterine growth retardation in the first trimester associated with triploidy. J Ultrasound Med. 1988; 17:153–154.

5. Bernashek G, Rudelstrofer R, Csaicsich P. Vaginal sonography versus serum human chorionic gonadotropin in early detection of pregnancy. Am J Obstet Gynecol. 1988; 158:608–612.

6. Blass H-G, Eik-Ness SH, Kiserud T, et al. Early development of the hindbrain: A longitudinal ultrasound study from 7 to 12 weeks of gestation. Ultrasound in Obstetrics and Gynecology. 1995; 5: 151–160.

7. Blumenfeld Z, Rottem S, Elgali S, et al. Transvaginal sonographic assessment of early embryological development. In: Timor-Tritsch IE, Rottem S, eds. Transvaginal Sonography. New York: Elsevier Science Publishing; 1988.

8. Brambatti B, Cislaghi C, Tului L, et al. First-trimester Down's syndrome screening using nuchal

translucency: A prospective study in patients undergoing chorionic villus sampling. Ultrasound in Obstetrics and Gynecology. 1995; 5:9–14.

9. Bromley B, Benacerraf B. Using the number of yolk sacs to determine amnionicity in early first trimester monochorionic twins. J Ultrasound Med. 1995; 14:415–419.

10. Bromley B, Harlow BL, Laboda LA, et al. Small sac size in the first trimester: A predictor of poor fetal outcome. Radiology. 1991; 178:375–377.

11. Bronshtein M, Blumenfeld Z. Transvaginal sonography: Detection of findings suggestive of fetal chromosomal anomalies in the first and early second trimesters. Prenat Diagn. 1992; 12:587–593.

12. Bronshtein M, Kushnir O, Ben-Rafael A, et al. Transvaginal sonographic measurement of fetal kidneys in the first trimester of pregnancy. J Clin Ultrasound. 1990; 18:299–301.

13. Bronshtein M, Rottem S, Yoffe N, et al. First-trimester and early second-trimester diagnosis of nuchal cystic hygroma by transvaginal sonography: Diverse prognosis of the septated from the nonseptated lesion. Am J Obstet Gynecol. 1989; 161:78–82.

14. Bronshtein M, Zimmer E, Gershoni-Baruch R, et al. First- and second-trimester diagnosis of fetal ocular defects and associated anomalies: Report of eight cases. Obstet Gynecol. 1991; 77:443–449.

15. Cacciatore B, Tiitnen A, Stenman U-H, et al. Normal early pregnancy: Serum hCG levels and vaginal ultrasonography findings. Br J Obstet Gynaecol. 1990; 97:899–903.

16. Cashner KA, Christopher CR, Dysert GA. Spontaneous fetal loss after demonstration of a live fetus in the first trimester. Obstet Gynecol. 1987; 70:827–830.

17. Chervenak FA, Isaacson G, Blakemore KJ, et al. Fetal cystic hygroma: Cause and natural history. N Engl J Med. 1983; 309:822–825.

18. Comas C, Martinez JM, Ojuel J, et al. First-trimester nuchal edema as a marker of aneuploidy. Ultrasound in Obstetrics and Gynecology. 1995; 5:26–29.

19. Cullen MT, Gabrielli S, Green JJ, et al. Diagnosis and significance of cystic hygroma in the first trimester. Prenat Diagn. 1990; 10:643–651.

20. Curtis JA, Watson L. Sonographic diagnosis of omphalocele in the first trimester of fetal gestation. J Ultrasound Med. 1988; 7:97–100.

21. Cyr DR, Mack LA, Schoenecker SA, et al. Bowel migration in the normal fetus: US detection. Radiology. 1986; 161:119–121.

22. Daya S. Accuracy of gestational age estimation by means of fetal crown–rump length measurement. Am J Obstet Gynecol. 1993; 168:903–908.

23. Dickey RP, Olar TT, Curole DN, et al. Relationship of first-trimester subchorionic bleeding detected by color Doppler ultrasound to subchorionic fluid, clinical bleeding, and pregnancy outcome. Obstet Gynecol. 1992; 80:415–420.

24. Dolkart LA, Rimers FT. Transvaginal fetal echocardiography in early pregnancy: Normative data. Am J Obstet Gynecol. 1991; 165:688–691.

25. Donald I. Sonar as a method of studying prenatal development. J Pediatr. 1969; 75:326.

26. Doubilet, PM, Benson CB. Embryonic heart rate in the early first trimester: What rate is normal? J Ultrasound Med. 1995; 14:431–434.

27. Fantel AG, Shepard TH. Basic aspects of early (first trimester) abortion. In: Iffy L, Kaminetzky HA, eds. Principles and Practices of Obstetrics and Perinatology. New York: John Wiley & Sons; 1981;1.

28. Finberg HJ, Birnholz JC. Ultrasound observation in multiple gestation with first-trimester bleeding: The blighted twin. Radiology. 1979; 132:137–142.

29. Giacomello F. Small sac size as a predictor of poor fetal outcome. Radiology. 1992; 184:578.

30. Goldstein SR. Early detection of pathologic pregnancy by transvaginal sonography. J Clin Ultrasound. 1990; 18:262–273.

31. Goldstein SR. Embryonic death in early pregnancy: A new look at the first trimester. Obstet Gynecol. 1994; 84:294–297.

32. Goldstein SR. Endovaginal Ultrasound. 2nd ed. New York: Alan R. Liss; 1991.

33. Goldstein SR, Subramanyam BR, Raghavenda BN, Nori SC, Hilton S. Subchorionic bleeding in threatened abortion: Sonographic findings and significance. Am J Roentgenol. 1983; 141:975–978.

34. Goldstein SR, Snyder JR, Watson C, et al. Very early pregnancy detection with endovaginal ultrasound. Obstet Gynecol. 1988; 72:200–204.

35. Green JJ, Hobbins JC. Abdominal ultrasound examination of the first trimester fetus. Am J Obstet Gynecol. 1988; 159:165–175.

36. Hill LM, Thomas ML, Kislak S, et al. Sonographic assessment of the first trimester fetus: A cautionary note. Am J Perinatol. 1988; 5:13–15.

37. Hobbins JC, Jones OW, Gottesfeld S, et al. Transvaginal ultrasonography and transabdominal embryoscopy in the first-trimester diagnosis of Smith-Lemli-Opitz syndrome, type II. Am J Obstet Gynecol. 1994; 171:546–549.

38. Hyett JA, Moscoso G, Nicolaides KH. First-trimester nuchal translucency and cardiac septal defects in fetuses with trisomy 21. Am J Obstet Gynecol. 1995; 172:1411–1413.

39. Jackson S, Porter H, Vyas S. Trisomy 18: First-trimester nuchal translucency with pathologic correlation. Ultrasound in Obstetrics and Gynecology. 1995; 5:55–56.

40. Johnson MP, Johnson A, Holgreve W, et al. First-

trimester simple hygroma: Cause and outcome. Am J Obstet Gynecol. 1993; 168:156–161.

41. Jurkovic D, Janiaux E, Campbell S, et al. Coelocentesis: A new technique for early prenatal diagnosis. Lancet. 1993; 341:1623–1624.

42. Kadar N, DeVore G, Romero R. Discriminatory HCG zone: Its use in the sonographic evaluation for ectopic pregnancy. Obstet Gynecol. 1981; 58:156–161.

43. Kurtz AB, Needleman L, Pennell RG, et al. Can detection of the yolk sac in the first trimester be used to predict the outcome of pregnancy? Am J Roentgenol. 1992; 158:843–847.

44. Levi CS, Lyons EA, Lindsay DJ. Early diagnosis of nonviable pregnancy with endovaginal US. Radiology. 1988; 167:383–385.

45. Levi CS, Lyons EA, Zheng XH, et al. Endovaginal US: Demonstration of cardiac activity in embryos of less than 5.0 mm in crown–rump length. Radiology 1990; 176:71–74.

46. Lindsay DJ, Lovett IS, Lyons EA, et al. Yolk sac diameter and shape at endovaginal US: Predictors of pregnancy outcome in the first trimester. Radiology. 1992; 183:115–118.

47. Maggio M, Callen NA, Hamod KA, et al. The first-trimester ultrasonographic diagnosis of conjoined twins. Am J Obstet Gynecol. 1985; 152:833–835.

48. McKenna KM, Feldstein VA, Goldstein RB, et al. The "empty amnion": A sign of early pregnancy failure. J Ultrasound Med. 1995; 14:117–121.

49. Montenegro N, Beiores J, Pereira L. Reverse end-diastolic umbilical artery blood flow at 11 weeks' gestation. Ultrasound in Obstetrics and Gynecology. 1995; 5:141–142.

50. Moore KL, Persaud TVN. The Developing Human. 5th ed. Philadelphia: WB Saunders, 1993:14–52, 473.

51. Nadal A, Bromley B, Benacerraf BR. Nuchal thickening or cystic hygromas in first- and early second-trimester fetuses: Prognosis and outcome. Obstet Gynecol. 1993; 82:43–48.

52. Nicolaides KH, Azar G, Byrne D, et al. Fetal nuchal translucency: Ultrasound screening for chromosomal defects in the first trimester of pregnancy. Br Med J. 1992; 304:867–869.

53. Nyberg DA, Filly RA, Filho DL, et al. Abnormal pregnancy: Early diagnosis by US and serum chorionic gonadotropin. Radiology. 1986; 158:393–396.

54. Nyberg DA, Filly RA, Mahony BS, et al. Early gestation: Correlation of hCG levels and sonographic identification. Am J Roentgenol. 1985; 144:451–454.

55. Nyberg DA, Laing FC, Filly RA, et al. Ultrasonographic differentiation of the gestational sac of early intrauterine pregnancy from the pseudogestational sac of ectopic pregnancy. Radiology. 1983; 146:755–759.

56. Nyberg DA, Laing FC, Filly RA. Threatened abortion: Sonographic distinction of normal and abnormal gestation sacs. Radiology. 1986; 158:397–400.

57. Nyberg DA, Mack LA, Harvey D, et al. Value of the yolk sac in evaluation early pregnancies. J Ultrasound Med. 1988; 7:129–135.

58. Pandya PP, Brizot ML, Kuhn P, et al. First-trimester fetal nuchal translucency thickness and risk for trisomies. Obstet Gynecol. 1994; 84:420–423.

59. Pandya PP, Goldberg H, Walton B, et al. The implementation of first-trimester scanning at 10–13 weeks' gestation and the measurement of fetal nuchal translucency thickness in two maternity units. Ultrasound in Obstetrics and Gynecology. 1995; 5:20–25.

60. Pandya PP, Kondylios A, Hilbert L, et al. Chromosomal defects and outcome in 1015 fetuses with increased nuchal translucency. Ultrasound in Obstetrics and Gynecology. 1995; 5:15–19.

61. Peisner DB, Timor-Tritsch IE. The discriminatory zone of β-hCG for vaginal probes. 1990. J Clin Ultrasound. 1990; 18:280–285.

62. Petrikovsky BM. First-trimester diagnosis of duodenal atresia. Am J Obstet Gynecol. 1994; 171:569–570.

63. Reese KA, Scioscia AL, Pinter E, et al. Prognostic significance of the human yolk sac assessed by ultrasonography. Am J Obstet Gynecol. 1988; 159:1191–1194.

64. Reuss A, Pipers L, van Swaaij E, et al. First-trimester diagnosis of recurrence of cystic hygroma using a vaginal ultrasound transducer. Eur J Obstet Gynecol Reprod Biol. 1987; 26:271–273.

65. Rottem S, Bronshtein M. Transvaginal sonographic diagnosis of congenital anomalies between 9 weeks and 16 weeks' menstrual age. J Clin Ultrasound. 1990; 18:307–314.

66. Sanders RC, James AE. The Principles and Practice of Ultrasonography in Obstetrics and Gynecology. 3rd ed. Norwalk, CT: Appleton-Century-Crofts; 1985.

67. Schats R, Jansen CAM, Wladimiroff JW. Embryonic heart activity: Appearance and development in early human pregnancy. Br J Obstet Gynaecol. 1990; 97:989–994.

68. Schmidt W, Yarkoni S, Crelin ES, et al. Sonographic visualization of physiologic anterior abdominal wall hernia in the first trimester. Obstet Gynecol. 1987; 69:911–915.

69. Shulman LP, Emerson DS, Felker RE, et al. High frequency of cytogenetic abnormalities in fetuses with cystic hygroma diagnosed in the first trimester. Obstet Gynecol. 1992; 80:80–82.

70. Siddiqi TA, Caligaris JT, Miodovnik M, et al. Rate of spontaneous abortion after first-trimester sonographic demonstration of fetal cardiac activity. Am J Perinatol. 1988; 5:1–4.

71. Szabo J, Gellen J. Nuchal fluid accumulation in trisomy-21 detected by vaginosonography. Lancet. 1990; 2:1133.

72. Szabo J, Gellen J, Szemere G. First-trimester ultrasound screening for fetal aneuploidies in women over 35 and under 35 years of age. Ultrasound in Obstetrics and Gynecology. 1995; 5:161–163.

73. Timor-Tritsch IE, Farine D, Rosen MG. A close look at early embryonic development with the high-frequency transvaginal transducer. Am J Obstet Gynecol. 1988; 159:676–681.

74. Timor-Tritsch IE, Peisner DB, Raju S. Sonoembryology: An organ-oriented approach using a high-frequency vaginal probe. J Clin Ultrasound. 1990; 18:286–298.

75. U.S. Department of Health and Human Services, Public Health Service, National Institutes of Health. Diagnostic Ultrasound Imaging in Pregnancy. NIH Publication no. 84-667. Washington, DC: U.S. Government Printing Office; 1984.

76. van Leeuwen I, Branch DW, Scott JR. First-trimester ultrasonography findings in women with a history of recurrent pregnancy loss. Am J Obstet Gynecol. 1993; 168:111–114.

77. Walderstrom U, Exelsson O, Nilsson S, et al. Effects of routine one-stage ultrasound screening in pregnancy: A randomized controlled trial. Lancet. 1988; 2:585–588.

78. Wilson RD, Kendrick V, Wittman BK, et al. Spontaneous abortion and pregnancy outcome after normal first-trimester ultrasound examination. Obstet Gynecol. 1986; 67:352.

79. Wilson RD, Venir N, Farquharson DF. Fetal nuchal fluid—physiological or pathological?—in pregnancies less than 17 menstrual weeks. Prenat Diagn. 1992; 12:755–763.

80. Wilson RL, Worthen NJ. Ultrasonic demonstration of myometrial contractions in intrauterine pregnancy. Am J Roentgenol. 1979; 132:243–247.

81. Yeh H, Rabinowitz J. Amniotic sac development: Ultrasound features of early pregnancy—the double bleb sign. Radiology. 1988; 166:97–103.

13

Sonographic Overview of Pregnancy

CAROL B. BENSON and PETER M. DOUBILET

First Trimester

Sonographic examination during the first trimester can be performed transabdominally, through a full bladder, or transvaginally. In the early part of the first trimester, transvaginal scanning, which offers higher resolution, is usually preferable to transabdominal scanning.[6] The vaginal transducer can be placed closer to the uterine cavity, so that transducers of higher frequency and resolution can be used. Furthermore, vaginal scanning does not require a full urinary bladder, saving the patient the time of filling and the discomfort of a distended bladder. In the latter part of the first trimester the advantages of transvaginal scanning become smaller. By this time the pregnant uterus has grown out of the pelvis, so that a full bladder is not needed and the structures to be imaged are larger.

Whichever method is selected, the entire uterus should always be imaged in two planes, with special attention given to the contents of the uterine cavity. Longitudinal and transverse images of the uterus and the gestational sac should be obtained, and measurements of the fetus as well as images of fetal anatomy should be included once the fetus is visible.

Both ovaries should be imaged. A simple ovarian cyst, the corpus luteum, is often seen in early pregnancy sonograms and is a normal finding. In some cases, it may become grossly enlarged (to as much as 10 cm) and may cause symptoms.[2] Com-plex or solid masses should be followed closely and may, in some cases, require surgery.

Approximately 5 to 6 days after fertilization (3 weeks' gestational or menstrual age), the developing embryo and gestational sac implant in the uterine cavity. The first sonographic evidence of an intrauterine pregnancy is the presence of a small anechoic collection within the uterus surrounded by two echogenic rings, termed the "double sac sign" (Fig. 13-1).[3] This finding is usually visible transvaginally at 5 weeks' gestational age. Within

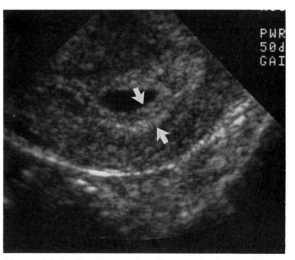

Figure 13-1. Double-sac sign. Transvaginal scan of intra-uterine gestation sac with fluid collection surrounded by two mildly echogenic rings (arrows).

233

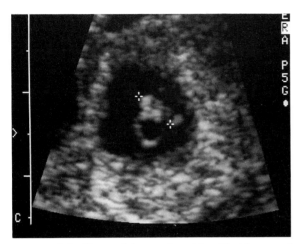

Figure 13-2. Six weeks' gestation. Magnified image of gestational sac with fetal pole (calipers) adjacent to yolk sac.

the developing gestational sac the yolk sac becomes visible at approximately 5.5 weeks' gestational age on transvaginal scan. Shortly thereafter (by 6.0 weeks with transvaginal scanning), a small fetal pole containing a beating fetal heart can be seen adjacent to or near the yolk sac (Fig. 13-2). With transabdominal scanning, each of these sonographic landmarks is visible approximately one-half week later than with transvaginal scanning. In particular, a visible fetal heartbeat should be seen transabdominally by 6.5 weeks' gestation.[1]

The gestational sac has two membranes: the

chorion, which encloses the entire gestational sac, and the amnion, which lies within it. The fetal pole develops within the amniotic cavity, whereas the yolk sac is located in the fluid space between the chorion and the amnion (Fig. 13-3). A distinct amniotic membrane can be seen sonographically as early as 7 weeks and remains visible until 13 to 15 weeks' gestation (Fig. 13-4), by which time the amnion has fused with the chorion. The chorion is visible only when there is fluid between the uterine wall and the chorion, as can occur with a subchorionic hematoma. The amnion appears as a smooth, thin membrane, whereas the chorion is thicker and more irregular in outline.

The fetal pole grows rapidly, about 2 mm per day, during the first trimester.[12] As the fetus differentiates and enlarges, its developing limbs, spine, and head can be recognized sonographically by 9 to 10 weeks' gestation (Fig. 13-5). By the end of the first trimester, much of the fetal anatomy may be visible, including spine, intracranial contents, stomach, and bladder. Transvaginal scanning in the late first trimester permits visualization of many fetal anatomic structures not seen transabdominally until several weeks later in the second trimester.[9]

As the conceptus grows, the placenta forms from chorionic villi and proliferating endometrium. As early as 7 to 8 weeks' gestation, the developing placenta is visible sonographically as a thickened area of increased echogenicity along one side of the gestational sac. Placental development may occur

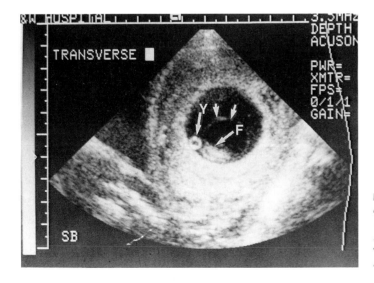

Figure 13-3. Eight weeks' gestation. Sonogram of gestational sac containing fetal pole (F, *arrow*) surrounded by the amnion (*arrowheads*). The yolk sac (Y, *arrow*) is located within the chorionic cavity, just outside the amniotic cavity.

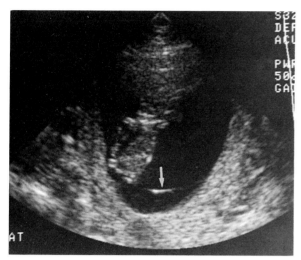

Figure 13-4. *The amniotic membrane (arrow) is visible within the gestational sac of this 12-week gestation.*

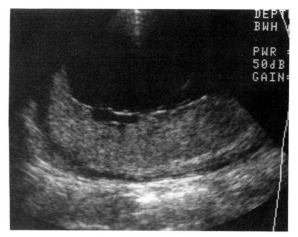

Figure 13-6. *Placenta. Sonogram of second trimester posterior placenta with characteristic homogeneous echo-pattern. The amniotic fluid in the cavity is anechoic.*

on any side of the gestational sac: anterior, posterior, fundal, or lateral. At first, placental limits are poorly defined, making it impossible to determine whether implantation is abnormally low, in which case there is potential for placenta previa. The placenta grows rapidly during the first trimester and in the early part of the second trimester to become a well defined, homogeneously textured crescentic mass on one surface of the gestational sac (Fig. 13-6). By the mid-second trimester (approximately 20 weeks), the now well defined margins of the

placenta permit a better assessment for placenta previa. The placenta continues to grow more slowly into the third trimester.[14]

The umbilical cord becomes visible during the latter half of the first trimester as a tortuous, echo-producing structure connecting the developing fetus to the placenta. The cord comprises three vessels, two small, spiraling umbilical arteries and a larger umbilical vein. The three components of the umbilical cord should be well visualized on ultrasound by 16 weeks' gestation (Fig. 13-7).

Second and Third Trimesters

During second and third trimesters the obstetric sonographic examination is usually performed transabdominally. The examination should include a full evaluation of the fetus, including assessment of fetal anatomy, size, position, and state, as well as examination of the uterus, placenta, and amniotic fluid. Although normal ovaries are often not visible in the second and third trimesters because the enlarging uterus obscures them, both adnexal areas should be scanned for residual corpus luteal cysts or disease. If the mother has flank pain or other symptoms or signs related to the kidneys, they should be included in the sonographic examination.

UTERUS: CERVIX AND LOWER SEGMENT

The cervix and lower uterine segment should be examined, looking for evidence of cervical incompetence or placenta previa. Evaluation of the lower segment and

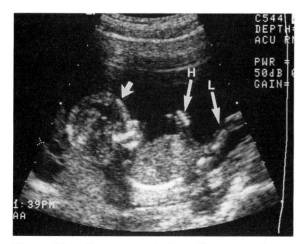

Figure 13-5. *Fourteen-week fetus. Sonogram demonstrating early fetal anatomy including the fetal head (arrowhead), hand (H, arrow), and leg (L, arrow).*

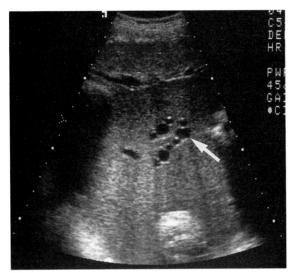

Figure 13-7. Three-vessel umbilical cord. Cross-sectional sonogram of umbilical cord (*arrow*) in echogenic amniotic fluid demonstrates a single umbilical vein with two smaller arteries.

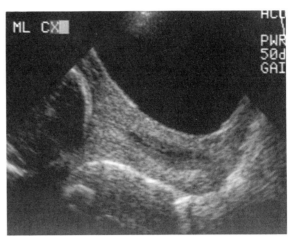

Figure 13-8. Normal cervix. Sagittal midline sonogram through a full maternal bladder demonstrates the long cervix with its hypoechoic cervical canal.

cervix is usually performed transabdominally through a partially full maternal bladder, but when the fetal head is low and obscures the cervix, transperineal or transvaginal scanning may be useful. Caution must be taken not to overfill the bladder because this may appose the anterior and posterior walls of the lower uterine segment, thereby creating the false appearance of placenta previa or causing a falsely long cervical measurement.

The cervix normally remains tightly closed until the time of delivery (Fig. 13-8). Dilatation of the cervix before term can lead to second trimester spontaneous abortion or premature delivery. If premature cervical dilatation, called cervical incompetence, is detected before the pregnancy is lost, a cerclage loop can be placed in the cervix to prevent further dilatation and permit the pregnancy to continue (Fig. 13-9). Several sonographic criteria have been proposed for early detection of cervical incompetence. Opening of the internal os or a cervical length less than 2.5 cm is suggestive of cervical incompetence.[5,7,10] Once a cerclage is in place, it is visible sonographically as several bright echoes within the muscle of the cervix (Fig. 13-10).

Marked dilatation of the cervix with bulging of membranes through the external os is a poor prognostic sign (Fig. 13-11). Special care should be taken to look at the contents of the fluid and

membranes protruding into the cervical canal. The presence of any part of the umbilical cord within the cervical canal is a serious threat to the fetus, an obstetric emergency requiring immediate intervention.[11]

THE UTERUS: BODY

The body of the uterus is made up predominantly of myometrium, a muscular layer. The uterine cavity is lined by an inner layer, the endometrium. During

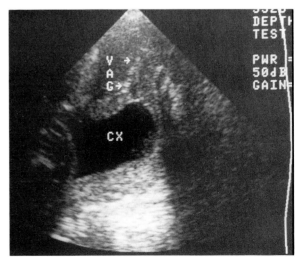

Figure 13-9. Dilated cervix. Transperineal scan demonstrating dilated cervix (CX) with bulging membranes toward the vagina (VAG, *arrows*).

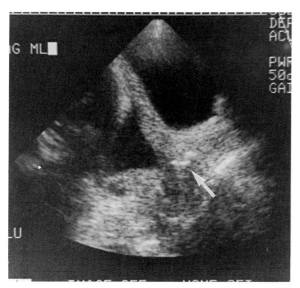

Figure 13-10. Incompetent cervix with cerclage. Longitudinal sonogram demonstrating dilated internal cervical os to level of cerclage (*arrow*), represented by bright echoes in distal cervix.

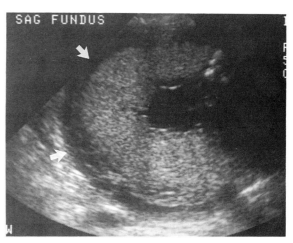

Figure 13-12. The myometrium appears as a thin, hypoechoic band (*arrows*) behind the placenta.

pregnancy, the smooth muscle of the myometrium stretches and hypertrophies rapidly. Myometrial vessels also proliferate and enlarge greatly.[11]

On sonographic examination, the myometrium appears as a band of tissue completely surrounding the gestational sac (Fig. 13-12) that is less echo-

genic than the placenta. The uterine vessels are most abundant along the lateral uterine wall and may alter the echogenic pattern of the myometrium as they enlarge (Fig. 13-13).

Myometrium thickness should be uniform around the gestational sac. Any evidence of thinning behind the placenta may indicate an abnormally adherent placenta, placenta accreta, increta, or percreta (Fig. 13-14).[8]

Throughout the pregnancy, focal areas of smooth muscle in the uterine wall contract, causing a bulging into the amniotic cavity. These con-

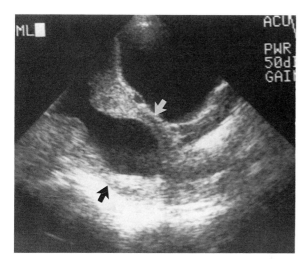

Figure 13-11. Dilated cervix with bulging membranes. Longitudinal sonogram of membranes containing amniotic fluid bulging through dilated cervix (*arrows*) to vagina.

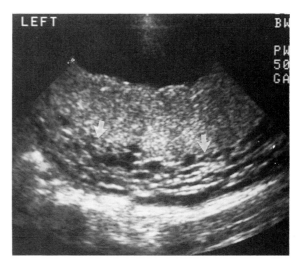

Figure 13-13. Many large uterine vessels (*arrows*) are visible along the lateral uterine wall behind the placenta.

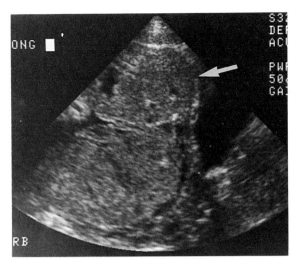

Figure 13-14. Placenta percreta. Sonogram of placenta and lower uterine segment demonstrating loss of the hypoechoic band of myometrium (*arrow*) normally seen beneath the placenta due to abnormal invasion of the placenta.

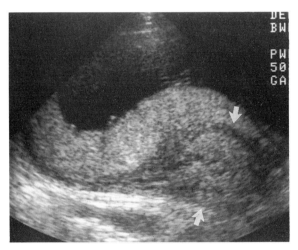

Figure 13-15. A focal contraction (*arrows*) is a homogeneous area of myometrium that bulges the placenta into the amniotic cavity.

tractions should not be confused with fibroids or altered placental patterns such as abruption or infarction. The muscle contractions appear homogeneous in echotexture and should disappear within 30 to 45 minutes (Fig. 13-15).[2]

Uterine leiomyomas, or fibroids, may be located in the wall of the uterus. They tend to be hypoechoic, round, and somewhat heterogeneous. They may distort the outer or inner contour of the uterus, but, unlike myometrial contractions, they do not change during the course of a sonographic examination (Fig. 13-16). Fibroids sometimes enlarge during pregnancy and may become symptomatic owing to degeneration or increased uterine irritability. Large fibroids positioned in the lower uterine segment may obstruct delivery.[2,13]

Occasionally a subchorionic hematoma produced by placental abruption may mimic a fibroid or uterine contraction. Within several days this subchorionic collection becomes cystic as the hematoma breaks down, and no longer confuses the diagnosis.[2]

AMNIOTIC FLUID

Amniotic fluid is normally anechoic (see Fig. 13-6) in the first and second trimesters. In the third trimester, it is normal to see floating echogenic particles within

the amniotic fluid, representing vernix, which is the result of sloughing of fetal skin.[4] If the vernix becomes highly concentrated, the amniotic fluid may become diffusely echogenic. Pathologic conditions, such as acute bleeding into the amniotic cavity or meconium staining, may also cause the amniotic fluid to appear echogenic. In the third trimester, it is impossible to differentiate these pathologic states sonographically from normally echogenic, vernix-filled amniotic fluid (Fig. 13-17).[4]

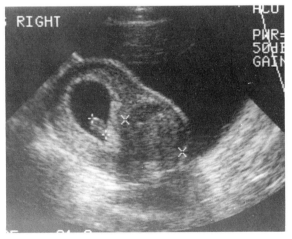

Figure 13-16. Fibroid. First trimester sonogram demonstrating heterogeneous round fibroid (× calipers) in anterior uterine wall adjacent to gestational sac containing small fetal pole (+ calipers).

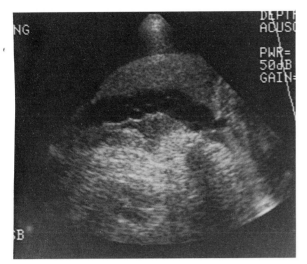

Figure 13-17. Echogenic amniotic fluid surrounds the anechoic umbilical cord.

Occasionally, a membranous structure may be seen floating in the amniotic cavity or extending across the cavity (Fig. 13-18). Membranes can be seen either with the amniotic band syndrome or as a result of a uterine synechia, a fibrous band or scar in the uterine cavity. In the former, the membranes adhere to the fetus and cause fetal malformations, often severe. In the latter, more common situation,

intact amnion and chorion are reflected over a synechia, producing a membrane that traverses part of the amniotic cavity. Such a membrane is characterized sonographically by a broad-based origin at the uterine wall and focal thickening of the membrane at its free edge, and by the fact that it does not adhere to the fetus.[15]

Altered amounts of amniotic fluid may be an indicator of abnormal fetal or maternal conditions. It is therefore important to include assessment of fluid volume as part of every sonographic examination. Experienced sonographers and sonologists find that subjective determination of the fluid volume is the best and most accurate method. This requires careful sonographic evaluation, comparing the observed amount of fluid with that expected at the current gestational age. Quantitative methods for volume assessment, which use measurements of pockets of amniotic fluid, have also proved accurate and would be the best approach for less experienced sonographers. The vertical depth of the best pocket of fluid is measured and correlated with gestational age, or the amniotic fluid index is calculated as the sum of the deepest pocket measurements from the four quadrants of the uterus.[4]

The volume of amniotic fluid increases to its maximum at 36 to 38 weeks, then decreases until delivery. The amniotic fluid volume surrounding

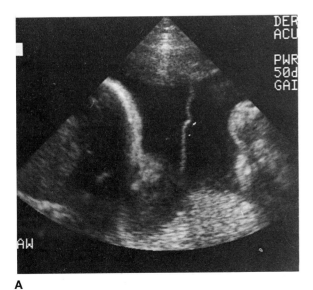

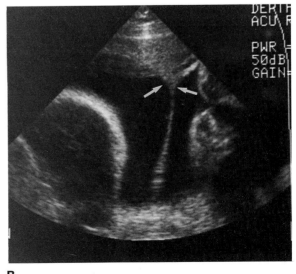

A   **B**

Figure 13-18. Amniotic sheet. (**A**) Sonogram demonstrating a membrane crossing a portion of the amniotic cavity. (**B**) The edge of the membrane at the uterine wall is broad based (*arrows*).

the fetus is maintained by a balance of several fetal and maternal factors. After 16 weeks' gestation, most of the fluid is produced by the fetal urinary system. Amniotic fluid is absorbed by fetal swallowing and gastrointestinal absorption. Abnormalities of either the genitourinary tract or the gastrointestinal tract, or of fetal swallowing can affect the amniotic fluid volume. Obstruction of the esophagus, duodenum, or proximal small bowel, or impairment of swallowing due to a central nervous system lesion or a thoracic mass, lead to polyhydramnios (Fig. 13-19). Diminished or absent urine output, which can result from bilateral renal agenesis, abnormal kidneys (e.g., autosomal recessive polycystic kidney disease), or urinary tract obstruction, leads to oligohydramnios. Other fetal factors that can alter the amniotic fluid volume include intrauterine growth retardation, which is associated with oligohydramnios, and fetal hydrops, which is often associated with polyhydramnios.[4]

Polyhydramnios is idiopathic in 60% of cases, and results from fetal structural anomalies in 20%. In the remaining 20% of cases, it is caused by maternal factors, the most common being maternal diabetes.

Oligohydramnios is rarely unexplained. The most common cause is premature rupture of membranes. Intrauterine growth retardation and fetal genitourinary anomalies account for most cases of oligohydramnios with intact membrane.[4]

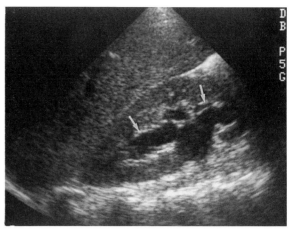

Figure 13-20. Moderate hydronephrosis of maternal right kidney (*arrows*) during pregnancy.

MATERNAL KIDNEYS

During pregnancy some degree of hydronephrosis of both kidneys is quite common, especially after the beginning of the second trimester, by which time the uterus has grown out of the pelvis and compresses the ureters (Fig. 13-20). In over 80% of cases the right renal collecting system is more dilated than the left. The dilated ureter can often be followed behind the uterus to the level of the pelvic brim.[11]

REFERENCES

1. Benson CB, Doubilet PM. Fetal measurements, normal and abnormal fetal growth. In: Rumack C, Charbonneau W, Wilson S, eds. Diagnostic Ultrasound. St. Louis: Yearbook Medical Publishers; 1990:723–738.
2. Benson CB, Jones TB, Lavery MJ, et al. Atlas of Obstetrical Ultrasound. Philadelphia: JB Lippincott; 1988.
3. Bradley WG, Fiske CE, Filly RA. The double-sac sign in early intrauterine pregnancy: Use in exclusion of ectopic pregnancy. Radiology. 1982; 148:223–226.
4. Doubilet PM, Benson CB. Amniotic fluid. In: Callen PW, ed. Ultrasonography in Obstetrics and Gynecology. 3rd ed. Philadelphia: WB Saunders; 1994:475–486.
5. Feingold M, Brook I, Zakut H. Detection of cervical incompetence by ultrasound. Acta Obstet Gynaecol Scand. 1984; 63:407–410.

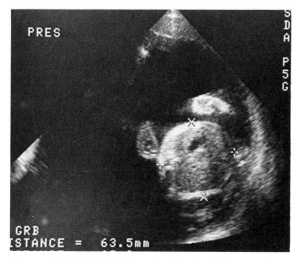

Figure 13-19. Polyhydramnios. Markedly increased amniotic fluid surrounds this fetal abdomen (calipers).

6. Fleischer AC, Kepple DM. Transvaginal sonography of early intrauterine pregnancy. In: Fleischer AC, Manning FA, Jeanty P, Romero R, eds. Sonography in Obstetrics and Gynecology: Principles and Practice. Stamford, CT: Appleton & Lange; 1996:53–81.

7. Hertzberg BS, Kliewer MA, Farrell TA, DeLong DM. Spontaneously changing gravid cervix: Clinical implications and prognostic features. Radiology. 1995; 196:721–724.

8. Litwin MS, Loughlin KR, Benson CB, et al. Placenta percreta invading the urinary bladder: Report of three cases and review of the literature. Br J Urol. 1989; 64:283–286.

9. Neiman HL. Transvaginal ultrasound embryography. Semin Ultrasound CT MR. 1990; 11:22–33.

10. Podobrik M, Bulic M, Smiljanic N, et al. Ultrasonography in detection of cervical incompetency. J Clin Ultrasound. 1988; 13:383–391.

11. Prichard JA, MacDonald PC, Gant NF. Williams' Obstetrics. 17th ed. Norwalk, CT: Appleton-Century-Crofts; 1985.

12. Robinson HP, Fleming JEE. A critical evaluation of sonar "crown–rump length" measurements. Br J Obstet Gynaecol. 1975; 82:702–710.

13. Rosati P, Exacoustos C, Mancuso S. Longitudinal evaluation of uterine myoma growth during pregnancy: A sonographic study. J Ultrasound Med. 1992; 11:511–515.

14. Spirt BA, Gordon LP. The placenta as an indicator of fetal maturity: Fact and fancy. Semin Ultrasound CT MR. 1984; 5:290–297.

15. Stamm E, Waldstein G, Thickman D, McGregor J. Amniotic sheets: Natural history and histology. J Ultrasound Med. 1991; 10:501–504.

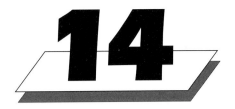

Sonographic Assessment of the Fetal Head, Neck, and Spine

JANE STRELTZOFF, EDITH D. GUREWITSCH, and FRANK A. CHERVENAK

A systematic approach to sonographic examination of the complex region of the head, neck, and spine is necessary to reveal the numerous possible abnormalities, which are among the most commonly diagnosed fetal malformations.

Because the membranous bones of the fetal cranium do not reflect sound waves to the extent that they do when they are more heavily calcified postnatally, real-time ultrasonography allows imaging of fetal intracranial contents in innumerable planes. Historically, serial axial scans had been preferred for antenatal ultrasound over the coronal and sagittal ones used by neonatal ultrasonographers and pathologists. This was a perceived limitation of the transabdominal approach because the fetal head is most often in an occiput-transverse position (i.e., the side of the head lies parallel to the mother's abdominal wall) and coronal and sagittal views were often technically difficult to image because of such factors as maternal obesity, abdominal wall scarring, or low-lying fetal head. Over the last several years, improvements in ultrasound technique and equipment, including use of high-frequency transvaginal probes, has made these coronal and sagittal planes accessible in the second and third trimesters through the acoustic window of the anterior fontanel.

In this chapter, we first outline a comprehensive method of examining the neural axis, pausing at various points to describe in detail what can be observed and the methods of approach that can be used. In the second part of this review, the various abnormalities of the fetal head, neck, and spine are discussed.

Anatomic Landmarks and Biometry

AXIAL VIEWS OF THE HEAD

The Biparietal Diameter Level

Perhaps the most intensely studied axial section of the fetal calvarium is at the level of the biparietal diameter (BPD). Several intracranial landmarks are located to define a plane approximately 15 degrees above the canthomeatal line and parallel to the base of the skull (Fig. 14-1). The two landmarks found most consistently are the paired hypoechoic thalami, which appear somewhat oval, and the cavum septi pellucidi, which is outlined by two short anterior lines parallel to the midline, thought to represent nearby white matter. Other structures commonly observed in the same plane and near the midline are, from posterior to anterior, the great cerebral vein, or vein of Galen, and its ambient cistern sitting above the cerebellum,[74] the mid-

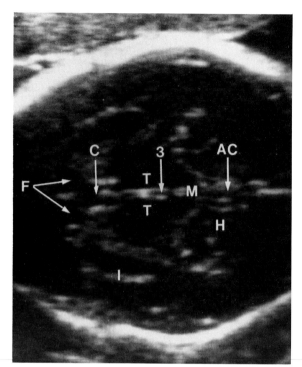

Figure 14-1. *Transverse scan of the fetal head at the level of the biparietal diameter demonstrating the frontal horns of the lateral ventricles (F), the cavum septi pellucidi (C), the thalamus (T), the third ventricle (3), the hippocampus (H), the insula (I), the midbrain (M), the great cerebral vein, and the ambient cistern (AC). (From Chervenak FA, Isaacson F, Lorber J. Anomalies of the Fetal Head, Neck, and Spine: Ultrasound Diagnosis and Management. Philadelphia: WB Saunders; 1988.)*

brain, the third ventricle between the thalami, and the frontal horns of the lateral ventricles. Laterally placed in the same plane are the spiral hippocampal gyri[63] posteriorly and the bright paired echoes of the insulae with pulsating middle cerebral arteries.

BIOMETRY. The BPD can be reproducibly measured in this plane as the distance from the proximal outer table to the distal inner table of the skull.[45,80] In addition, the head perimeter can be determined by direct measurement or calculated by adding the BPD and occipitofrontal diameter, measured from the midpoint of frontal and occipital echo complexes, and multiplying by 1.62.[56] The ratio of BPD to occipitofrontal diameter defines the cephalic index (normal range, 75 to 85). A higher value suggests brachycephaly and a lower value, dolicho-

cephaly. When these often normal variants of head shape are noted, BPD is considered inaccurate in determining gestational age, and head circumference is used instead.

MICROCEPHALY. "Microcephaly" means "small head." Its diagnosis, therefore, is based on biometry rather than on morphology. Consequently, without accurate menstrual history, microcephaly can be a difficult diagnosis to make. In general, a small head is the product of an underdeveloped brain, whether as a primary defect or as part of a more extensive malformation syndrome. The BPD (the biometric parameter most commonly measured by sonography) is unreliable in the prediction of microcephaly, yielding a 44% false-positive rate in one study.[25] Compression of the fetal head in normal pregnancies, with resultant dolichocephaly, accounts for many of these errors. A nomogram of head circumference as a function of gestational age, which corrects for such compressive changes, has proved to have greater predictive value. Although different biometric standards have been described to define microcephaly, a head perimeter three standard deviations or more below the mean for gestational age is considered a reliable indicator, and the correlation with mental retardation is very high.[85] Further aids to diagnosis include nomograms of ratios of head circumference to abdominal perimeter and of femur length to head circumference. Multiple fetal measurements should be used for greater accuracy.[25,26]

The prognosis for microcephaly varies, but most affected children are mentally retarded. In general, the smaller the head, the worse the prognosis. As with other malformations, the association with other anomalies increases the likelihood of a poor outcome. Risk of recurrence depends on underlying causes.

MACROCEPHALY. Macrocephaly is defined as a head circumference two to three standard deviations above the mean for gestational age and sex. Most often, macrocephaly is associated with an enlarged ventricular system (hydrocephalus) or other intracranial anomalies. A rare condition, megalocephaly, is an increase in brain mass in the absence of hydrocephalus. Most of these fetuses are normal. Even more rare is the association of megalocephaly with pathologic states, such as lipid storage diseases.

In such diseases, the person is usually severely retarded.[87]

The Internal Carotid Artery Level

Another important area for evaluation located at a plane parallel but inferior to the BPD is the level of the internal carotid artery. From the BPD, if the transducer is moved in a parallel fashion toward the base of the skull until the cerebral peduncles, the most rostral portions of the midbrain, are visualized, an oblique cross-section of the internal carotid artery can be obtained as it divides into the middle and anterior cerebral arteries anterior to the cerebral peduncles.

Doppler sampling of the fetal internal carotid artery, using 3.5- to 5.0-MHz transducers and a sample volume size not greater than 4 mm, displays a typical low-resistance pattern. The sonographer is cautioned that the pulsatility index of the internal carotid artery is affected by fetal activity and breathing movements. For accurate clinical study, Doppler sampling should be performed only when the fetus is inactive and apneic.[84] Doppler evaluation of the cerebral circulation is a useful adjunct in the evaluation of the growth-restricted fetus, particularly when the pulsatility index of the internal carotid artery is compared to that of the umbilical artery. High-resistance umbilical artery blood flow appears to precede a compensatory, or brain-sparing, cerebral vasodilatation seen in intrauterine growth restriction caused by placental insufficiency. The presence of a normal pulsatility index in the carotid artery with a high-resistance umbilical artery waveform suggests maintenance of normal cerebral circulation. As fetal hypoxia worsens, a decrease in the pulsatility index of the internal carotid artery is found.[88,89]

The Cerebellar Level

The cerebellum may also be visualized in a plane parallel and inferior to the BPD plane (Fig. 14-2). Once located, the cerebellar structures are best studied by rotating the ultrasound transducer inferior to the plane of the BPD. In this plane, the cerebellum, with its brightly echogenic, centrally placed vermis and two relatively nonechogenic hemispheres resembling a peanut, may be evaluated and measured. The midbrain may be seen in front of the vermis. The cisterna magna is seen and can

be measured anteroposteriorly in the midline between the vermis and the inner table of the occipital bone.[82] A normal measurement should not exceed 10 mm.

BIOMETRY. Between 16 and 24 weeks of gestation, the transcerebellar diameter measured in millimeters correlates 1:1 with the gestational age. Even in cases of suspected intrauterine growth retardation, the relationship of this diameter to gestational age holds steady and can be relied on for dating. Measurement of skin thickness behind the occipital bone, termed nuchal fold, can also be obtained in this view (Fig. 14-2). It is measured in the midline, from the outer table of the occiput to the outer portion of the skin. To maintain consistency in measurement of the nuchal skinfold, we advocate that care be taken to ensure that the cavum septi pellucidi appears in the same view as the cerebellum when nuchal skinfold thickness is measured. If the measurement is greater than 5 mm, the sonographer should check whether the neck is extended because that might increase the nuchal fold thickness. A nuchal skinfold thickness of 6 mm or greater

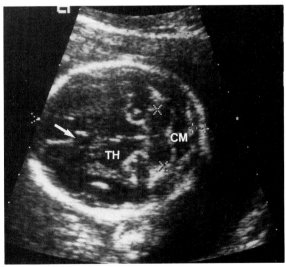

Figure 14-2. *Transverse scan through the fetal head at the level of the biparietal diameter but angled posteriorly and inferiorly to demonstrate the cerebellum, the cisterna magnum (CM), the thalamus (TH), and the cavum septi pellucidi (arrow). Measurements of the transcerebellar diameter (caliper x's) and the nuchal skinfold (caliper pluses) are demonstrated.*

has been reported to be associated with Down's syndrome.[8]

The Lateral Ventricle Level

Using the transabdominal approach, the lateral ventricles can be readily identified by 16 weeks' gestation as paired anechoic areas within the brain substance. The far-field ventricle, the one farthest from the ultrasound transducer, is more readily studied because reverberation artifacts often obscure the anatomy of the near-field hemisphere. The lateral wall of the ventricle may be visualized consistently as the first echogenic line on the distal edge of the echo-spared ventricle. The medial wall of the ventricle is visualized less consistently. A prominent echogenic area is often seen within the lateral ventricle, which represents the choroid plexus, a highly vascular epithelial proliferation arising within the ependyma of the ventricle that produces and resorbs cerebrospinal fluid.

In early fetal life, the ventricular system fills a large portion of the developing brain and has the form of two smooth, curved tubes joined above the third ventricle. As gestation progresses, the shape of the ventricular system increasingly resembles that found in the normal adult brain, and it occupies a decreasing proportion of the brain's volume. This evolution has been documented sonographically by several authors who have generated nomograms comparing the width of the lateral ventricle to the width of the cerebral hemisphere at various gestational ages.[54,58,75]

BIOMETRY. In the past, assessment of ventricle size was made by determining the ratio of lateral ventricular width to that of the cranial hemisphere. The lateral ventricular width would be measured from the midline echo to the echo of the lateral wall of the lateral ventricle at the point where the ventricular wall runs parallel to the midline. In the same image, the hemispheric width was measured as the longest distance between the midline and the inner edge of the skull perpendicular to the midline (Fig. 14-3). These values were then expressed as a ratio and compared to a nomogram. However, because the normal lateral ventricular-to-hemispheric ratio varies with gestational age, this technique was limited in that it required accurate menstrual dating. A more significant limitation of this method was

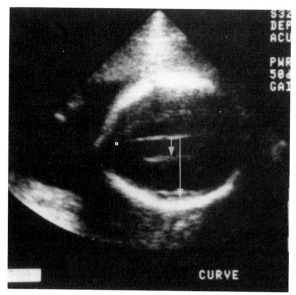

Figure 14-3. Transverse scan of the fetal head at the level of the lateral ventricle demonstrating the measurement of the lateral ventricular-to-hemispheric ratio.

the discovery that the echogenic landmark once thought to represent the lateral wall of the lateral ventricle represented a tract within the normal brain substance.[12,47]

In 1988, Cardoza and colleagues introduced the measurement of the lateral ventricle's width at its atrium, which is located at an axial plane angled just superiorly to the BPD.[16] Because atrial width does not change during pregnancy, this technique obviates the need for accurate menstrual dating. It also is the earliest site of ventricular dilatation in developing hydrocephalus. The atrium can be readily seen at the level of the BPD; however, its widest measurement is usually obtained in a view that demonstrates the continuity of the atrium of the lateral ventricle with its occipital horn. The widest diameter of the atrium is measured through the choroid plexus (Fig. 14-4). A normal measurement should not exceed 10 mm,[16] which is said to be at two to three standard deviations from the norm. Some authors now say that the upper limits of normal may be as great as 12.3 mm, which has led some to use 10 to 12.3 mm as a "gray zone." Mahony and coworkers have determined that the distance between the medial wall of the lateral ventricle and the medial margin of the choroid plexus

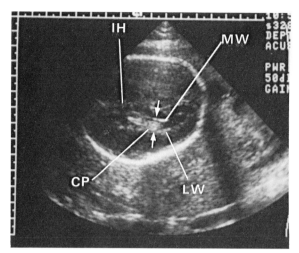

Figure 14-4. *Transverse scan of the fetal head demonstrating the lateral ventricle's atrium in continuity with the occipital horn. This is usually the view in which the widest diameter of the atrium can be measured (arrows) through the choroid plexus (CP). The medial wall (MW), lateral wall (LW), and interhemispheric fissure (IH) can be seen.*

should be less than 5 mm at the level of the atrium.[65]

The Base of the Skull Level

The base of the skull level may be identified by an echogenic "X" formed by the lesser wings of the sphenoid bone and the petrous pyramid. These bony ridges demarcate the anterior, middle, and posterior fossae (Fig. 14-5).

CORONAL AND SAGITTAL VIEWS OF THE HEAD

Coronal and sagittal views of the fetal intracranial anatomy are most often obtained transabdominally; however, these studies may be limited by maternal or fetal factors previously described. In recent years, proponents of transvaginal sonography have been able to obtain intracranial images in coronal and sagittal planes similar to those used for years in the evaluation of neonates. In a technique described by Monteagudo and colleagues, a 5.0- to 6.5-MHz transvaginal probe is advanced slowly into the vagina until the fetal head is imaged. The probe is then maneuvered to align its tip with the anterior fontanel. The examiner's free hand placed on the abdomen just above the symphysis pubis can be

used to manipulate the fetal head until a sharp image of the fetal brain through the anterior fontanel is obtained. Rotating the probe 90 degrees about its axis produces coronal and sagittal sections[68] (Fig. 14-6).

Coronal Sections

A series of consecutive coronal sections from anterior to posterior can be used to visualize the corpus callosum, the ventricular system, and the normal interhemispheric relationships. A coronal section passing through the level of the anterior horns of the lateral ventricles demonstrates the interhemispheric fissure, the corpus callosum crossing the midline, the cavum septi pellucidi, and the third ventricle straddled by the thalami (Fig. 14-7). Early in the second trimester, the fissure appears relatively straight. As new sulci and gyri develop with advancing gestation, the interhemispheric fissure becomes more irregular. The hypoechoic area between the skull and the cerebral cortex represents the subarachnoid space. This space diminishes in size throughout gestation as the cerebral cortical matter expands to fill the cranial vault. A posterior coronal

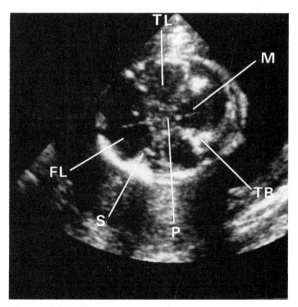

Figure 14-5. *Transverse scan through the base of the fetal skull demonstrating the bony ridges that demarcate the anterior, middle and posterior fossae. FL, frontal lobe; TL, temporal lobe; S, greater wings of sphenoid; TB, temporal bone; P, pituitary stalk; M, medulla.*

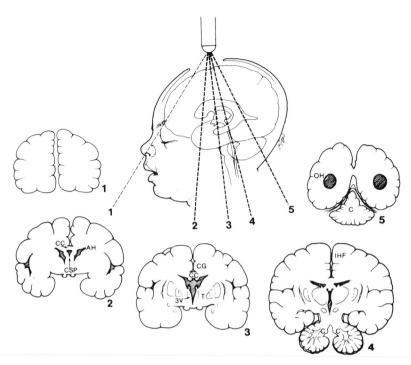

Figure 14-6. Schematic representation of the transvaginal technique for obtaining sagittal and coronal scans of the second and third trimester fetal head through the acoustic window of the anterior fontanel. Plane 1: anterior to the corpus callosum; plane 2: at the level of the anterior horns of the lateral ventricle; plane 3: at the level of the third ventricle; plane 4: posterior plane through the peduncles; plane 5: the posterior coronal plane through the occipital horns. CC, corpus callosum; AH, anterior horns of the lateral ventricle; CSP, cavum septi pellucidi; 3V, third ventricle; C, cerebellum; OH, occipital horn of the lateral ventricle; CG, cingulate gyrus. (Reprinted with permission from Monteagado A, Timor-Tritsch IE, Reuss ML, et al. Transvaginal sonography of the second- and third-trimester fetal brain. In: Timor-Tritsch IE, Rottem S, eds. Transvaginal Sonography. 2nd ed. New York: Elsevier; 1991:393–426.)

plane can be used to image the occipital horns of the lateral ventricles. In this last view, the cerebellum can be visualized between the fourth ventricle above it and the cisterna magna below it.

Sagittal and Parasagittal Sections

By 18 to 20 weeks' gestation, the corpus callosum is nearly fully developed. In a midsagittal section, it appears as a prominent, semilunar structure composed of three parts, from front to back: the genu, the body, and the splenium (Fig. 14-8). Above and below the corpus callosum are the cingulate gyrus and the sonolucent cavum septi pellucidi, respectively. The posterior fossa contains the cerebellum, the fourth ventricle, and the cisterna magna. The midsagittal view can also be used to evaluate the contour of the surfaces of the cerebral hemispheres. During the second trimester, the surface is smooth. However, as new gyri and sulci develop in the third trimester, echodense lines covering the cerebral cortex can be appreciated.

Parasagittal sections taken to the right or left of midline allow study of the anterior horns and bodies of the lateral ventricles. Normally, all the various segments of the lateral ventricle—the body

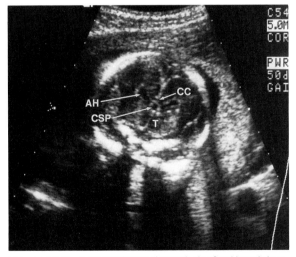

Figure 14-7. A coronal scan through the fetal head demonstrating the corpus callosum (CC) crossing the midline, the anterior horns of the lateral ventricles (AH), and the thalami (T) straddling the third ventricle. CSP, cavum septi pellucidi.

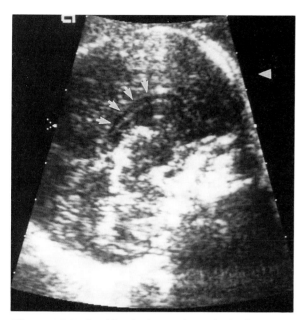

Figure 14-8. *A midsagittal scan through the fetal head demonstrating the corpus callosum (*arrows*), and the cavum septi pellucidi below it. Arrowhead = anterior.*

technique for obtaining these measurements is illustrated in Figure 14-10. The outer orbital distance is the more valuable measurement because it is the larger of the two measurements and thus has a greater range of normal variation across gestational age compared to the inner orbital distance. This allows for less controversy concerning the normality of a given measurement.

The ciliaris muscles and zonular fibers outlining the lens of the fetal eye may be visualized as a circular area on the front of the globe (Fig. 14-11). On occasion, the vitreous humor, the extraocular muscles, and the ophthalmic artery may be recognized.[57]

Ears

The pinna of the ear and the development of its cartilages have been observed sonographically.[10] The pinna is initially smooth but becomes increasingly ridged as gestation progresses (Fig. 14-12). Occasionally, even the basal turn of the cochlea or superior semicircular canal found within the petrous portion of the temporal bone may be imaged.[53]

and the anterior, posterior, and temporal horns—cannot be seen in a single plane. If all segments are seen in a single plane, this suggests ventricular dilatation. In the parasagittal view, a bright, echogenic arc that separates the caudate nucleus from the thalamus can also be imaged. This is known as the caudothalamic groove and is used as a landmark for the germinal matrix, which lies anterior to it (Fig. 14-9). The germinal matrix, a highly vascular tissue in the ependyma of the lateral ventricle, is not typically visualized unless it is abnormal. It is the site of origin of most of the intracranial hemorrhages seen in the preterm neonate.

THE FACE

Orbits and Eyes

Measurement of the distance between the bony orbits may be useful for determining gestational age as well as for searching for anomalies characterized by abnormal orbits spaced either narrowly or widely apart, defined as hypotelorism or hypertelorism, respectively.[55,66] Depending on the position of the fetal head, the inner and outer orbital distances can be measured in coronal or transverse planes and compared to nomograms. The

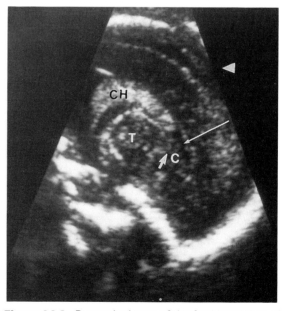

Figure 14-9. *Parasagittal scan of the fetal head demonstrating the thalamus (T), caudate nucleus (C), the choroid plexus (CH), the anterior horn of the lateral ventricle (*long arrow*), and the caudothalamic groove (*short arrow*), a landmark for the germinal matrix located anterior to it. Arrowhead = superior.*

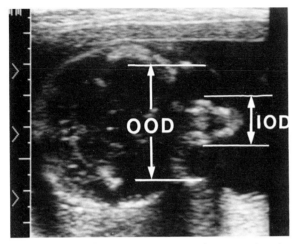

Figure 14-10. Transverse sonogram demonstrating the technique for measuring outer orbital and inner orbital diameters. (From Chervenak FA, Isaacson F, Lorber J. Anomalies of the Fetal Head, Neck, and Spine: Ultrasound Diagnosis and Management. Philadelphia: WB Saunders; 1988.)

Lower Face

The nares and upper lip can be visualized in a coronal scan (Fig. 14-13) and the face searched for cleft lip or palate. The tongue and its motion may be observed and the act of swallowing may be studied. The fetal profile (i.e., a midline sagittal view) is useful for verifying the shape and position of the nose and chin, as well as the contour of the face (Fig. 14-14). Isaacson and Birnhoz have described a way of documenting normal fetal breathing by demonstrating color flow due to amniotic fluid motion through the fetal nares.[52]

THE NECK

The neck should be examined with particular attention to its surface contours because a variety of lesions may protrude from this area. The centrally located trachea and the more peripherally located carotid bifurcation may be seen within the substance of the neck (Fig. 14-15). Visualization of the carotid artery may be difficult, however, because of the often curved position of the neck. Doppler evaluation of the common carotid artery has been performed to evaluate the cerebral circulation, but it is less representative of cerebral circulation than its internal carotid branch because the common ca-

rotid artery also gives rise to another branch, the external carotid artery.[88,89]

THE SPINE

An appreciation of the variability in the shapes of the vertebral bodies and the changing sonographic appearance of the spine during gestation is necessary to differentiate small defects of the spine from normal anatomic variations.[11] By 16 weeks' gestation, individual vertebrae may be identified by the observation of three echogenic ossification centers in the transverse plane. Two of these ossification centers are posterior to the spinal canal and are within the laminae; one is anterior and within the vertebral body itself (Fig. 14-16). If the spine is scanned sagittally, a line of vertebral bodies and a line of posterior elements may be seen on either side of the anechoic spinal canal. All three ossification centers cannot be imaged in the same plane on a sagittal view. In the coronal plane, the two echogenic posterior ossification centers can be followed progressively from the cervical region to the base of the spine (Fig. 14-17). The posterior ossification centers are normally parallel to each other or converge as they are followed from the lumbar to the

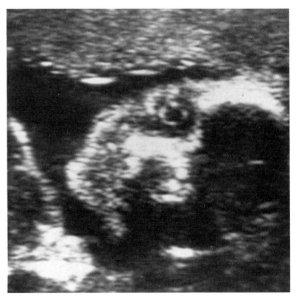

Figure 14-11. Coronal view of the fetal face. (From Chervenak FA, Isaacson F, Lorber J. Anomalies of the Fetal Head, Neck, and Spine: Ultrasound Diagnosis and Management. Philadelphia: WB Saunders; 1988.)

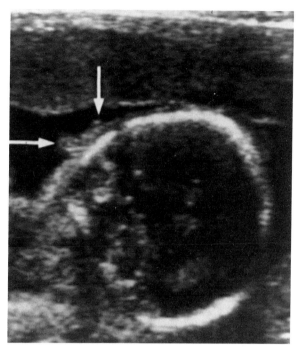

Figure 14-12. Smooth pinna of the fetal ear *(arrow)* at 18 weeks' gestation. (From Chervenak FA, Isaacson F, Lorber J. Anomalies of the Fetal Head, Neck, and Spine: Ultrasound Diagnosis and Management. Philadelphia: WB Saunders; 1988.)

sacral regions. Divergence of the posterior elements suggests abnormality, probably a meningocele or meningomyelocele.

The vertebral body, pedicles, transverse processes, posterior laminae, and spinous process all may be identified as echogenic structures on transverse scans. Imaging improves as gestation progresses. In addition, the spinal canal and intervertebral foramina may be seen as anechoic areas. In the sagittal plane, a line of vertebral bodies is still seen, but the posterior echoes are more complex, with spinous processes seen jutting from the line of other posterior elements (Fig. 14-18).

Anomalies of the Fetal Head, Neck, and Spine

There are a myriad of schemes for grouping and reviewing abnormalities of the fetal head, neck, and spine. We prefer the sonographer's-eye view, whereby characterization of what is visualized on the screen

forms the basis for developing a diagnosis. In this section, the anomalies are grouped in the following four categories: (1) those in which there is absence of a structure normally present; (2) those in which there is a herniation of internal contents through a defect in a normal structure; (3) those in which a normally small, even imperceptible structure is abnormally enlarged, representing dilatation behind an obstruction; and (4) those in which the presence of an abnormal structure is noted.

ABSENCE OF A STRUCTURE NORMALLY PRESENT

Anencephaly

Anencephaly, a congenital anomaly in which the cerebral hemispheres and overlying skull and scalp are entirely absent, is the most obvious and dramatic of the "absence" anomalies. The diagnosis of anencephaly is made when the upper portion of the cranial vault cannot be visualized. This bony structure normally can be seen after 14 weeks if the

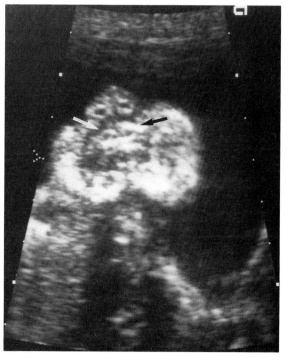

Figure 14-13. Oblique coronal scan of the fetal face demonstrating the nares, the upper lip *(white arrow)*, and the hard palate *(black arrow)*.

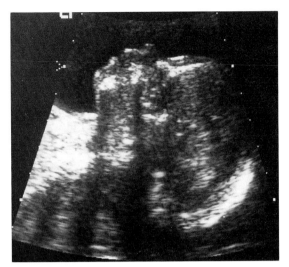

Figure 14-14. A midline sagittal view of the fetal face demonstrating the contour of the fetal forehead, nose, and chin.

head is not hidden in the mother's pelvis. It can be seen as early as 9 or 10 weeks by transvaginal sonography. The area of the cerebrovasculosa, a vascular malformation of the primitive brain stem seen in anencephaly, may appear as an ill-defined mass of heterogeneous density above the level of the orbits (Fig. 14-19). Polyhydramnios due to poor fetal swallowing may complicate these pregnancies. The diagnosis of anencephaly can be made with extraordinary accuracy. In the combined experiences of six centers, over 130 cases have been detected with no false-positive diagnoses.[19,69] Thus, anencephaly was the first malformation diagnosed with sufficient certainty by ultrasound that physicians were willing to perform elective abortion on the basis of sonographic images.[15,51,62,86]

Anencephaly is one of the most common congenital disorders in the world. Its incidence varies with geography, race, and sex. Anencephaly occurs most frequently in areas where spina bifida is also common. In 1984, its incidence in Northern Ireland was as high as 4.7 cases among 10,000 deliveries, whereas in the United States it was 2.6. It is a lethal anomaly. The risk of recurrence in subsequent pregnancies, as with most polygenic or multifactorial anomalies, increases with the number of previously affected fetuses.

Hydranencephaly

Hydranencephaly, a severe destructive insult, exists when no cerebral cortex can be seen. It is believed to result from bilateral occlusion of the internal carotid arteries. Sonographic findings include macrocephaly with a large, fluid-filled cranial vault. The midbrain, basal ganglia, thalamus, and cerebellum are usually spared.[42,77]

Lissencephaly, Pachygyria, and Microgyria

These disorders result from interruptions in the normal migration of neuroblasts into the cerebral cortex. Depending on the point in gestation at which the disruption takes place, the fetal cortex can completely lack sulci and gyri (lissencephaly), can have very few gyri (pachygyria), or have very small gyri (microgyria). All neonates with these disorders have severe neurologic sequelae.[3,5,36,37] Microcephaly, ventriculomegaly, a widened Sylvian fissure, and a blunted operculum of the insular cortex can be seen in lissencephaly.[3,36,37] Although the disruption in normal migration causing lissencephaly occurs between 12 and 24 weeks' gestation, prenatal diagnosis unfortunately cannot be made

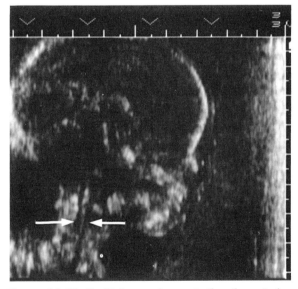

Figure 14-15. Sagittal scan demonstrating the anterior contour of the neck and the carotid artery bifurcation (*arrows*). (From Chervenak FA, Isaacson F, Lorber J. Anomalies of the Fetal Head, Neck, and Spine: Ultrasound Diagnosis and Management. Philadelphia: WB Saunders; 1988.)

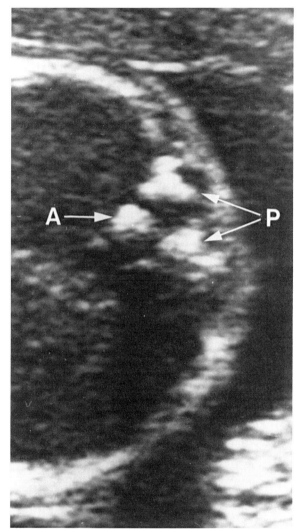

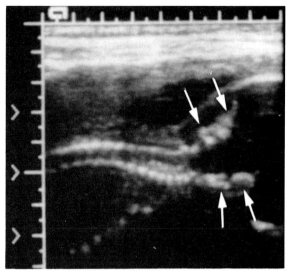

Figure 14-17. Coronal scan of the fetal spine demonstrating the normal divergence of the cervical spine (*arrows*) at the base of the skull.

Holoprosencephaly is divided into alobar, semilobar, and lobar varieties, defined by the degree of separation of the cerebral hemispheres (Fig. 14-20). The alobar form is the worst, showing no evidence of division of cerebral cortex into separate hemispheres. Thus, the falx cerebri and interhemi-

Figure 14-16. Transverse scan of the thoracic fetal spine at 18 weeks' gestation demonstrating the two posterior (P) and one anterior (A) ossification centers. (From Chervenak FA, Isaacson F, Lorber J. *Anomalies of the Fetal Head, Neck, and Spine: Ultrasound Diagnosis and Management.* Philadelphia: WB Saunders; 1988.)

with confidence until approximately 28 weeks. This is because the normal gyri and sulci cannot be well visualized until the third trimester.[67]

Holoprosencephaly

Holoprosencephaly describes a variety of abnormalities of the brain and face that result from incomplete cleavage of the primitive prosencephalon.

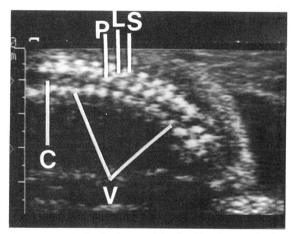

Figure 14-18. Sagittal scan of the fetal lumbosacral spine demonstrating the vertebral bodies (V), the spinal cord (C), the pedicles (P), laminae (L), and spinous processes (S). (From Chervenak FA, Isaacson F, Lorber J. *Anomalies of the Fetal Head, Neck, and Spine: Ultrasound Diagnosis and Management.* Philadelphia: WB Saunders; 1988.)

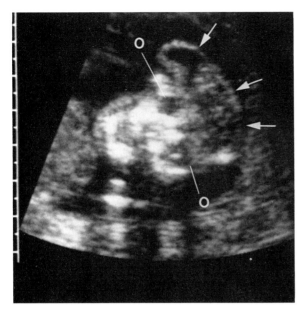

Figure 14-19. Coronal sonogram of fetal anencephaly demonstrating the area of the cerebrovasculosa (*arrows*) above the level of the orbits (O).

of the alobar type of holoprosencephaly. Cyclopia, the presence of a single median bony orbit with a fleshy proboscis above it, is the most severe malformation. In cebocephaly, hypotelorism is associated with a normally placed nose but with a single nostril (Fig. 14-23). Hypotelorism with a midline facial cleft also predicts the presence of alobar holoprosencephaly. Holoprosencephaly may also be associ-

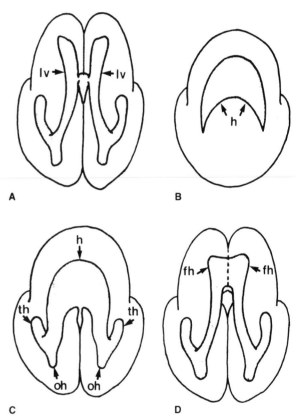

Figure 14-20. Schematic representation of the alobar, semilobar, and lobar forms of holoprosencephaly. (**A**) Normal brain. Both the cerebral hemispheres and the lateral ventricles (lv) are separated. (**B**) Alobar holoprosencephaly. There is an absence of the normal division of the cerebral hemispheres and a single ventricular cavity. (**C**) Semilobar holoprosencephaly. There is an incomplete separation of the cerebral hemispheres in the occipital area and partial development of the occipital (oh) and temporal horns (th) of the lateral ventricles. (**D**) Lobar holoprosencephaly. Nearly complete separation of the cerebral hemisphere and lateral ventricles except for the frontal portions. The frontal horns (Fh) of the lateral ventricles are usually mildly dilated. (Reprinted with permission from Pilu G, et al. Am J Perinatol. 1987; 4:41.)

spheric fissures are absent, there is a single common ventricle, and the thalami are fused (Fig. 14-21). The semilobar and lobar varieties represent greater degrees of brain development. The semilobar type demonstrates partially separated brain, whereas the lobar type shows almost complete separation of the hemispheres, although the frontal horns of the lateral ventricles are fused, as are the thalami. Microcephaly is usually present owing to decreased cortical mass, but macrocephaly may be seen if hydrocephalus develops.

The prechordal mesoderm, an embryonic connective mass between the oral cavity and the undersurface of the neural tube, is thought to be responsible for both the division of the prosencephalon and the production of the nasofrontal process. Failure of the sagittal division of the prosencephalon is thought to result in holoprosencephaly[35] (Fig. 14-22). The nasofrontal process gives rise to the ethmoid, nasal, and premaxillary bones and to the vomer and the nasal septum. Failure of these structures to develop normally can result in varying degrees of hypotelorism, cleft lip and palate, and nasal malformation. Indeed, individuals with holoprosencephaly often have associated midline facial anomalies, and certain facies predict the presence

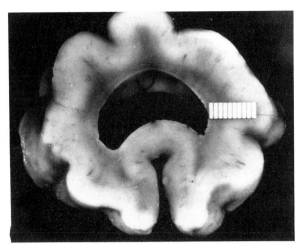

Figure 14-21. A postmortem example of alobar holoprosencephaly demonstrating the absence of the interhemispheric fissure and a single common ventricle. (From Chervenak A, Isaacson G, Hobbins JC, et al. The diagnosis and management of fetal holoprosencephaly. Obstet Gynecol. 1985; 66:322.)

ated with milder forms of midline facial dysplasia or with normal facies.[35]

Some cases of alobar holoprosencephaly may be missed, and the pathologic changes of lobar and semilobar holoprosencephaly may be too subtle to be detected by antenatal ultrasound.[22]

The alobar forms of holoprosencephaly carry a poor prognosis. More subtle forms may be associated with minimal neurologic deficits. Recurrence rates increase with associated chromosomal abnormalities or autosomal recessive and, rarely, autosomal dominant genetic syndromes. Prognosis is also related to associated anomalies.

FACIAL CLEFTS. Failure of lip fusion, normally complete by 35 days of intrauterine life, may impair subsequent closure of the palatal shelves, leading to cleft lip and cleft palates.[81] To demonstrate a facial cleft before birth, the lower portion of the face must be anterior (nearer the transducer) and clearly visualized (Fig. 14-24). Both sagittal and oblique coronal imaging planes may be useful. Undulating tongue movements,[28] hypertrophied tissue at the edge of the cleft,[27] and hypertelorism[27] have all been described as useful adjunctive findings in the diagnosis of a facial

cleft. Nevertheless, clefts are subtle changes in the face, and their diagnosis can be difficult and inconsistent. Most recently, evaluation of the fetal face has improved with use of three-dimensional ultrasonography to represent on a single image information normally requiring multiple two-dimensional planes of the face.[76]

Agenesis of the Corpus Callosum

Agenesis of the corpus callosum can occur as an isolated anomaly, but 80% of cases are associated with other anomalies such as hydrocephalus, Dandy-Walker syndrome, Arnold-Chiari malformation, and holoprosencephaly.[1,4,28,59] Because the normal development of the corpus callosum proceeds craniocaudally, partial agenesis of the corpus callosum usually involves the posterior portion. However, secondary dysgenesis can result from destructive insults occurring later in gestation.[9] The diagnosis of agenesis of the corpus callosum can require several planes of study. At the BPD level, the cavum septi pellucidi is absent and the third ventricle, now occupying the usual space of the cavum septi pellucidi, appears widened. Because of the absence of the corpus callosum, the third ventricle rides high, and may be visualized at the lateral ventricle level. The lateral ventricles may exhibit a characteristic tear-drop appearance, with laterally displaced medial walls and widened atria (Fig.

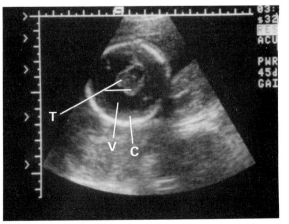

Figure 14-22. Transverse scan of the fetal head in alobar holoprosencephaly demonstrating a single common ventricle (V), compressed cerebral cortex (C), and prominent thalamus (T).

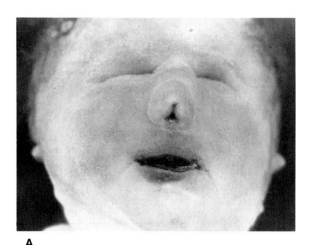
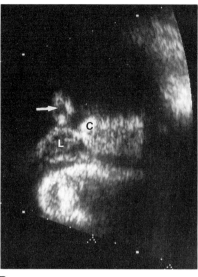

A   **B**

Figure 14-23. (**A**) Cebocephaly with hypotelorism and a single nostril. (From Chervenak FA, Isaacson G, Mahoney MJ, et al. The obstetric significance of holoprosencephaly. Obstet Gynecol. 1984; 63:115.) (**B**) Coronal oblique sonogram of fetus with cebocephaly demonstrating single nostril (*arrow*). L, lips; C, cheek.

14-25). Transvaginal sonography has proved a useful adjunct to improve the diagnosis of complete or partial agenesis of the corpus callosum. The pathognomonic lesion is the "sunburst" lesion seen on midsagittal section, representing radial orientation of the gyri and sulci to the third ventricle rather than paralleling the corpus callosum, which is absent.[2,33,46,48]

Dandy-Walker Malformation

Classically, the Dandy-Walker malformation consists of dysgenesis of the cerebellar vermis, cystic dilatation of the fourth ventricle—thought to be the result of obstruction of the foramina of Luschka and Magendie—and lateral displacement of the cerebellar hemispheres (Fig. 14-26). It is often associated with hydrocephalus and other structural anomalies such as agenesis of the corpus callosum. An enlarged cisterna magna, greater than 10 mm, should raise the suspicion of Dandy-Walker malformation, or a variant thereof. It may also represent an arachnoid cyst.[7,30,31,60]

Caudal Regression Syndrome

The caudal regression syndrome, a range of "absence" abnormalities resulting in absent vertebrae below the thorax and rudimentary pelvis (Fig.

14-27), is strongly associated with maternal diabetes mellitus. Other abdominal wall, genitourinary, and cardiac anomalies may also be found. An embryologic defect thought to occur in the third week of gestation allows for fusion of the lower limb buds with complete absence of the caudal structures, a condition known as sirenomelia—the most severe

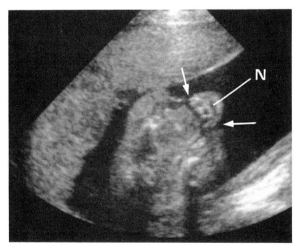

Figure 14-24. Oblique coronal scan of the fetal face demonstrating bilateral cleft lip (*arrows;* N, nose).

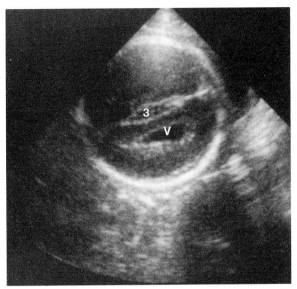

Figure 14-25. Transverse scan of a fetus with agenesis of the corpus callosum at the level of the interhemispheric fissure demonstrating the high-riding third ventricle (3) and lateral displacement of the medial wall of the lateral ventricle (V).

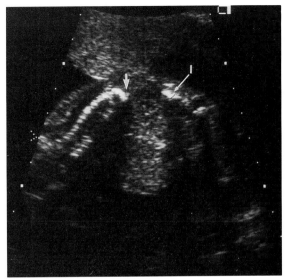

Figure 14-27. Coronal sonogram of a fetus with the caudal regression syndrome demonstrating the absence of the vertebral bodies (*arrow*) below the level of the thorax. I, iliac crest.

of the caudal regression syndromes. The incidence if sirenomelia is 1 in 60,000 neonates.[38,61,81]

Other Spinal Deformities

Hemivertebrae, caused by aplasia or dysgenesis of one of the two chondrification centers forming the vertebral bodies, may be identified sonographically by lateral displacement of the anterior ossification centers or improperly aligned vertebral bodies (Fig. 14-28). These may occur as an isolated entity but are more often seen in association with neural tube defects. Scoliosis, which may also be seen with hemivertebrae and meningomyelocele, may occur as an isolated defect of the spine. However, because the fetal skeleton is very flexible and subject to significant deformation forces in utero, certain criteria should be met before the diagnosis is made. In the absence of other anomalies, bends in the vertebral column should reach the extreme of 90 degrees and should be unchanging in serial scans.[41,72]

HERNIATION THROUGH A STRUCTURAL DEFECT

Cephalocele

Cephaloceles are protrusions of the meninges and frequently of brain substance through a defect in the cranium. Encephaloceles contain brain tissue

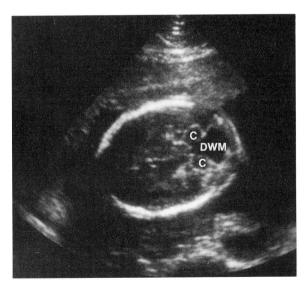

Figure 14-26. Transverse scan of a fetus with the Dandy-Walker malformation (DWM), comprising dysgenesis of the cerebellar vermis, cystic dilatation of the fourth ventricle communicating with the cisterna magnum, and lateral displacement of the cerebellar hemispheres (C).

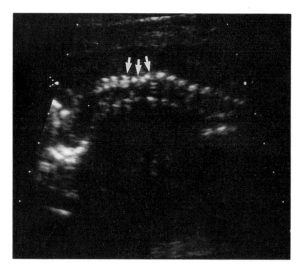

Figure 14-28. Sonogram of a fetus with hemivertebrae demonstrating the improperly aligned ossification centers of the vertebral bodies (*arrows*).

and cranial meningoceles do not. In the Western world, 75% of these lesions have been reported as occipital, but cephaloceles may also occur in other areas, including parietal, frontal, or nasopharyngeal areas of the calvarium.

Although cephaloceles usually result from a defect in neural tube closure, they may be seen in the amniotic band syndrome or in association with various malformation syndromes (e.g., Meckel's syndrome).[32]

Sonographically, cephaloceles appear as sac-like protrusions about the head that are not covered with bone. The diagnosis can be made with certainty only if an associated defect in the skull is imaged (Fig. 14-29). However, such a defect may be small and difficult to visualize. When a defect is present, its position may be determined using the bony structures of the face and spine, as well as intracranial anatomy, for orientation. Extrusion of a large amount of brain substance may result in microcephaly. Cephaloceles are commonly associated with hydrocephalus.[23] When brain tissue has herniated, it gives the sac a complex appearance because of the contained solid brain tissue. Ultrasound has not been particularly reliable in differentiating between meningoceles and encephaloceles when there is only a small amount of contained brain tissue. Routine sonography, occa-

sionally aided by transvaginal technique, must attempt to differentiate cephaloceles from such simulators as cystic hygroma, hemangiomas, teratomas, and branchial cleft cysts.[68] Encephaloceles, in general, carry a poor prognosis. Pure meningoceles may have a more favorable prognosis.

Iniencephaly

Iniencephaly is a rare anomaly in which there is a defect in the occiput of the cranium involving the foramen magnum with marked retroflexion of the fetal head and frequently a shortened spine. The malformation is thought to represent an arrest in embryonic development during the third week of gestation.[34] Diagnosis is based on visualization of the markedly retroflexed neck, such that the cranium may still be viewed during transverse scanning of the fetal thorax, and on an inability to visualize the entire spine[39] (Fig. 14-30). Other associated anomalies, including hydrocephalus, Dandy-Walker malformation, encephalocele, diaphragmatic hernia, and omphalocele, are seen in as many as 84% of fetuses with iniencephaly.[34]

Spina Bifida and Meningomyelocele

Spina bifida refers to a defect in the spine resulting from a failure of the two halves of the vertebral arch to fuse. These lesions usually occur in the lumbosacral and cervical regions. If the meninges protrude

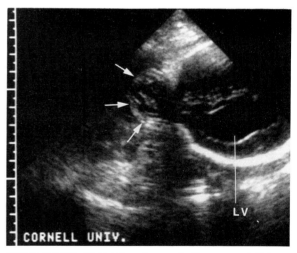

Figure 14-29. Sonogram demonstrating an occipital encephalocele with protruding brain tissue (*arrows*) and hydrocephalus, with an enlarged lateral ventricle (LV).

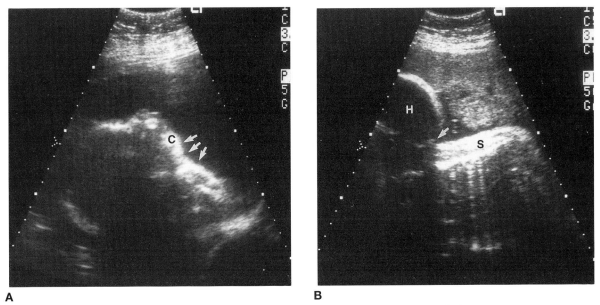

Figure 14-30. Sonogram of fetus with iniencephaly demonstrating (**A**) the marked retroflexion of the fetal neck (*arrows*; C, chin) and (**B**) the severely shortened spine (S). H, head (*arrow*).

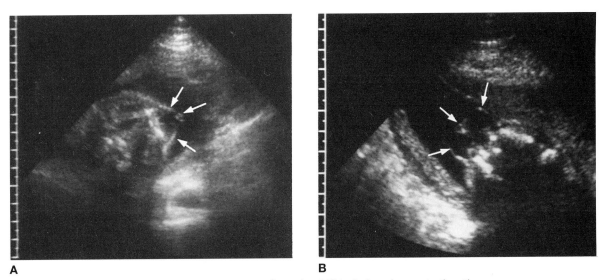

Figure 14-31. (**A** and **B**) Transverse sonograms of a spina bifida lesion demonstrating the splayed posterior ossification centers resulting from the lack of fusion of the two halves of the vertebral arch and the meningomyelocele (*arrows*).

through the defect, the lesion is designated a meningocele; if neural tissue is included, it is a meningomyelocele.

Sonographically, spina bifida is seen as a splaying of the posterior ossification centers of the spine, giving the vertebral segment a "U" or "V" shape (Fig. 14-31). The posterior ossification centers are more widely spaced than those in vertebral segments above and below the defect. A normal, mild progressive widening of the spinal canal is seen in the cervical region. Although the defect of spina bifida may be visualized on longitudinal scanning, meticulous transverse examination of the entire vertebral column is necessary to detect smaller defects. When a meningocele or a meningomyelocele is present and intact, a protruding sac may be detected (Fig. 14-32). Although detection of small spina bifida defects remains a challenge,[49,73] diagnosis of meningomyelocele has been aided tremendously by its nearly 100% association with the Arnold-Chiari malformation. Viewing of the actual meningomyelocele, however, is the only definitive way to make the diagnosis.[6,50]

Although spina bifida may be detected during routine ultrasound examination, many are found as a result of careful ultrasound examinations performed in pregnancies found to have elevations of maternal serum α-fetoprotein levels. Because elevated maternal serum α-fetoprotein can be elevated in anterior abdominal wall, as well as open neural tube, defects, if a spinal defect is not visualized in these circumstances, amniotic fluid α-fetoprotein and acetylcholinesterase determinations may have an adjunctive role in the diagnosis of smaller lesions.[64]

The prognosis for spina bifida depends on the level of the lesion. Bowel and bladder dysfunction, inability to walk, and complications due to associated hydrocephalus may occur.

Arnold-Chiari Malformations

The Arnold-Chiari malformations are a group of anomalies of the hindbrain, the most important of which is the Chiari II malformation. Most, if not all, cases of spina bifida are complicated by the Arnold-Chiari malformation, specifically the Chiari II malformation. Almost all of these patients show hydrocephalus.[6,50] In the Chiari II malformation, there is a variable displacement of a tongue of tissue derived from the inferior cerebellar vermis into the upper cervical spinal canal. Displacement of the cerebellum inferiorly changes its shape and effaces the cisterna magna, thereby producing the characteristic sonographic finding, the banana sign, referring to the flattened, centrally curved, banana-like appearance of the cerebellar hemispheres. There is a simi-

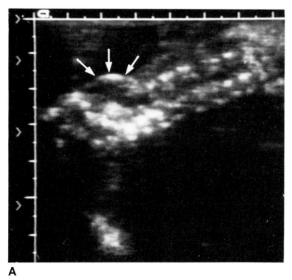
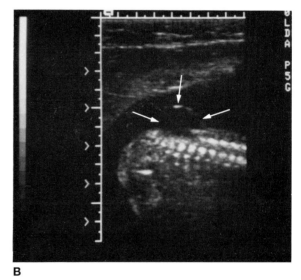

A **B**

Figure 14-32. (**A** and **B**) Longitudinal scans of the fetal spine demonstrating a meningomyelocele (*arrows*).

lar caudal displacement of the medulla and fourth ventricle. In extreme cases, the cerebellar hemispheres may be absent from view during fetal head scanning.

A second sonographic sign, the lemon sign, has been described in the Arnold-Chiari malformation. During the second trimester, a scalloping of the frontal bones can be seen in axial section of the head, giving a lemon-like configuration to the skull of an affected fetus. The caudal displacement of the cranial contents within the pliable fetal skull is thought to produce this scalloping effect. Unlike the banana sign, the lemon sign is not definitive because it can be seen in 1 in 250 otherwise normal fetuses and can be associated with intracranial or extracranial abnormalities other than meningomyelocele or encephalocele. Nevertheless, these charac-

teristic signs should alert the sonographer to search for spina bifida, and have led to its diagnosis in a fetus not previously suspected of having the disorder[70] (Fig. 14-33).

DILATATION BEHIND AN OBSTRUCTION

Ventriculomegaly and Hydrocephalus

Ventriculomegaly, an abnormal increase in the volume of the cerebral ventricles, has many different causes. Ventriculomegaly may be caused by intraventricular or extraventricular obstruction, a relative decrease in the amount of brain substance, or, rarely, an increase in cerebrospinal fluid production. The term "hydrocephalus" is often reserved for ventriculomegaly in which macrocephaly is present.

The overall incidence of congenital hydroceph-

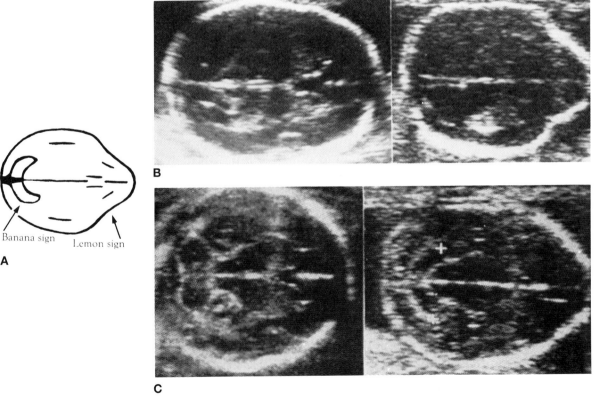

Figure 14-33. (**A**) Schematic representation of the "lemon" and "banana" signs in the Chiari II malformation. (**B**) Transverse sonogram of a normal fetal head (*left*) and the scalloped frontal bones ("lemon" sign) in a fetus with spina bifida (*right*). (**C**) Suboccipital bregmatic view of the fetal head in a normal fetus (*left*) and the elongated, effaced cerebellar hemispheres ("banana" sign) in a fetus with spina bifida (*right*). (Nicolaides KM, Campbell S, Gabbe SG, et al. Ultrasound screening for spina bifida: Cranial and cerebellar signs. Lancet. 1986; 2:72.)

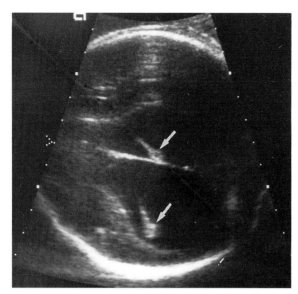

Figure 14-34. *Transverse scan of the fetal head in a fetus with hydrocephalus demonstrating the enlarged lateral ventricles, each with a "dangling choroid plexus" (arrows) within it.*

alus has been estimated to be between 0.5 and 3 per 1000 live births. Hydrocephalus is frequently associated with spina bifida. The incidence of isolated hydrocephalus is between 0.39 and 0.87 per 1000 live births.[44] Aqueductal stenosis, a congenital obstruction to flow of cerebrospinal fluid through the aqueduct of Sylvius connecting the third and fourth ventricles, accounts for 43% of cases, communicating hydrocephalus accounts for 38%, and Dandy-Walker malformations account for 13%. Other causes include agenesis of the corpus callosum, arachnoid cysts, and arteriovenous malformations such as a vein of Galen aneurysm.[14]

Although an abnormally increased head circumference or BPD may suggest the diagnosis of ventriculomegaly, examination of the intracranial contents is necessary for accurate diagnosis. This is particularly true because enlargement of the ventricles and cerebrospinal fluid displacement of the choroid plexus, termed the "dangling choroid plexus," within the enlarged lateral ventricle precedes cranial enlargement (Fig. 14-34).

The absence of ventriculomegaly early in gestation does not preclude its later development. Serial examinations are indicated for a pregnancy at risk, such as those in which an intrauterine infection is

suspected. With ventriculomegaly, the atria of the lateral ventricles dilate first; afterward, dilatation of other parts of the ventricular system, such as the frontal horns and occipital horns, as well as the third and fourth ventricles if there is communicating hydrocephalus, can be seen (Fig. 14-35). Qualitative assessment of ventriculomegaly can also be made transvaginally. On coronal section, progressive rounding and bulging of the superior and lateral angles of the frontal horns can be appreciated. On parasagittal section, dilatation of the occipital horns of the lateral ventricles can be seen.[68]

Certain pitfalls in the early detection of fetal ventriculomegaly have been described.[17] These include an artifactual hypoechoic area of sonographic "dropout" in the farfield's temporal brain and reverberation artifacts that obscure the nearfield of the image.[78]

Because the natural history of any case of ventricular enlargement is uncertain early in gestation,[20] the diagnosis and evaluation of ventriculomegaly and assessment of progressive ventricular enlargement may be documented by serial sonography. Once fetal ventriculomegaly is diagnosed, it is essential to search for associated anomalies, which have been reported to occur in as many as 83% of cases.[18] Although spina bifida

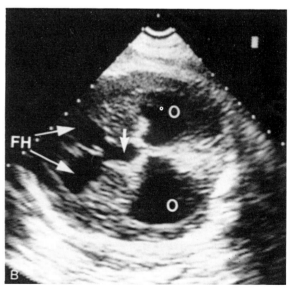

Figure 14-35. *Transverse sonogram of a fetus with severe hydrocephalus demonstrating dilatation of the frontal (FH) and occipital horns (O) of the lateral ventricles, as well as dilatation of the third ventricle (arrow).*

is the most common one, associated structural anomalies may affect any organ system. In addition to meticulous real-time sonographic evaluation, amniocentesis should be performed to determine the fetal karyotype, because approximately 10% of hydrocephalus is associated with aneuploidy.[18]

The prognosis for hydrocephalus depends not only on its severity, but on the associated anomalies. The outcome for children diagnosed in utero with isolated hydrocephalus ranges from normal mentation to severe retardation. One study showed a 75% survival rate for fetuses with isolated, nonprogressive ventriculomegaly; 59% of these survivors had normal intelligence.[43]

Cystic Hygroma

Fetal lymphatic vessels normally drain into two large sacs lateral to the jugular veins. If these jugular lymph sacs fail to communicate with the venous system, they may enlarge as they fill with lymph and form cystic hygromas. This failure in lymphatic drainage may also result in the generalized edema of hydrops fetalis[21,81] (Fig. 14-36). Cystic hygromas appear as either single or multiloculated cavities filled with fluid. Although they can be seen in the chest, axillae, and other areas, cystic hygromas arise most often about the neck.

Several sonographic features aid in the diagnosis of fetal cystic hygromas. Hygromas are usually

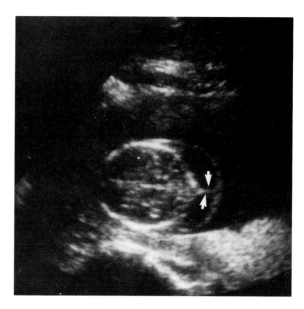

Figure 14-37. Transverse sonogram of a cystic hygroma demonstrating a midline septum (*arrows*).

located on the posterolateral neck, are cystic in appearance, and are frequently divided by random septa. Because they arise from paired jugular lymph sacs, which may enlarge to meet at the posterior midline, a septum representing the nuchal ligament may be visualized (Fig. 14-37). Associated hydrops is manifest sonographically as ascites, pleural effusion, pericardial effusion, and skin edema.[24] Other craniocervical masses that must be differentiated from cystic hygromas include cystic teratomas, cephalocele, hemangioma, branchial cleft cyst, and nuchal edema.[79]

Prognosis for cystic hygroma varies. If the hygroma is detected along with fetal hydrops, the condition is fatal and frequently is associated with abnormal karyotype. An isolated hygroma may have a good outcome. If redevelopment or drainage of the lymphatics to the venous system occurs, a cystic hygroma may disappear. Some believe the classic webbed neck of patients with Turner's syndrome is the result of reabsorption of their cystic hygroma.

PRESENCE OF AN ADDITIONAL STRUCTURE

Choroid Plexus Cysts

Small cysts may be noted in the choroid plexus of the lateral ventricles of 1% to 2% of all fetuses (Fig. 14-38). These lesions are usually transient and

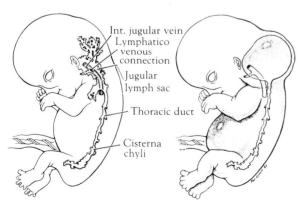

Figure 14-36. Schematic representation of the lymphatic drainage system in the normal fetus (*left*) and the failed lymphaticovenous connection in cystic hygroma (*right*). (Chervenak FA, Isaacson G, Blakemore KJ, et al. Fetal cystic hygroma: Cause and natural history. N Engl J Med. 1983; 309:822.)

Labels in figure 14-36: Int. jugular vein / Lymphatico venous connection / Jugular lymph sac / Thoracic duct / Cisterna chyli

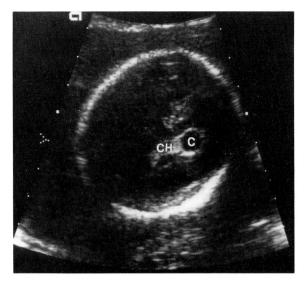

Figure 14-38. Transverse scan of the fetal head demonstrating a choroid plexus cyst. CH, choroid plexus; C, cyst.

without clinical significance, resolving before the end of the second trimester without sequelae.[29] Approximately 5%, however, are associated with trisomy 18 and another 1% have other karyotypic abnormalities.[71] Many of these fetuses may have other structural anomalies. Most authorities agree that fetuses with bilateral choroid plexus cysts measuring greater than 10 mm and other structural anomalies should have amniocentesis to rule out abnormal karyotype. However, abnormal karyotypes have been found in fetuses with choroid plexus cysts less than 10 mm, those with unilateral cysts, and those without associated structural anomalies. Because amniocentesis has a 0.5% rate of miscarriage, further studies are necessary to determine the true risk:benefit ratio of amniocentesis for fetuses with an imaged choroid plexus cyst and no other structural anomalies.

Intracranial Hemorrhage

Intracranial hemorrhage is most frequently seen in the preterm and occasionally even in the term neonate 48 to 72 hours after birth. Antenatal identification of intracranial hemorrhage by ultrasound has been reported. Most of these reports noted intraventricular or subependymal hemorrhage in fetuses under 32 weeks' gestation. There have been two reports of subdural hemorrhages diagnosed antenatally. Another case of subependymal hemorrhage was reported to have occurred near term and was associated with evidence of ischemic injury, which resulted in fetal death.[40] A typical antenatal hemorrhage is seen as an echogenic mass in the region of the germinal matrix or within the lateral ventricles (Fig. 14-39). Although a well established, prognostic grading system exists for neonatal intracranial hemorrhage,[13] the literature regarding the prognosis for antenatally diagnosed hemorrhages is limited. Although it is likely that a grading system such as that used for neonates may be applicable to fetal intracranial hemorrhage, follow-up of survivors of in utero intracranial hemorrhage is needed to determine the incidence of hydrocephalus, mental retardation, and cerebral palsy.

Porencephaly

Porencephaly is a destructive lesion of the brain that appears as one or several hypoechoic, cystic areas in the cerebral cortex, usually communicating with the ventricle (Fig. 14-40), believed to be related to an in utero ischemic event. It is thought that areas of prior intracranial hemorrhage or tissue necrosis resorb, leaving behind porencephalic cysts.

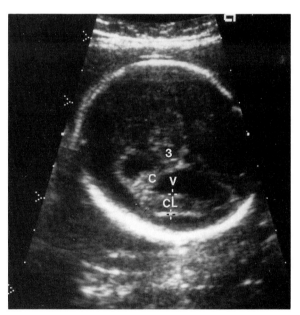

Figure 14-39. Transverse sonogram of a fetus with an intracranial hemorrhage demonstrating the presence of an echogenic mass (calipers and CL, clot) within the lateral ventricles (V). C, choroid plexus; 3, third ventricle.

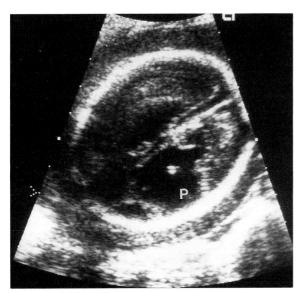

Figure 14-40. Transverse sonogram of a fetus with a resolved intracranial hemorrhage that has left behind a porencephalic cyst (P) communicating with the lateral ventricle.

Aneurysm of the Vein of Galen

Doppler imaging has significantly improved the diagnosis of arteriovenous malformations. Such malformations typically appear as cystic structures representing the dilated, end-to-end arteries and veins that have no intervening capillaries. Doppler studies can be used to demonstrate the blood flow through these structures. An aneurysm or arteriovenous malformation of the vein of Galen is often imaged behind the third ventricle. Its Doppler spectrum demonstrates a typically irregular and biphasic pattern. Increased intracranial blood flow may lead to cardiomegaly, and even hydrops in the affected fetus.[83]

REFERENCES

1. Atlas SW, Skolnik A, Naidich TP. Sonographic recognition of agenesis of the corpus callosum. Am J Neuroradiol. 1985; 6:369.
2. Atlas S, Skolnik A, Naidich T. Sonographic recognition of agenesis of the corpus callosum. Am J Roentgenol. 1985; 145:167–173.
3. Babcock DS. Sonography of congenital malformations of the brain. Neuroradiology. 1986; 28:428.
4. Barkovich AJ, Norman D. Anomalies of the corpus callosum: Correlation with further anomalies of the brain. Am J Roentgenol. 1988; 151:171.
5. Bauman ML. Neuroembryology: Clinical aspects. Semin Perinatol. 1987; 11:74–84.
6. Bell JE, Gordon A, Maloney AFJ. The association of hydrocephalus and Arnold-Chiari malformation with spina bifida in the fetus. Neuropathol Appl Neurobiol. 1980; 6:29.
7. Benaceraff B. Fetal central nervous system anomalies. Ultrasound Quarterly. 1990; 8:1–42.
8. Benaceraff BR, Barss VA, Laboda LA. A sonographic sign for the detection in the second trimester of the fetus with Down's syndrome. Am J Obstet Gynecol. 1985; 153:49.
9. Bertino RE, Nyberg DA, Cyr DR, et al. Prenatal diagnosis of agenesis of the corpus callosum. J Ultrasound Med. 1988; 7:251.
10. Birnholz JC. The fetal external ear. Radiology. 1983; 147:819.
11. Birnholz JC. Fetal lumber spine: Measuring axial growth with ultrasound. Radiology. 1986; 158:805.
12. Bowerman RA, DiPietro MA. Erroneous sonographic identification of fetal lateral ventricles: Relationship to the echogenic periventricular "blush." Am J Neuroradiol. 1987; 8:661.
13. Burstein J, Burstein R, et al. The incidence and evolution of subependymal and intraventricular hemorrhage. J Pediatr. 1978; 92:529–534.
14. Burton BK. Recurrence risks for congenital hydrocephalus. Clin Genet. 1979; 16:47.
15. Campbell S, Johnstone FD, Hold EM, et al. Anencephaly: Early ultrasonic diagnosis and active management. Lancet. 1972; 2:1226.
16. Cardoza JD, Goldstein RB, Filly RA. Exclusion of fetal ventriculomegaly with a single measurement: The width of the lateral ventricular atrium. Radiology. 1988; 169:711–717.
17. Chervenak FA, Berkowitz RL, Tortora M, et al. Diagnosis of ventriculomegaly before fetal viability. Obstet Gynecol. 1984; 64:652.
18. Chervenak FA, Berkowitz RL, Tortora M, et al. The management of fetal hydrocephalus. Am J Obstet Gynecol. 1985; 151:933.
19. Chervenak FA, Farley MA, Walter L, et al. When is termination of pregnancy during the third trimester morally justifiable? N Engl J Med. 1984; 310:501.
20. Chervenak FA, Hobbins JC, Wertheimer I, et al. The natural history of ventriculomegaly in a fetus without obstructive hydrocephalus. Am J Obstet Gynecol. 1985; 152:574.

21. Chervenak FA, Isaacson G, Blakemore KJ, et al. Fetal cystic hygroma: Cause and natural history. N Engl J Med. 1983; 309:822.

22. Chervenak FA, Isaacson G, Hobbins JC, et al. The diagnosis and management of fetal holoprosencephaly. Obstet Gynecol. 1985; 66:322.

23. Chervenak FA, Isaacson G, Mahoney MJ, et al. Diagnosis and management of fetal cephalocele. Obstet Gynecol. 1984; 64:86.

24. Chervenak FA, Isaacson G, Tortora M. A sonographic study of fetal cystic hygroma. J Clin Ultrasound. 1985; 5:311.

25. Chervenak FA, Jeanty P, Cantraine F, et al. The diagnosis of fetal microcephaly. Am J Obstet Gynecol. 1984; 149:512.

26. Chervenak FA, Rosenberg J, Brightman R, et al. A prospective study of the accuracy of ultrasound in predicting fetal microcephaly. Obstet Gynecol. 1984; 69:908.

27. Chervenak FA, Tortora M, Mayden K, et al. Antenatal diagnosis of median cleft face syndrome: Sonographic demonstration of cleft lip and hypertelorism. Am J Obstet Gynecol. 1984; 149:94.

28. Christ JE, Meininger MG. Ultrasound diagnosis of cleft lip and cleft palate before birth. Plast Reconstr Surg. 1981; 6:854.

29. Chudleigh P, Pearce JM, Campbell S. The prenatal diagnosis of transient cysts of the fetal choroid plexus. Prenatal Diag. 1984; 4:135.

30. Cohen HL, Haller JO. Advances in perinatal neurosonography. Am J Roentgenol. 1994; 163:801–810.

31. Cohen HL, Haller JO, Gross B. Diagnostic sonography of the fetus: A guide to evaluation of the neonate. Pediatr Ann. 1992; 21:87–99.

32. Cohen MM, Lemire RJ. Syndromes with cephaloceles. Teratology. 1982; 25:161.

33. Comstock C, Culp D, Gonzalez J, Boal D. Agenesis of the corpus callosum in the fetus: Its evolution and significance. J Ultrasound Med. 1985; 4:613–616.

34. David TJ, Nixon A. Congenital malformations associated with anencephaly and iniencephaly. J Med Genet. 1976; 13:263.

35. DeMeyer W, Zeman W. Alobar holoprosencephaly (arrhinencephaly) with median cleft lip and palate. Confin Neurol. 1963; 23:1.

36. Dobyns WB. Developmental aspects of lissencephaly and the lissencephaly syndromes birth defects. 1987; 23:225.

37. Dobyns WB, Kirkpatrick JB, Hittner HM, et al. Syndromes with lissencephaly: II. Walker-Warburg and cerebro-oculo-muscular syndromes and a new syndrome with type II lissencephaly. Am J Med Genet. 1985; 22:157.

38. Elejalde MM, Elejalde BF. Visualization of the fetal spine: A proposal of a standard to increase reliability. Am J Med Genet. 1985; 21:445.

39. Fiske CE, Filly RA, Golbus MS. Prenatal ultrasound diagnosis of amniotic band syndrome. J Ultrasound Med. 1982; 1:45.

40. Fogarty K, Cohen HL, Haller JO. Sonography of ultrasound fetal cranial hemorrhage: Unusual cases and a review of the literature. J Clin Ultrasound. 1989; 17:366–370.

41. Goldstein I, Winn HN, Hobbins JC. Prenatal diagnosis criteria for body stalk anomaly. Am J Perinatol. 1989; 6:84.

42. Greene MF, Benaceraff B, Crawford JM. Hydranencephaly: US appearance during in utero evolution. Radiology. 1985; 156:779.

43. Gupta JK, Bryce FC. Management of apparently isolated fetal ventriculomegaly. Obstet Gynecol Investigation. 1994; 49:716–721.

44. Habib Z. Genetics and genetic counselling in neonatal hydrocephalus. Obstet Gynecol Surv. 1981; 36:529.

45. Hadlock FP, Deter RL, Harrist RB, et al. Fetal biparietal diameter: Rational choice of plane of section for sonographic measurement. Am J Roentgenol. 1982; 138:871.

46. Hernanz-Schulman M, Dohan FC, Jones T, et al. Sonographic appearance of callosal agenesis: Correlation with radiologic and pathologic findings. Am J Neuroradiol. 1985; 6:361.

47. Hertzberg BS, et al. The three lines: Origin of sonographic landmarks in the fetal head. Am J Roentgenol. 1987; 149:1009.

48. Hilpert PL, Kurtz AB. Prenatal diagnosis of agenesis of the corpus callosum using endovaginal ultrasound. J Ultrasound Med. 1990; 9:363.

49. Hobbins JC, Grannum PAT, Berkowitz RL, et al. Ultrasound in the diagnosis of congenital anomalies. Am J Obstet Gynecol. 1979; 134:331.

50. Hobbins JC, Venus I, Tortora M, et al. Stage II ultrasound examination for the diagnosis of fetal abnormalities with an elevated amniotic fluid alpha-fetoprotein concentration. Am J Obstet Gynecol. 1982; 142:1026.

51. International Clearinghouse for Birth Defects Monitoring Systems. Annual Report. 1983.

52. Isaacson G, Birnhoz J. Human fetal upper respiratory tract function as revealed by ultrasonography. Ann Otol Rhinol Laryngol. 1991; 100(9 pt 1):743–747.

53. Isaacson G, Mintz MC. Prenatal sonographic visualization of the inner ear. J Ultrasound Med. 1986; 5:409.

54. Jeanty P, Dramaix-Wilmet M, Delbeke D, et al. Ultrasonic evaluation of fetal ventricular growth. Neuroradiology. 1981; 21:127.

55. Jeanty P, Dramaix-Wilmet M, Delbeke D, et al. Fetal ocular biometry by ultrasound. Radiology. 1982; 143:513.

56. Jeanty P, Romero R. Obstetrical Ultrasound. New York: McGraw-Hill; 1984:87–90.

57. Jeanty P, Romero R, Staudach A, et al. Facial anatomy of the fetus. J Ultrasound Med. 1986; 5:607.

58. Johnson ML, Dunne MG, Mack LA, et al. Evaluation of fetal intracranial anatomy by static and real-time ultrasound. J Clin Ultrasound. 1980; 8:311.

59. Kendall BE. Dysgenesis of the corpus callosum. Neuroradiology. 1983; 25:239.

60. Knutzon RK, McGahan J, Salamat M, Brant W. Fetal cisterna magna septa: A normal anatomic finding. Radiology. 1991; 180:799–801.

61. Loewry JA, Richards DG, Toi A. In-utero diagnosis of the caudal regression syndrome: Report of three cases. J Clin Ultrasound. 1987; 15:469.

62. Lorber J, Ward AM. Spina bifida: A vanishing nightmare? Arch Dis Child. 1985; 60:1086.

63. McGahan JP, Phillips HE, Ellis WG. The fetal hippocampus. Radiology. 1983; 147:201.

64. McIntosh R. The incidence of congenital malformations: A study of 5964 pregnancies. Pediatrics. 1954; 14:505.

65. Mahony BS, Nyberg DA, Hirsch JH, et al. Mild idiopathic lateral cerebral ventricular dilatation in utero: Sonographic evaluation. Radiology. 1988; 169:715–721.

66. Mayden KL, Tortora M, Berkowitz RL, et al. Orbital diameters: A new parameter for prenatal diagnosis and dating. Am J Obstet Gynecol. 1982; 144:289.

67. Monteagudo A, Reuss ML, Timor-Tritsch IE. Imaging the fetal brain in the second and third trimester using transvaginal sonography. Obstet Gynecol. 1991; 77:27–32.

68. Monteagudo A, Timor-Tritsch IE, Reuss ML, et al. Transvaginal sonography of the second- and third-trimester fetal brain. In: Timor-Tritsch IE, Rottem S, eds. Transvaginal Sonography. 2nd ed. New York: Elsevier; 1991:393–426.

69. Murken JD, Stengel-Rutkowski S, Schwinger E. Prenatal Diagnosis of Genetic Disorders. Stuttgart: Ferdinand Enke; 1979:94–192.

70. Nicolaides KM, Campbell S, Gabbe SG, et al. Ultrasound screening for spina bifida: Cranial and cerebellar signs. Lancet. 1986; 2:72.

71. Nicolaides KM, Rodeck CH, Gosden CM. Rapid karyotyping in nonlethal malformations. Lancet. 1986; 1:283.

72. Patten RM, et al. Limb-body wall complex: In utero sonographic diagnosis of a complicated fetal malformation. Am J Radiol. 1986; 146:1019.

73. Pearce JM, Little D, Campbell S. The diagnosis of abnormalities of the fetal central nervous system. In: Saunders RC, James AE, eds. The Principles and Practice of Ultrasonography in Obstetrics and Gynecology. 3rd ed. Norwalk, CT: Appleton-Century-Crofts; 1985:246–248.

74. Pilu G, DePalma L, Romero R, et al. The fetal subarachnoid cisterns: An ultrasound study with report of a case of congenital communicating hydrocephalus. J Ultrasound Med. 1986; 5:365.

75. Pretorius DH, Drose JA, Marco-Johnson ML. Fetal lateral ventricular ratio determination during the second trimester. J Ultrasound Med. 1986; 5:121.

76. Pretorius DH, Nelson TR. Fetal face visualization using three-dimensional ultrasonography. J Ultrasound Med. 1995; 14:349–356.

77. Pretorius DH, Russ PD, Rumack CM, Manco-Johnson ML. Diagnosis of brain neuropathology in utero. Neuroradiology. 1986; 28:386.

78. Reuter KL, D'Orsi CJ, Raptopoulos VD, et al. Sonographic pseudosymmetry of the prenatal cerebral hemispheres. J Ultrasound Med. 1982; 1:91.

79. Sabbagha RE, Tamura RK, Dal Campo S, et al. Fetal cranial and craniocervical masses: Ultrasound characteristics and differential diagnosis. Am J Obstet Gynecol. 1980; 138:511.

80. Shepard M, Filly RA. A standardized plane for biparietal diameter measurement. J Ultrasound Med. 1982; 1:145.

81. Smith DW. Recognizable Patterns of Human Malformation: Genetic, Embryologic and Clinical Aspects. 3rd ed. Philadelphia: WB Saunders; 1982.

82. Smith PA, Johansson D, Tzannatos C, et al. Prenatal measurement of the fetal cerebellum and cisterna cerebellomedullaris by ultrasound. Prenat Diagn. 1986; 6:133.

83. Trudinger BJ. Obstetric Doppler applications. In: Fleischer AC, et al, eds. The Principles and Practice of Ultrasonography in Obstetrics and Gynecology. 4th ed. Norwalk, CT: Appleton & Lange; 1991:171–191.

84. Van Eyck, Wladimiroff JW, Wijnigaard JAGW vd, et al. The blood flow velocity waveform in the fetal internal carotid and umbilical artery: Its relationship

to fetal behavioural states in normal pregnancy at 37–38 weeks of gestation. Br J Obstet Gynaecol. 1987; 94:736–741.

85. Warkany J. Microcephaly: Congenital Malformations. Chicago: Year Book Medical Publishers; 1971:237–244.

86. Warkany J. Congenital Malformations. Notes and Comments. Chicago: Year Book Medical Publishers; 1971:189–200.

87. Warkany J, Lemire RJ, Cohen MM. Mental Retardation and Congenital Malformations of the Central Nervous System. Chicago: Year Book Medical Publishers; 1981:101–122.

88. Wladimiroff JW, Tonge HM, Stewart PA. Doppler ultrasound assessment of cerebral blood flow in the human fetus. Br J Obstet Gynaecol. 1986; 93:471–475.

89. Wladimiroff JW, Wijnigaard JAGW vd, Degani S, et al. Cerebral and umbilical arterial blood flow velocity waveforms in normal and growth retarded pregnancies. Obstet Gynecol. 1987; 69:705–709.

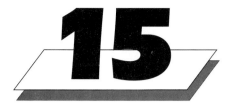

Ultrasound of the Normal Fetal Chest, Abdomen, and Pelvis

HARRIS L. COHEN, JEAN TORRISI, and JUDY SCHWARTZ

Ultrasound is the predominant imaging technique for the fetus. In the early 1970s, the diagnosis of as gross an abnormality as anencephaly was at the leading edge of sonographic capability. Real-time imaging, introduced in the late 1970s and early 1980s, allowed rapid changes in transducer positioning and angulation, enhancing fetal imaging. More recent improvements in machine and transducer hardware and software have resulted in improved contrast resolution, allowing visualization of small differences in fetal soft tissue structures, as well as improved spatial resolution, allowing improved definition of smaller fetal structures. High-resolution transducers, image memory (cineloop), as well as color Doppler and transvaginal probes have further improved fetal imaging. Improved technology, along with greater clinical experience and expertise, have allowed more sophisticated interpretations. The identification, and especially the early identification, of fetal abnormalities allows critical decisions to be made with regard to the continuation of a pregnancy or the preparation of the parents and the perinatal team for a difficult delivery or possible clinical problems during neonatal life.[13,14,35]

Knowledge of what is normal for the fetus permits recognition of variations in normal as well as the diagnosis of abnormality. In this chapter, we concentrate on the normal fetal chest, abdomen, and pelvis.

Scanning Technique and Principles

Principles for the sonographic evaluation of the fetus are to a large extent similar to those used in evaluating newborn infants. Transverse (transaxial), sagittal (longitudinal), and coronal views enhance the three-dimensional image that can be envisioned. The following are considerations that limit us imaging of the fetus.

AMNIOTIC FLUID LEVELS

An adequate amount of surrounding amniotic fluid must separate the fetus from the adjacent uterine wall, especially in the evaluation of the anterior and posterior skin surfaces of the thorax and abdomen. The fluid acts as a window for ultrasonic evaluation of internal fetal anatomy.

FETAL MOTION

Fetal position may vary from moment to moment due to movement of the fetus, particularly before the third trimester. The fetus must, typically, be evaluated while flexed within a compartment (the uterus) that is smaller than its length.

FETAL LIE

The examiner must be aware of the fetus' orientation with respect to the uterus. Various organs present different screen images depending on the fetal position and presentation.[66] Shadowing deep to bony elements makes the evaluation of some structures such as the spine easier in one position (e.g., spine up, or prone) than another (e.g., spine down, or supine). Structures deep to the transducer's focal points are seen less well than structures that fall within the focal points. Because penetration is affected by transducer frequency, this information is of particular note when using the higher-frequency (usually 5.0 to 7.5 MHz) transvaginal transducers.

Technique must be rigorous; the operator must maintain a constant vigil on fetal position and transducer position. Special techniques may be necessary to visualize adequately the fetus. These can range from subtle corrections of transducer angulation to broad shifting of transducer position on the maternal abdomen, shifting the mother's position on the table, having the mother walk about the department, or, in unusual circumstances, postponing evaluation to another day. Transvaginal and less "invasive" translabial imaging may aid in the evaluation of structures found within that portion of the fetus that is low within the maternal pelvis, at the time of ultrasound examination. These two techniques may also be used when fetal anatomic information is obscured by maternal obesity or abdominal wall scarring.[14,49]

The Thorax

The routine examination includes the thorax and its contents from the thoracic inlet at the base of the neck (the level of the clavicles) to the diaphragms separating the lung base from the abdominal contents. Transverse and longitudinal views are taken. Information to be assessed includes symmetry of the bony elements of the thorax; chest size in relation to the fetus in general and the fetal abdomen in particular; evaluation of the fetal heart; and the pulmonary echotexture and presence of the diaphragms.[27] With additional effort, smaller structures such as the fetal trachea, thyroid, and esophagus can be noted.

BONY ELEMENTS OF THE THORAX

The bony thorax consists of the clavicles, ribs, scapulae, vertebral bodies, and sternum surrounding the lungs, heart, and mediastinum. In the early stages of pregnancy, only ossified portions of the fetal skeleton are imaged directly as areas of increased echogenicity. With time, more echopenic, purely cartilaginous structures are also visualized. Knowledge of the timing of ossification center development may help in determining gestational age. Clavicular ossification is noted as early as 8 to 9 weeks, that of the ribs and scapulae at 10 to 11 weeks, and the sternum between 21 and 27 weeks.[65]

The clavicles are seen as bright echoes at the junction of the fetal neck and thorax. Their hypoplasia or complete absence (aplasia) may be noted as part of several clinical syndromes (e.g., cleidocranial dysostosis).[68] In a true transverse section the clavicles should be symmetric. Owing to their natural curvature it is difficult to image them, at all times, in their entirety,[3] especially in older fetuses. Clavicular growth is directly related to gestational age.[74]

Ribs appear as echogenic bands projecting in a fan-like pattern from the spine.[65] Their curvilinear shape makes it difficult to image large portions of several adjacent ribs (Fig. 15-1).[3] Ribs may be assessed for symmetry, and their symmetry may be used as an indication that the plane of the scan is suitable for biometric measurement (e.g., thoracic circumference). Particularly thick or thin ribs suggest abnormality (e.g., the ribs of a patient with osteogenesis imperfecta may be particularly thin).

The scapula is seen external to the ribs and surrounded by hypoechoic muscles.[3] The scapular echo, which, like that of other bones, does not correspond to the true size of the bone, is typically Y- or V-shaped, depending on the angle of insonation.[3,65]

The typical single anterior and paired posterior echoes of the ossification centers of the developing vertebral body are assessed for convergence of the posterior elements toward the nonossified spinous process (see Fig. 14-21). The posterior skin surface is evaluated to rule out the possibility of a break in the skin surface associated with myelomeningocele. The sternum is highly variable with respect to the development of its ossification centers. It is unusual to note the typical radiographic "string of beads" appearance of the normal sternal ossification cen-

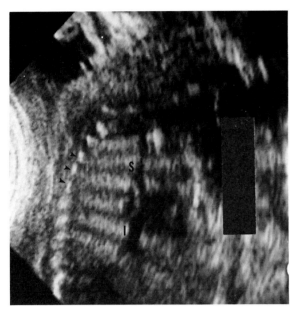

Figure 15-1. Oblique right parasagittal plane shows portions of the posterior right ribs (*arrowheads*) as echogenic densities between the heart and the thoracic periphery. Incidentally noted are the superior (S) and inferior (I) vena cavae.

ters, because this requires a coronal or coronal oblique view of the most anterior portion of the thoracic wall. These ossifications may appear as single anterior circular echoes when imaged in a transverse plane.[65]

SOFT TISSUE STRUCTURES OF THE CHEST

The muscles of the chest wall are hypoechoic and thin. They become somewhat more evident as the pregnancy progresses through the third trimester. The soft tissues may appear thick in general anasarca of the fetus or because of subcutaneous fat deposits in infants of diabetic mothers. Anterior chest wall masses consistent with fetal breasts under the influence of maternal hormone stimulation may be seen in fetuses of either sex.[22,28]

CHEST BIOMETRY

Various investigators have taken different thoracic measurements in attempts to see whether such information can be used to assess gestational age or to rule out pulmonary hypoplasia. Thoracic diameter measurements are obtained from outer edge to outer edge of the thorax on a true transverse view at the level of cardiac motion or just above the diaphragm.[40,56] Thoracic circumference measurements are taken along the outer limits of the thoracic cage at the level of the atrioventricular valve during fetal diastole. Both measurements increase as the pregnancy progresses. Kurtz and Goldberg believe the usefulness of thoracic diameter measurements in estimating gestational age is limited because of the great standard deviations noted in the accumulated biometric studies.[38] Nimrod and colleagues found a 0.87 correlation of thoracic circumference measurements with gestational age. Although this correlation is not as high as the 0.93, 0.92, and 0.95 correlations obtained with biparietal diameter, abdominal circumference, and femur length, respectively, the necessity for a useful measurement to avoid missing pulmonary hypoplasia makes such data important.[52]

Because the major components of the thorax are the heart and lungs, a significant decrease in lung volume, as would be found with pulmonary hypoplasia, should be reflected by thoracic circumference measurements that are low for the patient's predicted gestational age. Many sonologists evaluate the thoracic circumference by gestalt. A more exacting approach to evaluating a fetus for pulmonary hypoplasia would be by analyzing the thoracic to abdominal circumference (TC/AC) ratio. Cases of pulmonary hypoplasia usually have a smaller than normal ratio.[52] Certainly, a TC/AC decline over several examinations suggests a lethal pulmonary hypoplasia.[18] Chitkara and colleagues noted the TC/AC ratio to have a normal mean of 0.89, and to change little during the course of a pregnancy.[10] D'Alton and associates noted that this ratio is greater than 0.80 in almost all normal pregnancies.[25] Not all low TC/AC ratios are caused by pulmonary hypoplasia. A low ratio may be the result of a small thorax, which may be associated with various skeletal dysplasias. A normal thoracic circumference also may be maintained in spite of pulmonary hypoplasia, if there are associated large pleural effusions or a diaphragmatic hernia maintaining intrathoracic space and hence TC.[25] Sonographic correlation of biometric measurements with the actual intrathoracic image is absolutely necessary for proper diagnosis. As a good rule of thumb in assessing the intrathoracic contents, at the level of the atrioventricular valves, a transverse view of the chest should show the heart as occupying about one third of the cross-sectional area of the thorax.[3] In the transverse view, if the heart appears to occupy more than its share of the thorax, pulmonary hypoplasia must be considered, as well as the more obvious possibility of cardiomegaly.

THE LUNG

During fetal life, the deflated lungs appear as solid, space-occupying masses between the heart and ribs.[58] On a transverse view of the thorax the lungs are typically echogenic, with few, if any, breaks in the homogeneity of this pattern (Fig. 15-2). Each lung may be compared to its counterpart. Longitudinal or coronal views allow the echogenicity of the lungs to be compared with that of the liver or spleen. The lungs are separated from these abdominal organs by the thin, smooth, hypoechoic diaphragm.[3,27] Early in gestation, lung echogenicity is equal to or slightly less than that of the liver. As the gestation progresses, lung echogenicity increases until it is greater than that of the liver (Fig. 15-3).[27] Some investigators claim that the lungs are always more echogenic than the liver.[66] Several authors have debated the use of fetal lung echogenicity patterns and the lungs' acoustic transmission and compressibility to assess lung maturity

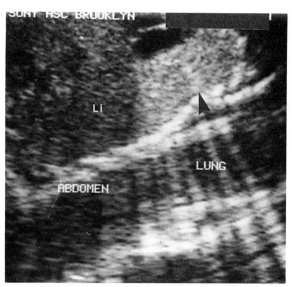

Figure 15-3. Coronal plane, right-side view of the normal chest and abdomen. The right lung is highly echogenic (*arrowhead*) compared to the subdiaphragmatic liver (Li).

and thereby avoid amniocentesis for biochemical analysis for fetal lung maturity. In theory, enhanced acoustic transmission and increased echogenicity, based on the known increase in lung fluid and the significant increase in the number of alveolar and terminal lung units that develop as a pregnancy progresses, most particularly between weeks 32 and 40, as well as the transformation of the alveolar cell lining from columnar to cuboidal, might aid in denoting lung maturity.[8] However, theory is not always clinical reality. The determination of fetal lung maturity is a crucial consideration in managing certain difficult pregnancies.[23] Current state-of-the-art technology as well as current imaging experience has shown that diagnostic ultrasonography cannot reliably indicate fetal lung maturity. Biochemical measurements of the lecithin–sphingomyelin ratio (ratios of 2.0 or greater are considered indicative of pulmonary maturity) and the presence of phosphatidyl glycerol remain the gold standard for the determination of fetal lung maturity.[7,8,23] Biparietal diameter measurements and placental grading have also proven unreliable for determining fetal lung maturity.[33]

THE DIAPHRAGM

The diaphragm (Fig. 15-4), noted as a thin hypoechoic band, was reliably imaged in only 3% of a group of normal 14-week fetuses evaluated in a

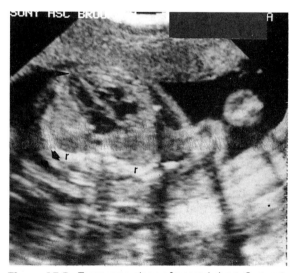

Figure 15-2. Transverse plane of normal chest. Symmetric homogeneous echogenicity of the lungs surrounds the echo-free cardiac chambers. The cardiac apex (*arrowhead*) points to the left side of this fetus in vertex presentation. Note the relatively symmetric posterior ribs (r) and the hypoechoic thoracic muscles (*arrows*).

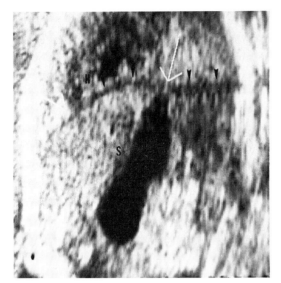

Figure 15-4. Left parasagittal view of chest, abdomen, and diaphragm. Arrowheads point to the hypoechoic band separating the thorax from the abdomen. Anteriorly is the heart (H) and posteriorly, the echo-free, fluid-filled stomach (S).

1988 study by Zador and colleagues. This percentage increased to 43% among fetuses of 20 weeks' gestation, and was as high as 81% in fetuses of 35 weeks' gestation.[75] It is possible that these percentages might vary if a study with more modern technology or one using transvaginal techniques in the younger fetal population were performed today. Imaging a diaphragm can help differentiate cystic intrathoracic masses of pulmonary origin from those that are of intraabdominal origin. However, as with all curved structures, even when the fetus is positioned optimally, the entire structure may not be visualized and small defects may be imagined or missed.

The Abdomen

By the beginning of the second trimester, the abdominal organs have attained their normal adult position and structure.[27] The liver, kidneys, and adrenal glands are readily identifiable. The echo-free fluid filling the gallbladder and stomach and the echo-free blood filling large vessels make them readily distinguishable. Visualization of the spleen is more variable, and the pancreas is seen far less often. Collapsed small bowel and, in the third tri-

mester, fluid or meconiumm-filled colon are often seen.

Examination of the abdomen is performed by transverse, coronal, and sagittal imaging of the fetus as a unit and, with proper angulation, its individual organs. Transverse views throughout the levels of the spine are evaluated for posterior elements that are parallel to each other or that meet centrally instead of diverging. The presence of an intact skin surface overlying the individual vertebral bodies is a helpful secondary sign to rule out myelomeningocele. Obviously, sufficient surrounding amniotic fluid and some distance from the uterine wall surface is needed to image any skin surface adequately. Images are usually recorded of a transverse view of the upper abdomen for abdominal circumference measurements. This view usually allows adequate images of the stomach and liver, as well as other nearby organs and structures. A more caudad transverse view is obtained to confirm the presence of two kidneys and to evaluate their anatomy. A sagittal view of the thorax, abdomen, and (usually) pelvis allows evaluation of the relative size of the thorax and abdomen as well as the relation of umbilical vessel entry to the anterior abdominal wall (Fig. 15-5). Umbilical vessel entry can also be readily noted on a transverse section of the abdomen taken at the level of the umbilicus. On both transverse and longitudinal–coronal views, the abdomen and its contents are checked for congenital abnormalities.

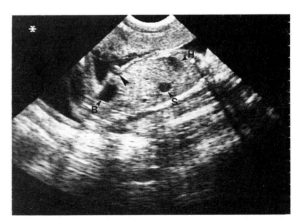

Figure 15-5. Left parasagittal plane view of normal anterior abdominal wall. The fetus is facing toward the left of the page. Evident are the echo-free heart (H), stomach (S), and bladder (B). Umbilical vessel entry is noted in the lower anterior abdominal wall (*large arrowhead*).

An optimal study should also include images through the orthogonal sagittal planes, as well. These views allow further evaluation of the fetal body surface and allow further observer orientation of the contained fetal structures. Sagittal views in right and left paramedian planes through the thorax and abdomen allow further comparison and evaluation of fetal lung and liver. Left parasagittal views denote the stomach, as well. Midline sagittal images allow evaluation of the umbilicus in relation to the fetal anterior abdominal wall. The umbilical vein can be followed in its course from the anterior abdominal wall into the liver's left portal vein (LPV).[64]

Transverse and, to a lesser extent, sagittal views can help determine the relationship of the abdominal organs (abdominal situs) to the intrathoracic organs, in particular, the position of the fetal heart and its apex. There is a 40% incidence of anomalies, particularly significant cardiac abnormalities, among fetuses and children with partial situs inversus (i.e., with their cardiac apex on the opposite side of the body from the fetal stomach). Mirror imaging of the thoracic and abdominal contents, also known as situs inversus totalis (e.g., with the heart in the right side of the thorax and the abdominal organs transposed, with the spleen and stomach on the right and the liver and gallbladder on the left side), has only a minimal increased incidence of abnormalities. It therefore is important to determine the arrangement of these structures in the fetus. When in cephalic presentation, a fetus with normal abdominal situs should have its spine, stomach, and umbilical vein imaged in a clockwise manner on a transverse image. These structures would be in a counterclockwise arrangement when imaged on a transverse view of a fetus in breech presentation. This information may be difficult to determine when a fetus is not well imaged or in transverse or indeterminate lie. A simple method of determining if there is situs inversus, in such cases, is to image the cardiac apex on transverse view and note if the stomach is on the same side as the apex when the transducer is angled toward the fetus' caudal structures. If it is, the situs is normal or, at the very least, there is situs inversus totalis, which, again, is cause for far less worry than partial situs inversus.[54]

As with the thorax, anatomic evaluation of the abdomen depends on fetal position, fetal flexion, and an adequate amount of surrounding amniotic fluid.[35] Significant maternal body fat limits evaluation.

ABDOMINAL SOFT TISSUES

Abdominal wall muscles are hypoechoic. Occasionally thin echogenic lines may be seen that represent fascial planes between the three main muscle groups, the internal oblique, transverse abdominal, and external oblique.[3] The echogenic skin line, highlighted by good sound transmission through surrounding amniotic fluid and the deeper hypoechoic muscle, may result in what Rosenthal and colleagues have described as the "pseudoascites sign" (see Fig. 24-12).[60]

UMBILICAL CORD AND ABDOMINAL VASCULATURE

A major difference between fetal and adult abdominal anatomy is the presence of patent umbilical vessels and ductus venosus acting as a conduit between the portal and systemic veins.[27]

The allantois, a caudal outpouching of the yolk sac that is not visible sonographically, is involved in early blood production. Its blood vessels become the umbilical artery and veins.[27,50] The umbilical

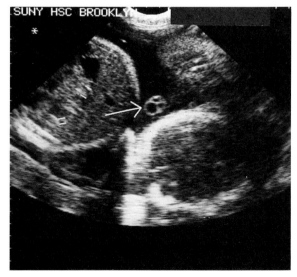

Figure 15-6. On transverse section, an arrow points to a normal umbilical cord. The two smaller umbilical arteries and the larger umbilical vein assume a mask-like or "Mr. Bill" configuration.

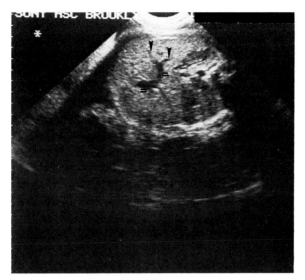

Figure 15-7. *Transverse oblique plane view of umbilical vein entry into left portal vein. The intrahepatic portion of the umbilical vein (U) is seen in its anteroposterior course to the portal venous system (P), running in a medial-lateral direction. The right portal vein bifurcation is marked by arrowheads.*

cord (Fig. 15-6) consists of two umbilical arteries with a mean width of 2.4 mm and one umbilical vein with a mean width of 8 mm. In 1% of pregnancies, the right umbilical artery regresses or does not form, and there is a single umbilical artery. Usually this is not significant, but it has been associated by various authors with an increased incidence of trisomy, low birth weight, twins, offspring of diabetic mothers, and stillborns.[36,37,51]

The thin-walled single umbilical vein enters the anterior abdomen, taking a cephalad oblique course, without branching, and enters the LPV (Fig. 15-7). Some fetal blood flows from the LPV into the narrow channel of the ductus venosus, bypassing the liver and entering the systemic venous system by the left hepatic vein or inferior vena cava, but, more typically, it flows medially into the right portal vein, perfusing the liver. Within 2 weeks after birth, the ductus venosus closes and is seen as an echogenic line in the fissure of the ligamentum venosum between the left and the caudate lobes.[9,27]

The two umbilical arteries, which carry most of the fetal aortic blood to the placenta, can be followed caudad from the anterior abdominal wall cord insertion site to the internal iliac arteries, which are just lateral to the bladder. The vessels can be followed to their origin at the iliac artery bifurcation. The abdominal aorta can often be seen throughout its course and is often an aid in noting the expected position of the kidneys on coronal views.[9,27,61,64]

BIOMETRY IN THE NORMAL ABDOMEN

The abdominal circumference has proved to be a key and accurate measurement in the evaluation of gestational age and fetal weight and in ruling out asymmetric growth retardation with its associated liver glycogen depletion and decreased liver size.[19,32,38] Its importance requires correct measurement. A true axial view of the abdomen is obtained at the level of umbilical cord entry into the LPV. Measurements are made along the outer perimeter of the abdomen. Indications of proper positioning include a circular abdominal outline, equidistant left- and right-side rib echoes, and visualization of the three ossification centers of the vertebral body (Fig. 15-8). A long segment of the intrahepatic portion of the umbilical vein, especially if it extends anteriorly, suggests an oblique rather than a true axial view. Angulated views that include lung are not acceptable. Shadowing from long bones, elliptical outlines due to myometrial contraction, and decreased amniotic fluid levels limit measure-

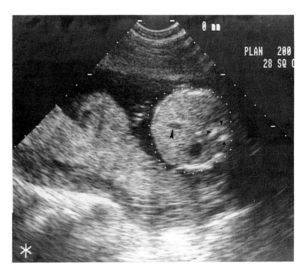

Figure 15-8. *Abdominal circumference is imaged in the transverse plane. A short segment of the intrahepatic portion of the umbilical vein (large arrowhead), the echo-free stomach, and the vertebral body ossification centers (small arrowheads) are seen. The ribs are equidistant.*

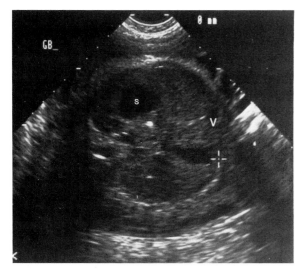

Figure 15-9. Transverse oblique plane shows the teardrop-shaped gallbladder to the right of the midline intrahepatic umbilical vein (V), stomach (S).

ment.[3,38,64] Abdominal circumference measurements are known to vary according to gender (males larger than females) and racial group (Europeans 30% larger than Asian Indians) and among offspring of diabetics, who have greater amounts of abdominal wall soft tissue.[47,55] To assess abdominal circumference measurements properly, therefore, the clinician must know his or her own clinical population.

LIVER, GALLBLADDER, PANCREAS, AND SPLEEN

The fetal liver is a large, homogeneously echogenic organ occupying the right upper quadrant and crossing midline to the left. It represents 10% of a fetus' weight at 11 weeks' gestation and represents 5% of the weight of the fetus at term.[27] Whereas in an adult the right lobe is much larger than the left lobe (ratio, 6:1), in the fetus the left lobe is as large as—and in fact slightly larger than—the right, possibly because it receives a greater percentage of oxygenated blood.[36] This may make it difficult to determine which side of the body is being imaged unless the fluid-filled, left-sided stomach is visible. The liver grows throughout pregnancy. Gross and coworkers describe a transverse ratio of the portion of the fetal liver that lies to the left of the umbilical part of the LPV to the portion that lies to the right

as 1.04 (range, 0.78 to 1.3). This ratio remains unchanged throughout gestation, even in the presence of intrauterine growth retardation.[31,38,70]

The gallbladder (Fig. 15-9), in its position to the right of midline, separates the right lobe from the medial left lobe, as does the middle hepatic vein. The fluid-filled gallbladder may appear similar to the tubular intrahepatic portion of the umbilical vein. Key differentiating points are the gallbladder's usually teardrop shape, its off-midline, rather than midline position, its extrahepatic location (posteroinferior to the liver), and the lack of communication between the gallbladder and vessels of the umbilical cord. Unlike the umbilical vein, the gallbladder does not reach the anterior abdominal wall.[3] The gallbladder is passive in fetal life and does not respond to fat ingested by the mother.[27] The fetal gallbladder was imaged in 84% of one studied group of 70 patients.[72] Absence of the gallbladder may be associated with several conditions, including biliary atresia.

The pancreas is rarely discretely imaged. Its echogenicity is similar to that of surrounding structures. Occasionally the fluid-filled stomach and the location of the pancreas anterior to the splenic vein may aid in its identification. Fetal pancreatic echogenicity is said to be slightly greater than that of the liver.[36]

The spleen is a well circumscribed, homoge-

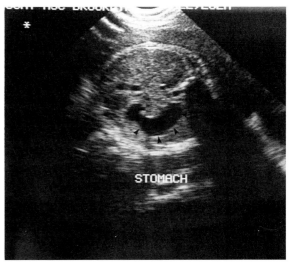

Figure 15-10. A more longitudinal view of the fluid-filled stomach is seen in this transverse plane of a normal fetus (*arrowheads*).

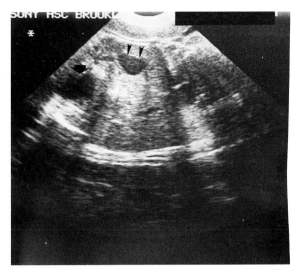

Figure 15-11. Gastric pseudomass is demonstrated in left parasagittal plane. Echoes fill the stomach (*arrowheads*). They were not seen on follow-up examination. The echo-free urine in the bladder (*arrow*) is seen inferiorly.

neous mass in the left upper abdomen. It can be seen at 18 weeks' gestation and thereafter.[27] We agree with Kurtz that it may be difficult to delineate in the absence of ascites. Landmarks used to identify it are the left hemidiaphragm and spine; the fluid-filled, usually anterior, stomach is the most consistent.[38] Best seen on transverse scans, the spleen is similar in echogenicity to the kidney and slightly less echogenic than the liver. Its size increases with the volume, reported as increasing approximately 18-fold during gestation.[62]

STOMACH AND BOWEL

The stomach (Fig. 15-10) should be imaged consistently in the second trimester. Occasionally, it is not visualized in normal fetuses in the early weeks of the trimester. However, absence of an imaged stomach after 18 weeks' gestation is associated with an abnormal outcome in 48% to 100% of cases.[42,48]

Typically, the stomach is filled with variable amounts of echo-free fluid.[3] Wladimiroff and colleagues have reported filling times of up to 45 minutes and emptying times that vary from a few minutes to (rarely) 30 minutes.[73] The stomach, if present, should therefore be seen at some point during a 60-minute examination. Filling volumes increase during the pregnancy: 1 ml is the mean at

20 weeks, 5 ml at 30 weeks, and 8 ml at 35 weeks. Volumes as great as 22 ml have been noted in a normal, nonobstructed stomach of a 35-week fetus.[69]

Echogenicity within the stomach fluid has been seen in cases of third-trimester placental abruption; this represents swallowed blood.[71] We have often seen what Fakhry and coworkers labeled a fetal gastric pseudomass (Fig. 15-11). Seen in 1% of a series of their cases, this idiopathic echogenicity within the stomach fluid, which is commonly seen in the second trimester and disappears on follow-up examination, may be caused by aggregates of swallowed cells and cell fragments. This seems logical, in that particles can be seen in normal amniotic fluid as early as week 16.[21] The stomach grows linearly during gestation in transverse, longitudinal, and anteroposterior planes.[26]

Early in gestation, small bowel normally herniates into the base of the umbilical cord as the bowel grows beyond abdominal capacity and undergoes part of its normal rotation about the superior mesenteric artery. Bowerman noted this normal temporary midgut herniation in the transabdominal images of all fetuses of 38 mm or less crown–rump length and two of six fetuses with a crown–rump length between 40 and 42 mm. The cord containing the normally herniated midgut can increase to a maximal dimension of 7 mm.[4] By week 14,

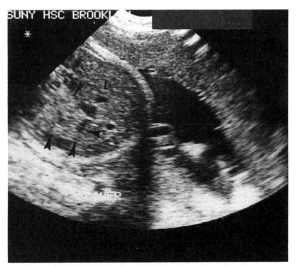

Figure 15-12. Transverse oblique plane view shows an echogenic pseudomass of collapsed small bowel (*arrowheads*) posterior and inferior to the liver (L).

this normal herniation has been reduced, and it is from 14 weeks on that pathologic abdominal wall defects may be definitively diagnosed.[17] Before significant amounts of fluid enter it, the small bowel appears as an echogenic pseudomass (Fig. 15-12), without shadowing, occupying a substantial portion of the abdomen. By 26 weeks this mass becomes less echogenic and sharply defined. By 29 to 30 weeks, the rate of fetal swallowing has overcome the resorptive capacity of stomach and proximal duodenum, allowing filling of distal small bowel and disappearance of the pseudomass.[46] Peristalsis may be seen in the small bowel that occupies the central abdomen. Normal fetal small bowel increases in diameter as gestational age increases. Normal small bowel diameter rarely exceeds 6 mm.[53,57] Nyberg and colleagues reported that no segment of imaged small bowel should be greater than 15 mm long.[53]

The colon is a long, continuous, tubular structure at the abdominal periphery (Fig. 15-13). Although it may be seen as early as 22 weeks, it is typically seen at 28 weeks and later. Nyberg and coworkers examined the colons of 130 fetuses and found linear increases in diameter throughout the third trimester. There is a maximal diameter of 23 mm at term for normal colon.[57] No peristalsis is seen. Meconium, which is less echogenic than

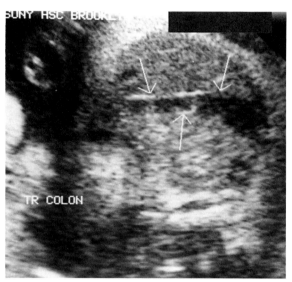

Figure 15-14. On this transverse oblique plane, arrows point to the fluid-filled transverse colon inferior to the liver.

bowel wall, may be routinely noted in discrete portions of colon. Transverse colon (Fig. 15-14) is seen most easily just caudad to the liver.[53] By the third trimester, normal bowel was seen in at least 80% of Zador and colleagues' 2389 examinations.[75]

KIDNEYS AND ADRENALS

The fetal kidneys can be seen as early as the 15th week after the last menstrual period. Most may be routinely imaged between weeks 17 and 22. Identification of the kidneys early in gestation is limited by the lack of significant contrast between the kidneys and the nearby soft tissues. This situation has been said to improve with the deposition of echogenic perirenal fat by the third trimesters.[12] Improvements in ultrasonographic equipment, particularly transducers, and increasing clinical experience are probably the key causes for improved fetal kidney visualization.[15]

On transverse images (Fig. 15-15), the kidneys are hypoechoic, ovoid masses on either side of the spine. The echogenic center of renal sinus fat is noted more consistently later in pregnancy. Grannum and colleagues have noted that the ratio of kidney circumference to abdominal circumference remains approximately 0.3 throughout pregnancy.[29,39]

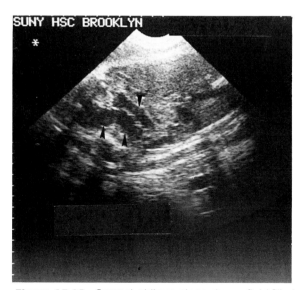

Figure 15-13. Coronal oblique plane shows fluid-filled normal colon (*arrowheads*), representing descending colon and sigmoid, at the abdominal periphery.

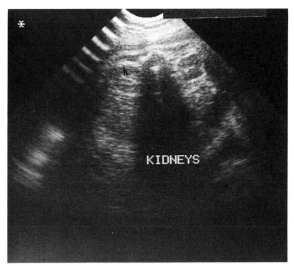

Figure 15-15. Echopenic normal kidneys (k, right kidney) flank the spine of this prone fetus (transverse plane view). Echogenicity at the center of the kidney is consistent with renal sinus fat. The echogenicity at the kidney periphery is consistent with perirenal fat.

Parasagittal views of each kidney show them to be paraspinous and bean-shaped. As in neonates, the normal hypoechoic renal pyramids (Fig. 15-16) may be seen arranged in anterior and posterior rows around the renal pelvis. They should not be mis-

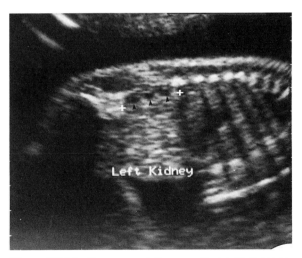

Figure 15-16. Crosses mark the superior and inferior extent of the kidney viewed in the left parasagittal plane. Echopenic pyramids (*arrowheads*) are noted along the posterior aspect of the kidney, the side closest to the transducer. In many cases, both the anterior and posterior row of pyramids can be visualized.

taken for renal cysts. Bertagnoli and colleagues, reporting on fetal renal lengths, found them to average about a millimeter per week of gestation. They noted average renal lengths of 3.0 cm at 32 weeks and 3.8 cm at 40 weeks. Our own reported measurements, but particularly our range of normal measurements for various gestational ages, are greater (Table 15-1).[1,15,43] This information would be of little clinical significance except for the fact that enlarged kidneys may be the first evidence of infantile (recessive) polycystic kidney disease and may be noted before imaging their associated increased echogenicity. Use of our wider range of normal measurements, which, compared to previous reports, are in greater agreement with measurements of the kidneys of neonates of equivalent age, can assuage clinical fears of polycystic kidney disease when a fetus is noted to have a somewhat prominent kidney of normal echogenicity.[15] Certainly,

TABLE 15-1. MEAN RENAL LENGTHS FOR VARIOUS GESTATIONAL AGES

Gestational Age (wk)	Mean Length (cm)	95% Confidence Interval (cm)
18	2.2	1.6–2.8
19	2.3	1.5–3.1
20	2.6	1.8–3.4
21	2.7	2.1–3.2
22	2.7	2.0–3.4
23	3	2.2–3.7
24	3.1	1.9–4.4
25	3.3	2.5–4.2
26	3.4	2.4–4.4
27	3.5	2.7–4.4
28	3.4	2.6–4.2
29	3.6	2.3–4.8
30	3.8	2.9–4.6
31	3.7	2.8–4.6
32	4.1	3.1–5.1
33	4	3.3–4.7
34	4.2	3.3–5.0
35	4.2	3.2–5.2
36	4.2	3.3–5.0
37	4.2	3.3–5.1
38	4.4	3.2–5.6
39	4.2	3.5–4.8
40	4.3	3.2–5.3
41	4.5	3.9–5.1

(Adapted from Cohen HL, Cooper J, Eisenberg P: Normal length of fetal kidneys: Sonographic study in 397 obstetric patients. Am J Roentgenol. 1991; 157:545–548.)

with continued clinical concern, follow-up examinations always help.

In one report, the contralateral kidneys of fetuses with nonfunctioning multicystic dysplastic kidneys were noted to undergo the phenomenon of compensatory hypertrophy. This has been a well-known growth phenomenon noted in the kidneys of children and at least younger adults, in which when one kidney is damaged or surgically removed, the remaining kidney grows to a greater degree to, in a sense, "compensate" for the absence of the contralateral kidney.[24]

The renal pelvis is typically collapsed (i.e., not urine filled) and therefore is not imaged. If filled with urine, an echo-free renal pelvis is noted. This renal pelvic dilatation is often evaluated by noting its anterior-to-posterior measurement. Grignon and associates reported fetuses with dilatations greater than 1 cm as being at risk for urinary abnormality requiring surgical correction 50% of the time. They considered pyelocalyceal dilatation of less than 1 cm to be physiologic.[12,30] There is some debate as to how worrisome it is and how closely fetuses with pyelocalyceal dilatation less than 1 cm in anteroposterior measurement should be monitored. This dilatation may be related to transient fetal urinary reflux or obstruction of pelvic urine outflow from a fluid-filled fetal bladder. Corteville and colleagues reported a greater degree of abnormal kidneys requiring corrective surgery in children with pyelocalyceal dilatation less than 1 cm. They suggest following, and we do follow fetuses with anteroposterior measurements as small as 4 mm if they are younger than 33 weeks' gestation, and as small as 7 mm if they are 33 weeks or older.[16,45] In cases without changing clinical conditions, we do follow-up examinations at no earlier than 4- to 6-week intervals. We obviously worry less if there is good bladder filling (evidence of at least one functioning and nonobstructed renal system) and normal amounts of amniotic fluid. Of key importance is the evaluation of this fetus and its kidneys when it is a neonate. This is best performed at day 2 or 3 of life. The fetal ureters are not normally visualized unless there is significant genitourinary system reflux or obstruction.

The adrenals are ovoid, triangular, or heart-shaped masses that are often imaged in the suprarenal area of the fetus. We have imaged the adrenals as early as the late first/early second trimester. They are easiest to note in relation to the kidney on longitudinal images. Lewis and colleagues reported being able readily to image the adrenal gland as separate from the adjacent renal parenchyma, as early as 1982. Certainly, if a fetus is positioned with its side up, evaluation of the side that is more distant from the transducer may be more difficult.[41]

On transverse view, the adrenals may appear reniform. This is particularly true in association with ipsilateral renal agenesis. There is an echogenic central medulla and a hypoechoic, thick outer cortex. Histopathologically the cortex is composed of a thick inner "fetal zone" and a thin outer permanent cortex (Fig. 15-17). The "fetal" portion of the adrenal is the portion that may be involved in adrenal hemorrhage. The fetal zone contributes to the adrenal gland reported as being proportionately 20 times the size of the adult adrenal. This fetal zone atrophies within the first 3 to 12 months of life.[59]

Although typically suprarenal in fetal life, by childhood the adrenal attains its more anterior and medial position in relation to the kidney.[11] The high retroperitoneal position of the adrenals can limit their imaging owing to obscuration from rib shadowing. Ratios of adrenal length to renal length have been reported as between 0.48 and 0.66.[38] Our work suggests that this ratio may be somewhat

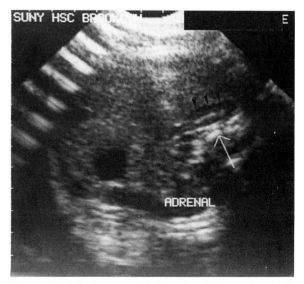

Figure 15-17. *A normal right adrenal (*arrowheads*) is seen to the side of the spine in a transverse oblique plane view. Note the echogenic central medulla and the hypoechoic periphery. (*White arrow *points to area of adrenal.)*

lower. The adrenals increase in size during pregnancy.[34,42] Human chorionic gonadotropin contributes to adrenal growth in the first half of pregnancy; thereafter adrenocorticotropic hormone controls adrenal growth.[43]

The Pelvis

The pelvis is a small structure in the fetus. Its sonographic image is made up predominantly of the bones of the pelvis, the pelvic muscles, and the bladder. The bony pelvis consists of echogenic iliac crests separated from the echogenic sacrum by the echopenic sacroiliac joint. Three ossification centers are noted along the sacrum. Although, as in the craniocervical region, there is some soft tissue prominence noted as hypoechoic density between skin and spine in the lumbosacral region, masses should not be seen. The hypoechoic gluteal muscles may be separated by thin fascial lines. The ischium and pubis are noted as echogenic anterior densities, and often the echogenic nonossified femoral head can be seen at the acetabular area.[3]

The bladder (Fig. 15-18) is seen as an echofree intrapelvic mass by 15 weeks' gestational age. It is circular to oblong in shape. Wall thickness cannot be appreciated in the normal bladder with-

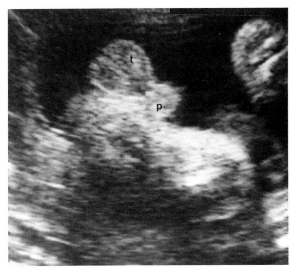

Figure 15-19. Coronal view of male genitalia. The penis (p) is seen in cross section. Echogenicity within the scrotum represents testes (t).

out the presence of ascites. It is a dynamic structure whose size varies with the degree of filling. At 32 weeks, the bladder's capacity is 10 ml, filling at the rate of 10 to 12 ml per hour. By week 40, capacity increases to 40 ml, filling at 27 ml per hour. The fetus voids about once per hour.[6] If the bladder fills, at least one functioning kidney is present. If no bladder is seen on examination, a repeat examination is performed. If necessary, the fetus may be challenged by injecting the mother intravenously with furosemide, which should induce diuresis within 15 to 45 minutes.[44] Occasionally the bladder may appear distended when there is no pathologic process. Waiting allows one to prove when the bladder empties. When distended, normally or pathologically, the bladder rises out of the narrow pelvis and into the upper abdomen.[12]

GENITALS

The identification of fetal genitalia requires adequate visualization of the perineum. A crossed thigh can readily hide a scrotum. Differences in genitalia are not very prominent before week 16.[12] In Elejalde and colleagues' work and literature review, the reported 3% error rate in gender identification occurred when gender assignment was made before the 24th week. His group identified the genitalia in 100% of cases after 20 weeks. This is not the

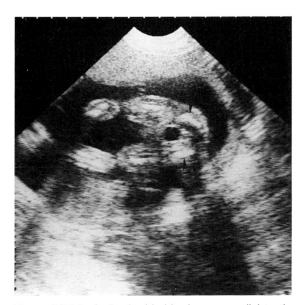

Figure 15-18. A circular bladder is seen medial to the echogenic iliac bones (*arrowheads*) of the pelvis in this coronal view.

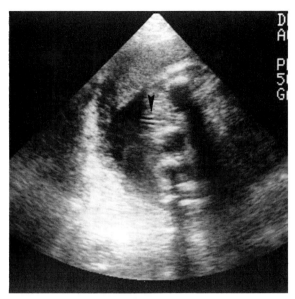

Figure 15-20. Coronal view of female genitalia. A central echogenic line represents the labia minora. To their side are the labia majora (*arrowhead,* right labia majora). The thighs are seen to a small extent, laterally.

universal experience. Of 3891 examinations reported in the literature, genitalia could not be visualized in 30%.[20] Birnholz reported a 3.3% error rate in gender assignment in fetuses before 24 weeks, and an overall error rate of 1.7%.[2]

Gender identification is of key clinical interest in diagnosing male fetuses affected by severe X-linked inherited disorders such as hemophilia or Duchenne's muscular dystrophy. Proof of different genitalia in twins can help prove dizygosity and rule out twin-to-twin transfusion syndrome and other problems associated with monozygotic twins. Rare intersex problems may be diagnosed if there is a discrepancy in karyotype gender from visualized genitals (e.g., testicular feminization syndrome, in which a fetus has a male karyotype and female genitalia).[12,43,67]

In the male fetus, the penis and scrotum (Fig. 15-19) are readily visualized between the thighs. On coronal or transverse views of the pelvis, the sonographer must be aware of the possibility of a nearby umbilical cord simulating a penis. Voiding into the amniotic fluid may be seen. Erections are not unusual. After 32 weeks, 93% of testicles have descended into the scrotum and are noted as echogenic masses.[2,12,63]

In female fetuses (Fig. 15-20), the labia majora are noted as masses of moderate echogenicity off the perineum. A central linear echogenicity between them represents the labia minora. The normal ovaries, uterus, and vagina are not typically visualized in a normal fetus.[12,20]

REFERENCES

1. Bertagnoli L, Lalatta F, Gallicchio R, et al. Quantitative characterization of the growth of the fetal kidney. J Clin Ultrasound. 1983; 11:349–356.
2. Birnholz J. Determination of fetal sex. N Engl J Med. 1983; 309:942–944.
3. Bowerman R. Thorax. In: Bowerman R, ed. Atlas of Normal Fetal Ultrasonographic Anatomy. Chicago: Year Book Medical Publishers: 1986.
4. Bowerman R. Sonography of fetal midgut herniation: Normal size criteria and correlation with crown rump length. J Ultrasound Med. 1993; 5:251–254.
5. Bowie J, Rosenberg E, Andreotti R, et al. The changing sonographic appearance of fetal kidneys during pregnancy. J Ultrasound Med. 1983; 2:505–507.
6. Campbell S, Wladimoroff J, Dewhurst C. The antenatal measurement of urine production. Journal of Obstetrics and Gynaecology of the British Commonwealth. 1973; 80:680–686.
7. Carson P, Meyer C, Bowerman R. Prediction of fetal lung maturity with ultrasound. Radiology. 1985; 155:533.
8. Cayea P, Grant D, Doubilet P, et al. Prediction of fetal lung maturity: Inaccuracies of study using conventional ultrasound instruments. Radiology. 1985; 155:473–475.
9. Chinn D, Filly R, Callen P. Ultrasonic evaluation of fetal umbilical and hepatic vascular anatomy. Radiology. 1982; 44:153–157.
10. Chitkara U, Rosenberg J, Chervenak F, et al. Prenatal sonographic assessment of the fetal thorax: Normal values. Am J Obstet Gynecol. 1987; 156:1069–1074.
11. Co C, Filly R. Normal fetal adrenal gland location. (Letter). J Ultrasound Med. 1986; 5:117.
12. Cohen H, Haller J. Diagnostic sonography of the fetal genitourinary tract. Urol Radiol. 1987; 9:88–98.
13. Cohen HL, Haller JO, Gross BR. Diagnostic sonography of the fetus: A guide to the evaluation of the neonate. Pediatr Ann. 1992; 21:87–89.
14. Cohen HL, Haller JO. Advances in perinatal neurosonography. Am J Roentgenol. 1994; 163:801–810.

15. Cohen HL, Cooper J, Eisenberg P, et al. Normal length of fetal kidneys: Sonographic study of 397 obstetric patients. Am J Roentgenol. 1991; 157: 545–548.

16. Corteville J, Gray D, Crane J. Congenital hydronephrosis: Correlation of fetal ultrasonographic findings with infant outcome. Am J Obstet Gynecol. 1991; 165:384–388.

17. Cyr D, Mack L, Schoenecker SA, et al. Bowel migration in the normal fetus: US detection. Radiology. 1986; 161:119–121.

18. D'Alton M, Mercer B, Riddick E, Dudley D. Serial thoracic versus abdominal circumference ratios for the prediction of pulmonary hypoplasia in premature rupture of the membranes remote from term. Am J Obstet Gynecol. 1992; 166:658–663.

19. Deter R, Harrist R, Hadlock F, et al. Fetal head and abdominal circumferences: I. Evaluation of measurement errors. J Clin Ultrasound. 1982; 10:357–363.

20. Elejalde B, de Elejalde M, Heitman T. Visualization of the fetal genitalia by ultrasonography: A review of the literature and analysis of its accuracy and ethical implications. J Ultrasound Med. 1985; 4:633–639.

21. Fakhry J, Shapiro L, Schechter A. Fetal gastric pseudomass. J Ultrasound Med. 1987; 6:177–180.

22. Fleischer A, Killam A, Boehm F, et al. Hydrops fetalis: Sonographic evaluations and clinical implications. Radiology. 1981; 141:163–168.

23. Fried A, Loh F, Umer M, et al. Echogenicity of fetal lung: Relation to fetal age and maturity. Am J Roentgenol. 1985; 145:591–594.

24. Glazebrook K, McGrath F, Steele B. Prenatal compensatory renal growth: Documentation with US. Radiology. 1993; 189:733–735.

25. Goldstein R. Ultrasound evaluation of the fetal thorax. In: Callen P, ed. Ultrasonography in Obstetrics and Gynecology. 3rd ed. Philadelphia: WB Saunders: 1994.

26. Goldstein I, Reece E, Yarkoni S, et al. Growth of the fetal stomach in normal pregnancies. Obstet Gynecol. 1987; 70:641–644.

27. Goldstein R, Callen P. Ultrasound evaluation of the fetal thorax and abdomen. In: Callen P, ed. Ultrasonography in Obstetrics and Gynecology. 2nd ed. Philadelphia: WB Saunders: 1988:207–239.

28. Graham D, Sanders R. Sonographic evaluation of the fetal chest. In: Sanders R, James A Jr, eds. The Principles and Practice of Ultrasonography in Obstetrics and Gynecology. 3rd ed. East Norwalk, CT: Appleton-Century-Crofts; 1985:219–228.

29. Grannum P, Bracken M, Silverman R, et al. Assessment of fetal kidney size in normal gestation by comparison of ratio of kidney circumference to abdominal circumference. Am J Obstet Gynecol. 1980; 136:249–254.

30. Grignon A, Filion R, Filiatrault D, et al. Urinary tract dilatation in utero: Classification and clinical applications. Radiology. 1986; 160:645–647.

31. Gross B, Harter L, Filly R. Disproportionate left hepatic lobe size in the fetus. J Ultrasound Med. 1982; 1:79–81.

32. Hadlock F, Deter R, Harrist R, et al. Fetal abdominal circumference as a predictor of menstrual age. Am J Roentgenol. 1982; 1339:367–370.

33. Hadlock F, Irwin J, Roecker E. Ultrasound prediction of fetal lung maturity. Radiology. 1985; 155:469–472.

34. Hata K, Hata T, Kitao M. Ultrasonographic identification and measurement of the human fetal adrenal gland in utero. Int J Gynaecol Obstet. 1985; 23:355–359.

35. Hatta R, Rees G, Johnson M. Normal fetal anatomy. Radiol Clin North Am. 1982; 20:271–284.

36. Hill L. Sonographic detection of fetal gastrointestinal anomalies. Ultrasound Quarterly 1988; 6:35–67.

37. Hill L, Kislak S, Runco C. An ultrasonic view of the umbilical cord. Obstet Gynecol Surv. 1987; 42:82–88.

38. Kurtz A, Goldberg B. Fetal body measurements. In: Kurtz A, Goldberg B, eds. Obstetrical Measurements in Ultrasound: A Reference Manual. Chicago: Year Book Medical Publishers; 1988:302–367.

39. Lawson T, Foley W, Berland L, et al. Ultrasonic evaluation of fetal kidneys: Analysis of normal size and frequency of visualization as related to stage of pregnancy. Radiology. 1981; 138:153–156.

40. Levi S, Erbsman F. Antenatal fetal growth from the nineteenth week: Ultrasonic study of 12 head and chest dimensions. Am J Obstet Gynecol. 1975; 121:262–268.

41. Lewis E, Kurtz A, Dubbins P, et al. Real-time ultrasonographic evaluation of normal fetal adrenal gland. J Ultrasound Med. 1982; 1:205–207.

42. McKenna K, Goldstein R, Stringer M. Small or absent fetal stomach: Prognostic significance. Radiology. 1995; 197:729–733.

43. Mahony B. The genitourinary system. In: Callen P, ed. Ultrasonography in Obstetrics and Gynecology. 2nd ed. Philadelphia: WB Saunders; 1988:254–276.

44. Mahony B, Filly R. The genitourinary system in utero. In: Hricak H, ed. Genitourinary Ultrasound. New York: Churchill Livingstone; 1986:1–2.

45. Mahony B. Ultrasound evaluation of the fetal genitourinary system. In Callen P, ed. Ultrasonography in Obstetrics and Gynecology. 3rd ed. Philadelphia: WB Saunders; 1994:389–419.

46. Manco L, Nunan F, Sohnen H, et al. Fetal small bowel simulating abdominal mass at sonography. J Clin Ultrasound. 1986; 14:404–407.

47. Meire H, Farrant P. Ultrasound demonstration of an unusual growth pattern in Indians. Br J Obstet Gynaecol. 1981; 88:260–263.

48. Millener P, Anderson N, Chrisolm R. Prognostic significance of non-visualization of the fetal stomach by sonography. Am J Roentgenol. 1993; 160:827–830.

49. Monteagudo A, Timor-Tritsch I, Moomjy M. Nomograms of the fetal lateral ventricles using transvaginal sonography. J Ultrasound Med. 1993; 12:265–269.

50. Moore K. The fetal membranes and placenta. In: Moore K, ed. The Developing Human. 3rd ed. Philadelphia: WB Saunders; 1982:111–139.

51. Morin F, Winsberg F. The ultrasonic appearance of the umbilical cord. J Clin Ultrasound. 1978; 6:324–326.

52. Nimrod C, Davies D, Iwanicki S, et al. Ultrasound prediction of pulmonary hypoplasia. Obstet Gynecol. 1986; 68:495–498.

53. Nyberg D, Mack L, Patten R, et al. Fetal bowel: Normal sonographic findings. J Ultrasound Med. 1987; 6:3–6.

54. Nyberg D. Intra-abdominal abnormalities. In: Nyberg D, Mahony B, Pretorius D, eds. Diagnostic Ultrasound of Fetal Anomalies. Text and Atlas (pp. 342–394). Chicago: Year Book; 1990.

55. Ogada E, Sabbagha R, Metzger B, et al. Serial ultrasonography to assess fetal macrosomia: Studies in 23 pregnancy diabetic women. JAMA. 1980; 243:2405–2408.

56. Pap G, Szoke J, Pap L. Intrauterine growth retardation: Ultrasonic diagnosis. Acta Paediatr Hung. 1983; 24:7–15.

57. Parulekar S. Sonography of normal fetal bowel. J Ultrasound Med. 1991; 10:211–220.

58. Romero R, Pilu G, Jeanty P, et al. The lungs. In: Romero R, Pilu G, Jeanty P, et al, eds. Prenatal Diagnosis of Congenital Anomalies. East Norwalk, CT: Appleton & Lange; 1988:195–208.

59. Rosenberg E, Bowie J, Andreotti R, et al. Sonographic evaluation of fetal adrenal glands. Am J Roentgenol. 1982; 139:1145–1147.

60. Rosenthal S, Filly R, Callen P, et al. Fetal pseudoascites. Radiology. 1979; 131:195–197.

61. Sanders R, Miner N, Martin J. Fetal anatomy. In: Sanders R, James A Jr, eds. The Principles and Practice of Ultrasonography in Obstetrics and Gynecology. 3rd ed. East Norwalk, CT: Appleton-Century-Crofts; 1985:123–140.

62. Schmidt W, Yarkoni S, Jeanty P, et al. Sonographic measurement of the fetal spleen: Clinical implications. J Ultrasound Med. 1985; 4:667–672.

63. Seeds J. Antenatal sonographic assessment of the genitourinary tract. In: Sanders R, Hill M, eds. Ultrasound Annual. New York: Raven Press; 1986:67–98.

64. Staudach A. Abdomen. In: Staudach A, ed. Sectional Fetal Anatomy in Ultrasonography. Berlin: Springer-Verlag; 1987:131–146.

65. Staudach A. Skeleton. In: Staudach A, ed. Sectional Fetal Anatomy in Ultrasonography. Berlin: Springer-Verlag; 1987:163–180.

66. Staudach A. Thorax (heart, lung, great vessels). In: Staudach A, ed. Sectional Fetal Anatomy in Ultrasonography. Berlin: Springer-Verlag; 1987:117–130.

67. Stephens J. Prenatal diagnosis of testicular feminization. Lancet. 1984; 2:1038.

68. Taybi H, Lachman R. Radiology of syndromes, metabolic disorders and skeletal dysplasias. 3rd Ed. Chicago: Year Book Medical Publishers, 1996:881.

69. Vandeberghe K, DeWolf F. Ultrasonic assessment of fetal stomach function: Physiology and clinic. In: Kurjak A, ed. Recent Advances in Ultrasound Diagnosis 2. Excerpta Medica International Congress Series 498. Amsterdam: Elsevier; 1980:275–282.

70. Vintzileos A, Neckles S, Campbell W, et al. Fetal liver ultrasound measurements during normal pregnancy. Obstet Gynecol. 1985; 66:477–480.

71. Walker J, Ferguson D. The sonographic appearance of blood in the fetal stomach and its association with placental abruption. J Ultrasound Med. 1988; 7:155–161.

72. Wei J, Haller J, Rachlin S, Berman M. Sonographic evaluation of the fetal gallbladder in utero: Incidence of visualization and morphology. JDMS 1993; 9:291–296.

73. Wladimiroff J, Legis R, Smith B. Human fetal stomach profile. In: Kurjak A, ed. Recent Advances in Ultrasound Diagnosis 2. Excerpta Medica International Congress Series 498. Amsterdam: Elsevier; 1980:552–558.

74. Yarkoni S, Schmitt W, Jeanty P, et al. Clavicular measurements: A new biometric parameter for fetal evaluation. J Ultrasound Med. 1985; 4:467–470.

75. Zador I, Bottoms S, Tse G, et al. Nomograms for ultrasound visualization of fetal organs. J Ultrasound Med. 1988; 7:197–201.

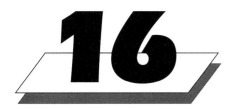

Abnormalities of the Fetal Chest, Abdomen, and Pelvis

HARRIS L. COHEN, DARA MULLER, and DANIEL L. ZINN

Knowledge of normal anatomy and biometry (discussed in Chap. 15), in combination with excellent equipment, sonologist/sonographer experience, and meticulous technique, allows for the superior diagnosis of abnormalities of the fetal thorax, abdomen, and pelvis. This chapter discusses these abnormalities and their diagnostic sonographic findings.

Thorax

The thorax should be evaluated for overall size and symmetry of its bony and soft tissue elements. Masses extending from beyond the thorax should be excluded. The normal intrathoracic contents should consist of homogeneous, relatively symmetric lung parenchyma surrounding the central heart and mediastinum (see Fig. 15-2). Evaluation of the sonographic image for assymetry, mass, or mediastinal shift is helpful in detecting possible intrathoracic pathology.

THE BONY THORAX AND ITS SOFT TISSUES

A few abnormalities long enough or large enough to appear to involve the thorax may actually extend from the head and neck. Encephaloceles, associated with calvarial defects, and myelomeningoceles, as-

sociated with defects of the vertebral column, are predominantly cystic masses with or without contained echogenic brain or spinal cord. The key differential diagnosis for a cystic mass in the region of the neck or upper thorax, when there is no abnormality of the spine or calvarium, includes fetal edema and cystic hygroma. Both of these abnormalities have a high association with karyotype abnormalities.[2,31,86]

Fetal edema may be focal at the neck but is more often associated with fetal hydrops and increased soft tissue thickness, forming a halo pattern around the neck, thorax, or abdomen (Fig. 16-1). Nuchal area edema has been associated with nonimmune fetal hydrops, fetal demise, and some skeletal dysplasias.[86,139] The presence of abnormal and excessive skin or soft tissue in the nuchal area is a well known clinical finding in many newborns with trisomy 21 (Down's syndrome). Benacerraf and colleagues were first to note this finding on antenatal ultrasound examination.[7] Gray and Crane showed that ultrasound screening for a nuchal fold thickness of 5 mm or greater (42% sensitivity) in the 14- to 18-week gestational age group and 6 mm or greater (83% sensitivity, positive predictive value of 1 in 38) in the 19- to 24-week group could be a more effective tool in diagnosing Down's syndrome than the use of maternal age greater than 35 years (20% sensitivity) or low maternal serum α-

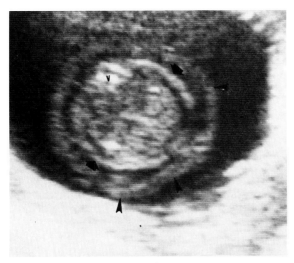

Figure 16-1. Fetal hydrops of upper abdomen is imaged in the transverse oblique plane. A halo of soft tissue (*arrowheads*) surrounds the fetal body (*arrows; V, vertebral body*).

fetoprotein levels (33% sensitivity).[56] Amniocentesis can certainly karyotype those fetuses with thick nuchal areas.[29]

Cystic hygromas, benign abnormalities of lymphatic origin occurring in 1 of every 6000 pregnancies, are thought to result from a failure in the development of normal lymphatic venous communication. The lymphatic sacs dilate, and sonographically they appear as unilocular or multilocular cystic masses. Most (80%) originate from the posterolateral neck (Fig. 16-2). At least half of cystic hygromas are evident in antenatal life; 10% are bilateral.[138] They may be seen extending to or originating from the thorax (Fig. 16-3) or the mediastinum, as well as the axilla or groin.[154] Internal solid elements seen on the sonographic image probably represent surrounding connective tissue or hemangiomatous elements.[29]

The differentiation of cystic hygroma from the statistically less likely thoracic wall hemangioma is difficult. Large hemangiomas may be associated with cardiac dilatation because of the presence of arteriovenous shunting and increased blood return to the heart.[154] Cystic hygromas may spontaneously resolve before birth, possibly owing to further development of lymphatic channel communication with the venous system. This is thought by some to be the cause of the webbed neck of patients with Turner's syndrome, a condition with an abnormal

fetal karyotype (XO) and a frequent association with cystic hygroma.[31] Cystic hygromas may also cause venous obstruction. In an affected fetus, ascites, pleural effusions, generalized edema, an enlarged edematous placenta, or cystic cutaneous lymphangiectasia may develop. The prognosis for such fetuses is poor.[125] In general, fetuses with cystic hygroma *and* hydrops succumb in utero or shortly after birth, but there have been occasional reports of the antenatal resolution of this finding.[20,29,31]

Other soft tissue masses involving the thorax are uncommon. The soft tissues of the thorax are normally thin, but they may be generally increased in fetuses of diabetic mothers, on the basis of subcutaneous fat deposition, or, as noted, in patients with fetal anasarca or edema, due to subcutaneous fluid.[45,55] Teratomas with combined cystic and solid components have been described. They may increase in size during pregnancy, growing more solid (echogenic) in appearance.[29] Hamartomas, benign, nonneoplastic overgrowths of the normal cellular elements of an affected area, often arise within a rib. They may have a disproportionately large intrathoracic component capable of displacing the fetal heart and causing respiratory insufficiency. Early diagnosis followed by complete resection in neonatal life is usually curative.[12]

The clavicles may be absent or hypoplastic in several syndromes, including cleidocranial dysplasia, Holt-Oram syndrome, and pyknodysostosis. Thick ribs may be noted in mucopolysaccharidoses as well as several skeletal syndromes, but diagnosis on prenatal ultrasound is often difficult.

Pulmonary Hypoplasia

Biometry allows evaluation of the thorax for pulmonary hypoplasia and syndromes involving the size of the chest wall. Pulmonary hypoplasia is associated with a poor prognosis. Pulmonary hypoplasia is rarely of primary origin. It is usually secondary to lung compression in utero. Causes are numerous (Table 16-1) and are related to compression from intrathoracic masses, but also from abdominal masses that prevent the downward movement of the diaphragm or have an intrathoracic component. The small thorax of several skeletal dysplasias is associated with lung hypoplasia. In oligohydramnios of any cause, the lack of transmitted fluid pulsations on the chest wall, said to be necessary for appropriate tracheobronchial tree

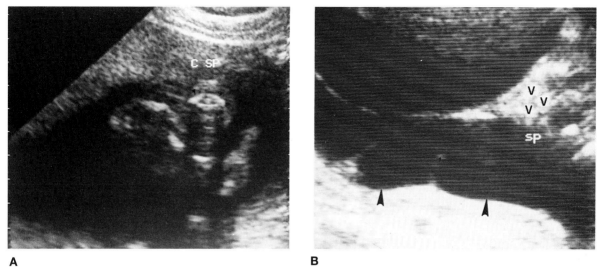

A   **B**

Figure 16-2. (**A**) Transverse view [fetal posterior is at upper portion of figure] of a normal cervical spine shows normally converging posterior elements (*arrows*). No masses are seen to extend from the neck. (**B**) Transverse view [left side of photo is posterior] shows a multilocular cystic mass (hygroma, *arrowheads*) posterior to the neck of the fetus. The hygroma is posterior and lateral to the three ossification centers (V) of the normal vertebral body seen at this level.

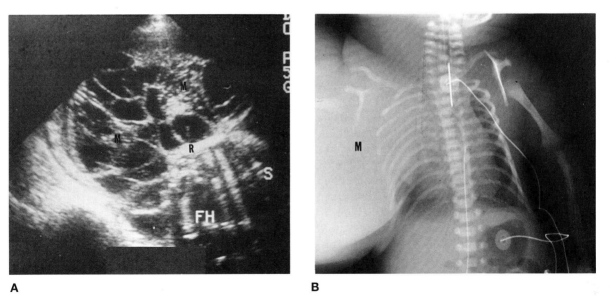

A   **B**

Figure 16-3. Cystic hygroma of the thoracic wall. (**A**) An ultrasound image in the coronal oblique plane shows a multilocular, predominantly cystic, mass (M) extending from the echogenic ribs (R) of the right thoracic wall (S, spine; FH, area of fetal heart). (**B**) Anteroposterior neonatal chest film reveals a soft tissue mass (M) off the right thorax.

▰▰▰▰ **TABLE 16-1. CAUSES OF PULMONARY HYPOPLASIA**

Intrathoracic masses that compress developing lung
   Pleural effusion
   Pulmonary cyst
   Teratoma
   Meningocele
   Hemangioma
Abdominal mass that prevents downward
     displacement of the diaphragm or compresses
     developing lung tissue
   Ascites
   Renal mass
   Diaphragmatic hernia and its contents
Oligohydramnios with a lack of transmitted fluid
     pulsation on the chest wall (said to be necessary
     for tracheobronchial tree development)
   Bilateral renal agenesis or obstruction
   Bilateral ureteral obstruction
   Bladder outlet obstruction, usually urethral atresia
   Prolonged rupture of membranes
Small thorax as part of a skeletal dysplasia
   Thanatophoric dwarfism
   Jeune's syndrome
   Ellis-Van Creveld syndrome
   Hypophosphatasia
   Cleidocranial dysostosis
   Metatrophic dwarfism
   Campomelic dwarfism

development, is thought to be the cause of the associated pulmonary hypoplasia. Prognosis is related to the degree of hypoplasia.[18,24,149]

Lung hypoplasia may be diagnosed by gestalt; a small chest cavity in relation to a larger abdominal cavity, or a prominent heart (taking up more than one third the area of the thorax on a transverse view) in a fetus without cardiac disease suggest pulmonary hypoplasia (Fig. 16-4).[24] Biometric methods for the evaluation of hypoplasia have been sought. Thoracic circumference-to-abdominal circumference ratios have been most helpful. The normal ratio has a mean of 0.89, and measurements under 0.77 (>2 SDs below the norm) are considered abnormal and suggestive of lethal pulmonary hypoplasia.[87,138,148]

THE MEDIASTINUM

Mediastinal masses are rare in the fetus and few have been imaged antenatally. These include mediastinal (including intrapericardial) teratoma,[32] enteric cyst,[111] lymphangioma, and mediastinal meningocele.[4] All may be associated with pleural effusion. Mass impression on the esophagus may lead to polyhydramnios because of gastrointestinal tract obstruction. Mass impression on the vena cava may compromise blood return to the fetal heart and lead to the development of fetal hydrops.[51]

THE LUNGS

Normal fetal lungs should be symmetrically echogenic. Half of all intrathoracic abnormalities noted on fetal examination are pleural effusions.[4] Imaged intrathoracic masses, excluding congenital diaphragmatic hernias, are usually cystic, but, at times, solid and echogenic. They can be found breaking up the homogeneity of the lung parenchyma or causing cardiac or mediastinal shift.[154] The predominant cystic masses of the lung include the typically unilocular bronchogenic cyst and the multicystic cystic adenomatoid malformation (CAM), types II and III. Other reported masses include pulmonary sequestration, congenital lobar emphysema, neurenteric cyst, bronchial atresia, and, in rare instances, teratoma.[51]

Bronchogenic Cyst

Several cases of bronchogenic cyst have been diagnosed antenatally.[3,4,154] Bronchogenic cysts may be unilocular (Fig. 16-5) or multilocular. They may

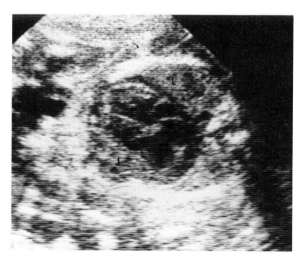

Figure 16-4. Hypoplastic lungs. A transverse oblique plane view through the thorax demonstrates that the heart takes up more than its usual one third of the intrathoracic space. Although the cause was initially thought to be cardiomegaly, autopsy revealed a normal-sized heart in a fetus with hypoplastic lungs related to oligohydramnios of renal origin (L, lung parenchyma).

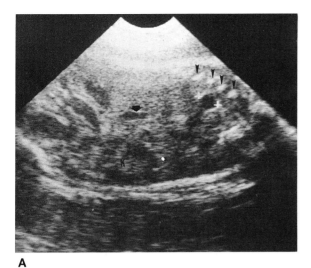
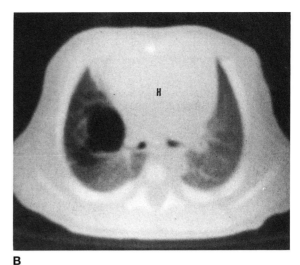

A   B

Figure 16-5. Bronchogenic cyst. (**A**) On a right parasagittal plane view of chest and abdomen, crosses mark off an echo-free mass within the normally echogenic lung. Ribs can be seen anteriorly (*small arrowheads*). The right kidney (K) as well as a small portion of the abdominal aorta (*large arrowhead*) may be noted in the abdomen. (**B**) Axial computed tomography view of neonate's thorax demonstrates a low-density area in the right thorax consistent with air filling the bronchogenic cyst (H, heart).

displace mediastinal structures, although this is an uncommon finding in neonatal life. Bronchogenic cysts result from abnormal budding of the ventral diverticulum of the primitive foregut and are lined by epithelium similar to that of a normal bronchus. They may contain cartilage, muscle, or mucus glands.[29] They may be found within the lung parenchyma or mediastinum. They often communicate with the trachea or mainstem bronchi.[3]

Cystic Adenomatoid Malformation

Excluding diaphragmatic hernias, CAM is the most frequently identified mass in the fetal chest.[29] Accounting for 25% of congenital lung malformations,[132] it is typically a unilateral disorder involving an entire lung lobe or part of one. Bilateral involvement may occur. Rarely, CAM may involve an entire lung.[43] It is characterized histologically as an adenomatoid increase in terminal respiratory elements leading to the development of a pathologic mass consisting of multiple cysts of different sizes (Table 16-2).[29,132]

Three forms of CAM have been described. Type I consists of a single cyst or multiple large cysts (usually 3 to 7 cm, but at least 2 cm) with a trabeculated wall and, often, smaller cystic out-

pouchings. Broad, fibrous septa and mucigenic cells may be responsible for areas of echogenicity within the mass. Type II CAM is a mass made up of multiple, uniform-sized cysts of about 1.5 cm in diameter. Types I and II appear cystic on ultrasound examination (Fig. 16-6). Type III consists of multiple, very small cysts (0.5 to 5.0 mm) that, like the multiple small cysts of infantile polycystic kidney disease, present numerous reflecting surfaces to the ultrasound beam. Because these small cysts cannot be resolved individually, they appear as a single, solid, homogeneously echogenic mass.[124,151] Patients with CAM may have associated renal, cardiac, or gastrointestinal malformations. As with all space-occupying lung masses, fetuses with CAM may have associated fetal hydrops, ascites, and polyhydramnios. The mass of CAM may expand and cause a greater-than-normal increase in thoracic diameter as well as inversion of the diaphragm. As with other lung masses, there have been reports of the significant decrease or the spontaneous resolution of CAMs antenatally.[44,93,132] Stillbirth and premature labor are common among these fetuses. Those with associated intrauterine hydrops have the poorest prognosis. Those whose lesions are imaged as cys-

◢▨▨▨◣ **TABLE 16-2.** CYSTIC ADENOMATOID MALFORMATIONS

Type	Histologic Findings	Sonographic Appearance[124,151]	Differential Diagnoses[29,132]
I	Single large cyst, usually 3–7 cm but at least 2 cm; trabeculated wall with smaller cystic outpouchings	Usually unilateral May involve a lung lobe or part of a lung lobe Rarely involves entire lung Can be bilateral Single large cyst with smaller cystic outpouchings visualized superior to the diaphragm in the fetal lung Can have echogenic areas within the cyst	Bronchogenic cyst Mediastinal mass Pleural and pericardial effusions Fluid-filled stomach and bowel in diaphragmatic hernia
II	Mass made up of multiple similar-sized cysts, 1.5 cm in diameter	Usually unilateral May involve a lung lobe or part of a lobe Rarely involves entire lung Can be bilateral Multiple similar sized cysts seen in the fetal lung replacing normal lung parenchyma	Same as type I
III	Multiple small cysts (0.5–5 mm)	Cysts too small to be resolved sonographically appear as a single solid echogenic mass in the fetal lung	Pulmonary sequestration Rhabdomyoma Mediastinal teratoma Herniated liver, spleen, or rarely kidney

tic appear to have a better prognosis than those with solid-appearing CAMs. Many neonates who survive with CAM have respiratory distress at birth, but most are asymptomatic. These patients usually do well after surgical excision of these masses.[29,51]

The differential diagnosis of the type III, solid-appearing CAM includes pulmonary sequestration, rhabdomyoma, mediastinal teratoma, and herniated abdominal contents, which may include liver, spleen, or, rarely, kidney.[29,132] The differential diagnosis of type I and II lesions includes cystic lung and mediastinal masses as well as pleural and pericardial effusions. Noting the position of the fluid-filled stomach and any fluid-filled bowel, if present, can help differentiate between types I or II CAM, in which the affected fetus has stomach and bowel in the normal subdiaphragmatic location, and a fetus with a diaphragmatic hernia, in which the fluid-filled stomach

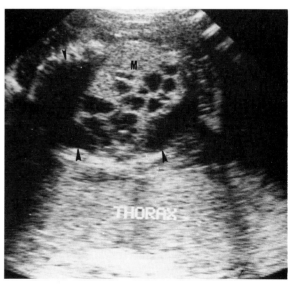

Figure 16-6. Transverse oblique plane. Multiple cysts are noted in the lung parenchyma of this patient with cystic adenomatoid malformation (M) and surrounding pleural effusion (*arrowheads*).

and bowel are in an intrathoracic location, simulating CAM.[132]

Pulmonary Sequestration

A pulmonary sequestration is a solid, nonfunctioning mass of lung tissue that lacks communication with the tracheobronchial tree and has a systemic arterial blood supply (and, in the extralobar type, a systemic venous drainage). Color Doppler has been used to image the abnormal vascular supplies and make the ultrasound diagnosis.[37] The lung mass of pulmonary sequestration is spherical, highly echogenic, and often found at the lung base. Occasional cases have been noted to resolve spontaneously in utero.[93] There is a bronchiectatic form that may simulate the ultrasound image of types I and II CAM.[29,102]

Pleural Effusion and Fetal Hydrops

Pleural effusion represents more than 50% of the intrathoracic disease diagnosed by ultrasound.[154] Any fluid in the pleural space of a fetus of any gestational age is abnormal. Overall mortality is reported to be 50%, and is highest when the pleural effusion is discovered before 33 weeks' gestation, is bilateral, or is associated with fetal hydrops.[51]

Pleural fluid may be an isolated finding, but more typically it is part of other fetal pathologic processes, which may or may not be imaged. It is most often seen in association with fetal hydrops, a condition associated with excessive fluid accumulations within the fetal soft tissues and body cavities.[99] The two types of hydrops are immune and nonimmune.

Immune hydrops (or erythroblastosis fetalis) usually occurs in a fetus whose mother has been sensitized, usually in previous pregnancies, by a blood factor histoincompatibility, typically Rhesus (Rh) factor, although potentially any of a myriad of fetal red blood cell antigens can serve as sensitizing agents. An immune reaction between maternal immunoglobulin G (IgG) and the fetal blood factor results. This reaction leads to significant fetal morbidity and mortality, with a small amount of ascites or pericardial effusion representing early signs of impending decompensation. Polyhydramnios is said to be more sensitive than placental thickening (>4 cm) as evidence of the severe fetal anemia that occurs before the development of frank immune hy-

drops. The sonographic findings of full-blown immune hydrops include profound skin thickening (>5 mm), significant pleural and pericardial effusions, ascites, hepatomegaly, and splenomegaly. At one time, Rh incompatibility was the cause of 98% of all immune hydrops. The development of RhoGam to protect the Rh-negative mother from histoincompatibility reactions with a future Rh-positive fetus reduced this to about 55%.[21]

Nonimmune hydrops is not a disease but a later result of different severe fetal diseases. It has a high incidence of mortality, ranging between 50% and 98%.[21] The sonographic findings are similar to those of immune hydrops. Causes include fetal cardiac arrhythmias or anomalies (e.g., hypoplastic left heart and supraventricular tachycardia, said to be the probable cause in many of the cases labeled idiopathic), intrauterine infection (any of the TORCH—*tox*oplasmosis, *r*ubella, *c*ytomegalovirus, *h*erpes—infections), chromosomal abnormalities (Turner's syndrome, trisomy 18 or 21), abdominal or pulmonary masses leading to venous obstruction (CAM or neuroblastoma), congenital hematologic disorders (α-thalassemia, a common cause in Asia), renal abnormalities (congenital nephrosis), and maternal causes (diabetes, toxemia).[21,32,131]

Hydrothorax (i.e., pleural effusion) unrelated to hydrops usually has an extrathoracic cause, but an intrathoracic lesion such as CAM has also been noted to play an etiologic role. On ultrasound examination, sonolucent fluid is seen within one or both hemithoraces, conforming to the shape of the chest cavity and its diaphragmatic contour (Fig. 16-7). If large, the pleural effusion may flatten or even evert the diaphragm.[51,77]

Mortality from pleural effusion is affected by the underlying cause as well as the degree of development of pulmonary hypoplasia, which may occur any time there is significant mass effect on the lung during its early development. In an attempt to decrease this possibility, mid-trimester thoracocentesis under ultrasound guidance was performed on a fetus who at birth had no lung abnormality.[6]

The typical isolated pleural effusion associated with respiratory distress in the newborn is chylous, but these effusions appear just as anechoic as serous pleural effusions owing to the absence of chylomicrons in the fetus.[51] Chylothorax is caused by overaccumulation of lymph. It is most often unilateral

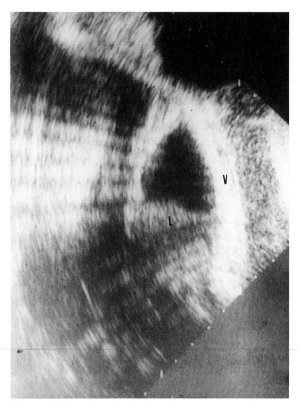

Figure 16-7. Pleural effusion. Right parasagittal plane view shows a triangular echo-free area above the liver (L) and anterior to the vertebral column (V).

and right sided. It occurs twice as often in male infants and is observed in association with congenital pulmonary lymphangiectasia, tracheoesophageal fistula, trisomy 21, and extralobar pulmonary sequestration.[121,134]

DIAPHRAGMATIC HERNIA

Congenital diaphragmatic hernia (CDH) has an incidence of 1 in every 2000 to 5000 live births. It results from defective formation or fusion of the diaphragm. These defects may result in the most common diaphragmatic abnormality, the postero-lateral Bochdalek hernia (92% of all), and in other types, including retrosternal and anteromedial (Morgagni) hernias as well as diaphragmatic eventration and, uncommonly, a complete absence of a diaphragm.[68,135] Left-sided involvement is five times more common than right-sided,[96] which may be because of the "protective" presence of the liver, whose mass is known to prevent craniad progres-

sion of bowel and thereby lessen symptoms and improve prognosis. CDH is unilateral 96% of the time and is found somewhat more commonly in male infants.[51,106,135]

Abdominal contents acting as an intrathoracic mass can lead to pulmonary hypoplasia. The hypoplasia may be bilateral despite a unilateral diaphragmatic lesion.[68] Overall mortality for CDH is 50% to 80%,[2] which includes a 35% rate of stillbirth. CDH is associated with major congenital anomalies of other body systems. Associated cardiovascular and central nervous system anomalies are the most lethal.[17]

There are familial forms of CDH. These occur bilaterally in 20% of cases (a far greater incidence compared to the 3% incidence found among sporadic cases), have a 2-to-1 male predominance, and fewer associated anomalies.[51,68] One Finnish study showed a 2% recurrence risk of CDH among subsequent siblings.[112]

On fetal ultrasound examination (Fig. 16-8), the stomach, bowel, or other organs of patients with CDH may be seen in the chest, often posteriorly. Fluid-filled structures are readily differentiated from normal echogenic lung parenchyma. Occasionally, peristalsis may be noted in the herniated small bowel. To rule out cystic abnormalities of the lung simulating CDH, the sonographer must search the abdomen to prove it contains no stomach. The fetus with CDH often has a smaller-than-normal abdominal circumference measurement. Often the heart and mediastinum shift away from the side of herniation. During fetal breathing, the abdominal organs may descend on the normal side and, paradoxically, ascend on the affected side. Polyhydramnios and pleural effusions may be noted. Polyhydramnios, in particular, is not a prognostically good sign because one series reported a 55% survival rate among patients with CDH without associated polyhydramnios, but only 11% survival in cases with associated polyhydramnios. Patients with smaller diaphragmatic defects or herniations that occur later in gestation have a better prognosis. A careful sonographic search should be made of fetuses with CDH for other congenital anomalies.[29,51,61,134]

The usual management of these cases includes karyotyping, fetal echocardiography, and delivery at a tertiary center. Experimental work with surgery in utero in fetal lambs[149] paved the way for similar

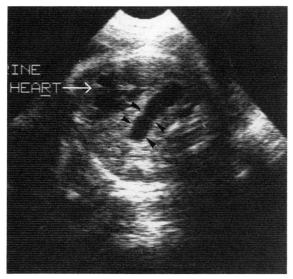
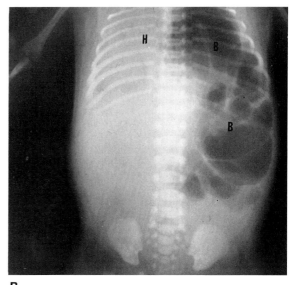

A   **B**

Figure 16-8. Diaphragmatic hernia. (**A**) On this transverse oblique view of a fetal chest, the heart has been shifted to the right chest (*arrow*). A tubular lucency (*arrowheads*) within the chest is a loop of bowel. (**B**) On anteroposterior film of the chest and abdomen, a radiolucency from air-filled bowel (B) is noted below the left hemidiaphragm and within the left chest of this neonate. The heart (H) has been shifted into the right chest, accounting for some of the "white-out" of the right lung field.

work in humans. It is hoped that removal of the compressing mass will allow the lung to grow and avoid the development of significant pulmonary hypoplasia. There has been no indication that early delivery improves the prognosis.[134] However, Harrison and colleagues have stated that they will attempt *fetal* surgery, and not wait for later delivery and increased time for lung maturity, if the CDH diagnosis is made before 24 weeks' gestation and the fetus's stomach or liver is imaged in the chest, and there is a low lung-to-thorax ratio as well as early evidence of polyhydramnios.[62]

Abdomen

SCANNING TECHNIQUES

A general fetal abdominal survey should evaluate the anterior abdominal wall to see that it is intact. This is most important at the site of umbilical cord entry. No masses should extend from the vertebral column or posteriorly (Fig. 16-9). The posterior elements of each vertebral body should converge or appear parallel to one another. Any divergence of the posterior elements, particularly in the pres-

ence of defects in the overlying skin or of posterior masses, suggests the presence of a meningocele or myelomeningocele. Protrusions from the abdominal sidewalls should also be searched for, although they are unusual. The soft tissues of the abdominal wall should not be thickened, a finding noted in hydrops fetalis but also in the offspring of diabetic (type C) mothers.[138]

Abdominal situs is determined by noting the liver's position on the side opposite the cardiac apex. This is best accomplished by caudad and craniad angulation of the transducer in the transverse plane. Complete situs inversus (cardiac apex on right and liver on left) can be diagnosed only by meticulous attention to fetal position and visualized anatomy.[142] In cases of correct abdominal situs, transverse images of the abdomen show the spine, stomach, and umbilical vein in clockwise relation when the fetus is in cephalic presentation and counterclockwise when the fetus is breech.

Abdominal circumference (AC) should be measured to assess conformity with accepted measurements for gestational age. Biometric evaluation

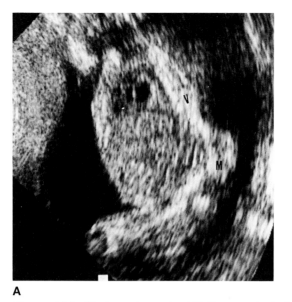
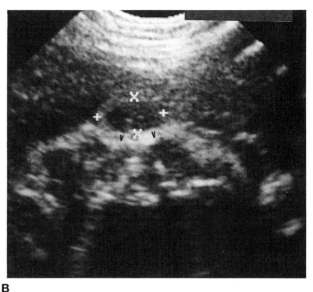

A   **B**

Figure 16-9. Myelomeningocele. (**A**) On a sagittal plane view a mass (M) consisting of a myelomeningocele is seen to extend posteriorly from the fetal vertebral column (V). (**B**) On the transverse plane view, crosses surround the mass, which lies posterior to divergent posterior elements of a vertebral body (v). No normal skin line was seen.

of AC allows assessment of the nutritional status of the fetus. Assymetric intrauterine growth retardation (IUGR; representing 80% of all cases of IUGR) shows a smaller AC, owing to loss of glycogen stores in the liver and the resultant decrease in liver size; there is no associated decrease in head circumference (HC) or femur length (FL) measurements. HC/AC and FL/AC ratios are, therefore, used to help determine IUGR.[87]

The remainder of the routine fetal abdominal survey includes evaluation of the transverse AC view for the presence of a fluid-filled stomach and assessment of the liver. A transverse view at the level of the kidneys may reveal renal obstruction. Coronal and longitudinal views may supplement the transverse views in further evaluating any area or organ of concern.

PERITONEUM AND ASCITES

Ascites (Fig. 16-10) represents fluid in the peritoneum. True fetal ascites is always abnormal. Depending on the amount, the fluid may be seen only in dependent portions of the fetus (e.g., the pelvis in a fetus in breech position) or, in large amounts, surrounding and shifting intraperitoneal structures superiorly, inferiorly, or laterally. Intraperitoneal

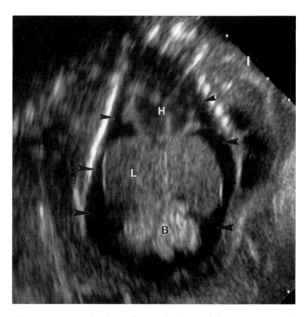

Figure 16-10. Ascites. Coronal view of fetal chest and abdomen. Ascitic fluid (*large arrowheads*) is seen to the side of the liver (L) and spleen as well as in the low abdomen and pelvis, where it surrounds echogenic collapsed bowel (B). Incidentally noted is pleural effusion (*small arrowheads*) surrounding the heart (H) in a fetus with an abnormal karyotype and an associated cystic hygroma. Pleural effusion and ascites in association with cystic hygroma predict a poor outcome.

fluid is seen best in the subhepatic space, flanks, and lower abdominal cavity or pelvis. The retroperitoneal structures such as the kidneys lie posterior to the free fluid. With patency of the processus vaginalis, ascitic fluid may extend into the scrotum as apparent hydroceles. In studies of intrauterine transfusions, the presence of at least 10 ml of intraperitoneal fluid at 22 weeks and 15 ml at 26 weeks is required before fetal ascites can be detected sonographically.[64]

Commonly noted in association with the multiple findings of fetal hydrops, fetal ascites may develop as an isolated finding in bowel perforation or as urinary ascites from bladder outlet obstruction or renal forniceal rupture.[98] Heart failure, infections, tumors, and twin–twin transfusions are other causes. Sonography typically demonstrates only 25% to 50% of the causes.[12]

If fetal ascites is detected, the sonographer and sonologist should investigate further, seeking bowel dilatation (indicating bowel obstruction), dilatation of the pyelocalyceal system or bladder (genitourinary problem), or intraabdominal cysts or peritoneal calcification indicative of bowel perforation and resultant meconium peritonitis or pseudocyst formation.[53] Because normal peristalsis is necessary to extrude meconium, this phenomenon usually is not seen until the fifth month of fetal life.[35]

If sterile meconium associated with bowel perforation is extruded into the peritoneal cavity, an intense foreign body reaction occurs. Punctate echogenicities develop over time, owing to the resultant irritative peritonitis caused by meconium and its subsequent calcification. This calcification is most easily detected around the liver (Fig. 16-11). Localized fibrotic reactions may cause walls to form about the areas of greatest meconium concentration within the peritoneum, forming meconium pseudocysts. These complex calcified masses may simulate retroperitoneal teratomas or calcified neuroblastomas. Other causes of peritoneal recess calcification include infections from TORCH (*to*xoplasmosis, *ru*bella, *cy*tomegalovirus, *he*rpes) organisms.[35,44,48,89]

PSEUDOASCITES

A hypoechoic band positioned along the inner aspect of the echo produced by the anterior abdominal wall and its subcutaneous tissue may simulate a

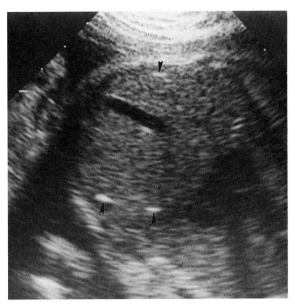

Figure 16-11. Peritoneal calcification. Transverse oblique plane view shows highly echogenic linear densities (*arrowheads*) at the liver periphery. This fetus probably had a bowel perforation.

small amount of ascites. This image of pseudoascites (Fig. 16-12) is created by the hypoechoic quality of the abdominal wall musculature sandwiched between the highly echogenic subcutaneous and preperitoneal fat. Unlike true ascites, it does not outline parts of the falciform ligament or umbilical vein, and it does not surround other abdominal organs.[63]

Liver and Spleen

The normal fetal liver has a homogeneous appearance. Although congenital anomalies are rare, atypical echogenicities can be seen in association with extramedullary hematopoiesis.[68] The fetal liver enlarges in association with immune or nonimmune causes of hydrops. If the longest liver length to the right of the aorta on a coronal image increases more than 5 mm in a week, isoimmunization must be ruled out.[87] The umbilical vein is enlarged in hydrops and in association with placental chorioangioma. Macrosomic fetuses have large livers, as do the fetuses of diabetic mothers, whereas growth-retarded infants have small livers.[68,133]

Solitary liver cysts may develop because of interruption of the development of the intrahepatic

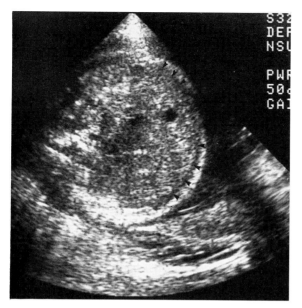

Figure 16-12. A hypoechoic band (*arrowheads*) at the inner aspect of the echogenic abdominal wall echoes represents the abdominal wall musculature, creating the image of pseudoascites.

biliary tree. A liver cyst as large as 10.5 cm has been reported.[22] There are several types of choledochal cysts. The most common is cystic dilatation of the common bile duct, which may be seen in an intrahepatic or subhepatic location, but other types include multiple intrahepatic and extrahepatic cysts or a common bile duct diverticulum. Antenatal detection and early surgery during infancy may prevent some severe clinical consequences, especially the development of biliary cirrhosis and portal hypertension.[34,39]

Diffuse liver calcification may be noted in fetuses with intrauterine infections, especially those caused by pathogens responsible for TORCH infections, and in particular toxoplasmosis and herpes simplex infection. There are also reported cases of fetal liver calcification due to ischemic, neoplastic, and idiopathic causes. Calcified portal thromboemboli have been reported on autopsy and plain films of newborn and stillborn infants. In a retrospective analysis of 25 fetuses with liver calcifications as their only imaged abnormality, prognosis was excellent, with 96% of the fetuses surviving.[11,52,150]

Liver masses are unusual but have been reported in the fetus. The most common vascular tumor of the neonatal liver is the infantile hemangioendothelioma, which may be associated with hepatomegaly, anemia, or high-output congestive heart failure. Sonography has shown these masses to be of variable, mixed echogenicity in neonates. There are reports of the antenatal detection of liver hemangiomas as well as a single case of focal nodular hyperplasia.[68,109,122,126]

Cases of echogenic masses within the fetal gallbladder that may or may not have shadowing have been diagnosed as gallstones in the fetus. Similar to sonographically imaged gallstones discovered in neonates, most are reported to disappear, possibly as a result of postnatal hydration or because they were not truly gallstones but tumefactive sludge. They seem to be unrelated to fetal well-being, and those that have not resolved appear to be asymptomatic in neonatal life.[9,15,80]

The fetal spleen is enlarged in cases of Rh and other isoimmunization (owing to extramedullary hematopoiesis or hydrops). A significant correlation has been noted between the perimeter measurement of the spleen and fetal hemoglobin deficit, allowing spleen size to predict severe fetal anemia.[115] The spleen may also be enlarged in chronic infections such as toxoplasmosis, cytomegalovirus, rubella, and syphilis, as well as in inborn metabolic errors, such as Gaucher's, Niemann-Pick, or Wolman's disease. The antenatal diagnosis of a congenital splenic cyst can be made if a cyst is noted in the left upper quadrant and can be separated from the imaged kidney and adrenal gland. Asplenia and polysplenia are associated with significant congenital heart disease, but the antenatal diagnosis of these entities is difficult.[38,68,91,144]

Kidney, Ureters, and Bladder

Fetal malformations are noted once in every 200 births. Urinary tract abnormalities represent between 35% and 50% of these.[24,67]

By 12 weeks' gestational age, the kidneys should have attained their normal position and the blood supply should be established. By 15 weeks' gestational age, the kidneys may be visualized sonographically as symmetric paraspinal masses. If no kidney is noted on one side, a search of the fetal abdomen, particularly of the embryologic "migratory path" of the kidney from the pelvis to the renal fossa, may reveal an ectopic kidney, which occurs in 1 in 2000 pregnancies. Asymmetry of renal tissue within or beyond the renal bed or an unusual kidney shape may be caused by a single horseshoe kidney, a duplicated system, a tumor, or fused or nonfused crossed renal ectopia.[24,49,69,76]

A renal pelvis greater than 1.0 cm in anteroposterior diameter is considered abnormal. Dilatations as small as 4 mm have been followed when presenting early in pregnancy (the second trimester) so as to avoid an abnormality that may be corrected in early life. Normal ureters are not imaged unless they are obstructed. The bladder, which may appear quite large in normal fetuses, should be seen either on initial or furosemide-enhanced follow-up examinations in all fetuses older than 15 weeks to rule out bilateral renal dysfunction or bilateral renal or ureteral obstruction. The bladder size, especially if enlarged, should be noted to decrease in size after fetal voiding to rule out bladder outlet obstruction. Bladder wall thickening, a sign of outlet obstruction, often caused by posterior urethral valves (PUV), should be excluded. A dilated posterior urethra in a male fetus suggests obstruction, usually PUV.[24,57,66]

AMNIOTIC FLUID

Amniotic fluid is a dialysate of maternal serum, essential for the maintenance of an even fetal temperature and biochemical homeostasis. Its presence allows fetal movement and growth and it is thought to be essential for the development of the tracheobronchial tree.[24] It is typically echoless, but can on occasion be filled with echogenic material. In one study of 19 fetuses with very echogenic amniotic fluid who soon after had third trimester amniocentesis, the echogenicity was caused by vernix caseosa in all but one case of fetal distress and intrauterine meconium passage.[16]

Amniotic fluid volume has been reported to average 60 ml at 12 weeks' gestation, increasing 20 to 25 ml per week until 16 weeks, and then increasing 50 to 100 ml per week until 20 weeks. The mean fluid volume at 20 weeks is 500 ml. The fetus may contribute to amniotic fluid volume by fluid transfer across the fetal skin surfaces, including skin, cord, chorion, and amnion. Fetal urine production begins at 12 weeks, but the amount is insignificant until the 18th to 20th weeks of gestation. By the late third trimester the fetus is producing approximately 450 ml of urine per day. Beyond 20 weeks, transudation of fluid across fetal surfaces is inade-

quate to maintain normal amniotic volume, and the fetus essentially modifies fluid volume and composition only by swallowing and urination.[24,146]

Normal amniotic fluid volume may be maintained by one functioning kidney and a nonobstructed genitourinary (GU) tract. Oligohydramnios of fetal origin results from abnormality of the GU tract, usually bilateral renal agenesis, urethral atresia, or bilateral nonfunctional renal dysplasia. The analysis of fetal anatomy is hindered, sometimes significantly, by oligohydramnios, which limits the imaging window about the fetus. The diagnosis of oligohydramnios is somewhat subjective and varies with fetal gestational age. Sonographically, the diagnosis can be made by gestalt, noting less fluid surrounding the fetus and crowding of fetal parts. Use of the amniotic fluid index (AFI) represents a more objective method of analyzing the fluid level. A measurement less than 7 cm is always abnormal and suggests oligohydramnios of any cause.[108] Some authors diagnose oligohydramnios if no fluid pocket greater than 2 cm can be found (polyhydramnios is evidenced by an AFI greater than 24 cm or the presence of a pocket larger than 8 cm). Compression of the fetal abdomen by decreases in surrounding amniotic fluid may cause a pseudoomphalocele image (Fig. 16-13), a finding that may also be simulated by uterine contractions.[24,108,140]

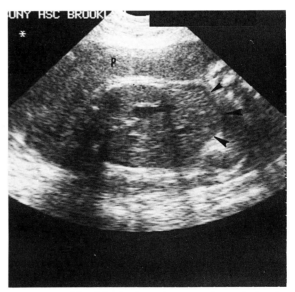

Figure 16-13. Oligohydramnios–pseudoomphalocele. On a transverse oblique view of fetal abdomen, no fluid surrounds the fetal abdomen or separates it from placenta (P). The pointed anterior abdominal wall (*arrowheads*) may simulate an omphalocele.

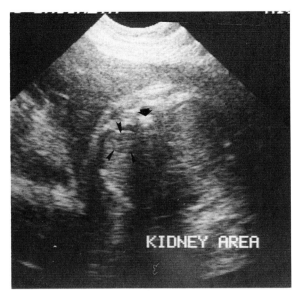

Figure 16-14. Renal agenesis. Kidney is simulated by normal adrenal gland. The image was made in the transverse plane at the level of the kidneys. Oval masses on either side of the vertebral body (*arrow*) look like kidneys. At autopsy there were no kidneys but prominent, normal adrenals (*arrowheads,* right adrenal).

RENAL AGENESIS

Bilateral renal agenesis is the most severe anomaly of the GU system. It occurs at the rate of 1 to 3 cases per 10,000 live births, predominantly in male infants. It has been noted to recur at a 5% rate within affected families.[24,36] Fetuses with bilateral renal agenesis have an increased incidence of other anomalies, especially involving the musculoskeletal system (in particular sirenomelia) in 40% and the cardiovascular system in 14% of cases.[97]

Severe oligohydramnios is noted between the 16th and 28th weeks of gestation. The most helpful sonographic finding of bilateral agenesis is the failure to detect the fetal bladder despite repeated examinations and furosemide challenge. In the presence of renal agenesis, the adrenal gland may take on, as discussed, a more globular shape (Fig. 16-14) and simulate the presence of a kidney on ultrasound examination.[24,94,156]

Early neonatal death associated with renal agenesis results from pulmonary hypoplasia. Affected infants are often in breech presentation, deliver prematurely, and have Potter's-type facies and features (flattened nose, epicanthic folds, low-set ears, receding chin, hypertelorism, brachycephaly,

and talipes equinovarus) owing to the lack of cushioning typically provided in utero by the surrounding amniotic fluid.[24,36,127] Evaluating a fetus for unilateral renal agenesis is difficult because the secondary signs—absent bladder filling and oligohydramnios—are not observable when the fetus has one functioning kidney.

FETAL HYDRONEPHROSIS

Sonography allows ready detection of fetal hydronephrosis. Small amounts of anechoic fluid may be seen in the renal pelvis, in sharp contrast with the normal echogenicity of the renal parenchyma.

After 24 weeks' gestation, it is common to see at least some dilatation of the central renal pelvis. One study showed anteroposterior measurements of the renal pelvis to be as wide as 1 to 2 mm in 41% and 3 to 11 mm in 18% of normal fetuses. Theories as to the cause include the influence of maternal hormones and maternal fluid volume expansion, although experimental work with sheep

 TABLE 16-3. GRADING SYSTEM FOR FETAL HYDRONEPHROSIS[57]

Grade I, Physiologic dilatation
    Renal pelvis: <1 cm in anteroposterior diameter
    Calyces: Not visualized
    Cortex: Unremarkable
Grade II
    Renal pelvis: 1.0–1.5 cm
    Calyces: Not visualized (normal)
    Cortex: Unremarkable
Grade III
    Renal pelvis: >1.5 cm
    Calyces: Slight dilatation
    Cortex: Unremarkable
Grade IV
    Renal pelvis: >1.5 cm
    Calyces: Moderately dilated
    Cortex: No significant abnormality
Grade V
    Renal pelvis: >1.5 cm
    Calyces: Severe dilatation
    Cortex: Atrophic
Percentage of patients that required surgery based on grade: Gr. I, 0%; Gr. II, 39%; Gr. III, 62%; Gr. IV, 100%; Gr. V, 100%

Because significant obstructions eventually requiring postnatal surgery have been found in younger fetuses with less than 1.0 cm anteroposterior measurements,[30] we follow older fetuses with dilatations of 7 mm or greater and, in cases of 23 weeks or younger, those with 4 mm or greater renal pelvic dilatation.

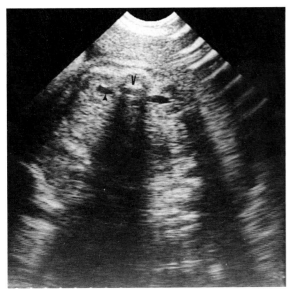

Figure 16-15. *Transverse plane view of bilateral physiologic dilatation of fetal renal pelvis. Echo-free urine is seen in each renal pelvis. Anteroposterior dimension of this dilatation is less than 5 mm. No postnatal abnormality was noted (V, vertebral body; arrowhead, right renal pelvis).*

has shown no change in fetal urine production with maternal volume expansion.[24,72,97,146] In some fetuses the degree of pelvic dilatation has been noted to change, usually decrease, with fetal bladder emptying, and this may be similar to the decrease or absence of renal pelvic dilatation (hydronephrosis) seen in adults after the emptying of full bladders.[123]

The diagnosis of fetal hydronephrosis is of great importance. There is much discussion, however, as to which group of fetuses to follow. A grading system (Table 16-3) developed by Grignon et al. assessed fetal hydronephrosis in relation to neonatal clinical outcome. Grade I dilatations (Fig. 16-15) were considered physiologic. Grade II (Fig. 16-16) and grade III were considered evidence of intermediate hydronephrosis. Fifty percent of these patients required postnatal surgical intervention. All patients with grade IV (Fig. 16-17) and grade V hydronephrosis, which consisted of anteroposterior measurements of the renal pelvis of 1.5 cm or greater, but with varying degrees of visualized renal parenchyma, required surgical intervention.[57] Corteville and associates reported abnormal kidneys requiring corrective surgery in children with pyelocalyceal dilatation less than 1 cm.[30] In an attempt

not to miss any lesion due to obstruction or another cause that may lead, if missed, to renal dysfunction later in childhood, we have tended to follow older fetuses with dilatations of 7 mm or greater. Because some fetuses, later proven to have significant urinary tract obstructions, have been reported in early pregnancy to have smaller renal pelvis anteroposterior measurements, we try to adhere to Corteville and associates' suggestion to follow fetuses with renal pelvis anteroposterior measurements as small as 4 mm, particularly if noted at 23 weeks' gestation or earlier. Corteville and associates' study noted 100% sensitivity, or the detection of all true-positive cases of fetal hydronephrosis, when a 4-mm or greater pelvic anteroposterior diameter measurement was used as evidence of abnormality. However, using this small a measurement, they had a false-positive group comprising greater than 42% of their cases. Using a 7-mm or greater measurement as evidence of abnormality, they noted only a 61% sensitivity for a true-positive diagnosis in 14- to 23-week-old gestations, but a 91% sensitivity among 24- to 32-week old gestations. Just over one third of both those groups of cases were false positive.[30,97]

We follow fetuses with dilated renal pelves ev-

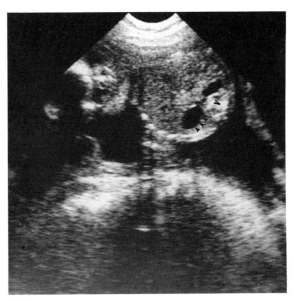

Figure 16-16. *Grade II dilatation. On transverse plane view arrowheads point to 1.3-cm dilatation of left renal pelvis. Dilatation on the right was physiologic. At birth, the baby had a ureteropelvic junction obstruction on the left and a normal right kidney (V, vertebral body).*

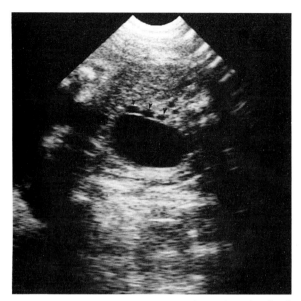

Figure 16-17. Grade IV dilatation. Longitudinal oblique plane view demonstrates a 3-cm dilatation of the renal pelvis with mild to moderate dilatation of calyces *(arrowheads)*. There was renal cortex, although it is difficult to see on this view.

ery 4 to 6 weeks, asking the clinicians to be wary of any impression of decreasing amniotic fluid. As long as there is a single functioning kidney, it is permissible to be less aggressive about follow-up until after birth. The postnatal confirmation of hydronephrosis should not be made within the first day or two of life because of the relative neonatal dehydration and relatively low glomerular filtration rate of young infants, which may contribute to a falsely normal appearance of the newborn renal pelvis.[24,88] Unless there is a clinical emergency, we save our neonatal renal assessment for day 2 to 3 of life. This is one of several cases in clinical ultrasound in which doing an immediate "emergency" examination does the patient a disservice.

A dilated renal pelvis can be caused by obstruction at any level of the urinary tract. It may be the result of vesicoureteral reflux, or may be related to prune belly syndrome. It may on rare occasions be caused by mass effect from a pelvic mass. Benacerraf and coworkers have linked mild fetal renal pelvis dilatation to Down's syndrome, but have not recommended amniocentesis when there is no other suspect finding for this karyotype abnormality. Most kidneys with antenatal pyelectasis (particularly when less than 1 cm) prove to be normal at birth.

The many cases of antenatally imaged fetal GU tract dilatation that have proven in neonatal life to be unrelated to either obstruction or vesicoureteral reflux have encouraged a decidedly conservative approach to intrauterine intervention, particularly for unilateral GU system dilatation.[8,24,57,97]

GENITOURINARY TRACT OBSTRUCTION

Early diagnosis of renal obstruction and subsequent early pediatric surgery for correction is necessary to ensure future renal function. A long-term follow-up study of patients with severe obstructive uropathy noted improvement or normalization of renal function when surgery was performed within the first year of life. If surgery was not performed until after age 2 years, patients experienced progressive deterioration of renal function.[5,24,103]

The most common cause of congenital obstructive hydronephrosis is ureteropelvic junction obstruction, which occurs in 1 of every 1258 newborns and is bilateral in almost one third of cases. Bilateral involvement is usually asymmetric; severe bilateral involvement is unusual. Progressive dilatation during antenatal life is common, particularly with the higher grades of obstruction.[58,146]

Ureterovesical junction obstruction is rare and is noted by dilatation of the ureter to the level of the bladder. Occasionally a partial renal obstruction may be noted antenatally due to a renal duplication anomaly consisting, unilaterally or bilaterally, of two renal collecting system moieties and their ureters. The upper pole (moiety) of the duplicated kidney often appears cyst-like because of obstruction, usually because of ectopic placement of its distal ureter, often in association with an ectopic ureterocele. The lower moiety often has associated vesicoureteral reflux and may, therefore, on occasion appear to have pyelocalyceal dilatation. The prenatal diagnosis of a duplicated kidney system is often limited by the small size of the upper moiety and the changing size of the ureterocele owing to intravesical pressures. Ureteroceles found outside the bladder may simulate any pelvic cystic mass, including ovarian cyst, anterior meningocele, and hydrocolpos. Primary megaureter can cause obstruction by lack of peristalsis in a focal portion of distal ureter. The ureter may appear dilated on ultrasound examination, but severe hydronephrosis is unusual.[24,58,113,145]

Bladder outlet obstructions are seen in patients with PUV, urethral atresia, and the caudal regression syndrome (a rare condition of variable severity that may range from sacral hypoplasia to complete absence of the sacrum and lumbar spine in association with genitourinary and gastrointestinal anomalies). In each case of bladder outlet obstruction there may be retrograde filling and dilatation of bladder, ureters, and renal pelvis. The bladder wall proximal to an area of obstruction may become trabeculated and appears thickened.

Posterior urethral valves (Fig. 16-18) is predominantly a male abnormality because of redundant membranous folds in the posterior urethra that lead to varying degrees of GU system obstruction. Typically, there is a thick-walled, dilated bladder, and often an apparent dilated posterior urethra. If the obstructed urine refluxes with pressure into the renal pelvis, there may be forniceal rupture and the development of a perirenal urinoma or urinary ascites. Severe hydronephrosis is seen in about 15% of cases. Severe hydronephrosis may lead to Potter's syndrome. Late, incomplete, or transient obstruction may lead to little, if any, renal damage. Female fetuses with dilated bladders may have caudal re-

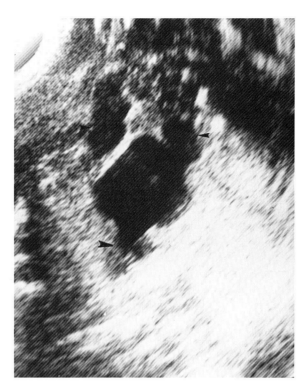

Figure 16-19. Urethral atresia. Coronal plane view shows dilated ureters (*small arrowheads*) leading to a dilated bladder with a conical outlet at the histopathologically proven point of urethral atresia (*large arrowhead*). This fetus died as a newborn of complications related to pulmonary hypoplasia.

gression syndrome, in which the presence of anal atresia and a persistent cloaca has been reported as a cause of obstruction of bladder and bowel.[50,66]

Complete urethral atresia (Fig. 16-19) is similar to severe PUV. Sonographic evidence of an enlarged bladder, dilated urethra, bilateral hydronephrosis, oligohydramnios, and cystic renal dysplasia (Potter's type IV) may be seen.[24,50]

PRUNE BELLY SYNDROME

Fetal ascites, when not caused by hydrops, may result from a GU system abnormality. Fetal ascites can distend the fetal abdomen and has been implicated in the development of the lax abdominal musculature of prune belly syndrome. Of 14 infants with posterior urethral obstruction reviewed by Hayden and colleagues, 77% had the prune belly triad of deficient abdominal musculature, cryptorchidism, and GU anomaly. Whether this represents

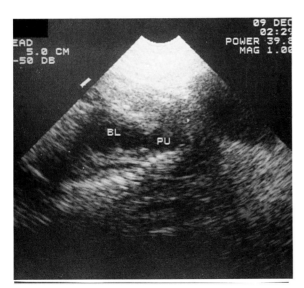

Figure 16-18. Posterior urethral valves. Transverse oblique view at level of bladder and posterior urethra shows urine in the bladder (BL) and the posterior urethra (PU), which normally is not imaged. There is some increased thickness to the bladder wall. The valve itself was not imaged antenatally but was noted on a neonatal voiding cystourethrogram.

truly prune belly syndrome, a sporadic mesodermal defect occurring in 1 in 40,000 births and usually associated with dilated, tortuous ureters and ineffective peristalsis, or pseudo-prune belly syndrome, is unknown. Both disorders may show undulation of the anterior abdominal wall of the fetus when the transducer is used to tap on the mother's abdominal wall.[66,70,157]

RENAL DYSPLASIA

Renal dysplasia is the result of abnormal metanephric tissue differentiation. Disorganized epithelial structures and fibrous tissue replace normally functioning glomeruli and tubules; dysplastic areas are irreversibly damaged. It is the cysts or cystic areas of these dysplasias that most readily allow their antenatal diagnosis.[97] Renal dysplasias are said to occur at the rate of 2 to 4 cases for every 1000 births. There is some controversy regarding their classification and pathogenesis. Osthanondh and Potter classified cystic dysplasias of the kidneys into four types: type I, autosomal recessive polycystic kidney disease (RPK), also known as infantile polycystic kidney disease; type II, multicystic dysplastic kidney (MDK); type III, autosomal dominant polycystic kidney disease, also known as adult polycystic kidney disease; and type IV, cystic renal dysplasia. Types II and IV are the most common (Table 16-4).[24,46,116]

Recessive polycystic kidney disease affects both kidneys, and its reported incidence is 2 cases in 110,000 births,[134] with a 25% recurrence rate in affected families. Saccular dilatations of the collecting tubules create multiple small cysts, typically, 1 to 2 mm and therefore too small to be resolved as cysts on sonography. The classic image is that of massively enlarged, homogeneously echogenic kidneys (Fig. 16-20) taking up most of the abdomen's space. Unlike in other dysplasias, there is no increase in connective tissue within these kidneys. Affected fetuses tend to have severe oligohydramnios because of bilateral renal dysfunction, and the bladder is not imaged. Neonatal death is usually caused by pulmonary hypoplasia. Cases have been reported of kidneys later proven to have RPK that appeared normal on early antenatal scans, and abnormal only on scans in later pregnancy. Surviving children with RPK often have associated hepatic fibrosis, with a severity inversely related to the severity of their renal disease.[24,97,100]

Multicystic dysplastic kidney is the most common of the cystic renal dysplasias. Some believe that MDK results from early ureteropelvic atresia. When, in the typical case, MDK is only a unilateral finding, the amniotic fluid level—and therefore fetal lung development—is unaffected. An abnormality in the contralateral kidney is not uncommon, and contralateral ureteropelvic junction obstructions are often seen. Bilateral MDK (19% incidence in one study of contralateral MDK disease) or MDK with contralateral renal agenesis (11%) is incompatible with life. There is a question of at least a partial genetic influence in this disorder, which has a 3% to 5% familial recurrence rate. The sonographic image (Fig. 16-21) consists of multiple, large anechoic cysts of variable size, the largest of which is *not* central (more typical of hydronephrosis). The kidney may vary in size from small to normal to large, but the reniform shape is often absent. Increased echogenicity between the cysts is usually the result of connective tissue proliferation. The renal pelvis and proximal ureter are absent or atretic. Histologically, these kidneys typically consist of thick-walled cysts, small groups of tubules, and poorly formed glomeruli. Nephrons, although few in number, can produce urine, which is why these dysplastic kidneys have been reported occasionally to increase in size. Many reports of disappearing MDKs may, in part, be related to eventual cessation of any urine production.[24,65,84,97,143]

Autosomal dominant (or adult) polycystic kidney disease is rarely seen in antenatal life. Case reports note cysts interspersed in the cortex and medulla of bilaterally enlarged kidneys. Small cysts may not be resolved and the kidneys may appear only echogenic. Although adult polycystic kidney disease is a bilateral disease, there may be asymmetry of involvement. Amniotic fluid levels may be normal or decreased.[46,101,129]

Type IV dysplasia is thought to be secondary to an early obstruction of the GU tract. Usually seen in severe cases of PUV, it is commonly seen in association with the more severe obstruction of urethral atresia (Fig. 16-22). It has been reported in the caudal regression syndrome with persistent cloaca and other obstructions. Focal and segmental dysplasia may be seen and are often caused by obstruction or atresia of one of the ureters extending from a duplicated kidney. Ultrasonographically, there is usually significant oligohydramnios and

▰▰▰ TABLE 16-4. FETAL RENAL DYSPLASIA

Type	Involvement	Sonographic Appearance	Associated Findings
TYPE I, Autosomal recessive polycystic kidney disease or infantile polycystic kidney disease	Bilateral	1- to 2-mm cysts too small to be seen sonographically; massively enlarged homogeneous echogenic kidneys taking up most of the abdomen's space	Oligohydramnios, bladder not visualized, neonatal death due to pulmonary hypoplasia
TYPE II, Multicystic dysplastic kidney (*most common*)	Usually unilateral	Multiple large anechoic cysts of varying size, the largest not being central; kidney size varies from small to normal to large; reniform shape is often lost; echogenicity between cysts results from proliferation of connective tissue	Amniotic fluid level and lung development unaffected in unilateral dysplasia
TYPE III, Autosomal dominant polycystic kidney disease or adult polycystic disease	Uncommon in neonatal life; bilateral disease usually presents in adult life		
TYPE IV, Cystic renal dysplasia	Occurs secondary to an early genitourinary tract obstruction; can be seen in severe cases of posterior urethral valves; commonly seen in urethral atresia	Moderately enlarged echogenic kidneys with scattered small cysts	Significant oligohydramnios

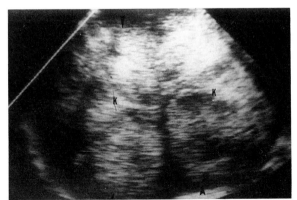

Figure 16-20. Autosomal recessive (infantile) polycystic kidney disease. Transverse oblique view of abdomen shows echogenic enlarged kidneys (K, *arrowheads*) taking up most of this newborn's abdomen. A high near-field gain setting is responsible for the apparent increase in the echogenicity of the anterior third of the kidneys.

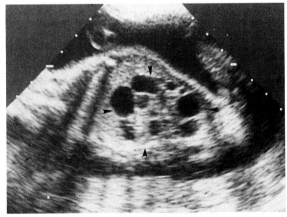

Figure 16-21. Multicystic dysplastic kidney. Longitudinal view shows multiple cysts of varying sizes in this right renal mass (*arrowheads*) that retains a relatively reniform shape. The left kidney was normal.

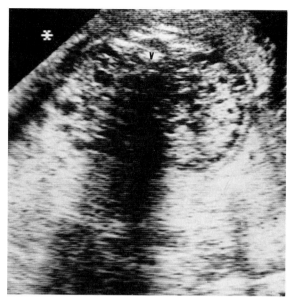

Figure 16-22. Cystic renal dysplasia, type IV. Transverse plane image shows scattered cysts, mostly peripheral, in these enlarged kidneys of a fetus with genitourinary tract obstruction due to urethral atresia (v, vertebral body).

13, and one tenth of those with trisomy 18 have associated renal cystic involvement.[97,158]

MISCELLANEOUS AND UNUSUAL FETAL RENAL FINDINGS

Fetal renal hamartomas (congenital mesoblastic nephromas) are the most common renal neoplasms of the first few months of life. They have been noted antenatally as unilateral echogenic masses. Bilateral fetal renal tumors may be simulated by the enlarged but functioning kidneys associated with tyrosinosis, glycogen storage diseases, and other congenital metabolic disorders. Renal vein thrombosis is a well-known entity in neonates that often presents with palpably enlarged kidneys and associated hematuria or varying degrees of renal failure. Theoretic etiologies include septicemia, maternal diabetes, prenatal steroid administration, and congenital renal defects. Linear echoes or densities within the kidneys suggest the pathognomonic intrarenal calcification within thrombosed renal vessels.[13,75,117]

moderately enlarged kidneys with small to medium capsular or parenchymal (usually peripheral) cysts. Other findings depend on the site and degree of obstruction. Obstructions at or distal to the bladder that are of long standing may show bladder wall thickening and enlargement as well as ureteral dilatation and a tortuous ureteral course when there is obstruction along the course of the ureter.[6,24,97,100]

OTHER DISEASES WITH RENAL CYSTS

Several inherited syndromes have nonobstructive cystic renal dysplasia as part of their findings. These include Zellweger, Ehlers-Danlos, and von Hippel-Lindau syndromes. Meckel-Gruber syndrome is one such entity with renal cysts (usually as part of bilateral MDK) associated with occipital encephalocele and polydactyly. It has a 25% recurrence rate in future pregnancies. Knowledge of the associated ultrasound findings of syndromes can aid in making more specific antenatal diagnoses. This is particularly true in assessing future pregnancies. Half of all patients with the VACTERL (*v*ertebral abnormalities, *a*nal atresia, *c*ardiac abnormalities, *t*racheo-*e*sophageal, *r*enal, and *l*imb [or *r*adius] abnormalities) association, one third of those with trisomy

SCROTUM

Fetal hydroceles (Fig. 16-23) are very common. A variable amount of fluid remaining from normal testicular descent into the scrotum can be seen surrounding the testes. These hydroceles do not in-

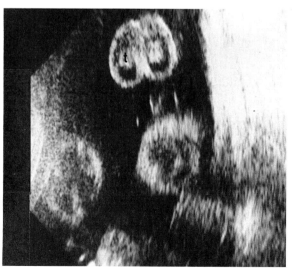

Figure 16-23. Hydrocele. In a coronal view, fluid surrounds each testicle (t, right testis) in this scrotum surrounded by amniotic fluid.

crease in size and tend to be resorbed within the first 9 months of life. Enlarging hydroceles indicate continued patency of the processus vaginalis and continued communication with the peritoneum, and are readily noted in fetal ascites. Increasing scrotal volume may indicate an inguinal hernia. Intrascrotal extension of meconium peritonitis may produce echogenic or calcified intrascrotal masses.[24,81,104] A heterogeneous testicle and occasionally one that may simulate a hydrocele, but is echopenic and not echoless, may suggest antenatal testicular torsion.[60]

ADRENAL GLANDS

The fetal adrenal gland, as previously mentioned, may assume a more circular shape and simulate a kidney in the presence of renal agenesis. The adrenal gland has also been described as appearing flat (the "lying down" adrenal sign) in other cases of fetal or neonatal renal agenesis or ectopia.[73] Anencephalic fetuses have small adrenal glands, allegedly because no adrenocorticotropic hormone is produced.[18] The adrenal gland is said to weigh less in the offspring of preeclamptic mothers and patients with antepartum hemorrhage.[42]

The diagnosis of congenital malignant neoplasms of the adrenal gland are very rare. Most of those discovered antenatally have been neuroblastomas, the most common extracranial solid malignancy of children. The sonographic patterns of those antenatally detected neuroblastomas have been nonspecific, with mixed cystic and solid, solid, and hyperechoic masses reported. The asymmetry of these masses from the contralateral adrenal gland may help differentiate them from enlargement due to fetal adrenal hemorrhage.[42]

The Intraluminal Gastrointestinal Tract

ESOPHAGUS

Rapid proliferation of the esophageal epithelium during the fetal embryonic period creates almost complete closure of the esophageal lumen. One infant in every 2500 live births, predominantly male infants, may have a complication thought to be caused by this esophageal maldevelopment or by unequal partitioning of the foregut into the esophagus and trachea, resulting in esophageal atresia.[68]

Several types are described. The most common consists of a proximal esophageal pouch with communication with the more distal gastrointestinal (GI) tract through a fistula between the tracheobronchial tree of the respiratory tract, usually at or near the tracheal bifurcation, and the more distal esophagus. Communication with the more distal GI tract significantly reduces the number of fetuses that present with polyhydramnios due to impaired swallowing. Polyhydramnios (Fig. 16-24) has been reported in 76% of affected fetuses but in only 8% of those with an associated fistula. Another helpful sign for the antenatal diagnosis of esophageal atresia is the absence of a fluid-filled stomach. Even fetuses with a fistula may have only partly filled stomachs. Cases have been reported of actual antenatal visualization of the area of esophageal atresia. This finding requires the fortuitous presence of fluid in the proximal esophagus at the time of imaging.[40,52,68,128]

Esophageal atresia is associated with Down's syndrome and other chromosomal abnormalities, and is part of the VACTERL association. Fetuses

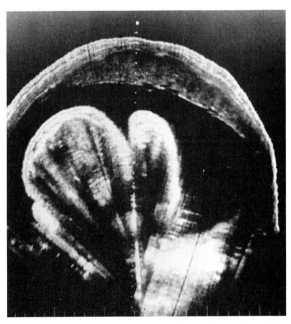

Figure 16-24. Polyhydramnios and esophageal atresia. Transverse plane view through gravid uterus demonstrates polyhydramnios. This fetus proved at birth to have esophageal atresia without distal gastrointestinal tract communication. The atresia itself was not imaged antenatally.

suspected of having esophageal atresia should be studied to note if any of these associated abnormalities are present.[155]

STOMACH

A fluid-filled stomach noted in the left upper quadrant may allow the sonographer or sonologist to image adjacent normal structures, such as the spleen, and to rule out abnormalities other than esophageal atresia without fistula (i.e., abdominal situs inversus, diaphragmatic hernia, and obstruction of the upper GI tract). The absence of stomach fluid can be seen on a physiologic basis in oligohydramnios or in the purported stress of nonimmune hydrops, despite polyhydramnios. However, absence of a stomach or the continuous imaging of an unusually small fetal stomach after 18 weeks' gestational age (in the absence of oligohydramnios) is associated with a guarded prognosis. McKenna and colleagues recorded associated structural abnormalities or intrauterine/neonatal death in 85% of a group of 27 fetuses with an absent stomach and 52% of a group of 52 fetuses with an unusually small stomach. Chromosomal abnormalities were noted in 38% of the absent stomach group that underwent karyotyping and in 4% of the small stomach group.[52,95]

Duplications of Stomach and Bowel

Duplications can exist throughout the bowel. They are probably caused by errors of GI lumen recanalization, and in the stomach in particular, by errors in the development of normal inpouching of the longitudinal folds. Stomach duplication is the least common, although 109 cases were reported in the literature through 1984.[10]

Antenatal diagnoses of duplications have been made in all parts of the GI tract. They are typically echoless cystic structures, occasionally filled with echogenic hemorrhagic or inspissated material. Echogenic inner walls may be seen, owing to their mucosal lining.[10,15,21,78,152]

MIDGUT VOLVULUS

The bowel attains its normal position and configuration after a 270° rotation, of which the first 180° occurs in the extraembryonic coelom at the base of the umbilical cord (in weeks 6 through 10). The remaining 90° occurs within the fetal abdomen. If the small bowel fails to enter the abdominal cavity and rotate properly, or if the long mesenteric attachments that fix the bowel to the posterior abdominal wall fail to develop, the bowel will be malrotated and may twist about the axis of the superior mesenteric artery, resulting in poor vascular flow to the small bowel distal to the point of obstruction or volvulus. If it is not untwisted surgically, infarction results.[23,26,68]

Midgut volvulus is usually diagnosed in the first days of life; the infant may present with distention or obstruction, but, most typically, with bilious vomiting. Antenatal diagnosis has been made by noting mild polyhydramnios, an echogenic mass under the fetal liver, and slightly dilated bowel loops. The sonographer may note, antenatally, the typical neonatal sonographic image of a fluid-filled proximal duodenum with an arrowhead twist at the point of descending or transverse duodenal obstruction.[23,26,141]

SMALL BOWEL OBSTRUCTION

Causes of small bowel obstruction include the aforementioned intestinal duplications as well as bowel atresia or stenosis, midgut volvulus and congenital peritoneal bands, internal hernias, and Hirschsprung's disease when it involves the entire colon.[114]

Duodenal atresia occurs in 1 in 10,000 births. As a result of failure of recanalization during the embryonic period, there is usually a membrane or diaphragm in the duodenum in its descending (second) or horizontal (third) portion. Less often, the duodenal atresia is caused by transverse diaphragms, blind-ending loops connected by a linear fibrous attachment, or unconnected blind loops. Fluid filling the stomach and the duodenum at the site of obstruction creates the classic "double-bubble" image of duodenal atresia (Fig. 16-25). The double-bubble image is nonspecific and can be seen in other entities, including duodenal stenosis (typically involving the third or fourth portion of the duodenum), annular pancreas (a ring of anomalously rotated pancreas encircling the descending portion of the duodenum), and in association with anomalous peritoneal bands (Ladd's bands) associated with abnormal bowel rotation, and often midgut volvulus.[53,68]

Almost half of all duodenal atresia cases are associ-

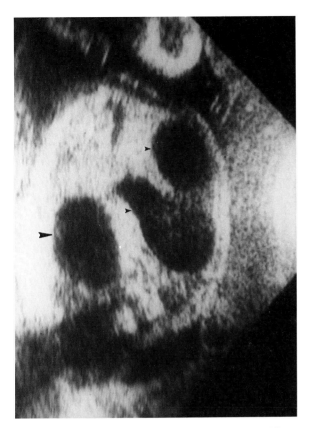

Figure 16-25. Double-bubble sign. Transverse oblique plane view shows fluid-filled stomach (*small arrowhead*), in this case visualized with a little more anatomic detail than the classic single bubble of stomach and second bubble of proximal duodenum (*large arrowhead*). Although typically it is caused by duodenal atresia, the double-bubble sign is nonspecific. In this case it was caused by a more distal jejunal atresia.

TABLE 16-5. PREVALENCE OF ANOMALIES ASSOCIATED WITH DUODENAL ATRESIA[47,52,68,110]	
Anomaly	**Prevalance (%)**
Cardiovascular	20
Bowel malrotation	22–40
Trisomy 21	33
Symmetric growth retardation	50
Polyhydramnios	45
Esophageal atresia or tracheoesophageal fistula	7

noileal atresia (Fig. 16-26) are more common, with the most common sites of involvement being the proximal jejunum or the distal ileum. Antenatal impairment of the blood supply to the jejunum and ileum is thought to be responsible. Jejunoileal atre-

ated with other anomalies (Table 16-5). One fifth are cardiovascular, 22% to 40% are bowel malrotations, and as many as one third are associated with trisomy 21. About 50% of affected fetuses show symmetric growth retardation, and, as with any high GI tract obstruction, many (45%) have polyhydramnios. Seven percent have associated esophageal atresia and tracheoesophageal fistula. Early neonatal surgery is associated with a good GI tract result.[47,52,68,110]

Duodenal atresia may be part of an uncommon, complex, and extensive small bowel atresia (known as apple-peel or Christmas tree atresia) that involves most of the small bowel to the proximal ileum. This is thought to be caused by prenatal obstruction of either the right colic or marginal branch of the superior mesenteric artery. Smaller areas of jeju-

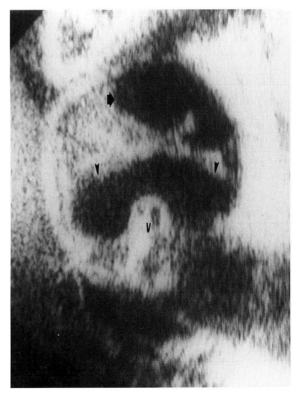

Figure 16-26. Jejunal atresia. Fluid fills a dilated transverse duodenum (*arrowheads*) noted crossing the midline vertebral body (V). This suggests normal bowel rotation. More distal bowel dilatation was noted, suggesting jejunal atresia, although the specific site of obstruction could not be determined antenatally (*arrow, stomach*).

sias occur sporadically once in every 3000 to 5000 births. Polyhydramnios associated with small bowel obstruction is usually seen only in the third trimester. Proximal lesions are associated with a higher incidence of polyhydramnios. In more distal obstructions, if they develop polyhydramnios, the increase in amniotic fluid occurs later and to a lesser degree. Although small bowel obstructions may be caused by one long atresia or multiple, smaller-length areas of atresia, the antenatal ultrasound image typically shows only one area of dilated fluid-filled loops proximal to the obstruction.[52,92]

Dilated bowel is also an antenatal sonographic sign of meconium ileus due to cystic fibrosis, an inherited (autosomal recessive) dysfunction of the exocrine and mucus-producing glands, most particularly of the pancreas, biliary tract, intestines, and bronchi, with associated disturbances of mucus and electrolyte secretion. It is the most common lethal genetic condition among whites, occurring at a frequency of 1 in 2000 live births. The meconium ileus that fetuses with cystic fibrosis may suffer consists of a small bowel obstruction due to impaction of the distal ileum with inspissated meconium. Meconium ileus, like other causes of small bowel obstruction, may lead to bowel perforation and the complications and findings of meconium peritonitis.[52,53,114]

The findings of polyhydramnios, a disproportionately dilated proximal small bowel (see Fig. 16-26), the failure to detect normal colon in late pregnancy, fetal ascites or peritoneal calcifications (see Fig. 16-11), decreased or absent peristalsis in dilated bowel loops noted over a period of time, and a large abdominal circumference for gestational age should make the examiner suspect a small bowel obstruction. Lack of bowel contents entering the large bowel can produce microcolon. Associated bowel perforations, which often close before birth, may be the cause of ascites and meconium peritonitis.[52] Peristalsis, which in postnatal work may highlight bowel just proximal to a point of early obstruction, is not always easy to determine in antenatal small bowel evaluation. Functional causes of bowel dilatation may simulate obstruction, including the rare congenital chloridorrhea, with its profuse chloride diarrhea, dilated small bowel, and microcolon.[59]

ECHOGENIC BOWEL

Clinical reports have noted that collapsed small bowel often appears as an echogenic "mass" in normal fetuses. This is an especially common finding among fetuses less than 20 weeks' gestational age. However, it also can be a normal finding at other points in pregnancy, particularly the late third trimester.[19,41] Increased bowel echogenicity has been associated with several pathologic conditions, including fetal viral (cytomegalovirus) infections, chromosomal abnormalities (triploidy and trisomy 21, 18, or 13), and mesenteric ischemia, but particularly meconium ileus with its hyperechoic intraluminal meconium. Increased intraluminal bowel echogenicity has also been linked to swallowed blood from intraamniotic bleeding, as well as an unusual case of intraluminal gas produced by bacteria associated with maternal amnionitis.[18,71,119,137] Exactly what represents increased echogenicity is highly subjective. Certainly, bowel echogenicity greater than the echogenicity of nearby fetal bone has been commonly acclaimed as indicating greater risk for meconium ileus/cystic fibrosis and the pathologic processes associated with increased bowel echogenicity. Because of the increased association with fetal demise and IUGR, these fetuses should be followed closely.[71,119,137]

In analyzing an area of increased echogenicity or possible calcification in the fetal abdomen, the clinician should consider the possibility that the increased echogenicity or calcification is neither in the parenchyma of an organ such as the liver nor within bowel lumen, but rather is on the peritoneal surface (see Fig. 16-11). Peritoneal echogenicity, often seen at the periphery but not within the liver, is caused by meconium peritonitis and the sterile chemical reaction that develops on peritoneal surfaces from contact with meconium that has leaked from small intrauterine bowel perforations. At least half of these perforations are thought to result from distal mechanical obstructions, whereas the remainder may be caused by viral infections such as cytomegalovirus or parvovirus B19. Only one fourth of cases of meconium peritonitis result from meconium ileus and cystic fibrosis.[137]

COLON OBSTRUCTION

Large bowel obstructions are more difficult to diagnose antenatally than those of the small bowel. They are not associated with increases in amniotic fluid. Normal colon tends to be seen only later in pregnancy (third trimester), and bowel peristalsis is not seen. The major causes of large bowel obstruction are imperforate anus, or anal atresia, and Hirschsprung's disease (an aganglionosis of part of or the entire colon). Focal bowel dilatation has been reported as an antenatal clue. Total colonic Hirschsprung's disease is a particularly difficult diagnosis to make because of the lack of a normal segment of bowel for comparison.[68,114,153]

A colon diameter (wall-to-wall measurement) greater than 23 mm in a preterm fetus is considered abnormal.[118] Fetal rectosigmoid colon, however, can reach a size of 2 to 3 cm when filled with meconium near term. Seen in as many as 6% of a group of third trimester fetuses, it can simulate a presacral mass.[79]

Abdominal Wall Defects

Abdominal wall defects vary in type and complexity. The two most common types, omphalocele and gastroschisis, have been well evaluated by sonography. Other abdominal wall defects range from the mundane umbilical hernia, with its linea alba defect and protruding bowel covered by skin and subcutaneous tissue, to the complex defects of cloaca or bladder extrophy, ectopia cordis, amniotic band syndrome, and the limb–body wall complex. The development of the anterior abdominal wall is based on fusion of four ectomesodermal folds, a cephalic, a caudal, and a pair of lateral folds. Abdominal wall defects are one of the causes of high α-fetoprotein levels in amniotic fluid or maternal serum, and should be searched for in such situations. Knowledge of the particular defect and its associated abnormalities is necessary for proper decision making with regard to continuation of pregnancy, method of delivery, and surgical treatment (Table 16-6).[68,135]

OMPHALOCELE

Omphalocele (Fig. 16-27) is a midline defect that occurs in 1 in 4000 births. It may be caused by failure of fusion of the lateral ectomesodermal folds or by persistence of the body stalk in an area normally occupied by abdominal wall.[54,135]

Sonography may reveal abdominal viscera, covered by an amnion/peritoneal sac, protruding through a midline defect (2 to 10 cm) into the base of the umbilical cord. The omphalocele typically contains liver, but it may contain other viscera, usually large or small bowel, and not contain liver. There is often associated fetal ascites.[54,68] Omphaloceles are often

(50% to 70%) associated with other anomalies whose presence affects prognosis for the worse. Gastrointestinal anomalies are found in 30% to 50% of cases—usually bowel malrotation, but sometimes atresia or stenosis of small bowel, bowel duplication, biliary atresia, tracheoesophageal fistula, and imperforate anus. Half of the anomalies are cardiovascular, including ventricular and atrial septal defects, tetralogy of Fallot, pulmonary artery stenosis, and abnormalities of the great vessels. Forty to 60% of patients have a chromosomal abnormality, including trisomies 13, 18, and 21 as well as Turner's, Klinefelter's, and triploidy syndromes.[54,68,82] The smaller the abdominal wall defect and the fewer the associated anomalies, the better the prognosis. Defects greater than 5 cm tend to a more adverse outcome. The presence of spleen or heart in the sac has been associated with a poor outcome.[107,135]

Omphaloceles are part of several significant fetal malformation syndromes. One seventh of omphalocele cases are associated with the Beckwith-Wiedemann syndrome (organomegaly, macroglossia, hypoglycemia, hemihypertrophy, and increased risk for Wilms' tumor). Cloacal extrophy involves a low omphalocele with cloacal or bladder extrophy and variable caudal abnormalities. Omphaloceles associated with ectopia cordis are part of the pentalogy of Cantrell.[54,68,135]

Proper imaging to rule out omphalocele requires evaluation of the anterior abdominal wall and noting, in normal patients, entry of the cord into an intact wall. Because of the normal physiologic herniation of bowel into the umbilical cord, the clinician must be cautious about the diagnosis of omphalocele before 12 weeks' gestational age, by which time the physiologic event has ended. A definitive first trimester diagnosis is made by some imagers only if the omphalocele is larger than the abdomen itself.[54] Bowerman reported that omphalocele may be suggested early in pregnancy, if the cord containing midgut has a maximal dimension of 7 mm or greater.[14] Occasionally, the antenatal evidence of a sac membrane enables an omphalocele to be differentiated from gastroschisis on the postnatal examination of an infant whose sac ruptured during delivery.

GASTROSCHISIS

Gastroschisis (Fig. 16-28) is a smaller abdominal wall defect (2 to 4 cm) that is off midline, typically just to the right of it, and unrelated to the

◢◤◢◤ **TABLE 16-6 ANOMALIES INVOLVING THE BODY WALL**

Type of Anomaly	Description	Sonographic Appearance	Diagnostic Considerations
Omphalocele	Herniation of abdominal viscera into the base of the umbilical cord; liver involvement common	Complex membrane-enclosed sac; midline anterior wall defect continuous with umbilical cord. Size varies with amount of involved viscera.	29%–66% association with other anomalies
Gastroschisis	Herniation of abdominal viscera through an off-midline defect in the abdominal wall, usually located just to the right of the umbilicus; liver involvement very unusual	Free-floating bowel loops not bound by a sac. Insertion of the umbilical cord is normal.	Associated gastrointestinal anomalies are common; anomalies of other systems are rarely seen
Umbilical cord hernia	Protrusion of a small amount of intestine at the umbilicus	Similar to omphalocele; covered by skin and subcutaneous tissue, usually less than 2–4 cm	Limited clinical significance; associated anomalies are unusual
Bladder extrophy	Congenital failure of abdominal wall to develop over bladder; urinary bladder may be everted (inside may protrude through abdominal wall)	Variable: May see a fluid-filled intrapelvic portion of bladder with a contiguous extraabdominal mass with echogenicity similar to that of soft tissue. More commonly, no fluid-filled intrapelvic bladder is seen.	Most common in boys; may be associated with gastrointestinal, genitourinary, and musculoskeletal anomalies; must be differentiated from urachal cyst
Ectopic cordis	Defect of the lower sternum and anterior abdominal wall; heart protrudes into extrathoracic sac covered by skin or a thin membrane	Beating heart protrudes through anterior abdominal wall into amniotic fluid	Often associated with amniotic band syndrome; other associated anomalies include craniofacial and limb deformities and omphalocele; very poor prognosis
Limb–body wall complex	Complex of anomalies including lateral body wall defects of thorax and abdomen with herniation of viscera; cranial, craniofacial, spinal, and limb anomalies common	Herniated viscera within a complex membrane-involved mass, severe scoliosis, cranial defects, spinal defects	A severe form of amniotic band syndrome is thought to play a major role in pathogenesis; no genetic predisposition has been identified; not compatible with life

umbilical cord. Theoretic causes include abnormal involution of the right umbilical vein and disruption of the omphalomesenteric artery.[33] Gastroschisis occurs once in every 2500 to 5800 pregnancies. Except for bowel malrotation and jejunal or ileal atresia, associated anomalies are probably related to vascular compromise of the malrotated bowel, and are far less common than with omphalocele.[54,68]

The herniated viscera, usually small or large bowel (rarely liver), are not covered by a sac. This fact leads to the development of a fibrinous coating

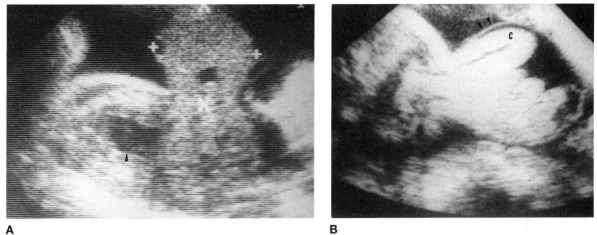

A   **B**

Figure 16-27. Omphalocele. (**A**) Coronal view. A large mass, marked off by crosses, is seen extending anterior to the abdomen. The abdominal cavity appears small owing to a decrease in its contents (*arrowhead, heart*). (**B**) Transverse oblique view of anterior abdominal wall shows that the omphalocele sac (*arrowheads*) contains colon (c). On another view the sac was seen to enter the umbilical cord. Matching images of anterior abdominal wall, omphalocele, and cord help to confirm the diagnosis, although this is sometimes difficult with large omphaloceles.

on the bowel, probably the result of chemical peritonitis produced by its contact with fetal urine in the amniotic fluid.[54,85,135] Although there is active debate over the method of delivery, most clinicians favor cesarean section to avoid further contamination of the uncovered, eviscerated bowel. Surgical closure is done primarily or in stages; a Silastic covering is placed over the bowel and abdominal wall defect between operations.[83,90]

Sonographically, this abnormality has been noted as early as 14 to 16 weeks. The diagnosis can typically be made by visualizing free-floating small bowel loops in the amniotic fluid. Sometimes the image may simulate that of an omphalocele, and

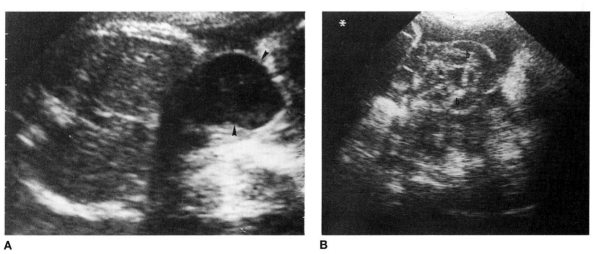

A   **B**

Figure 16-28. Gastroschisis. (**A**) In this transverse oblique view, the stomach (*arrowheads*) is seen extending through an off-midline anterior wall defect. (**B**) In the transverse view, several loops of small bowel (b), without a covering sac, are seen in the amniotic fluid surrounding the fetus.

the imager must attempt to rule out omphalocele by proving that the mass is not associated with the umbilical cord.

PATENT URACHUS AND BLADDER EXTROPHY

The urachus connects the allantoic stalk to the anterior cloaca. Normally, around week 12, patency is obliterated and the urachus becomes the median vesicular ligament. Partial obliteration can lead to cystic masses between the bladder and umbilicus along the anterior abdominal wall. A urachal cyst (cystic mass along the duct's course without bladder communication), urachal sinus (cystic mass that communicates with the anterior abdominal wall but not with the bladder), or partially patent urachus (cystic tubular area communicating with the bladder but not the abdominal wall) may be noted. Rarely, patent urachus (complete communication between bladder and anterior abdominal wall at the umbilicus) may occur (1 to 2.5 per 100,000 deliveries, twice as often in boys as in girls). It has been noted antenatally as a cystic mass extending from the bladder apex to the anterior abdominal wall at the umbilicus. The abnormality is limited and is not associated with other significant congenital abnormalities. The mass may be noted extraabdominally and therefore may require differentiation from the more serious problem of bladder extrophy.[97,120]

Bladder extrophy is a more common (1 in 25,000 to 40,000 births, three times more common in boys) and serious anomaly, associated with other GU, GI, and musculoskeletal abnormalities. Failure of development of a primitive streak of mesoderm in the allantoic extension of the cloacal membrane leads to variable presentations of bladder extrophy, including split bony symphysis, divergent rectus muscles, and exteriorization of the bladder. The extraabdominal mass, in variants that have an intrapelvic portion of fluid-filled bladder, are said to be echogenic, simulating omphalocele more than patent urachus.[97,105,120]

Pelvis

The normal fetal pelvis is small, and masses within it typically extend into the abdomen. The only routinely visualized normal organ is the fluid-filled bladder. In the third trimester, the meconium-filled, echopenic, and tubular rectosigmoid may be noted. Normal muscle groups are often seen to be separated by echogenic fascial lines. The two major groups of abnormality in this area are those of the female genital system, seen as pelvic masses that may extend beyond the pelvis and into the abdomen, and sacrococcygeal teratomas (SCT), noted as predominantly external masses with variable internal pelvic extension. A good check to determine that there is no external SCT is to look for symmetry of the soft tissues of the fetal rump without evidence of an associated mass (see Fig. 15-18).

FEMALE GENITAL SYSTEM

Despite maternal hormone stimulation, antenatal visualization of vagina, uterus, or ovary is possible only if there is abnormal enlargement or a pelvic

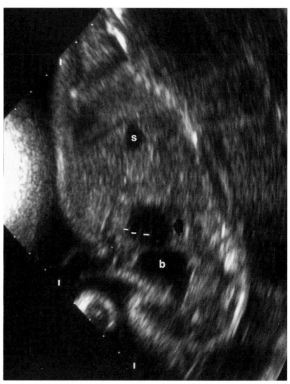

Figure 16-29. Cystic ovary. Longitudinal view of fetal chest, abdomen, and pelvis. A multiseptated cystic structure (*arrow*) is seen superior to the bladder (b). In a female fetus, the possibility must be considered that this represents a normal, albeit hyperstimulated ovary due to significant stimulation by circulating maternal hormones. That is what this proved to be. White lines point to apparent septations, which actually represented cyst walls (s, stomach).

▰▰▰ TABLE 16-7. CLASSIFICATION OF SACROCOCCYGEAL TERATOMA

Type I	Predominantly *external* component, minimal presacral or intrapelvic extension
Type II	Predominantly *external* component, significant *intrapelvic* extension
Type III	Small external component, significant *intrapelvic/intraabdominal* component
Type IV	No apparent external component, predominantly *presacral* or *intrapelvic* tumor

(Data from Hogge W, Thiagarajah S, Barber V, et al. Cystic sacrococcygeal teratoma: Ultrasound diagnosis and management. J Ultrasound Med. 1987; 6:707–710.)

mass.[97] Hydrometrocolpos, a cystic dilatation of the vagina and uterus due to fluid and mucus accumulation proximal to a point of obstruction, is noted as a hypoechoic mass posterior to the bladder that may occasionally compress the lower ureters, leading to hydronephrosis. When the obstruction is caused by vaginal atresia or a vaginal membrane, there may be associated genitourinary tract abnormalities.[1,25,29,97] Fetal ovarian cysts are noted infrequently on ultrasound examination and are nearly always benign. They probably develop in response to maternal hormonal stimulation. Small follicular cysts not visualized on fetal examination are found in many autopsy specimens and are certainly a common finding in the ovaries of the neonate.[27]

Fetal ovarian cysts may be unilocular or multiseptate cystic masses (Fig. 16-29) that, when enlarged, may rise out of the pelvis and into the abdomen. These cystic masses may be simulated by urachal cysts, enteric duplications, or mesenteric cysts. Bilateral multiseptate cystic pelvic masses in a female fetus suggest an ovarian origin. Internal echogenicity may be noted within the ovarian cysts due to hemorrhage. This may be evidence of ovarian torsion. An ovarian mass on a pedicle can present in a high abdominal location, or in varying locations on follow-up examinations, thus obscuring its site of origin.[27,29,97,130] Cystic ovaries are not of unusual concern in the neonate and are often followed clinically when there are no symptoms. However, surgeons operate on a neonate with a cystic ovary on a pedicle, because they are at risk for torsion, and cystic ovaries with hemorrhage/fluid levels or with contained clot or multiple septations suggesting that torsion has already occurred.[28]

Ovarian cysts, unlike hydrometrocolpos, are said not to compress the GU system, although they can compress bowel. This may be responsible for the reported 1 case in 10 of polyhydramnios associated with large ovarian cysts. These large cysts may cause dystocia.[29,97]

Sacrococcygeal Teratoma

The SCT is the most common tumor noted in neonatal life. Most cases are asymptomatic and discovered after birth. There may be associated morbidity and mortality related to prematurity, dystocia, traumatic delivery, and intratumoral hemorrhage. Antenatal diagnosis is therefore important. In a few cases, placentomegaly and fetal hydrops may occur and are associated with fetal demise. In those few cases discovered in a fetus too young to deliver (less than 28 weeks) and "amenable to easy resection," Harrison and colleagues suggest the consideration

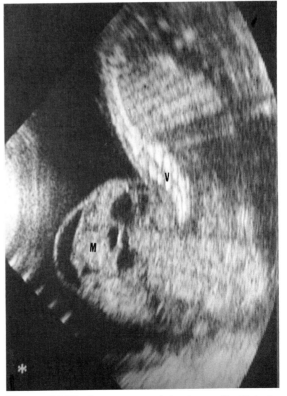

Figure 16-30. Sacrococcygeal teratoma. Sagittal view shows a predominantly solid mass (M) extending from the patient's sacral area. No vertebral column (v) abnormality was noted.

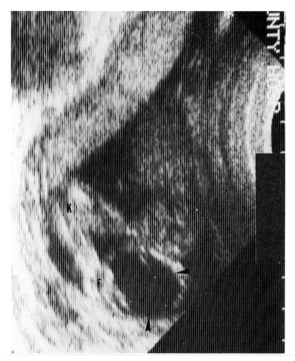

Figure 16-31. Cystic sacrococcygeal teratoma. On the sagittal view a cystic mass (*arrowheads*) extends from this fetus' rump as if the fetus were sitting on it (K, knee; F, foot).

of intrauterine resection.[62] The increased incidence (2% to 4% in newborns, 60% in 4-month-old infants) of malignant components discovered in SCTs, as time goes on, suggests the need for early diagnosis and excision in neonatal life to prevent malignant degeneration.[29,74]

Typically noted as a large mass off the fetal rump, SCT occurs in 1 in every 40,000 births, more often in twin gestations. Affected girls outnumber boys by a ratio of four to one. SCT develops during fetal life, and its growth tends to parallel that of the fetus. The pregnancy is often large for gestational age. These masses may have significant intrapelvic extensions and have been classified according to the degree of exterior component or intrapelvic extension (Table 16-7). There are no associated sacral vertebral anomalies, although the incidence of associated vertebral anomalies in other locations is increased.[74,145]

On antenatal examination, those with external masses are easiest to diagnose. The tumors may be solid or of mixed (Fig. 16-30) echogenicity, with interspersed or peripheral cystic components.

About 15% of SCTs are cystic (Fig. 16-31). There is little correlation between size and consistency and ultimate prognosis. The imaging of increased echogenicity or echogenicity and shadowing due to contained calcification is variable. The intrapelvic mass may be noted when mass effect causes bowel or ureteral dilatation, or anterior compression of the bladder. Cystic intrapelvic SCTs may simulate anterior meningocele, ovarian cyst, or the normal bladder. They may be simulated by normal, near-term, meconium-filled rectosigmoid.[29,74,79,147]

REFERENCES

1. Abraham D, Koenigsberg M, Hoffman-Tretin J. The prenatal ultrasound appearance of hydrometrocolpos. J Diagn Med Sonogr. 1985; 1:115–116.
2. Adzick N, Harrison M, Glick P, et al. Diaphragmatic hernia in the fetus: Prenatal diagnosis and outcome in 94 cases. J Pediatr Surg. 1985; 20:357–361.
3. Albright E, Crane J, Schakelford G. Prenatal diagnosis of bronchogenic cyst. J Ultrasound Med. 1988; 7:91–95.
4. Avni E, Vanderelst A, Van Gansbeke D, et al. Antenatal diagnosis of pulmonary tumours: Report of two cases. Pediatr Radiol. 1986; 16:190–192.
5. Beck A. The effect of intrauterine urinary obstruction upon the development of the fetal kidney. J Urol. 1971; 105:784–789.
6. Benacerraf B, Frigoletto F Jr. Mid-trimester fetal thoracentesis. J Clin Ultrasound. 1985; 13:202–204.
7. Benacerraf B, Brass V, Laboda L, et al. A sonographic sign for detection of Down syndrome. Am J Obstet Gynecol. 1985; 151:1078–1079.
8. Benacerraf B, Mandell J, Estroff J, et al. Fetal pyelectasis: A possible association with Down syndrome. Obstet Gynecol 1990; 76:58–60.
9. Beretsky I, Lankin D. Diagnosis of fetal cholelithiasis using real-time high resolution imaging employing digital detection. J Ultrasound Med. 1983; 2:381–383.
10. Bidwell J, Nelson A. Prenatal ultrasonic diagnosis of congenital duplication of the stomach. J Ultrasound Med. 1986; 5:589–591.
11. Blanc W, Berdon W, Baker D, et al. Calcified portal vein thromboemboli in newborn and stillborn infants. Radiology. 1967; 88:287–292.
12. Brar M, Cubberley D, Baty B, et al. Chest wall hamartoma in a fetus. J Ultrasound Med. 1988; 7:217–220.
13. Brill P, Mitty H, Strauss L. Renal vein thrombosis:

A cause of intrarenal calcification in the newborn. Pediatr Radiol. 1977; 6:172–175.

14. Bowerman R. Sonography of fetal midgut herniation: Normal size criteria and correlation with crown rump length. J Ultrasound Med. 1993; 12:251–254.

15. Brown D, Teele R, Doubilet P, et al. Echogenic material in the fetal gallbladder: Sonographic and clinical observations. Radiology. 1992; 182:73–76.

16. Brown D, Polger M, Clark P, et al. Very echogenic amniotic fluid: Ultrasonography–amniocentesis correlation. J Ultrasound Med. 1994; 13:95–97.

17. Butler N, Claireaux A. Congenital diaphragmatic hernia as a cause of perinatal mortality. Lancet. 1962; 1:659–663.

18. Callan N, Colmorgen H, Weiner S. Lung hypoplasia and prolonged preterm ruptured membranes: A case report with implication for possible prenatal ultrasonic diagnosis. Am J Obstet Gynecol. 1985; 151:756–757.

19. Caspi B, Hagay Z, Hellman Y, et al. Echogenicity of the fetal bowel due to gas accumulation. J Ultrasound Med. 1993; 4:231–233.

20. Chervenak F, Isaacson G, Blakemore KJ, et al. Fetal cystic hygroma: Cause and natural history. N Engl J Med. 1983; 309:822–825.

21. Chinn D. Ultrasound evaluation of hydrops fetalis. In: Callen P, ed. Ultrasonography in Obstetrics and Gynecology. 3rd ed. Philadelphia: WB Saunders; 1994:420–439.

22. Chung W. Antenatal detection of hepatic cyst. J Clin Ultrasound. 1986; 14:217–219.

23. Cloumer M, Fried A, Selke A. Antenatal observation of midgut volvulus by ultrasound. J Clin Ultrasound. 1983; 11:286–288.

24. Cohen H, Haller J. Diagnostic sonography of the fetal genitourinary tract. Urol Radiol. 1987; 9:88–98.

25. Cohen H, Haller J. Pediatric and adolescent genital tract abnormalities. In: Babcock D, ed. Neonatal and Pediatric Ultrasonography. New York: Churchill Livingstone; 1989:187–215.

26. Cohen H, Haller J, Mestel A, et al. Neonatal duodenum: Fluid-aided US examination. Radiology. 1987; 164:805–809.

27. Cohen HL, Shapiro M, Mandel F, Shapiro M. Normal ovaries in neonates and infants: A sonographic study of 77 patients 1 day to 24 months old. AJR Am J Roentgenol. 1993; 160:583–586.

28. Cohen HL. The female pelvis. In: Siebert J, ed. Syllabus: Current Concepts: A Categorical Course in Pediatric Radiology. Chicago: RSNA Publications; 1994:65–72.

29. Comstock C. Fetal masses: Ultrasound diagnosis and evaluation. Ultrasound Quarterly. 1988; 6:229–256.

30. Corteville J, Gray D, Crane J. Congenital hydronephrosis: Correlation of fetal ultrasonographic findings with infant outcome. Am J Obstet Gynecol. 1991; 165:384–388.

31. Crane J. Ultrasound evaluation of fetal chromosomal disorders. In: Callen P, ed. Ultrasonography in Obstetrics and Gynecology. 3rd ed. Philadelphia: WB Saunders; 1994:35–51.

32. Cyr D, Guntheroth W, Nyberg D, et al. Prenatal diagnosis of an intrapericardial teratoma: A cause for nonimmune hydrops. J Ultrasound Med. 1988; 7:87–90.

33. DeVries P. The pathogenesis of gastroschisis and omphalocele. J Pediatr Surg. 1980; 15:244–251.

34. Dewbury K, Aluwihare M, Birch S, et al. Prenatal ultrasound demonstration of a choledochal cyst. Br J Radiol. 1980; 53:906–907.

35. Dillard J, Edwards D, Leopold G. Meconium peritonitis masquerading as fetal hydrops. J Ultrasound Med. 1987; 6:49–51.

36. Dubbins P, Kurt A, Wapner R, et al. Renal agenesis: Spectrum of in utero findings. J Clin Ultrasound. 1981; 9:189–193.

37. Eisenberg P, Cohen HL, Coren C. Color Doppler in pulmonary sequestration diagnosis. J Ultrasound Med. 1992; 11:175–176.

38. Elieser S, Ester F, Ehud W, et al. Fetal splenomegaly, ultrasound diagnosis of cytomegalovirus infection: A case report. J Clin Ultrasound. 1984; 12:520–521.

39. Elrad H, Mayden K, Ahart S, et al. Prenatal ultrasound diagnosis of choledochal cyst. J Ultrasound Med. 1985; 4:553–555.

40. Eyheremendy E, Fister M. Antenatal real-time diagnosis of esophageal atresia. J Clin Ultrasound. 1983; 11:395–397.

41. Fakhry J, Reisner M, Shapiro L, et al. Increased echogenicity in the lower fetal abdomen: A common normal variant in the second trimester. J Ultrasound Med. 1986; 5:489–492.

42. Ferraro E, Fakhry J, Aruny J, et al. Prenatal adrenal neuroblastoma: Case report with review of the literature. J Ultrasound Med. 1988; 7:275–278.

43. Fine C, Adzick N, Doubilet P. Decreasing size of a congenital cystic adenomatoid malformation in utero. J Ultrasound Med. 1988; 7:405–408.

44. Fleischer A, Davis R, Campbell L. Sonographic detection of a meconium-containing mass in a fetus: A case report. J Clin Ultrasound. 1983; 11:103–105.

45. Fleischer A, Killam A, Boehm F, et al. Hydrops

fetalis: Sonographic evaluation and clinical implications. Radiology. 1981; 141:163–168.

46. Fong K, Rahmani M, Rose T, et al. Fetal renal cystic disease: Sonographic–pathologic correlation. AJR Am J Roentgenol. 1986; 146:767–773.

47. Fonkalsrud E, DeLorimer A, Hays M. Congenital atresia and stenosis of duodenum: A review compiled from members of the surgical section of the American Academy of Pediatrics. Pediatrics. 1969; 43:79–83.

48. Foster M, Nyberg D, Mahony B, et al. Meconium peritonitis: Prenatal sonographic findings and their clinical significance. Radiology. 1986; 165:661–665.

49. Giulian B. Prenatal ultrasonographic diagnosis of fetal renal tumors. Radiology. 1984; 152:69–70.

50. Glazer G, Filly R, Callen P. The varied sonographic appearance of the urinary tract in the fetus and the newborn with urethral obstruction. Radiology. 1982; 144:563–568.

51. Goldstein R. Ultrasound evaluation of the fetal thorax. In: Callen P, ed. Ultrasonography in Obstetrics and Gynecology. 3rd ed. Philadelphia: WB Saunders; 1994:333–346.

52. Goldstein R. Ultrasound evaluation of the fetal abdomen. In: Callen P, ed. Ultrasonography in Obstetrics and Gynecology. 3rd ed. Philadelphia: WB Saunders; 1994:347–369.

53. Goldstein R, Filly R, Callen P. Sonographic diagnosis of meconium ileus in utero. J Ultrasound Med. 1987; 6:663–666.

54. Goncalves LF, Jeanty P. Ultrasound evaluation of fetal abdominal wall defects. In: Callen P, ed. Ultrasonography in Obstetrics and Gynecology. 3rd ed. Philadelphia: WB Saunders; 1994:370–388.

55. Graham D, Sanders R. Sonographic evaluation of the fetal chest. In: Sanders R, James A Jr, eds. The Principles and Practice of Ultrasonography in Obstetrics and Gynecology. 3rd ed. Norwalk, CT: Appleton-Century-Crofts; 1985:219–228.

56. Gray D, Crane JP. Optimal nuchal skin-fold threshold based on gestational age for prenatal detection of Down syndrome. Am J Obstet Gynecol. 1994; 171:1282–1286.

57. Grignon A, Filion R, Filiatrault D, et al. Urinary tract dilatation in utero: Classification and clinical applications. Radiology. 1986; 160:645–647.

58. Grignon A, Filiatrault D, Homsy Y, et al. Ureteropelvic junction stenosis: Antenatal ultrasonographic diagnosis, postnatal investigation and follow-up. Radiology. 1986; 160:649–651.

59. Groli C, Zucca S, Cesaretti A. Congenital chloridorrhea: Antenatal ultrasonographic appearance. J Clin Ultrasound. 1986; 14:293–295.

60. Gross B, Cohen HL, Schlessel J. Perinatal diagnosis of bilateral testicular torsions: Beware of torsions simulating hydroceles. J Ultrasound Med. 1993; 12:479–482.

61. Harrison M, Adzick N, Nakayama D, et al. Fetal diaphragmatic hernia: Fatal but fixable. Semin Perinatol. 1985; 9:103–112.

62. Harrison M, Adzick N, Flake A. Prenatal management of the fetus with a correctable defect. In: Callen P, ed. Ultrasonography in Obstetrics and Gynecology. 3rd ed. Philadelphia: WB Saunders; 1994:536–547.

63. Hashimoto B, Filly R, Callen P. Fetal pseudoascites: Further anatomic considerations. J Ultrasound Med. 1986; 5:151–152.

64. Hashimoto B, Filly R, Callen P. Sonographic detection of fetal intraperitoneal fluid. J Ultrasound Med. 1986; 5:203–204.

65. Hashimoto B, Filly R, Callen P. Multicystic dysplastic kidney in utero: Changing appearance on US. Radiology. 1986; 159:107–109.

66. Hayden S, Russ P, Pretorius D, et al. Posterior urethral obstruction: Prenatal sonographic findings and clinical outcome in fourteen cases. J Ultrasound Med. 1988; 7:371–375.

67. Helin I, Persson P. Prenatal diagnosis of urinary tract abnormalities by ultrasound. Pediatrics. 1986; 78:879–883.

68. Hill L. Sonographic detection of fetal gastrointestinal anomalies. Ultrasound Quarterly. 1988; 6:35–68.

69. Hill L, Gryzbek P, Mills A, Hogge W. Antenatal diagnosis of fetal pelvic kidneys. Obstet Gynecol. 1994; 83:333–336.

70. Hill L, Breckle R, Gehrking W. The prenatal detection of congenital malformations by ultrasonography. Mayo Clin Proc. 1983; 5:805–826.

71. Hill L, Fries J, Hecker J, Gryzbek P. Second-trimester echogenic small bowel: An increased risk for adverse perinatal outcome. Prenat Diagn. 1994; 14:845–850.

72. Hoddick W, Filly R, Mahony B, et al. Minimal renal pyelectasis. J Ultrasound Med. 1985; 4:85–89.

73. Hoffman C, Filly R, Callen P. The "lying down" adrenal sign: A sonographic indicator of renal agenesis or ectopia in fetuses and neonates. J Ultrasound Med. 1992; 11:533–536.

74. Hogge W, Thiagarajah S, Barber V, et al. Cystic sacrococcygeal teratoma: Ultrasound diagnosis and management. J Ultrasound Med. 1987; 6:707–710.

75. Jayogopal S, Cohen H, Brill P, et al. Neonatal renal vein thrombosis: Demonstration by CT and US. Pediatr Radiol. 1990; 20:2.160–162.

76. Jeffrey R Jr, Laing F, Wing V, et al. Sonography of the fetal duplex kidney. Radiology. 1984; 153:123–124.

77. Jouppila P, Kirkinen P, Herva R, et al. Prenatal diagnosis of pleural effusions by ultrasound. J Clin Ultrasound. 1983; 11:516–519.

78. Kangerloo H, Sample W, Harven G, et al. Ultrasonic evaluation of abdominal gastrointestinal duplication in children. Radiology. 1979; 131:191–194.

79. Karcnik T, Rubenstein J, Swayne L. The fetal presacral pseudo-mass: A normal sonographic variant. J Ultrasound Med. 1991; 10:579–581.

80. Keller M, Markle B, Laffey P, et al. Spontaneous resolution of cholelithiasis in infants. Radiology. 1985; 157:345–348.

81. Kenney P, Spirt B, Ellis D, et al. Scrotal masses caused by meconium peritonitis: Prenatal sonographic diagnosis. Radiology. 1985; 154:362.

82. Kim S. Omphalocele. Surg Clin North Am. 1976; 56:361–371.

83. Kirk E, Wah R. Obstetric management of the fetus with omphalocele or gastroschisis: A review and report of one hundred and twelve cases. Am J Obstet Gynecol. 1983; 146:512–518.

84. Kleiner B, Filly R, Mack L, et al. Multicystic dysplastic kidney: Observations of contralateral disease in the fetal population. Radiology. 1986; 161:27–29.

85. Kluck P, Tibboel D, van der Kamp A, et al. The effect of fetal urine on the development of the bowel in gastroschisis. J Pediatr Surg. 1983; 18:47–50.

86. Knochel J, Lee T, Melendez M, et al. Fetal anomalies involving the thorax and abdomen. Radiol Clin North Am. 1982; 20:297–310.

87. Kurtz A, Goldberg B. Fetal body measurements. In: Obstetrical Measurements in Ultrasound: A Reference Manual Chicago: Year Book Medical Publishers; 1988:302–367.

88. Laing F, Burke V, Wing V, et al. Postpartum evaluation of fetal hydronephrosis: Optimal timing for follow-up sonography. Radiology. 1984; 152: 423–424.

89. Lauer J, Craddock T. Meconium pseudocyst: Prenatal sonographic and antenatal radiologic correlation. J Ultrasound Med. 1982; 1:333–335.

90. Lenke R, Hatch E Jr. Fetal gastroschisis: A preliminary report advocating the use of cesarean section. Obstet Gynecol. 1986; 67:395–398.

91. Lichman J, Miller E. Prenatal ultrasonic diagnosis of splenic cyst. J Ultrasound Med. 1988; 7:637–638.

92. Lyrenis S, Cnattingius S, Lingberg B. Fetal jejunal atresia and intrauterine volvulus: A case report. J Perinatol Med. 1982; 10:247–248.

93. MacGillivray T, Harrison M, Goldstein R, Adzick N. Disappearing fetal lung lesions. J Pediatr Surg. 1993; 28:1321–1324.

94. McGahan J, Myracle M. Adrenal hypertrophy: Possible pitfall in the sonographic diagnosis of renal agenesis. J Ultrasound Med. 1986; 5:265–268.

95. McKenna K, Goldstein R, Stringer M. Small or absent fetal stomach: Prognostic significance. Radiology 1995; 197:729–733.

96. McNamara J, Eraklis A, Gross R. Congenital posterolateral diaphragmatic hernia in the newborn. J Thorac Cardiovasc Surg. 1968; 55:55–59.

97. Mahony B. Ultrasound evaluation of the fetal genitourinary system. In: Callen P, ed. Ultrasonography in Obstetrics and Gynecology. 3rd ed. Philadelphia: WB Saunders; 1994:254–290.

98. Mahony B, Callen P, Filly R. Fetal urethral obstruction: US evaluation. Radiology. 1985; 157:221–224.

99. Mahony B, Filly R, Callen P, et al. Severe non-immune hydrops fetalis: Sonographic evaluation. Radiology. 1984; 151:757–761.

100. Mahony B, Filly R, Callen P, et al. Fetal renal dysplasia: Sonographic evaluation. Radiology. 1984; 152:143–146.

101. Main D, Mennuti M, Cornfeld D, et al. Prenatal diagnosis of adult polycystic kidney disease. Lancet. 1983; 2:337.

102. Mariona F, McAlpin G, Zador I, et al. Sonographic detection of fetal extrathoracic pulmonary sequestration. J Ultrasound Med. 1986; 5:283–285.

103. Mayor G, Genton N, Torado A, et al. Renal function in obstructive nephropathy: Long-term effects of reconstructive surgery. Pediatrics. 1975; 56: 740–743.

104. Meizner I, Katz M, Zamora E, et al. In utero diagnosis of congenital hydrocele. J Clin Ultrasound. 1983; 11:449–451.

105. Mirk P, Calisti A, Fileni A. Prenatal sonographic diagnosis of bladder extrophy. J Ultrasound Med. 1986; 5:291–293.

106. Moore K. Body cavities, primitive mesenteries, and diaphragm. In: Before We Are Born: Basic Embryology and Birth Defects. 3rd ed. Philadelphia: WB Saunders; 1989:126–133.

107. Moore T. Gastroschisis and omphalocele: Clinical differences. Surgery. 1977; 82:561–568.

108. Moore T, Cayle J. The amniotic fluid index in normal human pregnancy. Am J Obstet Gynecol. 1990; 162:1168–1173.

109. Nakamoto S, Dreilinger A, Dattel B, et al. The sonographic appearance of hepatic hemangioma in utero. J Ultrasound Med. 1983; 2:239–241.

110. Nelson L, Clark C, Fishburne J, et al. Value of serial sonography in the in utero detection of duodenal atresia. Obstet Gynecol. 1982; 59:657–660.

111. Newnham J, Crues J, Vinstein A, et al. Sonographic diagnosis of thoracic gastroenteric cyst in utero. Prenat Diagn. 1984; 4:467–471.

112. Norio R, Kaarininen H, Rapola J, et al. Familial congenital diaphragmatic defects: Aspects of etiology, prenatal diagnosis and treatment. Am J Med Genet. 1984; 17:471–483.

113. Nussbaum A, Dorst J, Jeffs R, et al. Ectopic ureterocele: Their varied sonographic manifestations. Radiology. 1986; 159:227–235.

114. Nyberg D, Hastrup W, Watts H, et al. Dilated fetal bowel: A sonographic sign of cystic fibrosis. J Ultrasound Med. 1987; 6:257–260.

115. Oepkes D, Meerman R, Vandenbussche F, et al. Ultrasonographic fetal spleen measurements in red blood cell-alloimmunized pregnancies. Am J Obstet Gynecol. 1993; 169:121–128.

116. Osthanondh V, Potter E. Pathogenesis of polycystic kidneys. Arch Pathol. 1964; 77:459–512.

117. Patel R, Connors J. In utero sonographic findings in fetal renal vein thrombosis with calcifications. J Ultrasound Med. 1988; 7:349–352.

118. Parulekar S. Sonography of normal fetal bowel. J Ultrasound Med. 1991; 10:211–220.

119. Paulson EK, Hertzberg BS. Hyperechoic meconium in the third trimester fetus: An uncommon normal variant. J Ultrasound Med. 1991; 10:677–680.

120. Persutte W, Lenke R, Kropp K, et al. Antenatal diagnosis of fetal patent urachus. J Ultrasound Med. 1988; 7:399–403.

121. Petres R, Redwine F, Cruikshank D. Congenital bilateral chylothorax: Antepartum diagnosis and successful intrauterine surgical management. JAMA. 1982; 248:1360–1361.

122. Petrikovsky B, Cohen HL, Scimeca P, Bellucci E. Prenatal diagnosis of focal nodular hyperplasia of the liver. Prenat Diagn. 1994; 14:406–409.

123. Petrikovsky B, Cohen HL, Cuomo M, et al. Degree of fetal hydronephrosis depends on the fetal bladder size. (Abstract) Am J Obstet Gynecol. 1994; 170:363.

124. Pezzuti R, Isler R. Antenatal ultrasound detection of cystic adenomatoid malformation of lung: Report of case and review of the recent literature. J Clin Ultrasound. 1983; 11:342–346.

125. Phillips H, McGahan J. Intrauterine fetal cystic hygromas: Sonographic detection. AJR Am J Roentgenol. 1981; 136:799–802.

126. Platt L, Devore G, Benner P, et al. Antenatal diagnosis of a fetal liver mass. J Ultrasound Med. 1983; 2:521–522.

127. Potter E. Bilateral absence of ureters and kidneys. Obstet Gynecol. 1965; 25:3–12.

128. Pretorius D, Meier P, Johnson M. Diagnosis of esophageal atresia in utero. J Ultrasound Med. 1983; 2:475–476.

129. Pretorius D, Lee M, Manco-Johnson M, et al. Diagnosis of autosomal dominant polycystic kidney disease in utero and in the young infant. J Ultrasound Med. 1987; 6:249–255.

130. Preziosi P, Fariello G, Moiorana A, et al. Antenatal sonographic diagnosis of complicated ovarian cysts. J Clin Ultrasound. 1986; 14:196–198.

131. Queenan J, O'Brien G. Diagnostic ultrasound in erythroblastosis fetalis. In: Sanders R, James EA Jr, eds. The Principles and Practice of Ultrasonography in Obstetrics and Gynecology. 3rd ed. Norwalk, CT: Appleton-Century-Crofts; 1985: 279–288.

132. Rempen A, Feige A, Wunsch P. Prenatal diagnosis of bilateral cystic adenomatoid malformation of the lung. J Clin Ultrasound. 1987; 15:3–8.

133. Roberts A, Mitchell J, Murphy C, et al. Fetal liver length in diabetic pregnancy. Am J Obstet Gynecol. 1994; 170:1308–1312.

134. Romero R, Pilu G, Jeanty P, et al. The lungs. In: Prenatal Diagnosis of Congenital Anomalies. East Norwalk, CT: Appleton & Lange; 1988:195–208.

135. Romero R, Pilu G, Jeanty P, et al. The abdominal wall. In: Prenatal Diagnosis of Congenital Anomalies. East Norwalk, CT: Appleton & Lange; 1988:209–232.

136. Romero R, Pilu G, Jeanty P, et al. The gastrointestinal tract and intraabdominal organs. In: Prenatal Diagnosis of Congenital Anomalies. East Norwalk, CT: Appleton & Lange; 1988.

137. Rypens F, Avni E, Abehsera M, et al. Areas of increased echogenicity in the fetal abdomen: Diagnosis and significance. Radiographics. 1995; 15: 1329–1344.

138. Sabbagha R, Sheik Z. Skeletal abnormalities. In: Sabbagha R, ed. Diagnostic Ultrasound Applied to Obstetrics and Gynecology. 3rd ed. Philadelphia: JB Lippincott; 1987:399–412.

139. Sabbagha R, Dalcampo S, Shkolnick A. Correlative anatomy. In: Sabbagha R, ed. Diagnostic Ultrasound Applied to Obstetrics and Gynecology. 3rd ed. Philadelphia: JB Lippincott; 1987:264–289.

140. Salzman L, Kuligowska E, Semine A. Pseudoomphalocele: Pitfall in fetal sonography. AJR Am J Roentgenol. 1986; 146:1283–1285.

141. Samuel N, Dicker D, Feldberg D. Ultrasound diagnosis and management of fetal intestinal obstruction and volvulus in utero. J Perinat Med. 1984; 12:333–337.

142. Sarti D. Ultrasound evaluation of normal and abnormal fetal anatomy. In: Sarti D, ed. Diagnostic Ultrasound: Text and Cases. 2nd ed. Chicago: Year Book Medical Publishers; 1987: 873–892.

143. Schifer T, Heller R. Bilateral multicystic dysplastic kidneys. Pediatr Radiol. 1988; 18:242–244.

144. Schmidt W, Yarkoni S, Jeanty P, et al. Sonographic measurements of the fetal spleen: Clinical implications. J Ultrasound Med. 1985; 4:667–672.

145. Schoenecker S, Cyr D, Mack L. Sonographic diagnosis of bilateral fetal renal duplication with ectopic ureteroceles. J Ultrasound Med. 1985; 4:617–618.

146. Seeds J. Antenatal sonographic assessment of the genitourinary tract. In: Sanders R, Hill M, eds. Ultrasound Annual 1986. New York: Raven Press; 1986:67–98.

147. Sheth S, Nussbaum A, Sanders R, et al. Prenatal diagnosis of sacrococcygeal teratoma: Sonographic–pathologic correlation. Radiology. 1988; 169:131–136.

148. Skiptunas S, Weiner S. Early prenatal diagnosis of asphyxiating thoracic dysplasia (Jeune's syndrome): Value of fetal thoracic measurement. J Ultrasound Med. 1987; 6:41–43.

149. Soper T, Pringle K, Schofield J. Creation and repair of diaphragmatic hernia in the fetal lamb: Techniques and survival. J Pediatr Surg. 1984; 19:33–40.

150. Stein B, Bromley B, Michlewitz H, et al. Fetal liver calcifications: Sonographic appearance and postnatal outcome. Radiology. 1995; 197:489–492.

151. Stocker T, Madewell J, Drake RT. Congenital cystic adenomatoid malformation of the lung: Classification and morphologic spectrum. Hum Pathol. 1977; 8:155–171.

152. van Dam L, deGroot C, Hazeborek F, et al. Intrauterine demonstration of bowel duplication by ultrasound. Eur J Obstet Gynecol Reprod Biol. 1984; 18:229–232.

153. Vermesh M, Mayden K, Confino E, et al. Prenatal sonographic diagnosis of Hirschsprung's disease. J Ultrasound Med. 1986; 5:37–39.

154. Weiss J, Cohen H, Haller J, et al. Cystic abnormalities of the fetal thorax: Sonographic evaluation. Journal of Diagnostic Medical Sonography. 1987; 3:172–176.

155. Witt D, Hall J. Multiple congenital anomaly syndromes. In: Rudolph A, Hoffman J, Axelrod S, eds. Pediatrics. 19th ed. East Norwalk, CT: Appleton & Lange; 1991:416–428.

156. Wladimiroff J. Effect of furosemide on fetal urine production. Br J Obstet Gynaecol. 1975; 82:221–224.

157. Woodard J. Prune belly syndrome. In: Kelalis P, King R, Belman A, eds. Clinical Pediatric Urology. 2nd ed. Philadelphia: WB Saunders; 1985:805–824.

158. Zerres K, Volpel M, Weif H. Cystic kidneys: Genetics, pathologic anatomy, clinical picture and prenatal diagnosis. Hum Genet. 1984; 68:104–135.

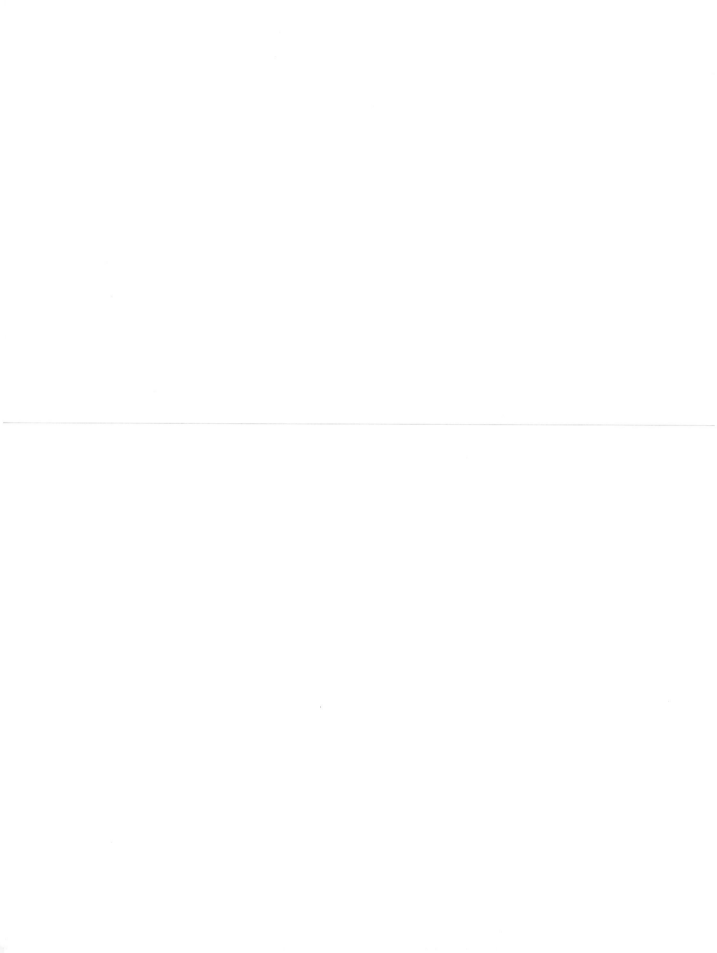

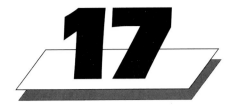

Fetal Echocardiography

DALE R. CYR, WARREN G. GUNTHEROTH, KARIN M. SMITH,
and THOMAS C. WINTER, III

Constant improvement in image resolution has been the basis for a multitude of ultrasonographic advances. No fetal ultrasound technique has been affected more by equipment advances than fetal echocardiography.[3,4,30,63] Fetal cardiac ultrasonography has evolved beyond obtaining only anatomic information in diagnosing congenital heart disease. Today, anatomic imaging is supplemented with hemodynamic information provided by Doppler techniques to enhance diagnostic capabilities in the fetal heart.[8,12,14,24,49,66,70]

This chapter discusses basic knowledge needed to perform this subspecialized sonogram and obtain useful anatomic and hemodynamic information.

Normal Development and Anatomy

In the first weeks of embryonic development, the cardiovascular system is one of the first to function. Blood begins to circulate within the embryo at the end of the third postconceptual week, consistent with 5 weeks' gestational (postmenstrual)

age.[53] With high-resolution endovaginal transducers, the embryonic heart may be seen beating at this time. The primitive heart tube is formed by partial fusion of the cardiogenic cords (Fig. 17-1). Once fusion occurs, the primitive heart tube thickens to form the myoepicardial mantle, which gives rise to the myocardium and epicardium. The inner portion of the heart tube goes on to form the endocardium.

During the fourth and fifth weeks of gestation, the heart tube elongates and begins to form three primary areas: the bulbus cordis, ventricle, and atrium. The truncus arteriosus, which also develops during this period, is contiguous with the bulbus cordis and supplies blood to multiple aortic arches that exist at this time in gestation (Fig. 17-2).

The atrioventricular canal is created by thickening of the ventral and dorsal walls of the bulboventricular loop, better known as the endocardial cushions.

The endocardial cushions continue to grow inward and fuse to form the septum of the atrioventricular canal, dividing the canal into right and left sides. The atrium divides into the left and right atria by the formation of the septum secundum and septum primum, which are fused with the septum of the atrioventricular canal. The venae cavae and pulmonary veins communicate with the right and left atria, respectively. The partitioning of the ven-

The authors dedicate this chapter to their friend and colleague Laurence A. Mack, MD. His mentoring, patience, and guidance in the development of the University of Washington's fetal echocardiography program will always be remembered.

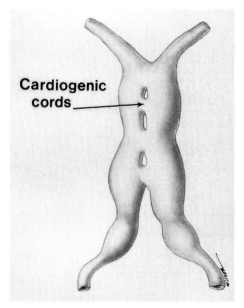

Figure 17-1. Cardiogenic cords at approximately 5 weeks' gestation.

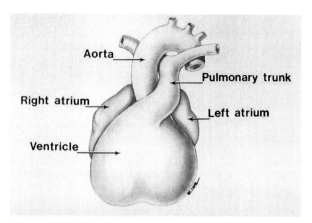

Figure 17-3. Fetal heart at approximately 8 weeks' postmenstrual gestation. At this point, the heart has conformed to traditional anatomy and is considered fully developed.

tricle begins at the apex, and moves superiorly toward the endocardial cushions with fusion, by the end of the seventh week. The cardiac valves form from subendocardial tissue at the orifices of the great vessels and atrioventricular (AV) canals.

At the end of the seventh week of gestation, ridges form within the wall of the bulbus cordis, as well as the truncus arteriosus. Both sets of ridges are in communication with each other, and eventu-

ally fuse to form the aorticopulmonary septum. This newly formed septum divides the bulbus cordis and truncus arteriosus into two channels, the aorta and pulmonary trunk. The bulbus cordis at this point becomes incorporated within the ventricular walls.[2]

Around the 40th day of gestation, or 7 weeks postmenstrual, the embryonic heart has completed its complex formation. The last developmental transformation allows the multiple aortic arches to conform to the normal aortic arch and its cranial branches, with which we are familiar. The embryonic heart can now be considered fully developed and will function the same throughout the rest of gestation (Fig. 17-3). Most congenital heart anomalies, which are in essence maldevelopments at various stages of cardiac embryogenesis, have developed by this time.

Fetal Circulation

The fetal circulation is fully developed after final embryogenesis, which is approximately 7 postmenstrual weeks.[67] It is at this point in gestation that the embryonic heart rate is at its slowest, averaging 90 bpm. This can be easily visualized using high-resolution, commercially available real-time units, by either transabdominal or transvaginal techniques. The embryonic heart rate then increases and plateaus after 9 weeks, with heart rates ranging from 135 to 170 bpm, with rates of approximately 140

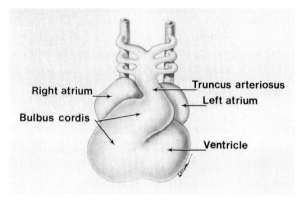

Figure 17-2. Fetal heart during the sixth and seventh weeks of gestation, demonstrating bulbus cordis, truncus arteriosus, ventricle, atria, and multiple aortic arches.

EMBRYONIC HEART RATES

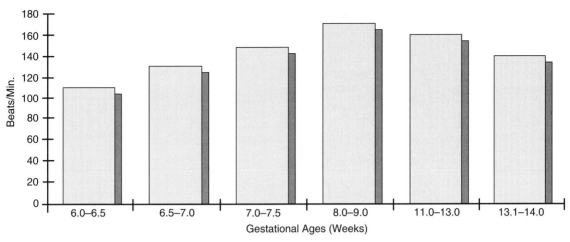

Figure 17-4. Embryonic heart rates. (From Cyr DR. Embryosonography. Presented at the 37th annual convention of the American Institute of Ultrasound in Medicine, Honolulu, Hawaii, 1993.)

bpm through the remainder of the first and second trimesters (Fig. 17-4).[18,67,72]

The fetus receives blood from the placenta through the umbilical vein. The umbilical vein enters the fetal abdomen, and supplies its blood flow to the liver. The intrahepatic umbilical vein anastomoses with the portal sinus (left portal vein), where blood may take two routes. Most blood volume passes through the fetal liver, and enters the inferior cava (IVC) through the hepatic veins. The remaining blood enters the ductus venosus, which bypasses the liver circulation, and enters either the hepatic veins draining into the IVC, or the IVC directly.[52]

Blood then enters the right atrium from the IVC and is channelled by the eustachian valve toward the foramen ovale and into the left atrium. The eustachian valve also reduces regurgitant flow during ventricular systole. The highly oxygenated IVC blood is directed across the atrial septum by the eustachian valve, which is in direct communication with the lower edge of the septum secundum of the interatrial septum, called the crista dividens. A small percentage of highly oxygenated blood remains in the right atrium, and mixes with deoxygenated blood returning to the heart, from the superior vena cava.[64]

Almost the entire blood volume returning to the heart by way of the superior vena cava traverses the tricuspid valve and enters the main pulmonary artery through the right ventricular outflow tract and pulmonary valve. Most of this blood flow continues down the ductus arteriosus and directly enters the descending aorta for systemic circulation. The ductus arteriosus acts to bypass the largely nonfunctioning fetal lungs, which receive only 30% of the right ventricular output. After birth, the ductus arteriosus constricts and permanently closes, becoming the ligamentum arteriosum.

The left atrium receives most of its blood from the IVC, by way of the foramen ovale, and the small amount of blood returning from the fetal lungs, by way of the pulmonary veins. The left atrial blood then traverses the mitral valve and exits the left ventricle through the left ventricular outflow tract and aortic valve. This highly oxygenated blood volume is mainly distributed to the cranial half of the fetus through brachiocephalic vessels arising from the aortic arch (Fig. 17-5).[53]

Sonographic Technique and Anatomy

When performing fetal echocardiography, the most important step is that of determining the anatomic orientation of the fetal heart. This is accomplished

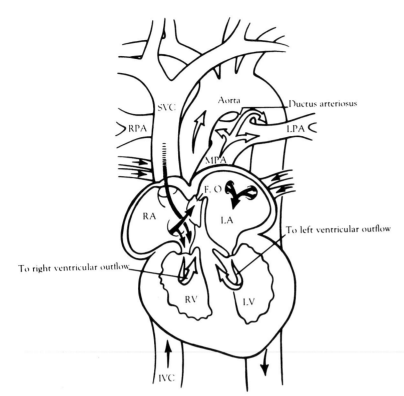

Figure 17-5. Normal fetal circulation. IVC, inferior vena cava; RV, right ventricle; LV, left ventricle; LA, left atrium; RA, right atrium; FO, foramen ovale; MPA, main pulmonary artery; RPA, right pulmonary artery; LPA, left pulmonary artery; SVC, superior vena cava.

by determining the fetal lie and fetal spine location. This information allows the sonographer to ascertain the left, right, cranial, caudal, dorsal, and ventral aspects of the fetal heart. The most important fetal echocardiographic view is the four-chamber view (Fig. 17-6).[16,21,58,68] This view allows the two atria, ventricles, atrioventricular valves (mitral and tricuspid valves), as well as interatrial and interventricular septa to be visualized. This view is obtained by imaging the fetal thorax in a transverse plane. In utero, the apex of the heart typically lies on an axis close to the perpendicular of the fetal spine.

In this imaging plane, it is important to distinguish the left from the right side of the heart. This may be accomplished by visualizing the foramen ovale flap moving in and out of the left atrium, caused by atrial shunting of blood from the right atrium to the left during systole. The identification of the moderator band in the apex of the right ventricle can also assist in fetal heart left–right orientation. The moderator band, which runs from the interventricular septum to the lower free wall of the right ventricle, should not be confused with an intraventricular tumor. Once left–right orientation has been accomplished, the appropriate AV valves and cardiac chambers can be identified.[17,19]

Additional cardiac anatomy may be elicited by subtle anterior transducer angulation from the four-chamber view, producing visualization of the left ventricular outflow tract as well as the proximal aortic root. This view may be referred to as the five-chamber view or extended four-chamber view (Fig. 17-7). The anatomic relationship between the interventricular septum and aorta is also appreciated in this view. Further anterior movement of the transducer brings the main pulmonary artery into view. The pulmonary valve may be seen within the pulmonary artery, arising from the right side of the fetal heart (Fig. 17-8). Thus, all major parts of the fetal intracardiac anatomy, as well as the great vessels, may be imaged, starting from the four-chamber view. Fortunately, the fetal four-chamber

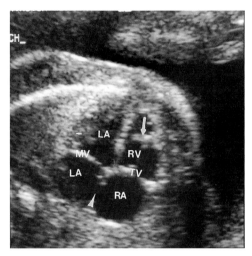

Figure 17-6. Sonogram of the four chamber view (*arrowhead,* foramen ovale; *arrow,* moderator band). LA, left atrium; MV, mitral valve; LV, left ventricle; RV, right ventricle; TV, tricuspid valve; RA, right atrium.

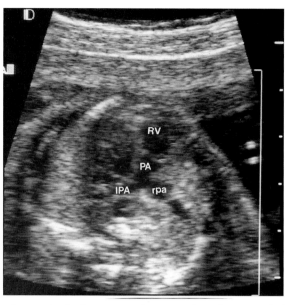

Figure 17-8. Sonogram demonstrating the extended four-chamber view of the right ventricular outflow tract/pulmonary artery. RV, right ventricle; PA, pulmonary artery; rpa, right pulmonary artery; lpa, left pulmonary artery.

view can be obtained in most cases throughout gestation. Reports have shown visualization rates with the four-chamber view of from 75% to 100% in the second and third trimesters.[22,23,58,68] Studies have shown that most abnormalities, approximately 65%,

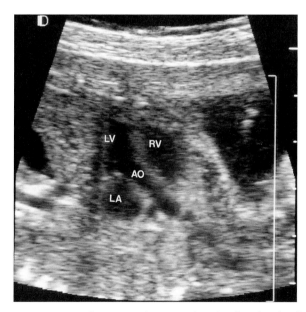

Figure 17-7. Sonogram demonstrating the five-chamber/extended four-chamber view. LA, left atrium; AO, aorta/aortic root; LV, left ventricle; RV, right ventricle.

can initially be detected from the four-chamber view, and 85% of cardiac anomalies were detected if the extended four-chamber view (great vessels) was imaged in association with the four-chamber view.[1,6,10]

The short-axis view is probably the second most important fetal echocardiographic plane. Typically, this view is imaged with the fetus in a sagittal plane (90-degree transducer rotation from four-chamber or long-axis views), remembering that the apex of the heart is approximately perpendicular to the fetal spine. Having imaged the fetal heart in cross section, the sonographer may sweep the heart from the apex to the superior aspect of the heart. Three distinct levels are described in the short-axis view. The first level is at the ventricular apices, demonstrating both ventricles and the inferior aspect of the muscular ventricular septum. Further transducer movement toward the left lateral aspect of the fetus (superior within the fetal heart) allows the aortic root to be imaged in a transverse plane with the pulmonary artery wrapping around the aortic root (Fig. 17-9). The pulmonary valve as well as the pulmonary bifurcation can be seen at this level. Slight transducer movement superiorly

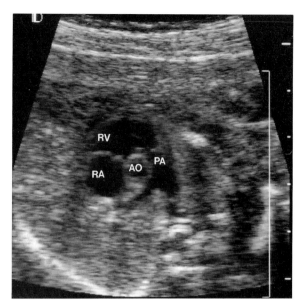

Figure 17-9. Sonogram of short-axis view at aortic/pulmonic level. RA, right atrium; RV, right ventricle; PA, pulmonary artery; AO, aorta in transverse axis at the level of aortic valve.

ductal arch and aortic arch, especially in cases where great vessel orientation is in question. The best way of determining which great vessel is being imaged is to identify the cepahlic vessels arising from the transverse aortic arch.

Technical Factors Affecting Imaging

The fetal echocardiographic views described allow a detailed anatomic examination of the fetal heart. The extent to which the sonographer is able to visualize the fetal heart depends on the position of the fetus, fetal gestational age, as well as maternal adipose tissue thickness and if the mother has had previous lower abdominal surgery. Ideal gestational ages in which to image the fetal heart are from 18 through 34 weeks, with peak visualization rates before 30 weeks' gestation (Table 17-1).[22,23,58,68]

Throughout gestation, the fetal heart is very small, allowing sound beam artifacts, such as "partial volum-

may image the ductus arteriosus arising from the main pulmonary artery and entering the descending aorta, demonstrating great vessel orientation. Although this view can be imaged in a high percentage of patients, it is best seen when the fetus is in a spine-posterior or spine-left lie.

Another important view when performing fetal echocardiography is the long-axis view. The transducer should be in a position so the fetus is imaged in a transverse plane. The transducer also needs to be angulated slightly lateral and cephalad to visualize the left ventricular outflow tract in relation to the interventricular septum. The left ventricle, left atrium, interatrial septum, right ventricle, and part of the right atrium may also be evaluated in this view. With further cranial angulation of the transducer, the aortic arch may be imaged (Fig. 17-10), including the carotid, subclavian, and brachiocephalic arteries. With subtle lateral transducer adjustment, the ductus arteriosus may be seen entering the descending aorta (Fig. 17-11). This view demonstrates the "ductal arch" and represents the most commonly imaged vascular arch within the fetal thorax. It is essential to differentiate between the

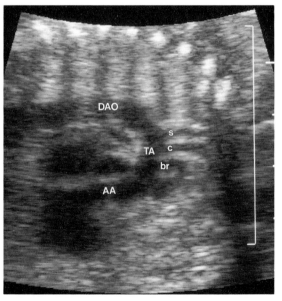

Figure 17-10. Sonogram of cephalically angled long-axis view demonstrating aortic arch and cephalic branch vessels. AA, ascending aortic arch; TA, transverse arch; DAO, descending aortic arch; br, brachiocephalic artery; c, carotid artery; s, subclavian artery.

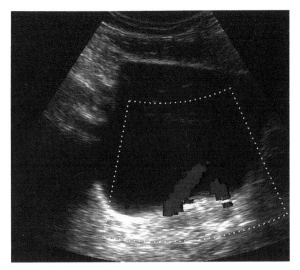

Color Plate 1. Color Doppler of the region of the ureteric orifices often shows dramatic plumes of color when the jets enter the urinary bladder. (See also Fig. 4-21D.)

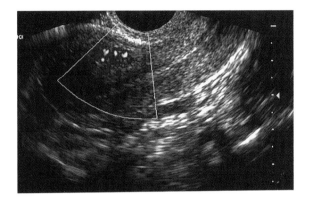

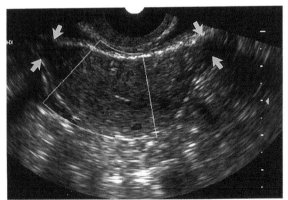

Color Plate 2. (*Top*) An endovaginal view of the uterus in sagittal plane with a power-Doppler sample box placed over the mid-corpus region. Power Doppler is not sensitive to direction of blood flow, but is more sensitive to the presence of flow. Note the rich vascularization of the middle layer of the myometrium, indicated by the bright spots of color where blood flow was detected. (*Bottom*) An endovaginal transverse scan of the same uterus, again illustrating the vascularization of the middle layer of the myometrium. These vessels are normally not visible on gray scale imaging alone. Also note the conical "ears" (*arrows*) which extend from the lateral margins of the uterus. These represent the cornua or "horns" of the uterus, where the fallopian tubes, the round ligaments, and the ovarian ligaments are attached to the uterus. (See also Fig. 4-37C,D.)

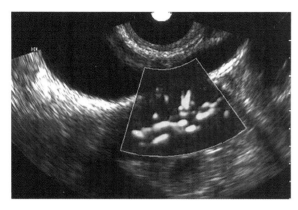

Color Plate 3. A power Doppler image of the ovary, in a medial plane. The color highlights blood flow in the abundant vessels in the ovarian hilus. Note the concentration of vessels in the hilus and the relative absence of large vessels in the cortex. (See also Fig. 4-50C.)

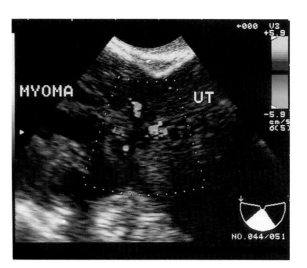

Color Plate 5. In this long-axis view, color flow Doppler shows vessels at the attachment site of the pedunculated myoma to the uterus. (See also Fig. 7-9B.)

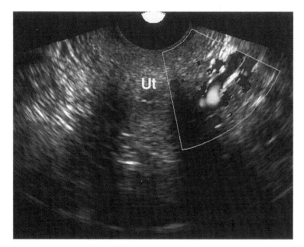

Color Plate 4. This transverse endovaginal scan of the region of the uterine isthmus (Ut) uses power Doppler imaging to demonstrate the abundant vessels which lie along the lateral cervical margins. Blood flow is indicated by the presence of color, with the volume of flow indicated by brighter shades of color. Power Doppler is not directional, so we cannot determine if flow in any specific vessel is toward or away from the transducer. (See also Fig. 4-58B.)

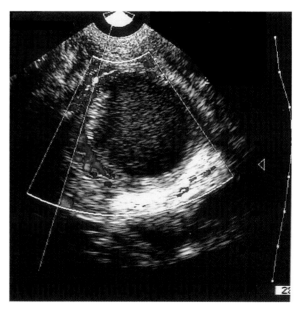

Color Plate 6. This solid-appearing adnexal mass displaying good through-transmission has multiple peripheral vessels displayed with color Doppler. The pulsed Doppler revealed an RI of 0.65 and a slight notch in early diastole. A tuboovarian abscess was found surgically. (See also Fig. 7-15A.)

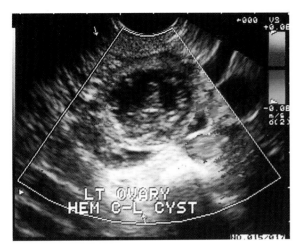

Color Plate 7. A ring of color is displayed with a hemorragic corpus luteum cyst. This hemorrhagic corpus luteum cyst is complex in appearance. (See also Fig. 7-18.)

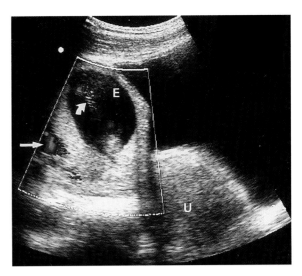

Color Plate 9. An ultrasound ordered because of a palpable adnexal mass reveals a viable 13-week tubal ectopic pregnancy (*E*). Color Doppler shows flow in the umbilical cord (*curved arrow*) and placental vessels (*straight arrow*). (See also Fig. 11-11.)

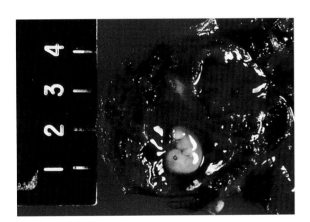

Color Plate 8. The embryo within the removed spleen. (See also Fig. 11-4B.) (Courtesy of Cynthia Hoeflinger, MD, PhD.)

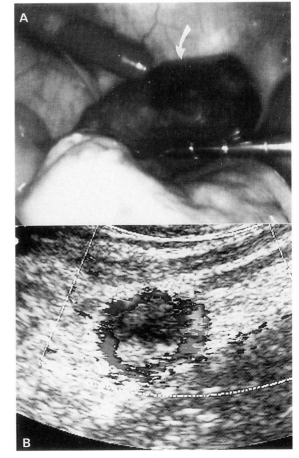

Color Plate 10. (**A**) a laparoscopy confirmed a tubal ectopic pregnancy (*curved arrow*) found on ultrasound. A salingostomy was performed. (**B**) The suspect area was scanned with Doppler showing the typical color pattern exhibited by trophoblastic tissue. (See also Fig. 11-16A,B.)

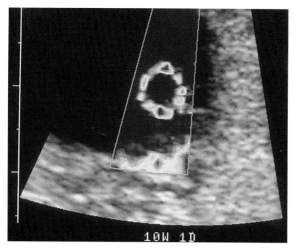

Color Plate 11. Low-velocity flow detected in the walls of the secondary yolk sac. The yolk sac plays a role in the transport of nutrients to the embryo and is the first site of blood cell formation. (See also Fig. 12-11B.)

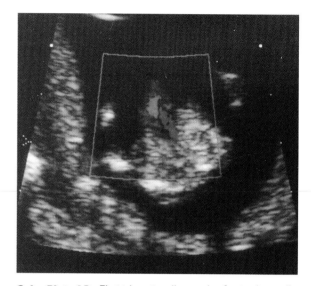

Color Plate 12. First trimester diagnosis of ectopic cordis. Color flow is seen in the heart, which is imaged beyond the confines of the thoracic cavity. (See also Fig. 12-37B.) (Courtesy of Patricia Mayberry, RT, RDMS, RVT; St. Luke's–Roosevelt Hospital Center, New York, NY.)

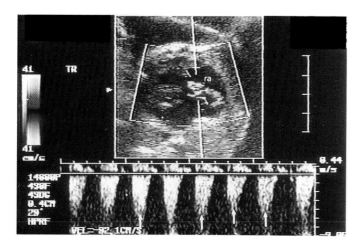

Color Plate 13. Triplex sonogram demonstrating a fetus with tricuspid regurgitation. The regurgitant jet is seen moving back into the right atrium (ra) and is demonstrated in blue. The Doppler spectral analysis shows the typical waveform of a regurgitant jet (below baseline/reversed flow) during systole (arrows). (See also Fig. 17-15.)

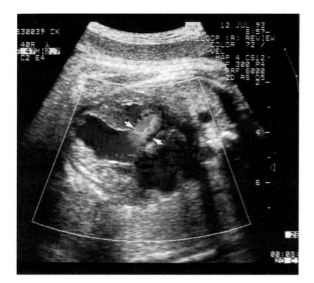

Color Plate 14. Color Doppler of a VSD demonstrates blood crossing from left to right through an interventricular septal defect (*arrowhead*). (See also Fig. 17-16*B*.)

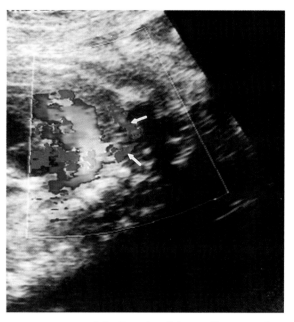

Color Plate 15. Color Doppler of descending aorta demonstrates reversed flow (red) toward transverse arch (*arrows*). (See also Fig. 17-18.) These findings are consistent with severe coarctation or interrupted aortic arch.

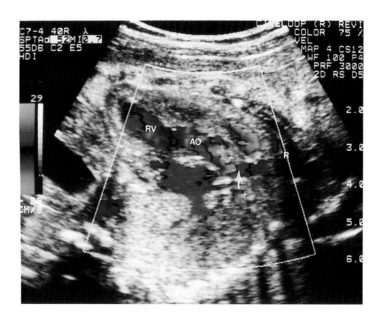

Color Plate 16. d-TGA. Color Doppler demonstrating continuity of flow of right ventricle to aorta to brachiocephalic artery. (See also Fig. 17-22*C*.)

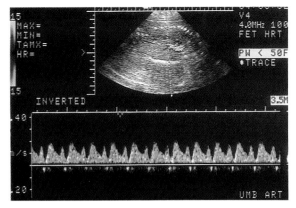

Color Plate 17. Normal inferior vena cava waveform. Note the characteristic triphasic pattern which is also seen when sampling the suctus venosus. The triphasic pattern is a result of the fetal cardiac cycle. Note the reverse blood flow, which dips below the baseline and is present in normal fetuses during atrial contraction. (See also Fig. 20-9.)

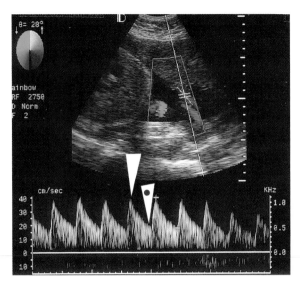

Color Plate 19. B-mode sonography with pulsed Doppler of the umbilical artery in normal fetus at ~34 weeks and without IUGR shows an S/D ratio of 2.23 (*arrow*, systole; *dotted arrow*, diastole). (See also Fig. 24-3A.)

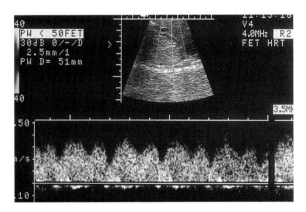

Color Plate 18. Ductus venosus blood flow pattern in a normally grown fetus. Note the characteristic triphasic pattern. The first spike seen is consistent with ventricular systole, the second is a result of ventricular diastole, and the sudden dip coincides with atrial systole. Also notice that there is high forward flow throughout the entire cardiac cycle. (See also Fig. 20-10.)

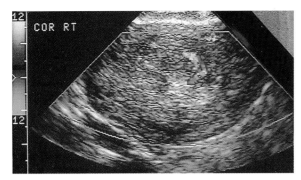

Color Plate 20. A color flow Doppler coronal endovaginal section demonstrates the nature of blood flow in residual trophoblast tissue. (See also Fig. 27-2C.) (Courtesy of Stephanie Ellingson, BA, RT(R), RDMS, The University of Iowa Hospital and Clinics, Iowa City, IA.)

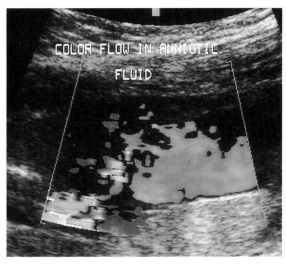

Color Plate 22. Color noise. Fetal movement caused this color flash in the amniotic fluid. (See also Fig. 30-22B.)

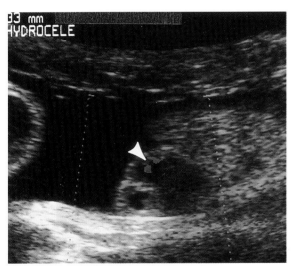

Color Plate 21. Color noise. Color noise occurred in this fetal hydrocele (*arrowhead*) because of fluid motion. (See also Fig. 30-22A.)

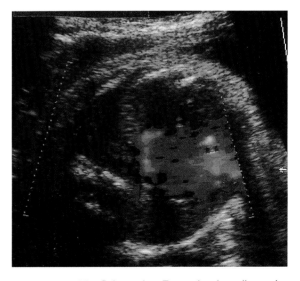

Color Plate 23. Color noise. Transmitted cardiac pulsations caused this color noise in the fetal heart. (See also Fig. 30-23.)

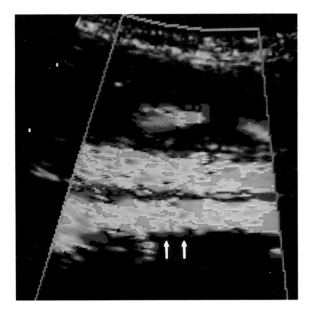

Color Plate 24. Color Doppler image shows color in both the true vessel (*arrowheads*) and the "ghost" vessel (*arrows*). (See also Fig. 30-25B.)

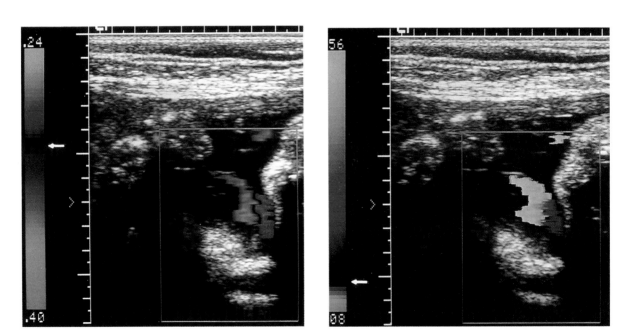

Color Plates 25 and 26. Operator-dependent artifact: incorrect baseline setting. Color Doppler images of the umbilical vessels emphasize the fact that incorrect baseline settings can depict a false direction of flow. As the baseline (*arrow*) is changed, the direction of flow appears to reverse. (See also Fig. 30-26A,B.)

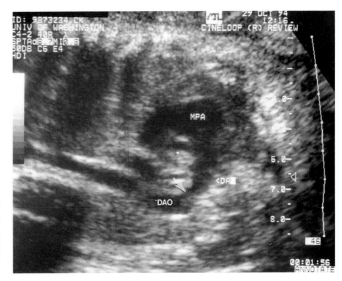

Figure 17-11. Sonogram demonstrating ductus arteriosus entering decsending aorta, "ductal arch." MPA, main pulmonary artery; <DA, ductus arteriosus; DAO, descending aorta. The arrowhead indicates the ductus arteriosus insertion in the descending aorta.

ing," which may falsely project normal cardiac structures as if they are in abnormal anatomic sites. Fetuses throughout the second trimester are also extremely mobile, which can cause significant problems in imaging the fetal heart. After 34 weeks' gestation, the fetal skeletal system matures, giving rise to significant shadowing artifacts and reducing the ability to use fetal intercostal sonographic windows. In contrast to the second trimester, the third trimester fetus does not move as extensively, which may leave the sonographer without an optimal imaging window, with little hope of productive fetal movement allowing improved visualization.

If the fetus is not in a suitable position for specific anatomic surveillance, gently jostling the maternal abdomen with the transducer to induce fetal movement may help the fetus move into a favorable position. If this technique fails, having the mother go for a walk may induce fetal movement. As a last resort, the exami-

nation may be rescheduled for another time in the hope that the fetus will be in a more favorable position. Table 17-2 demonstrates the basic fetal echocardiographic views that should be attempted in every screening obstetric examination. Advanced fetal echocardiographic views that may be used for further evaluation of the fetal heart are also outlined.

M-Mode

The use of M-mode sonography in conjunction with two-dimensional imaging is not routine in most obstetric ultrasound centers. The use of M-mode is essential when evaluating the fetal heart for arrhythmias and subtle contractile abnormalities. Fetal arrhythmias are thought to account for approximately 30% of fetal cardiac referrals.[38,51,59] Information derived from fetal M-mode allows individual chamber sizes and ventricular wall thick-

TABLE 17-1. VISUALIZATION (%) OF FETAL FOUR-CHAMBER VIEW

Gestational Age (wk)	Persutte & Jones, 1996[58]	Schultz et al., 1994[68]	Cyr et al., 1988[22]
16–20	70%	80%	—
20–24	81%	94%	95%
25–29	82%	98%	96%
30–34	78%	98%	100%
35–40	72%	100%	100%

TABLE 17-2. ROUTINE VIEWS FOR EVALUATING THE FETAL HEART

View	Anatomy Visualized
SCREENING	
Four chamber	All four chambers
	Atrioventricular valves
	Atrioventricular septum
Five chamber (extended four chamber)	Left ventricular outflow
	Aortic root. Demonstrates aortic, left ventricular continuity.
Pulmonary artery view (anterior movement from five-chamber/extended four-chamber view)	Demonstrates right ventricular outflow in continuity with right ventricle.
	Main pulmonary artery can be seen.
ADVANCED IMAGING OF FETAL HEART	
Four chamber	Same as above
Five chamber/extended four chamber (anterior movement from four chamber)	Same as above
Right ventricular outflow tract/pulmonary artery view from four chamber (anterior transducer movement from five-chamber/extended four-chamber view)	Same as above
Short-axis view, apical level	Demonstrates right and left ventricle in transverse plane. Ventricular septum and papillary muscles can also be seen.
Pulmonary/aortic level	Demonstrates aorta in cross section with main pulmonary artery lying anterior to aorta. Right ventricle can also be seen.
Long-axis view	Demonstrates left ventricular outflow tract (LVOT), left atrium, left ventricle, aortic root, ventricular septum. Demonstrates aortic, LVOT continuity.
Aortic arch view	Demonstrates ascending aorta, aortic arch, descending aorta with cephalic vessels.
Right ventricular inflow view	Demonstrates right atrium, tricuspid valve, right ventricle and ventricular septum.
Right atrial inflow view	Demonstrates inferior and superior venae cavae, right atrium.

nesses to be evaluated in relation to gestational age, or in comparison to other cardiac chambers; nomograms of specific areas of cardiac anatomy in relation to gestational size are available.[7,13]

M-mode can give the fetal echocardiographer the rate of atrial and ventricular contractions, independently or together, providing the opportunity to diagnose a variety of arrhythmias, as well as congenital heart block.

The ideal position for M-mode interrogation is a four-chamber view with the fetal spine toward either maternal side. This allows the M-line to be placed perpendicularly through both atria and, with repositioning of the M-line, through both ventricles. Occasionally, it may be necessary to visualize atrial and ven-

tricular contractions simultaneously. This is most easily accomplished with the fetal heart apex either pointing toward or away from the transducer, with the M-line traversing atrium and ventricle. Some equipment allows dual M-modes to be used, alleviating the need for such specific fetal heart positioning. Both systolic and diastolic ventricular measurements should be made on all M-modes, although two-dimensional measurements may suffice. These measurements can be made by using hand-held calipers on hard-copy images, or by using ultrasound machine calipers available on-line during the real-time examination, or off-line at independent workstations. During maximal ventricular contraction (systole), measurements should be made from the endocardial wall of the ventricle to the coexisting contraction on the interventricular septum. The same process is repeated during the diastolic cycle, measuring from the endocardial ventricular wall to its corresponding diastolic septal component. Care should be taken not to include the chordae tendonae in either measurement. Atrial measurements are usually performed to determine size, not function, and thus only one measurement is required. Measuring from either the left or right atrial wall (depending on which atrium is being interrogated) to the atrial septum is all that is required.[19]

The most common arrhythmias identified in the fetus are premature atrial contractions (PACs). These arrhythmias are benign and are usually seen between the gestational ages of 25 to 35 weeks, and account for nearly 75% of all fetal arrhythmias (Fig. 17-12).[74] PACs may or may not have transmission (conduct) to the ventricle. Premature ventricular contractions are also common in utero (8%), and are also benign in healthy fetuses. These arrhythmic events usually show a classic compensatory pause caused by the ventricular refractory period. It is not uncommon to have coexistent PACs and premature ventricular contractions.[19,25] Supraventricular tachyarrhythmias (SVTs) are of great concern to the clinician; if they persist and have heart rates greater than 230 bpm, fetal death can occur from heart failure (Fig. 17-13).[35] Because of fetal heart failure, fetal hydrops is a common finding with persistent SVT.[25,37,48,51] Treatment and conversion of SVTs have been well documented in the literature us-ing such medications as digoxin, verapamil, and quinidine.[15,30,37,45,75]

Doppler Echocardiography

Pulsed Doppler has become an indispensible diagnostic tool in studying the fetal heart.[20,32,44] Recent improvements in equipment, namely smaller sample volumes and higher pulsed repetition frequencies, have allowed fetal echocardiographers to interrogate specific areas of the fetal heart to analyze intracardiac and intravascular flow characteristics. The most common use of Doppler in the fetal heart is to note valve regurgitation, to evaluate flows through septal defects, and to detect the presence or absence of flow, as in valvular or vessel atresias.[32,36,62] It is important to keep in mind that the pressures and pressure gradients, which help determine flow velocities and turbulence, are quite different in the fetus. The two ventricles have pressures that are approximately equal in the fetus; consequently, ventricular septal defects (VSD) in utero may not demonstrate the typical high-velocity jets noted on Doppler in children or adults.[64]

Although Doppler in the fetal heart has its special applications, traditional Doppler principles still hold true. The fetal echocardiographer must continually be aware of exactly where he or she is relative to the heart at all times. The rapid heart rate as well as fetal movement change sample volume

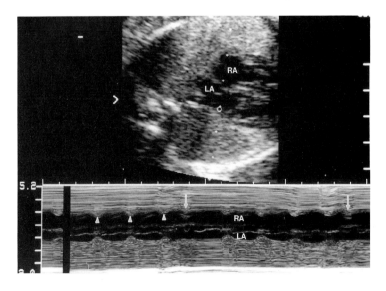

Figure 17-12. Duplex M-mode with M-line traversing the right atrium (RA) and left atrium (LA) in a fetus with premature atrial contractions. Arrowheads demonstrate normal atrial contractions and arrows depict the premature atrial beat.

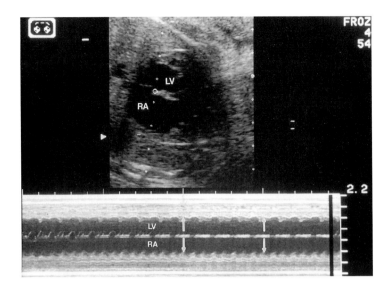

Figure 17-13. Duplex M-mode demonstrating a fetus with supraventricular tachycardia. The M-line is traversing the left ventricle (LV) and right atrium (RA). On the M-mode, the arrows define a 1-second duration. The LV has a rate of 240 bpm, whereas the atrium is in flutter with a rate of 480 bpm.

position frequently. It is also important to realize how big the sample volume size is in relation to the structure that is being interrogated. Typical chamber and great vessel sizes are routinely under 1 cm, and caution should be used to rule out "partial voluming" artifacts. It is also important constantly to be aware of the velocity scale (Nyquist limit), to avoid mistaking normal velocities for abnormal flows or vice versa. Doppler filters, which affect sensitivity, should be used cautiously to avoid "flooding" the Doppler spectra with excess noise, which may give a false impression of turbulence (a potential indication of stenosis). On the other hand, too much of a Doppler filter may eliminate turbulence

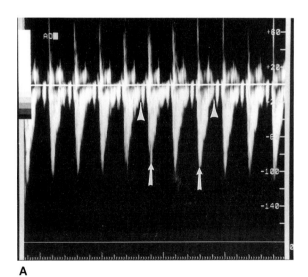

A

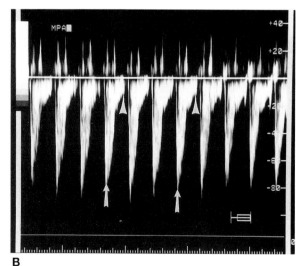

B

Figure 17-14. Spectral analysis demonstrating typical velocity waveforms of the fetal ascending aorta (AO) (**A**) and main pulmonary artery (MPA) (**B**). Note similar systolic (*arrows*) and diastolic (*arrowheads*) patterns of the two great arteries. Distinguishing between the two great vessels may be difficult by spectral analysis and Doppler audio signals.

TABLE 17-3. INTRACARDIAC DOPPLER VELOCITIES (CM/SEC) IN THE NORMAL FETUS

Parameter	Aorta	Main Pulmonary Artery	Mitral Valve	Tricuspid Valve
Maximum velocity	70 ± 3	60 ± 4	47 ± 4	51 ± 4
Mean velocity	18 ± 2	16 ± 2	11 ± 1	12 ± 1

(Modified from Reed KL, Meijboom EJ, Sahn DJ, et al. Cardiac Doppler flow velocities in human fetuses. Circulation. 1986; 73:41–46.)

or regurgitant jets, giving a false-negative impression. It is essential to understand how each piece of equipment displays and processes these important variables.[19]

Several studies have published normal ranges of velocities and volume flows through all cardiac valves (mitral, tricuspid, pulmonic, aortic) (Fig. 17-14).[60,61,71] These values seem to be consistent throughout gestation (Table 17-3). Velocities may be displayed as meters/second or centimeters/second, and volume flows (Q) may be calculated using the formula Q = velocity × area. Calculating the area of valve orifices gives rise to very high intraobserver and interobserver variability, and small measurement differences can lead to significant errors in calculations because the area formula uses the square of diameter. Extreme caution is therefore advised when relying on these calculations. Ratios using peak velocities during systole and diastole have also been formulated in the hope of determining abnormal intracardiac blood flow.[42,61]

The role of Doppler color flow mapping in fetal echocardiography has shown some utility and is highly favored by some investigators in specific clinical circumstances. Reports have focused on visualizing septal defects and regurgitant jets (Fig. 17-15).[14,24,62] Inherently, color flow Doppler has slower pulse repetition rates than standard pulsed Doppler, which may lead to unique artifacts, especially in the types of flow rates with rapid acceleration and deceleration that are seen within fetal hearts. For example, the threshold for "turbulence" is relatively low in color Doppler, and normal, high-velocity flow may be confused with disturbed flow. The sonographer must also beware of the fusion of two flow paths that may suggest defects where none exist.

Direction of flow is important information, and is relatively easy to determine, either by pulsed or color Doppler mapping. For example, the determination of normal ductal flow in the fetus, which is right to left (pulmonary artery to aorta), can quickly

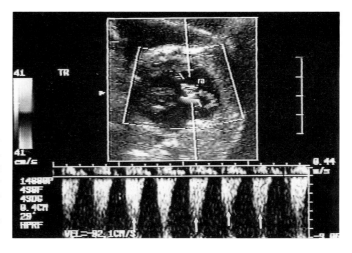

Figure 17-15. Triplex sonogram demonstrating a fetus with tricuspid regurgitation. The regurgitant jet is seen moving back into the right atrium (ra) and is demonstrated as blue/green. The Doppler spectral analysis shows the typical waveform of a regurgitant jet (below baseline/reversed flow) during systole (arrows). (See also Color Plate 13.)

rule out significant pulmonary artery disease such as severe pulmonary stenosis or atresia.[36] Similarly, reversed flow in the ascending aorta indicates aortic atresia and reversed flow in the distal aortic arch indicates interrupted aortic arch, or severe coarctation.

The Abnormal Fetal Heart

Given state-of-the-art equipment and sophisticated personnel, most serious congenital heart lesions can be identified in utero. This is important when considering sonography as a screening tool for the detection of congenital heart disease (CHD) in the general population. Fetuses with CHD may be more common than previously thought. Published rates of CHD prevalence in live newborns are 8 per 1000, but are 27 per 1000 among stillbirths.[54,55] This discrepancy is a result of the high perinatal mortality, which is, in part, associated with a 25% extracardiac anomaly rate that includes an abnormal karyotype rate of 50% to 71%. Among fetuses with isolated CHD, there is a 29% rate of chromosomal abnormalities.[28,34,57]

The diagnosis of CHD in utero can affect medical management of mother or fetus, or both, as well as mode and site of delivery. Determining postpartum care of the infant may be the most important factor in diagnosing CHD in the fetus.[30]

When imaging the fetal heart, the fetal echocardiographer must evaluate several conditions. The first and most important is whether the left and right sides of the heart are symmetric. Given that the fetal right heart measures only slightly larger than the left, the two sides should appear nearly symmetric. Actual measurement and comparison with published nomograms for chamber or great vessel size is important, because a subjectively "small" chamber may measure normal, and a subjectively "normal" chamber may, in fact, measure large. Cardiac rate and rhythm should also be documented. When imaging the great vessels, ensuring that their origin is from the proper side of the heart is of extreme importance. Imaging the fetus in multiple echocardiographic planes, including those previously described, allows the sonographer to determine normal versus abnormal cardiac morphology.[19,26]

Beam width artifact may give a false impression of vessel origin, but multiple views usually resolve questions concerning the true situs of the great vessels. It is important when determining cardiac situs that the sonographer not only orient to the fetal heart, as discussed earlier, but to the fetal abdomen. Extreme caution should be used when observing the fetal stomach or liver for fetal orientation. The position of the imaged abdominal contents (particularly the liver and stomach) can be reversed from side to side in situs inversus abdominalis totalis. The actual fetal position and fetal spine location should be noted to help determine fetal left and right sides.[17]

When abnormalities are seen using the described systematic imaging approach, congenital heart disease must be considered. We describe the most common forms of fetal congenital defects, and their sonographic appearances.

ISOLATED SEPTAL DEFECTS

Visualizing isolated VSDs depends on the size of the defect. Obviously, the larger the defect the better chance of its visualization. Caution must be observed when the fetal cardiac apex is anterior, or facing the transducer. This particular position allows "dropout" of the membranous ventricular septum, which could lead to a false-positive diagnosis of a VSD. If there is a question of a VSD being present, the ventricular septum should be imaged in a plane perpendicular to the insonating beam (Fig. 17-16).

Atrial septal defects are difficult to diagnose because the foramen ovale is normally patent throughout gestation. In our experience, only large defects, primum defects, or complete septal agenesis can be reliably diagnosed. A thorough understanding of this anatomy helps distinquish normal from abnormal findings.[33,41]

VENTRICULAR HYPERTROPHY

In utero ventricular hypertrophy is most commonly associated with severe outlet stenosis or obstruction, but may also indicate a cardiomyopathy, including the type associated with maternal diabetes. Using M-mode or two-dimensional imaging, the ventricular sizes and myocardial thickness can be measured and plotted and assessed throughout gestation against published nomograms.[31,65]

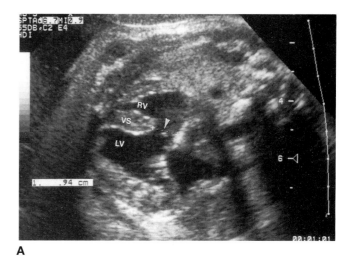

A

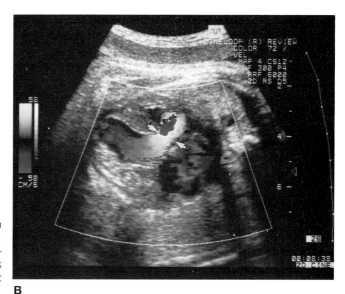

B

Figure 17-16. (**A**) Sonogram demonstrating a ventricular septal defect (VSD, *arrowhead*). RV, right ventricle; LV, left ventricle; VS, ventricular septum. (**B**) Color Doppler of the VSD demonstrates blood flow pattern through the VSD, which is left to right. (See also Color Plate 14.)

HYPOPLASTIC HEART SYNDROMES

The Hypoplastic Left and Hypoplastic Right Heart Syndromes

Hypoplastic heart syndrome is a potentially lethal lesion that most commonly affects the left side of the heart, although hypoplastic right hearts do occur. It is characterized by hypoplasia of the ventricle, atrium, atrioventricular valve, semilunar valve, and great vessel of the affected side. It is important to note that not all of the affected cardiac structures may be hypoplastic, particularly early in fetal life. Chamber sizes have been documented to change from normal to hypoplastic or from normal to enlarged in the course of a few months. The unaffected side will, ultimately, be enlarged and the fetus may or may not have associated hydrops, depending on the severity of the hypoplasia, whether it is obstructive to pulmonary venous return, and whether the other ventricle is able to assume the function of pump for both the systemic and pulmonic circulations.[29,46] When only one side of the heart can be visualized in the four-chamber view, a hypoplastic heart anomaly must be considered.[5,9] It is imperative that the affected side be imaged in detail. Typically, the ventricle, atrium, and, most important, the AV valve, semilunar valve, and great vessel are concurrently hypoplastic. It is not uncommon for the unaffected AV valve to have significant insufficiency, because the enlargement of that side causes stretching of the annulus. Figure 17-17 demonstrates the classic appearance of a hypoplastic left heart.

Hypoplastic Ventricles

Isolated hypoplastic ventricles are frequently associated with atresia of the concordant AV valve. If the right ventricle is hypoplastic, the condition is commonly referred to as tricuspid atresia, rather than hypoplastic right ventricle. In tricuspid atresia, the right ventricular outflow tract is usually present, although small. The right ventricular outflow tract

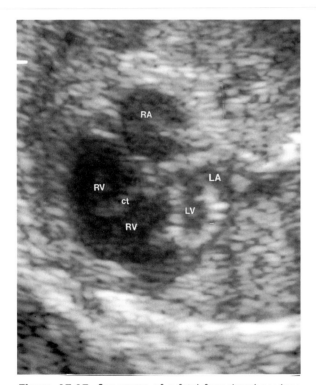

Figure 17-17. Sonogram of a fetal four-chamber view demonstrating left hypoplastic heart. Note significant discrepancy between left and right sides. RA, right atrium; RV, right ventricle; ct, chordae tendinae; LA, left atrium; LV, left ventricle.

usually receives its blood supply from a ventricular septal defect, allowing systemic and pulmonary blood flow. The left-sided correlate is that of mitral atresia, which is far less common in utero. Similar atresia of the semilunar valve may occur with or without hypoplasia of the ventricle on that side. Pulmonary atresia, for example, may be associated with a hypoplastic right ventricle, but may also be found with a relatively normal-sized right ventricle. Pulmonary atresia is usually seen with marked tricuspid regurgitation and marked enlargement of the right atrium.[50,62]

COARCTATION OF THE AORTA AND THE INTERRUPTED AORTIC ARCH

Coarctations of the aorta typically occur distal to the origin of the left subclavian artery, close to the entry of the fetal ductus arteriosus. Fetal diagnosis of this entity is difficult because the ductal flow normally is right to left, and normal fetal flow may mask the coarctation site. Interrupted aortic arch, an entity in which there is an atretic segment of the aortic arch, is almost always associated with a ventricular septal defect, which serves as a warning to examine the arch carefully. The interruption most frequently occurs proximal to the left subclavian origin, and color Doppler examinations can demonstrate cephalic (reversed) flow from the ductus back to the left subclavian.[56] Sharland and colleagues found only the most severe forms of coarctation had consistent sonographic findings: a relatively small left ventricle and ascending aorta, with right-to-left blood flow through the ductus arteriosus.[69] These sonographic findings are also consistent with interrupted aortic arch, and differentiation between coarctation and interruption of the aorta may be difficult (Fig. 17-18). In both circumstances, the neonate is duct dependent, and the neonatologist and pediatric cardiologist should be alerted to this fact before delivery.

ENDOCARDIAL CUSHION DEFECTS

Failure of the common AV orifice to separate into the mitral and tricuspid valves and failure of both septa to close give rise to a range of endocardial cushion defects (ECD) of varying severity. These may also be referred to as AV septal defects.[52,74]

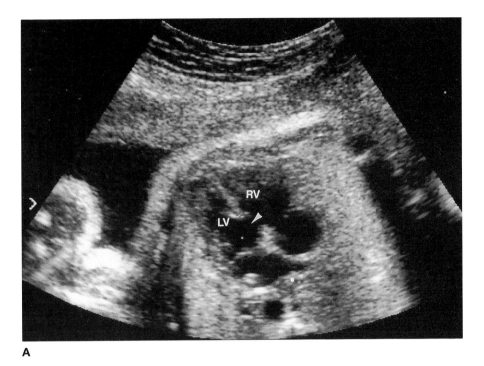

A

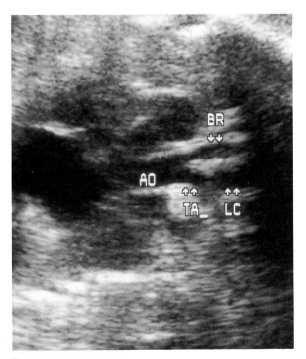

B

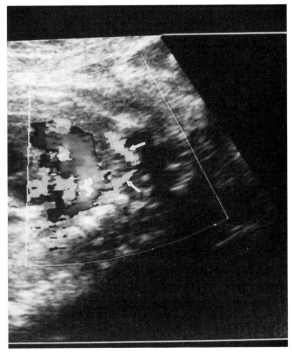

C

Figure 17-18. (A) Four-chamber view demonstrating large ventricular septal defect (*arrow-head*). RV, right ventricle; LV, left ventricle. **(B)** Sagittal section of the fetal thorax demonstrating the aortic arch, which measured significantly small for gestational age. AO, ascending aorta; TA, transverse arch; BR, brachiocephalic artery; LC, left carotid. Note the aortic arch could not be imaged distal to left carotid takeoff. **(C)** Color Doppler of descending aorta demonstrates reversed flow (red) toward transverse arch (*arrows*). (See also Color Plate 15.) These findings are consistent with severe coarctation or interrupted aortic arch.

The two major forms of ECD are the complete AV canal and partial AV canal.[27]

Complete AV canal, which is the most common form of ECD, has a large combined AV septal defect with a common septal leaflet of the AV valve. There may be absence of the interatrial septum, and a large ventricle that has an incomplete septum. There usually is a cleft of the septal leaflet of the mitral valve, and there may be mitral and tricuspid regurgitation. Valvular regurgitation is an ominous sign, and may lead to the development of fetal hydrops and death. This defect is commonly associated with Down's syndrome. Figure 17-19 demonstrates an example of a complete ECD.

The partial AV canal usually has two AV valves present, although they are deformed. There is a low primum atrial septal defect and there may be a small VSD. Both forms demonstrate a cleft in the septal leaflet of the mitral valve, which may or may not allow regurgitation.[74]

TETRALOGY OF FALLOT

The tetralogy of Fallot consists of a large VSD, overriding aorta, and infundibular stenosis, with the possibility of pulmonary valvular stenosis or atresia. All of these findings may vary in severity.[11,38] The most common abnormal sonographic finding is the demonstration of the overriding aorta, and visualization of the septal defect(s). Even using Doppler techniques, pulmonary stenosis may not be apparent early in gestation. The chambers may or may not be symmetric, depending on the severity of the pulmonary stenosis and size of the septal defects. Abnormalities may be overlooked unless great care is taken at the time of the initial scan. Figure 17-20 demonstrates a fetus diagnosed with tetralogy of Fallot.

EBSTEIN'S ANOMALY

Ebstein's anomaly is defined as inferior displacement of the tricuspid valve, causing atrialization of the right ventricle (Fig. 17-21). However, the tricuspid annulus is not displaced and, since the valvular leaflets are thin, their displacement can be easily missed. The degree of tricuspid incompetence varies considerably, and the prognosis depends on the severity of the compromise.[76] Sonographic appearances show variable asymmetry of the chambers on the four-chamber view.[72] Doppler interrogation of the tricuspid valve is essential in determining if regurgitation is present, because this may lead to right heart failure and hydrops. The association of Ebstein's anomaly and maternal lithium exposure is controversial.[40]

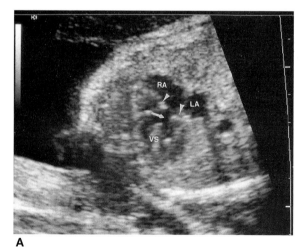
A

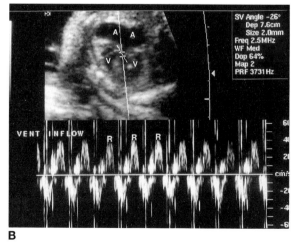
B

Figure 17-19. (**A**) Four-chamber view demonstrating complete endocardial cushion defect (*arrow*). RA, right atrium; LA, left atrium; VS, ventricular septum. Arrowheads point to common atrioventricular valve. (**B**) Doppler interrogation of the common atrioventricular valve shows valve incompetence (regurgitation). A, atria; V, ventricles; R, regurgitation jets.

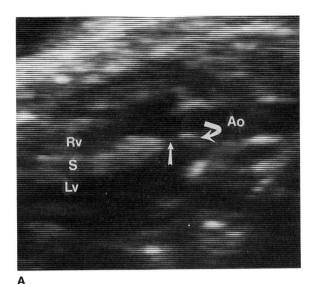
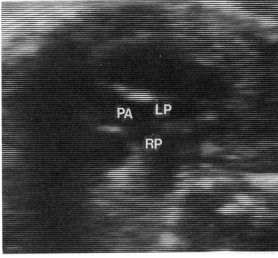

A   **B**

Figure 17-20. Four-chamber view and short-axis view demonstrating an overriding aorta with ventricular septal defect (*straight arrow*) consistent with tetralogy of Fallot. (**A**) Four-chamber view. RV, right ventricle; S, intraventricular septum; LV, left ventricle; AO, aorta; aortic valve (*curved arrow*). (**B**) Short-axis view demonstrating normal-appearing pulmonary artery (PA) and bifurcation. LP, left pulmonary artery; RP, right pulmonary artery. After birth, the newborn was found to have moderate infundibular pulmonary stenosis. (Courtesy of John Denny, MD, Swedish Hospital, Seattle, Washington.)

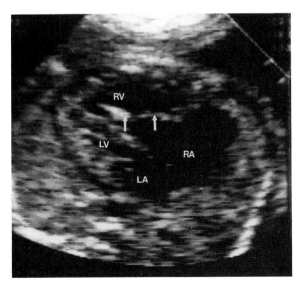

Figure 17-21. Four-chamber view in a 24-week fetus demonstrating atrialization of the right ventricle, and inferior displacement of tricuspid valve (*arrows*) consistent with Ebstein's anomaly. RA, right atrium; LA, left atrium; LV, left ventricle; RV, right ventricle.

TRANSPOSITION OF THE GREAT ARTERIES

Transposition of the great arteries (TGA) may be seen as an isolated entity or associated with other cardiac defects. Two types of TGA exist, dextro-transposition (d-TGA), which is the most common form (80%), and levo-transposition (l-TGA). Both types of TGA have great vessel–ventricular discordance, and the sonographer must guard against partial voluming artifacts with the limited angles permitted in fetal echocardiography, which may create false-positive and false-negative diagnoses.

It is of the utmost importance to be certain of fetal heart orientation (left, right) when considering this diagnosis. Because both arteries have similar sizes in the fetus, and have almost identical Doppler signals, careful two-dimensional imaging defining the great vessel in relation to a particular ventricle proves or disproves this particular diagnosis.

The classic appearance of d-TGA of the great arteries shows the aorta arising from the normal right side of the heart, but anteriorly from the morphologic right ventricle instead of from its normal mid-cardiac exit from the posterior ventricle. The pulmonary artery arises from the left ventricle posterior to the aorta (Fig. 17-22). In corrected transposition or l-TGA, the great vessels (aorta and pulmonary) arise from the anatomically correct side, but the ventricles are morphologically reversed (inversion). The "parallel arteries" sign, originally described in the pediatric echocardiography literature, may be helpful in diagnosing TGA. This sign is seen when the aorta and pulmonary arteries, in the extended four-chamber views, parallel each other when exiting the heart, rather than exhibiting the normal "crossing" of the great arteries. False-positive parallel artery signs are common because it is possible to image the ductus arteriosus and ascending aorta simultaneously. Views from different positions are needed to confirm this suspicion. Another helpful scanning technique is to try to trace the aortic arch back to the originating ventricle. If these signs are not

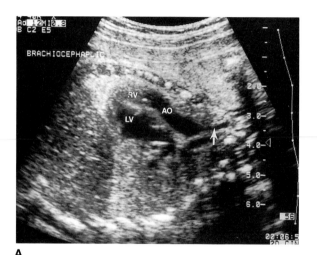

A

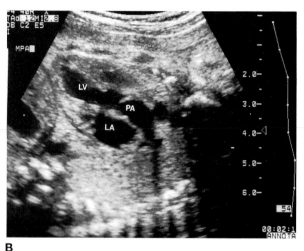

B

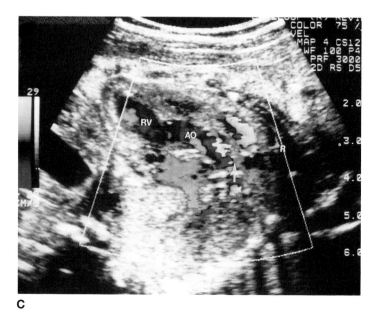

C

Figure 17-22. (**A**) Sagittal section through 28-week fetus demonstrating the aorta arising anteriorly from the right ventricle. AO, aorta; RV, right ventricle; LV, left ventricle. Arrowhead points to the brachiocephalic artery arising from transverse arch. (**B**) Modified four-chamber view demonstrates the posterior great vessel arising from the left ventricle (LV), which was the pulmonary artery (PA). LA, left atrium. (**C**) Color Doppler demonstrating continuity of flow of right ventricle to aorta to brachiocephalic artery. (See also Color Plate 16.)

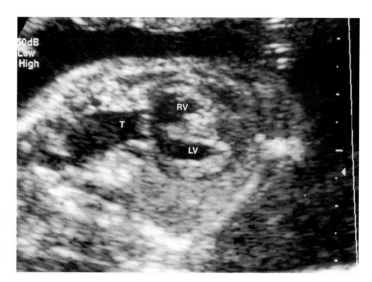

Figure 17-23. Extended four-chamber view showing common truncus (T) great vessel, arising from both right ventricle (RV) and left ventricle (LV). This is consistent with truncus arteriosus.

noted and the techniques cannot be performed, then the diagnosis cannot be ruled in or out. It is relatively common for a septal defect to be associated with TGA.[43,74]

TRUNCUS ARTERIOSUS

Truncus arteriosus occurs when the embryonic truncus arteriosus does not partition into a separate aorta and pulmonary artery, thus maintaing some degree of continuity between the channels (Fig. 17-23). Three major types of truncus occur, although only two forms can be diagnosed with ultrasound. Truncus can range from a common conduit that functions as both aorta and pulmonary artery, from which the left and right pulmonary arteries arise, to almost complete cleavage of the two arteries. (A fourth type, with no identifiable pulmonary arteries, is now considered a form of pulmonary atresia.[47]) Sonographically, the demonstration of continuity between the two great vessels should give rise to suspicion of a truncus arteriosus. A ventricular septal defect is almost always present. Using Doppler, turbulence or high velocities may or may not be noted within the common vessel or at the roots of the aorta or pulmonary arteries.[73] This is a subtle lesion that may not be diagnosed antenatally because of limitations of fetal position, age, and size.[19,74]

CARDIAC TUMORS

Although rare, congenital cardiac tumors or masses have been diagnosed in the fetus. The most common tumors are rhabdomyomas and, very rarely, rhabdomyosarcomas, which cannot be differentiated sonographically (Fig. 17-24). They appear as echogenic masses that may be seen within any or all of the cardiac chambers. These lesions are commonly associated with tuberous sclerosis. Other

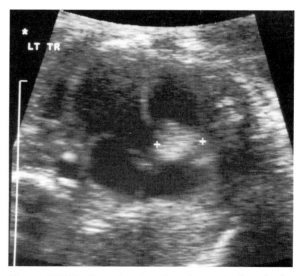

Figure 17-24. Four-chamber view demonstrating classic appearance of rhabdomyoma, which is located within the right ventricle at the level of the tricuspid annulus.

▰▰▰ **TABLE 17-4. OUTLINE OF FETAL CONGENITAL HEART DEFECTS AND SONOGRAPHIC APPEARANCES**

Heart Defect	Sonographic Appearances
Univentricular heart	Left/right heart asymmetry; normal-sized great vessels. VSD/ASD may be present.
Pulmonary atresia	Increased right side of heart if no VSD present. Nonvisualization of pulmonary artery in specific views (ant. four-chamber, short-axis). Careful duplex scanning may help in demonstrating no right ventricular outflow.
Double-outlet right ventricle	Both great arteries arising from right ventricle. VSD/ASD may be present.
Total anomalous pulmonary venous return	Several forms exist, very difficult diagnosis in utero. Important to follow pulmonary veins that may empty into right atrium or ventricle. Right chambers usually increase. Both great vessels appear normal.
Situs inversus	Important to be absolutely sure of left–right orientation of fetal heart in relation to fetal position. The fetal heart may appear normal. Abdominal structures may also be inversed.
Ectopia cordis	Fetal heart is partially or totally outside fetal thorax, usually through sternal defect. Important to look for congenital heart disease as well as other fetal abnormalities.
Valvular atresia	Chamber dilatation proximal to atretic valve. Contralateral dilatation if no VSD is present to decompress volume overload.
Interrupted aortic arch	Slight increase in right ventricle size. Abnormally small ascending aorta. Doppler/color may show reversed flow in ductus arteriosus.
Coarctation of the aorta	Possibly slight right ventricular enlargement. Possible turbulent descending aortic flow distal to ductus arteriosus entrance. Doppler/color may show reversed flow in ductus arteriosus in severe forms of coarctation.

ASD, atrial septal defect; VSD, ventricular septal defect.

considerations for fetal intracardiac tumors are fibromas, myxomas, and teratomas, which often are pericardial in origin.[39]

It is important for the fetal echocardiographer to determine if imaged masses are within the heart or outside the heart but within the pericardium.[21] Congenital lung masses such as cystic adenomatoid malformation and pulmonary sequestration may also give the false impression of cardiac masses because they may displace and indent the cardiac space. Fetal hydrops may or may not occur depending on how large these masses are, and if obstruction to blood flow occurs.

Other congenital heart anomalies that are diagnosable in utero are outlined in Table 17-4, with probable echocardiographic appearances.

In summary, the ability to image the fetal heart using sonography has become more sophisticated over the last few years. It can be a difficult and time-consuming examination but, given personnel expertise, the information given to the clinical perinatologist can aid in the care of both mother and fetus. It is imperative that the sonographer know the equipment being used, with its capabilities and limitations, in great detail. It is also imperative to have a good understanding of fetal development and congenital heart disease so that proper interrogation of the fetal heart can be made.

REFERENCES

1. Achiron R, Glaser J, Gelernter I, Hegesh J, Yagel S. Extended fetal echocardiographic examination for detecting cardiac malformations in low risk pregnancies. Br Med J. 1992; 304:671–674.
2. Adams FH. Fetal and neonatal circulation. In: Adams FH, Emmanouilides GC, eds. Heart Disease in Infants, Children and Adolescents. 3rd ed. Baltimore: Williams & Wilkins; 1983:11–17.

3. Allan L, Sharland G, Cook A. Color Atlas of Fetal Cardiology. London: Mosby-Wolfe; 1994.

4. Allan LD. Fetal diagnosis of fatal congenital heart disease. J Heart Lung Transplant. 1993; 12:S159–S161.

5. Allan LD, Cook A, Sullivan I, Sharland GK. Hypoplastic left heart syndrome: Effects of fetal echocardiography on birth prevalence. Lancet. 1991; 337:959–961.

6. Allan LD, Chita SK, Sharland GK, Fagg NL, Anderson RH, Crawford DC. The accuracy of fetal echocardiography in the diagnosis of congenital heart disease. Int J Cardiol. 1989; 25:279–288.

7. Allan LD, Joseph MC, Boyd EG, et al. M-mode echocardiography in the developing human fetus. Br Heart J. 1982; 47:573–583.

8. Benacerraf BR, Sanders SP. Fetal echocardiography. Radiol Clin North Am. 1990; 28:131–147.

9. Blake DM, Copel JA, Kleinman CS. Hypoplastic left heart syndrome: Prenatal diagnosis, clinical profile, and management. Am J Obstet Gynecol. 1991; 165:529–534.

10. Bromley B, Estroff JA, Sanders SP, et al. Fetal echocardiography: Accuracy and limitations in a population at high and low risk for heart defects. Obstet Gynecol. 1992; 166:1473–1481.

11. Callan NA, Kan JS. Prenatal diagnosis of tetralogy of Fallot with absent pulmonary valve. Am J Perinatol. 1991; 8:15–17.

12. Callan NA. Fetal echocardiography. Curr Opin Obstet Gynecol. 1991; 3:255–258.

13. Cartier MS, Davidoff A, Warnecke LA, et al. The normal diameter of the fetal aorta and pulmonary artery: Echocardiographic evaluation in utero. Am J Roentgenol. 1987; 149:1003–1007.

14. Copel JA, Morotti R, Hobbins JC, Kleinman CS. The antenatal diagnosis of congenital heart disease using fetal echocardiography: Is color flow mapping necessary? Obstet Gynecol. 1991; 78:1–8.

15. Copel JA, Kleinman CS. Fetal echocardiography in the diagnosis and management of fetal heart disease. Clin Diagn Ultrasound. 1989; 25:67–83.

16. Copel JA, Pilu G, Green J, et al. Fetal echocardiographic screening for congenital heart disease: The importance of the four-chamber view. Am J Obstet Gynecol. 1987; 157:648–655.

17. Cordes TM, O'Leary PW, Seward JB, Hagler DJ. Distinguishing right from left: A standardized technique for fetal echocardiography. J Am Soc Echocardiogr. 1994; 7:47–53.

18. Cyr DR, Nghiem HV, Mack LA. Sonography of the first trimester. In: Hagan-Ansert S, ed. Textbook of Ultrasonography. 4th ed. St. Louis: Mosby–Yearbook; 1994.

19. Cyr DR, Guntheroth WG, Mack LA. Fetal echocardiography. In: Berman M, Craig M, Kawamura D, eds. Diagnostic Medical Sonography, Vol. 2. Philadelphia: JB Lippincott, 1990;249–271.

20. Cyr DR. Intracardiac fetal Doppler. In: Proceedings of the 6th Annual Spring SDMS Conference, Anaheim, California, 1988.

21. Cyr DR, Guntheroth WG, Nyberg DA, Smith JR, Ek M. Prenatal diagnosis of an intrapericardial teratoma: A cause for nonimmune hydrops. J Ultrasound Med. 1988; 7:87–90.

22. Cyr DR, Komarniski CA, Guntheroth WG, Mack LA. The prevalence of imaging fetal cardiac anatomy. J Diagn Med Sonogr. 1988; 6:299–304.

23. DeVore GR, Medearis AL, Bear MB, Horenstein J, Platt LD. Fetal echocardiography: Factors that influence imaging of the fetal heart during the second trimester of pregnancy. J Ultrasound Med. 1993; 12:659–663.

24. DeVore GR, Horenstein J, Siassi B, Platt LD. Fetal echocardiography: VII. Doppler color flow mapping: A new technique for the diagnosis of congenital heart disease. Am J Obstet Gynecol. 1987; 156:1054–1064.

25. DeVore GR, Siassi B, Platt L. Fetal echocardiography: III. The diagnosis of cardiac arrhythmias using real-time—directed M-mode ultrasound. Am J Obstet Gynecol. 1983; 146:792.

26. Drose JA, Cyr DR. Fetal echocardiography. In: DuBose TJ, ed. Fetal Sonography. Philadelphia: WB Saunders; 1996:253–261.

27. Feldt RH, Edwards WD, Puga FJ, et al. Atrial septal defects and atrioventricular canal. In: Adams FH, Emmanouilides GC, eds. Heart Disease in Infants, Children and Adolescents. 3rd ed. Baltimore: Williams & Wilkins; 1983:118–133.

28. Fogel M, Copel JA, Cullen MT, Hobbins JC, Kleinman CS. Congenital heart disease and fetal thoracoabdominal anomalies: Associations in utero and the importance of cytogenetic analysis. Am J Perinatol. 1991; 8:411–416.

29. Freedom RM. Hypoplastic left heart syndrome. In: Adams FH, Emmanouilides GC, eds. Heart Disease in Infants, Children and Adolescents. 3rd ed. Baltimore: Williams & Wilkins; 1983:411–421.

30. Friedman AH, Copel JA, Kleinman CS. Fetal echocardiography and fetal cardiology: Indications, diagnosis and management. Semin Perinatol. 1993; 17:76–88.

31. Gandhi JA, Zhang XY, Maidman JE. Fetal cardiac hypertrophy and cardiac function in diabetic pregnancies. Am J Obstet Gynecol. 1995; 173:1132–1136.

32. Gembruch U, Hansmann M, Redel DA, Bald R. Fetal two-dimensional Doppler echocardiography (colour flow mapping) and its place in prenatal diagnosis. Prenat Diagn. 1989; 9:535–547.

33. Graham TP, Bender HW, Spach MS. Ventricular septal defect. In: Adams FH, Emmanouilides GC, eds. Heart Disease in Infants, Children and Adolescents. 3rd ed. Baltimore: Williams & Wilkins; 1983:134–153.

34. Greenwood RD, Rosenthal A, Parisi L, et al. Extra-cardiac abnormalities in infants with congenital heart disease. Pediatrics. 1975; 55:485–492.

35. Guntheroth WG, Cyr DR, Shields LE, Nghiem HV. Rate-based management of fetal supraventricular tachycardia. J Ultrasound Med. 1996; 15:453–458.

36. Guntheroth WG, Cyr DR, Winter T, Easterling T, Mack LA. Fetal Doppler of pulmonary atresia. J Ultrasound Med. 1993; 5:281–284.

37. Guntheroth WG, Cyr DR, Mack LA, et al. Hydrops from reciprocating A-V tachycardia in a 27 week fetus requiring quinidine for conversion. Obstet Gynecol. 1985; 66:295–300.

38. Guntheroth WG, Kawabori I, Baum D. Tetralogy of Fallot. In: Adams FH, Emmanouilides GC, eds. Heart Disease in Infants, Children and Adolescents. 3rd ed. Baltimore: Williams & Wilkins; 1983:215–227.

39. Holley DG, Martin GR, Brenner JI, et al. Diagnosis and management of fetal cardiac tumors: A multicenter experience and review of published reports. J Am Coll Cardiol. 1995; 26:516–520.

40. Jacobson SJ, Jones K, Johnson K, et al. Prospective multicentre study of pregnancy outcome after lithium exposure during first trimester. Lancet. 1992; 339:530–533.

41. Kachalia P, Bowie JD, Adams DB, Carroll BA. In utero sonographic appearance of the atrial septum primum and septum secundum. J Ultrasound Med. 1991; 10:423–426.

42. Kenny JF, Plappert T, Doubilet P. Changes in intracardiac blood flow velocities and right and left ventricular stroke volumes with gestational age in the normal human fetus: A prospective Doppler echocardiographic study. Circulation. 1986; 74:1208–1216.

43. Kirklin JW, Colvin EV, McConnell ME, Bargeron LM Jr. Complete transposition of the great arteries: Treatment in the current era. Pediatr Clin North Am. 1990; 37:171–177.

44. Kleinman CS, Huhta JC, Silverman NH. Doppler echocardiography in the human fetus. J Am Soc Echocardiogr. 1988; 1:287–290.

45. Kleinman CS, Weinstein EM, Talner NS, et al. Fetal echocardiography: Applications and limitations. Ultrasound Med Biol. 1984; 10:747–755.

46. Lang P, Norwood WI. Hemodynamic assessment after palliative surgery for hypoplastic left heart syndrome. Circulation. 1983; 68:104–108.

47. Mair DD, Edwards WD, Fuster V, et al. Truncus arteriosus. In: Adams FH, Emmanouilides GC, eds. Heart Disease in Infants, Children and Adolescents. 3rd ed. Baltimore: Williams & Wilkins; 1983:400–410.

48. Martin GR, Ruckman RN. Fetal echocardiography: A large clinical experience and follow-up. J Am Soc Echocardiogr. 1990; 3:4–8.

49. McCurdy CM Jr, Reed KL. Basic technique of fetal echocardiography. Semin Ultrasound CT MR. 1993; 14:267–276.

50. McGahan JP, Choy M, Parrish MD, Brant WE. Sonographic spectrum of fetal cardiac hypoplasia. J Ultrasound Med. 1991; 10:539–546.

51. Meijboom EJ, van-Engelen AD, van-de-Beek EW, Weijtens O, Lautenschutz JM, Benatar AA. Fetal arrhythmias. Curr Opin Cardiol. 1994; 9:97–102.

52. Moore KL, Persaud T, eds. The Developing Human. 5th ed. Philadelphia: WB Saunders; 1993:304–353.

53. Moore KL, ed. The Developing Human: Clinically Oriented Embryology. 3rd ed. Philadelphia: WB Saunders; 1982.

54. Nora JJ, Nora AH. Update on counseling the family with a first degree relative with a congenital heart defect. Am J Med Genet. 1988; 29:137–142.

55. Nora JJ, Nora AH. Maternal transmission of congenital heart disease: New recurrence risk figures and the question of cytoplasmic inheritance and vulnerability to teratogens. Am J Cardiol. 1987; 59:459–463.

56. Norwood WI, Lang P, Hansen DD. Physiologic repair of aortic atresia–hypoplastic left heart syndrome. N Engl J Med. 1983; 308:23–30.

57. Paladini D, Calabro R, Palmieri S, D'Andrea T. Prenatal diagnosis of congenital heart disease and fetal karyotyping. Obstet Gynecol. 1993; 81:679–682.

58. Persutte WH, Jones OW. The four-chamber view of the fetal heart: How achievable is it? J Diagn Med Sonogr. 1996; 12(2):69–71.

59. Reed KL. Fetal arrhythmias: Etiology, diagnosis, pathophysiology and treatment. Semin Perinatol. 1989; 13:294–304.

60. Reed KL, Meijboom EJ, Sahn DJ, et al. Cardiac Doppler flow velocities in human fetuses. Circulation. 1986; 73:41–46.

61. Reed KL, Sahn DJ, Scagnelli S, et al. Doppler echocardiographic studies of diastolic function in the hu-

man fetal heart: Changes during gestation. J Am Coll Cardiol. 1986; 8:391–395.

62. Respondek ML, Kammermeier M, Ludomirsky A, Weil SR, Huhta JC. The prevalence and clinical significance of fetal tricuspid valve regurgitation with normal heart anatomy. Am J Obstet Gynecol. 1994; 171:1265–1270.

63. Rice MJ, McDonald RW, Reller MD, Sahn DJ. Pediatric echocardiography: Current role and a review of technical advances. J Pediatr. 1996; 128:1–14.

64. Rudolph AM. Distribution and regulation of blood flow in the fetal and neonatal lamb. Circ Res. 1985; 57:811–821.

65. Rustico MA, Benettoni A, Bussani R, Maieron A, Mandruzzato G. Early fetal endocardial fibroelastosis and critical aortic stenosis: A case report. Ultrasound in Obstetrics and Gynecology. 1995; 5:202–205.

66. Sahn D, Kisslo J. Report of the Council on Scientific Affairs: Ultrasonic imaging of the heart. Report of the Ultrasonography Task Force. Arch Intern Med. 1991; 151:1288–1294.

67. Schats R, Jansen CAM, Wladimiroff JW, et al. Embryonic heart activity: Appearance and development in early human pregnancy. Br J Obstet Gynaecol. 1990; 97:989–994.

68. Schultz SM, Pretorius DH, Budorick NE. Four-chamber view of the heart: Demonstration related to menstrual age. J Ultrasound Med. 1994; 13:285–289.

69. Sharland GK, Chan KY, Allan LD. Coarctation of the aorta: Difficulties in prenatal diagnosis. Br Heart J. 1994; 71:70–75.

70. Sharland GK, Chita SK, Allan LD. The use of colour Doppler in fetal echocardiography. Int J Cardiol. 1990; 28:229–236.

71. Shenker L, Reed KL, Marx GR, et al. Fetal cardiac Doppler flow studies in perinatal diagnosis of heart disease. Am J Obstet Gynecol. 1988; 158:1267–1273.

72. Shenker L, Astle C, Reed K, Anderson C. Embryonic heart rates before the seventh week of pregnancy. J Reprod Med. 1986; 31:333–335.

73. Silverman NH, Golbus MS. Echocardiographic techniques for assessing normal and abnormal fetal cardiac anatomy. J Am Coll Cardiol. 1985; 5:20S–29S.

74. Stamm ER, Drose JA, Thikman D. The fetal heart. In: Rumack CM, Wilson SR, Charbenau JW, eds. Diagnostic Ultrasound. St. Louis: Mosby–Yearbook; 1991:800–827.

75. van Engelen AD, Weijtens O, Brenner JI, et al. Management outcome and follow-up of fetal tachycardia. J Am Coll Cardiol. 1994; 24:1371.

76. van Mierop LHS, Schiebler GL, Victorica BE. Ebstein's anomaly. In: Adams FH, Emmanouilides GC, eds. Heart Disease in Infants, Children and Adolescents. 3rd ed. Baltimore: Williams & Wilkins; 1983:283–295.

18

Normal and Abnormal Fetal Limbs

BIRGIT BADER-ARMSTRONG

The femur and the humerus are the two fetal long bones routinely measured during an ultrasound examination conducted to determine gestational age (GA). The femur is usually the easier of the two to measure because the humerus is quite often wedged between the fetal chest and the uterine wall. When it is impossible to obtain accurate measurements of these bones, the radius and ulna or the tibia and fibula can be measured. GA estimation nomograms are available for most bones from the 12th week to term (see Appendixes).

In addition to dating the pregnancy, measurement and evaluation of fetal long bones also documents their existence or absence, whether they are properly mineralized and formed, and how they are positioned in relation to the rest of the limb. A skeletal abnormality is often a characteristic of a syndrome involving other organs. Such a finding alerts the sonographer to proceed with a more detailed fetal anatomic examination and to obtain a family history for any genetically transmitted skeletal abnormalities.

In this chapter, we explain normal and abnormal development and sonographic assessment of fetal limbs, and the most prevalent fetal limb malformations with their associated anomalies (Table 18-1).

Normal Fetal Limbs

ANATOMY

It is the calcium content of the bones that generates the high-amplitude reflection on ultrasound and permits imaging of the fetal skeleton. The shaft of the long bone is the primary ossification center and may be especially well visualized in the first trimester using a transvaginal approach (Fig. 18-1). The epiphysis is the secondary ossification center and is separated from the shaft by a layer of cartilage (Fig. 18-2). The two epiphyseal centers seen most often in fetal ultrasound are the distal femoral epiphysis (visible at 32 to 35 weeks) and the proximal tibial epiphysis (visible by 34 or 35 weeks). The proximal humeral epiphysis may not form until term. It is never seen in normal fetuses before term.

The metacarpals and phalanges of the fetal hand are visible in the second trimester (Fig. 18-3); the carpal bones ossify after birth. The talus, calcaneus, metatarsals, and phalanges of the foot begin to calcify during the second trimester.

SONOGRAPHIC TECHNIQUE

To image the femur, position the transducer in a transverse plane through the fetal trunk and scan toward the bladder. The bright, short, linear echoes on either side of the bladder are the iliac bones. The femur is found lateral and caudad to the ilium. Slowly rotate the transducer until the longest axis of the shaft is obtained. This is a hand–eye coordination task that requires practice. A normal shaft is fairly straight, symmetric, and evenly ossified. The sonographer should rock the transducer gently to be sure the femur and not one of the paired lower leg bones is being visualized. In the lower leg, the tibia (the medial shaft) is thicker than the fibula.

Care must be taken to ensure that the longest

TABLE 18-1. SKELETAL DYSPLASIAS AND THEIR ASSOCIATED ANOMALIES

Dysplasia	Curved or Bowed Long Bones	Hypomineralization	Bone Fractures	Radial Aplasia	Polydactyly	Macrocephaly	Heart Disease	Narrow Thorax
Achondrogenesis		X	X					X
Achondroplasia						X		X
Asphyxiating thoracic dysplasia								X
Camptomelia	X	X			X	X	X	X
Ellis-van Creveld syndrome					X		X	
Holt-Oram syndrome				X			X	
Hypophosphatasia	X	X	X					
Osteogenesis imperfecta	X	X	X					
Short rib–polydactyly syndrome		X			X		X	X
Thrombocytopenia– absent radius syndrome				X				
Thanatophoric dwarfism	X	X			X	X		X
VACTERL associations				X	X		X	

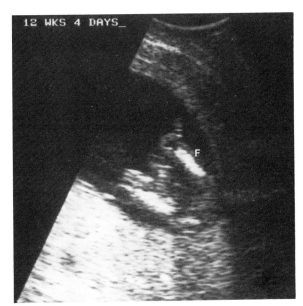

Figure 18-1. Femur (F) was imaged at 12.5 weeks using a transvaginal probe.

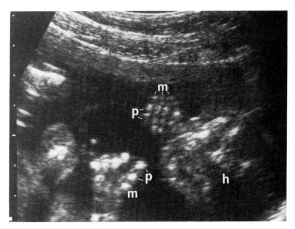

Figure 18-3. Fetal hands at 19 weeks show the phalanges (p) and metacarpals (m); h, fetal head.

dimension of the femoral shaft is visualized and that the ends of the image are sharply defined. The ends may appear blunted or slightly curved. In a normal pregnancy, mild bowing of either femoral shaft may be produced by the curved medial border of the femur after 18 weeks' GA. The posterior-lying femur often has a more pronounced bowing, mimick-

ing skeletal dysplasia (Fig. 18-4). Mild artifactual bowing should not cause the examiner to obtain an inaccurate measurement. If the transducer is not perpendicular to the shaft, an oblique view is obtained and the measurement is artificially shortened. Acoustic shadowing should fall perpendicular to and behind the long bone to verify the correctness of the scanning plane. The femur length can be overestimated by several millimeters by including the "distal femur point." This thin white line most likely represents a reflection from the smooth sur-

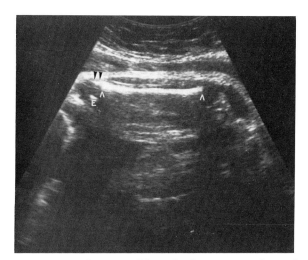

Figure 18-2. Femur at 37 weeks demonstrates the end points of the ossified shaft (*white arrows*), reflections from the lateral aspect of the distal femoral cartilage (*black arrows*), and the distal femoral epiphysis (E).

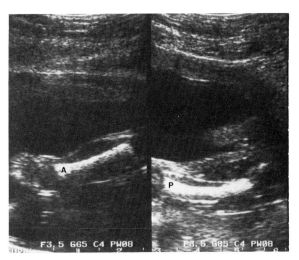

Figure 18-4. Femurs at 21 weeks' gestation. The shaft of the anterior femur (A) has slight normal curvature. The posterior femur (P) exhibits a more pronounced artifactual bowing.

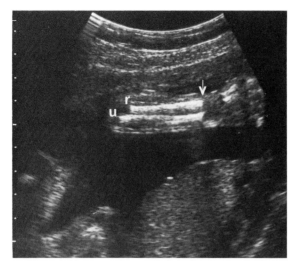

Figure 18-5. Radius (r) and ulna (u) at 25 weeks' gestation. Note that the distal radius and ulna end at the same point (arrow).

face of the lateral aspect of the distal femoral epiphyseal cartilage, and is therefore not part of the ossified femoral shaft itself (see Fig. 18-2).[12] Normal growth patterns of the long bones have been established to determine GA.[15,16] Serial measurements of fetal long bones are useful in the diagnosis of certain skeletal dysplasias. With achondroplasia, the femur length may be appropriate during the early pregnancy, and then drop below the 10th percentile for GA in the second trimester as the syndrome progresses and manifests itself sonographically.

To measure the humerus, place the transducer in a transverse plane at the level of the fetal shoulders and rotate the transducer on the scapula until the longest length of the humerus is imaged. Rock the transducer gently back and forth to be certain the humerus is actually being visualized and not the radius or ulna. Obtaining a diagnostic image of the humerus in late pregnancy requires more patience than imaging the femur, because the upper arm is often wedged between the trunk and the uterine wall. When evaluating the lower arm, document that the distal radius and ulna end at the same point (Fig. 18-5). This is a helpful landmark for assessing lower arm reductions. The ulna is the longer of the two bones.

Several technical factors may limit the sonographer's ability to visualize limbs. Limbs located in the near field are often difficult to delineate. The

sonographer may use an acoustic standoff pad to shift the focal zone of the transducer to the region of interest. Oligohydramnios results in a poor overall resolution of the crowded fetus. Limbs may be tucked under the trunk or lie in a bizarre position. A transvaginal approach may be helpful in an early pregnancy complicated by severe oligohydramnios (Fig. 18-6). With polyhydramnios, the fetus is often very active or may lie beyond the focal range of the transducer. If the patient can be positioned on her elbows and knees, the fetus will naturally fall to the lowest point and the sonographer can attempt to scan the mother's abdomen from below.

Patience is often the key to obtaining a good diagnostic scan. A fetus that remains in an unfavorable position may move after the mother empties her bladder or takes a short walk. As a last resort, the patient can be rescheduled to complete her examination the next day.

Abnormal Fetal Limbs

Skeletal dysplasia is the abnormal development of the cartilaginous and osseous tissues, resulting in bones that appear shortened, thin, or deformed, or that fail to form at all. Fetuses with long bone measurements more than 2 standard deviations be-

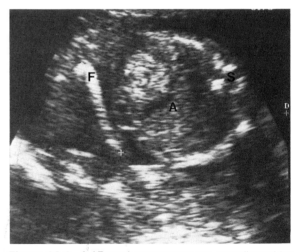

Figure 18-6. A 17-week pregnancy was complicated by severe oligohydramnios. An initial transabdominal scan was unable to identify and accurately measure any fetal limbs. A transvaginal approach demonstrated a femur length (F) consistent with 16 weeks' gestation. Fetal abdomen (A) and spine (S) are seen in cross section.

TABLE 18-2. LETHAL DYSPLASIAS

Achondrogenesis
Asphyxiating thoracic dysplasia*
Camptomelic dysplasia*
Ellis-van Creveld syndrome*
Homozygous achondroplasia
Hypophosphatasia*
Osteogenesis imperfecta Type II
Short rib–polydactyly syndrome
Thrombocytopenia–absent radius syndrome*
Thanatophoric dysplasia
VACTERL associations*

*Mildly affected patients may survive.

low normal require a more detailed anatomic scan. Some syndromes are uniformly lethal, and others are lethal in their more severe forms (Table 18-2).

Most forms of short-limbed dwarfism are inherited. In autosomal dominant forms of dwarfism, such as achondroplasia, there is a 50% chance that an affected parent will pass the trait on to offspring. When both parents are affected, the fetus has a 25% chance of not inheriting the gene from either parent and being normal; a 50% chance of receiving the gene from one parent and being heterozygously affected; and a 25% chance of inheriting the abnormal gene from both parents and being homozygously affected. This homozygous genotype is associated with the most severe form of dysplasia. When both parents are carriers of the gene for an autosomal recessive trait, there is a 25% chance that the fetus will receive two genes for that trait and inherit the dysplasia. When unaffected parents have a child with a skeletal dysplasia as the result of spontaneous mutation, the risk of recurrence in subsequent pregnancies is minimal.

As a group, skeletal dysplasias are rare and are not always detectable prenatally by ultrasound. For example, the manifestations of osteogenesis imperfecta types I, III, and IV may not be severe enough in utero to be demonstrated by ultrasound examination. Fetuses affected by heterozygous achondroplasia may exhibit normal long bone growth patterns until 21 to 26 weeks' GA.[18] A sporadic occurrence of this form of dwarfism may be missed if the patient's solitary examination occurs before 26 weeks' GA.

Short-limbed dysplasias are classified into four descriptive categories. A rhizomelic dwarf's greatest bone shortening is the proximal extremity (i.e., the humerus and femur). Mesomelia is predominantly middle segment limb shortening involving the radius, ulna, tibia, and fibula. Acromelia involves shortening of the distal extremities (i.e., the bones of the hands and feet). Micromelia is the shortening of an entire extremity.

SONOGRAPHIC TECHNIQUE

Skill, patience, and a complete and accurate patient history are the major ingredients for a thorough ultrasound examination, especially when there is a suspicion of skeletal dysplasia. A finger and toe count is beyond the time restrictions in most laboratories for routine ultrasound examinations for dating. However, a closer look at the fetal hands and feet is indicated when a patient presents with a family history of genetically transmitted skeletal abnormalities or whenever a long bone abnormality is noted on routine examination.

When attempting to scan a fetus at risk, the sonographer should document and measure each limb that can be imaged. True bowing of a limb, which may result in a short-for-GA measurement, should be distinguished from mild artifactual bowing. Any sharply angulated midshaft indicates a fracture (Figs. 18-7 and 18-8). Shadowing from overlying fetal limbs may artificially shorten a long bone

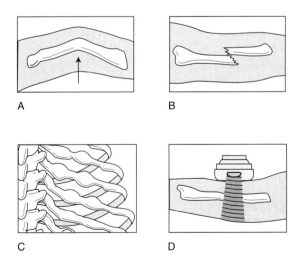

Figure 18-7. Appearance of fractures. (**A**) Highly angled shaft. (**B**) Overlapping segments of bone. (**C**) Beading of the ribs caused by the callus formation at the fracture site. (**D**) Sonographic pitfall. "Gap" caused by shadowing from fetal limb is not a fracture.

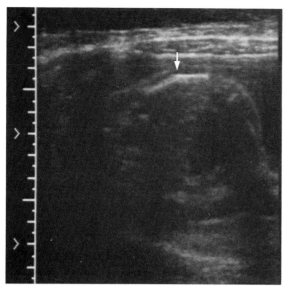

Figure 18-8. Sonogram of fracture site (*arrow*) in a femur. (Filly RA, Golbus MS. Ultrasonography of the normal and pathologic fetal skeleton. Radiol Clin North Am. 1982; 20:321.)

third trimesters. Often, the prognosis for the fetus is the determining factor in the parent's decision whether to terminate the pregnancy. Should the pregnancy continue, an accurate diagnosis is helpful for planning subsequent obstetric care and mode and place for obstetric delivery.

SKELETAL DYSPLASIAS

Skeletal dysplasias are complex disorders. The following brief paragraphs describe several of the more commonly seen dysplasias. Fetal sonography may or may not show some or all of these reported features. A thorough examination will aid in the diagnosis of a general skeletal dysplasia and may on occasion even provide a definitive diagnosis.

Thanatophoric Dysplasia

Thanatophoric means "death-producing." It occurs in approximately 1 in 6400 deliveries,[33] and is one of the more common forms of lethal short-limbed dwarfism seen. Its etiology is unknown. It presents

or even create a gap that mimics a fracture (Fig. 18-9). Abnormal skeletal mineralization may make the cranium or long bones difficult to visualize, or make them appear thin or unevenly mineralized (Fig. 18-10).

The sonographer should determine the dominant type of limb shortening (Table 18-3). In a normal fetus, the distal radius and ulna should end at the same point, and this rules out radial hypoplasia (see Fig. 18-5). Calculate the thoracic circumference–abdominal circumference ratio (normal ratio, 0.89)[7] to rule out an abnormally narrow thorax, which may result in respiratory distress at birth. Document any other associated abnormalities observed, such as polyhydramnios, polydactyly, club foot, prominent skin thickening in the neck and limb areas, cleft lip or palate, cardiac defects, or the presence of a two-vessel umbilical cord.

Table 18-4 lists skeletal dysplasias by their ultrasound findings. When a genetically transmitted skeletal dysplasia is suspected, a genetic amniocentesis for chromosomal analysis may be indicated to confirm the diagnosis. Transvaginal ultrasound or fetoscopy may be used to image or visualize limbs of suspected fetuses in early pregnancy. A flat film of the abdomen for fetal bone mineralization and configuration may be helpful in the second and

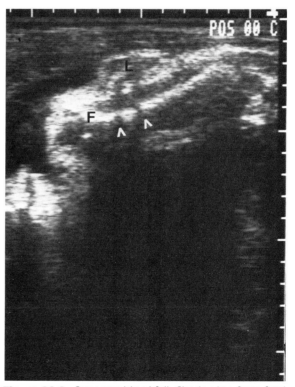

Figure 18-9. Sonographic pitfall. Shadowing from fetal limb (L) may artificially shorten a femur (F) or may create gaps mimicking fractures (*arrowheads*).

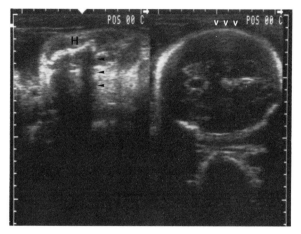

Figure 18-10. Osteogenesis imperfecta Type II. The humerus (H) is short, misshapen, and shows uneven acoustic shadowing due to faulty mineralization (*black arrowheads*). The cranium is poorly mineralized.

sonographically as extreme micromelia, bowed long bones, a narrow thorax and protruding abdomen giving a "champagne cork" appearance, short ribs, flattened vertebral bodies, and general hypomineralization of all bones (Fig. 18-11).[4,13,20] Associated abnormalities of the head are macrocephalus secondary to hydrocephalus and frontal bossing (protruding forehead). Thanatophoric dwarfism with cloverleaf skull (Kleeblattschadel) occurs when pre-

////// TABLE 18-3. DOMINANT CATEGORY OF LIMB SHORTENING IN SKELETAL DYSPLASIAS

Skeletal Dysplasia	Dominant Category
Achondrogenesis	Micromelia*
Achondroplasia	Rhizomelia†
Asphyxiating thoracic dysplasia	Mesomelia‡
Camptomelic dysplasia	Mesomelia, rhizomelia
Congenital hypophosphatasia	Micromelia
Ellis-van Creveld syndrome	Rhizomelia
Hypophosphatasia	Micromelia
Osteogenesis imperfecta	Micromelia
Radial aplasia, hypoplasia	Mesomelia
Short rib–polydactyly syndrome	Micromelia
Thanatophoric dysplasia	Micromelia

* Shortening of entire extremity.
† Shortening of proximal extremity.
‡ Middle segment limb shortening (radius, tibia).

////// TABLE 18-4. SONOGRAPHIC FINDINGS IN SKELETAL DYSPLASIA

Curved or bowed long bones
  Camptomelic dysplasia
  Hypophosphatasia
  Osteogenesis imperfecta
  Thanatophoric dysplasia
Hypomineralization
  Achondrogenesis
  Camptomelic dysplasia
  Hypophosphatasia
  Osteogenesis imperfecta
  Short rib–polydactyly syndrome
  Thanatophoric dysplasia
Narrow thorax
  Achondrogenesis type I
  Achondroplasia
  Asphyxiating thoracic dysplasia
  Camptomelic dysplasia
  Short rib–polydactyly syndrome
  Thanatophoric dysplasia
Polydactyly
  Asphyxiating thoracic dysplasia*
  Ellis-van Creveld syndrome
  Short rib–polydactyly syndrome
  VACTERL association*
Radial aplasia or hypoplasia
  Holt-Oram syndrome
  Thrombocytopenia–absent radius syndrome
  VACTERL associations
Bone fractures
  Achondrogenesis
  Hypophosphatasia
  Osteogenesis imperfecta
Heart disease
  Asphyxiating thoracic dysplasia
  Ellis-van Creveld syndrome
  Holt-Oram syndrome
  Short rib–polydactyly syndrome*
  VACTERL association*
Macrocephaly
  Achondroplasia
  Camptomelic dysplasia*
  Thanatophoric dysplasia

* Does not occur in all cases.

mature closure of the coronal and lambdoid sutures causes the temporal bones to bulge out. This creates the trilobular, or cloverleaf, calvarial shape (Fig. 18-12).[35,37] Massive polyhydramnios is a prominent feature that may lead to premature labor.[36] The infant dies shortly after birth from cardiorespiratory failure. Differential diagnosis includes achondrogenesis, Ellis-van Creveld syndrome, and Jeune's syndrome.

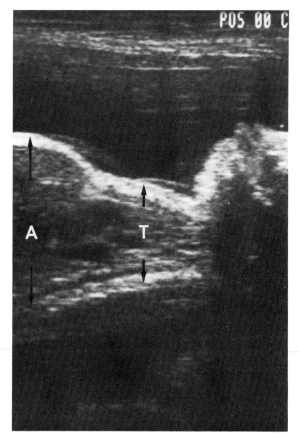

Figure 18-11. Longitudinal view of a thanatophoric dwarf. The thorax (T) is narrow and the abdomen (A) protrudes, giving a "champagne cork" appearance.

Achondroplasia

Achondroplasia is inherited in an autosomal dominant manner, but it frequently appears as a spontaneous disorder. It is the most common nonlethal type of dwarfism. There is rhizomelic limb bowing and frontal bossing. One characteristic finding for heterozygous achondroplasia is a three-pronged "trident" configuration of the fingers.[14] Occasional associated findings are macrocephalus and hydrocephalus. Serial femur length measurements may fall within the normal range up to 24 to 26 weeks' GA. A normal intelligence and life expectancy is possible, although the person may suffer from spinal problems, pulmonary compromise, and difficulties during pregnancy due to a small pelvis. Adult heights average 49 inches for women and 52 inches for men. The homozygous form, inherited from two parents who are heterozygous achondroplastic dwarfs, is a lethal condition.

Achondrogenesis

Achondrogenesis types I and II may be autosomal recessive conditions or may occur spontaneously. Type I is characterized by micromelia, a narrow thorax with extremely short ribs, and polydactyly. Type II is more severe and presents with extreme micromelia, a short thorax, and protruding abdomen. Although the entire skeleton shows varying degrees of hypomineralization, the spinal column is especially affected.[21] The short, thin fetal ribs may show "beading" (see Fig. 18-7), which is evidence of multiple healing fractures. Achondrogenesis is associated with severe polyhydramnios and edema of the soft tissues (Fig. 18-13)[2]; however, excess skin folds over a shortened frame may also give the appearance of hydrops.[23] Achondrogenesis results in stillbirth or neonatal death because of pulmonary hypoplasia. Differential diagnosis includes congenital hypophosphatasia. Rib fractures may also be seen in osteogenesis imperfecta type II.

Short Rib–Polydactyly Syndrome

This syndrome may have a similar appearance to achondrogenesis. It is differentiated by additional findings of cardiac and genitourinary anomalies,

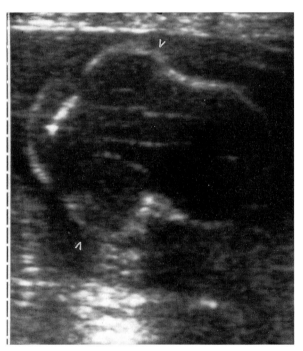

Figure 18-12. Bulging of the temporal bones of a cloverleaf skull (*arrows*). (Courtesy of Glenn A. Rousse, MD, Marie DeLange, BS, RDMS, Loma Linda University Medical Center, Loma Linda, CA.)

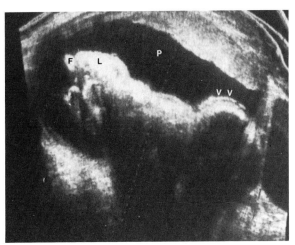

Figure 18-13. Fetus affected by achondrogenesis. The lower limbs (L) are short, and the foot (F) is seen. There is scalp edema (*arrowheads*) and marked polyhydramnios (P).

and cleft lip.[8,11,28] Transmission is autosomal recessive. Manifestations of the dysplasia vary, and four types of short rib–polydactyly syndrome have been identified. Each has a fatal prognosis.

Asphyxiating Thoracic Dysplasia

This is a rare, autosomal recessive disease also known as Jeune syndrome. Major findings on ultrasound examination are shortening of the extremities, funnel-shaped chest with short, horizontal ribs, and renal dysplasia.[9,19] Occasionally, polydactyly occurs. Severity of the disease varies. Most affected infants die within the first year of life from respiratory failure and infections; a few survive through early adulthood.

Ellis-van Creveld Syndrome

This is a rare chondroectodermal dysplasia and its features vary widely. There is an autosomal recessive mode of inheritance. Most often, only the femurs are shortened with normal appearing humeri. An atrial septal defect occurs in over 50% of the affected fetuses. Postaxial polydactyly (an extra digit on the medial side) may also be seen, especially if the extra digit contains a bony structure. The affected fetus may have a partial or pseudo-cleft lip. Approximately half of those affected can survive into adulthood.[24] Differential diagnosis includes thanatophoric dwarfism and Jeune's syndrome.

Osteogenesis Imperfecta

This dysplasia is an inherited connective tissue disorder characterized sonographically by varying degrees of hypomineralization of the entire skeleton. Bones are fragile and are easily fractured, leading to deformity. Sillence and coworkers classified osteogenesis imperfecta (OI) into four groups.[32]

Type I occurs most frequently and is autosomal dominant. Sonographic diagnosis in utero is difficult because mineralization is grossly normal and fractures usually occur after birth.

Type II, the most severe form, has an autosomal recessive transmission pattern. Its major sonographic landmarks include long bones and ribs that are shortened, bowed, or fractured, and decreased acoustic shadowing behind hypomineralized long bones.[1,5,27] The outline of the skull may be irregular and intracranial structures may be unusually well visualized owing to a thin cranium (see Figs. 18-8 and 18-10). The decrease in mineralization allows the skull to be easily deformed when compressed by the transducer. Early prenatal diagnosis can be obtained by chorionic villus sampling. Amniocentesis may be considered in the second and third trimester to evaluate the amniotic pyrophosphate level; a high value may indicate OI.[34] Most fetuses are stillborn or die early in the neonatal period of cardiorespiratory complications and infections. Differential diagnosis includes achondrogenesis and congenital hypophosphatasia.

Type III may be either autosomal recessive or autosomal dominant. Long bone fractures may be present at birth or may not appear until the child begins to walk. Although the child may survive into adulthood, the long bones and spine become progressively deformed.

Type IV is an autosomal dominant condition. It is the mildest form of the disease and unlikely to be diagnosed by ultrasound examination. A normal life span is possible; however, the person is likely to be short of stature.

Camptomelic Dysplasia

The term *camptomelic,* coined from the Greek word for "bent limb," describes the characteristic findings of bowed long bones. The tibia and fibula are most severely affected. However, some fetuses affected with camptomelic dysplasia do not exhibit bowed limbs sonographically. Associated abnormalities include shortened and poorly ossified long bones, and a narrow, barrel-shaped thoracic cage.[6,8,10] Occasional findings include hydrocephalus, macrocephalus, cleft palate, and polyhydramnios. This is a rare form of short-limbed dwarfism. Many cases are sporadic; however, autosomal recessive transmission is suggested. Most affected children die in early infancy from respiratory failure. Camptomelic dysplasia can mimic nonlethal forms of OI.[31]

Congenital Hypophosphatasia

Hypophosphatasia is an autosomal recessive metabolic disorder. The principal sonographic finding is severe hypomineralization of the entire skeleton. The calvarium is especially difficult to demonstrate and is easily compressed by its environment. Ribs are short and have a beaded appearance. Limbs are bowed, fractured, and shortened. Polyhydramnios may be present.[8,21,38] There is a wide variation in the severity of this syndrome. Those who are severely affected die early in infancy from respiratory failure. Differential diagnoses include OI Type II and achondrogenesis.

LIMB ABNORMALITIES

Individual limb abnormalities are often features of more complex genetic disorders, or result from other causes, including maternal teratogen exposure and amniotic band syndrome. Limb abnormalities are not life threatening in themselves. The prognosis for the fetus depends on whether other disorders are involved.

The Fetal Hand

Sonographic demonstration of some fetal hand malformations may allow a specific prenatal diagnosis to be made. Overlapping fingers have been associated with trisomy 18, and the three-pronged (trident) appearance of the second, third, and fourth digits is a characteristic finding in heterozygous achondroplasia. Club hand may be seen with conditions such as radial aplasia and prolonged oligohydramnios. Optimal evaluation of the fetal hand occurs at 20 weeks. Assessing its posture and the number and appearance of the digits should be attempted in pregnancies at risk for genetic disorders, skeletal dysplasias, and limb reduction defects.[30]

Polydactyly

Polydactyly is the presence of extra fingers or toes, either on the medial aspect (postaxial) or lateral aspect (preaxial). It is a frequent finding in several genetic syndromes such as trisomies 13, 18, and 21, short rib–polydactyly syndrome, and asphyxiating thoracic dystrophy. The extra digit may usually be visualized sonographically at about 18 weeks' GA if it contains a bony structure.

Limb Reduction Abnormality

Limb reduction is the congenital absence of one or more limbs or segments of limbs. The following terms are often used:

Aplasia: absence of a bone
Hypoplasia: incomplete development of a bone
Amelia: absence of one or more limbs
Hemimelia: absence of one or more extremities below elbow or knee
Acheiria: absence of one or more hands
Apodia: absence of one or more feet
Adactyly: absence of one or more digits from hands or feet
Phocomelia: absence of proximal portion of extremity with hand or foot attached to trunk

Approximately 25 syndromes are characterized by aplasia or hypoplasia of the radius. Some, such as trisomies 13, 18, and 22, have genetic origins (Fig. 18-14). Other causes include maternal expo-

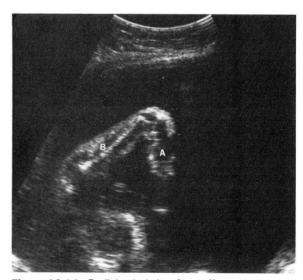

Figure 18-14. Radial aplasia in a fetus affected by trisomy 18. The hand (A) is seen attached to the humerus (B).

sure to illicit drugs or medications. Some appear spontaneously. To determine whether the radius is hypoplastic, the sonographer should note whether the distal end of the radius lines up with the distal end of the ulna, or whether it is shorter than the ulna (see Fig. 18-5). Aplasia would show no radius present. Care should be taken to note a single ulna as separate and different from the humerus, which may be followed to its articulation at the shoulder. Also, the hand on the affected limb is radially deviated (club hand; Fig. 18-15).

Holt-Oram Syndrome

This is an autosomal dominant disorder in which there is an absence of the thumbs. Care should be taken not to confuse a triphalangeal thumb, which contains three phalanges instead of the normal two, with the second digit of the hand. Holt-Oram syndrome is associated with congenital heart disease and phocomelia.

Thrombocytopenia–Absent Radius (TAR) Syndrome

This is an autosomal recessive blood disorder associated with decreased platelets and absence of the radius, usually bilateral. The sonographic feature in this syndrome that differentiates it from other absent radius syndromes is the presence of five fully formed digits. In other syndromes, the thumb may not be formed. Unilateral or bilateral absence of the ulna and humerus may occur. Occasional findings

include heart defects or renal anomalies. Infant mortality is approximately 40%, owing to hemorrhage early in infancy.

VACTERL Association

The VACTERL association is the finding in some patients of associated *v*ertebral anomalies, *a*nal atresia, *c*ardiac anomalies, *t*racheo*e*sophageal fistula, *re*nal anomalies, and *l*imb dysplasia. At least three features have to be found before this association may be considered in an abnormal neonate. A single umbilical artery has been reported in these patients, but it is most often an incidental finding associated with congenital or other abnormalities.

Club Foot

Club foot is characterized by medial deviation and inversion of the sole of the foot. Although club foot is seen in genetic syndromes such as trisomy 18, the fetus may have simply inherited a genetic predisposition to laxity of joint ligaments. Club feet are also associated with spina bifida and nongenetic conditions such as caudal regression syndrome, lead poisoning, oligohydramnios, and positional constraint. On ultrasound, the club foot is imaged on the same frontal plane as the lower leg and is almost at a right angle with the ankle (Fig. 18-16*B*). A normal foot is seen in transverse section and perpendicular to the lower leg (see Fig. 18-16*A*).

Amniotic Band Syndrome (ABS)

The exact explanation for the formation of amniotic bands is unknown. It is thought that the fibrous bands probably form after rupture of the amnion in early pregnancy. Some authors have reported a few cases of fetal anomalies suggestive of amniotic band syndrome after invasive procedures such as chorionic villus sampling and amniocentesis.[3,17] Bands imaged on ultrasound appear as linear densities attached from one uterine wall to another or from the uterine wall to a fetal part (Fig. 18-17). These strands may entangle and amputate fetal limbs and digits. Those that attach themselves or cross and compress an area of the fetus can cause mutilating craniofacial, limb, and visceral deformities.[22,25,26] Some amniotic bands detected by ultrasound have been reported to disappear as the pregnancy continued, leaving little or no evidence of their formation at delivery.[29]

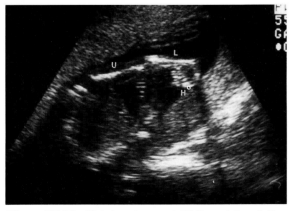

Figure 18-15. Club hand seen at 19.5 weeks' gestation. U = humerus (upper portion of limb); L = radius (lower portion of limb). (Courtesy of Catherine Carr-Hoefer, RDMS, Good Samaritan Hospital, Corvallis, OR.)

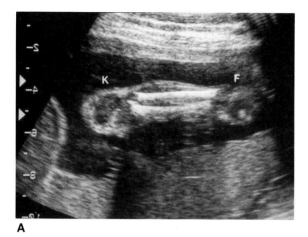

A

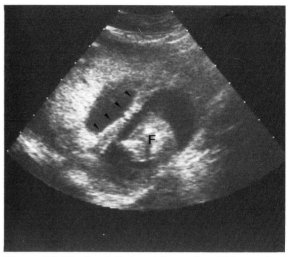

Figure 18-17. Amniotic band (*arrowheads*) is attached from uterine wall to uterine wall. Fetal parts (F) are seen on one side of the band.

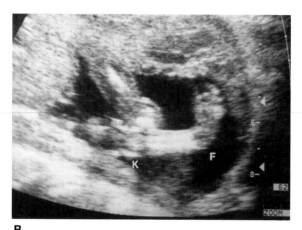

B

Figure 18-16. (*A*) Normal lower leg with the foot (F) seen in transverse section and perpendicular to the lower leg and knee (K). (*B*) Medial deviation of a club foot (F). The lower leg and knee (K) are seen on the same plane.

Sirenomelia Sequence

Sirenomelia is an embryonic defect that results in the fusion of the lower extremities (Fig. 18-18). It is associated with monozygotic twinning and pregnancies that are complicated by poorly controlled diabetes. Other anomalies include absence of the urinary bladder, genital defects, renal agenesis, and oligohydramnios.

MATERNAL CONDITIONS AND ASSOCIATED LIMB ABNORMALITIES

Obtaining a detailed and accurate medical and social history from the mother is very important. Maternal disease processes, medications, substance abuse, and exposure to radiation or industrial chemicals affect the environment of the developing fetus and may result in skeletal growth abnormalities.

Limb measurements below the 10th percentile may represent severe intrauterine growth retardation, fetal alcohol syndrome, or illicit drug abuse. However, if both the mother and father are short

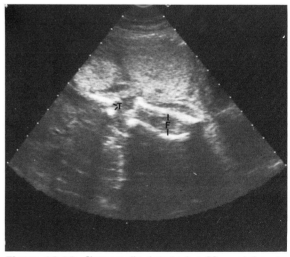

Figure 18-18. Sirenomelia detected at 23 weeks' gestation in the fetus of a diabetic mother. The proximity of the two femurs (F) and the proximal ends of both tibias (T) indicate fusion of the lower extremities.

in stature, the fetus may simply be a normal, genetically petite baby. Environmental compression due to oligohydramnios or uterine tumors can deform limbs. Toxic agents have also resulted in skeletal deformities. As a historical note, pregnant women in Europe used thalidomide in the 1960s as a remedy for nausea. Many of these pregnancies resulted in fetuses affected with phocomelia. The Food and Drug Administration never approved its sale for pregnant women in the United States.

The sonographer can detect sonographic signs of skeletal dysplasias on routine, complete examinations and look for associated anomalies. When evidence of dysplasias is found, it is often recommended that the patient be referred to a tertiary sonographic laboratory for confirmation of the diagnosis.

REFERENCES

1. Bader B, Warner RW. Osteogenesis imperfecta type II: A review for sonographers. J Diagn Med Sonogr. 1987; 3:275–280.
2. Benacerraf B, Osathanondh R, Bieber FR. Achondrogenesis type I: Ultrasound diagnosis in utero. J Clin Ultrasound. 1984; 12:357.
3. Boyd PA, Keeling JW, Selinger M, et al. Limb reduction and chorion villus sampling. Prenat Diagn. 1990; 10:437–441.
4. Brandon PS, Rouse GA, DeLange M. Sonography of thanatophoric dwarfism: A review. J Diagn Med Sonogr. 1990; 1:24–28.
5. Bulas DI, Stern HJ, Rosenbaum KN, et al. Variable prenatal appearance of osteogenesis imperfecta. J Ultrasound Med. 1994; 13:419–427.
6. Carlan SJ, Parsons MT, Flasher J. Camptomelic skeletal dysplasia with a narrow thorax. J Diagn Med Sonogr. 1990; 1:40–42.
7. Chitkara U, Rosenberg J, Chervenak FA, et al. Prenatal sonographic assessment of the fetal thorax: Normal values. Am J Obstet Gynecol. 1987; 156:1069–1074.
8. Donnenfeld AE, Mennuti MT. Second-trimester diagnosis of fetal skeletal dysplasias. Obstet Gynecol Surv. 1987; 42:199–217.
9. Elejalde BR, deElejalde MM, Pansch D. Prenatal diagnosis of Jeune syndrome. Am J Med Genet. 1985; 21:433.
10. Fryns JP, van den Berghe K, van Assche A, et al. Prenatal diagnosis of camptomelic dwarfism. Clin Genet. 1981; 19:199.
11. Gembruch U, Hansmann M, Fodisch HJ. Early pre-

12. Goldstein RB, Filly RA, Simpson G. Pitfalls in femur length measurements. J Ultrasound Med. 1987; 6:203–207.
13. Griffis WS. Thanatophoric dysplasia: A case study. J Diagn Med Sonogr. 1994; 10:24–27.
14. Guzman ER, Day-Salvatore D, Westover T, et al. Prenatal ultrasonographic demonstration of the trident hand in heterozygous achondroplasia. J Ultrasound Med. 1994; 13:63–66.
15. Hadlock FP, Harrist RB, Deter RL, et al. Ultrasonically measured fetal femur length as a predictor of menstrual age. Am J Roentgenol. 1982; 138:875–878.
16. Jeanty P, Rodesch F, Delbeke D, et al. Estimation of gestational age from measurements of fetal long bones. J Ultrasound Med. 1984; 3:75–79.
17. Kohn G. The amniotic band syndrome: A possible complication of amniocentesis. Prenat Diagn. 1987; 7:303–305.
18. Kurtz AB, Filly RA, Wapner RJ, et al. In utero analysis of heterozygous achondroplasia: Variable time of onset as detected by femur length measurements. J Ultrasound Med. 1986; 5:137–140.
19. Lipson M, Waskey J, Rice J, et al. Prenatal diagnosis of asphyxiating thoracic dysplasia. Am J Med Genet. 1984; 18:273.
20. Loong EPL. The importance of early prenatal diagnosis of thanatophoric dysplasia with respect to obstetric management. Eur J Obstet Gynecol Reprod Biol. 1987; 25:145–152.
21. McGuire J, Manning F, Lang I, et al. Antenatal diagnosis of skeletal dysplasia using ultrasound. Birth Defects. 1987; 23:367–384.
22. Mahony BS, Filly RA, Callen PW, et al. The amniotic band syndrome: Antenatal sonographic diagnosis and potential pitfalls. Am J Obstet Gynecol. 1985; 152:63–68.
23. Mahony BS, Filly RA, Copperberg PL. Antenatal sonographic diagnosis of achondrogenesis. J Ultrasound Med. 1984; 3:333.
24. Mahoney MJ, Hobbins JC. Prenatal diagnosis of chondroectodermal dysplasia (Ellis-van Creveld syndrome) with fetoscopy and ultrasound. N Engl J Med. 1977; 297:258.
25. Malinger G, Rosen N, Achiron R, et al. Short communications: Pierre Robin sequence associated with amniotic band syndrome. Ultrasonographic diagnosis and pathogenesis. Prenat Diagn. 1987; 7:455–459.
26. McFerrin-Richardson S, Gill K, Arcement L. Amniotic band syndrome. J Diagn Med Sonogr. 1994; 10:137–143.
27. Metz E, Goldhofer W. Sonographic diagnosis of le-

thal osteogenesis imperfecta in the second trimester: Case report and review. J Clin Ultrasound. 1986; 14:380–383.

28. Naumoff P, Young LW, Mazler J, et al. Short rib–polydactyly syndrome type III. Radiology. 1977; 122:443–447.

29. Papp Z, Toth Z, Csecsei K, et al. Are there "innocent" amniotic bands? [Letter] Am J Med Genet. 1986; 24:207–209.

30. Reiss RE, Foy PM, Mendiratta V, et al. Ease and accuracy of evaluation of fetal hands during obstetrical ultrasonography: A prospective study. J Ultrasound Med. 1995; 14:813–820.

31. Sanders RC, Greyson-Fleg RT, Hogge WA, et al. Osteogenesis imperfecta and camptomelic dysplasia: Difficulties in prenatal diagnosis. J Ultrasound Med. 1994; 13:691–700.

32. Sillence DO, Rimoin DL, Danks DM. Clinical variability in osteogenesis imperfecta: Variable expressivity or genetic heterogenity. Birth Defects. 1979; 15:113–129.

33. Smith DW. Recognizable Patterns of Human Malformation. 3rd ed. Philadelphia: WB Saunders; 1982:242.

34. Solomons CC, Gottesfeld K. Prenatal biochemistry of osteogenesis imperfecta. Birth Defects. 1979; 15:69.

35. Stamm ER, Pretorius DH, Rumack CM, et al. Kleeblattschadel anomaly: In utero sonographic appearance. J Ultrasound Med. 1987; 6:319–324.

36. Thompson BH, Parmley TH. Obstetric features of thanatophoric dwarfism. Am J Obstet Gynecol. 1971; 109:396.

37. Weiner CP, Williamson RA, Bonsib SM. Sonographic diagnosis of cloverleaf skull and thanatophoric dysplasia in the second trimester. J Clin Ultrasound. 1986; 14:463–465.

38. Wladimiroff JW, Niermeijer MF, van der Harten JJ, et al. Early prenatal diagnosis of congenital hypophosphatasia: Case report. Prenat Diagn. 1985; 5:47.

19

Assessment of Fetal Age and Size: Techniques and Criteria

TERRY J. DuBOSE

A large portion of any obstetrical sonographic examination involves measuring various parameters of the pregnancy. These measurements have two objectives: to determine the size and development of the fetus and to estimate the fetal age. Both objectives are interrelated; fetal size can be an indicator of the dates of the pregnancy, assuming the fetus is growing normally.

The earliest work in fetal sonographic biometry was reported by Dr. Ian Donald, of Glasgow, Scotland. In the late 1950s and early 1960s, Dr. Donald used a borrowed A-mode scanner to measure gestational sacs and the biparietal diameters (BPDs) of fetal heads.[55,57] From this modest beginning it is now possible to find published reports of the sonographic measurement of virtually every major fetal organ, from calvarial volume to the foot length.[17]

This chapter on sonographic fetal biometry describes the commonly used and most accurate fetal parameters. The physical principles and instrumentation that influence the measurement of these dimensions are also explained and advice is offered on how to obtain the most accurate measurements.

The estimated date of confinement (EDC) is the term generally used to indicate the expected birth date. This date is often called the gestational age, although it is actually counted from the last menstrual period (LMP) and not from the date of conception. The dates of the pregnancy are important for planning the mode and date of delivery, determining dates of possible termination, gauging fetal growth, and suggesting whether or not the pregnancy is progressing normally. Fetal size is an important indicator of fetal health. In general, reasonably large babies are considered healthier than relatively smaller babies of the same gestational age. Fetal measurements also provide information about the normalcy of fetal proportions.

Fetal size and dates of the pregnancy are estimated from sonographic measurements. The parameters discussed were selected because they are relatively accurate and easy to obtain. Several measurements are presented because no one magic parameter is consistently accurate in all fetuses. Using more than one or two fetal parameters also improves the accuracy in assessing dates and fetal size.[17,42,52,64,93] Nomograms for estimating fetal size and age by multiple parameters are given on pages 356 to 360 (Tables 19-1 and 19-2).

General Scanning Methodology and Use of Fetal Age Charts

All normal fetuses originate from a single fertilized egg and grow to a birth size that varies from infant to infant. The most accurate measurements of fetal age are those made early in the pregnancy, before individual growth patterns have had much effect on

359

◢◢◢ TABLE 19-1. FIRST-TRIMESTER AGE TABLE

Age (days)		Age (weeks)		hCG Mean (mIU/ml)	CRL (mm)	EHR (B/M)	FHR (B/M)	Chorionic Cavity	
LMP	C age	LMP	C age					(3D mean) GSD (mm)	(2D mean) GSD (mm)
26	12	3.7	1.7	100					
29	15	4.1	2.1	233					4
32	18	4.6	2.6	533		84			9
33	19	4.6	2.6	2,796		89			10
35	21	5.0	3.0	4,151	1	94		10	12
38	24	5.4	3.4	4,794	2	105		13	15
41	27	5.9	3.9	6,429	3	115		16	17
42	28	6.0	4.0	7,510	5	121		18	19
44	30	6.3	4.3	10,117	6	126		19	20
47	33	6.7	4.7	13,397	8	136		22	24
50	36	7.1	5.1	21,526	10	147		25	27
53	39	7.6	5.6	39,164	14	157		28	31
55	41	7.9	5.9	56,211	15	163		30	33
56	42	8.0	6.0	75,000	16	168		31	34
59	45	8.4	6.4		22	178		34	39
62	48	8.9	6.9		26	189		37	44
65	51	9.3	7.3		28		180	40	48
68	54	9.7	7.7		29		173	43	54
71	57	10.1	8.1		32		168	46	57
74	60	10.6	8.6		37		167	49	62
77	63	11.0	9.0		45		166	52	68
80	66	11.4	9.4		46		164	55	74
83	69	11.9	9.9		52		162	58	79
86	72	12.3	10.3		57		160	60	82
89	75	12.7	10.7		63		158		88
92	78	13.1	11.1		68		155		89

This table can be used to compare various embryo/fetal parameters to age by days and weeks. C Age, conceptual age = LMP −14 days. The 3D mean GSDs are the average of three perpendicular diameters of the chorionic sac and the 2D mean GSDs are the average of the two greatest diameters from a single image. The hCG (Second International Standard) column is a composite of five published tables.[31,80,81,83,97] CRL, crown−rump length; EHR, embryonic heart rate; FHR, fetal heart rate; GSD, gestational sac diameter.

From DuBose TJ: Fetal Sonography. Philadelphia, WB Saunders, 1996; p 113.

the fetus. Such individuation takes place later in gestation.

Earlier measurements tend to produce the most accurate dates of the pregnancy.[30] Transvaginal or endovaginal transducers produce detailed images of the early embryo allowing what proponents have called "sonoembryology"[102] and "sonomicroscopy."[39] These detailed images have modified some attitudes in relation to imaging and dating in early pregnancy.[87]

Normal human fetuses tend to be uniform in morphology.[41,90,95] Although there may be some differences in various normal growth parameters due to altitude, genetics, maternal smoking, and other influences, such differences are small in most cases. This is especially true of the average fetus early in gestation. Variations in any single parame-

ter's prediction of age will usually be less than ±10% of the age at any given time in pregnancy (±2 weeks at mid-pregnancy and ±4 weeks at term). This means that virtually any published chart derived with valid scientific methodology can be used to estimate fetal age. It is important that the user know how the measurements were generated to compose a given chart. If, for example, the chart was created using BPD measurements that were taken from the outer edge to the inner edge of the skull, it will produce valid age estimates only if the BPD for the fetus being examined is measured in the same manner. In other words, if the sonographer does not know how the author of a particular chart took the measurements and did the calculations to produce that chart, then use of that chart may lead to error.

Some experts recommend measuring a parameter several times and averaging for the measurement of record,[6] and others believe that one single "correct" measurement is sufficient.[58] The former of these methods is preferred. Multiple measurements (three, four, or more) are made of any given parameter and are observed for a "cluster" with a range of <2 or 3 mm. Any measurements that fall outside the cluster are discarded and the remaining measurements are averaged for the measurement of record.

There are generally two ways of listing fetal age in charts. One is to list the estimated age in weeks and days; the other is to use weeks and tenths of weeks. Either method is valid. In this chapter the latter method is used because it is easier to compute average ages and to determine the number of weeks for serial studies using weeks and tenths. Also, using weeks and days implies an accuracy that sonography does not possess. Few sonographic parameters have an accuracy better than ±1 week. Fetal age is usually computed in "menstrual weeks" because of the historical precedent of using the date of the LMP for calculating the dates of the pregnancy. Normally conception takes place about 2 weeks after the LMP. Birth normally occurs 40 weeks from the LMP (a 38-week gestation ± 2 to 3 weeks). In this chapter embryonic and fetal ages are given as the number of weeks since the LMP, unless otherwise stated (i.e., *28 weeks LMP* means the pregnancy has completed the 28th but not the 29th week after the LMP). The term *last normal menstrual period* (LNMP) is used only for the first day of the last period as reported by the woman.

Accuracy of Sonographic Measurements

Image resolution determines the biometric accuracy of any sonogram. Two factors govern the resolution of a sonographic beam.[63,78,104] Axial resolution is one aspect of image resolution and the beam width or lateral resolution is the other (Fig. 19-1). Axial resolution involves measurements along the axis or path of the beam. Lateral resolution governs any dimension measured transversely, or across the path of the beam. The focal range of a sonographic transducer is the depth at which the sound beam width (lateral resolution) is narrowest or best focused.

Axial resolution is related directly to the frequency of the sound and the pulse length and re-

production rate of those pulses producing the sonographic beam. Short and frequent pulses yield the greatest axial resolution. An ultrasound system cannot distinguish the echoes from two structures separated by less than the length of a single pulse. This explains why transducers that produce higher frequency sound usually produce shorter pulses, and therefore have better axial resolution.[108] Accordingly, a sonographer should use the highest-frequency transducer that produces adequate penetration and diagnostic-quality images.

Lateral resolution is related to beam width. In general, the wider the beam of sound, the wider a single echo in the image will appear. An ultrasound system cannot separate echoes that are closer together than the width of the beam. A beam width artifact tends to make measurement points a bit fuzzy.[98,109] Cursors should be placed at the edge of the most definite echo observed but should not include the beam width artifact (see Fig. 19-1).

It is important for the sonographer to understand how the orientation of a measured fetal structure affects fetal measurement accuracy with regard to axial and lateral resolution. In general, images obtained along the beam axis using the axial resolution have the least measurement error, whereas measurements taken transversely to the beam using lateral resolution have the greatest errors. Usually only the BPD and the diameters of the gestational sac and abdomen that are parallel to the beam can take advantage of the lesser measurement errors obtained using axial resolution. Almost all other parameters are measured using lateral resolution and exhibit some indistinctness at the edges owing to beam width artifact. To obtain measurements of the greatest accuracy the sonographer must exercise judgment and skill to select the appropriate transducer, obtain images, and place cursors for measurements.

Although any modern real-time transducer can be used effectively for fetal measurements, curvilinear and linear-array transducers, with their larger near field of view, make measurements easier to obtain in advanced pregnancy.[3,43] In early pregnancy (before 8 to 9 weeks LMP) transvaginal transducers provide much clearer images, especially in cases of ectopic pregnancy.

All transducers used to obtain measurements should be tested for accuracy. Sonographers can test for proper equipment function using an AIUM Standard Test Object or other acceptable phantoms. If measurements on the test object appear

TABLE 19-2. FETAL AGE AND AGE RANGE ANALYSIS—BASIC BABY II

Age (weeks)	E/FHR	GSD	CRL	3-D BPD	BPD	FOD	VCD	CV	THC	CHC	CERB	BiOD	FSL	FemL	HumL	ADA	AC	LNMP	MFP AA	Age AA	Range
41				96	100	123	66	482	349	260			74	79	70	120	376	39.7	40.75	41	
40				96	97	119	70	451	339	264			73	77	67	118	371	38.0	39.84	40	
39				93	95	116	66	421	330	252	43	60	71	76	67	116	365	38.5	38.78	39	
38				91	93	116	65	397	328	249	44	58	69	73	65	114	359	36.1	37.94	38	
37				90	91	113	65	376	320	244	47	60	67	73	63	110	342	38.0	36.99	47	
36				88	89	111	64	351	314	240	51	59	65	71	62	103	325	35.4	36.00	36	
35				86	87	109	63	329	307	234	46	59	63	68	60	99	310	35.2	34.96	35	
34				84	85	106	62	307	299	230	40	57	61	66	58	95	299	35.0	34.02	34	
33				82	83	104	60	289	294	224	38	55	59	64	56	92	289	33.2	33.04	33	
32				80	80	101	58	260	285	217	40	52	56	62	55	89	281	32.2	31.99	32	
31				78	78	98	57	243	277	212	38	51	54	59	53	85	268	30.2	31.02	31	
30				75	75	95	55	220	268	205	36	50	52	57	51	81	253	30.2	29.99	30	
29				73	73	93	55	204	260	200	35	48	49	55	50	77	243	30.1	29.00	29	
28				71	71	89	52	181	251	192	33	46	47	53	48	74	231	28.3	28.00	28	
27				68	68	86	51	166	242	187	32	46	45	50	46	71	221	26.4	27.04	27	
26				66	65	83	49	146	233	178	30	44	43	48	44	68	212	26.7	26.01	26	
25				63	62	79	47	127	221	171	28	43	41	46	43	65	205	26.3	25.01	25	
24				60	59	76	45	110	211	163	27	41	39	43	40	61	191	23.4	24.00	24	
23				56	56	71	42	93	199	154	25	40	37	40	38	58	181	23.8	23.00	23	
22				53	53	67	40	78	188	146	24	38	34	37	36	54	170	22.4	22.00	22	
21				50	49	62	38	65	175	137	22	36	32	35	34	51	160	21.1	21.02	21	
20				47	46	59	35	54	165	129	21	34	30	32	31	47	149	20.7	20.02	20	
19			130	44	44	55	33	44	155	121	19	32	28	29	29	44	138	19.5	19.05	19	
18			121	40	40	50	31	35	142	112	19	30	25	26	26	40	126	18.6	17.99	18	
17		115	113	37	37	46	29	28	131	104	18	28	22	23	23	36	113	16.7	17.03	17	
16		112	104	34	34	42	25	20	118	93	17	25	20	20	20	33	103	16.6	16.02	16	
15		104	92	30	30	37	23	14	105	83	15	23	17	16	16	29	91	15.4	15.01	15	
14	150	93	83	26	27	33	20	10	93	73	14	21	15	13	13	25	78	14.8	14.01	14	
13	152	80	71	23	23	28	17	6	81	63	12	17	13	10	10	21	68	15.0	13.01	13	
12	159	76	58	20	20	24	14	3.8	69	54	10	13	11	7	7	18	57	12.1	12.02	12	

																AA Weeks	LNMP Weeks
11	163	63	46	16	17	20	13	13	2.4	56	46	6	5	15	48	12.4	11.00	11
10	167	53	37	13	13	17	9	9	1.2	42	46	4	4	13	40	12.0	9.99	10
9	175	46	25	11	11	13	8		0.7	31	30			10	30	10.4	9.01	9
8	165	35	17	7	7	9	5		0.2	19	19			7	22	10.2	8.01	8
7	142	26	10	5	7	5										9.2	7.00	7
6	114	18	5		5											8.0	6.01	6
5	98	11	2													6.7	4.94	5
4		5														6.2	4.01	4

Age range analysis summary:
  Growth interval:
    Last exam #n
    − First exam
      Difference:

Instructions

To perform age range analysis (ARA) for each examination:
Take measurements and calculate values for each parameter using the formulas below. Circle the table values, determine each parameter age, and average all parameter ages; interpolate for more accuracy. Enter the examination average age in tenths of weeks under AA. Subtract the examination's smallest parameter age from the largest and enter the difference under RANGE.

ARA: The range of ages should not be more than 20% ($\pm 10\% = \pm 2$ SD) of the average age. Single parameters should not be more than $\pm 10\%$ from the average age. To determine the relative location of any parameter in the time-series distribution, use the following formula:

$$(\text{Parameter age} - AA)/(AA \times 0.05) = \text{location in standard deviation (SD)}$$

$$(\underline{\hspace{1cm}} - \underline{\hspace{1cm}})/(\underline{\hspace{1cm}} \times 0.05) = \underline{\hspace{1cm}} \text{ SD}$$

For growth intervals in serial studies:
Take measurements and calculate values for each parameter, and determine average age for each examination. Place the mother's reported LNMP in weeks and average age for each examination in the blanks at the bottom of the table. Subtract the LNMP and average ages of the first (dating) examination from the last (comparative) examination ($LNMP_n$ and AA_n).

Interpretation: If the $LNMP_n - LNMP_1$ and $AA_n - AA_1$ differences (time intervals) are approximately equal, then appropriate growth has occurred. In general, the difference between the LNMP and AA time intervals should not be greater than 10% of the fetal age. If the LNMP difference is greater than the AA difference, then less growth than expected has occurred (possible intrauterine growth restriction). If the LNMP difference is less than the AA difference, then accelerated growth has occurred.

▰▰ TABLE 19-2. (Continued)

Measurements & Calculations

Circumferences may be calculated from two diameters: circumference = $(d_1 + d_2) \times 1.57$
Cranial volume is calculated from three diameters: $CV = FOD \times BPD \times VCD \times 0.000555$

Acronym	Description	Measurement or Calculation	Unit
E/FHR	Heart rate	M-mode {age < 9.2 LMP weeks = ((EHR × .3) + 6)/7}	B/M
GSD	Gestational sac diameter	Largest diameter of chorionic cavity	mm
CRL	Crown-rump length	Top of head to rump: do not include legs	mm
BPD	Biparietal diameter	Leading edge to leading edge (outer to inner)	mm
3-D BPD	3-D BPD correction	Average (FOD + BPD + VCD)/3 = BPD	mm
FOD	Fronto-occipital diameter	Middle of frontal to middle of occipital bones	mm
VCD	Vertical cranial diameter	Middle of cranial vertex to middle of hippocampal base line	mm
CV	Cranial volume	Use CV calculation above, mm diameters for CV in milliliters	ml
THC	Transverse head circumference	THC = (FOD + BPD) × 1.57	mm
CHC	Coronal head circumference	CHC = (VCD + BPD) × 1.57	mm
CERB	Cerebellar transverse diameter	Transverse cerebellar diameter	mm
BiOD	Binocular diameter	Distance between outer edges of the ocular globes	mm
FSL	Fractional spine length	Seven complete thoracolumbar vertebral bodies and spaces	mm
FemL	Femur length	Length of femoral diaphysis	mm
HumL	Humerus length	Length of humeral diaphysis	mm
ADA	Abdominal diameter average	Average of transverse (TAD) and AP (AAD) abdominal diameters	mm
AC	Abdominal circumference	AC = (TAD + AAD) × 1.57	mm
LNMP	Last normal menstrual period	Mean of mothers' reported LNMPs for this population	week
Average	Average age	Mean of all exam AAs for each week (± 0.25 week)	week
Age	Age in weeks	Age on day 1 of week	week
AA	Average age in LMP weeks	Blank for average of parameter ages for current exam	week
Range	Range of ages	Subtract smallest parameter age from largest parameter age	week

Table 19-2 and its instructions and legend facilitates the manual calculation of the mutiple fetal parameter average age (MFP AA) and age range analysis (ARA). It was developed over a period of 10 years (1984–1994) and the population includes >10,000 sets of fetal measurements and observations. The use of these analyses will produce results similar to those produced by computer software shown in Figures 19-2 and 19-3.
(Reprinted with permission from DuBose, TJ: Fetal Sonography. Philadelphia: WB Saunders, 1996: pp 97–99.)

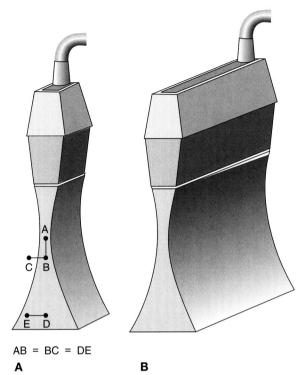

AB = BC = DE

A   **B**

Figure 19-1. *Axial and lateral resolution. A stylized drawing of the shape of a linear array transducer beam and the resulting field of view. The focal range is at the location where the beam is most narrow. In this image the distance between various points are equal, AB = CB = ED. Points C & B and E & D are imaged with lateral resolution; however, D & E will not appear as separate echoes on the monitor because there is less distance between them than the beam width at that distance. Points A & B will be resolved as two echoes with axial resolution. (From DuBose TJ: Fetal Sonography, Philadelphia, WB Saunders, 1996; p 73.)*

inaccurate, the machine should be recalibrated by an authorized service person. Generally, sonographic measurement errors in the range of 1% to 2% (1 or 2 mm/10 cm) may be expected.[75] These standard errors may be due to beam width, machine calibration, and cursor placement variation.[20,74,107]

Multiple Fetal Parameters Technique

Because all fetuses are proportioned differently, it must be recognized that any single fetal parameter, used alone, may not be as specific an indicator of fetal age as desired. This is especially true later in pregnancy. This can be an important consideration

with serial studies for fetal growth and development, because in subsequent examinations fetal position or other changing conditions may preclude exact replication of a set of fetal measurements used in earlier examinations. It has been found that in cases of premature rupture of the membranes, the external uterine pressure on the fetal skull can produce measurement errors in BPD as well as the transverse cephalic index in as many as 45% of the cases.[15,66,84]

Other problems may occur in progressive diseases such as hydrocephalus or maternal diabetes. Figure 19-2 shows examples of a computer analysis of fetal parameters, illustrating the advantage of using multiple fetal parameters. If only one or two measurement parameters are used, then in the event of progressive abnormalities or changing fetal or intrauterine conditions, one may have difficulty comparing biometric information on follow-up examinations. For this reason it is recommended that the following measurements be obtained routinely as a minimum: head measurements, abdominal circumference (AC), and the length of at least one extremity long bone, preferably the femur. As a rule, the more measurements that are taken and averaged, the more accurate the fetal age estimate will be.

In 1981, Bovicelli and coworkers suggested that using the combined crown-rump length (CRL) and BPD improved the estimation of fetal age in the first trimester.[8] In 1983, Hadlock and coworkers[46] found that throughout pregnancy an average gestational age determined from multiple fetal parameters [BPD, transverse head circumference (THC), AC, and the femoral diaphysis length (FemL)] yielded a more accurate estimation of fetal age throughout gestation than any single parameter used alone. They referred to this average age as the multiple fetal parameter (MFP) average age.[46,47] This research was replicated and confirmed in 1986 by Ott.[86] The average of MFPs is a more accurate indicator of fetal age for two reasons. Fetal parameters obtained early in gestation are so small that any error in measurement due to the limits of resolution in the sonographic instrument used or to operator error will be relatively larger. In addition, late in gestation there is more molding of the fetal skull leading at times to relative dolichocephaly and brachycephaly, and other individuation of fetal proportions (i.e., some fetuses are fatter, some thinner, some longer, and some shorter). Using multiple parameters tends to minimize these errors and average out normal individual variations.[21]

Inherent in the concept of estimating age

```
EXAM DATE:   1   6   86              EXAM# = 1  By: TD   BB#: 1115
PT:                                   AGE:      PT.#
DR.:                                  LMP = (M) = 7  4  85 = 26.6 Wks
════════════════════════════════════ BASIC BABY (c) ═══════════════════
Probable  Sex F  BPD/FOD =0.78         Fetal Heart = 171 B/M
      HistoG  Calc    Week +/- SD
BPD  =(B) = 67 mm.= 26.5   0.0         SUMMARY:  Ave.WKS Range  n  SD  Min  Max
THC  =(T) =239 mm.= 26.7   0.2         ALL AGE  (A) 26.5    1.3   8  0.5  25.7 27.0
CHC  =(C) =188 mm.= 27.0   0.4         BRAIN AGE(b) 26.7    0.5   5  0.2  26.5 27.0
CV   =(V) =168  cc.= 26.9   0.3        BODY AGE     26.0    1.0   3 -0.3  25.7 26.7
TriCD =(>) = 67 mm.= 26.6  0.1            (b)=EDC (MM DD)= 4 8 ( 40 LMP WKS.Term)
HumL =(H)= 44 mm.= 25.8  -0.5             SHEPARD.WT. (Ba) =   950 Gm.+- 190 Gm.
FemL =(F)= 47 mm.= 25.7  -0.6             HADLOCK.WT. (Fa) =   911 Gm.+- 182 Gm.
AC   =(a) =218 mm.= 26.7   0.1            HADLOCK.WT. (TFa) =  898 Gm.+- 135 Gm.

                                             B
                                             >
                                             TC
                                            FHaV
───────────────────────────────────────  ││ @  ││ ────────────────────────
M=A=b=(@) ──────────────────────────────
MENSTRUAL WKS>1   1   1   1   1   2   2   2   2      2   3   3   3   3   3   4   4
       2   4   6   8   0   2   4   6   8   0   2   4   6      8   0   2   4   6   8   0   2
                                       ↑   MFP  ↑
                                       ↑   AA   ↑
                              ─2SD────┘  ↑ └+2SD──────
```

A

```
EXAM DATE:  11   7   84              EXAM# = 1  By: TD   BB#: 207
PT:                                   AGE:      PT.#
DR.:                                  LMP = (M) = 5  3  84 = 26.9 Wks
════════════════════════════════════ BASIC BABY (c) ═══════════════════
Probable  Sex F  BPD/FOD =0.78         Fetal Heart = 152 B/M
      HistoG  Calc    Week +/- SD      SUMMARY:  Ave.WKS Range  n  SD  Min  Max
BPD  =(B) = 69 mm.= 27.2   0.1         ALL AGE  (A) 27.1    3.7   7  1.4  25.0 28.7
THC  =(T) =248 mm.= 27.7   0.4         BRAIN AGE(b) 28.0    1.5   4  0.7  27.2 28.7
CHC  =(C) =199 mm.= 28.7   1.2         BODY AGE     25.9    2.8   3 -0.9  25.0 27.8
CV   =(V) =195  cc.= 28.4   0.9           (b)=EDC (MM DD)= 1 30 ( 40 LMP WKS.Term)
HumL =(H)= 42 mm.= 25.0  -1.6             SHEPARD.WT. (Ba) =   909 Gm.+- 182 Gm.
FemL =(F)= 52 mm.= 27.8   0.5             HADLOCK.WT. (Fa) =   918 Gm.+- 184 Gm.
AC   =(a) =203 mm.= 25.0  -1.6            HADLOCK.WT. (TFa) =  923 Gm.+- 138 Gm.




                                           H      C
LMP=ALL AGE= (*)──────────────────────     a __BTFV_____
                                        │ │ * b   │
MENSTRUAL WKS>1   1   1   1   1   2   2   2   2 ↑ 2   3   3   3   3   3   4   4
       2   4   6   8   0   2   4   6   8   0   2   4   6 ↑ 8   0   2   4   6   8   0   2
                                       ↑   MFP  ↑
                                       ↑   AA   ↑
                              ─2SD────┘      └+2SD──────
```

B

Figure 19-2.

from an average of MFPs is the idea that no single parameter is a perfect indicator of fetal age.[22,92] This is because all people have slightly different proportions.

The sonographer measures and calculates the age suggested by each parameter (Tables 19-1 and 19-2).[25] Because all fetal parameters cannot be measured throughout pregnancy, the following chart (Table 19-3) can be used to determine which parameters are best used during progressive weeks of the pregnancy. Although it may be possible to obtain many of these measurements earlier or later than this Table 19-3 illustrates, the recommended times of parameter measurement are based on both the ease of obtaining the measurement and its relative accuracy. The use of transvaginal transducers may allow measurements 1 to 4 weeks earlier than the recommended weeks in this chart.

Fetal parameter ages can also be estimated using polynomial formulas.[17] Sonographic equipment often use these complex formulas as built-in software to estimate fetal ages and weights. The operator only needs to take the parameter measurement and the formula calculations are invisible to the sonographer. Figure 19-3 shows selected dating curves for various parameters from Table 19-2.

Measurement Techniques in the First Trimester

GESTATIONAL SAC DIAMETER (GSD)

The earliest measurement of the gestational sac diameter (GSD) for dating pregnancy was made by Ian Donald, using an average of three diameters.[55] The shape of the early gestational sac can vary greatly, depending on many factors such as presence of uterine fibroids, shape of the uterus (degree of retroflexion or anomalies), presence of pelvic pathology, and pressure from a full urinary bladder. Using transvaginal transducers avoids the latter problem but does not alleviate the effects of the others.

For these reasons the GSD measurements are of limited reliability and are seldom used after 6 or 7 LMP weeks when fetal structures can be imaged and measured.[67] If one can observe an intrauterine sac with a "double ring" sign (Fig. 19-4) and if the human chorionic gonadotropin (hCG) titer is appropriate (Table 19-1), an intrauterine gestation is presumed to exist.[11,73,107]

A single GSD measurement may be obtained by measuring the longest inside diameter. Two diameters may be measured using the average of the two greatest perpendicular diameters from the same image (Table 19-1), or a three-diameter average of three inside perpendicular diameters.

A general rule of thumb is that the GSD, in centimeters, plus 4 (some authors use 3)[73] nearly equals the age in menstrual weeks.

CROWN-RUMP LENGTH (CRL)

Once the embryo is clearly visible in the gestational sac, its CRL can be measured. The CRL has been called "the single most accurate method of assessing fetal age because of its minimal biologic variation in size in the first trimester and the rapid growth of this measurement at this stage of pregnancy."[36] Properly taken, this measurement usually is considered accurate to within 3 to 5 days.[51,76,89] One study has shown that the CRL age charts de-

(Text continues on page 375)

◄

Figure 19-2. Computer printout for Fetal Growth Analysis. Computer screens from two fetuses at approximately the same age (A = 26.6 weeks and B = 26.9 weeks). The heading of each screen has patient information (identification deleted). Below the headings on the left is a tabular form of fetal parameter measurements, estimated ages and ± SD in weeks, on the right is the summary of the fetal parameter ages and estimated weight by three methods. Across the bottom of each screen is the age range analysis symbolic histogram showing the relative location of each parameter in the distribution by its character (*symbol*). (**A**) A normal fetus at 26.6 LMP weeks with normally distributed (bell curve) parameters. This fetus delivered at 39.8 LMP weeks weighing 3255 g (7.16 lb), and 51 cm (20 in) long, a normal baby. (**B**) A fetus with intrauterine growth restriction (IUGR) at 26.9 LMP weeks. Note that the abdomen and humerus are well below the −1 SD for age in the distribution. This fetus delivered at 40 LMP weeks weighing 2586 g (5.7 lb) and was 45.7 cm (18 in) long, a small baby. (MFP AA, multiple fetal parameter average age; b, average cranial age; B, BPD; T, transverse head circumference; C, coronal head circumference; V, cranial volume; H, humeral length; F, femoral length; a, abdominal circumference.) (From DuBose TJ (ed): Fetal Sonography. Philadelphia, WB Saunders, 1996; p 146.)

▰▰▰ **TABLE 19-3. MEASUREMENTS TIMETABLE**

Parameter	Advantages	Disadvantages	When to Use	Accuracy ± 2 SD ± % AA
Gestational sac diameter (GSD)	Easiest measurement early in gestation	High variability of measurements, low accuracy	Before 8 weeks LMP	± 2 weeks ± 0.9 week ± 11.5% AA
Crown-rump length (CRL)	Highest accuracy early in gestation; easy to obtain	Not available after first trimester	5–15 weeks LMP	± 3–5 days ± 0.7 week ± 3.2% AA
Embryonic heart rate (EHR) before 9.2 LMP	High accuracy, easy; predictive of first trimester outcome	Not available after 9.2 weeks LMP; requires M-mode	5–9.2 weeks LMP	± 6 days ± 0.8 week ± 10.0% AA
3D BPD correction three cranial diameter average	High accuracy in late pregnancy; encourages close neurologic observation	Requires three cranial measurements	Use when head shape or molding affects cranial measurements	± 1 week ± 0.9 week ± 3.6% AA
Transverse head circumference (THC)	Requires only two measurements; accepted as standard	Does not reflect vertical cranial diameter molding	12 weeks LMP to term if cranial shape is normal	± 1 week ± 1.0 week ± 3.7% AA
Biparietal diameter (BPD)	Easy to obtain; low interoperator variability	Affected by cranial shape and molding	9–33 weeks LMP if cranial shape is normal	± 2 weeks ± 1.2 weeks ± 4.3% AA
Binocular distance (BiOD)	Occasionally easy when fetus faces up and BPD is difficult	Relatively low accuracy; fetal position can make measurements impossible	15–30 weeks LMP	± 3.3 weeks ± 1.7 weeks ± 6.6% AA
Cerebellum (CERB)	Encourages close neurologic observation	Relatively low accuracy; difficult to obtain early or late in gestation	18–35 weeks LMP	± 3 weeks ± 2.7 weeks ± 6.5% AA
Abdominal circumference (AC)	Important for fetal weight and health	Interoperator variability and fetal position may affect accuracy	12 weeks LMP to term	± 3.5 weeks ± 1.8 weeks ± 5.9% AA
Femoral length (FemL)	Relatively easy to obtain	Fetal motion may make measurements difficult	14 weeks LMP to term	± 3.4 weeks ± 1.7 weeks ± 6.2% AA
Humeral length (HumL)	Relatively easy to obtain	Fetal motion may make measurements difficult	14 weeks LMP to term	± 3.8 weeks ± 1.8 weeks ± 6.4% AA
Fractional spine length (FSL): seven thoracolumbar vertebral spaces and bodies	Easy when fetus in prone position	Relatively low accuracy; fetal position can make measurements impossible	15 weeks LMP to term	± 3.5 weeks ± 3.4 weeks ± 13.1% AA
Last normal menstrual period (LNMP) by menstrual history	Often the only independent date available for a pregnancy	Very low accuracy; often unknown or unreliable	When available, use only for comparative ages	± 4.0 weeks ± 4.9 weeks ± 33.7% AA

Accuracy, accuracy of fetal measurements as generally accepted; ± 2 SD, variation of ages in mean standard deviations. Deviations will be less earlier in gestation and greater later. Calculated from 1993 BBII data, n = 2728.[17] ± % AA, as a general rule of thumb, the normal fetal parameter ages exhibit more variation with increasing age. Here the residuals of parameter ages (PA) were calculated as a percentage of the average age (AA) of multiple fetal parameters ({PA − AA/ AA} × 100). Note that in general cranial parameters have less variation than those of the body, and all except for the LNMP, GSD, and FSL are < ±10% of the AA. The LNMP variation was large in this population (1993 data, n = 1685 with reported LNMP), probably because many referrals were for uncertain dates.

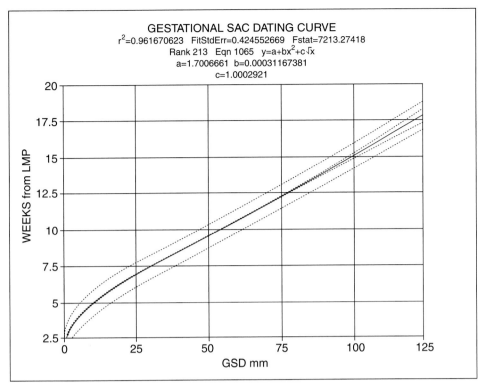

A

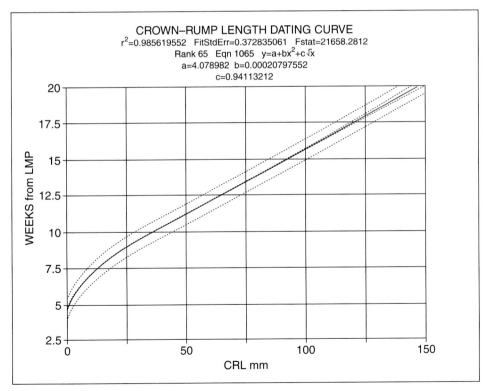

B

Figure 19-3. Fetal dating curves. Selected dating curves for fetal parameter ages shown in Table 19-2. Data are from 2728 consecutive referral cases in 1993. All measurements were taken, as appropriate to time in gestation, by more than 12 sonographers in four different laboratories in Austin, Texas. (**A**) Gestational sac diameters (GSD). Two greatest diameters averaged from a single image. The GSD is actually the chrionic sac. (**B**) Crown-rump length (CRL). CRL excluding extremities or yolk sac. (*continued*)

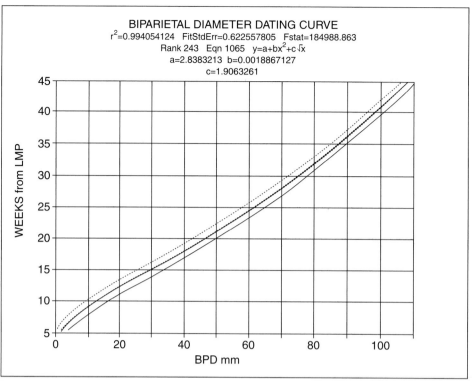

C

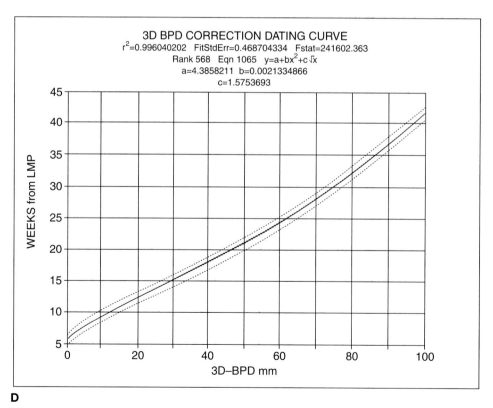

D

Figure 19-3. (CONTINUED) (**C**) Biparietal diameter (BPD). Standard BPD, transverse head circumference. (**D**) Three-dimensional (3D) BPD correction. 3D BPD is the average of three cranial diameters: (FOD + BPD + VCD)/3. The 3D BPD can be substituted for BPD in age or weight estimations in case of head molding or variation in shape. (*continued*)

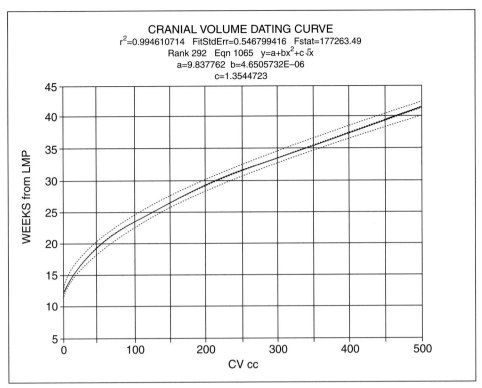

E

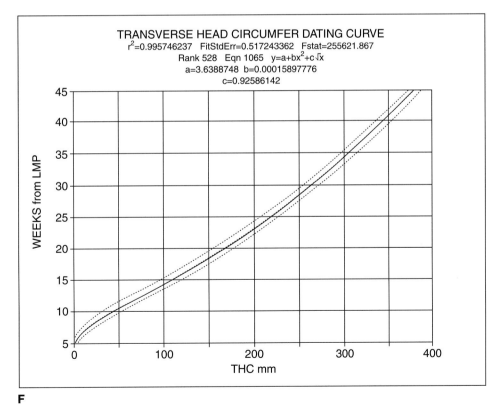

F

Figure 19-3. (Continued) (E) Cranial volume (CV). The CV is accurate in late pregnancy for estimating age. CV = FOD × BPD × VCD × 0.000555. Millimeter measurements will result in milliliter volume with this formula. **(F)** Transverse head circumference (THC): This is the standard head circumference in common usage. (*continued*)

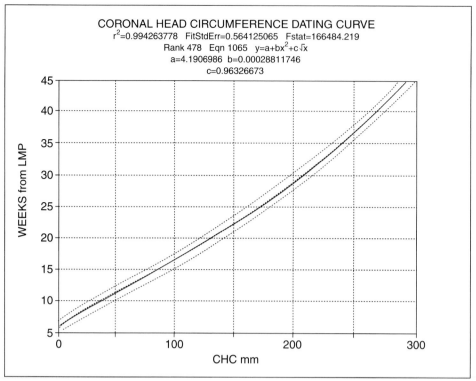

G

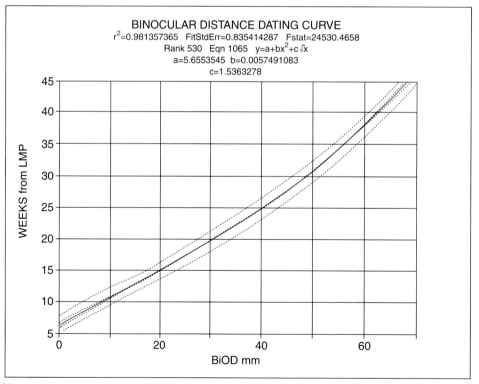

H

Figure 19-3. (CONTINUED) (**G**) Coronal head circumference (CHC): The CHC is a perfect circle in normally shaped heads. If the THC and CHC are normal in appearance, then a BPD alone will suffice for age and weight estimates. (**H**) Binocular distance (BiOD): The BiOD is the distance between the outer edges of the orbits of the eyes. Note the wide variation in comparison to cranial parameters. (*continued*)

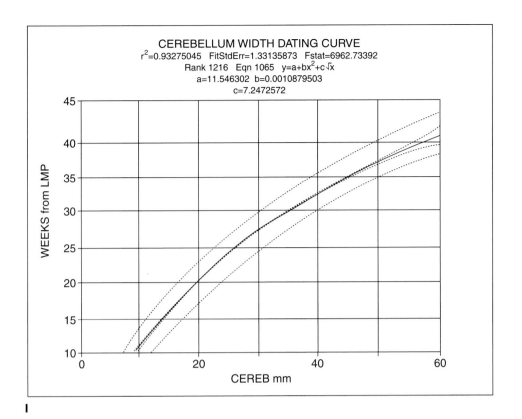

CEREBELLUM WIDTH DATING CURVE
r^2=0.93275045 FitStdErr=1.33135873 Fstat=6962.73392
Rank 1216 Eqn 1065 $y=a+bx^2+c\sqrt{x}$
a=11.546302 b=0.0010879503
c=7.2472572

I

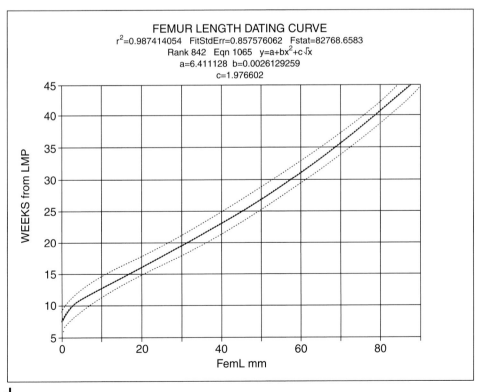

FEMUR LENGTH DATING CURVE
r^2=0.987414054 FitStdErr=0.857576062 Fstat=82768.6583
Rank 842 Eqn 1065 $y=a+bx^2+c\sqrt{x}$
a=6.411128 b=0.0026129259
c=1.976602

J

Figure 19-3. (CONTINUED) (**I**) Cerebellum width (Cerb): Widest measurement of the transverse cerebellum. Again, compare the variance with other cranial parameters. (**J**) Femur length (FemL): Femur length as commonly used. (*continued*)

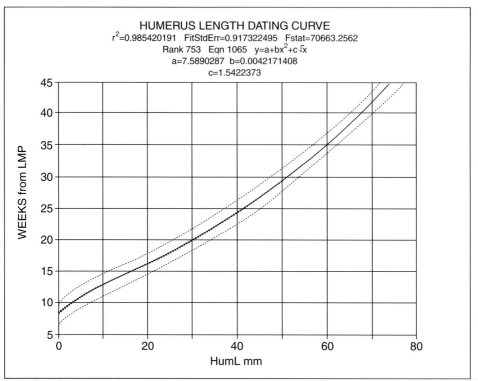

K

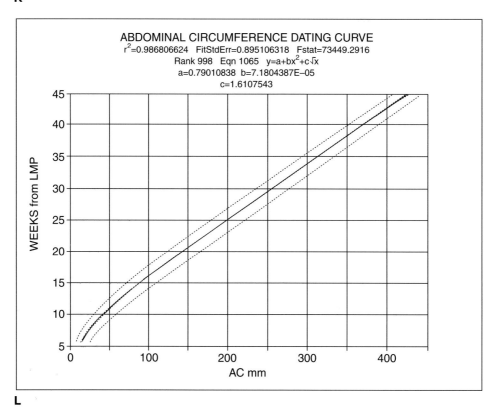

L

Figure 19-3. (Continued) (**K**) Humerus length (HumL): Humerus length, note similarity to the FemL. (**L**) Abdomen circumference (AC): The AC is important in weight estimates. Note increased variation in last trimester.

rived from transabdominal images are also valid for transvaginal measurements.[12,94]

Methods of Measuring Crown-Rump Length

The fetal CRL is measured from the top of the head to the bottom of the rump. It excludes the legs (Figs. 19-4, 19-5). When measuring early in the first trimester (6 to 8 weeks LMP) care should be taken to avoid including the yolk sac (which will usually be very close to the embryo) in the measurement. The embryonic period of development lasts until the eighth conceptual (10th menstrual) week. From that time until term the baby is a fetus, although the terms embryo and fetus are often used interchangeably.[79]

Identification of the body can easily be made if cardiac motion can be observed with real-time ultrasonography. The fetal pole should be visible when the gestational sac reaches

≥2.5 cm as measured with modern real-time equipment.[69,82,83]

More accurate measurements can be made if the image is enlarged as much as possible while keeping the entire CRL in view. This makes cursor placement easier and more uniform. The CRL is less accurate beyond the first trimester because of variations in fetal position and flexion.

Measurement Techniques in the Second and Third Trimester

FETAL HEAD MEASUREMENTS

Biparietal Diameter (BPD)

The fetal BPD has long been a primary sonographic measurement for determining fetal age. The BPD is usually easy to obtain, has a distinctive appearance, and provides a relatively accurate measurement.

The BPD measurement carries a small interob-

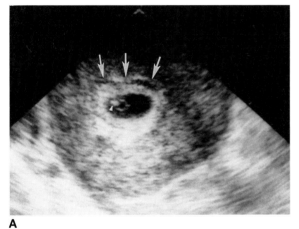
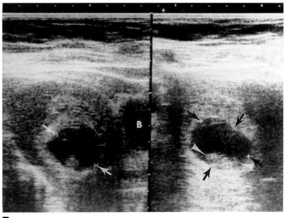

A   B

Figure 19-4. *Gestational sac diameter.* (**A**) *Transvaginal scan of a normal 5.1-week (LMP) gestational sac with a double-ring sign (arrows). The small, circular yolk sac can be seen adjacent to the embryonic pole (small arrowhead). The largest diameter of the sac is 15.7 mm; and the CRL of the embryonic pole is 4.0 mm, both of which are the equivalent of 5.1 weeks. The embryonic heart rate (FHR) was measured at 97 bpm by motion mode using the transvaginal transducer. The FHR correlates with 5.0 weeks LMP. (**B**) Linear array split image demonstrating the three-dimensional measurement of a gestational sac (GS). The left side image, a midsagittal plane view, shows the uterus, maternal urinary bladder (B), and one dimension of the GS (white arrows). The right side image is a transverse plane with cephalic angulation making it perpendicular to the measurement on the sagittal (left) image. Two dimensions of the GS are measured in the right image (black arrows); a valid CRL was also obtained from the right image (white arrowheads). The three GSD measurements resulted in a mean GSD of 30 mm, or 7.0 weeks LMP. The single largest GSD was 39 mm, or 7.8 weeks. The CRL was 18.0 mm, or 8.1 weeks; BPD was 7.3 mm, or 8.3 weeks; the CV was 0.2 ml, or 8.1 weeks; the FHR was 169 bpm, or 8.2 weeks; and the average age for five cranial and for all eight parameters was 8.2 weeks LMP, with a range of ages from 7.8 to 8.7 weeks.*

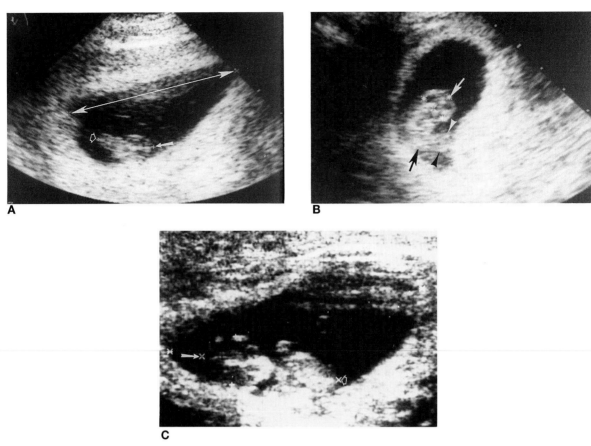

Figure 19-5. Crown-rump length. (**A**) Transabdominal, real-time, sector image of a gestational sac containing an 8.3-week embryo. The largest GSD (X's at each end of long, double arrow) and CRL were taken from this image (crown, *small white arrow;* rump, *open white arrow*). The coronal head and interhemispheric fissure are well demonstrated. The average age of seven parameters was 8.3 weeks LMP, with a range of 8.0 (CRL) to 8.7 (GSD); the FHR was 159 bpm, which correlated to 7.7 weeks LMP. The cranial volume (CV) was 0.2 ml, or 8.1 weeks LMP. (**B**) Transvaginal scan of an 8.2-week LMP embryo in a coronal view. The CRL (*arrows*) measured 18.7 mm, which indicates 8.2 weeks LMP. The electronic calipers are marking the coronal triangle and vertical cranial diameter (VCD). The umbilical cord (*arrowheads*), which is relatively large, might represent normal midgut herniation. Seven fetal parameters were evaluated for age during this examination as follows in weeks LMP: GSD, 8.1; CRL, 8.2; BPD, 8.6; THC, 8.4; CHC, 8.2; CV, 8.2; TriCD, 8.6; and FHR 177 bpm, 8.4 weeks. The average age of all seven parameters and the five head parameters were 8.3 and 8.4 weeks, respectively; age range was 0.4 weeks between the minimum and maximum parameter ages. The reported LMP was 8.4 weeks prior to the examination. (**C**) Transabdominal, linear-array image of the CRL (*arrows*) of a 9.7-week LMP embryo; the CRL was 32 mm or 9.9 weeks LMP. The white arrow points to the fetal head, in which the midline can be seen. The open arrow marks the rump. The crosshatches measure this BPD as 12.2 mm, or 9.6 weeks. The CRL was 32.0 mm, or 9.9 weeks. The average age using nine parameters was 9.7 weeks LMP, with an overall range from 9.1 weeks (THC) to 10.2 weeks (GSD). The CV was 1.1 m, or 10.0 weeks.

server variance or error (usually <2 mm), but molding and normal morphologic variations of the fetal head have a greater effect on the accuracy of BPD in assessing age. These effects and the lesser reliability of the BPD measurements tend to be greatest after the 33rd menstrual week when extrinsic pressure on the fetal skull is greatest. The resulting fetal skull molding makes the BPD a less accurate parameter for fetal age after that time. The BPD can also be affected by oligohydramnios, which can enhance molding of the skull.[66,84,96] If there is any molding of the head the three-dimensional BPD correction method below may be used to improve biometric accuracy.[15]

Two of the most notable BPD fetal age charts were published by Sabbagha and Hughey in 1978[91,95] and by Kurtz and associates in 1980.[68] Each group used meta-analysis.[88] Sabbagha's group developed a composite BPD–age chart from four previously published reports. Kurtz's group reviewed 25 BPD charts published worldwide. They found that 17 of these studies were devised by sound scientific methods and therefore used the data from these studies to produce a single chart, which they estimated was valid for ~90% of the world's population. Both of these BPD charts produce virtually identical results. These two charts are probably the most widely used in the world to estimate sonographic fetal age.

Most of the published BPD charts, including the ones discussed above, were created using leading edge measurements (outer skull table to inner skull table) obtained in a transverse view with a lateral approach (Figs. 19-6 to 19-9). The plane of this transverse view has been widely described. It produces accurate measurements because the leading edges of the parietal bones reflect very sharp, specular echoes enhanced by the axial resolution of the sound beam. The normally circular shape of the skull in the coronal plane makes the BPD easy to obtain and relatively accurate in normally shaped heads.[15]

MEASUREMENT METHODS. The BPD can be measured routinely from 12 weeks' gestation and occasionally earlier. The sonographer must first identify the fetal lie. Beginning transversely at the base of the fetal cranium the sonographer locates the base X formed by the sphenoid bones (bilateral anteriorly) and petrous bones (bilateral posteriorly) (see Fig. 19-8*A*). The proper plane for the BPD lies parallel to and above this base X.[2,9,33] From the base X scan the plane of view is moved higher in the

skull until the thalamus and cavum septi pellucidi are located.[2,9,21,33,66] For an optimal measurement, the entire calvarium should be seen as a complete oval. A transverse plane that includes the top of the cerebellum is too low in the posterior portion of the image (see Fig. 19-8*B,C*).[77]

The BPD is measured from the fetal parietal bones that form the lateral walls of the skull (see Figs. 19-6, 19-8). The BPD is measured at the widest transverse diameter of the skull, just above the ears. The view for the BPD measurement should be made perpendicular to the interhemispheric fissure (midline) in either the transverse or coronal plane and should include the thalamus (see Figs. 19-7 to 19-9).[2,9,21,32,33] When measuring from the leading edge of the parietal bone the soft tissue of the scalp should be excluded (see Figs. 19-8, 19-9). Lowering the system gain helps distinguish soft tissue from bone; the bone echoes persist at lower gain settings.

If the fetus' face is turned directly toward or away from the maternal spine or if the fetus' head is low in the pelvis, behind the maternal pubic bone, measurement of the BPD may be difficult. When the fetus' head is low in the pelvis a slight Trendelenburg position (maternal pelvis elevated, head lowered) sometimes helps to bring the head out of the mother's pelvis. The fetus may move to a more convenient position in response to the mother's changing position or if the sonographer proceeds with other parts of the examination and returns later to try the measurement again. As uncooperative as fetuses may be, an experienced sonographer should be able to obtain accurate BPD measurements at least 95% of the time. In the rare event of an extremely uncooperative fetus when no satisfactory BPD can be obtained other fetal parameters may serve as indicators of fetal age. If the fetal head is very low in the pelvis a transvaginal transducer may allow BPD measurements.[15,106]

The accuracy of the predictive value of the BPD has been reported by some authors as ±3 weeks from 29 weeks LMP to term.[96] However, many consider the BPD reliable to (±2 weeks) only until about 33 weeks LMP.[66] Consequently, if the BPD is going to be used to estimate fetal age, the measurement has to be obtained before 33 weeks LMP.[66] Near term, or in case of head molding or abnormal head shape at any time during ges-

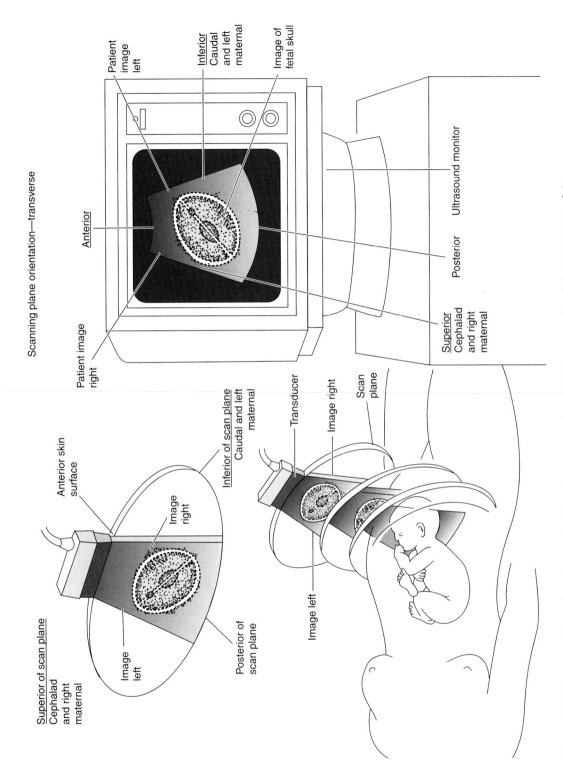

Scanning plane orientation—transverse

Patient image left

Inferior
Caudal and left maternal

Image of fetal skull

Anterior

Posterior   Ultrasound monitor

Patient image right

Superior
Cephalad and right maternal

Superior of scan plane
Cephalad and right maternal

Anterior skin surface

Inferior of scan plane
Caudal and left maternal

Image right

Transducer

Image right

Scan plane

Image left

Image left

Posterior of scan plane

Figure 19-6. Sonographic sectional geometry. The planar geometry of fetal sonography. This is an image of the transverse fetal head. (From DuBose TJ: Fetal Sonography. Philadelphia, WB Saunders, 1996; p 158.

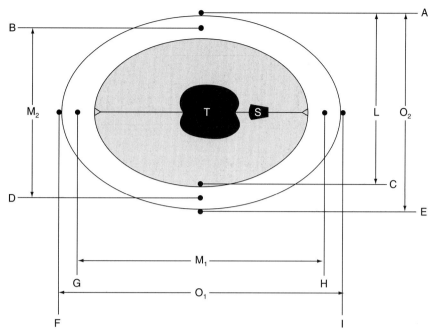

Figure 19-7. Transverse head circumference. Various locations in which fetal skulls have been measured sonographically. Here O_1 = outer-to-outer FOD; M_1 = mid-to-mid FOD; O_2 and M_2 = outer-to-outer and mid-to-mid BPDs, respectively; L = leading-edge to leading-edge BPD; thalamus = T and S = cavum septum pellucidi. Algebraically $O_2/O_1 = M_2/M_1$ and $L = M_2$; therefore, $O_2/O_1 = L/M_1$. Because the leading-edge to leading-edge BPD (L) is the most common and sonographically logical, it is recommended. Because the outer-to-outer FOD tends to be exaggerated due to beam width artifacts, and because the mid-to-mid FOD (M_1) preserves the more normal BPD/FOD ratio the M_1 measurement is recommended. If ellipse drawing tools are used, then the ellipses AHCG or BHDG are recommended for the same reasons. (From DuBose TJ: Fetal Sonography. Philadelphia, WB Saunders, 1996; p 161.)

tation, the three-dimensional BPD correction is recommended.

Transverse Head Circumference

The transverse head circumference (THC) was first suggested as an indicator of fetal age by Levi and Erbsman in 1975.[70] Many authors have suggested that the BPD may be inaccurate owing to normal variations in head shape and molding.[2,21,22,33,44,45,53,56,66,70,96] The consistency of the fetal head has been referred to as plastic.[29] If pressure against the external lateral wall(s) of the skull shortens the BPD, then the long and/or vertical axis will be displaced and lengthened. Likewise, if the long and/or vertical axis is compressed, the width (BPD) of the skull will be enlarged to compensate. Therefore, two-dimensional circumferences of the fetal skull are more accurate than one-dimensional diameters, and three-dimensional measurements are more accurate than two-dimensional ones because three-dimensional measurements are better estimates of the cranial volume.[15,66]

Hadlock and colleagues[50] found that using the two diameters in the formula for the circumference resulted in essentially the same measurement as direct outlining methods, if the BPD and frontal occipital diameter (FOD) are measured outer edge to outer edge. Because hand tracing outlining methods are tedious and slow, the use of ellipse drawing tools or the two-diameter method to calculate the circumference is generally recommended. Whatever method is employed, a chart that was generated using the same method should be used to evaluate fetal age (see Table 19-2). If one wishes to measure the THC using the perimeter tracing method, the measurement should be made around the outer edge of the calvarium. Table 19-2 is recommended for fetal age determination. The THC for this table was generated from leading edge to leading edge

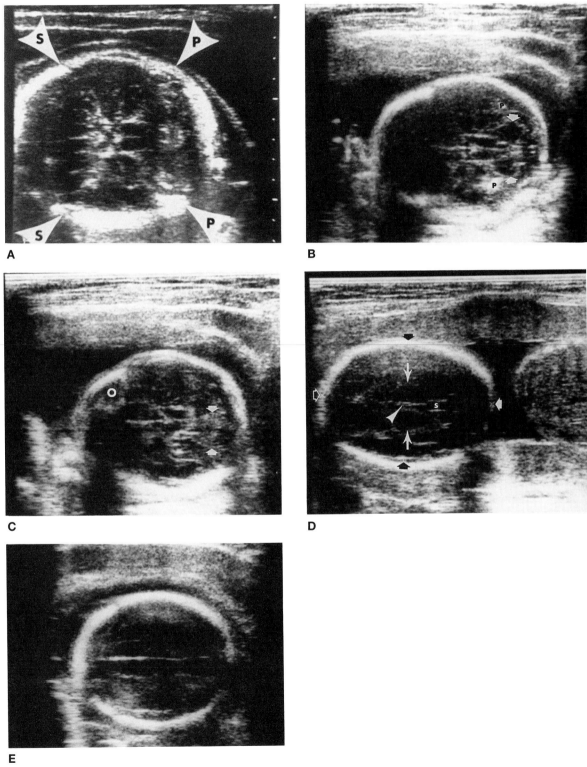

Figure 19-8.

BPDs and mid-edge to mid-edge FODs (see Fig. 19-7).[33] The same anatomic landmarks should be seen in the transverse section where the FOD is measured as in the BPD section. This transverse view should include the cavum septi pellucidi, interhemispheric fissure (midline), and thalamus. The greatest source of error in measuring the THC is selection of a calvarial image in an improper or angled plane. A shortened THC measurement can result if the proper transverse plane is not used (Figs. 19-8, 19-9).

MEASUREMENT METHODS. The THC can be measured directly from the photographed image using a map measurer (planimeter), by using an ellipse drawing function to trace the outline of the skull on the display screen, or by measuring two perpendicular diameters and calculating the circumference. The average of two diameters of the fetal skull, the BPD and long axis, is used in the following formula for the circumference of a circle:

$$\text{Circumference} = \pi(d_1 + d_2)/2 = (d_1 + d_2)1.57$$

where d_1 and d_2 represent the two diameters and the constant, π, is 3.14159.

The FOD has been measured two ways, outer edge to outer edges, and middle of the frontal bone and the occipital bone echoes (Fig. 19-7).[21,96] Because the use of outer edge to outer edge FOD measurements results in a slightly larger variation than the use of the middle of echo to middle of echo FOD, the latter method is recommended.[21]

This larger variance in the outer to outer measurements is thought to be due to the inclusion of the beam width artifact or lateral resolution of the beam, which causes a bit of fuzziness to the echoes from the edges of the frontal and occipital bones.[50]

Cephalic Index

Normal skulls have variable shapes. The cephalic index (CI = BPD/FOD × 100) is used to determine if the shape of the transverse fetal skull can allow a reliable BPD measurement. The CI does not address the variation of the vertical axis of the head.[22] Usually the normal CI is ~80% (±9%) in about 95% of fetuses. These percentages vary somewhat from investigator to investigator, depending on how the head measurements are taken.[21,44,50,61,66]

A fetus with a long and narrow or dolichocephalic head will have a relatively short BPD measurement, and the CI will be below normal. A fetus whose BPD is relatively wide and whose FOD is short is called brachycephalic; the CI is greater than normal and again suggests an unreliable BPD measurement (CI > 89%). Other fetal head dysmorphisms such as acrocephaly, turricephaly, and oxycephaly in which the calvarium is relatively high (a sort of "cone-headedness") may be missed using the CI, in that all have vertical diameters of the cranium which are greater or less than normal.[15,23,66,84] An apparent reverse oxycephaly is called platycephaly. It often occurs late in pregnancy or when crowding of the fetus puts pressure

◄

Figure 19-8. Various transverse heads. (**A**) Scan of the base of the fetal skull shows the base X formed by the bilateral sphenoid bones (S) anteriorly and the bilateral petrous (P) bones posteriorly. This plane is parallel to the plane of the transverse head circumference (THC) but is much too low for a BPD measurement. The plane is perpendicular to the plane of the coronal head circumference (CHC).[1,6,7,17] The optic chiasm (hypoechoic X) and pons can be observed at the center of the image. (**B**) A scan taken slightly higher in the fetal skull but still too low in the posterior skull for a BPD measurement. The cerebellum (*white arrows*) can be seen in the posterior portion of the skull between the petrous bones (P). (**C**) The anterior aspect of the image is too low for a valid BPD measurement. This can be determined because the sphenoid bone over the orbit of the eye (O) is visualized. The top of the cerebellum is between the arrows. (**D**) The correct plane for a BPD measurement. This is confirmed by the central midline and the visualization of the thalamus (*white arrows inside skull*) and the cavum septi pellucidi (S). Note that in this image the frontal bone is on the right near the cavum septi pellucidi (*white arrowhead*). The BPD leading edge-to-leading edge measurement is indicated by the wide, black arrows. The FOD, taken from the middle of the echo from the edge of the frontal bone (*solid white, wide arrow*) to the middle of the echo from the edge of the occipital bone (*open wide arrow*) is also shown. The very narrow "double midline" of the third ventricle (*white arrowhead*) lies at the exact center of the thalamus. (**E**) Scan is too high in the skull for a BPD measurement, as demonstrated by the long, continuous midline and absence of the midbrain structures.

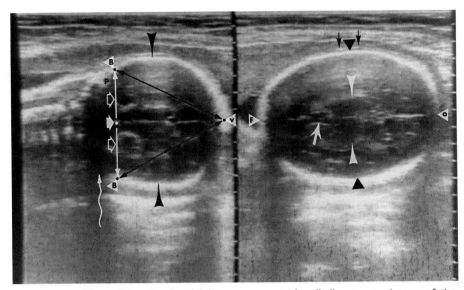

Figure 19-9. Three-dimensional cranial measurement. A split linear-array image of the coronal view of the head on the left and the transverse view on the right. The right image shows the correct plane for the BPD; thalamus (*white arrowheads inside skull*) and the cavum septi pellucidi (*white arrow*). The BPD is measured from leading edge-to-leading edge (black triangles) of the parietal bones. The two small, black arrows mark the scalp. The FOD is measured between the white triangles (F, frontal; O, occipital). The left image is a coronal image showing the measurement of the vertical cranial diameter (VCD), which is between the vertex of the skull (white triangle with v) and the base of the skull (*wide, white arrow*). The VCD is the height of a triangle described by the white triangles (B-B-V). The base of the triangle is an imaginary line (B-B) (hippocampal baseline, HBL), which is tangential to the circles around the bilateral hippocampal gyri (*open arrows*) and the tops of the petrous bones (P), which cause the acoustic shadow (*wavy arrow*). The VCD is measured from the midpoint of the HBL along the interhemispheric fissure to the vertex of the skull.[15] The coronal circumference around the triangle (B-B-V) will be a nearly perfect circle in normally shaped heads, and its diameter (TriCD) will be equal to the BPD (*black arrowheads*).[15-17] The computation for the circumference around the triangle and its diameter is a complex mensuration formula that is best left to computers.[4] The bodies of the lateral cerebral ventricles extend superolateral (~45 degrees) on either side of the cavum verge and after 18 LMP weeks fit wholly within the apex of the coronal triangle. The average of the BPD, FOD, and VCD is equal to the BPD in normally shaped heads. This three-dimensional average has been called the three-dimensional BPD correction and will yield more accurate dates near term than the BPD or THC used alone.[17] The three-dimensional average can be used in a standard BPD fetal age table for fetal ages near term, regardless of the skull shape or molding.

on the vertex of the skull, causing shortening of the vertical dimension of the skull and widening of both diameters of the transverse plane (BPD and FOD), which may not affect the CI.

Three-Dimensional Head Measurements and the Three-Dimensional BPD Correction

By using the BPD, FOD, and vertical cranial diameter (VCD) in a formula for the volume of a sphere, an approximate cranial volume (CV) can be ob-

tained that is more closely correlated with the fetal age than BPD or THC, but this formula is more difficult to calculate and is less desirable for routine use without a computer (Figs. 19-2, 19-10; Table 19-2).[4,15,21,66]

A new method that is easier to calculate than the CV and is as accurate is the simple average of the three diameters of the skull[15,21,23] (Figs. 19-9 and 19-10):

$$\text{3-D BPD} = (\text{BPD} + \text{FOD} + \text{VCD})/3$$

It is coincidental that this three-dimensional

average of the fetal skull (3-D) is equal to the BPD in normally shaped heads (ratio of BPD/ 3-D = 0.99, ±2 SD = 0.08).[23] This means that if the head is abnormally shaped due to morphologic variation or normal molding, the 3-D average will be equal a "corrected BPD" for that fetus (see Appendix E), regardless of degree of brachycephaly, dolichocephaly, oxycephaly, or platycephaly.[13,15,21,23,56,62,66,71,78,84,85] This assumes, of course, that the head is simply abnormally shaped and not microcephalic or megalocephalic. The three-dimensional average can be used to correlate with the estimated fetal age or weight on a standard chart that uses the BPD.[15,23]

The average three-dimensional BPD correction is more accurate than the BPD or the THC for estimating fetal age but not significantly more accurate if the fetus has a normally shaped head. This method is most useful for obviously abnormal head shapes and is particularly useful after about 33 to 35 weeks LMP or with premature rupture of membranes, when the head is more likely to be molded.[84] If high accuracy in fetal dates and growth is desired in serial studies, then the three-dimensional BPD correction method is recommended for routine use.[15]

MEASUREMENT METHODS. The coronal view of the fetal skull used for the VCD measurement is perpendicular to the transverse plane used for the BPD and FOD. The VCD is measured from the middle of the echoes at the vertex of the skull to the midpoint of an imaginary line that is tangential to the bases of the circles around the bilateral hippocampal gyri (hippocampal baseline, HBL; see Figs. 19-9 through 19-11). This imaginary line is also in the plane of the base X (Fig. 19-8*A*).[2,9,15,21,33]

The anatomic structures that are often visualized with this view are the interhemispheric fissure (falx cerebri), the bodies and temporal

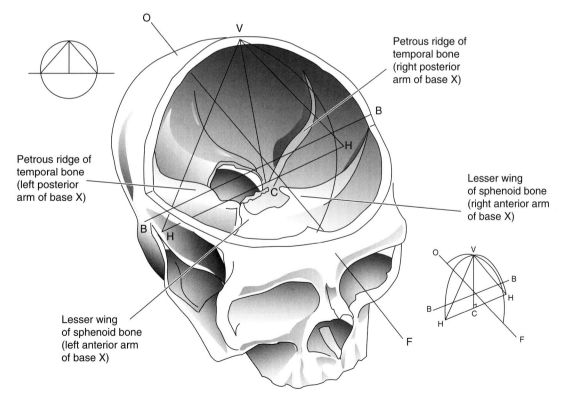

Figure 19-10. *Fetal skull. Solid geometry of fetal skull discussed in this chapter. BPD = B-B′, FOD = F-O, VCD = VC, HBL = H-H′, and the coronal triangle (TriCD) = H-H′-V. (Drawing by Victoria Vescovo Alderman, M.A., RDMS.) (From DuBose TJ: Fetal Sonography. Philadelphia, WB Saunders, 1996; p 159.)*

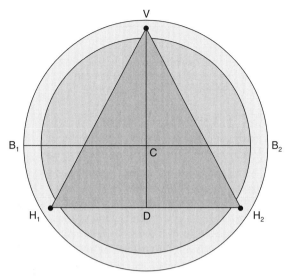

Figure 19-11. Fetal head coronal circle. This drawing shows all the measurements from the circle of the coronal head (see Fig. 19-9). The BPD is leading-edge to leading-edge or outer-to-inner between B_1 and B_2. The hippocampal baseline (HBL) is between H_1 and H_2, the VCD is from the vertex (V) of the triangle to the middle (D) of the HBL, and the two sides of the triangle are between H_1 and H_2 and V. A complex mensuration formula will calculate the circumference of the circle from the length of the HBL and the two sides. From this calculation the coronal triangle circumference diameter (TriCD) can be derived, which will be equal to the BPD in normally shaped heads (r = 0.994, n = 1736). (From DuBose TJ: Fetal Sonography. Philadelphia, WB Saunders, 1996; p 169.)

horns of the lateral ventricles, the third ventricle, the thalamus, the petrous and squamous portions of the temporal bones, the midbrain, the hippocampus, both parietal bones, and the cervical spine. This coronal plane may be used to obtain five different dimensions of the fetal skull (Figs. 19-7 through 19-11). The coronal view is obtained simply by rotating the transducer 90 degrees from the transverse view of the fetal skull to the vertical coronal view. In a normal fetal head the coronal plane of the skull forms a perfect circle (Figs. 19-9 through 19-11).[15]

FETAL BODY MEASUREMENTS

Abdominal Circumference

Abdominal circumference (AC) is a valuable indicator of fetal growth because it reflects the development of abdominal organs such as the liver and spleen. Few other fetal parameters are so often mis-

measured, however, as is the AC. Because most modern formulas for estimating fetal weight rely heavily on this measurement, its importance cannot be overemphasized. Abdominal measurements can also be affected by the degree of spinal flexion, fetal breathing motion, sonographic technique, and accurate visualization of the skin line.

The measurement of the AC is performed at the standard transverse abdominal level where the umbilical and portal veins are confluent. This is usually the largest transverse section of the abdomen and is also reflective of the size of the spleen, and particularly the liver, which are indicators of fetal health and well-being. The liver is proportionately larger in the fetus than in the adult.[37,40] The AC measurement also reflects the amount of subcutaneous fat, which has a large influence on fetal weight. The AC is considered more important as an indicator of fetal weight and health than as an indicator of fetal age.[1,15]

MEASUREMENT METHODS. The standard view for obtaining the AC is at the level of the umbilical vein junction with the portal vein and perpendicular to the spine.[54] The AC should be circular in shape. If the plane used to measure the AC is oblique to the spine, one axis will be elongated, resulting in an erroneously large measurement.

A successful measuring technique for obtaining the fetal AC is to first visualize the long axis of the fetal spine. After the lie of the spine is observed, the transducer field of view is turned perpendicular to the midportion of the spine; the fetal stomach and umbilical vein are then located. The favored view will demonstrate the confluence of the umbilical and portal veins in the fetal liver, called the "hockey stick" view by some (Fig. 19-12). If these veins cannot be visualized owing to fetal position or maternal obesity, then a section demonstrating the fluid-filled fetal stomach is acceptable. It is important, however, when using the stomach as a landmark, not to mistake fluid in the lower gastrointestinal tract for the stomach. Measurements above or below the standard hockey stick view may produce an erroneously small AC.[54] Observation of heart motion indicates a plane superior to the proper AC plane. Visualization of both fetal kidneys is an indication that the section is too low for accurate AC measurement.[65,71] The lower ribs may normally be observed bilaterally but, if seen, should be symmetric.

After the AC view is obtained and the image

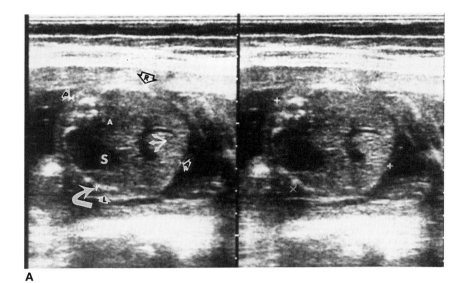

A

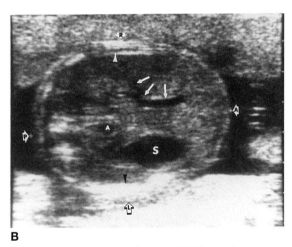

B

Figure 19-12. Fetal abdominal circumference. (**A**) The abdomens are nearly perfect circles. The anteroposterior abdominal diameter (AAD) is indicated by the wide white arrows with A and P. The transverse abdominal diameter (TAD, left) is actually measured incorrectly to the edge of a rib (*curved arrow*) rather than to the more appropriate skin line (*white arrows* L and R). The fluid-filled stomach (S) lies just distal to the fetal spine. The umbilical-portal vein confluence is marked by the three white arrows. (**B**) The AC appears slightly elongated front to back, owing to compression between the placenta and the maternal spine. Good judgment had to be exercised to be sure that the plane of section was appropriate and not simply an oblique plane. The confluence of the umbilical and portal veins is marked by three white arrows. The AC measurement in this image was 177.4 mm, or 22.2 weeks LMP, which is −0.1 week less than the average brain (cranial) age. This would place the approximate fetal weight very near the 50th percentile of normal weights for a 22.3-week LMP fetus and was well within −1 SD of fetal weights.

frozen, two perpendicular abdominal diameters are obtained. Both are measured from the outer skin lines. The transverse abdominal diameter (TAD) is measured from side to side and the anteroposterior abdominal diameter (AAD) is taken from the skin line above the umbilical cord insertion to the skin line just behind the spine. Care must be taken to measure to the skin line so that the resulting circumference is not underestimated. Acoustic shadowing from extremities or the spine can also make the skin line difficult to see in some segments of the AC. The ellipse drawing function of modern machines can also be used. It often helps to look at the "full circle" of the abdomen rather than to focus attention on a single area. Measurements should be taken several times and observed for a cluster range, eliminating any measurements falling outside of the "best" cluster. The best measurements are then averaged for the measurement of record.

While ACs have been measured and calculated using the same techniques as the THC, some use ellipse drawing functions or trace the circumference directly on the image and others use two diameters and the formula for the circumference of a circle. The two-diameter calculation of the circle circumference method is recommended here for the same reasons as for the THC: The results are similar and tracing the circumference is tedious, time-consuming, and subject to operator error. The formula is:

$$AC = 1.57 \times (d_1 + d_2),$$

where d_1 and d_2 are the two diameters of the abdomen. The resulting AC will be in the same units as the diameters (i.e., diameters measured in millimeters will yield an AC in millimeters).

Sonographers should be sure that the measurements extend to the outer abdominal wall and not just to the fetal peritoneal lining. This error is most common when a lateral approach to the abdomen is used and when positioning the caliper for the deep abdominal wall. The peritoneal cavity wall and ribs often generate very strong specular echoes. This may lead to errors resulting in underestimation of the AC by excluding the hypoechoic skin, muscle, and baby fat from the measurement (Fig. 19-12).

FETAL EXTREMITIES MEASUREMENTS

Long Bones

The fetal long bones are good indicators of fetal growth. Although the head and abdomen may be subject to changes in shape due to molding or position,

the long bones are not. A limiting factor in using long bones for measurements is that they are affected by the genetic pool; tall parents tend to have long babies. The accuracy of the humerus, tibia, and ulna measurements in predicting fetal age are considered by some researchers to be approximately ±3 weeks at term, and for the femur, about ±2.2 weeks near term, and less earlier in gestation.[60] Fetal femur length has been shown to correlate both with fetal age and crown-heel length at birth.[48] Other research has found the long bones to have a variation that follows the age range analysis (ARA, see below) rule of just <±10% of the age throughout pregnancy.[17,27]

Visualization and measurement of any fetal long bone or other linear structure with sonography require some mental gymnastics involving eye–hand coordination. The greatest source of error in measuring any long bone occurs when the transducer is positioned slightly oblique to the bone rather than along its axis and, therefore, does not include both ends of the bone. An attempt to exclude the effects of beam width artifacts at the ends of linear structures must be made whenever measurements are taken.

The measurement of the long bones is best accomplished by obtaining several measurements and averaging them for the measurement of record. Usually the average measurement of a single bone is all that is necessary for estimating fetal age. However, all fetal extremities should be visually examined to confirm symmetry and normal morphology.

Femoral Length (FemL)

The femur is among the most commonly used parameters for estimating fetal age and may be more accurate than the BPD late in pregnancy.[60,105] It is usually called a femur length measurement (FemL), but this is a misnomer. The femoral measurement used in obstetric sonography is actually the length of the osseous femoral diaphysis, or shaft, of the bone. This measurement does not include the cartilaginous femoral head or distal femoral condyles. In Figure 19-13 a small but distinct echo is visible continuing from the shaft toward the distal end of the femoral condyles. This echo is not a beam width artifact. It is a specular echo reflected from the proximal edge of the epiphyseal cartilage, which Goldstein and coworkers[38] called the distal femur point (DFP). The DFP is always seen on the side of the condyles nearest the transducer and should not be included in the diaphysis measurements.

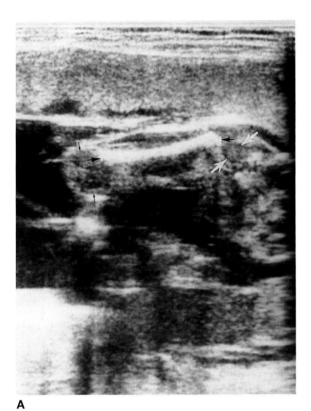
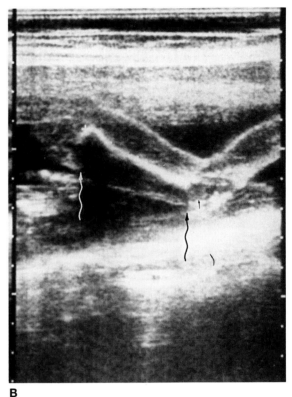

A   **B**

Figure 19-13. Femoral length. Coronal (**A**) and sagittal (**B**) images of the femur. (**A**) The ossified portion of the femoral diaphysis is measured between the large black arrows. The hypoechoic condyles of the distal femur are shown between the small black arrows and the echopenic femoral head is circular (*white arrows*). (**B**) The fetal thigh, calf, and slightly bent knee are imaged from a posterior view. The diaphysis of the femur creates an acoustic shadow (*wavy arrows*); the length of the diaphysis is commonly referred to sonographically as the femur length (FemL). The distal, hypoechoic femoral condyle is marked by the small arrow at the knee.

MEASUREMENT METHODS. To locate the femur, it is first necessary to determine the fetal position (head, spine, and rump). The sonographer can locate the femurs by scanning transversely along the spine until the echogenic, obliquely oriented iliac bones are visible. Then the transducer is moved along the iliac bone until the echogenic linear echo produced by the femur is seen. Once the femur's general location is identified, it becomes necessary to angle the transducer until a linear echo with a clean acoustic shadow is generated. The femur (Fig. 19-13) may have a slightly curved or bowed appearance when viewed from the posteromedial aspect, but this does not normally affect its length relative to age.[19,38] For additional discussion of fetal limbs see Chapter 18.

Humeral Length

The humerus nearest to the transducer is usually easy to find in relationship to the head and spine, but the humerus deep to the transducer is often obscured by the fetal ribs or spine. The humerus has similar measurements to the femur.[60]

MEASUREMENT METHODS. The humerus is best located by first imaging the fetal head and spine to assess the fetal lie. The transducer is then moved caudal from the head until the neck region is located. As the transducer is moved in a caudal direction, the shoulder will appear. At this point the transducer should be rotated until a well-defined linear echo is imaged from the shoulder to the elbow. To make sure that this is the single bone of the humerus, cross-plane rocking[16] of the transducer from side to side is used to avoid confusion with the two linear bone echoes of the forearm, representing the radius and ulna.

In some projections the distal end of the humerus appears to have a split or relatively echo-free, central Y-shaped portion (Fig. 19-14). The Y shape is caused by scanning coronally through the hu-

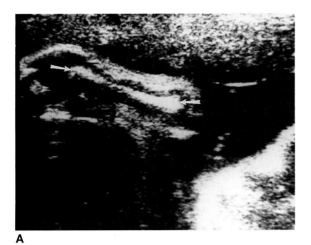

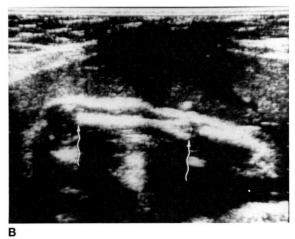

A   **B**

Figure 19-14. Humeral length. (**A**) The humeral length shown is from a sagittal scan plane. White arrows mark either end of the humerus measurement. (**B**) A coronal projection with a Y-shaped distal humerus. The white arrows here show the acoustic shadow marking the ends of the humeral shaft. Measurement is made to the longest of the split ends or the Y of the epicondyles.

merus, showing the coronoid fossa between the lateral and medial epicondyles. The recommended measurement includes the entire ossified portion of the humerus to the end of the longest epicondyle. At the proximal end of the humerus a proximal humeral point (PHP)[19] may be observed as specular echoes from the near side of the cartilaginous humeral head. This is analogous to the DFP of the femur and should not be included in the humeral measurements (Fig. 19-15).

Distal Extremity Bones

The distal long bones of the arms and legs can be difficult to measure because the fetus, particularly if active, may move them frequently and not allow a reliable prediction as to their relationship to the spine or head. Once the bone is located, measuring it is not difficult. If one encounters a fetus with a disparity in the more often measured parameters, the distal bone measurements can be used to resolve any conflict in age estimates. Routine measurements of the distal long bones are not necessary for most sonographic examinations, but the bones should be observed for normal morphology and contralateral symmetry.

Ulna

To measure the ulna the sonographer should do a survey scan of the fetus to locate the head, spine, and humerus. The sonographer follows the hu-

merus out to the elbow. There it can be determined whether the elbow is flexed or extended, and the ulna can be followed out to the hand. The sonographer should be aware that there are two bones in the forearm, the ulna and radius. The ulna is the larger of the two and is anatomically medial in location. The increased length of the ulna over the length of the radius is most obvious at the proximal or elbow end of the bones (Fig. 19-16). If the fetal

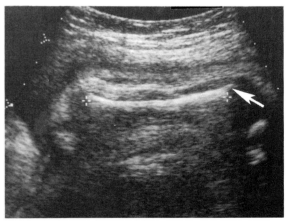

Figure 19-15. Proximal humeral point and humeral length. Humerus measurement (56.5 mm) at 35 LMP weeks by MFP average age. Arrow points to the proximal humeral point (HPH). This is a specular echo from the near side of the cartilaginous humeral head and should not be included in the humeral length.

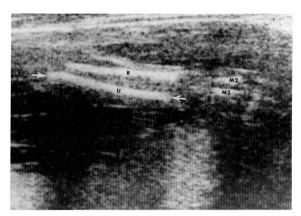

Figure 19-16. *Ulna and radius. The parallel bones of the ulna (U) and radius (R) and a portion of the hand. The two hand bones are the second and third metacarpals (M2, M3); the fourth and fifth metacarpals lie in the acoustic shadow of the second and third metacarpals. The first metacarpal, or thumb, is not in the plane of the image. The ulna is the larger of the two bones in the forearm, and its measurement is indicated by the arrows.*

wrist and hand are rotated, the ulna and radius will be crossed rather than parallel.[60]

Tibia

The tibia, like the ulna, can be imaged in a variety of locations, depending on fetal position and activity. To locate the tibia, the sonographer follows the femur from the hip out to the knee and determines whether the knee is flexed or extended. The tibia is the larger of the two bones in the lower leg and is located medially (Fig. 19-17).[60]

Embryo/Fetal Heart Rate (E/FHR)

Early in the first trimester, before 8 weeks LMP, the GSD and CRL are the primary sonographic measurements that can be used for dating the pregnancy. During this early time (before 9.2 weeks LMP) the embryonic heart rate (EHR) can also be used to estimate the embryo's age.[17,18,25,28,35] From about the early fifth week LMP, the EHR accelerates from ~85 beats per minute (bpm) to a peak of about 175 bpm during the early ninth week LMP[7] (Fig. 19-18). This is a rate of acceleration of 3.3 bpm per day, or an increase of about 10 bpm every 3 days, or a 100 bpm increase during the first month of cardiac activity. Until recently the EHR has not been used for dating, and it is not as accurate as the CRL, but it is more accurate than the GSD and can be especially helpful to cor-

roborate the early dates when using a vaginal transducer.[14,24,25,26,34]

The estimation of embryonic age from the EHR uses a simple linear regression formula (Fig. 19-18):

$$\text{Age from conception in days } (\pm 6)$$
$$= (\text{FHR} \times 0.3) - 8$$

OR

$$\text{Age in menstrual days } (\pm 6) = (\text{FHR} \times 0.3) + 6$$

This formula is accurate within ± 6 days if an accurate EHR is used before 9.2 weeks LMP.[24,25] The EHR should be determined using M-mode sonography for greater accuracy. Attempting to count an EHR that may normally exceed 170 bpm during the ninth and 10th weeks LMP, while watching a clock, can yield large errors.[7,18,99]

In one population it was found that if the EHR age was less than the CRL age by 8 days or more before the ninth LMP week, there was a 67% to 83% chance of first trimester loss[18] (Fig. 19-18). Another way of looking at this issue is to estimate a lower threshold for the EHR (EHRt).

$$\text{EHR} < \text{EHRt} = \{7 + [(\text{CRL weeks} - 2)21]\}$$

If the EHR is less than the EHRt, then there is a

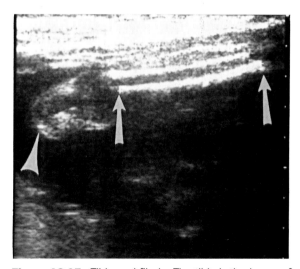

Figure 19-17. *Tibia and fibula. The tibia is the larger of the two bones, the shin bone, in the lower leg of the fetus. This measurement is not difficult to make once the tibia is located (arrows). Location is often varied owing to fetal position. The large, white arrowhead marks the fetal heel.*

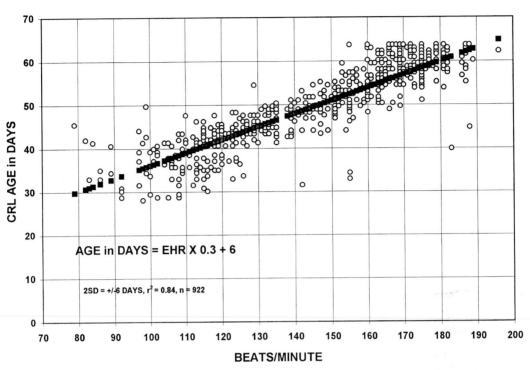

DAYS AGE from EMBRONIC HEART RATE

AGE in DAYS = EHR X 0.3 + 6

2SD = +/-6 DAYS, r² = 0.84, n = 922

Figure 19-18. Embryofetal heart rate. This graph shows the fetal age in days (LMP) calculated from the CRL (Y axis) plotted against the embryonic heart rate (EHR, X axis) 9.2 LMP weeks (64.4 days). The linear regression formula will estimate the fetal age in days to within ± 6 days in 95% of the cases (±2 SD). EHR estimated ages that are more than −8 days less than the age by CRL have been found to have a high probability of 1st trimester miscarriage.[17]

high likelihood of first trimester loss (100% in this population).

Binocular Measurement

The distance from the outer edges of the left and right fetal eyes is called the binocular distance (BiOD).[59] The BiOD is useful when fetal position makes the BPD or other measurements difficult to obtain. To measure the BiOD, both orbits must be imaged at their greatest diameters. The outer orbit to outer orbit distance is measured from the outside of the globes or the insides of the skeletal orbit (Fig. 19-19). It must be pointed out that this measurement may also be difficult to obtain at times owing to the fetus' position. Late in gestation, fetal nasal bones tend to shadow the detail of the eye farthest from the transducer during lateral scans. These shadowing effects of the nasal bones may cause the observer to measure to the inside of the

lateral retina at times or to the inner surface of the zygoma at other times.

The diameters of the individual globes of the eyes and the interocular (between the eyes) distance have also been used to estimate fetal growth.[53] Because these measurements are relatively small, any error in cursor placement will cause a relatively large percentage error. For this reason, the larger BiOD is favored.

Other Measurements

FETAL WEIGHT

Calculation from Measurement Parameters

Weight is one of the most often sought parameters of fetal growth in obstetrics.[17,43,49,100,103] This is because low birth weight, or intrauterine growth restriction (IUGR), has been associated

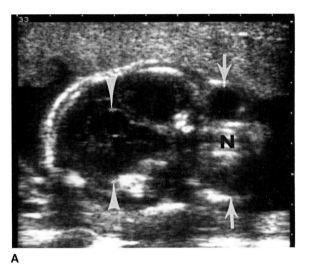 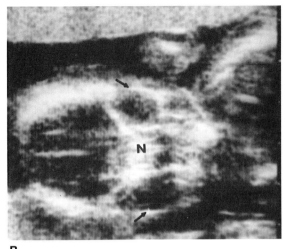

A **B**

Figure 19-19. Binocular distance and cerebellar diameter. BiOD, the binocular distance between the outsides of the ocular globes is demonstrated (*arrows*). (**A**) The cerebellum can often be observed from the same transverse image as the BiOD (between the white arrowheads). (**B**) In a coronal plane view through the fetal facial bones and orbits (*black arrows*) the interhemispheric fissure of the frontal lobes of the brain can also be observed. In both images the echogenic nasal bones (N) are seen between the orbits. The zygomatic bones form the major portion of the lateral echoes of the orbits, and the BiOD is measured to the inside of the bilateral zygomas (*arrows*).

with higher incidences of neonatal morbidity and death, whereas normal to slightly higher birth weights are usually associated with healthy neonates. Therefore, an estimate of the relative fetal weight is important to alert the obstetrician to developing problems and to assist in subsequent management of the pregnancy. An indication of the importance of this parameter is the fact that more than 19 different studies of sonographic fetal weight estimates had been published by 1986.[43,89] Appendix L is an abbreviated table that uses the BPD and average diameter of the abdomen to estimate fetal weight. Appendix O is a table that uses the BPD and AC for estimating fetal weight. If the head exhibits any molding, then the three-dimensional BPD correction or the corrected Biparietal Diameter Formula in Appendix E should be substituted in the table.

Recent research has found that the mean fetal weight varies in populations. This research studied birth weights for >38,000 singleton, sonographically dated, term pregnancies. Using stepwise multiple regression analysis the researchers found that, "*Apart from gestational age and sex, the maternal height,*

weight at first visit, ethnic group, parity and smoking all have significant and independent effects on birth weight."[35] This means that much of the variation and standard errors in fetal weight estimates can be accounted for by these variables. It also means that in the future new and much more complex calculations using computers will be required to achieve these more accurate weight estimates.

Most of the multiple-parameter fetal weight estimation formulas are a variation of a theme that uses parameters of the fetal head or abdomen or other somatic parameters to estimate the relative fat content, as well as the size of the head and liver and the fetus' length. This works because the brain is the most uniform organ of human growth, whereas the size of the abdomen indicates fat content and liver size, and the femur length is usually proportional to fetal length.[48] The caveat for these methods is that they cannot detect "symmetric IUGR" in a single examination. The sonographer should be particularly careful when taking measurements to be used in weight estimates, particularly those involving abdominal diameter and AC. It is easy to err on the small side and underestimate fetal weight. A discussion estimating fetal weight can be found in Chapter 24.

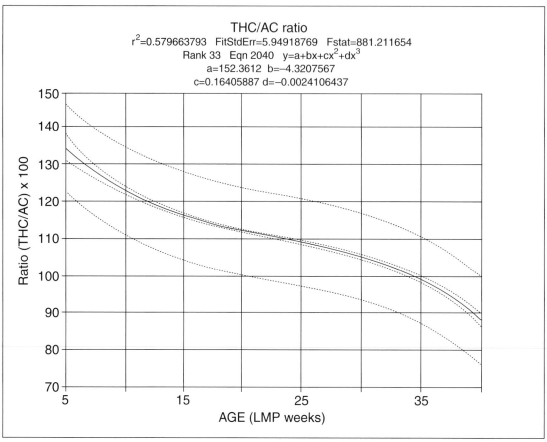

Figure 19-20. Head and abdominal circumferences ratios. Ratios of the transverse head and abdominal circumferences. This graph demonstrates the more standard HC:AC ratio; here it is called the transverse head circumference/abdominal circumference ratio (THC/AC). With the THC/AC ratio as the fetal abdomen gets larger, the ratio is smaller. Also, as the fetal age increases the ratio becomes smaller.

FETAL PARAMETER RATIOS

Ratios of various parameters have been historically used to assess fetal proportionality. The ratio or index is a powerful statistical tool for comparing the relative sizes of two parameters. This is because many fetal parameters grow at different rates and it is difficult to compare their sizes directly. However, at any given time in gestation the ratio of their sizes will normally be fairly consistent. This means that calculating the ratio of the two measurements will provide an idea of their relative sizes, one to the other.

In a ratio the parameter that is the so-called "standard" is usually the denominator.[101] As the comparative numerator becomes larger, the ratio also increases, and vice versa. This standard is not always followed and either parameter can be used as the numerator as long as the observer understands the relationships in the ratio.[10] It is best if ratios compare like measurements; that is to say, compare linear to linear measurements, circumferences to circumferences or volumes to volumes. A consideration for the use of ratios to evaluate proportions is in the case where a particular ratio is abnormal. The observer must then determine if the numerator or the denominator of the ratio is the abnormal parameter.

$$\text{Ratio} = \text{numerator/denominator}$$

$$\text{Percentage} = 100(\text{numerator/denominator})$$

ABDOMEN TO HEAD RATIO

Many ratios have been proposed to evaluate the proportionality of fetal parameters. One of the most common is the transverse head circumference/

TABLE 19-4. RATIOS

LMP (Weeks)	THC/AC			ADA/FemL			ADA/3D BPD			FemL/3D BPD			LMP (Weeks)
	+2 SD	Mean	−2 SD	+2 SD	Mean	−2 SD	+2 SD	Mean	−2 SD	+2 SD	Mean	−2 SD	
10	1.4	1.2	1.0	3.7	2.8	1.8	1.0	0.9	0.8				10
11	1.4	1.2	1.0	2.9	2.3	1.7	1.1	0.9	0.8	0.4	0.3	0.2	11
12	1.4	1.2	1.1	2.4	2.0	1.6	1.1	1.0	0.8	0.5	0.4	0.3	12
13	1.3	1.2	1.1	2.1	1.8	1.5	1.1	1.0	0.9	0.6	0.5	0.4	13
14	1.3	1.2	1.1	1.9	1.7	1.4	1.1	1.0	0.9	0.6	0.5	0.5	14
15	1.3	1.2	1.0	1.8	1.6	1.4	1.1	1.0	0.9	0.7	0.6	0.5	15
16	1.3	1.2	1.0	1.8	1.6	1.3	1.1	1.0	0.9	0.7	0.6	0.5	16
17	1.3	1.1	1.0	1.7	1.5	1.3	1.1	1.0	0.9	0.7	0.6	0.6	17
18	1.3	1.1	1.0	1.7	1.5	1.3	1.1	1.0	0.9	0.7	0.6	0.6	18
19	1.2	1.1	1.0	1.7	1.5	1.3	1.1	1.0	0.9	0.7	0.7	0.6	19
20	1.2	1.1	1.0	1.6	1.5	1.3	1.1	1.0	0.9	0.8	0.7	0.6	20
21	1.2	1.1	1.0	1.6	1.5	1.3	1.1	1.0	0.9	0.8	0.7	0.6	21
22	1.2	1.1	1.0	1.6	1.4	1.3	1.1	1.0	0.9	0.8	0.7	0.6	22
23	1.2	1.1	1.0	1.6	1.4	1.3	1.1	1.0	0.9	0.8	0.7	0.6	23
24	1.2	1.1	1.0	1.6	1.4	1.2	1.1	1.0	0.9	0.8	0.7	0.7	24
25	1.2	1.1	1.0	1.6	1.4	1.3	1.1	1.0	0.9	0.8	0.7	0.7	25
26	1.2	1.1	1.0	1.6	1.4	1.3	1.1	1.0	1.0	0.8	0.7	0.7	26
27	1.2	1.1	1.0	1.6	1.4	1.3	1.1	1.0	1.0	0.8	0.7	0.7	27
28	1.2	1.1	1.0	1.6	1.4	1.3	1.1	1.0	1.0	0.8	0.7	0.7	28
29	1.2	1.1	1.0	1.6	1.4	1.3	1.1	1.0	1.0	0.8	0.7	0.7	29
30	1.2	1.1	1.0	1.6	1.4	1.3	1.1	1.0	1.0	0.8	0.8	0.7	30
31	1.1	1.0	0.9	1.6	1.4	1.3	1.2	1.1	1.0	0.8	0.8	0.7	31
32	1.1	1.0	0.9	1.6	1.4	1.3	1.2	1.1	1.0	0.8	0.8	0.7	32
33	1.1	1.0	0.9	1.6	1.4	1.3	1.2	1.1	1.0	0.9	0.8	0.7	33
34	1.1	1.0	0.9	1.6	1.4	1.3	1.2	1.1	1.0	0.9	0.8	0.7	34
35	1.1	1.0	0.9	1.6	1.5	1.3	1.3	1.2	1.0	0.9	0.8	0.7	35
36	1.1	1.0	0.9	1.7	1.5	1.3	1.3	1.2	1.1	0.9	0.8	0.7	36
37	1.0	0.9	0.8	1.7	1.5	1.3	1.3	1.2	1.1	0.9	0.8	0.7	37
38	1.0	0.9	0.8	1.8	1.5	1.3	1.4	1.2	1.1	0.9	0.8	0.7	38
39	1.0	0.9	0.8	1.8	1.5	1.3	1.4	1.2	1.1	0.9	0.8	0.7	39
40	1.0	0.9	0.8	1.7	1.5	1.3	1.4	1.2	1.1	0.9	0.8	0.7	40

Various ratios for comparing relative sizes of two parameter measurements in millimeters. The first and last columns are the fetal ages. Each ratio has a column for the means and ± 2 standard deviations (2 SD), which accounts for ~95% of the population (n = 2728). In this table circumferences are compared with circumferences and linear measurements are compared with linear measurements. Transverse head circumference to abdominal circumference (THC/AC) ratio: as the AC becomes relatively larger, the ratio becomes smaller. Average diameter of the abdomen to the femur length (ADA/FemL): as the abdomen becomes larger, the ratio increases. ADA to 3D BPD: as the average diameter of the abdomen becomes relatively larger, the ratio also becomes larger. FemL/3D BPD: as the femur length becomes relatively longer, the ratio becomes larger.

abdominal circumference ratio (THC/AC) (Fig. 19-20).[10,17,101] With this ratio, as the abdomen becomes larger, relative to the head, the ratio becomes smaller, and vice versa. The THC/AC ratio will normally be a 1:1 ratio (299 mm/299 mm = 1.0) at ~34 LMP weeks. This ratio should normally be >100% before 34 weeks and less after that time.

OTHER BODY RATIOS

Other ratios that are useful in the study of fetal proportions are ratios comparing the femur length, the BPD or three-dimensional BPD, and the abdominal diameter average (ADA) (Table 19-4). In all ratios using the BPD as the comparative standard, the three-dimensional BPD correction is recommended if there is any head molding.

AGE RANGE ANALYSIS (ARA)

Another method of evaluating fetal parameter proportionality is the age range analysis (ARA).[17] The ARA method is based on the concept that the age determined from the size of any single parameter is the equivalent of the measurement expressed in time, or the fourth dimension. For example, a normal, relatively short, fat fetus could have a femur that measures as a 19-week size-age while the AC could equate to a 22-week size-age. It is absurd to assume that the abdomen was conceived 3 weeks before the femur. A more logical view is that the age is the mean (20.5 weeks) and consider the femur and AC as residing under the extreme tails of the normally distributed bell curve. The statistical logic of the ARA is explained elsewhere[17] (Table 19-2).

From the ARA two rules of thumb can be postulated: (1) No two fetal parameter size-ages for the same examination should be different by >20% of the mean fetal age. (2) No single fetal parameter size-age should be >±10% different from the average age of multiple fetal parameters.

If either of these two rules is not satisfied, then the sonographer should determine that the parameters were correctly measured and that the age calculations are correct. If all measurements and calculations are correct, then fetal disproportion must be considered.

Summary

Factors of which the sonographer should be particularly aware are as follows:

1. To use any fetal parameter size-age chart the user must know how the measurements were taken and must take measurements by the methods used by the author to construct the chart.

2. The use of multiple fetal parameter average ages and the range of the ages will produce more accurate dates and will be more likely to expose abnormal parameters or erroneous measurements than will the use of single fetal parameters.

3. Any two fetal parameter ages from the same examination should not have a range in weeks >20% of the fetal age (range of ages = maximum age − minimum age).

4. All parameter ages from an examination should be within ±10% of the average fetal parameter age.[17]

5. Age estimates from fetal head parameters normally have about half the error (variance) of body parameter ages.

6. Long bone (femur, humerus) sonographic measurements should include only the osseous portions of the bone diaphysis (shaft). The sonographer should be careful not to include beam width artifacts or the DFP or PHP in the measurement.

7. If the transverse cephalic index is normal and the coronal skull shape is a circle, then the BPD is a good estimator of dates; otherwise, the three-dimensional BPD correction is recommended as head molding increases.

8. When taking measurements the sonographer should always use the transducer and focal range that will give the highest resolution.

REFERENCES

1. American Institute of Ultrasound in Medicine. AIUM guidelines. J Ultrasound Med. 1991; 10:576–578.
2. Athey PA, Hadlock FP. Ultrasound in Obstetrics and Gynecology. St. Louis, CV Mosby, 1981; 23–36.
3. Bartrum RJ, Crow HC. Real-Time Ultrasound: A Manual for Physicians and Technical Personnel, 2nd ed. Philadelphia, WB Saunders, 1983; 147.
4. Beyer WH, ed. CRC Standard Mathematical Tables, 28th ed. Boca Raton, FL, CRC Press, 1987; p 122.
5. Birnholz JC. Fetal lumbar spine: Measuring axial growth with US. Radiology. 1986; 158:805–807.
6. Birnholz JC. Ultrasonic measurements. In Deter RL, Harrist RB, Birnholz JC, et al, eds. Quantita-

tive Obstetrical Ultrasonography. New York, John Wiley & Sons, 1986; p 10.

7. Blaas H-G, Eik-Nes SH, Kiserud T, Hellevik LR. Early development of the abdominal wall, stomach and heart from 7 to 12 weeks of gestation: A longitudinal ultrasound study. Ultrasound Obstet Gynecol. 1995; 6:248–249.

8. Bovicelli L, Orsins LF, Rizzo N, et al. Estimation of gestational age during the first trimester by real-time measurement of fetal crown-rump length and biparietal diameter. Clin Ultrasound. 1981; 9:71–75.

9. Bowie JD. Real-time ultrasonography in the diagnosis of fetal anomalies. In Winsburg F, Cooperberg PL, eds. Clinics in Diagnostic Ultrasound. New York, Churchill, Livingstone, 1982; p 228.

10. Campbell S, Thomas A. Ultrasound measurements of the fetal head to abdomen circumference in assessment of growth retardation. Br J Obstet Gynaecol. 1977; 84:164–174.

11. Chilcote WS, Asokan S. Evaluation of first-trimester pregnancy by ultrasound. Clin Obstet Gynecol. 1977; 20:253–263.

12. Cullinan JA, Wilson S, Toi A, et al. Validation of transvaginal crown-rump length measurements (abstr). J Ultrasound Med. 1988; 7:S108.

13. Deter RL, Harrist RB, Hadlock FP, et al. Longitudinal studies of fetal growth using volume parameters determined with ultrasound. J Clin Ultrasound. 1984; 12:313–324.

14. Doubilet PM, Benson CB. Embryonic heart rate in the early first trimester: What rate is normal? J Ultrasound Med. 1995; 14:431–434.

15. DuBose TJ. Fetal cranial biometry. In Fetal Sonography. Philadelphia, WB Saunders, 1996; pp 157–199.

16. DuBose TJ. Physics and methodology of obstetrical sonography. In Fetal Sonography. Philadelphia, WB Saunders, 1996; pp 58–64.

17. DuBose TJ. Fetal size/age analysis. In Fetal Sonography. Philadelphia, WB Saunders, 1996; pp 95–156.

18. DuBose TJ. Embryo/fetal heart rates. In Fetal Sonography. Philadelphia, WB Saunders, 1996; pp 263–274.

19. DuBose TJ. Fetal extremities. In Fetal Sonography. Philadelphia, WB Saunders, 1996; pp 237–244.

20. DuBose TJ. A simple test of excessive B scanner transducer ring. Med Ultrasound. 1983; 7:169–172.

21. DuBose TJ. Fetal biometry: Vertical calvarial diameter and calvarial volume. J Diagn Med Ultrasound. 1985; 1:205–217.

22. DuBose TJ. Basic Baby II Instruction Manual. Austin, TX, Mind's Eye Images, 1987; pp 24–25.

23. DuBose TJ. 3D BPD Correction. J Ultrasound Med. 1988; 7:S97.

24. DuBose TJ, Cunyus JA, Johnson L. Embryonic heart rate and age. J Diag Med Sonogr. 1990; 6:151–157.

25. DuBose TJ, Cunyus JA, Dickey DK, et al. Fetal gestational days = (fetal heart rate 0.3) + 7. J Diag Med Ultrasound. 1989; 4:198.

26. DuBose TJ, Dickey DK, Butschek CM, et al. Fetal heart rate communication. J Ultrasound Med. 1988; 7:237–238.

27. DuBose TJ, Poole E, Butschek CM, et al. Range of multiple fetal parameters. J Ultrasound Med. 1988; 7:S205.

28. DuBose TJ, Porter L, Dickey DK, et al. Sonographic correlation of fetal heart rate and gender. J Diagn Med Sonogr. 1989; 5:49–53.

29. Eastman NJ, Hellman LM. Williams' Obstetrics. New York, Appleton-Century-Crofts, 1961; pp 416–417.

30. Filly R. Editorial. Radiology. 1988; 166:274–275.

31. Filly RA. Ultrasound evaluation during the first trimester. In Callen PW, ed. Ultrasound in Obstetrics and Gynecology, 3rd ed. Philadelphia, WB Saunders, 1993; p 89.

32. Finberg HJ. Fetus power (lecture). Radiol Today. 1987; 1.

33. Fiske CE, Filly RA. Ultrasound evaluation of the normal and abnormal fetal neural axis. In Callen PW, ed. Ultrasonography in Obstetrics and Gynecology. Philadelphia, WB Saunders, 1983; p 100.

34. Fine C, Cartier M, Doubilet P. Fetal heart rates: Values throughout gestation. J Ultrasound Med. 1988; 7:S105.

35. Gardosi J, Mongelli M, Willcox M, Chang A. An adjustable fetal weight standard. Ultrasound Obstet Gynecol. 1995; 6:168–174.

36. Goldberg BB, Wells PNT. Ultrasonics in Clinical Diagnosis, 3rd ed. New York, Churchill Livingstone, 1983; p 32.

37. Goldstein RB. Ultrasound evaluation of the fetal abdomen. In Callen PW, ed. Ultrasonography in Obstetrics and Gynecology, 3rd ed. Philadelphia, WB Saunders, 1993; pp 351–355.

38. Goldstein RB, Filly RA, Simpson G. Pitfalls in femur length measurements. J Ultrasound Med. 1987; 6:203–207.

39. Goldstein RS. New Insights Into Early Pregnancy and Its Failure: Society of Diagnostic Medical Sonographers, 12th Annual Conference, Atlanta, 1995, Official Conference Proceedings. pp 179–199.

40. Gross BH, Harter P, Filly RA. Disproportionate left hepatic lobe size in the fetus: Ultrasonic demonstration. J Ultrasound Med. 1982; 1:79–81.

41. Hadlock FP. Evaluation of fetal dating studies. In Deter RL, Harrist RB, Birnholz JC, et al (eds): Quantitative Obstetrical Ultrasonography. New York, John Wiley & Sons, 1986; p 39.

42. Hadlock FP. Evaluation of fetal dating studies. In Deter RL, Harrist RB, Birnholz JC, et al, eds. Quantitative Obstetrical Ultrasonography. New York, John Wiley & Sons, 1986; pp 42–43.

43. Hadlock FP. Evaluation of fetal weight estimating procedures. In Deter RL, Harrist RB, Birnholz JC, et al, eds. Quantitative Obstetrical Ultrasonography. New York, John Wiley & Sons, 1986; pp 115–117.

44. Hadlock FP, Deter RL, Carpenter RJ, et al. Estimating fetal age: Effect of head shape on BPD. Am J Roentgenol. 1981; 137:83–85.

45. Hadlock FP, Deter RL, Harrist RB, et al. Fetal head circumference: Relation to menstrual age. Am J Roentgenol. 1982; 138:649–653.

46. Hadlock FP, Deter RL, Harrist RB, et al. Computer-assisted analysis of fetal age in the third trimester using multiple growth parameters. J Clin Ultrasound. 1983; 11:313–316.

47. Hadlock FP, Deter RL, Harrist RB, et al. Estimating fetal age: Computer-assisted analysis of multiple fetal growth parameters. Radiology. 1984; 152:497–501.

48. Hadlock FP, Deter RL, Roecker E, et al. Relation of fetal femur length to neonatal crown-heel length. J Ultrasound Med. 1984; 3:1–3.

49. Hadlock FP, Harrist RB, Sharman RS, et al. Estimation of fetal weight with the use of head, body, and femur measurements: A prospective study. Am J Obstet Gynecol. 1985; 151:333–337.

50. Hadlock FP, Kent WR, Loyd JL, et al. An evaluation of two methods for measuring fetal head and body circumferences. J Ultrasound Med. 1982; 1:359–360.

51. Hadlock FP, Shah YP, Kanon DJ, et al. Fetal crown-rump length: Reevaluation of relation to menstrual age (5–18 weeks) with high-resolution real-time US. Radiology. 1992; 182:501–505.

52. Hansmann M, Hackeloer BJ, Staudach A. Normal fetal anatomy in the second and third trimester. In Hansmann M, Hackeloer BJ, Staudach A, eds. Ultrasound Diagnosis in Obstetrics and Gynecology. Berlin, Springer-Verlag, 1985; p 113.

53. Hansmann M, Hackeloer BJ, Staudach A. Normal fetal anatomy in the second and third trimester. In Hansmann M, Hackeloer BJ, Staudach A, eds. Ultrasound Diagnosis in Obstetrics and Gynecology. Berlin, Springer-Verlag, 1985; pp 169–175.

54. Hansmann M, Hackeloer BJ, Staudach A. Normal fetal anatomy in the second and third trimester. In Hansmann M, Hackeloer BJ, Staudach A, eds. Ultrasound Diagnosis in Obstetrics and Gynecology. Berlin, Springer-Verlag, 1985; pp 124–130.

55. Hellman LM, Kobayashi M, Fillisti L, et al. Growth and development of the human fetus prior to the twentieth week of gestation. Am J Obstet Gynecol. 1969; 103:789–800.

56. Hill LM, Breckle R, Gehrking WC. The variable effects of oligohydramnios on the biparietal diameter and the cephalic index. J Clin Ultrasound. 1984; 3:93–95.

57. Holmes JH. Diagnostic ultrasound during the early years of A.I.U.M. J Ultrasound Med. 1980; 8:299–308.

58. Jeanty P. Basic baby II. J Ultrasound Med. 1987; 6:548.

59. Jeanty P, Cantraine F, Cousaert E, et al. The binocular distance: A new way to estimate fetal age. J Ultrasound Med. 1984; 3:241–243.

60. Jeanty P, Rodesch F, Delbekd D, et al. Estimation of gestational age from measurements of fetal long bones. J Ultrasound Med. 1984; 3:75–79.

61. Jordaan HVF. The differential enlargement of the neurocranium in the full-term fetus. S Afr Med J. 1976; 50:1978–1981.

62. Jordaan HVF, Dunn LJ. A new method of evaluating fetal growth. Obstet Gynecol. 1978; 51:659–665.

63. Kremkau FW. Diagnostic Ultrasound: Physical Principles & Exercises. New York, Grune & Stratton, 1980; pp 47–50.

64. Kurtz AB, Goldberg BB. Combined fetal head and body measurements. In Kurtz AB, Goldberg BB, eds. Obstetrical Measurements in Ultrasound: A Reference Manual. Chicago, Year Book Medical Publishers, 1988; p 137.

65. Kurtz AB, Goldberg BB. Fetal body measurements. In Kurtz AB, Goldberg BB, eds. Obstetrical Measurements in Ultrasound: A Reference Manual. Chicago, Year Book Medical Publishers, 1988; p 91.

66. Kurtz AB, Goldberg BB. Fetal head measurements. In Kurtz AB, Goldberg BB, eds. Obstetrical Measurements in Ultrasound: A Reference Manual. Chicago, Year Book Medical Publishers, 1988; pp 22–35.

67. Kurtz AB, Shaw W, Wapner RJ, et al. The inaccuracy of total intrauterine volume: Sources of errors and proposed solution (abstr). J Ultrasound Med. 1983; 2:101.

68. Kurtz AB, Wapner RJ, Kurtz RH, et al. Analysis of biparietal diameter as an accurate indicator of gestational age. J Ultrasound Med. 1980; 8:319–326.

69. Laing FC. First trimester bleeding: The role of ultrasound (lecture). SDMS Spring Symposium, Orlando FL, 1986.

70. Law RG, MacRae KD. Head circumference as an index of fetal age. J Ultrasound Med. 1982; 1:281–288.

71. Lawson TL, Foley WD, Berland LL, et al. Ultrasonic evaluation of fetal kidneys. Radiology. 1981; 138:156.

72. Li DFH, Woo JSK. Fractional spine length: A new parameter for assessing fetal growth. J Ultrasound Med. 1986; 5:379–383.

73. Lyons EA, Levi CS. Ultrasound in the first trimester of pregnancy. Radiol Clin North Am. 1982; 20:261.

74. McDicken WN. Diagnostic Ultrasound: Principles and Use of Instruments, 2nd ed. New York, John Wiley & Sons, 1981; pp 31–32.

75. McDicken WN: Diagnostic Ultrasound. Principles and Use of Instruments, 2nd ed. New York, John Wiley & Sons, 1981; p 34.

76. MacGregor SN, Tamura RK, Sabbagha RE, et al. Underestimation of gestational age by conventional crown-rump length dating curves. Obstet Gynecol. 1987; 70:344–348.

77. McLeary RD, Kuhns LR, Barr M. Ultrasonography of the fetal cerebellum. Radiology. 1984; 151:439–442.

78. Martinez DA, Barton JL. Estimation of fetal body and fetal head volumes: Description of technique and nomograms for 18 to 41 weeks of gestation. Am J Obstet Gynecol. 1980; 137:78–84.

79. Moore KL. The Developing Human, 3rd ed. Philadelphia, WB Saunders, 1982; pp 70–92.

80. Nyberg DA, Filly RA, Filho DLD, et al. Abnormal pregnancy: Early diagnosis by ultrasound and serum chorionic gonadotropin levels. Radiology. 1986; 158:393–396.

81. Nyberg DA, Hill LM. Normal early intrauterine pregnancy: Sonographic development and hCG correlation. In Nyberg DA, Hill LM, Bohm-Velez M, et al, eds. Transvaginal Ultrasound. St. Louis, Mosby/Year Book, 1992; pp 80–82.

82. Nyberg DA, Laing FC, Filly RA. Threatened abortion: Sonographic distinction of normal and abnormal gestation sacs. Radiology. 1986; 158:397–400.

83. Nyberg DA, Mack LA, Laing FC, et al. Distinguishing normal from abnormal gestational sac growth in early pregnancy. J Ultrasound Med. 1987; 6:23–27.

84. O'Keeffe DF, Garite TJ, Elliott JP, et al. The accuracy of estimated gestational age based on ultrasound measurements of biparietal diameter in preterm premature rupture of the membranes. Am J Obstet Gynecol. 1985; 151:309–312.

85. Olmstead WW, Smirniotopoulos JG. Congenital dysplasias primarily involving the skull. In Putnam CE, Ravin CE, eds. Textbook of Diagnostic Imaging. Philadelphia, WB Saunders, 1988; p 110.

86. Ott WJ. Accurate gestational dating. Obstet Gynecol. 1985; 66:311.

87. Persutte WH. First Trimester Prenatal Diagnosis: The Next Frontier. Society of Diagnostic Medical Sonographers, 12th Annual Conference, Atlanta, 1995, Official Conference Proceedings. pp 119–233.

88. Ramírez G. Statistics. In DuBose TJ, ed. Fetal Sonography. Philadelphia, WB Saunders, 1996; pp 53–54.

89. Rose BI. Abbreviated tables for estimating fetal weight with ultrasound. J Reprod Med. 1988; 33:298–300.

90. Ruvolo KA, Filly RA, Callen PW. Evaluation of fetal femur length for prediction of gestational age in a racially mixed obstetric population. J Ultrasound Med. 1987; 6:417.

91. Sabbagha RE. Gestational age. In Sabbagha RE, ed. Diagnostic Ultrasound, Applied to Obstetrics and Gynecology, 3rd ed. Philadelphia, JB Lippincott, 1994; p 165.

92. Sabbagha RE. Gestational age. In Sabbagha RE, ed. Diagnostic Ultrasound, Applied to Obstetrics and Gynecology, 2nd ed. Philadelphia, JB Lippincott, 1987; pp 96–107.

93. Sabbagha RE. Gestational age. In Sabbagha RE, ed. Diagnostic Ultrasound, Applied to Obstetrics and Gynecology, 3rd ed. Philadelphia, JB Lippincott, 1994; pp 176–177.

94. Sabbagha RE. Gestational age. In Sabbagha RE, ed. Diagnostic Ultrasound, Applied to Obstetrics and Gynecology, 3rd ed. Philadelphia, JB Lippincott, 1994; pp 162–167.

95. Sabbagha RE, Hughey M. Standardization of sonar cephalometry and gestational age. Obstet Gynecol. 1978; 52:402–406.

96. Sabbagha RE, Barton FB, Barton BA. Sonar biparietal diameter I. Analysis of percentile growth differences in two normal populations using same methodology. Am J Obstet Gynecol. 1976; 126:479–484.

97. Sabbagha RE, Choen LS, Karins ML, et al. Early pregnancy evaluation. In Sabbagha RE, ed. Diagnostic Ultrasound Applied to Obstetrics and Gynecology, 3rd ed. Philadelphia, JB Lippincott, 1994; p 596.

98. Sarti DA. Diagnostic Ultrasound, 2nd ed. Chicago, Year Book Medical Publishers, 1987; pp 14–15.

99. Schats R, Jansen CAM, Waldimiroff JW. Embryonic heart activity: Appearance and development in early human pregnancy. Br J Obstet Gynaecol. 1990; 97:989–994.

100. Shepard MJ, Richards VA, Berkowitz RL, et al.

An evaluation of two equations of predicting fetal weight by ultrasound. Am J Obstet Gynecol. 1982; 142:47.

101. Sokal RR, Rohlf FJ: Biometry. The Principles and Practice of Statistics in Biological Research, 2nd ed. New York, WH Freeman, 1981; pp 17–19.

102. Timor-Tritsch IE, Peisner DB, Raju S. Sonoembryology: An organ-oriented approach using a high-frequency vaginal probe. J Clin Ultrasound. 1990; 18:286–298.

103. Warsof SL, Gohari P, Berkowitz RL, et al. The estimation of fetal weight by computer-assisted analysis. Am J Obstet Gynecol. 1977; 128:881.

104. Winter J, Kimme-Smith C, King W III. Measurement accuracy of sonographic sector scanners. Am J Roentgenol. 1985; 144:645–648.

105. Wolfson RN, Peisner DB, Chik LL, et al. Comparison of biparietal diameter and femur length in the third trimester: Effects of gestational age and variation in fetal growth. J Ultrasound Med. 1986; 5:145.

106. Yaghoobian J. Simplified method for estimation of fetal age by biparietal measurement. J Diagn Med Sonogr. 1987; 3:33–35.

107. Zador IE, Sokol RJ, Chik L. Interobserver variability: A source of error in obstetric ultrasound. J Ultrasound Med. 1988; 7:245–249.

108. Zagzebski JA. Physics and Instrumentation. In Sabbagha RE, ed. Diagnostic Ultrasound, Applied to Obstetrics and Gynecology, 3rd ed. Philadelphia, JB Lippincott, 1994; pp 13–14.

109. Zagzebski JA. Physics and Instrumentation. In Sabbagha RE, ed. Diagnostic Ultrasound, Applied to Obstetrics and Gynecology, 3rd ed. Philadelphia, JB Lippincott, 1994; pp 14–18.

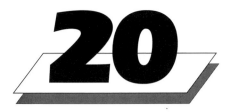

Doppler Ultrasound of the Normal Fetus

JOANNE C. ROSENBERG

History of Doppler Ultrasound Technique

In 1842, an Austrian professor of mathematics and geometry, Dr. Christian Johann Doppler, first described in detail the effect that now bears his name.[14] Dr. Doppler did not observe the effect of motion on sound frequencies but on shifts in light frequencies emitted from double stars.

Before the application of the Doppler effect to evaluating the vasculature, research of the circulatory system entailed surgery and radiology. In the 1930s, Barcroft and associates performed radiographic studies on fetal lambs and goats to establish the circulatory pathways.[4] Lind and Wegelius in 1954 used cardiographic techniques to describe the arterial and venous circulation in human fetuses and found it was similar to that of fetal sheep. Numerous other investigators reported on highly invasive procedures on preabortive fetuses.[29]

Satomura first described the clinical application of Doppler ultrasound technology in 1959.[43] The simplest type of Doppler is continuous wave (CW). Early CW transducers were not very specific because they were unable to distinguish whether flow moved toward or away from the transducer. This deficit was overcome with the addition of spectrum analyzers and audible signals, which allowed estimation of the frequency of the Doppler shift and the direction of flow.

Pulsed-wave (PW) Doppler, which adds information on the location of a moving target, was introduced in the late 1960s almost simultaneously by two independent laboratories. Baker in Washington studied transcutaneous blood flow measurements in humans,[2,3] whereas Peronneau and colleagues in France used their system initially on animals.[39,40] Duplex Doppler imaging—PW Doppler used in conjunction with two-dimensional ultrasound imaging—helps guide the Doppler sampling from the ultrasound vessel visualized.

Color flow mapping and color power Doppler provide color-coded flow direction and aid in vessel identification. Contrast agents, the most recent development, are increasing the signal strength to make imaging small vessels much easier.[44]

Bioeffects

To date, Doppler and real-time ultrasound have not been associated with any ill effects to fetus or mother. This assessment has been arrived at independently by every consensus group that has reviewed the literature and research findings in this area.

The U.S. Food and Drug Administration (FDA) guidelines state that there are no known risks associated with use of Doppler ultrasound at the recommended power levels. There are specific

399

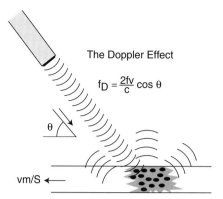

Figure 20-1. An incident ultrasound beam of frequency (*f*) is scattered by moving red blood cells. As a result of the Doppler effect, the back-scattered echo has a center of frequency that is higher by f_D. $f_D = 2fv \cos \theta/c$, where f_D is the change in ultrasound frequency, also known as the Doppler shift frequency; *f* is the frequency of the incident ultrasound; *v* is the relative velocity between the target and the transducer; θ is the angle between the beam and the direction of the movement of the target; and *c* is the velocity of sound in the medium.

Reflections of blood flow can be studied with two basic Doppler techniques. The simplest technique is CW Doppler; the other, PW, is discussed later. With CW Doppler, a single transducer has two separate piezoelectric crystals, one that continuously emits sound and another that simultaneously receives it (Fig. 20-2). The frequency of the received echo is compared to the frequency of the transmitted echo to derive the Doppler shift.

Because the crystals are continuously emitting sound waves and receiving them, CW Doppler cannot identify the location of sound reflection. No imaging is available with this system, but it may be used in conjunction with real-time imaging to locate or confirm the vessel sampling site.

CW is limited to the study of superficial vessels because it cannot discriminate between signals arising from different structures along the beam path, but it is inexpensive, portable, and simple to operate.

FDA guidelines for fetal ultrasound, including that the Doppler spatial peak-temporal average intensity (SPTA) be less than 94 mW/cm^2 in situ.[1] SPTA is a unit used to measure ultrasound energy intensity. Most commercial equipment uses variable acoustic power outputs between 1 and 46 mW/cm^2. The power output of a given Doppler unit should be known before it is used on a fetus.

The Principles of Doppler Ultrasound

A complete discussion of the physics of Doppler ultrasound can be found in textbooks such as Kremkau's[30] and Hykes and colleagues'.[20] The following is an overview of these principles.

CONTINUOUS-WAVE DOPPLER ULTRASOUND

The Doppler effect is a change in frequency resulting from motion of the sound source (Fig. 20-1). The Doppler effect has applications in everyday life, ranging from home burglar alarms to police radar detectors. In medicine, Doppler ultrasound is used to detect and measure blood velocity and flow.

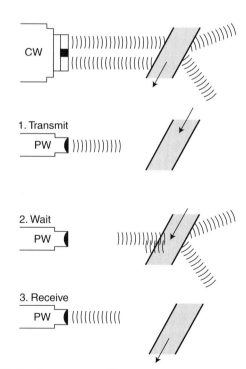

Figure 20-2. (A) Continuous-wave (CW) Doppler transducer that continually transmits and receives reflections to and from the target. **(B)** Pulsed-wave (PW) Doppler transducer (1) transmits a single pulse, and (2) waits for it to return. (3) The time it takes to return is determined by the depth of the target.

PULSED-WAVE DOPPLER

In PW Doppler, short bursts of ultrasound energy are emitted at regular intervals (see Fig. 20-2). The same piezoelectric crystal both sends and receives the signals, allowing for range or depth discrimination. The depth of the target is calculated from the elapsed time between transmission of the pulse and reception of its echoes, assuming a constant speed of sound in tissues. With PW, a sample volume, which is a selected area to be studied, can be designated by manipulating the joystick on the Doppler keyboard. This allows the operator to obtain a reading of a vessel at a certain depth. This is done by adjusting the depth of the sample volume. The area inside the sample volume site is commonly known as the gate (Fig. 20-3). The gate can be adjusted between 1 and 15 mm according to the size of the vessel being studied.

Duplex Doppler sonography combines PW Doppler with real-time imaging, allowing the sampling of vessels at specific anatomic locations. With direct visualization of the vessel, the direction of the insonating Doppler beam can be adjusted to obtain optimal waveforms with maximum velocities. The gate depth and width can also be selected under direct visualization. For example, if no image is available to differentiate between them, an abnormal uterine artery waveform can produce the same Doppler signal as a normal common iliac artery waveform.

The angle of insonation is the angle at which the Doppler beam encounters or intersects the vessel to be sampled. Mirror imaging or other artifacts can occur when the angle of insonation is close to 90 degrees. If this happens, the system cannot distinguish direction of flow and produces the same waveform above and below the baseline. The optimal angle for PW Doppler is 30 to 60 degrees.[30]

Aliasing is a phenomenon that occurs in PW systems when the pulse repetition frequency (PRF) is less than two times the Doppler shift frequency (see Fig. 20-3). This occurs during attempts to sample high-velocity blood flow. PRF is the number of pulses sent out by the transducer per second. The Nyquist limit is the minimum PRF required to register a frequency without aliasing.[38] This proves to be one half the frequency. For example, to detect a frequency of 10 kHz, the PRF must be 20 kHz. It is the speed of sound in tissue that basically limits the PRF. Aliasing can be avoided by increasing the PRF, increasing the angle of insonation, using a lower-frequency transducer, or switching to CW (CW Doppler has no range resolution).[30]

In a study by Mehalek and colleagues,[34] CW and PW flow velocity waveforms were compared using the patient as the control. The systolic-to-diastolic (S/D or A/B) ratios obtained with CW and PW Doppler systems were found to be comparable. Therefore, a laboratory can use either a CW or PW Doppler system effectively.

COLOR FLOW MAPPING

Color flow imaging involves the addition of color to overwrite the gray-scale ultrasound image to indicate movement such as blood flow. A bar of preselected colors is displayed on the left side of the ultrasound screen. As with CW and PW Doppler, the color bar has a baseline. The baseline on the color bar is the black line that separates the two main colors. The color above this baseline indicates blood flow toward the transducer, and the color below the baseline indicates flow away from the transducer. Color flow mapping does not distinguish or code arteries versus veins; rather, it simply assigns color to flow toward or away from the transducer. Two arbitrary primary colors are selected and assigned to differentiate blood flow. Typically, red is assigned for blood flow toward the transducer, and blue is assigned to blood flowing away. The colors can be changed by the operator. Once an appealing color scheme has been selected, the ex-

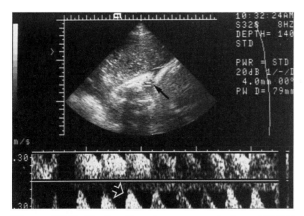

Figure 20-3. Duplex Doppler sonogram demonstrates aliasing. Note the wraparound of the peak systolic peaks (*open arrow*). The area inside the opened gate is the sample volume site (*arrow*).

aminer should use the same combination of colors to ease the recognition of flow abnormalities. Positive velocities (when red is selected as the flow toward the transducer) can go from dark red to white or bright yellow. Negative velocities (when blue is selected as flow away from the transducer) can range from dark blue to white or light cyan. The color white is commonly used to represent an increase in blood velocity. Darker colors represent slower velocities. The color green represents flow disturbances. Turbulence is represented by a mixture of colors such as red, green, and blue.

The disadvantage of using color is that to obtain a high-quality color image, the gray-scale image is usually compromised or degraded, or vice versa. This is because the computer divides its processing time to generate one image into generating two separate images, one in gray scale and the other in color. Quality is therefore compromised. In addition, color flow is angle dependent, which means that color shadings become darker as the angle of insonation approaches 90 degrees. A tortuous vessel may change from red to blue even though it is the same vessel with constant flow. When the angle of insonation hits that same vessel, the area at 90 degrees to the beam will have no color assigned and will image as a black line. The optimal angle to sample with color flow is 30 to 60 degrees. Another potential error when using color is that flashes of color may be displayed by aberrant tissue motions. This produces frequency shifts and may result in confusing color displays. To avoid this, as with CW and PW Doppler, there is a "thump" filter, also known as a velocity or wall filter, built into every machine. A wall filter minimizes the flash artifacts by filtering out the low-level velocities without losing valuable information.

COLOR POWER DOPPLER

Color power Doppler (CPD) is the newest addition to the Doppler evaluation family. CPD calculates the random noise in the CPD mode instead of the mean Doppler frequency shift. Random noise in the CPD mode is different from that in other Doppler modes because the noise has a uniformly low power because of the standard signal-to-noise ratio. The color scale is calculated on the intensity or power of the signal, which displays indirectly the number of blood cells insonated by the Doppler beam. CPD was initially developed to provide an alternate method for assessing low flow velocities because they have a large number of reflectors moving at low velocities. Particles with low velocities are represented by colors of brighter intensity levels. Advantages over standard color Doppler are that CPD is angle independent and does not alias because the integral of the power spectrum is the same regardless of whether the signal wraps around. CPD also increases the usable dynamic range of the Doppler image because it extends the imaged flow down to the noise floor.

There are some drawbacks to using CPD; because the entire color scale is used, there is no differentiation in flow direction or speed. CPD cannot distinguish blood flow reversal; it also cannot differentiate between arterial and venous blood flow. CPD is extremely sensitive to low blood flow, which makes it very sensitive to motion artifacts. Because of this, CPD cannot be used near the fetal heart or great vessels.

ANALYSIS OF THE DOPPLER SIGNAL

Doppler ultrasound has many uses in examining the maternal–fetal circulation. Qualitative Doppler allows us to identify the direction of blood flow and detect flow disturbances such as stenosis or turbulence. More important, Doppler allows the sonographer to isolate abnormal flow patterns that help to identify pregnancies at risk of poor fetal outcome. Quantitative flow measurements include blood velocity and flow. Qualitative measurements look at characteristics of the waveforms, which indirectly give an approximation of flow and resistance to flow. These include the S/D ratio,[45] the resistance index (RI),[41] and the pulsatility index (PI)[18] (Fig. 20-4). Waveform appearance is affected by cardiac contractility, blood viscosity, elasticity of the vessel wall, the peripheral resistance in the circulation, the distance of the sampling site from the heart, and the presence or absence of turbulence.[19]

INTERPRETATION OF WAVEFORMS

After a waveform is obtained, there are standard definitions used to report the Doppler findings. Most fetal and maternal vessels such as the uterine and arcuate arteries have ranges of normal previously established. The range may actually vary with the patient's gestational age. Any S/D, PI, or

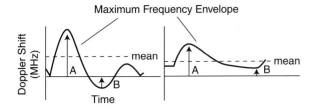

$$\text{A/B Ratio} = \frac{A}{B} \quad \text{(Stuart et al 1980)}$$

$$\text{Resistance Index (modified)} = \frac{A - B}{A} \quad \text{(Pourcelot 1974)}$$

$$\text{Pulsatility Index} = \frac{A - B}{\text{mean}} \quad \text{(Gosling 1975)}$$

Figure 20-4. *Diagram of Doppler waveform and the indices used to describe them. (A, systole; B, diastole.)*

RI in those normal ranges should be reported as within normal limits. High flow ratios, which is flow that indicates a slight resistance in the circulation, should be reported as such. Absent end-diastolic velocity describes the absence of blood flow during the diastolic part of the cardiac cycle.

Reversal of blood flow is defined as flow that actually extends under the Doppler baseline. "Shunting" is a term used when blood flow in the fetal middle cerebral artery, normally a high-resistance circulation, is increased, resulting in low-resistance circulation. This happens in severe cases of fetal growth restriction because blood is shunted from other organs to protect the fetal brain. Notching is a common finding associated with the maternal uterine artery. A uterine artery notch is an extra bump seen between the systolic peak and diastole. In the fetal venous system there may be indentations in the umbilical vein that occur consistently with every diastole; these findings should be described as venous pulsations.

QUANTITATIVE DOPPLER INDICES

Quantitative Doppler can quantify flow disturbances, estimate absolute blood flow, assess vascular impedance, and help characterize tissue. Quantitative Doppler indices include velocity and flow measurements. Velocity is defined as the maximum Doppler shift over a cardiac cycle; flow is defined as the average velocity times the lumen area of a vessel. If the vessel is circular, the area can be deter-

mined from one diameter, whereas if it is an ellipse, two diameters are required.

Several potential errors are inherent in measuring fetal blood flow volume. One source of error is the inaccurate measurement of the angle of the vessel to the insonating ultrasonic beam. The estimate of velocity is strongly dependent on the magnitude of the angle. A linear-array transducer with a Doppler offset at a fixed angle gives an accurate measurement of the angle. If the insonating beam angle is 30 degrees, there is a 3% to 4% error in the Doppler velocity measurement; a 60-degree angle produces a 15% error; but an 80-degree angle produces a 50% error. (Error rates given include a 5% error in measuring the angle.[17]) The need to measure the angle of insonation limits this method to vessels whose axis lies in the same plane for a few centimeters of their course. The intraabdominal umbilical vein or the fetal descending aorta is suitable. Yet another error in estimating flow volume can arise in measuring the vessel diameter. Small measurement errors in vessels of small diameter create huge errors. For example, a 1-mm error in the measurement of an 8-mm vessel produces a 25% error variation in the flow calculation.[11] The diameter of vessels—especially the fetal aorta—may vary 20% over the cardiac cycle. The sample volume must embrace the entire lumen, to ensure that it is uniformly insonated.

QUALITATIVE DOPPLER INDICES

Qualitative measurements of flow velocity waveforms are angle independent and are therefore easier to obtain. The A/B or S/D ratio was first described by Stuart and colleagues[45] in 1980. This is the ratio of the peak systolic velocity to the end-diastolic velocity. In 1974, Pourcelot[41] first described the RI as a mathematical derivative of the simple S/D ratio. RI is the difference between systolic and diastolic pressure divided by the systolic pressure. Gosling and King[18] in 1975 showed that, analyzed in a certain way, time–velocity waveforms are sensitive to changes in impedance. They proposed the PI, the difference between peak systolic pressure and end-diastolic pressure divided by the mean maximum frequency over the entire cardiac cycle. A microcomputer is required to outline the maximum envelope of the waveform.

In 1983, Campbell and colleagues[10] developed

a new index for waveform analysis, the frequency index profile (FIP). Developed specifically for the uteroplacental arteries, the FIP consists of a complicated computerized analysis of the standard waveform. The maximum Doppler shift (f_D) is measured every 0.04 seconds throughout the cardiac cycle. Each value of f_D is divided by the mean of all the measured frequencies throughout the cardiac cycle. This is expressed as a percentage of the mean f_D. The FIP was designed to detect subtle changes in waveforms.

Clinical Applications

PLACENTAL CIRCULATION

Pregnancy places tremendous stress on the maternal circulation. Cardiac output increases in early pregnancy, reaching a peak of 30% to 50% above non-pregnant values at 20 to 24 weeks' gestation.[23] This increase in the maternal cardiac output is caused by the dramatic increase in uterine blood flow needed to satisfy the metabolic demands of the fetus. The maternal blood volume normally expands by approximately 40% to compensate for the slight drop in the mean arterial pressure.

In the placental circulation, blood enters the placenta from the fetus through the paired umbilical arteries. The blood is distributed throughout the chorionic plate to the chorionic villi, where it passes through villous capillaries and drains into a network of veins that are parallel to the arteries. Exchange of oxygen, carbon dioxide, nutrients, and waste products occurs across the villous capillaries. The blood is then returned to the fetus by way of the umbilical vein.

UMBILICAL CORD

The umbilical cord is the crucial intrauterine link between the fetal and the placental circulation. It is normally composed of two arteries and a single large vein ensheathed in Wharton's jelly for protection.

The umbilical arteries are a single-layered intima of endothelial cells resting on a medium of smooth muscle cells. Fine elastic fibrils are scattered throughout the arterial walls. The umbilical vein consists of a thin intima and a well defined internal elastic lamina. The medial subintimal smooth muscle fibers are arranged longitudinally.[13] The vessels

are arranged spirally to reduce torsion and knots that would occur if they were floating free. Doppler ultrasound can be used to determine adequacy of umbilical cord blood flow (Table 20-1).

UTERINE VASCULATURE

The blood supply to the pregnant uterus is derived chiefly from the uterine arteries. The ovarian arteries also contribute, but to a lesser degree. The main uterine artery derived from the internal iliac artery branches off once it reaches the uterus to form the arcuate arteries. The main uterine arteries circle the anterior and posterior surfaces, forming anastomoses with the arcuate arteries on the opposite side. The radial arteries branch off the arcuates and are directed into the uterine lumen to form the spiral arteries, which pass into the uterine decidua to feed the intervillous space (Fig. 20-5).

Early in pregnancy, the trophoblast invades the spiral artery in the decidua to form lakes of maternal blood. At 16 to 24 weeks, the placental cytotrophoblasts invade the spiral arteries in the

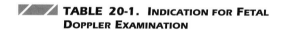

TABLE 20-1. INDICATION FOR FETAL DOPPLER EXAMINATION

Maternal disease
    Hypertension (chronic or pregnancy-induced)
    Collagen vascular disease
    Renal disease
    Diabetes (classes B, C, R, F)
    Malnutrition
    Rh or Kell sensitization
    Anemia
Suspected IUGR
    Estimated fetal weight ≤10th percentile
    Incorrect dates versus IUGR
    Unexplained oligohydramnios
Risk Factors for IUGR
    Previous IUGR infant
    Smoker >1 pack/day cigarettes
    Drug or alcohol ingestion
    Elevated maternal serum α_2-fetoprotein
    Discordant growth of multiple gestations
Other
    Umbilical cord anomaly
    Previous fetal demise
    Fetal chromosomal anomaly
    Inadequate placentation

IUGR, intrauterine growth retardation.

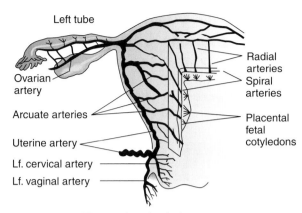

Figure 20-5. *The uterine circulation.*

Left tube

Ovarian artery

Arcuate arteries

Uterine artery

Lf. cervical artery

Lf. vaginal artery

Radial arteries

Spiral arteries

Placental fetal cotyledons

myometrium, eroding their walls and producing dilated vessels with low resistance. If this does not occur, the vessels remain constricted and exhibit increased resistance. This may place the patient at risk for preeclampsia and intrauterine growth retardation (IUGR). Early changes in uterine and arcuate artery blood flow can be detected and followed by serial Doppler flow studies.

Scanning Technique

CONTINUOUS-WAVE STUDY OF THE UMBILICAL ARTERY

Because CW Doppler systems are blind to the exact location of the Doppler signal, they may be used in conjunction with a real-time ultrasound system to aid in vessel identification. Real-time ultrasound may be useful for determining the origin of an abnormal signal, but each vessel has its own unique waveform and sound and can often be identified without real-time imaging.

The fetal umbilical artery and the maternal uterine and arcuate arteries are the vessels studied most commonly with CW Doppler. While the blood vessels are examined, the patient lies in a semirecumbent position to prevent supine hypotension.[33] To reduce Doppler scanning time, the umbilical cord can be identified with real-time sonography to guide the placement of the beam for Doppler scanning. It has been documented that arterial resistance is greater at the insertion of the umbilical cord into the fetal abdomen than at the placental cord insertion.[35] If

the placental cord insertion cannot be identified, a free loop midcord is sampled. The angle of the transducer is manipulated slightly until a strong signal is obtained.

The signal should be sharp and easily distinguished. If the borders of the peak and troughs are not clear, the gain can be raised or lowered until a distinguishable signal is obtained. The normal waveform signal looks identical to the pulsed wave Doppler waveform (Fig. 20-6). Wall filters, which filter out low-level echoes, should be set as low as possible. If the gain is lowered too much, the end-diastolic velocity may be falsely obliterated. The arterial signal should be visualized on one side of the baseline, with the steady nonpulsatile venous flow in the opposite direction. Because fetal breathing activity can alter flow ratios, it is good practice to wait until breathing stops.[33] Breathing can be identified either by an undulating venous Doppler signal or by fetal chest wall movements. Once three or four waveforms of equal height are obtained, the image is frozen while the necessary measurements are taken. A single waveform should never be used for quantitative assessment; rather, a number of sequential waveforms should be averaged to minimize beat-to-beat variation.[33]

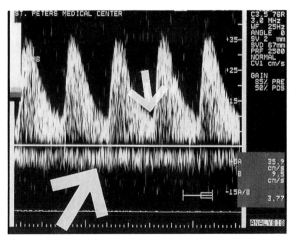

Figure 20-6. *Typical umbilical artery and vein waveform. The arterial blood flow is above the baseline. Note the clear systolic peaks of the artery with the small arrow pointing out the diastolic trough. Below the baseline is normal continuous venous flow (large arrow).*

UTERINE ARTERY

To evaluate the maternal uterine or arcuate artery with CW Doppler, the transducer should be placed parauterine in the maternal iliac fossa. Slight medial and caudal angulation may be necessary to obtain the correct signal. Slight moves are made with the transducer until the much slower maternal pulse is audible. The normal uterine arterial waveform is distinct and should have sufficient diastolic blood flow (Fig. 20-7*A*), whereas the iliac arteries will have reversed end-diastolic flow or none. Abnormal uterine arteries can give a similar waveform to that of the internal iliac artery, so care must be exercised.

Arcuate arteries are located between the umbilicus and the iliac crest on the lateral side of the uterine fundus, although the exact location varies with gestational age. Having the patient lie in the semirecumbent position makes obtaining the signal quicker and easier. The transducer can be angled medial until the proper signal is obtained (see Fig. 20-7*B*).

Pulsed-Wave Doppler

UMBILICAL ARTERY WAVEFORMS

Imaging the umbilical artery with a duplex system is fairly easy. The cord is located with the real-time transducer; a loop is identified at midcord or at the placental umbilical cord insertion,[35] and the Doppler cursor is dropped into the umbilical vessels. Because S/D, PI, and RI are angle-independent measurements, it is not necessary to correct for the angle of insonation. The umbilical waveform should demonstrate clean peaks of equal height, and umbilical vein flow should be visible in the opposite direction (see Fig. 20-6).

UMBILICAL VEIN WAVEFORMS

Umbilical venous blood flows from the placenta, through the ductus venosus, into the inferior vena cava, across the right atrium, through the foramen ovale into the left atrium, and out the left ventricle.

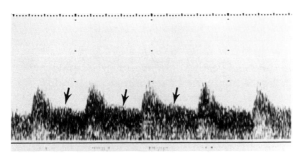

A

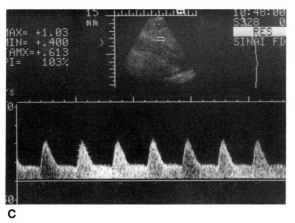

C

B

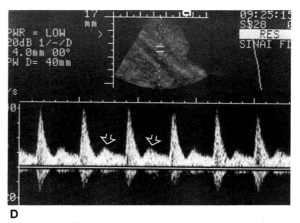

D

Figure 20-7. (**A**) Normal uterine artery waveform demonstrates a normal S/D ratio. Note the high diastolic flow (*arrows*). (**B**) Normal arcuate artery waveform on the same patient. (**C**) Duplex image of normal uterine artery. (**D**) An abnormal uterine artery at 32 weeks' gestation. Note the high S/D ratio and the arrow demonstrating the persistence of the "notch."

The rate of umbilical vein flow steadily increases with advancing gestational age and parallels fetal growth until approximately 37 weeks, after which there is a reduction. Animal studies have suggested that a major determinant of umbilical venous flow is resistance in the fetal–placental circulation.[12] Indik and Reed[22] showed that umbilical arterial flow returning to the placenta affects the flow velocity of the umbilical venous blood flow returning to the fetus, and vice versa. Umbilical venous flow should be constant and nonpulsatile (see Fig. 20-6), which means the diameter of the waveform should remain the same throughout the entire fetal cardiac cycle. When alterations in flow are noticed, it should be ascertained that the fetus is not breathing because this causes fluctuations in the flow. Umbilical vein pulsations have been associated with adverse fetal outcomes.[21] Umbilical vein pulsations are described as repetitive, persistent decreases in venous velocity that are coincident with the fetal cardiac cycle (Fig. 20-8).

UTERINE WAVEFORMS

To image the uterine artery with PW Doppler, the external iliac artery is first visualized with real-time equipment. The external iliac artery most commonly appears in the maternal iliac fossa as a large, long vessel running parallel to the uterus. The uterine artery is seen branching around the external iliac

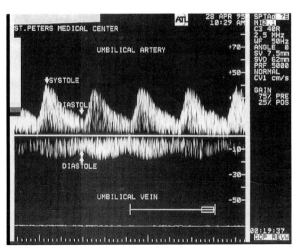

Figure 20-8. Umbilical artery and vein waveform demonstrating persistent repetitive umbilical vein pulsations (seen below the baseline) that coincide with the cardiac cycle. The double arrows point to the diastolic cycle.

artery and is located medial to the iliac artery but lateral to the uterus. The operator should try to identify the vessel first on real-time, to save actual Doppler time. If it is technically impossible to get good duplex images, the sonographer must search up and down the medial aspect of the external iliac artery until the proper signal is obtained (see Fig. 20-7C,D). Color flow can aid in quick vessel identification.

In early pregnancy and in nonpregnant women, the uterine artery waveform has a notch at the beginning of the diastolic phase of the cardiac cycle. A true notch represents a deceleration of at least 50 Hz below the maximum diastolic velocities, and rarely occurs after the 20th week of gestation. In nonpregnant women and in early pregnancy, the uterine artery waveform has a high pulsatility with reduced diastolic velocity. In the second trimester there is a decrease in impedance that continues until 24 weeks' gestation.[9] One reason for this is the invasion in the myometrial portion of the spiral arteries, which occurs around 16 weeks' gestation.[9] The presence of a notch or persistently elevated ratios may imply that the pregnancy suffers from inadequate nutrition and oxygenation. Yet another explanation may be a maternal vasospasm causing increased resistance inside the vessel.

FETAL DESCENDING AORTA

Most studies of fetal blood flow have evaluated volume flow and velocity in the aorta. In 1979, Gill used a modified eight-transducer water-path transducer to perform the first flow studies. He estimated that he achieved errors of less than 10%.[17]

Various investigators have used a linear-array transducer with a pulsed Doppler probe at a fixed angle of 45 degrees. The fixed angle helps ensure that the angle of insonation of the Doppler beam is less than 60 degrees from the direction of flow of the red blood cells.[47] The fetal descending aorta and umbilical vein are the vessels most often studied with flow velocity. The descending aorta should be examined just above the level of the diaphragm. The transducer should be parallel to the aorta. The sample gate should be opened beyond the lumen walls, to ensure even insonation of the vessel.

Gill[16] has shown that for low beam–flow angles, increasing the gate to exceed the lumen diameter compensates in part for the inadequate beam width.

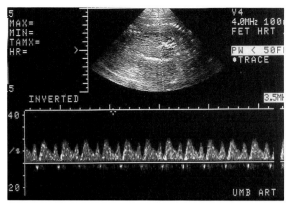

Figure 20-9. Normal inferior vena cava waveform. Note the characteristic triphasic pattern which is also seen when sampling the ductus venosus. The triphasic pattern is a result of the fetal cardiac cycle. Note the small amount of reverse blood flow which dips below the baseline in normal fetuses due to atrial contraction. (See also Color Plate 17.)

The aortic flow velocity waveform shows rapid acceleration during systole. From peak systole to end-diastole there is rapid deceleration. There is no reversal of flow during diastole in normal fetuses. At 12 to 13 weeks, there is absent end-diastolic blood flow. Diastolic flow gradually appears, suggesting a lowering of systemic vascular resistance. After 17 to 18 weeks, there is no significant decrease in the PI with advancing gestational age. The S/D, RI, and PI show little change in the third trimester, except for a slight increase in end-diastolic flow. The aortic blood flow velocity changes with increasing distance from the fetal heart.[32] This index is affected significantly by changes in the fetal heart rate and fetal behavioral state such as fetal breathing; therefore, sampling should not be done during these times.

INFERIOR VENA CAVA

In the fetal inferior vena cava (IVC), blood flows in three phases. This is demonstrated in the Doppler waveform (Fig. 20-9). The first spike is consistent with systole because forward flow occurs when the atrium relaxes. During diastole, a second peak occurs as the atrioventricular valves open. The third phase is characterized by reverse flow during late diastole. In a healthy fetus there is a significant decrease of reverse flow as the gestational age advances.

The IVC Doppler sampling should be taken immediately distal to its widening, which is its entrance into the right atrium. This site allows a truer sample of the IVC to be taken without reverberation interference from the adjacent hepatic veins and ductus venosus.

In a normal, healthy fetus, the highest peak and time–velocity integral occur during systole, followed by a smaller peak and time–velocity integral during diastole.

DUCTUS VENOSUS

The fetal ductus venosus functions exclusively in the fetal circulation. The ductus venosus forms a shunt between the umbilical vein and the IVC, allowing blood to bypass the hepatic circulation. The ductus venosus Doppler waveform should be sampled mid-sagitally immediately above the umbilical sinus or obliquely, transecting the upper fetal abdomen. The waveform is characterized by the classic triphasic pattern that is also seen in the IVC (Fig. 20-10). The ductus venosus and IVC waveforms both have triphasic patterns but are differentiated from each other first by the location of the Doppler sampling site, and second by the waveform architecture itself. The ductus venosus waveform has a high diastolic flow component, whereas the IVC does not. The waveform pattern has a systolic and early dia-

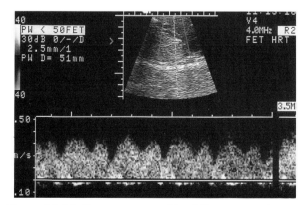

Figure 20-10. Ductus venosus blood flow pattern in a normal fetus. Note the characteristic triphasic pattern. The first spike seen is consistent with ventricular systole, the second is a result of ventricular diastole, and the sudden dip coincides with atrial systole. Also notice that there is high forward flow throughout the entire cardiac cycle. (See also Color Plate 18.)

stolic forward component with a late diastolic reverse component. Because the ductus venosus has a narrow lumen, it can demonstrate very high velocities. The average velocity in the ductus venosus is approximately three to four times higher than in the IVC and umbilical vein. Blood flow velocities in the ductus venosus increase with advancing gestational age. When evaluating the waveform, the sonographer should look at the peak systolic velocity, minimum velocity during atrial contractions, and time–average velocity.

CEREBRAL BLOOD FLOW

In a normal pregnancy, there is continuous forward flow in the fetal middle cerebral artery throughout the cardiac cycle. This high-resistance circulation results in a high Doppler reading in a normal fetus, which is actually the opposite of the case in other fetal vessels. With fetal growth retardation, there is a marked increase in internal carotid and a decrease in cerebral resistance.[50] This decrease in cerebral resistance results in a low Doppler ratio. Intrauterine asphyxia alters blood flow to the fetal organs and brain, which may ultimately cause brain damage.

To sample the middle cerebral artery, a biparietal diameter is first obtained with duplex sonography. The middle cerebral artery appears anterior to the thalamus on either side of the midline. This is the level of bifurcation into the middle and anterior cerebral arteries (Fig. 20-11 *A,B*). In normal pregnancy, the middle cerebral S/D ratio and PI decrease with advancing gestational age, signifying decreasing resistance (Fig. 20-12 *A,B*). In the face of IUGR and hypoxic stress, a drop in the middle cerebral S/D ratio and PI signify a marked decrease in resistance, and perhaps increased blood flow to the brain. This is believed to be a brain-sparing effect.

Factors That Affect Waveforms

Most investigators perform fetal Doppler studies with the patient supine or semirecumbent. According to Marsal and colleagues,[33] the patient should be semirecumbent to avoid supine hypotension. When fetal breathing occurs, flow patterns in the umbilical vein and artery are modulated (Fig. 20-13). This is because the increase in tracheal or intrapleural pressure increases venous return to the heart. Fetal breathing may be associated with an irregular heart rate, owing to respiratory sinus arrhythmia. Doppler sampling should not be performed during episodes of fetal breathing movements.

Because fetal blood flow is affected by irregularities in the fetal heart rate pattern, Doppler examination should not be performed during episodes of fetal bradycardia or tachycardia. Normal waveforms

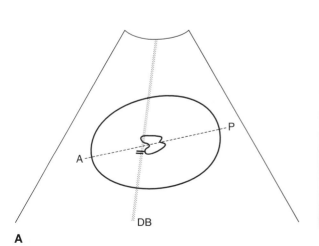

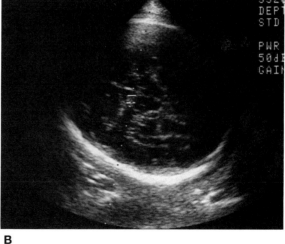

A   **B**

Figure 20-11. (**A**) Diagrammatic representation and (**B**) sonographic representation of Doppler sampling site to obtain a middle cerebral arterial waveform.

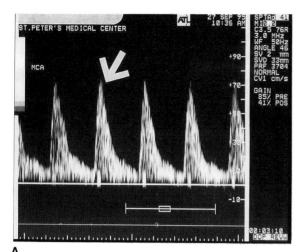

A

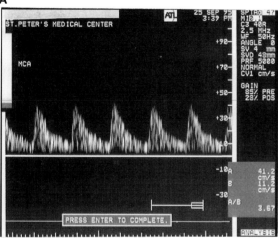

B

Figure 20-12. (**A**) A normal fetal middle cerebral artery waveform. The fetal middle cerebral artery is normally a high-resistance circuit. Note the normally high systolic peaks (*arrow*) and the low diastolic trough. In the face of fetal growth restriction or hypoxic stress, the fetal mechanism of brain sparing takes effect in an effort to protect and conserve the fetal brain, and blood is shunted away from vital organs and sent to the fetal brain (**B**), thereby creating a low-resistance circuit. Note the low systolic peak and the high diastolic flow.

are altered by changes in heart rate or rhythm. With extrasystolic beats, there is a lower peak and mean velocity. The first post-extrasystolic beat shows an increase in blood velocity that does not fully compensate for the extrasystolic beat. Compensation does occur, however, over the next three or four beats.[31,33]

The influence of pharmacologic agents on uterine and fetal blood flow is variable and controversial. Joupilla and others have observed no major change in umbilical vein flow associated with the mother's smoking or being administered oxygen, caffeine, labetolol, alcohol, or anesthesia.[25-29] Medications that alter heart rate, such as β-mimetics (Ritodrine, terbutaline) used for tocolysis, may lower Doppler S/D ratios in the fetal aorta and uterine artery, thus confusing interpretation of the waveforms.[36]

Identifying Placental and Fetal Insertion

Investigators have noted the clinical significance of the effect of waveform sampling site on Doppler ratios. This is more pronounced in the fetal umbilical circulation than in the maternal uterine circulation. The uterine circulation is composed of multiple vessels that branch and that are fed by collateral vessels, whereas the umbilical circulation consists of the umbilical cord itself. Because resistance to blood flow is greater at the fetal umbilical cord insertion than at the placental cord insertion (Fig. 20-14),[35] it is important to obtain a fetal umbilical waveform sample as close to the placental cord insertion as possible.

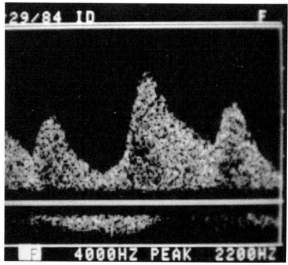

Figure 20-13. Continuous-wave Doppler waveform demonstrating alterations in the umbilical artery and vein caused by an episode of fetal breathing.

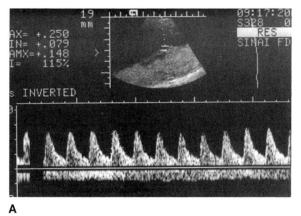
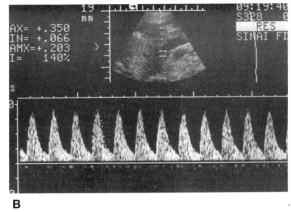

A   B

Figure 20-14. Duplex sonogram demonstrates differences in umbilical Doppler waveform depending on sampling location. (**A**) Umbilical placental insertion (mean S/D ratio, 3.1) and (**B**) fetal umbilical insertion (mean S/D ratio, 5.3).

Several theories might explain the lower ratio at the placental cord insertion than at the fetal cord site. One is that the changes in arterial diameter or wall elasticity may alter the waveform. Another is that pressure changes across the fetal abdominal wall lead to changes in resistance. The third explanation is that the decrease in the ratio may be the result of dampening and attenuation of the propagated wave. If the sampling location is not known and ratios are high, the examiner should take multiple samples at different locations along the cord to see whether the results are consistent. The accuracy of Doppler measurements depends on consistent and uniform measurement techniques.

Future Directions

Doppler ultrasound is gaining acceptance in the surveillance and management of the fetus at risk for poor perinatal or neonatal outcome. Since Doppler has been introduced, various investigators have acknowledged its usefulness as a screening tool to aid in the prediction of subsequent pregnancy complications.[6-8,11,21,37] Very high umbilical S/D ratios, absent end-diastolic flow, and complete reversal of flow have been associated with fetal and neonatal death.[5,42,48,49]

Doppler ultrasound has shown that in fetuses with asymmetric IUGR, vascular resistance increases in the aorta and umbilical artery and decreases in the middle cerebral artery. This phenom-

enon ensures blood flow to the brain at the expense of the extremities, reinforcing the head-sparing theory. Increased vascular resistance is reflected by diminished or absent umbilical diastolic flow, leading to an increased S/D ratio or PI. Extreme cases of elevated resistance causing absent or reversed umbilical end-diastolic flow velocity waveforms are associated with high rates of morbidity and mortality[42] (Fig. 20-15).

It is just as important to evaluate the maternal vessels as it is to evaluate the fetal side of the circulation. Abnormal waveform readings can be early signs of a predisposing condition and should not be ignored.[9,15,24,46] The finding of an abnormal fetal or uterine waveform necessitates careful monitoring, which should include repeated Doppler examinations, growth scans, and tests of fetal well-being. These tests may be suggested to the attending obstetrician. Doppler evidence of disease is thoroughly covered in the chapter discussing fetal abnormalities.

The advent of duplex Doppler sonography permits the sonographer to be very specific as to which vessels to study. Vessels from the umbilical cord to the intricate circle of Willis have been studied. Technology has now made it possible to study vessels with very low flow. Color flow mapping and color power Doppler have helped further our understanding of the complicated fetal circulatory pathways—not only of the vessels but of the organs they supply. It is anticipated that Doppler studies will help the clinician to

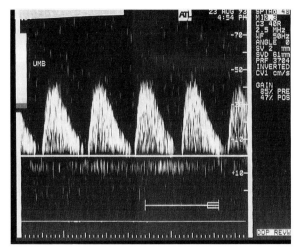

A

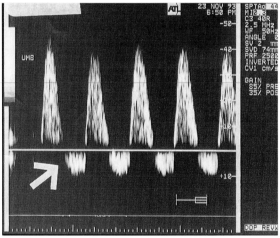

B

Figure 20-15. (**A**) Absent end-diastolic velocity (AEDV) in umbilical artery. Note the absolute lack of flow in the diastolic cycle. A high wall filter can give a false reading and mimic AEDV. (**B**) Complete reversal of blood flow in an umbilical artery. Note how the blood flow actually dips below the baseline (*arrow*) during the diastolic cycle. This is a severe finding and should be reported immediately.

take better care of the fetus in addition to providing a noninvasive means of studying the pathophysiology of disease states.

REFERENCES

1. American Institute of Ultrasound in Medicine. Bioeffect considerations of the safety of diagnostic ultrasound. J Ultrasound Med. 1988; 7(Suppl):1–6.

2. Baker DW. Pulsed ultrasonic Doppler blood flow sensing. IEEE Transsonics-Ultrasonics. 1970; 17: 170.

3. Baker DW, Watkins D. A phase-coherent pulsed Doppler system for cardiovascular measurement. In: Proceedings of the 20th Alliance for Engineering in Medicine and Biology, Stockholm. 1967; 27:2.

4. Barcroft J, Flexner LB, McClurkin T. The output of the fetal heart in the goat. J Physiol. 1934; 82:498–508.

5. Berkowitz GS, Chitkara U, Rosenberg J, et al. Sonographic estimation of fetal weight and Doppler analysis of umbilical artery velocimetry in the prediction of intrauterine growth retardation: A prospective study. Am J Obstet Gynecol. 1988; 5:1149–1153.

6. Bewley S, Cooper D, Campbell S, et al. Doppler investigation of the uteroplacental blood flow resistance in the second trimester: A screening study for pre-eclampsia and intrauterine growth retardation. Br J Obstet Gynaecol. 1991; 98:871–879.

7. Bower S, Bewley S, Campbell S. Improved prediction of pre-eclampsia by two stage screening of uterine arteries using the early diastolic notch and color Doppler imaging. Obstet Gynecol. 1993; 82:78–83.

8. Bower S, Schuchter K, Campbell S. Doppler ultrasound screening as part of routine antenatal scanning: Prediction of pre-eclampsia and intrauterine growth retardation. Br J Obstet Gynaecol. 1993; 100:989–994.

9. Campbell S, Cohen-Overbeek TE. Doppler investigation of the uteroplacental circulation during pregnancy. In: Maulick D, McNellis D, eds. Doppler Ultrasound Measurement of Maternal–Fetal Hemodynamics. New York: Perinatology Press; 1987.

10. Campbell S, Diaz-Recasens J, Griffin DR, et al. New Doppler technique for assessing uteroplacental blood flow. Lancet. 1983; 1:675–677.

11. Chan F, Pun T, Lam C, et al. Pregnancy screening by uterine artery Doppler velocimetry: Which criterion performs best? Obstet Gynecol. 1995; 85:596–602.

12. Dawes GS. The umbilical circulation. Am J Obstet Gynecol. 1962; 84:1634–1648.

13. DeSa DJ. Pathology of the placenta. In: Perrin E, ed. Pathology of the Placenta. 2nd ed. New York: Churchill Livingstone; 1984.

14. Doppler CJ. Uber das farbige Licht der Dopplersterne. Abhand Lungen der Koniglishen Bohmischen Gesellschaft der Wissenchaften. 1842; 2:465.

15. Fleisher A, Schulman H, Farmikides G, et al. Uterine artery velocimetry in pregnant women with hypertension. Am J Obstet Gynecol. 1986; 154:806–813.

16. Gill RW. Accuracy calculations for ultrasonic pulsed

Doppler blood flow measurements. Austral Phys Eng Sci Med. 1982; 5:51–57.

17. Gill RW. Measurement of blood flow by ultrasound accuracy and sources of error. Ultrasound Med Biol. 1985; 11:625–641.

18. Gosling RG, King DH. Ultrasound angiography. In: Marcus AW, Adamson L, eds. Arteries and Veins. Edinburgh: Churchill Livingstone; 1975.

19. Hill M, Lande I, Grossman J. Duplex evaluation of fetoplacental and uteroplacental circulation. In: Grant EG, White EM, eds. Duplex Sonography. New York: Springer-Verlag; 1988.

20. Hykes D, Hedrick WR, Starchman DE. Ultrasound Physics and Instrumentation. New York: Churchill Livingstone; 1995.

21. Indik J, Reed K. Umbilical venous pulsations can indicate problems with forward blood flow through the heart. In: Arduini D, Rizzo G, Romanini C, eds. Cardiac Function. New York: Parthenon Publishing Group; 1995.

22. Indik J, Reed KL. Variation and correlation in human fetal umbilical Doppler velocities with fetal breathing: Evidence of the cardiac placental connection. Am J Obstet Gynecol. 1990; 163:1792–1796.

23. Itzkovitz J. Maternal–fetal hemodynamics. In: Maulik D, McNellis D, eds. Ultrasound Measurements of Maternal–Fetal Hemodynamics. New York: Perinatology Press; 1987.

24. Jacobson SL, Inhof R, Manning N, et al. The value of Doppler assessment of the uteroplacental circulation in predicting pre-eclampsia or intrauterine growth retardation. Am J Obstet Gynecol. 1990; 162:110–114.

25. Joupilla P, Kirkinen P, Eik-Nes S. Acute effect of maternal smoking on the human fetal blood flow. Br J Obstet Gynaecol. 1983; 90:7.

26. Joupilla P, Kirkinen P, Koivula A, et al. The influence of maternal oxygen inhalation on placental and umbilical venous blood flow. Eur J Obstet Gynecol Reprod Biol. 1983; 16:151.

27. Joupilla P, Kirkinen P, Koivula A, et al. Ritodrine infusion during late pregnancy: Effects on fetal and placental blood flow, prostacyclin and thromboxane. Am J Obstet Gynecol. 1985; 151:1028.

28. Joupilla P, Kirkinen P, Koivula A, et al. Labetolol does not alter the placental and fetal blood flow or maternal prostanoids in preeclampsia. Br J Obstet Gynaecol. 1986; 93:543.

29. Kirkinen P, Joupilla P, Koivula A, et al. The effect of caffeine on placental and fetal blood flow in human pregnancy. Am J Obstet Gynecol. 1983; 147:939.

30. Kremkau F. Doppler Ultrasound. 2nd ed. Philadelphia: WB Saunders; 1995.

31. Lingman G, Dahlstrom JA, Eik-Nes SH, et al. Haemodynamic evaluation of fetal heart arrhythmias. Br J Obstet Gynaecol. 1984; 91:647.

32. Lingman G, Marsal K. Fetal central blood circulation in the third trimester of normal pregnancy: II. Aortic blood velocity waveform. Early Hum Dev. 1986; 13:151–159.

33. Marsal K, Lindblad A, Lingman G, et al. Blood flow in the fetal descending aorta: Intrinsic factors affecting movements and cardiac arrhythmias. Ultrasound Med Biol. 1984; 10:339–348.

34. Mehalek K, Berkowitz G, Chitkara U, et al. Comparison of continuous-wave and pulsed-wave S/D ratios of umbilical and uterine arteries. Am J Obstet Gynecol. 1988; 72:603.

35. Mehalek K, Rosenberg J, Berkowitz GS, et al. Umbilical and uterine artery flow velocity wave forms: Effect of the sampling site on Doppler ratios. J Ultrasound Med. 1989; 4:171–176.

36. Nimrod C, Davies D, Harder J, et al. Doppler evaluation of the impact of beta mimetic therapy on human fetal aortic and umbilical blood flow. In: Proceedings of the Society of Perinatal Obstetricians. Sixth Annual Meeting, San Antonio, February 1986.

37. North RA, Ferrier C, Long D, et al. Uterine artery Doppler flow velocity wave forms in the second trimester for the prediction of pre-eclampsia and fetal growth retardation. Obstet Gynecol. 1994; 83:378–386.

38. Nyquist H. Certain topics in telegraph transmission theory. Transactions of the American Institute of Electrical Engineering. 1928; 47:617–644.

39. Peronneau P, Deloche A, Bui-Mong-Hung H, et al. Debitmetrie ultrasonore: Developpements et applications experimentales. Eur Surg Res. 1969; 1:147.

40. Peronneau P, Hinglais H, Pellet M, et al. Velocimetre sanguin par effet Doppler a l'emission ultrasonore pulsáe. L'onde Electrique. 1970; 59:369.

41. Pourcelot L. Application clinques de l'examen Doppler transcutanie. In: Peronneau P, ed. Velometric Ultrasonor Doppler. Paris: 10 Inserm; 1974; 34:625.

42. Rochelson BL, Schulman H, Farmakides G, et al. The significance of absent end-diastolic velocity in umbilical artery velocity wave forms. Am J Obstet Gynecol. 1987; 156:1213–1218.

43. Satomura S. A study on examining the heart with ultrasonics: I. Principles. II: Instruments. Jpn Circ J. 1956; 20:227.

44. Schleif R. Ultrasound contrast agents. Current Opinion in Radiology. 1991; 3:198–207.

45. Stuart B, Drumm J, Fitzgerald DE, et al. Fetal blood velocity wave forms in normal and complicated pregnancies. Br J Obstet Gynaecol. 1980; 87:780.

46. Todros T, Ferrazz E, Arduini D, et al. Performance of Doppler ultrasonography as a screening test in low risk pregnancies: Results of a multicentic study. J Ultrasound Med. 1995; 14:343–348.

47. Tonge HM, Wladimiroff JW, Noordam MJ, et al. Blood flow velocity wave forms in the descending fetal aorta: Comparison between normal and growth-retarded pregnancies. Obstet Gynecol. 1986; 67:851–855.

48. Trudinger BJ, Giles WB, Cook CM. Flow velocity wave forms in the maternal uteroplacental and fetal umbilical placental circulation. Am J Obstet Gynecol. 1985; 152:155–163.

49. Trudinger BJ, Giles WB, Cook CM, et al. Fetal umbilical artery flow velocity wave forms and placental resistance. Br J Obstet Gynaecol. 1985; 92:23.

50. Wladimiroff JW, Tonge HM, Stewart PA. Doppler ultrasound assessment of cerebral blood flow in the human fetus. Br J Obstet Gynaecol. 1986; 93:471–475.

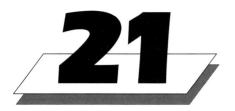

The Placenta and Umbilical Cord

LINDA M. CHASE

Accurate assessment of the placenta and umbilical cord is of considerable importance in today's ultrasound laboratory. The sonographer now has the tools to perform detailed evaluation of placental morphology and fetoplacental hemodynamics as well as placental localization. There are few "absolute associations" in placental pathology.[32] Changes in vascular resistance within the placenta can be caused by structural lesions, such as umbilical cord compression, placental tumor, or lesions consequent to maternal disease, such as hypertension or diabetes. These changes can severely compromise the fetus. Moreover, the morphology and vascular condition of the placenta and umbilical cord may suggest the presence of coincident fetal anomalies.

The extensive technological advances that have facilitated detailed sonographic study of the placenta include Doppler spectral analysis, color flow Doppler, and transvaginal and transperineal ultrasound. Many laboratories now consider transvaginal sonography to be a routine part of first trimester evaluation, and it has also become a staple in the evaluation of complications such as placenta previa and vasa previa, late in pregnancy. Color flow Doppler and conventional Doppler, used judiciously, have revolutionized fetoplacental sonography and greatly increased our understanding of normal and abnormal gestational hemodynamics. A further benefit of these advances has been to render established techniques, such as amniocentesis,

quicker, safer, and easier to perform. In addition, a variety of newer ultrasound-guided invasive procedures such as percutaneous umbilical blood sampling, chorionic villus sampling, and placental biopsy have added to the fetal diagnostic repertoire.

Placenta

PLACENTAL STRUCTURE AND FUNCTION

Placental Function

The placenta is the link between the mother and the fetus. It is where all nutritional, respiratory, and excretory exchanges that ensure fetal growth and development take place. Fetal well-being depends on an intact and uncompromised uteroplacental vascular supply.[23] Maternal disease or vascular abnormalities can affect the size, vascularization, and function of the placenta, which in turn may compromise fetal well-being.

Size, Shape, and Location

The placenta is a flattened, circular, vascular organ that weighs about 500 to 600 g at term (one sixth to one seventh of fetal weight). Attachment to the uterine wall can occur anywhere within the uterine cavity. At the fetal side is a fused layer of amnion and chorion (choroid plate) with underlying fetal vessels. At the maternal side are about 20 functional lobes, or cotyledons, composed of maternal sinusoids and chorionic villous structures (Fig. 21-1).[67] It is a relatively homogeneous organ that may exhibit varying degrees of calcification and anechoic spaces (lacunae) in later pregnancy.

The final shape attained by the placenta can be first noted by the end of the fourth month of gestation. It is almost always discoid. The cord usually inserts centrally, but it may insert eccentrically near the margins (battledore placenta) or into membranes (velamentous insertion) (Fig. 21-2).[17] In general, the wider the base of attachment, the thinner the placenta. Normally the placenta is between 1.5 and 5 cm thick,[30] although placentas thicker than 4 cm are considered abnormal by some authorities.[27] Placental volume increases linearly as pregnancy progresses, reaching a maximum well before term.[79] The ratio of placental to fetal weight is approximately 1:6.[31]

Placental Circulation

The maternal and fetal circulations are separate.[31] Oxygenated maternal blood is pumped through spiral arterioles that terminate at the base of the placenta, and enters the intervillous spaces (sinus) surrounding and bathing the villi. Gases and nutrients are exchanged across the walls of the villi, allowing nutrition, respiration, and waste removal to take place. Deoxygenated fetal blood, carried to the placenta by the umbilical arteries, circulates through capillaries in the chorionic villi within the placental lobes. The resulting oxygenated blood within the villous capilliaries returns to the fetus through the umbilical vein (see Fig. 21-1).[40,68]

During pregnancy, maternal blood volumes are increased to satisfy fetal needs. The many vascular channels and sinusoidal structure of the placenta create a low-impedance system, even lower than other fetal vascular beds, at least until late in pregnancy.[75] Doppler investigation of maternal and fetal vessels demonstrates the low-resistance nature of the placenta. Anything that causes increased placental resistance or placental insufficiency can have profound effects on the developing fetus. The term "placental insufficiency" is often used with reference to nonspecific placental deficiencies. These usually relate to increased vascular resistance within

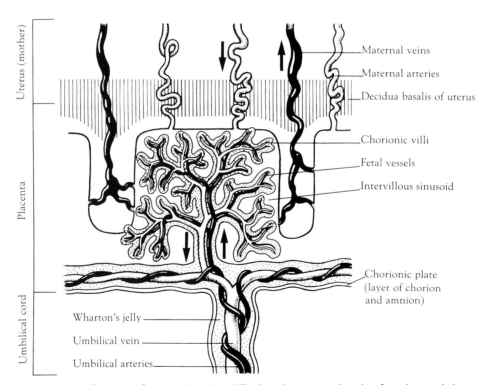

Figure 21-1. Diagram of placental and umbilical cord structure showing fetoplacental circulation. Note that the darker-appearing vessels in the diagram contain deoxygenated blood.

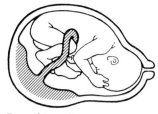

A Central insertion

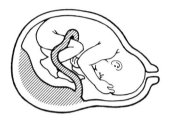

B Battledore placenta (marginal insertion)

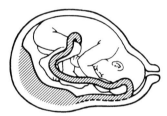

C Velamentous insertion

Figure 21-2. Umbilical cord insertions. (**A**) Central insertion of cord into placenta. (**B**) Battledore insertion. Cord is inserted near the margin or edge of the placenta. (**C**) Velamentous insertion. Cord is inserted into chorioamniotic membranes, which extend beyond the placental parenchmya and lie along the uterine wall. Location of this type of insertion near the lower uterine segment can lead to complications such as vasa previa.

the placenta, caused by either maternal or placental alterations. Doppler evaluation in compromised pregnancies provides much needed information leading to improved management of these patients. Fetoplacental Doppler is discussed in depth in Chapter 20.

SCANNING TECHNIQUES

Transabdominal, Transvaginal, and Transperineal Imaging and Doppler

Transabdominal scanning with either a sector or linear transducer provides excellent delineation of placental structure and location. Use of a sector

scanner with an anterior placenta only allows the imaging of small portions of superficial structures. The linear transducer provides a larger field of view (particularly if a dual image mode is available; Fig. 21-3). With transvaginal transducers, visualization of the placenta and umbilical cord is obtained with great clarity at a much earlier time in gestation than with transabdominal scanning. In addition, because the transducer is placed within the vagina, directly adjacent to the uterus, there is no need for a full bladder. The proximity to the os, and an empty bladder, make the transvaginal approach ideal for evaluating questionable previas late in pregnancy (Fig. 21-4).

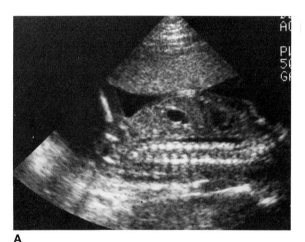

A

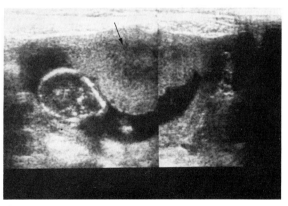

B

Figure 21-3. (**A**) Real-time sector scan of anterior placenta. Only a small portion of placenta is visualized because of small field of view provided by sector shape. (**B**) Dual-format linear scan of anterior placenta. A wider field of view than that from a static scan can be obtained. Note the subplacental uterine contraction (*arrow*).

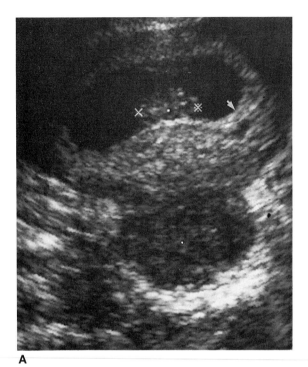

A

B

Figure 21-4. Comparison of transabdominal and transvaginal scans. (**A**) Transabdominal scan of an early pregnancy (about 8 weeks). The placental tissue is poorly defined (*arrow*). Note the fibroid located posterior to the uterus. (**B**) Transvaginal scan of the same gestation clearly defines focal thickening of the early placenta (*arrow*).

Transperineal ultrasound is a relatively new procedure that is proving to be a valuable adjunct to obstetric ultrasound protocols when transvaginal imaging is not available or contraindicated, particularly in assessing low-lying placentas.[25,33] Often in late second or third trimester pregnancies, the endocervical canal is obscured transabdominally, because of obstructive fetal parts and the inability to maintain a full bladder. With transperineal ultrasound, this area can be clearly imaged in most cases. With the transducer placed directly on the maternal perineum, it is possible to obtain an image similar to that obtained transvaginally, with less discomfort to the patient.[26,77]

In the past few years, valuable information has been obtained from conventional and color flow Doppler studies of the umbilical cord and placenta. For example, evaluation of the systolic–diastolic ratio in the uterine artery and evaluation for the persistence of an early diastolic notch have been demonstrated to be effective predictors of perinatal outcome, because they relate directly to increased placental or umbilical impedence.[53] Use of pulsed-wave Doppler may expose the fetus to higher energy intensities than are consistent with safety. It is suggested that Doppler be used on the fetus only when a study is clinically indicated, and that power output, color sector size, and examination time be kept to a minimum.[35]

Is a Full Bladder Important?

For most transabdominal applications, the answer is a qualified "yes." A properly full bladder enhances placental visualization in early pregnancy and improves imaging of the lower uterine segment later in gestation (Fig. 21-5). This latter point is particularly relevant when a diagnosis of placenta previa is being considered. An empty bladder may preclude visualization of the cervical os, but an overdistended bladder can cause a false-positive appearance of placenta previa (Fig. 21-6). A very full bladder causes close apposition of the anterior and posterior walls of the lower uterine segment, producing what appears to be the internal cervical os at a falsely superior location. The sonographer can improve patient comfort and reduce the possibility of false-positive images of placenta previa by varying the degree of bladder distention during the examination (i.e., start with full bladder, then have the patient empty 1 cup of urine at a time).[43] In general, a bladder is

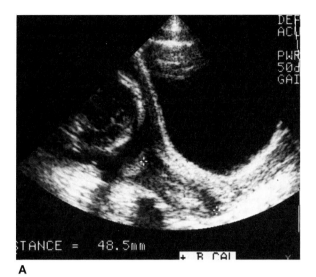
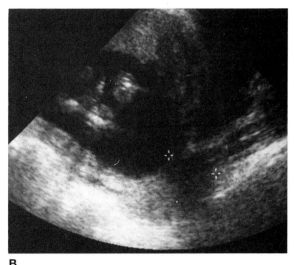

A   **B**

Figure 21-5. (**A**) Sector scan of the lower uterine segment showing an adequately full bladder. The cervix measures 4.8 cm, which is within normal limits. (**B**) Sector scan of the lower uterine segment with an inadequately full bladder. The entire lower segment, including the cervix, is difficult to visualize.

considered adequately full when cervical length is between 3 and 5 cm.[39] To relieve severe discomfort in late second and third trimester pregnancies, once the cervical area has been evaluated, the patient may void before the remainder of the examination is performed.

Because the transvaginal examination is best performed with an empty bladder,[73] it may be better tolerated in late pregnancy and can be a valuable tool in assessing placenta previa. It should be noted, however, that although no adverse effects of the use of transvaginal imaging have been confirmed,[38] in some laboratories transvaginal scanning is prohibited if vaginal bleeding has occurred during the

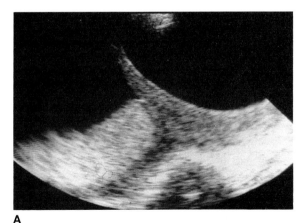
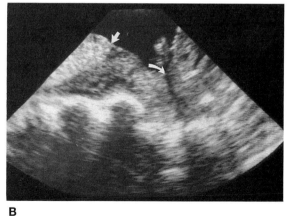

A   **B**

Figure 21-6. (**A**) Sector scan of overdistended bladder. The cervix is not easily measured and the position of the internal os is unclear. Because of the compression of the lower uterine segment, the edge of the placenta appears to cover the internal os. (**B**) Postvoid scan of same patient. The internal os (*curved arrow*) is now seen to be clearly separate from the edge of the placenta (*straight arrow*).

pregnancy. In such cases, transperineal scanning may suffice.

Transducer, Angle, Frequency, and Gain Settings

A 3- or 3.5-MHz transducer is adequate for most routine imaging of the placenta. A lower-frequency transducer may be needed to improve visualization in large patients, late in the third trimester, or when the fetus lies over a posterior placenta. Most newer-generation, real-time units allow the user to control electronically the focal zone of the transducer.

When scanning the placenta, the beam should be as perpendicular as possible to the chorionic plate, especially when measuring thickness. Gains should be adjusted so that the placenta has a uniform and homogeneous granular texture. Both the sharp, linear acoustic interface of the chorionic plate and the hypoechoic retroplacental zone should be seen clearly (Fig. 21-7). Differentiation of placental tissue from that of a uterine contraction or myoma depends on clear visualization of these structures, particularly because posterior contractions may appear as echogenic as pla-

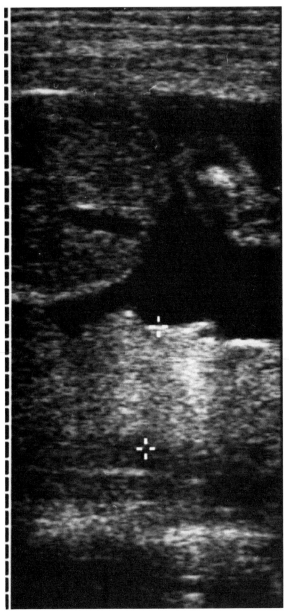

Figure 21-8. Real-time linear scan of posterior placenta showing placement of cursors for measurement of placental thickness. Beam is perpendicular to the midpoint of the placenta, and the retroplacental complex is not included in the measurement.

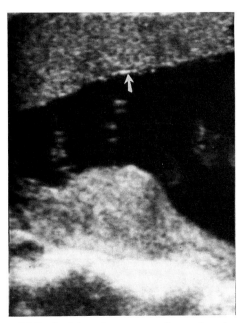

Figure 21-7. Real-time linear scan of anterior placenta showing distinct chorionic plate (*arrow*). Note increased echogenicity of posterior uterine contraction due to the transsonicity of the amniotic fluid.

cental tissue. In such cases, other than waiting 20 to 30 minutes for disappearance of a contraction, the only way to prove that a particular tissue mass is placental is to demonstrate areas of placental demarcation.[20,68] The gains may have to be reduced with posterior placentas to offset enhanced acoustic trans-

▨▨▨▨ **TABLE 21-1. DISEASE STATES IN RELATION TO PLACENTAL APPEARANCE**[17,61,68]

Increased Placental Thickness (>5 cm)	Decreased Placental Thickness (<1.5 cm)	Early Placental Maturation	Delayed Placental Maturation
Diabetes (nonvascular types)	Preeclampsia	IUGR	Gestational diabetes
Rh disease (hydropic changes)	IUGR	Hypertension	Rh disease
Cytomegalovirus infection	Juvenile diabetes (vascular forms)		
Abruption*	Placentation abnormality		
Chorioangioma	(membraneous placenta)		
Multiple gestation			
Syphillis			
Chrosomal abnormality (triploidy)			

* Apparent thickening due to retroplacental clot, isoechoic with placenta.[17]
IUGR, intrauterine growth retardation.

mission from the overlying amniotic fluid. It is also important not to confuse a retroplacental contraction (see Fig. 21-3*B*) with the retroplacental complex of maternal veins. Increasing the gain to visualize flowing blood during real-time observation can be useful in distinguishing placental lakes or retroplacental vascular structures from other hypoechoic placental or retroplacental masses. The use of color Doppler aids in this evaluation.

Measurement of Placental Thickness

The sonographer should first identify the placentomyometrial interface in a midpoint position that (in a posterior placenta) is as free of fetal shadowing as possible. The measurement should exclude the myometrium and retroplacental complex, and the transducer should be perpendicular to the placenta, lest the resultant measurement be falsely high (Fig. 21-8).[27] Evaluation of this measurement should take into consideration the shape of the placenta. For example, a broad-based placenta may be thinner

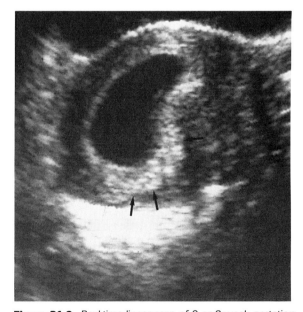

Figure 21-9. Real-time linear scan of 8 or 9-week gestation showing focal thickening along one side of gestational sac (*arrows*), representing early placental formation.

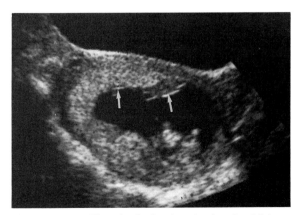

Figure 21-10. The chorionic plate is already visible as bright linear echoes on this sector scan of an early placenta (*arrows*). A smaller portion of this membrane can be appreciated in a sector scan than in a static or linear scan (see Fig. 21-7*B*) because the beam is perpendicular to less of this specular reflector at any point in a sector scan.

and a narrow-based placenta thicker, without indicating the presence of any lesion.

NORMAL SONOGRAPHY OF THE PLACENTA

Scanning Protocol

Placental evaluation should be part of every obstetric scan. The location of the placenta must be noted, especially its relation to the internal cervical os. If there is an accessory, or succenturiate lobe, its location must be noted as well, along with the position of the connecting tissue or membranes. Structural texture and morphology of the placenta and the insertion site of the cord should be evaluated, and any abnormalities noted. Placental thickness should be determined and correlated with clinical data (Table 21-1). If there has been any vaginal bleeding or abdominal pain, the retroplacental area should be carefully assessed for possible areas of elevation.

Morphology

The early placenta is usually visualized by 8 to 10 weeks as focal thickening of the decidua surrounding the gestational sac (Fig. 21-9). By 12 weeks, the placenta is clearly visualized as a discoid structure with a homogeneous granular texture. The sharp, linear acoustic interface of the chorionic plate on the fetal side of the

placenta can usually be identified at this stage (Fig. 21-10).[17] Other than the site of cord insertion, the subchorionic area usually appears smooth and uninterrupted throughout most of pregnancy. However, later in pregnancy this chorionic interface becomes less smooth as more fetal vessels develop just below the placental surface.[51] Work with transvaginal probes with color flow Doppler has demonstrated the low-resistance, high diastolic blood flow characteristic of the normal placenta as early as 5 weeks' gestation.[28] Even without use of Doppler, red blood cell movement may be demonstrated by scanning at increased gain settings. In this manner, subchorionic and intraplacental vascular structures may be differentiated from other, nonvascular, pathologic entities.[17,30,64] Turning the transducer 90 degrees to demonstrate the tubular nature of an unknown structure provides another clue to suggest that it is vascular (Fig. 21-11). Occasionally, an area of the chorionic plate may be seen that appears separated from the placenta. This could represent an area of prior placental (subchorionic) hemorrhage and may be correlated with a previous episode of vaginal bleeding.

Intraplacental Texture

Placental texture changes from an echogenic focal thickening of the wall of the gestational sac early in pregnancy, to the fine, granular, homogeneous

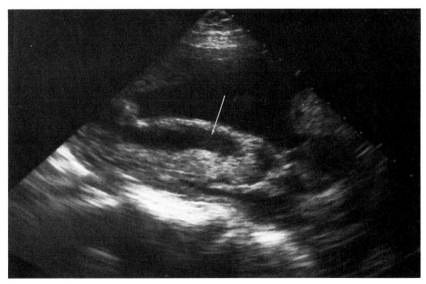

Figure 21-11. Sector scan of subchorionic tubular, lucent space in posterior placenta (*arrow*). Real-time scanning, showing movement of red blood cells, confirmed its vascular nature.

texture seen from the end of the first trimester. This texture continues throughout most of the pregnancy and is usually retained in the older placenta. However, in the second and third trimesters, intraplacental and subchorionic vascular spaces may sometimes be seen and should be assessed carefully. Although they usually have no clinical significance (Fig. 21-12*A*), any areas of varied echogenicity; a multiple cystic or vesicular appearance; irregular, hypoechoic areas; or highly echogenic areas with hypoechoic margins should be carefully documented. When very large, some of these placental findings have been seen in association with increased levels of maternal serum α-fetoprotein. A late third trimester placenta may exhibit cystic areas located centrally within clearly delineated lobes. These are not vascular and are thought to represent areas of necrosis (see Fig. 21-12*B*).[9]

The Retroplacental Complex

No assessment of the placenta is complete without evaluation of the retroplacental complex (RPC). This zone is composed of the decidua basalis and portions of the myometrium, including maternal veins draining the placenta. It is consistently imaged after 21 weeks regardless of placental position,[20,40,54] and mea-

sures on average 9.5 mm (Fig. 21-13).[54] Proper identification of this area is important. A prominent anterior RPC can lead to excessive bleeding during invasive procedures such as amniocentesis or cesarean section. In addition, the RPC can mimic abruptio placentae, degenerating fibroids, or hydatidiform mole. Real-time visualization of blood flow in this area helps distinguish the normal RPC from the aforementioned pathologic conditions.[20,40]

Sonographically, the RPC appears as a hypoechoic subplacental region containing many horizontal linear echoes representing venous channels.[40,45,68] Large venous channels may be visualized within the complex, most commonly in posteriorly located placentas, where the effects of gravity-induced pressure can overdistend the veins.[40,68] The appearance of large venous channels may also occur when the beam strikes tangentially, as with a fundal or lateral placenta.[68]

Normal Placental Calcification

Placental calcium deposition is a normal physiologic process occurring throughout pregnancy. More than 50% of placentas show some degree of macroscopic calcification after 33 weeks.[64,68] Although the degree of normal calcification is variable, it usu-

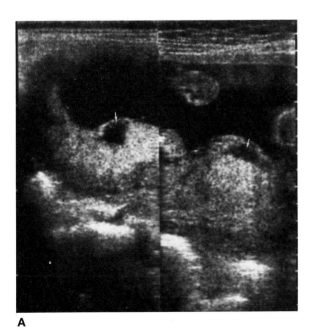
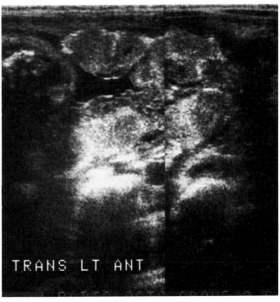

A   **B**

Figure 21-12. **(A)** Dual-format linear scan showing two views of a large subchorionic venous lake (*arrows*). **(B)** Dual-format linear scan of a mature placenta demonstrating calcifically delineated cotyledons with centrally located sonolucent areas.

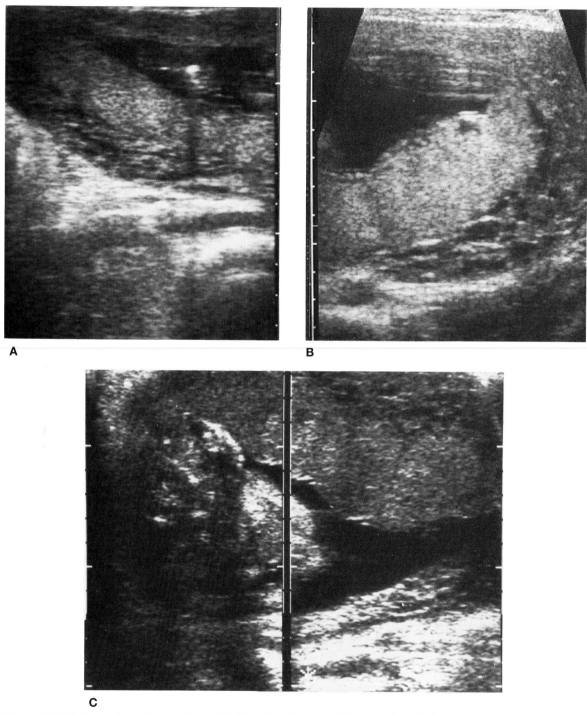

A

B

C

Figure 21-13. Retroplacental complexes. (**A**) Posterior placenta, (**B**) posterolateral placenta, and (**C**) anterior placenta showing the convoluted, tubular maternal draining veins that are part of the retroplacental complex.

ally increases throughout pregnancy, becoming more prominent as first the basal area and then the interlobar septa calcify (Fig. 21-14).[17] Calcium may also be found in the villous, perivillous, and subchorionic spaces.[17,68] Intraplacental calcifications are imaged sonographically as strong acoustic echoes without significant acoustic shadowing.[68]

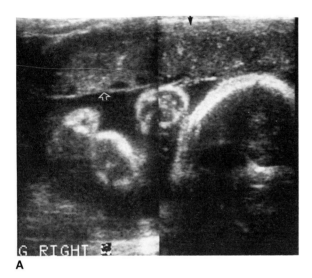

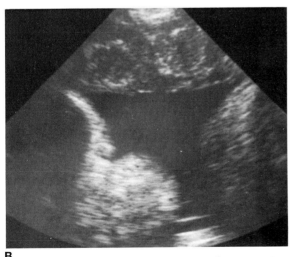

Figure 21-14. (**A**) Dual-format linear scan of an anterior grade II placenta with basal echogenicities (*arrow*) and comma-like densities (*open arrow*). (**B**) Sector scan of grade III placenta showing septal calcifications delineating cotyledons. Note the more sonolucent appearance of the central echoes. These sonolucencies are better visualized in Figure 21-12*B*.

PLACENTAL GRADING

A grading system based on the degree of placental calcification (Table 21-2) was at one time thought to be an indicator of fetal pulmonary maturity. It is now known that multiple factors, including smoking, low maternal age, parity, and even season of the year can affect the degree of placental calcification,[30,49,57,65,68] and it is no longer considered a marker for lung maturity.

More to the point, assessment of placental calcification is important in certain serious maternal and fetal conditions. For example, premature placental calcification can occur in maternal hypertensive states and in association with intrauterine growth retardation; and other conditions such as gestational diabetes or fetal cardiopulmonary disorders may retard the rate of placental calcification. Therefore, evaluating placental maturity in relation to the age of gestation can give additional, important input to the entire clinical picture.[50,61]

ABNORMALITIES OF THE PLACENTA

Table 21-3 lists the common placental abnormalities and their sonographic appearances.

Abnormal Shape and Configuration

BILOBED PLACENTA (SUCCENTURIATE LOBE). Although it usually consists of one mass, the placenta may be bilobed or have a smaller accessory, succenturiate lobe. This occurs in 0.14% to 3.0% of cases (Fig. 21-15).[68] The accessory lobe is connected to the main placental mass either by vessels within a membrane or by a bridge of chorionic tissue.[68] Delineation of the umbilical cord insertion into the placenta identifies the main placental mass.[51] Identification of an accessory lobe is clinically relevant due to the high risk of postpartum hemorrhage associated with retained accessory lobes.[17,64] There is also a risk of massive intrapartum fetal bleeding secondary to rupture of connecting vessels between the lobes.[67] This may lead to fetal anemia, shock, and even death.[51] Therefore, sonographic delineation of placental tissue in more than one area of the uterus, and if possible the connecting bridge between the two placental masses, especially if it overlies the os, is a valuable contribution to management of the obstetric patient.[17,30] Care should be taken not to confuse a fold in the placenta with an extra lobe.

▰▰▰▰ **TABLE 21-2. PLACENTAL GRADING BASED ON PLACENTAL CALCIFICATIONS**

1. Placental Grading[17,18]
     Grade 0 No calcifications (to about 31 wk)
              I Scattered calcifications (31–36 wk)
              II Basal calcifications (36–38 wk)
              III Basal and interlobar septal calcifications (38 wk to term)
2. The placenta matures considerably after the 40th week.
3. Two parts of the placenta may have different grades,[18] in which case the highest grade is assigned.
4. Most term pregnancies have grade I or II placentas.
5. Only about 10%–15% of term placentas are grade III.

CIRCUMVALLATE PLACENTA. In 1% to 7% of deliveries, the area of placental implantation extends beyond the limits of the chorionic plate. A rim forms around this margin of placenta that does not have associated chorion (Fig. 21-16). The rim consists of fibrinoid tissue with hyaline degeneration of villi. Presence of circumvallate placenta may be associated with maternal bleeding, and may be one cause of amniotic band or sheet development.[41,51] Sonographically, circumvallate placenta may be seen as irregular subchorionic or subamniotic marginal cystic structures or infolding of the placental margin.[51]

ABNORMAL MEMBRANES/AMNIOTIC BANDS. Before fusion at about 16 weeks' gestation, the amnionic and chorionic membranes are separated by the extraembryonic coelom. A floating membrane seen before this time is thought to represent the not-yet-fused amnion. Floating membranes seen after 16 weeks may represent a separation of the fused membranes or separation of both membranes from the decidua. This may be present without complications or may be associated with vaginal bleeding of varying degrees. Before 16 weeks, the amnion itself may rupture and collapse, leaving the fetus to develop as an "extraamniotic pregnancy" within the extraamniotic coelom.[51]

Sonographically, a collapsed amnion may be seen as multiple, wavy linear echoes in the dependent portion of the uterus. Amniotic bands, on the other hand, are seen as linear echoes traversing the amniotic cavity (Fig. 21-17). The consequences of amniotic bands to the fetus vary widely. Although in most cases they do not disturb the fetus, fetal entanglement with these membranes, refered to as the amniotic band syndrome, can result in limb deformities and spine and facial abnormalities of varying degrees of severity, and may even result in

amputation of compromised body parts.[51] A variant of the amniotic band, the amniotic sheet or shelf, is seen as a thicker and broader floating membrane with only one free edge. This is thought to represent a deep fold of the chorion and may also restrict fetal movement.[51] Follow-up sonographic evaluation to document any fixation of fetal parts is necessary.

ANNULAR PLACENTA AND PLACENTA MEMBRANACEA. Annular placenta refers to a ring-shaped placenta that attaches circumferentially to the myometrium. Placenta membranacea refers to a rare condition in which there is no differentiation of chorion frondosum from chorion laeve, and placental villi cover all or most of the surface of the gestational sac. The placenta is usually much thinner than normal.[51] Both the annular placenta and placenta membranacea have been associated with antepartum and postpartum hemorrhage. Neither has been detected sonographically,[48] but there is no reason why antenatal visualization may not be possible in the future. A placenta membranacea would be diagnosed if placental tissue were seen over most of the uterine cavity.[68]

Abnormal Placental Size

Variation in placental size may be indicative of several important fetal and maternal pathologic conditions (see Table 21-1). Much research has been conducted to determine the best sonographic means of assessing placental size in relation to gestational age. Although surface area and volumetric measurements show this relationship best, their determination is extremely time consuming, cumbersome, and impractical,[17,64] requiring serial images of the placenta no more than 2 cm apart and the application of complicated equations.[17,79] Thick-

Abnormality	Description	Sonographic Characteristics	Differential Diagnosis
Placenta previa	Placental tissue obstructing internal os. Most common cause of bleed in 2nd and 3rd trimester	Placental tissue seen to cover internal os—whether completely, partially or marginally.	Uterine contraction, fibroid, overdistended bladder may falsely suggest previa
Abruption	Premature separation of all or part of the placenta	Elevated portion of placenta or extramembraneous[18] retroplacental, subchorionic, or intraplacental,[64] hypoechoic or complex, transsonic mass of varying echogenicity.[45] May appear as normal placenta. May appear as thickened placenta.[45]	Retroplacental thrombosis, normal placenta, abnormally thick placenta, normal retroplacental complex
Placenta accreta	Decidual formation defect with abnormal placental attachment to uterine wall[61]	Normal retroplacental hypoechoic area not visualized.	Myometrial scar
HYPOECHOIC LESIONS			
Fibrin depositions	Secondary to vascular thrombosis and cystic degeneration of fibrin	Anechoic areas in intervillous spaces beneath chorion. Lack of real-time evidence of blood flow.[17,64]	Venous lakes, hematoma
Hematoma	Area of retroplacental or intraplacental clot	May be hypoechoic or of varied echogenicity depending on age of clot. Lack of real-time evidence of blood flow.	Venous lakes, fibrin deposition
Intervillous thrombi	Interplacental areas of hemorrhage and pooling of blood; increase in Rh isoimmunization[17,68]	Hypoechoic areas of varying size throughout placenta.	Hematoma
Breus' mole	Massive subchorionic thrombosis—rare—secondary to extreme venous obstruction; unrelated to fibrin deposition[17,68]	Extensive hypoechoic hematoma without evidence of venous flow.[68]	Placental tumor, fibroid, hematoma[17,68]
Infarct[51]	Result of obstruction of spiral arteries	No confirmed sonographic appearance, but necrotic infarct may appear hypoechoic or show placental thinning.	Retroplacental hematoma, fibrin deposition
Placental lake	Subchorionic blood-filled spaces	Subchorionic, anechoic, tubular spaces. Flow may be demonstrated.	Fibrin depositions
NEOPLASTIC LESIONS			
Chorioangioma	Tumor resulting from vascular malformation[68]; most common placental tumor—benign—may be multiple, small or single large; associated with fetal edema[56,67,78]	Usually isoechoic; placenta may show as placental thickening without discrete mass.[17,56] Large mass may extend from fetal surface of placenta. Associated with hydramnios—may see vascular channels within mass.	Fibroid, Breus' mole
Teratoma	Rare, benign to highly malignant germ cell tumor	Complex, heterogeneous mass; may have calcifications.	Fibroid

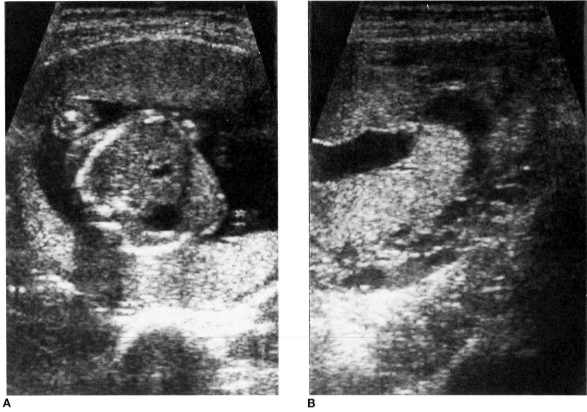

A   **B**

Figure 21-15. (**A**) A bilobed placenta showing both an anterior and posterior component. The connecting membrane is not visible. (**B**) Posterior placenta with anterior accessory lobe. The connecting membrane is well visualized.

ness is more variable and less accurate than volume, being a function of gestational age, placental location, and transducer angle; however, because it is easier to measure, thickness is used routinely.

As a general rule, after 23 weeks the placenta should be no thinner than 1.5 cm or thicker than 5.0 cm. An abnormally thick placenta can be seen in association with maternal gestational diabetes (due to villous edema) or in any case of placental hydrops, which is associated with fetal cardiac overload. A thin placenta (≤1.5 cm) may be seen in pregnancies complicated by essential maternal hypertension and preeclampsia, and with intrauterine growth retardation and placental infarction.[68]

PLACENTAL HYDROPS. The abnormal thickness of a hydropic placenta is due to fluid overload, usually secondary to high-output cardiac failure in the fetus. This can occur in erythroblastosis fetalis (immune hydrops; Fig. 21-18), fetomaternal and twin-to-twin transfusion syndromes, chorioangioma (in which fetal blood is shunted through the placental circulation), and vascular obstruction such as umbilical vein thrombosis.[7,8] Sonography of the hydropic placenta shows it to be abnormally thick (usually ≥5.0 cm—it may reach 8 to 10 cm), and it assumes a more rigid, bulbous appearance. The normal placental architecture is lost and a "ground-glass" appearance is seen.[22,58]

Abnormal Placental Location (Placenta Previa)

When the placenta partially or completely covers the internal cervical os, the patient is said to have placenta previa. Total placenta previa occurs when implantation of the placenta crosses the internal os. Sonographically, the body of the placenta is seen to cover the os completely (Fig. 21-19). When just the edge of the placenta is seen to abut or cover

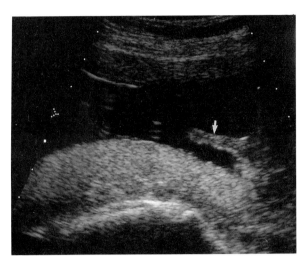

Figure 21-16. Linear scan of circumvallate placenta. Note infolding of the rim of the placenta (*arrow*), representing the portion of placental tissue not covered by chorion. (Courtesy of Catherine Carr-Hoefer, RT, RDMS, RDCS, RVT, Sonographer Coordinator, Good Samaritan Hospital, Corvallis, Oregon.)

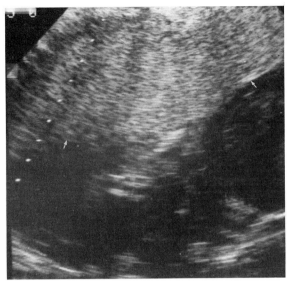

Figure 21-18. Sector scan of an enlarged anterior placenta (*arrows*) in a confirmed Rh-immunosensitive pregnancy. The perpendicular thickness measurement is over 5 cm. Note the increased echogenicity of the placental tissue.

the os, it is described as a marginal, or partial placenta previa (Fig. 21-20). In these cases, implantation does not cross the os. If the edge of the placenta is near but not abutting the os, it is classified as a low-lying placenta (Fig. 21-21).

Although clinically significant placenta previas are uncommon (less than 1% of deliveries[68]), placenta previa is frequently seen in clinical sonography. Up to 93%

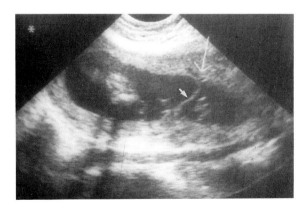

Figure 21-17. Gestational sac with amniotic band (*arrow*) extending from two portions of a lateral placenta, which gives the appearance of being both anterior and posterior in this plane. No limb entanglement was evidenced at this time.

of these patients experience significant, painless vaginal bleeding requiring sonographic evaluation.[36] Indeed, placenta previa is said to be the cause of most third trimester bleeding.[20,68,72] Most authorities agree (although there is some dissension[21]) that placenta previa is the result of an abnormally low implantation of the conceptus. It is more common in patients with previous lower uterine incisional scars for cesarean section or myomectomy. Placenta previa seems to be more prevalent in older women and in multiparas. It is thought that myometrial scarring leads to the development of a poorly vascularized, thinner placenta, which occupies a greater uterine surface area, increasing the probability of encroachment on the cervical os.[36]

Although a sonographic diagnosis of placenta previa can be made with considerable accuracy,[20] it is important that the sonographer bear several facts in mind. This diagnosis cannot be made before 34 to 36 weeks, unless more than one third of the placenta covers the internal os.[30] The reason for this is that in most suspected second trimester placenta previa cases, apparent "placental migration" (caused by late second and early third trimester differential growth of the lower uterine segment) results in a normal implantation at term (63% to 91% of cases).[30,34,74] On the other hand, a persistent placenta previa may be diagnosed as

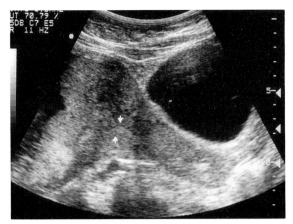

Figure 21-19. Sector scan of complete placenta previa. Placental tissue is attached to uterine wall on both sides of the os and completely covers the os. The slightly echogenic mucosa of the endocervical canal is outlined by the arrows. (Courtesy of Harris L. Cohen, MD, Professor of Radiology and Director of Division of Diagnostic Ultrasound, State University of New York University Hospital at Brooklyn/Kings County Hospital Center, Brooklyn, New York.)

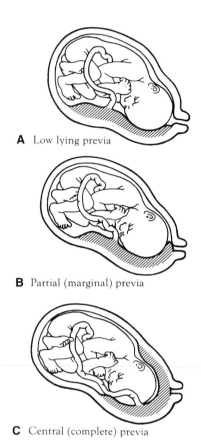

A Low lying previa

B Partial (marginal) previa

C Central (complete) previa

Figure 21-21. Diagram of three types of placentae previa. (**A**) In low-lying placenta, the edge of the placenta is visualized near the os. (**B**) In marginal or partial previa, placental tissue may cover the os but is not attached to the wall at the other side. (**C**) In complete previa, placental tissue completely covers the internal os and is attached to the uterine wall on both sides of the os.

early as 20 weeks, if the placenta is shown completely to cover the internal os.

The clinical course and outcome of placenta previa are related to the degree of cervical os encroachment. It is important for the sonographer to

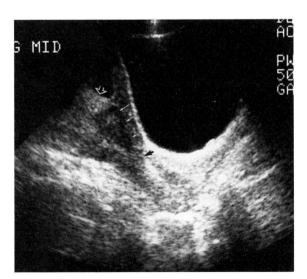

Figure 21-20. Sector scan of a marginal previa. Note that the placenta (*open arrow*) covers the area of the os (*closed arrow*) but is not attached to the uterine wall on the other side. The edge of the placenta has been elevated by a marginal hematoma (*small arrows*).

try to establish the degree of previa that is present. A placenta located less than 2 cm from the internal os usually requires a cesarean section because of maternal bleeding.[51]

The knowledge of several technical points and ultrasound techniques can help in the diagnosis of placenta previa. A focal, symmetric, lower uterine segment contraction can be mistaken for placenta previa.[36] Repeat scanning after waiting for a half hour should show in the case of a contraction that it has subsided. The sonographer can vary the degree of bladder distention to decrease the rate of false-positive diagnosis. This technique can also help to determine more accurately the type of previa present. In late pregnancy, it may be necessary to scan through a fairly empty bladder, making transabdominal visualization of the cervical area difficult; however, as a rule of thumb, if a third trimester placenta is shown to cover the fundus, chances of a previa are small, because most placentas are unlikely to extend from the fundus to the cervix.[30] Exceptions to this may occur if the placenta is thin and flat, covering a greater area of the intrauterine surface, or if an accessory lobe is present in association with the lower segment. In these cases, transvaginal or transperineal scanning can usually provide additional diagnostic information.

When in doubt, it is most important to err on the side of caution and assume the presence of placenta previa. A false-positive diagnosis early in pregnancy, to be reassessed at a later date, does not harm the mother or fetus, whereas a missed diagnosis is potentially catastrophic. The usual causes of missed diagnosis are poor technique and poor visualization of a posterior placenta obscured by an overlying fetal head. It has been suggested that a measurement of less than 1.0 cm between the fetal head and the maternal sacrum, measured in a mid-sagittal plane, rules out placenta previa (Fig. 21-22), and a measurement of less than 1.5 cm makes a previa unlikely.[51] In the case of a questionable anterior placenta previa, the same measure-

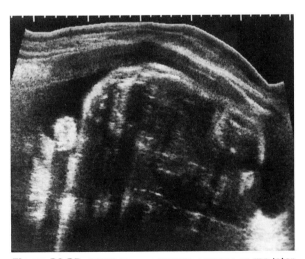

Figure 21-22. Static scan of placenta previa. In the later stages of pregnancy, especially with a posterior placenta, it is not always easy to visualize the cervical area. In those cases, the sonographer should measure the distance from the presenting part (in this case, the fetal back) to the bright echoes of the maternal sacrum. A measurement of over 1.5 cm indicates the possibility of intervening placental tissue. The measurement here is about 4 cm.

ments apply between the presenting area and the maternal bladder.[18] But if the placenta is compressed or lateral in location, this distance can be smaller, and placenta previa is still not excluded.

Retroplacental Hemorrhage (Placental Abruption)

Placental abruption refers to the premature separation of all or part of the placenta from the underlying myometrium. Abruption has been associated with, among other things, maternal vascular disease, maternal hypertension, trauma, a short umbilical cord, as well as increased maternal age.[67] Abruption may manifest itself in three ways: as external bleeding without significant intrauterine hematoma, as the development of a retroplacental or marginal hematoma with or without external bleeding, and as formation of a submembranous clot at a distance from the placenta, with or without external bleeding.[68] Clinically, patients may be asymptomatic, or may be quite ill with acute hemorrhage and shock, presenting with a rigid abdomen and severe uterine contractions. Fetal death may occur.[51] It is important to recognize that the bleeding associated with abruption is usually painful (especially when retroplacental in location). Although it is classically described as a cause of up to one third of third trimester bleeding, it can occur earlier in pregnancy as well.[68,76]

The sonographic appearance of retroplacental hemorrhage is varied, depending on its location, size, and age.[20,45,68] The hematoma is usually hypoechoic or of mixed echogenicity, and its echogenicity increases as the clot becomes more organized.[52,56,68,76] As the hematoma matures, it may appear isoechoic with the placenta. In such cases, the placenta at first glance may appear to be abnormally thick; however, differentiation of the placenta from the underlying clot can often be made by having the patient lie on her side. This provides a different angle of access to the ultrasound beam and may allow for visualization of the interface between the hematoma and the placenta. If the hematoma is near the lower uterine segment, transperineal ultrasound may provide more diagnostic information (Fig. 21-23).[24,45]

The diagnosis of retroplacental abruption is usually based on clinical symptoms such as abnormal bleeding, fetal distress, acute abdominal pain,

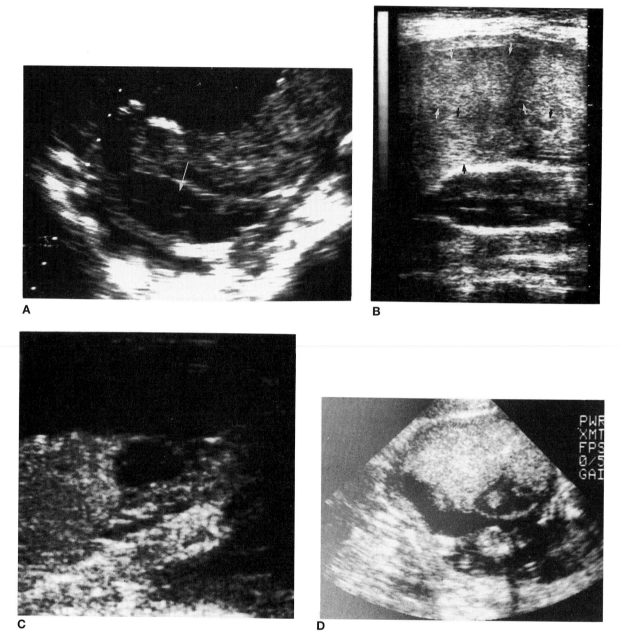

Figure 21-23. Placental abruption. (**A**) Subplacental abruption (*arrow*) in which a large portion of placental tissue has lifted away from the subjacent myometrium. The sonolucent appearance of the hematoma would indicate that the damage was very recent, although the presence of a few internal echoes might indicate that some clotting has taken place. (**B**) Linear scan of placental abruption, which has the appearance of a hydropic placenta because the acoustic texture of the subplacental hematoma (*white arrows*) is isodense with that of the placental tissue (*black arrows*). The echogenic appearance of the hematoma indicates a clot of several days' standing. (**C**) Linear scan of marginal hematoma, showing an area of recent bleeding. (**D**) Sector scan of a subchorionic hematoma. This was secondary to bleeding after amniocentesis.

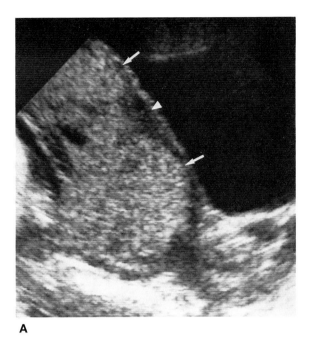

A

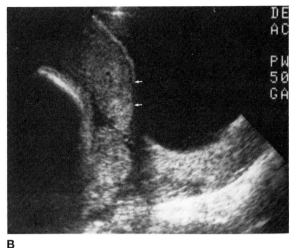

B

Figure 21-24. (**A**) Sector scan of a full placenta previa with coincident placenta percreta. Placental tissue appears to extend right to the external portion of the uterine wall in several places (*arrows*), with small patches of intervening myometrium (*arrowhead*). At delivery, placental tissue was actually found to have invaded the maternal urinary bladder. (**B**) Sector scan of a low anterior placenta with focal placenta acreta. Note the gradual thinning of the basal plate (*arrows*). (**C**) Transvaginal scan of placenta percreta. The placenta, which was a complete previa, has completely invaded the myometrium and extended to, and possibly through, the bladder wall. This gestation was 27 weeks by dates, 35 weeks by sonographer. (Courtesy of Yansheng Wei, Department of Obstetrics and Gynecology, Methodist Hospital, Brooklyn, New York.)

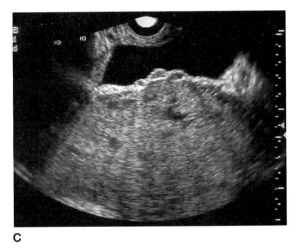

C

and tense and tender uterus. Sonography is diagnostic only if a clot or elevation of part of the placenta can be visualized.[40,63] An interesting example of a secondary finding that might alert the sonographer to look for evidence of an abruption is a case report of an echogenic mass within the fetal stomach in a patient with retroplacental hemorrhage.[76] Presumably, some intraamniotic bleeding must have occurred from the abruption, which was then ingested by the fetus. However, many normal fetuses may have intraluminal debris in their stomach from ingested vernix caseosum. It should be emphasized that sonography cannot be relied on to exclude the diagnosis if no hematoma is seen.[8,17,56] Many cases of abruption of the placenta may look normal, especially late in pregnancy.[40,58]

The clinical outcome depends on the size of the abruption and its location. For example, a paraplacental (marginal) clot has much less clinical importance than a large retroplacental hematoma associated with placental separation, which has a far

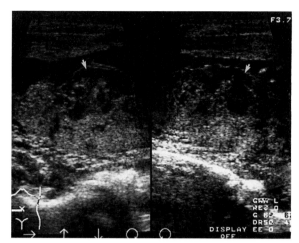

Figure 21-25. Dual-image linear scan of posterior placenta showing two views of an area of large, abnormal vascular spaces (*arrows*). This was thought to be a Breus' mole, but pathologic confirmation was not available.

greater likelihood to lead to premature delivery or miscarriage. The differential diagnosis of a retroplacental hemorrhage includes normal maternal veins in the retroplacental complex, hydatidiform mole, and chorioangioma.[56]

Abnormal Placental Attachment (Placenta Acreta, Increta, Percreta)

Some relatively uncommon conditions are the result of defective decidua formation causing abnormal attachment of the placenta to the uterine wall. In these cases, there is no decidua basalis between the trophoblast and the myometrium.[51] As with placenta previa, the presence of uterine scarring seems to predispose patients to the development of this condition. In fact, up to two thirds of cases occur in association with placenta previa, and in patients with a history of prior cesarean section. In placenta acreta, the chorionic villi are in direct contact with the myometrium. Placenta increta and percreta are more severe forms. With increta, the villi invade the myometrium as far as the serosa, and with percreta, the villi penetrate the uterine wall, and their presence can lead to uterine rupture.[17,36,51]

Sonography may reveal obliteration or focal disruption of the normal retroplacental hypoechoic complex, perhaps with a focal mass-like extension of placental tissue into the uterine wall, or even the bladder wall (Fig. 21-24).[36,51] Antenatal detection of this condition is difficult but extremely important. If it is not

treated (usually by hysterectomy), it can lead to maternal exsanguination.[30,36] Recently, the effective diagnostic use of transvaginal sonography and color flow Doppler in demonstrating these conditions has been reported.[38] Patients with persistent placenta previa at term were evaluated for suspected placenta acreta. All cases of placenta acreta exhibited several placental lacunae and, on Doppler examination, showed marked or turbulent blood flow extending from within the placental tissue into the surrounding myometrium. These findings correlated with subsequent diagnosis of placenta acreta.[38]

Abnormalities of Placental Echogenicity— Hypoechoic Placental Lesions

SUBCHORIONIC LAKES. These are tubular, anechoic lesions found beneath the chorionic plate that correspond to blood-filled spaces found at delivery. There is some question as to whether these represent normal mature villi or an early stage of intervillous thrombosis or fibrin deposition. It has been

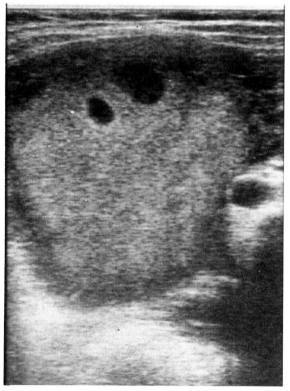

Figure 21-26. Linear scan of a placenta with two hypoechoic areas containing fibrin streaks.

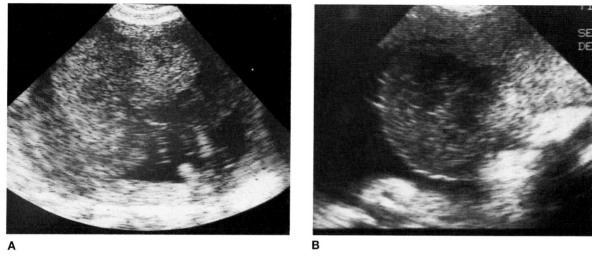

A   **B**

Figure 21-27. Sector scans of placental chorioangiomas (**A,B**). Both show inhomogeneous texture caused by numerous vascular channels and stroma. Vascular channels are seen in (**B**).

suggested that increased flow in these areas is related to decreased fibrin deposition.[51,68]

INTERVILLOUS THROMBOSIS. Intervillous thrombosis represents an intraplacental area of hemorrhage and clot. It is probably the result of a tear in the villi causing leakage of fetal red blood cells, which in turn stimulate maternal coagulation.[68] These areas of thrombosis appear sonographically as hypo-echoic lesions of varying sizes that may contain linear echogenicities representing fibrin deposits. They are most commonly found midway between the subchorionic and basal areas of the placenta and are present in up to 50% of term pregnancies.[51,68] More extensive, heterogenous and hypoechoic lesions may represent massive subchorionic hematoma or thrombosis (Breus' mole), a rare occurrence secondary to venous obstruction (Fig.

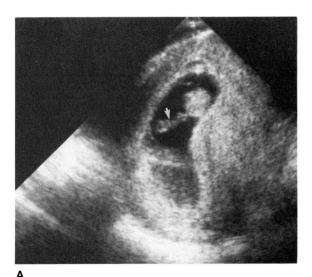
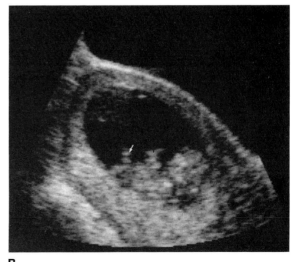

A   **B**

Figure 21-28. (**A**) Transvaginal scan of early gestation showing the umbilical cord extending from the fetus (*large arrow*). The twisted nature of the cord is evident. (**B**) Transabdominal scan at about the same age shows less definition, with the cord appearing as a series of short, linear echogenicities (*small arrow*).

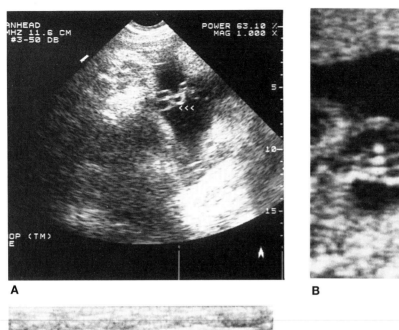

A

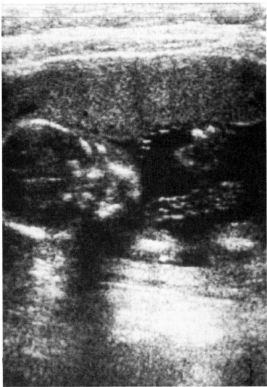

C

B

Figure 21-29. (**A**) Linear scan of umbilical cord in transverse plane showing the large vein and two smaller arteries. This is commonly called the "Mickey Mouse sign." (**B**) The cord in longitudinal section commonly appears as parallel, bright linear echoes. (**C**) In this scan, the twisted nature of the vessels within the cord is apparent.

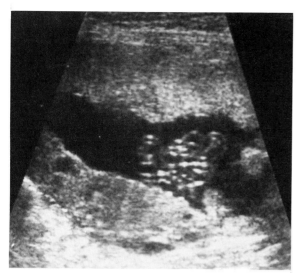

Figure 21-30. *When several portions of the cord are folded on top of one another, this "stack of coins" appearance is seen.*

21-25).[17,51,68] These lesions often separate the chorionic plate from the underlying villous tissue and may bulge into the amniotic cavity. The blood in these cases is generally of maternal origin and there is an associated large placenta.[13,51] These are usually found in abortuses, missed abortions, or premature deliveries.[4]

FIBRIN DEPOSITION. Fibrin deposition is an apparently insignificant clinical event that is probably the end result of intervillous and subchorionic thrombosis,[64] which results from pooling and stasis of maternal blood in the perivillous and subchorionic spaces.[17,68] Fibrin deposits have been variously reported as sonographically hypoechoic lesions in the subchorionic area or within the placental mass,[68] and as linear echogenic streaks within an anechoic lesion[51] (Fig. 21-26), possibly representing different degrees of deposition.

PLACENTAL INFARCTION. It is thought that placental infarcts result from obstruction of the spiral arterioles and are usually found at the periphery of the placenta.[51] They may be associated with retroplacental hemorrhage and may occur in up to 25% of term placentas.[68] Although they usually have no clinical significance, they appear to be more common in association with intrauterine growth retardation (IUGR) and mothers with preeclampsia.[68] There has been little confirmed sonographic evidence of placental infarcts,[1,51] but the demonstration of areas of placental thinning might suggest this condition.

Nontrophoblastic Placental Tumors

Chorioangioma and teratoma represent the two primary nontrophoblastic tumors of the placenta.

CHORIOANGIOMA. A chorioangioma is a benign vascular malformation found in about 1% of examined placentas.[66] Small chorioangiomas may be nonsymptomatic, whereas large chorioangiomas may result in the development of maternal toxemia, premature labor, IUGR, fetal hydrops, or fetal demise.[51,68] In addition, there may be significant shunting of blood through the tumor, which has been documented with Doppler.[20,64,66]

Sonographically, small chorioangiomas are usually seen as clusters of small tumors that may be isoechoic to the placenta, and therefore appear only as areas of focal thickening of the placenta.[17,19,56,78] They may, however, be less echogenic than placental tissue.[66] The single, large chorioangioma, seen less often, may appear as a well circumscribed, complex mass on the fetal surface of the placenta, adjacent to the cord insertion[78] or protruding into the amniotic cavity (Fig. 21-27).[51,56,68] It has been associated with polyhydramnios in 35% of cases.[66] One study showed that chorioangiomas may be sonographically indistinguishable from placental hemorrhage.[3] Vascular channels may be seen within the mass.[67]

TERATOMA. Teratomas of the placenta are very rare. They are usually benign but can be highly malignant.[17,68] Although no description has been documented,[66] sonographically they would appear as a complex mass.

Gestational Trophoblastic Disease

Gestational trophoblastic disease (GTD) is a designation given to several disorders arising from either normal or abnormal fertilization of an ovum, resulting in neoplastic changes in the trophoblastic elements of the developing blastocyst. GTD is classified into hydatidiform mole, either complete or partial; nonmetastatic disease or invasive mole; and metastatic disease or choriocarcinoma.[12,51] GTD is treated extensively in Chapter 25. Table 22-1 describes the sonographic features of these conditions.

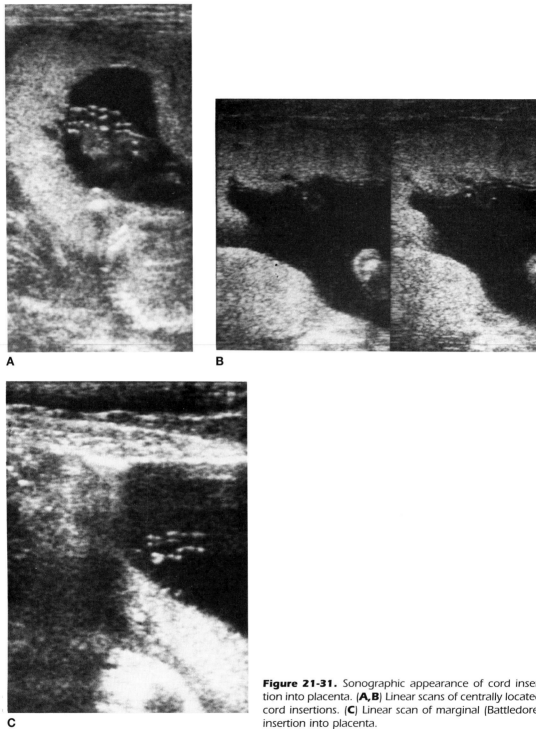

A

B

C

Figure 21-31. Sonographic appearance of cord insertion into placenta. (**A,B**) Linear scans of centrally located cord insertions. (**C**) Linear scan of marginal (Battledore) insertion into placenta.

Abnormality	Description	Sonographic Characteristics	Differential Diagnosis
Excessive Wharton's jelly	Diffuse or focal deposits of excess Wharton's jelly[2,60]; may liquefy and get very large	Variably echogenic, soft tissue mass with three vessels visible within, usually near fetal abdomen, may be cystic if liquified.	Hernia, tumor, hematoma, cysts
Umbilical hernia	Small protrusion of abdominal contents into umbilical cord seen after 17 wk	Small mass adjacent to abdomen. Usually regresses spontaneously.	Small omphalocele
Omphalocele	Protrusion of abdominal structures (liver, bowel) into base of cord—covered by peritoneum; high incidence of associated congenital abnormalities	Mass adjacent to anterior abdominal wall, covered by membrane, into apex of which cord appears to insert. Sac may be distended by ascites.	Gastroschisis, hematoma
False knot	Folding of vessels that are longer than covering membrane,[2] or simple dilatation of vessels	Irregular protrusion from cord.[2]	
True knot	Results from excessive fetal movement, especially with a long cord, or polyhydramnios[62]; may become tightened and occlude umbilical vessels[2]; associated increased incidence of congenital anomalies[62]	Irregular protrusion from cord.[62]	May see cloverleaf pattern of cord.[51]
Stricture	Localized narrowing of cord, disappearance of Wharton's jelly, torsion of cord or thickening of vessel walls with narrowing of lumen	Narrowing of cord close to fetus with edematous area distal.[62]	
Umbilical vein thrombosis	Occlusion of umbilical vein secondary to localized increase of resistance in umbilical circulation; associated with maternal diabetes, arthritis, nonimmune hydrops[1,3]	Increased echogenicity of umbilical vessels or echoic material within lumen.	Artifact
Cystic masses Allantoic cyst (developmental urachal cyst)	Fluid-filled remnant of allantoid duct[60,62] associated with patent urachus and lower tract obstructions	Usually small, mild focal dilatation of cord.	Omphalomesenteric cyst
Omphalomesenteric cyst	Vestigal patency and dilatation of duct seen after 16 wk[60,62]	Cystic dilatation up to 6 cm, usually located close to fetus.	Hematoma, liquefied Wharton's jelly
Solid masses Hemangioma	Benign tumor of vessels or Wharton's jelly—if large, can cause vascular obstruction[60]; may be associated with increased amniotic fluid and α-fetoprotein and nonimmune hydrops[62]	Varied appearance— hyperechoic mass with smooth, lobulated contours, up to 15 cm; may have small, ovoid lucencies or numerous, small, highly echoic reflectors. Surrounding cord may appear edematous—usually located near placental margin.[47,62]	Hematoma, teratoma

(continued)

◢◢◢◢ **TABLE 21-4.** (Continued)

Abnormality	Description	Sonographic Characteristics	Differential Diagnosis
Complex masses			
Hematoma	Rare; result of extravasation of blood into Wharton's jelly[62] from rupture of umbilical vein[2,60]; may be due to congenital weakness of vessel wall, or iatrogenic; associated with perinatal loss	May be septated, hyperechoic or hypoechoic depending on age of clot, may be more irregular than other cystic lesions. May appear as enlargement of cord with constriction of vessels.[60] Has been reported as large, hypoechoic, septated mass ajacent to fetal abdomen.[2,62]	Tumors, cysts
Teratoma	Rare germ cell tumor	Disorganized, heterogeneous mass, up to 9 cm in diameter, may have calcifications, found at any point along the cord.[62]	Hemangioma, hematoma[62]

The Umbilical Cord

STRUCTURE AND FUNCTION

The umbilical cord normally contains two arteries and one vein surrounded by a mucoid connective tissue (Wharton's jelly), all enclosed in a layer of amnion.[16] The vein brings fresh, oxygenated blood to the fetus and the arteries carry deoxygenated blood from the fetus to the placenta. The umbilical arteries are longer than the vein and wind around it. All the vessels are longer than the cord itself, resulting in twisting and bending of the cord and vessels (see Fig. 21-1).[16] The arteries have thicker walls and smaller cross-sectional areas (4 mm) than the vein (1.0 cm).[62] At term, the mean length of the cord is about 55 cm (range, 30 to 120 cm), with a mean circumference of 3.6 cm.[2,58]

SCANNING TECHNIQUE

The umbilical cord is best visualized in the late second and early third trimester, when amniotic fluid volume is at its peak. Owing to the extreme length of the cord it is unlikely, on a routine basis, to scan it in its entirety to rule out abnormalities. If a lesion is suspected, every effort must be made to view as much of the cord as possible. Changing the mother's position from side to side may help shift the position of the fetus in relation to the cord. The placental insertion site of the cord, as well as its entry site to the fetus (to rule out, for example, omphalocele) should be imaged and documented routinely. The presence of three vessels within the cord should also be documented. Visualization of the number of cord vessels is difficult when there is oligohydramnios, and may be troublesome in the third trimester even in the normal fetus, due to the relative lack of fluid and the presence of potentially obstructing fetal parts.[16] Any abnormality in cord size, position, degree of coiling, or attachment sites to placenta or fetus should be noted.[10]

NORMAL SONOGRAPHIC APPEARANCE

In early pregnancy, the umbilical cord may appear as a series of short, linear echoes extending from the fetus to the placenta (Fig. 21-28). It can be seen soon after visualization of the fetal pole.[10] As pregnancy progresses, transverse images through the cord reveal the three circles representing the larger vein and two smaller arteries. Longitudinal images at this stage reveal a series of parallel linear echoes within the amniotic fluid that may exhibit the characteristic twisted appearance of the cord (Fig. 21-29). The "stack of coins" appearance refers to visualization of several portions of cord folded on each other (Fig. 21-30).[12] Arterial pulsations may be demonstrated within the umbilical arteries. The insertion of the umbilical cord into the placenta appears as a V- or U-shaped hypoechoic area just beneath the chorionic plate (Fig. 21-31).[62]

ABNORMALITIES OF THE UMBILICAL CORD

Table 21-4 lists the common umbilical cord abnormalities and their sonographic appearances.

Absence of Umbilical Cord

Complete absence of the umbilical cord (body stalk anomaly) or presence of a very short cord has been associated with the limb–body wall complex, a syndrome of severe fetal structural anomalies.[14,51] Body stalk anomaly is a fatal condition. It has been linked to maternal cocaine abuse.[51] Sonographically, no cord would be seen, but rather an extraembryonic membranous sac in direct apposition to the chorionic plate.[14]

Abnormalities of Cord Insertion

The umbilical cord usually inserts in the center of the placenta; however, it may be marginal or velamentous (see Fig. 21-2). In the latter case, vessels are found lying on the surface of the chorioamniotic membranes. This condition is associated with various fetal anomalies, a lower birth weight, and more intrapartum complications, often due to umbilical cord malpresentation, such as vasa previa.[11,62] For this reason, careful examination of the placental insertion site is important.

True and False Knots

As previously described, the differences in umbilical vein, umbilical artery, and cord stromal length give rise to bending and twisting of the umbilical cord. Sometimes this twisting may appear as a false knot, which has no clinical significance. It can, however, be sonographically confused with a true knot of the cord, which occurs when the fetus actually passes through a loop of cord. This potentially hazardous situation occurs in about 1% of deliveries.[62] It is difficult to detect sonographically, but has been associated with a cloverleaf pattern of the cord.[51] Color Doppler may aid in the diagnosis.

Abnormal Cord Position

NUCHAL CORD. In about 24% of all deliveries, the umbilical cord is looped around the neck of the fetus one or more times.[46,69] Multiple looping has been associated with increased incidence of complications, such as decreased fetal breathing, movement, and birth weight.[29,37,46] Meconium-stained amniotic fluid has also been associated with nuchal cord, usually when coincident with oligohydramnios.[71] In most cases, however, the cord is loosely looped around the fetal neck, and is clinically insignificant. Only rarely is nuchal cord associated with significant perinatal complications.[29,37,46,69] The presence of a nuchal cord can be demonstrated during routine sonography (Fig. 21-32). Color Doppler is helpful in differentiating cord from other neck masses.[10] This diagnosis should be considered whenever the umbilical cord is imaged around or near the fetal neck.

CORD PROLAPSE AND VASA PREVIA. There are several forms of umbilical cord prolapse. Occult prolapse refers to loops of cord adjacent to the fetal presenting part.[21] Vasa previa refers to a situation in which a segment of umbilical cord is located between the presenting fetal part and the lower

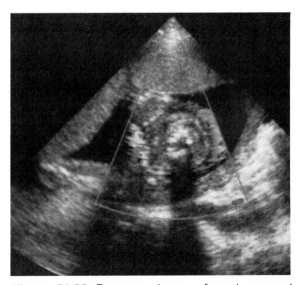

Figure 21-32. *Transverse image of cord wrapped around the fetal neck (nuchal cord). This is a black and white image produced with a color flow Doppler transducer. The visualization of color flow greatly enhanced the ability to see this structure clearly.*

pole of intact membranes (Fig. 21-33). Frank prolapse refers to cord protrusion into the cervix, usually through ruptured membranes.[15,21,62] Vasa previa, although rare, can be responsible for severe fetal complications during delivery.[42] In some instances, prolapse or vasa previa may be due to velamentous insertion of the cord into membranes that do not overlie placental tissue and that may cross the cervical os before joining the placenta. Prolapse may also be due to abnormal vessels extending from the placental surface.[51]

Sonographic detection of prolapse is clinically important because it may lead to cord compression and fetal vascular compromise, a potentially fatal situation. It can also place these vessels at risk for laceration.[51] Visualization of loops of cord between the presenting part and the cervix or within the cervical canal is greatly improved by use of the transvaginal probe and color flow

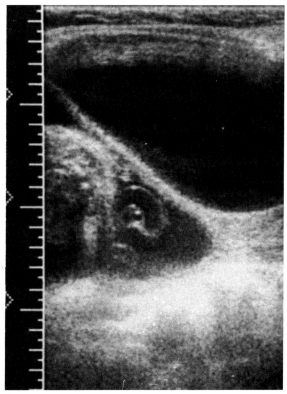

Figure 21-33. *Linear scan of vasa previa. Loops of cord are visualized between the cervix and the presenting fetal part. This situation can present grave complications during delivery.*

Doppler.[42,44] If there is associated velamentous insertion of the umbilical cord or a low-lying placenta, they should be documented.[15] Predisposing factors to the development of umbilical cord prolapse are fetal malpresentation, polyhydramnios, premature rupture of membranes, excessive cord length, multiple gestation, and cephalopelvic disproportion.[21]

Single Umbilical Artery

A two-vessel cord representing an umbilical vein and a single umbilical artery (SUA) is seen in 0.5% to 1.0% of all pregnancies, and is thought to be due to either primary agenesis of one of the embryonic umbilical arteries or atrophy of a previously normal umbilical artery.[15,64] A small percentage of fetuses with SUA have associated IUGR, or anomalies of the central nervous, cardiovascular, and genitourinary systems.[51] On sonographic investigation (which is better made closest to the fetal end of the cord[51]), the cord has lost its braided appearance[62] and only two vessels are viewed transversely (Fig. 21-34). Often, the SUA measures more than 4.0 mm in diameter.[55]

Two related studies are noteworthy. One case study documented an umbilical cord with three arteries in association with conjoined twins.[5] The other study looked at fetuses with noncoiled umbilical cords, which is often associated with a two-vessel cord. The combined incidence of fetal anomalies or death in this group (16%) was significantly greater than in the control group (3.5%).[70]

Umbilical Cord Size

THINNING OF THE UMBILICAL CORD. Segmental thinning of the cord is an infrequent finding. It is usually caused by absence of a portion of the muscle in the wall of the artery. The placentas in these cases may contain similar vascular lesions. Marked segmental thinning may be associated with increased congenital anomalies and perinatal distress.[59]

ENLARGEMENT OF THE UMBILICAL CORD. Enlargement of the cord is very rare. It may be a normal variant, but can be due to tumors or cysts, or be an indicator of possible isoimmune sensitivity. In the latter case, umbilical vein dilatation (varix) in the fetal abdomen usually precedes dilatation in the cord.[58] When this happens, a large cystic mass (rep-

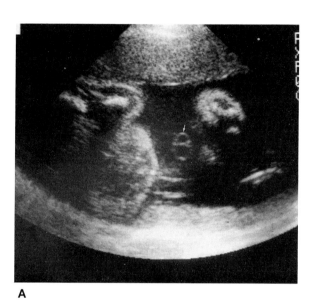

A

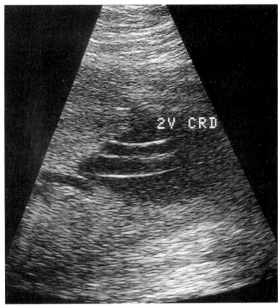

B

C

Figure 21-34. Sector scans of two-vessel cord. (**A**) Transverse image of two-vessel cord. The arrow points to the single artery, which is slightly smaller than the vein, although somewhat larger than an artery in a three-vessel cord. The two vessels may also appear to be the same size. (**B**) Longitudinal image of two-vessel cord. Note the lack of twisting of the cord. (**C**) Transverse black and white image of two-vessel cord with color Doppler image of blood flowing in opposite directions, suggesting that one vessel is the vein, and the other the artery. (**B** and **C** courtesy of Catherine Carr-Hoefer, RT, RDMS, RDCS, RVT, Sonographer Coordinator, Good Samaritan Hospital, Corvallis, Oregon.)

resenting the umbilical vein) may be seen in the fetal abdomen near the umbilicus. There may be associated fetal hydrops and fetal death, but the fetus can also be perfectly normal.[16,51]

Diffuse enlargement of the cord may be due to edema,[2] or excessive deposits of Wharton's jelly.[2,60] Focal enlargement may be due to umbilical hernia, omphalocele, false or true knot, and various cystic and solid lesions.

Umbilical Cord Masses

CYSTIC MASSES. Cystic masses of the cord are usually related to the vestigial patency of an embryonic structure (Fig. 21-35),[60,62] or, rarely, to an aneu-

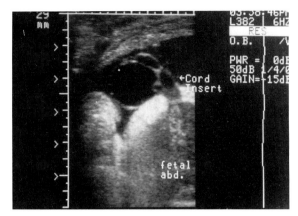

Figure 21-35. Allantoid cyst located near the fetal insertion of the cord. These cystic structures on the umbilical cord are usually seen close to the fetal abdomen and represent dilatation of a fetal remnant. Often they are associated with a patent urachus. They may be confused with umbilical cord hematomas. (Courtesy of Catherine Carr-Hoefer, RT, RDMS, RDCS, RVT, Sonographer Coordinator, Good Samaritan Hospital, Corvallis, Oregon.)

rysm of an umbilical artery or vein.[51] Excessive deposits of Wharton's jelly, which appears as a soft tissue mass, may liquefy and present as a large, cystic mass.[51] If a cyst is discovered, serial examinations should be performed to verify normal fetal growth and to note any change in the size of the cyst, because an expanding cyst (or any mass on the cord) may compress blood vessels. Doppler evaluation may be helpful in such cases.

Umbilical cord hematomas are rare and have been associated with increased maternal serum α-fetoprotein, nonimmune hydrops, cord torsion, and perinatal death.[51,68] Hematomas appear echogenic when acute, but may also appear hypoechoic or even cystic later on. Differentiation from other cystic masses may be difficult, but hematomas are often irregular, septated, and more complex than other cystic lesions. They may also appear as an edematous portion of the cord.

SOLID MASSES. Solid masses of the umbilical cord include hemangiomas, angiomyxomas, dermoids, and teratomas.[9] Although precise sonographic diagnosis of hemangioma is not possible, the presence of a heterogeneous, solid umbilical cord mass near the placental end of the cord (Fig. 21-36) should suggest the diagnosis. When any mass on the cord is visualized, careful examination of the anterior abdominal wall of the fetus should be made to rule out associated abnormalities of abdominal wall formation. The sonographer should also examine the mass for the presence of vessels within. With any mass of the cord, mechanical compression and impairment of circu-

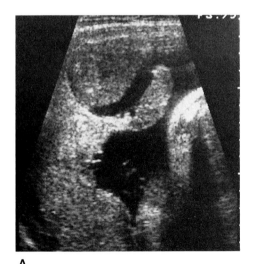

A

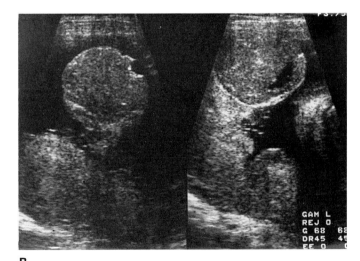

B

Figure 21-36. Umbilical cord hemangioma. In the images in (**A**) and the right side of (**B**), it is difficult to determine whether the hemangioma is of placental or umbilical origin. In the left-hand image of (**B**), however, the entire hemangioma is visualized separate from the placenta, and the tubular lucency in the other frames was determined to represent the umbilical vein.

lation is a possible consequence, especially if the mass arises from the vascular tissue itself.[9,47,62] The presence of calcifications in a disorganized, heterogeneous mass anywhere along the length of the cord is suggestive of a teratoma.[62]

Umbilical Vein and Arterial Thrombosis

Umbilical vein thrombosis and occlusion is a serious condition associated with nonimmune fetal hydrops and has associated prenatal mortality. Thrombosis may also occur in the umbilical arteries, with associated aneurysmal dilatation.[62] The incidence of primary thrombosis increases in diabetic mothers.[1] Secondary, or reactive thrombosis (with associated hydrops and even cardiac failure) may result from a mechanical cord impairment such as torsion, knotting, compression, or hematoma.[1,6] Sonographically, the thrombus may present as increased echogenicity of the umbilical vessels.[62]

REFERENCES

1. Abrams SL, Callen PW, Filly RA. Umbilical vein thrombosis: Sonographic detection in utero. J Ultrasound Med. 1985; 4:283–285.

2. Allen M. Diagnostic challenge: I. Excessive amount of Wharton's jelly. J Diagn Med Sonogr. 1987; 3:27, 29, 30.

3. Bromley B, Benacerraf BR. Solid masses on the fetal surface of the placenta: Differential diagnosis and clinical outcome. J Ultrasound Med. 1994; 13:883–886.

4. Cavanagh D. Spontaneous abortion. In: Danforth DN, ed. Obstetrics and Gynecology. 4th ed. Philadelphia: Harper & Row; 1982:378–393.

5. Cohen HL, Shapiro ML, Haller JO, Schwartz D. The multivessel umbilical cord: An antenatal indicator of possible conjoined twinning. J Clin Ultrasound. 1992; 10:278–282.

6. Collins JH. Prenatal observation of umbilical cord torsion with subsequent premature labor and delivery of a 31-week infant with mild nonimmune hydrops. Am J Obstet Gynecol. 1995; 172:1048–1049.

7. Crane JP. Sonographic evaluation of multiple frequency. Semin Ultrasound CT MR. 1984; 5:144–156.

8. Cyr D. Fetal umbilical Doppler. In: SDMS 5th Annual Conference Proceedings. Dallas: Society of Diagnosis Medical Sonographers; 1988:51–53.

9. DuBose TJ. Extrafetal structures of pregnancy. In: Fe-

tal Sonography. Philadelphia: WB Saunders; 1996: 345–374.

10. Dudiak CM, Salomon CG, Posniak HV, Olson MC, Flisak ME. Sonography of the umbilical cord. Radiographics. 1995; 15:1035–1050.

11. Eddleman KA, Lockwood CJ, Berkowitz GS, Lapinski RH, Berkowitz RL. Clinical significance and sonographic diagnosis of velamentous umbilical cord insertion. Am J Perinatol. 1992; 9:123–126.

12. Fleischer AC, Gordon AN. Sonography of trophoblastic diseases. In: Fleischer AC, Romero R, Manning MD, Jeanty P, James AE, eds. The Principles and Practice of Ultrasonography in Obstetrics and Gynecology. 4th ed. Norwalk, CT: Appleton-Century-Crofts; 1991:501–508.

13. Fox H. Pathology of the placenta. In: Chervenak FA, Isaacson GA, Campbell S, eds. Ultrasound in Obstetrics and Gynecology. Vol. 2. Boston: Little, Brown; 1993:1211–1221.

14. Giacola GP. Body stalk anomaly: Congenital absence of the umbilical cord. Obstet Gynecol. 1992; 80(3 pt 2):527–529.

15. Gianopoulos J, Carver T, Tomich PG, et al. Diagnosis of vasa previa with ultrasonography. Obstet Gynecol. 1987; 69:488–491.

16. Graham D, Fleischer AC, Sacks GA. Sonography of the umbilical cord and intrauterine membranes. In: Fleischer AC, Romero R, Manning MS, Jeanty P, James AE, eds. The Principles and Practice of Ultrasonography in Obstetrics and Gynecology. 4th ed. Norwalk, CT: Appleton-Century-Crofts; 1991:159–170.

17. Graham D, Guidi S, Sanders RC. Sonography of the placenta. In: Sanders RC, Hill MC, eds. Ultrasound Annual. New York: Raven Press; 1984:121–137.

18. Grannum P, Hobbins JC. The placenta. In: Callen PW, ed. Ultrasonography in Obstetrics and Gynecology. Philadelphia: WB Saunders; 1983:141–157.

19. Grundy HO, Byers L, Walton S, et al. Antepartum ultrasonographic evaluation and management of placental chorioangioma: A case report. J Reprod Med. 1986; 31:520–522.

20. Hadlock FP. The placenta. In: Athey PA, Hadlock FP, eds. Ultrasound in Obstetrics and Gynecology. 2nd ed. St. Louis: CV Mosby; 1985.

21. Hales ED, Westney LS. Sonography of occult cord prolapse. J Clin Ultrasound. 1984; 12:283–285.

22. Harmon C. Ultrasound in the management of the alloimmunized pregnancy. In: Fleischer AC, Manning FA, Jeanty P, Romero R, eds. The Principles and Practice of Ultrasonography in Obstetrics and Gynecology. 5th ed. Stamford, CT: Appleton and Lange; 1996:583–610.

23. Harris RD, Barth RA. Sonography of the gravid

uterus and placenta: Current concepts. Am J Roentgenol. 1993; 160:455–465.

24. Hertzberg BS, Bowie JD, Carroll BA, Kliewer MA, Weber TM. Diagnosis of placenta previa during the third trimester: Role of transperineal sonography. Am J Roentgenol. 1992; 159:83–87.

25. Hertzberg BS, Bowie JD, Weber TM, Carroll BA, Kliewer MA, Jordan SG. Sonography of the cervix during the third trimester of pregnancy: Value of the transperineal approach. Am J Roentgenol. 1991; 157:73–76.

26. Hertzberg BS, Kliewer MA, Baumeister LA, McNally PB, Fazekas CK. Optimizing transperineal sonographic imaging of the cervix: The hip elevation technique. J Ultrasound Med. 1994; 13:933–936.

27. Hoddick WK, Mahony BS, Callen PW, et al. Placental thickness. J Ultrasound Med. 1985; 4:479–482.

28. Jaffe R, Warsof SL. Transvaginal color Doppler imaging in the assessment of uteroplacental blood flow in the normal first-trimester pregnancy. Am J Obstet Gynecol. 1991; 164:781–785.

29. Jauniaux E, Ramsay B, Peellaerts C, Scholler Y. Perinatal features of pregnancies complicated by nuchal cord. Am J Perinatol. 1995; 12:255–258.

30. Jeanty P, Romero R. Obstetrical Ultrasound. New York: McGraw-Hill; 1984.

31. Kaiser IH. Fertilization and the physiology and development of fetus and placenta. In: Danforth DN, ed. Obstetrics and Gynecology. 4th ed. Philadelphia: Harper & Row; 1982.

32. Kaplan C. Placental pathology for the nineties. Pathol Annu. 1993; 28(Pt 1):15–72.

33. Karis JP, Hertzberg BS, Bowie JD. Sonographic diagnosis of premature cervical dilatation: Potential pitfall due to lower uterine segment contractions. J Ultrasound Med. 1991; 10:83–87.

34. Khan AT, Stewart KS. Ultrasound placental localization in early pregnancy. Scot Med J. 1987; 32:19–21.

35. Kremkau FW. Doppler Ultrasound: Principles and Instruments. 2nd ed. Philadelphia: WB Saunders; 1995.

36. Laing FC. Ultrasound evaluation of obstetric problems relating to the lower uterine segment and cervix. In: Sanders RC, James AE Jr, eds. The Principles and Practice of Ultrasonography in Obstetrics and Gynecology. 3rd ed. Norwalk, CT: Appleton-Century-Crofts; 1985:355–367.

37. Larson JD, Rayburn WF, Crosby S, Thurnau GR. Multiple nuchal cord entanglements and intrapartum complications. Am J Obstet Gynecol. 1995; 173:1228–1231.

38. Lerner JP, Deane S, Timor-Tritsch IE. Characterization of placenta accreta using transvaginal sonography and color Doppler imaging. Ultrasound in Obstetrics and Gynecology. 1995; 5:198–201.

39. Mahony BS, Nyberg DA, Luthy DA, et al. Translabial ultrasound of the third trimester uterine cervix: Correlation with digital examination. J Ultrasound Med. 1990; 9:717–723.

40. Marx M, Casola G, Scheible W, et al. The subplacental complex: Further sonographic observations. J Ultrasound Med. 1985; 4:459–461.

41. McCarthy J, Thurmond AS, Jones MD, et al. Circumvallate placenta: Sonographic diagnosis. J Ultrasound Med. 1995; 14:21–26.

42. Megier P, Desroches A, Esperandieu O, Mekari B. [Prenatal diagnosis of vasa previa with velamentous cord insertion using Doppler color echography.] [French] J Gynecol Obstet Biol Reprod. 1995; 24:415–417.

43. de Mendonia LK. Sonographic diagnosis of placenta accreta: Presentation of six cases. J Ultrasound Med. 1988; 7:211–215.

44. Meyer WJ, Blumenthal L, Cadkin A, Gauthier DW, Rotmensch S. Vasa previa: Prenatal diagnosis with transvaginal color Doppler flow imaging. Am J Obstet Gynecol. 1993; 169:1627–1629.

45. Mintz MC, Kurtz AB, Arenson R, et al. Abruptio placentae: Apparent thickening of the placenta caused by hyperechoic retroplacental clot. J Ultrasound Med. 1986; 5:411–413.

46. Miser WF. Outcome of infants born with nuchal cords. J Fam Pract. 1992; 34:441–445.

47. Mishriki YY, Vanyshelbaum Y, Epstein H, et al. Hemangioma of the umbilical cord. Pediatr Pathol. 1987; 7:43–49.

48. Molloy CE, McDowell W, Armour T, et al. Ultrasonic diagnosis of placenta membranacea in utero. J Ultrasound Med. 1983; 2:377–379.

49. Monaghan J, O'Herlihy C, Boylan P. Ultrasound placental grading and amniotic fluid quantitation in prolonged pregnancy. Obstet Gynecol. 1987; 70: 349–352.

50. Montan S, Jorgensen C, Svalenius E, et al. Placental grading with ultrasound in hypertensive and normotensive pregnancies: A prospective, consecutive study. Acta Obstet Gynaecol Scand. 1986; 65:477–480.

51. Nelson LH. Ultrasonography of the Placenta: A Review. An AIUM Monograph. Laurel, MD: American Institute of Ultrasound in Medicine; 1994.

52. Nyberg DA, Mack LA, Benedetti TJ, et al. Placental abruption and placental hemorrhage: Correlation of sonographic findings with fetal outcome. Radiology. 1987; 164:357–361.

53. Park YW, Cho JS, Kim HS, Song CH. The clinical implications of early diastolic notch in third trimester Doppler waveform analysis of the uterine artery. J Ultrasound Med. 1996; 15:47–51.

54. Persutte WH, Lenke RR. Maternal urinary bladder

filling for middle- and late-trimester ultrasound: Is it really necessary? J Ultrasound Med. 1988; 7:203–206.

55. Persutte WH, Lenke RR. Transverse umbilical arterial diameter: Technique for the prenatal diagnosis of single umbilical artery. J Ultrasound Med. 1994; 13:763–766.

56. Price SA. Ultrasound visualization of abruptio placentae with massive hemorrhage protruding into the amniotic cavity. Journal of Diagnostic Ultrasound. 1986; 2:161–163.

57. Proud J, Grant AM. Third-trimester placental grading by ultrasonography as a test of fetal well-being. Br Med J. 1987; 294:1641–1644.

58. Queenan JT, O'Brien GD. Diagnostic ultrasound in erythroblastosis fetalis. In: Sanders RC, James AE Jr, eds. The Principles and Practice of Ultrasonography in Obstetrics and Gynecology. 3rd ed. Norwalk, CT: Appleton-Century-Crofts; 1985:279–287.

59. Qureshi F, Jacques SM. Marked segmental thinning of the umbilical cord vessels. Arch Pathol Lab Med. 1994; 118:826–830.

60. Ramanathan K, Epstein S, Yaghoobian J. Localized deposition of Wharton's jelly: Sonographic findings. J Ultrasound Med. 1986; 5:339–340.

61. Reece EA, Hobbins JC. Ultrasonography and diabetes mellitus in pregnancy. In: Sanders RC, James AE Jr, eds. The Principles and Practice of Ultrasonography in Obstetrics and Gynecology. 3rd ed. Norwalk, CT: Appleton-Century-Crofts; 1985:297–320.

62. Romero R, Pilu G, Jeanty P, et al. The umbilical cord. In: Romero R, Pilu G, Jeanty P, Ghidini A, Hobbins JC, eds. Prenatal Diagnosis of Congenital Anomalies. Norwalk, CT: Appleton & Lange; 1988:385–402.

63. Sauerbrei EE, Pham DII. Placental abruption and subchorionic hemorrhage in the first half of pregnancy: Ultrasound appearance and clinical outcome. Radiology. 1986; 160:109–112.

64. Sauerbrei EE, Nguyen KT, Nolan RL. A Practical Guide to Ultrasound in Obstetrics and Gynecology. New York: Raven Press; 1987.

65. Shah YG, Graham D. Relationship of placental grade to fetal pulmonary maturity and respiratory distress syndrome. Am J Perinatol. 1986; 3:53–55.

66. Shalev E. The placenta and umbilical cord. In: Chervenak FA, Isaacson GA, Campbell S, eds. Ultrasound in Obstetrics and Gynecology. Vol. 2. Boston: Little, Brown; 1993:1083–1098.

67. Spirt BA, Kagen EH. Sonography of the placenta

(obstetrical ultrasound update). Semin Ultrasound. 1980; 1:293–310.

68. Spirt BA, Gordon LP, Kagen EH. Sonography of the placenta. In: Fleischer AC, Manning FA, Jeanty P, Romero R, eds. The Principles and Practice of Ultrasonography in Obstetrics and Gynecology. 5th ed. Stamford, CT: Appleton and Lange; 1996:173–202.

69. Steinfeld JD, Ludmir J, Eife S, Robbins D, Samuels P. Prenatal detection and management of quadruple nuchal cord: A case report. J Reprod Med. 1992; 37:989–991.

70. Strong TH, Finberg HJ, Mattox JH. Antepartum diagnosis of noncoiled umbilical cords. Am J Obstet Gynecol. 1994; 170:1729–1731.

71. Strong TH, Sarno AP, Paul RH. Significance of intrapartum amniotic fluid volume in the presence of nuchal cords. J Reprod Med. 1992; 37:718–720.

72. Timor-Tritsch IE, Monteagudo A. Diagnosis of placenta previa by transvaginal sonography. Ann Med. 1993; 25:279–283.

73. Timor-Tritsch IE, Rottem S, Elgalis S. How transvaginal sonography is done. In: Timor-Tritsch IE, Rottem S, eds. Transvaginal Sonography. New York: Elsevier; 1988:15–25.

74. Townsend RR, Laing FC, Nyberg DA, et al. Technical factors responsible for "placental migration": Sonographic assessment. Radiology. 1986; 160:105–108.

75. Trudinger GJ. Obstetric Doppler applications. In: Flesicher AC, Romero R, Manning MD, Jeanty P, James AE, eds. The Principles and Practices of Ultrasonography in Obstetrics and Gynecology. 4th ed. Norwalk, CT: Appleton-Century-Crofts; 1991:173–191.

76. Walker JM, Ferguson DD. The sonographic appearance of blood in the fetal stomach and its association with placental abruption. J Ultrasound Med. 1988; 7:155–161.

77. Weber TM, Hertzgberg BS, Bowie JD. Transperitoneal ultrasound: Alternative technique to improve visualization of the presenting fetal part. Radiology. 1991; 179:747–750.

78. Willard DA, Moeschler JB. Placental chorioangioma: A rare cause of elevated amniotic fluid alpha-fetoprotein. J Ultrasound Med. 1986; 5:221–222.

79. Wolf H, Oosting H, Treffers PE. Placental volume measurement by ultrasonography: Evaluation of the method. Am J Obstet Gynecol. 1987; 156:1191–1194.

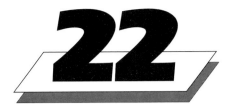

22

Observing Fetal Maturation Through Fetal Movement and Fetal Breathing

CATHERINE A. WALLA and LAWRENCE D. PLATT

Interest in the nature of fetal activity has led to the scientific study of fetal movements and breathing over the last 100 years. Noninvasive, in utero observations regarding the qualitative, as well as the quantitative, aspects of fetal motor behavior throughout the course of pregnancy have been achieved only recently, however, with linear-array real-time ultrasonography. The visualization of fetal activity in terms of the current status of that activity as well as its development has proven vital to the assessment of fetal condition. Recent basic and clinical investigations have indicated that not only the presence of fetal movement and breathing, but their development, are direct reflections of the status of the fetal central nervous system (CNS). The ultimate goal of clinical studies investigating fetal motor behavior has been the antenatal identification of the fetus with a compromised CNS to allow for reaching a more informed diagnosis concerning either the therapy or the timely delivery of that fetus. The purpose of this chapter is to address the clinical applications of fetal movements and breathing in the determination of fetal health.

Fetal Body Movements

The study of fetal movements in pregnancy is important in that they reflect the development of the fetal CNS. As such, fetal motor activity can be seen as a function controlled by the CNS and can reflect both the neural development of and possible disturbances in the CNS.[39] As early as 1885, Preyer[58] studied fetal movements on aborted living fetuses with intact gestational sacs, as well as by palpation of the maternal abdomen. He was convinced that spontaneous limb movement of the fetus occurred before 16 and probably even 12 weeks' gestation. More detailed studies of fetal movements have been carried out on exteriorized fetuses, but the impact of determination of the physiologic state of the fetus was not known. Other methods that have been used in the detection and analysis of fetal movements have included maternal perception of fetal movement,[9,20,59,67,75] piezoelectric crystals,[68,74] surface electrodes,[24] tocodynamometers,[18] and unprocessed Doppler signals.[82] Although these methods provided methods of the quantification of prenatal motor behavior, they were unable to define either the quality of fetal movements or the correlation of one type of movement to another. Ultrasound imaging techniques have permitted the opening of a new vista for analysis of fetal motor behavior.

FETAL MOVEMENT IN EARLY GESTATION

A detailed classification of individual movement patterns of the fetus was developed by three independent research groups: Birnholz and colleagues,[4]

449

Ianniruberto and Tanjani,[26] and deVries and associates.[15] A comparison of these studies of early fetal motor activity has demonstrated that although there are some discrepancies in the observed time of onset of the various types of movements, all three studies demonstrated a successive development from simple movements involving the whole fetal body to more complex movements (Table 22-1). DeVries and associates'[15] examination of the qualitative aspects of the development of fetal movement determined a specific sequence of emergence of the movements that was evident in all fetuses studied. It was discovered that all movements that could be identified in the term fetus were present by the age of 15 weeks. The morphologic appearance (Table 22-2) of movement patterns has little variance throughout pregnancy once these patterns emerge.

As discerned from these studies, the earliest movement of the fetus can be appreciated as early as 6 to 7 weeks. By 8 weeks, general movements of the limbs, trunk, and head can be identified. Concomitantly, a "startle" motion was seen in this period. Hiccoughs were observed as early as 9 weeks. Fetal breathing movements, both regular and irregular in pattern, have been identified as early as 10 weeks as solitary movements or in combination with jaw opening or swallowing. Identification of the rotation of the fetus (Fig. 22-1) as well as active locomotion resulting in position change was made at 10 weeks.

TABLE 22-1. CLASSIFICATION AND WEEK OF ONSET OF FETAL MOVEMENTS

de Vries, et al, 1982[15]		Birnholz, et al, 1978[4]		Ianniruberto and Tajani, 1981[26]	
Week of Onset	Movements	Week of Onset	Movements	Week of Onset	Movements
7	Just-discernible movements			6–7	Vermicular movements
8	Startle	7–16	Twitch	8–18	Jerky global flexion and extension
8	General movements	12–16	Combined/repetitive simultaneous or serial movements of head, trunk, and limbs	11–18	Jumps, with change of lying position
9	Hiccough	24	Vigorous diaphragmatic excursions	22	Sudden rhythmic diaphragm movements
10	Breathing movements	24	Respiratory	13–14	Breathing movements
9	Isolated arm or leg movement	10–12	Independent limb movements	12–13	Isolated or independent movement of limbs
9	Isolated retroflexion of the head	14	Isolated extension of head		
9–10	Isolated rotation of head	14	Isolated rotation of head	12–13	Head rotation
10	Isolated anteflexion of head	14	Isolated flexion of head		
10–11	Jaw movements			13–14	Opening of mouth
12	Sucking and swallowing	24	Probable thumb sucking	13–14	Swallowing
10	Hand–face contact	16	Hand–face contact	12–13	Hands in contact with hand, face, or mouth
10	Stretch			16	Global extension
11	Yawn				
10	Rotation of fetus			12–13	Rotation, with change in lying position

(Modified from DeVries JIP, Visser GH, Prechtl HFR. Fetal motility in the first half of pregnancy. Clin Develop Med. 1984; 94:46–64.)

◢◢◢◢ **TABLE 22-2.** CLASSIFICATION OF FETAL MOVEMENT PATTERNS

Movement	Description
Just-discernible movements	Slow and small shifting of the fetal contour, lasting from 0.5 to 2 sec.
Startle	Quick, generalized movement always initiated in limbs and sometimes spreading to neck and trunk. Flexion or extension of limbs usually of large amplitude, but can be small or just discernible. Movements last about 1 sec.
General movements	Applicable if the whole body is moved but no distinctive pattern or sequence of body parts can be recognized.
Hiccoughs	Consists of a jerky contraction of diaphragm; abrupt displacement of diaphragm, thorax and abdomen.
Breathing movements	"Inspiration" consists of fluent, simultaneous movement of diaphragm (caudal direction), leading to movements of thorax (inward) and abdomen (outward).
Isolated arm or leg movements	May be rapid or slow movements and may involve extension, flexion, external and internal rotation, or abduction and adduction of an extremity without movements in other body parts.
Isolated retroflexion of the head	Displacement of the head can be small or large. Large movements may cause overextension of the fetal spine.
Isolated rotation of the head	Head may turn from a midline position to one side and back. This movement is often associated with hand–face contact.
Isolated anteflexion of the head	Carried out at a slow velocity. May occur alone or together with hand–face contact, when sucking can be observed.
Sucking and swallowing	Rhythmic bursts of regular jaw opening and closing at rate of about 1 per second may be followed by swallowing. Swallowing consists of displacements of tongue or larynx
Hand–face contact	Hand slowly touches face and fingers frequently extend and flex.
Stretch	Carried out at a slow speed. Consists of forceful extension of back, retroflexion of head, and external rotation and elevation of arms.
Yawn	Prolonged wide opening of jaws, followed by quick closure, often with retroflexion of head and sometimes elevation of arms.
Rotation of fetus	Rotation occurs around sagittal or transverse axis. Complete change around transverse axis is achieved by complex general movement including alternating leg movements. Rotation around longitudinal axis can result from leg movements with hip rotation or from rotation of head followed by trunk rotation.

(DeVries JIP, Visser GHA, Prechtl HFR. The emergence of fetal behavior: I. Qualitative aspects. Early Hum Dev. 1982; 7:301–322.)

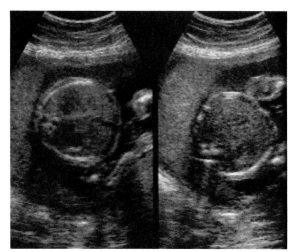

Figure 22-1. Two cross-sectional scans of a 15-week fetus demonstrates rotation of its body.

As can be seen in Table 22-3, an inverse relationship exists between both the incidence and the mean number of fetal movements, and gestational age. A decrease in the number as well as the incidence of movement is exhibited by the fetus as gestational age increases.[18,43,44,48,57] Thus, as the fetus matures during the second half of pregnancy, the incidence of motor activity decreases from a maximum of 21% in the 20- to 22-week fetus,[14] to 10% in the 30- to 40-week fetus.[48] A similar decrease in the average number of movements observed in an hour can also be demonstrated with increasing gestational age. The fetus at 24 to 26 weeks moves an average of 53 times per hour, as opposed to the 26- to 28-week fetus, who has a mean of 46 movements,[43] and the 30- to 40-week fetus with 31 hourly movements.[48]

Although an increased number of movements occur in the younger fetus, these movements have a shorter duration than movements observed at a later gestational age.[43] This aspect of fetal motor behavior can be related to the gradual maturation of the CNS. Dobbing and Sands[20] have reported that by the beginning of the third trimester, the number of neurons in the CNS has reached adult levels. These existing neurons, however, continue to exhibit hypertrophy, with an increase in dendritic arborization and synaptic connections. This second phase of brain growth is associated with glial cell hyperplasia and neuron myelination. Based on this evidence, Nasello-Paterson and coworkers[43] have thus suggested that the fetus at 24 to 28 weeks might experience a "short-circuit" effect in transmission of nerve impulses to the neuromuscular junction. Alternatively, these fetuses may have rela-

Quantitatively, the very young fetus has been found gradually to increase the amount of time spent moving. By 11 weeks, the fetus moves approximately 21% to 30% of the time observed (Table 22-3), with a wide range of activity demonstrated between individual fetuses (25% to 91%).[16]

FETAL MOVEMENT IN LATE GESTATION

Analysis of fetal movement patterns during the second half of pregnancy is characterized by the development of (1) periodicity of individual movements, (2) a fixed combination of individual movements, and (3) the association of fetal heart rate patterns with fetal movement. These facets of movement can be related to the maturation of the CNS.

◢◢◢◢ **TABLE 22-3.** SUMMARY OF THE CHARACTERISTICS OF FETAL MOVEMENT ACCORDING TO GESTATIONAL AGE

Study Population	Period of Observation	Gestational Age	Incidence of Movement	Number of Movements/Hour	Diurnal* Pattern
de Vries, et al, 1988[13]	1 hr	11 wk	21%–30%	—	—
de Vries, et al, 1987[14]	6 hr	20–22 wk	5%–21%	—	2200–2400
Nasello-Paterson, et al, 1988[43]	24 hr	24–26 wk	13%	53	2300–0800
Nasello-Paterson, et al, 1988[43]	24 hr	26–28 wk	12%	46	2300–0800
Patrick, et al, 1982[48]	24 hr	30–40 wk	10%	31	2100–0100

*Greatest increase in number of movements to time of day.

tively few motor units innervated. Transmission of nerve impulses to muscle would result in uncontrolled, sporadic movements.[43]

The second half of pregnancy is also characterized by the establishment of a diurnal pattern of motility (see Table 22-3). Twenty-four-hour observations of fetal movements have demonstrated that the 24- to 28-week fetus has an increase in the incidence of movement during the late night to early morning hours (11 PM to 8 AM).[43] The 30- to 40-week fetus, however, has a more limited diurnal pattern in which an increase of movement is seen only from 9 PM to 1 AM.[48]

Correlation of fetal movements with fetal heart rate has been found as early as at 20 to 22 weeks.[14] The interaction between movements and heart rate accelerations becomes more evident by 32 weeks' gestation. The number and amplitude of fetal heart rate accelerations associated with movements increase as the fetus approaches 32 weeks.[48] It appears, therefore, that as the fetus nears this gestational age, there is an increasing probability that a nonstress test (NST) will be reactive.

There was no significant evidence of change in movements that could be associated with maternal meals.[43,48] Thus, feeding a patient before an ultrasound examination will not increase the opportunity of observing fetal movements. Cigarette smoking does not alter the incidence of fetal movements; however, it has been reported that the periodicity pattern of movements is modified.[70] Maternal caffeine use does not appear to have an effect on general fetal body movements.[40]

Fetal Breathing Movements

Fetal breathing movements were first described by Ahlfeld in 1888.[1] This early investigation involved the observation of periodic rhythmic intrauterine fetal movements in the periumbilical area of pregnant women. Whether breathing movements were actually a part of the fetus's repertoire of motor behavior was held in doubt until direct evidence was provided by Dawes and colleagues,[10,11] who performed studies on chronic lamb preparations. This basic research performed on fetal lambs aroused clinical interest in the use of fetal breathing movements as a variable in the determination of fetal condition. Both A-mode ultrasound[5] and tocodynamometers[73] have been used in the detection

of human fetal respiratory movements. As with fetal movements, however, real-time ultrasound has proven to be the method of choice in the qualitative and quantitative investigation of fetal breathing.

Several clinical studies have been performed using real-time ultrasonography. In the human fetus, Connors and associates[8] studied the effects of maternal inhalation of various concentrations of carbon dioxide mixtures. It was discovered that the percentage of time of the incidence of fetal breathing movements correlated significantly with maternal end-tidal P_{CO_2}. Fetal breathing movements increased during periods of hypercapnia, but decreased with maternal hyperventilation.

In addition, human fetal breathing movements have been observed during maternal hypoxemia and its resolution. Manning and Platt[37] have reported a cessation of fetal respirations in the presence of a maternal P_{O_2} less than or equal to 40 mm Hg. Conversely, when the maternal P_{O_2} was greater than or equal to 60 mm Hg, fetal breathing movements were present 23% to 80% of the observed time.

A reduction of human fetal breathing movements can be attributed to causes other than those stated previously. For example, operative manipulation of the human fetus can be a causative agent in significantly decreasing the incidence of fetal breathing movements. It has been observed that fetal breathing movements are partially inhibited up to 2 days after an amniocentesis.[33]

Human fetal breathing movements have also been found to be decreased or abolished with the maternal ingestion of sedatives[5,37] and alcohol.[41] Long-term use of caffeine, however, causes an increased incidence of fetal breathing.[40]

CHARACTERISTICS OF FETAL BREATHING IN EARLY PREGNANCY

In general, movement patterns have an obvious effect on the development of the fetus. Fetal breathing movements have been considered as a "preparatory exercise" for extrauterine breathing.[56] These particular movements are considered essential for fetal lung growth. Fetal respiratory activity permits both the neuromuscular and skeletal development of the respiratory system to occur, and enables the appropriate respiratory epithelial development of the gas-exchanging surfaces of the lung.[29]

Breathing can easily be visualized in the fetus by obtaining a longitudinal sectional view with a real-time scanner. These movements consist of a movement of the diaphragm in a caudal direction, leading to an inward movement of the anterior chest wall and a simultaneous outward movement of the anterior abdominal wall (Fig. 22-2). The earliest such movements have been observed is at 10 weeks' gestation, with a tendency for these movements to have a regular pattern. Fetal breathing at this gestational age may be observed alone or in combination with jaw opening or swallowing, as well as with general body movements.[14] Fetal hiccoughs, which can be considered as a particular pattern of fetal breathing, have been recognized as early as 9 weeks. These movements consist of a jerky contraction of the fetal diaphragm. On sonographic scans, hiccoughs are seen as an abrupt displacement of the diaphragm, thorax, and abdomen. They may occur as single events, but most frequently follow each other in regular succession.[14] Other researchers have not observed these movements until 22 to 24 weeks[4,26] (see Table 22-1).

DeVries and colleagues[13] have observed that in fetuses from 7 to 19 weeks, a high incidence of hiccoughs is present during early gestation (9 to 13 weeks). The incidence of this particular movement, however, decreases with an increase in gestational age. In contrast, the incidence of breathing movements has been found to have a positive correlation with gestational age. Although a relatively low incidence of breathing was seen in the early stages of gestation, fetal respiration was found to increase with advancing fetal age. Fetal breathing movements in early gestation were not found to have any diurnal patterns.[14]

FETAL BREATHING IN LATE GESTATION

Manning and Platt[34] have described five patterns of fetal breathing that can be recognized in the second half of pregnancy (Table 22-4). These patterns include regular, irregular, irregular slow, and periodic accelerated breathing as well as hiccoughs. The fetus younger than 26 weeks' gestation was characterized especially by a pattern of irregular slow breathing.

Overall, the incidence of fetal breathing has a positive correlation with gestational age, that is, the incidence of breathing increases with increasing maturity of the fetus (Table 22-5). Twenty-four-hour observations of respiratory movement have demonstrated a nadir of 13.7% incidence in the 24- to 26-week fetus,[44] as opposed to a high of 31% incidence in the fetus of 30 to 40 weeks' gestation.[49,50,64,65] This incidence of breathing, however, dramatically decreases not only during labor, but up to 3 days before the initiation of the labor process (Table 22-6).[6,64]

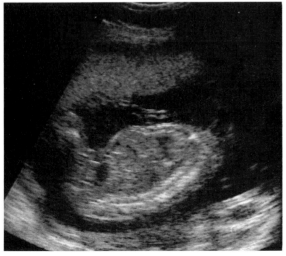
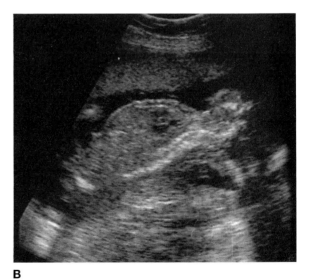

A   **B**

Figure 22-2. Fetal breathing movements of an 18-week fetus. Compare the inward location of the chest wall (**A;** inspiration) to its outward location during expiration (**B;** expiration).

TABLE 22-4. PATTERNS OF FETAL BREATHING MOVEMENTS

Pattern	Characteristics of Patterns	Rate
Regular	Regular in rate and amplitude	40–60 breaths/min
Irregular	Observed in the fetus <26 wk gestational age; highly irregular in rate and amplitude	20–100 breaths/min
Irregular slow	Slow, large amplitude	6–20 breaths/min
Periodic accelerated	Crescendo–decrescendo changes in rate and amplitude	30–90 breaths/min
Hiccoughs	Irregular, intermittent, large-amplitude breaths; short duration of individual breaths	20–60 breaths/min

(Manning FM, Platt LD. Fetal breathing movements: Antepartum monitoring of fetal condition. Clin Obstet Gynecol. 1979; 6:335–349.)

The length of periods of apnea have a similar positive relationship with gestational age in that as the fetus matures, the apneic intervals increase (see Table 22-5). The longest apneic interval in the 24- to 26-week fetus was observed to be a relatively brief period of 12 minutes,[44] compared to the 122-minute apneic interval of the 38- to 39-week fetus.[49]

This positive correlation was not observed between fetal hourly respiratory rate and gestational age, however. It was found that the number of breaths per hour gradually increased from 24 to 31 weeks' gestation. However, as the fetus approached term, this number was found to decrease (see Table 22-5).

A diurnal pattern of fetal breathing appears early in the second half of pregnancy. At 24 to 26 weeks, the fetus shows an increase in the frequency of breathing movements between 11 PM and 2 AM.[44] This peak of fetal breathing may be a maturation change in the fetal brain, allowing central receptors to become more sensitive to raised maternal carbon dioxide tension associated with sleep.[68] As the fetus matures, it gradually alters the timing of this pattern so that by 30 to 39 weeks, the greatest number of fetal respiratory movements are observed between 4 and 7 AM.[49]

In contrast to the findings observed in fetal

TABLE 22-5. SUMMARY OF THE CHARACTERISTICS OF FETAL BREATHING MOVEMENTS ACCORDING TO GESTATIONAL AGE

Study Population	Gestational Age	Incidence	Mean Hourly Respiratory Rate	Longest Apneic Interval	Diurnal Pattern*
de Vries, et al, 1987[14] (6-hr observation period)	20–22 wk	1%–40%	—	—	1300–1500 2200–2400
Natale, et al, 1988[44] (24-hr observation period)	24–26 wk	13.7%	42.8	12 min	2300–0200
Natale, et al, 1988[44] (24-hr observation period)	26–28 wk	14.2%	43.9	14 min	0200–0500
Patrick, et al, 1980[49] (24-hr observation period)	30–31 wk	31%	58.3	68 min	0400–0700
Patrick, et al, 1978[50] (8-hr observation period)	34–35 wk	31.8%	49.1	—	—
Patrick, et al, 1980[49] (24-hr observation period)	38–39 wk	31%	47	122 min	0400–0700

*Greatest increase in number of fetal breathing movements according to time of day.

TABLE 22-6. INCIDENCE OF FETAL BREATHING MOVEMENTS OBSERVED BEFORE AND DURING LABOR IN THE TERM FETUS

Study Population	Observational Period	Incidence
Carmichael, et al, 1984[6]	3 d before onset of labor	22.2%
Carmichael, et al, 1984[6]	12 hr before onset of labor	11.4%
Richardson, et al, 1979[64]	Latent phase of labor	8.3%
Richardson, et al, 1979[64]	Active phase of labor	0.8%

movement investigations, a significant increase in fetal breathing after a maternal meal was seen in the fetus of 30 to 32 weeks' gestation.[46]

Clinical Significance of Fetal Movements and Breathing Movements

Motor behavior of the fetus, including both fetal movements and breathing movements, has been demonstrated to be a normal fetal function throughout the course of pregnancy. It has been suggested that a decrease, cessation, or change in fetal motor behavior may be an indication of fetal condition. Before the use of real-time ultrasonography in the detection of fetal motor behavior, maternal perception of fetal movements was the main determinant in assessing fetal movements.

Clinical applications of the results of investigational studies of fetal movements and respiratory activity have revolved around attempts to find more accurate methods for the assessment of fetal health. In early pregnancy, in patients with a threatened abortion, simply the presence of fetal movements is considered to be a positive sign.[27] In later pregnancy, maternal perception and recognition of fetal movement has been found to be an early indicator of fetal well-being. Fetal movement counting techniques[47,51] have been found to be easy to introduce to patients and are routine methods for fetal surveillance. Moore and Piacquadio have reported that fetal movement counting can decrease the incidence of unexplained term stillbirths.[42] The quantification of fetal movements has also been used in the assessment of fetal well-being in pregnancies that may be complicated by factors such as diabetes[17] and congenital malformations.[60] In diabetic pregnancy, for example, it was discovered that the

length of active periods did not increase with increasing gestational age, as found in normal pregnancies, thus indicating a maturational delay in the fetus of a diabetic mother. With regard to the malformed fetus, it was observed that evidence of fetal inactivity was more common among fetuses with anomalies than among those with no defects.

Fetal breathing has been considered to be an indicator of fetal condition in that it is a component of the normal fetal motor behavioral repertoire. Platt and coworkers[56] demonstrated a significant relationship between the presence or absence of fetal breathing movements in the last observation before delivery and the resulting Apgar score. In the presence of respiratory activity, the fetus was found to be more likely to have an Apgar score greater than or equal to 7. Manning and colleagues[35] conducted a similar investigation in which the presence or absence of breathing movements was correlated with Apgar scores. This study, however, included the additional factor of the NST, which was observed in relation to Apgar scores as a sign of neonatal distress. It was discovered that each test taken separately was of equal strength in predicting neonatal outcome. However, when the tests were used in combination with one another, the results, when abnormal, led to significant improvement in predicting fetuses likely to have an abnormal outcome.

FETAL BIOPHYSICAL PROFILE

Manning and Platt's findings culminated in the development of the fetal biophysical profile.[31] A combination of five variables was used to develop a fetal test to diagnose the fetus in utero. These variables include fetal breathing movement, fetal movements, fetal tone, amniotic fluid volume, and the NST (indicating fetal heart rate reactivity). These variables were chosen because they are initiated and regulated by the fetal CNS, and it is thought that the presence of any given variable is indirect evidence of a functioning and intact neurologic system.

Because nervous tissue is highly dependent on adequate oxygenation, the presence or absence of these biophysical activities may reflect the state of fetal oxygenation. It has been theorized that an asphyxial insult, regardless of cause, elicits adaptive protective fetal responses that are manifest in consistent changes in biophysical variables. With regard to short-term biophysical variables that reflect immediate fetal condition (heart rate reactivity, fetal movement, fetal breathing, and fetal tone), the fetal response is a suppression of some or all of these activities, which may in turn reduce fetal oxygen consumption.[32] Further, it is hypothesized that fetal asphyxia induces a chemoreceptor reflex redistribution of cardiac output toward essential fetal organs (brain, heart, and placenta) at the expense of the kidneys and lungs. A prolonged or repeated episode of hypoxia initiating a redistribution of blood flow would lead to a near-cessation of perfusion of the fetal lung and kidney, resulting in decreased urine and lung fluid production that leads to oligohydramnios, a reduction in amniotic fluid volume.[7] The fifth biophysical variable, amniotic fluid volume, is therefore thought to reflect chronic fetal condition.

Variations in sensitivity to hypoxemia of specific areas of the brain responsible for the initiation of biophysical activities have been suggested, possibly indicating that increasing degrees of hypoxemia result in a progressive loss of biophysical function. It has been proposed that during fetal neurodevelopment a higher oxygen level is required for newly developing CNS and for reflex biophysical activities. The biophysical activities that become active first in fetal development appear to be the last to disappear when asphyxia arrests all biophysical activities. In terms of development, the fetal tone center is the earliest to function during intrauterine life (7.5 to 8.5 weeks), followed by the fetal movement, fetal breathing movement, and heart rate reactivity centers.[77] Clinical studies have demonstrated that the NST results and fetal breathing movements are the first biophysical variables to become abnormal in the asphyxiated fetus, followed by fetal movements, and finally by fetal tone.[54,63,79] It should be noted, however, that the absence of any one of these variables does not necessarily imply that the CNS is not intact and functioning. Because of the cyclic nature of many of these factors, absence of any one of the variables may reflect a sleep–rest state rather than a neurologic depression.

The methods used in fetal assessment by the fetal biophysical profile included measurements of fetal breathing movements, fetal movements, amniotic fluid volume, fetal tone, and the NST during the same observation period. Except for the NST, all variables were recorded using real-time ultrasound. For each observation period, each variable was coded as normal or abnormal according to specific criteria. The criteria as originally[31] reported were:

> NST: reactive (normal) if two or more heart rate accelerations of at least 15 beats per minute in amplitude and at least 15 seconds duration associated with fetal movements(s) in a 10-minute period
>
> Fetal breathing movements: present (normal) if at least one episode of fetal breathing of at least 60 seconds' duration within a 30-minute observation period
>
> Fetal movements: present (normal) if at least three discrete episodes of fetal movements within a 30-minute observation period
>
> Fetal tone: normal if upper and lower extremities in position of full flexion and head flexed on chest; at least one episode of extension of extremities with return to position of flexion or extension of spine with return to position of flexion
>
> Amniotic fluid volume: normal if fluid evident throughout the uterine cavity; largest pocket of fluid greater than 1 cm in vertical diameter

Current usage of the biophysical profile (Table 22-7) reflects the reassessment of the value of decreased amniotic fluid in evaluating fetal condition. The amniotic fluid index (AFI) has replaced the use of one pocket of amniotic fluid. In an analysis of this method, Phelan and associates[52] have suggested that an AFI of 5.0 cm or less is indicative of oligohydramnios. An advantage of using the AFI is that ultrasound practitioners have the ability to follow quantitative changes of the amniotic fluid with advancing gestational age. Thus, serial measure-

▰▰▰ **TABLE 22-7.** Characteristics of the Fetal Biophysical Profile

Parameter	Score 2 (Normal)	Score 0 (Abnormal)
Nonstress test	Reactive: Two or more fetal heart rate accelerations of at least 15 bpm in amplitude and at least 15 sec duration in 10 min within a 40-min testing period.	Nonreactive: One or no fetal heart rate accelerations of at least 15 bpm and 15 sec duration in 10 min within a 40-min testing period.
Fetal breathing movements	The presence of at least one episode of sustained fetal breathing of at least 30 sec duration within a 30-min observation period.	The absence of fetal breathing or the absence of an episode of breathing of at least 30 sec duration during a 30-min observation period.
Fetal body movements	The presence of at least three discrete episodes of fetal movements in a 30-min period. Simultaneous limb and trunk movement counted as a single movement.	Two or less discrete fetal movements in a 30-min observation period.
Fetal tone	Upper and lower extremities in position of full flexion and head flexed on chest. At least one episode of extension of extremities with return to position of flexion or extension of spine with return to position of flexion.	Extemities in position of extension or partial flexion. Spine in position of extension. Fetal movement not followed by return to flexion.
Amniotic fluid volume	Amniotic fluid index >5.0 cm.	Amniotic fluid index ≤5.0 cm.
Maximum score	10	
Minimum score		0

Interpretation: Score 10 or 8: Normal test—repeat in 4–7 days (dependent on indication). Score 6: Equivocal test—repeat within 12 hr. Score 4, 2, or 0: Abnormal test—consider delivery.

ments of the AFI may be an effective means of assessing fetal status throughout pregnancy.[53,66]

A second alteration in the original criteria of the biophysical profile is in the duration of fetal breathing. Currently, a 30-second observation period of regular fetal breathing within a 30-minute testing period is considered a normal parameter in the profile, as opposed to the original 60-second observation period. This modification was instituted subsequent to assessing Manning and co-workers'[38] use of a decreased duration of fetal breathing.

The fetal biophysical profile is used primarily in patients with high-risk factors. Initiation of testing is set at a gestational age identical to that used in other methods of fetal surveillance (the contraction stress test and the NST), that is, the minimal gestational age at which the physician would be willing to intervene should an abnormal test be observed (see Table 22-7). The patient is put in a semi-Fowler's position during the testing period in which the NST is performed, followed by the sonographic observation of biophysical activities. Various criteria have been applied for interpreting the NST. The occurrence of five accelerations of greater than 15 beats per minute for more than 15 seconds in 20 minutes was initially required for a normal or reactive test. More recent studies have suggested that fewer accelerations of the same magnitude may be adequate. Many institutions define a reactive NST as the occurrence of two qualifying accelerations within a 10-minute period. Failure to demonstrate a reactive pattern owing either to lack of accelerations with movement or to lack of fetal movement is termed a nonreactive NST. Amniotic fluid volume is determined by dividing the maternal abdomen into four quadrants, using the umbilicus and linea nigra as the horizontal and vertical reference points of division, respectively. Holding the ultrasound transducer perpendicular to the floor, the vertical diameter of the largest pocket of amniotic fluid is identified and measured. The numbers from each quadrant are summed, and the result is the AFI (see Fig. 24-8). Each biophysical variable is coded as normal whenever fixed criteria are reached, regardless of the duration of observation, up to a maximum of 30 minutes for the ultrasound variables, and up to 40 minutes when determining fetal heart rate reactivity. An arbitrary score of 2 is given if a variable is normal, and 0 if abnormal. The fetal biophysical profile score is the result of adding each score of all five variables. The highest possible score obtainable is 10; the lowest score that can be observed when all the parameters are abnormal is 0. A combined score of 10 or 8 is regarded as normal. A score of 6 is equivocal and indicates that the profile should be repeated within 12 hours. A score of 4, 2, or 0 is indicative of fetal compromise and delivery of the fetus should be considered. A deviation from this system applies in the case of oligohydramnios. In any fetus with decreased amniotic fluid and intact membranes, and with all other biophysical profile variables normal, delivery is considered at many institutions.

RELATIONSHIP OF THE BIOPHYSICAL PROFILE SCORE TO FETAL WELL-BEING

Clinical experience with the fetal biophysical profile as a measure of fetal compromise has yielded encouraging results. A number of prospective studies have reported on the biophysical profile results of more than 26,000 high-risk patients, demonstrating that a significant exponential rise in perinatal morbidity as well as mortality occurs with decreasing profile scores.[2,12,30,54,55,69,77] Further, the value of the biophysical profile in assessing the fetus at risk for asphyxia has been substantiated in a number of clinical studies that have revealed a strong relationship between the fetal biophysical profile score and umbilical venous pH.[32,62,79,81,83,84] Manning and colleagues[32] compared fetal biophysical profile scores with umbilical venous pH values measured in blood obtained by immediate percutaneous umbilical blood sampling. They discovered that there was a highly significant linear correlation between biophysical profile score and umbilical venous pH, with a score of 0 out of 10 always associated with a pH less than 7.20, and a score of 8 or 10 was always found to be associated with a pH greater than 7.25. Further, the umbilical venous pH fell significantly as the biophysical profile score fell.

Studies by Vintzileos and colleagues[76,78,80] have suggested the use of a modified fetal biophysical profile as an early predictor of fetal infection in patients with premature rupture of the membranes. It was discovered that a biophysical profile score of 7 or lower (out of a possible score of 12) was a good predictor of impending fetal infection in this particular group of patients. The absence of fetal breathing and a nonreactive NST were the first signs of impending infection, whereas decreased tone and fetal movement were late manifestations of this obstetric complication.

In analyzing the profile in relation to gestational age, Baskett[3] has determined that a decreasing number of abnormal NSTs as well as abnormal detections of abnormal fetal breathing movements occur with advancing gestational age. The profile was found more likely to be equivocal at 26 to 33 weeks because it is possible that either the NST or fetal breathing may be observed as abnormal compared to those parameters in fetuses who are at 34 to 41 weeks' gestational age. It is suggested, therefore, that the biophysical profile should be interpreted in relation to the gestational age of the fetus being tested. These results, however, have not been investigated by other researchers and thus have not been confirmed. Currently the biophysical profile is being utilized in the assessment of high risk pregnancies ranging from 25 weeks gestational age to 44 weeks.[36,55,80]

VIBROACOUSTIC STIMULATION

Vibroacoustic stimulation has been used as an adjunct in fetal heart rate assessment (NST) since the mid-1980s. Although the reactive NST has been found to be a safe and reliable indicator of fetal well-being, a nonreactive NST is a less sensitive indicator of fetal compromise. Episodes of nonreactivity are often related to fetal behavioral state. One of the problems with antepartum fetal heart rate testing is the difficulty in separating healthy fetuses at rest from sick fetuses who are not moving because of asphyxia. Various attempts to stimulate the fetus have proven ineffective. These include the administration of orange juice before testing and manual manipulation of the maternal abdomen.[21,22] Vibroacoustic stimulation is performed as an adjunct to improve the efficacy of antepartum fetal heart rate testing. It is used to reduce the incidence of falsely nonreactive tests presumably secondary to fetal sleep states and overall testing time. After 25 weeks of gestation, it was discovered that the normal fetus has developed auditory startle behavior,[26] a behavior that is distinguished from but similar to the neonatal Moro reflex. On stimulation with sound, it was found that the fetus also responded with a significant increase in fetal movements that were associated with a corresponding increase of basal fetal heart rate and fetal heart rate accelerations.[25,61] The stimulus is generated by an artificial larynx or a similar commercially produced device that provides both acoustic and vibratory stimuli. This device emits fundamental tones of approximately 85 to 100 dB with a fundamental frequency of 850 Hz. When applied to the maternal abdomen, the fetus changes state and reacts with a startle response. The vibroacoustic stimulator has received U.S. Food and Drug Administration approval for antepartum use between 28 and 42 weeks' gestation.

Vibroacoustic stimulation is initiated in NST after 10 minutes of nonreactivity. The stimulator is applied to the maternal abdomen for 1 second and fetal heart rate response is observed for 1 minute. If the criteria for adequate accelerations are not met, the fetus is stimulated for 2 seconds. If accelerations are not achieved after an additional 1-minute observation, a third application of stimulation is performed for 3 seconds. The fetal heart rate is then observed until it becomes reactive or 40 minutes have elapsed. Several studies have reported that the use of vibroacoustic stimulation results in a signifi-

cant reduction in the number of nonreactive NSTs and a decrease in the time required for a reactive test to occur.[71,72] Reactivity achieved with stimulation was found to have a predictive value equal to that of a spontaneously reactive NST.

As with other antepartum fetal assessment techniques such as the NST or the contraction stress test, the fetal biophysical profile has proven to have a high specificity but a relatively low sensitivity. To improve the sensitivity of the biophysical profile, Divon and colleagues[19] recommended that sound stimulation be added to assess fetal tone. Tone assessment is made by the ultrasonic observation of the presence or absence of spontaneous fetal limb extension–flexion movements (Fig. 22-3). It has been suggested that this is a subjective and qualitative measurement because postnatally, tone is determined by observing an active resistance by the neonate in response to a straightening of the extremities. Through the use of real-time ultrasound, it was discovered that the startle response, expressed as extension and return to flexion of the fetal forearm, could be evoked each time the sound–vibratory stimulus was applied to the maternal abdomen. This provoked response was considered to be a more objective evaluation of fetal tone than previously thought. In addition, sound stimulus may assist in altering the behavioral state of the fetus (i.e., awaken the fetus from a quiet sleep state to an active, awake state). In an active, awake state, the positive responses the biophysical profile at-

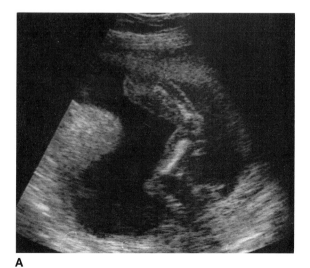

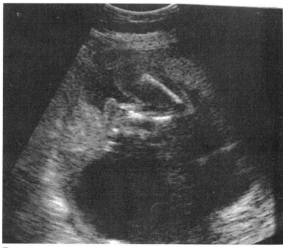

A   **B**

Figure 22-3. (**A**) Extension and (**B**) flexion of the leg of an 18-week fetus.

tempts to identify are more likely to be recognized in a neurologically normal fetus. Vibroacoustic stimulation, however, can cause a decrease in fetal breathing movements that can persist for up to an hour after the stimulus.[23]

Kuhlman and associates[28] have used sound stimuli to evoke a startle response in the fetus. They identified a facial startle reaction, however, in contrast to the startle response suggested by Divon and colleagues. All normal fetuses who were older than 27 weeks' gestational age and were subjected to sound stimuli had startle responses. However, when a group of hydrocephalic fetuses was subjected to the sound stimuli, all of the fetuses who failed to demonstrate startle responses either died in utero or within several months after birth, and had the most severe CNS defects.

In general, measurements of the biophysical profile parameters have been made as objective as possible to eliminate the possibility of any qualitative judgments in assessment of the fetus.

Summary

The human fetus has completely developed its repertoire of motor behavior by 16 weeks' gestational age, including both fetal movements and breathing movements. As the fetus advances in age, however, these behaviors are altered both in frequency as well as in their relationship to each other, as regulated by the maturation of the fetal CNS. Thus, diagnosis of fetal condition based on motor behavior must be made with regard to not only possible adverse intrauterine conditions to which the fetus may be subjected, but also to the particular gestational age of that fetus.

The development of the fetal biophysical profile has become an important diagnostic tool for assessing fetal well-being. It is, however, less predictive of fetal jeopardy. It may be possible that the analysis of additional variables (such as the sound-stimulated startle response) or the refinement of existing variables can increase the sensitivity of this testing scheme.

REFERENCES

1. Ahlfeld F. Uber Bisher Noch Nicht Beschriebene Intrauterine Bewegungen des Kindes. In: Verhandlungen der Deutschen Gesellschaft der Gynakologie. Leipzig: Breitkopf & Hartel; 1888.

2. Baskett TF, Allen AC, Gray JH, Young DC, Young LM. Fetal biophysical profile and perinatal death. Obstet Gynecol. 1987; 70:357–360.

3. Baskett TF. Gestational age and fetal biophysical assessment. Am J Obstet Gynecol. 1988; 158:332–334.

4. Birnholz JC, Stephens JC, Faria M. Fetal movement patterns: A possible means of defining neurologic developmental milestones in utero. Am J Roentgenol. 1978; 130:537–540.

5. Boddy K, Dawes, GS. Fetal breathing. Br Med Bull. 1975; 31:3–7.

6. Carmichael L, Campbell K, Patrick J. Fetal breathing, gross fetal body movements, and maternal fetal heart rates before spontaneous labor at term. Am J Obstet Gynecol. 1984; 148:675–679.

7. Cohn HE, Sacks EJ, Heymann MA, et al. Cardiovascular responses to hypoxemia and acidemia in fetal lambs. Am J Obstet Gynecol. 1974; 120:817–824.

8. Connors G, Hunse C, Carmichael L, et al. The role of carbon dioxide in the generation of human fetal breathing movements. Am J Obstet Gynecol. 1988; 158:322–327.

9. Connors G, Natalie R, Nasello-Paterson C. Maternally perceived fetal activity from twenty-four weeks' gestation to term in normal and at risk pregnancies. Am J Obstet Gynecol. 1988; 158:294–299.

10. Dawes GS. Breathing before birth in animals and man. N Engl J Med. 1974; 290:557–559.

11. Dawes GS, Fox HE, Leduc BM, et al. Respiratory movements and rapid eye movement sleep in the foetal lamb. J Physiol. 1972; 220:119–143.

12. DeVoe LD, Castillo RA, Searle N, et al. Prognostic components of computerized fetal biophysical testing. Am J Obstet Gynecol. 1988; 158:1144–1148.

13. DeVries JIP, Visser GHA, Prechtl HFR. The emergence of fetal behavior: III. Individual differences and consistencies. Early Hum Dev. 1988; 16:85–103.

14. DeVries JIP, Visser GHA, Mulder EJH, et al. Diurnal and other variations in fetal movement and heart rate patterns at 20–22 weeks. Early Hum Dev. 1987; 15:333–348.

15. DeVries JIP, Visser GHA, Prechtl HFR. The emergence of fetal behavior: I. Qualitative aspects. Early Hum Dev. 1982; 7:301–322.

16. DeVries JIP, Visser GH, Prechtl HFR. Fetal motility in the first half of pregnancy. Clin Develop Med. 1984; 94:46–64.

17. Dierker LJ, Pillay S, Sorokin Y, et al. The change in fetal activity periods in diabetic and nondiabetic pregnancies. Am J Obstet Gynecol. 1982; 143:181–185.

18. Dierker LJ, Rosen MG, Pillay S, et al. The correla-

tion between gestational age and fetal activity periods. Biol Neonate. 1982; 42:66–72.

19. Divon MY, Platt LD, Cantrell CJ. Evoked fetal startle response: A possible intrauterine neurological examination. Am J Obstet Gynecol. 1985; 154:454–456.

20. Dobbing J, Sands J. Quantitative growth and development of human brain. Arch Dis Child. 1973; 48:757–767.

21. Druzin ML, Gratacos J, Paul RH, et al. Antepartum fetal heart rate testing: XII. The effect of manual manipulation of the fetus on the nonstress test. Am J Obstet Gynecol. 1985; 151:61–64.

22. Eglinton GS, Paul RH, Broussard PM, et al. Antepartum fetal heart rate testing: XI. Stimulation with orange juice. Am J Obstet Gynecol. 1984; 150:97–99.

23. Gagnon R, Hunse C, Carmichael L, Fellows F, Patrick J. Effects of vibratory acoustic stimulation on human fetal breathing and gross fetal body movements near term. Am J Obstet Gynecol. 1986; 155:1227–1230.

24. Granat M, Lavie P, Adar D, et al. Short term cycles in human fetal activity: I. Normal pregnancies. Am J Obstet Gynecol. 1979; 134:696–701.

25. Grimwade JC, Walker DW, Bartlett M, et al. Human fetal heart rate changes and movement in response to sound and vibration. Am J Obstet Gynecol. 1971; 109:86–90.

26. Ianniruberto A, Tajani E. Ultrasonographic study of fetal movements. Semin Perinatol. 1981; 5:175–181.

27. Jouppila P. Fetal movements diagnosed by ultrasound in early pregnancy. Acta Obstet Gynaecol Scand. 1976; 55:131–135.

28. Kuhlman K, Burns K, Sabbagha R, et al. Real time ultrasonographic imaging of fetal response decrement to external acoustic stimulation. Presented at the meeting of the Society of Perinatal Obstetricians, San Antonio, Texas, January, 1986.

29. Maloney JE, Alcorn D, Bowes G, et al. Development of the future respiratory system before birth. Semin Perinatol. 1980; 4:251–260.

30. Manning FA, Harman CR, Morrison I, Menticoglou SM, Lange IR, Johnson JM. Fetal assessment based on fetal biophysical profile scoring: IV. An analysis of perinatal morbidity and mortality. Am J Obstet Gynecol. 1990; 162:703–709.

31. Manning FA, Platt LD, Sipos L. Antepartum fetal evaluation: Development of fetal biophysical profile. Am J Obstet Gynecol. 1980; 136:787–795.

32. Manning FA, Snijders R, Harman CR, Nicolaides K, Menticoglou S, Morrison I. Fetal biophysical profile score: VI. Correlation with antepartum umbilical ve-nous fetal pH. Am J Obstet Gynecol. 1993; 169:755–763.

33. Manning FH, Platt LD, LeMay M. Effect of amniocentesis on fetal breathing movements. Br Med J. 1972; 2:1582–1583.

34. Manning FM, Platt LD. Fetal breathing movements: Antepartum monitoring of fetal condition. Clin Obstet Gynecol. 1979; 6:335–349.

35. Manning FA, Platt LD, Sipos L, et al. Fetal breathing movements and the nonstress test in high risk pregnancies. Am J Obstet Gynecol. 1979; 135:511–515.

36. Manning FA, Morrison MB, Harman CR, et al. Fetal assessment based on fetal biophysical profile scoring: Experience in 19,221 referred high risk pregnancies. Am J Obstet Gynecol. 1987; 157:880–884.

37. Manning FA, Platt LD. Maternal hypoxemia and fetal breathing movements. Obstet Gynecol. 1977; 53:758–760.

38. Manning FA, Baskett TF, Morrison I, Lange I. Fetal biophysical profile scoring: A prospective study in 1,184 high-risk patients. Am J Obstet Gynecol. 1981; 140:289–294.

39. Marsal D. Fetal activity. In: Chervenak FA, Isaacson GC, Campbell S, eds. Ultrasound in Obstetrics and Gynecology. Boston: Little, Brown & Co.; 1993: 463–470.

40. McGowan J, Devoe LD, Searle N, Altman R. The effects of long- and short-term maternal caffeine ingestion on human fetal breathing and body movements in term gestation. Am J Obstet Gynecol. 1987; 157:726–729.

41. McLeod W, Brien J, Loomis C, et al. Effect of maternal ethanol ingestion on fetal breathing movements, gross body movements, and heart rate at 37 to 40 weeks gestational age. Am J Obstet Gynecol. 1983; 145:251–257.

42. Moore TE, Piacquadio K. A prospective evaluation of fetal movement screening to reduce the incidence of antepartum fetal death. Am J Obstet Gynecol. 1989; 160:1075–1080.

43. Nasello-Paterson C, Natale R, Connors G. Ultrasonic evaluation of fetal body movements over twenty-four hours in the human fetus at twenty-four to twenty-eight weeks gestation. Am J Obstet Gynecol. 1988; 158:312–316.

44. Natale R, Nasello-Paterson C, Connors G, et al. Patterns of fetal breathing activity in the human fetus at 24 to 28 weeks of gestation. Am J Obstet Gynecol. 1988; 158:317–321.

45. Natale R, Nasello C, Turliuk R. The relationship between movements and accelerations in fetal heart rate at twenty-four to thirty-two weeks gestation. Am J Obstet Gynecol. 1984; 148:591–595.

46. Natale R, Nasello-Paterson C, Turliuk R. Longitudi-

nal measurements of fetal breathing, body movements, heart rate, and heart rate accelerations at 24 to 32 weeks of gestation. Am J Obstet Gynecol. 1985; 151:256–263.

47. Neldam S. Fetal movements as indicator of fetal wellbeing. Lancet. 1980; 1:1222–1224.

48. Patrick J, Campbell K, Carmichael L, et al. Patterns of gross fetal body movements over 24-hour observation intervals during the last 10 weeks of pregnancy. Am J Obstet Gynecol. 1982; 142:363–371.

49. Patrick J, Campbell K, Carmichael L, et al. Patterns of human fetal breathing during the last 10 weeks of pregnancy. Obstet Gynecol. 1980; 56:24–30.

50. Patrick J, Fetherston W, Vick H, et al. Human fetal breathing movements and gross fetal body movements at weeks 34 to 35 gestation. Am J Obstet Gynecol. 1978; 130:693–699.

51. Pearson JF, Weaver JB. Fetal activity and fetal wellbeing. Br Med J. 1976; 1:1305–1307.

52. Phelan JP, Smith CV, Broussard P, Small M. Amniotic fluid volume assessment with the four-quadrant technique at 36–42 weeks' gestation. J Reprod Med. 1987; 32:540–542.

53. Phelan JP, Ahn MO, Smith CV, Rutherford SE, Anderson E. Amniotic fluid index measurements during pregnancy. J Reprod Med. 1987; 32:601–604.

54. Platt LD, Eglinton GS, Sipos L. Further experience with the fetal biophysical profile score. Obstet Gynecol. 1983; 61:480–485.

55. Platt LD, Walla CA, Paul RH, et al. A prospective trial of the fetal biophysical profile versus the nonstress test in the management of high-risk pregnancies. Am J Obstet Gynecol. 1985; 153:624–633.

56. Platt LD, Manning FA, Lemay M, et al. Human fetal breathing: Relationship to fetal condition. Am J Obstet Gynecol. 1978; 132:514–518.

57. Prechtl HFR. Continuity and changes in early neural development. Clin Develop Med. 1984; 94:1–15.

58. Preyer W. Spezielle Physiologie des Embryo. Leipzig: Grieben; 1885.

59. Rayburn WF, Motley ME, Stempel LE, et al. Antepartum prediction of the postmature infant. Obstet Gynecol. 1982; 60:148–153.

60. Rayburn WF, Barr M. Activity patterns in malformed fetuses. Am J Obstet Gynecol. 1982; 142:1045–1048.

61. Read JA, Miller JC. Fetal heart rate acceleration in response to acoustic stimulation as a measure of fetal well being. Am J Obstet Gynecol. 1977; 129:512–517.

62. Ribbert LSM, Snijders RJM, Nicolaides KH, Visser GH. Relationship of fetal biophysical profile and blood gas values at cordocentesis in severely growth-retarded fetuses. Am J Obstet Gynecol. 1990; 163:569–571.

63. Ribbert LSM, Nicolaides KH, Visser GHA. Prediction of fetal acidaemia in intrauterine growth retardation: Comparison of quantified fetal activity with biophysical score. Br J Obstet Gynaecol. 1993; 100:653–656.

64. Richardson B, Natale R, Patrick J. Human fetal breathing activity during electively induced labor at term. Am J Obstet Gynecol. 1979; 133:247–255.

65. Roberts AB, Little D, Cooper D, et al. Normal patterns of fetal activity in the third trimester. Br J Obstet Gynaecol. 1979; 86:4–9.

66. Rutherford SE, Smith CV, Jacobs N, Phelan JP. The four-quadrant assessment of amniotic fluid "volume": An adjunct to antepartum fetal heart rate testing. Presented at the meeting of the Society of Perinatal Obstetricians, San Antonio, Texas, January, 1986.

67. Sadovsky E, Polishuk WZ. Fetal movements in utero. Obstet Gynecol. 1977; 50:49–55.

68. Sadovsky E, Polishuk WZ, Mahler Y, et al. Fetal movements recorder: Use and indications. Int J Gynaecol Obstet. 1977; 15:20–24.

69. Schifrin BS, Guntes V, Gergely RC, et al. The role of real-time scanning in antenatal fetal surveillance. Am J Obstet Gynecol. 1981; 140:525–530.

70. Eriksen PS, Gennser G, Lofgren O, Nilsson R. Acute effects of maternal smoking on fetal breathing and movements. Obstet Gynecol. 1983; 61:367–372.

71. Smith CV, Phelan JP, Broussard PM, et al. Fetal acoustic stimulation testing: A retrospective analysis of the fetal acoustic stimulation test. Am J Obstet Gynecol. 1985; 153:567–569.

72. Smith CV, Phelan JP, Broussard PM, et al. Fetal acoustic stimulation testing: III. Prediction value of a reactive test. J Reprod Med. 1988; 33:217–218.

73. Timor-Tritsch IE, Dierker LJ, Hertz RH, et al. Regular and irregular human fetal respiratory movement. Early Hum Dev. 1980; 4:315–324.

74. Valentin L, Marsal K. Fetal movement in the third trimester of normal pregnancy. Early Hum Dev. 1986; 14:295–306.

75. Valentin L. Lofgren O, Marsal K, Grillberg B. Subjective recording of fetal movements: I. Limits and acceptability in normal pregnancies. Acta Obstet Gynaecol Scand. 1984; 68:223–228.

76. Vintzileos AM, Campbell WA, Nochimson DJ, Connolly ME, Fuenfer MM, Hoehn GJ. The fetal biophysical profile in patients with premature rupture of the membranes: An early predictor of fetal infection. Am J Obstet Gynecol. 1985; 152:510–516.

77. Vintzileos AM, Campbell WA, Ingardia CJ, et al. The fetal biophysical profile and its predictive value. Obstet Gynecol. 1983; 62:271–278.

78. Vintzileos AM, Campbell WA, Nochimson DJ,

Weinbaum PH, Minochnick MH, Escoto DT. Fetal biophysical profile versus amniocentesis in predicting infection in preterm premature rupture of the membranes. Obstet Gynecol. 1986; 68:488–494.

79. Vintzileos AM, Gaffney SE, Salinger LM, Campbell WA, Nochimson DJ. The relationship between fetal biophysical profile and cord pH in patients undergoing cesarean section before the onset of labor. Obstet Gynecol. 1987; 70:196–201.

80. Vintzileos AM, Bors-Koefoed R, Pelegaro JF, et al. The use of the fetal biophysical profile improves pregnancy outcome in premature rupture of the membranes. Am J Obstet Gynecol. 1987; 157:236–240.

81. Vintzileos AM, Gaffney SE, Salinger LM, Kontopoulos VG, Campbell WA, Nochimson DJ. The relationships among the fetal biophysical profile, umbilical cord pH, and Apgar scores. Am J Obstet Gynecol. 1987; 157:627–631.

82. Wheeler T, Roberts K, Peters J, et al. Detection of fetal movements using Doppler ultrasound. Obstet Gynecol. 1987; 70:251–254.

83. Yoon BH, Romero R, Roh CR, et al. Relationship between the fetal biophysical profile score, umbilical artery Doppler velocimetry, and fetal blood acid–base status determined by cordocentesis. Am J Obstet Gynecol. 1993; 169:1586–1594.

84. Yoon BH, Syn HC, Kim SW. The efficacy of Doppler umbilical artery velocimetry in identifying fetal acidosis: A comparison with fetal biophysical profile. J Ultrasound Med. 1992; 11:1–6.

85. Junge HD. Behavioral states and state related fetal heart rate and motor activity patterns in the newborn infant and the fetus antepartum: A comparative study. J Perinat Med. 1979; 7:85.

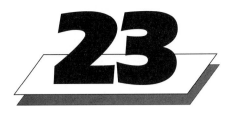

Multiple Gestations

JULIA A. DROSE and MARK A. DENNIS

In our sonography practice we have seen many an unsuspecting couple react with excitement at the discovery of a twin pregnancy. Members of the medical community respond in a more tempered fashion, being aware of the numerous problems and complications that may accompany multiple-gestation pregnancies. Although multiple gestations account for approximately 1% of all live births, the associated perinatal mortality rate may be as much as 5 to 10 times higher than in singleton births, principally because of prematurity, and thus the 1% also accounts for 10% to 13% of all neonatal deaths.[13,27] These alarming statistics may be altered through early diagnosis and ultrasound monitoring. Although in prospectively screened populations ultrasound is 98% sensitive in diagnosing multiple gestations, because ultrasound screening in the community is not performed routinely on all pregnancies, many multiple gestations may go undiagnosed until later in pregnancy. Late diagnosis is associated with elevated mortality and morbidity rates. Once they are diagnosed and closely monitored, the probability of an unfavorable outcome in multiple gestations may actually be reduced from 60% to 25%.[31] The role of the sonographer therefore is to diagnose accurately a multiple-gestation pregnancy and to follow the pregnancy regularly to detect associated fetal complications.

Clinical Information

The most common reason for suspecting a multiple-gestation pregnancy is the physical finding of "large for gestational age fetus." The differential diagnosis for this clinical presentation includes polyhydramnios, uterine fibroids, molar pregnancy, erroneous dates, macrosomic fetus, or extrauterine masses (i.e., ovarian). On physical examination, the diagnosis of multiple gestations may be suspected through the palpation of two or more fetuses or when two or more fetal heart beats varying in location and by more than 10 beats per minute in rate are discovered by auscultation or Doppler examination. Early increases in maternal blood pressure and anemia, greater than would be expected with a singleton gestation, may also be found.

Laboratory values may indicate multiple gestations as well. Routine maternal serum α-fetoprotein (MSAFP) determination is performed in most centers today. Twenty to 30% of pregnant women have an MSAFP level greater than the 95th percentile.[40] About 10% of these pregnancies are multiple gestations. Quantitation of human serum placental lactogen (HPL) is a less common but more sensitive test for detecting multiple gestations. Ninety-five percent of twin pregnancies fall within the group of HPL levels greater than one standard deviation (SD) above the mean for gestational age in singleton pregnancies.[22] A combined increase in MSAFP and HPL can raise the twin detection rate to approximately 80% without imaging. The maternal serum human chorionic gonadotropin level may also be higher in multiple gestations.[23]

The level of clinical suspicion for multiple gestation is elevated by maternal history. The two major types of twinning are monozygotic (MZ) and

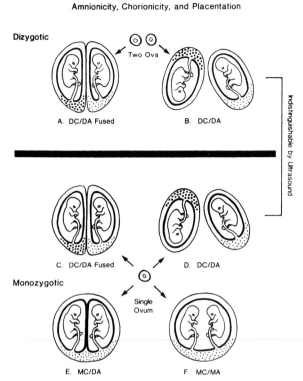

Amnionicity, Chorionicity, and Placentation

Dizygotic

Two Ova

A. DC/DA Fused   B. DC/DA

Indistinguishable by Ultrasound

C. DC/DA Fused   D. DC/DA

Monozygotic

Single Ovum

E. MC/DA   F. MC/MA

Figure 23-1. Dizygotic twinning is depicted above the horizontal bar and monozygotic twinning, below. *A–D* are dichorionic–diamniotic (DC/DA) twins; monozygosity and dizygosity cannot be differentiated by evaluation of placentation or membranes alone. The appearance of a single placenta results from fusion of separate placentas and may be distinguished from *E* and *F* (monochorionic [MC] pregnancies with diamniotic and monoamniotic [MA] membranes, respectively) by the presence of a thick membrane. Note the thick membranes in *A* and *C* and the thin membrane in *E*.

advancing maternal age as well, peaking at 35 to 39 years. There is an overall twinning rate in the United States of approximately 1 in 90 births. Blacks have the highest incidence of multiple births (1/76), Asians the lowest rate (1/92), and the probability of whites bearing DZ twins is 1 in 86. With regard to geographic differences, the highest global DZ twinning rate is in Chile (1/51) and the lowest is in Venezuela (1/294). Finally, pharmacologic ovulation induction variably increases the probability of multiple births.[13]

Anatomy and Physiology

The placental membranes are composed of two layers, the outer layer (chorion) and the inner layer (amnion). Three types of placentation or combinations of membranes and placentas are possible with twin gestations (Fig. 23-1). In dichorionic–diamniotic gestations, the fetuses have separate placentas and chorions, and therefore their own separate amniotic sacs. As pregnancy progresses, the placentas may fuse, giving the sonographic appearance of a single placenta. Monochorionic–diamniotic fetuses are enclosed in separate amniotic sacs but share one placenta and one chorion. In the third category, the monochorionic–monoamniotic pregnancy, both fetuses share the same placenta, chorion, and amniotic sac. All DZ twins are of the dichorionic–diamniotic variety, but the type of placentation in MZ twins depends on the stage of embryonic development at which separation occurs (Table 23-1). In MZ gestations, the mortality rate can range from 9% in dichorionic cases to 50% in

dizygotic (DZ). Thirty percent of all twins are of the MZ type, in which a single ovum divides after fertilization. This type of event appears to be random and independent of clinical and epidemiologic factors except in rare instances.[13] Nearly 70% of all twin gestations are of the DZ type, the result of the fertilization of two ova. This type of event depends on polyovulation, which in turn is related to maternal medical history and environmental factors. DZ twinning is increased if there is a history of DZ twinning on the maternal side of the family. Women who are themselves DZ twins have 1 chance in 58 of delivering twins. Women who have borne DZ twins previously have 1 chance in 40 of repeating this in a subsequent pregnancy. The incidence of multiple births appears to increase with

TABLE 23-1. Association of Placentation of MZ Twins with Timing of Zygote Division

Time of Zygote Division (days)	MZ Placentation	Approximate Frequency
3	DC/DA	33%
4–7	MC/DA	66%
8–13	MC/MA	3%
13+	Conjoined (MC/MA)	1/50,000– 1/100,000

MZ, monozygotic; DC, dichorionic; DA, diamniotic; MC, monochorionic; MA, monoamniotic.

(Adapted from Crane JP. Sonographic evaluation of multiple pregnancy. Semin Ultrasound CT MR. 1984; 5:144–156.)

monoamniotic cases.[5] The differing risks associated with different types of MZ placentation make it desirable to determine amnionticity and chorionicity by ultrasound examination in all cases of multiple gestation (Table 23-2).[17,30]

Examination Techniques and Imaging

SCANNING PROTOCOL

When scanning multiple gestations, it is of utmost importance to be thorough. The evaluation of each fetus should be performed as if it is a completely separate examination, thereby avoiding oversights (Table 23-3). The sonographer should resist the tendency to condense the multiple-gestation examination into the time normally allotted for a singleton examination, and, if possible, appropriate time should be reserved in advance. The examination should begin with scanning of the uterus in either a transverse or a longitudinal plane, from one side to the other, to determine the number of fetuses. Next, the lower uterine segment is scanned again

to identify the presenting fetus. The fetus with the lowest presenting part should be labeled fetus A. Unusually, two fetuses may coexist at the same level, in which case they should be labeled "left fetus" or "right fetus." It may also be helpful to identify the fetus' sex. If the twins are DZ, 50% will be of opposite sexes. In this situation, should the fetuses change in relative position (fetus A become fetus B), follow-up growth measurements will still be possible. Because it is very rare for MZ twins to be of different sexes (a chromosome abnormality must be involved), if two separate fetal sexes are identified, this virtually guarantees dizygosity. Twins of the same sex may be DZ or MZ.

Once the presenting fetus (A) has been identified, the fetal spine should be followed to connect the appropriate head with its corresponding body. After fetus A's body parts have been identified and its position determined, a routine fetal anatomy examination and documentation, as set forth by the American Institute of Ultrasound in Medicine,[3] the American College of Radiology,[2] and the American College of Obstetrics and Gynecology[1] should be

TABLE 23-2. ASSOCIATION OF PLACENTATION AND COMPLICATIONS

Ultrasound Findings	Placentation	Significance
Single placenta, thin membrane	MC/DA	Intrapartum jeopardy of second twin after first twin delivered
		Only necessary to aspirate one sac on amniocentesis
		Twin–twin transfusion is possible and periodic ultrasound is recommended beginning wk 25
		Contraindication to selective termination of one twin
		Complications possible in surviving twin if one twin dies
Single placenta, no membrane	MC/MA	High mortality rate if MC/MA due to entanglement or twin–twin transfusion
	Fused DC/DA or MC/DA	Always rescan later if no membrane is detected early
Entangled fetuses or cords	MC/MA	Extremely high risk
No membrane with stuck twin	MC/DA with one placenta	Both fetuses at risk due to vascular communications
	DC/DA with two placentas	Lower risk for nonstuck twin (excludes twin–twin transfusion as a cause)
Single placenta, thick membrane	MZ or DZ, DC/DA	Low risk
Two placentas with or without membrane	DZ, DC/DA	Low risk
Two fetal sexes	DC/DA	Low risk

DC, dichorionic; DA, diamniotic; MC, monochorionic; MA, monoamniotic; MZ, monozygotic; DZ, dizygotic.

▰▰▰ **TABLE 23-3.** Sonographic Protocol
for Sonographic Examinations of Multiple Gestation

- Identify number of fetuses present
- Identify fetal position
- Label presenting fetus "A"
- Identify presence and thickness of membrane
- Identify number of placentas
- Show similar fetal parts on same scan to demonstrate the number of fetuses present and to prove those parts are not conjoined
- Biometry of both fetuses: biparietal diameter, head circumference, abdominal circumference, femur length
- Fetal survey of both fetuses, including cranium, ventricles, cerebellum, spine, four-chamber heart, umbilical cord insertion site, stomach, bladder, kidneys, extremities

performed. After this is completed, fetus B should be identified and its head and body connected in the manner described previously. The anatomy of this fetus should then be documented. When multiple pregnancies are documented, both heads should be recorded on one scan and both bodies on another, if possible, to prove that it is a multiple gestation and that the fetuses are not conjoined.

It is important to identify the number of placentas and to identify a membrane, if there is one separating the fetuses, as well as to characterize the membrane. Essentially, if two placentas are identified, the pregnancy is dichorionic–diamniotic, and the fetuses are in the lowest risk category for complications (Fig. 23-2).[30,37] Dichorionic–diamniotic pregnancies are said to have a thick dividing membrane consisting

of four layers (two amnions and two chorions). If only one placenta is identified and the membrane appears thick, again, this may indicate a dichorionic–diamniotic pregnancy with fused placentas (Fig. 23-3). In either of these two situations, the appearance may be associated with DZ or MZ twins. In the event that only one placenta is identified and the dividing membrane is thin, indicative of only two layers (two amnions) being present, the pregnancy is probably monochorionic–diamniotic (Fig. 23-4) and is at higher risk for fetal complications. If no membrane is readily visualized, it is important to search for one thoroughly and carefully because membranes may be difficult to find later in gestation, even when present. In general, membranes are seen in 90% of all twins at some point in pregnancy, and

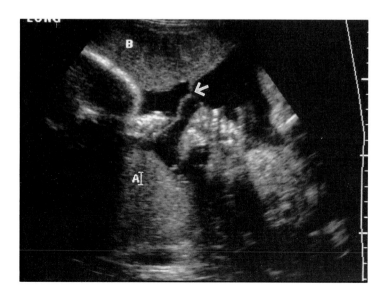

Figure 23-2. Longitudinal image of a dichorionic–diamniotic pregnancy as demonstrated by two fetuses separated by a membrane (*arrow*), and two separate placentas, one anterior (B) and one posterior (A).

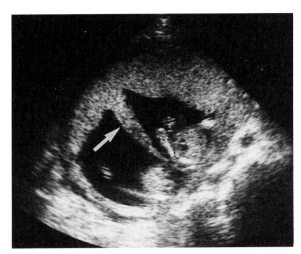

Figure 23-3. *Real-time image of early twin diamniotic–dichorionic pregnancy as demonstrated by a thick membrane (arrow) separating two fetuses. It is difficult to separate the two placentas, and in this instance, the thickness of the membrane differentiates a dichorionic pregnancy with a fused placenta from a monochorionic pregnancy and only one placenta, because in the latter case, the membrane would be thin.*

only 10% of the remainder may be monochorionic–monoamniotic gestations (Fig. 23-5). Therefore, although failure to identify a membrane late in the third trimester when a single placenta is present cannot be considered strong evidence of a monochorionic–monoamniotic pregnancy, it must be suspected, and other signs of monochorionic–monoamniotic twinning, such as fetal entanglement or cord entanglement, should be sought. The highest fetal morbidity and mortality rates are associated with monochorionic–monoamniotic twins. Finally, intrauterine bands, synechiae, amniotic "sheets,"[46] or uterine septa may look similar to and should not be mistaken for membranes. Usually the distinction is straightforward: a free edge is visible in the aforementioned entities, whereas a membrane separating fetuses is uninterrupted.

As in routine singleton scans, the amount of amniotic fluid should be determined. A previously held concept that polyhydramnios is common in twin gestations has not been confirmed in more recent studies. It occurs in only 5% to 10% of twin gestations.[26] Although two amniotic cavities with normal amounts of amniotic fluid may initially give the impression of increased fluid on ultrasound, true polyhydramnios is not a common finding.[26] It is important to assess amniotic fluid quantity as

objectively as possible. As with singleton gestations, amniotic fluid can be assesed by a variety of methods. The single largest pocket of fluid can be measured in a vertical diameter, with a measurement of greater than 8 cm considered polyhydramnios.[21] A subjective assessment of amniotic fluid can be accomplished by real-time scanning through the entire uterus and observing the amount of fluid surrounding the fetus.[8] This method is quick and efficient and very reliable in the hands of experienced operators. The amniotic fluid index, which sums the deepest vertical fluid pocket measurements of the four quadrants of the uterus, cannot be used with multiple-gestation pregnancies if they are diamniotic.[38]

In uncomplicated twin and high-order multiple gestations, interval scanning should be planned every 3 to 4 weeks in the third trimester, to detect complications as they arise and to allow appropriate management. If the placentation is monochorionic, more frequent scanning may be necessary, because these fetuses are at high risk for complications of discordance (twin–twin transfusion) or entanglement.[17]

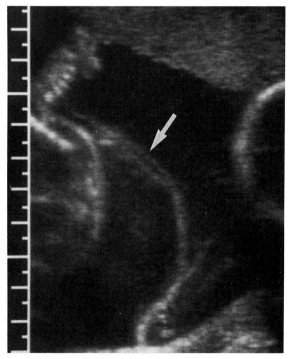

Figure 23-4. *A monochorionic–diamniotic twin gestation with a thin membrane composed of two layers separating the fetuses. The arrow points to two layers in the diamniotic membrane.*

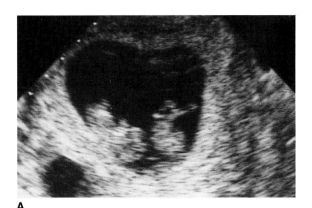
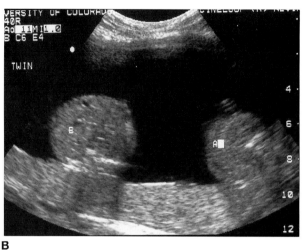

A   **B**

Figure 23-5. *Real-time images of monochorionic–monoamniotic gestations, early in pregnancy* (**A**) *and in the second trimester of pregnancy* (**B**), *show two fetuses in close proximity with no separating membrane.*

THE VANISHING TWIN

The actual prediction of fetal number at term depends on technical factors as well as the probability of fetal survival. Interestingly, a significant number of pregnancies that begin with multiple sacs demonstrated on ultrasound end as singleton gestations at term. In a study by Gindoff and coworkers,[20] 23 multiple pregnancies were identified in a total of 300 prospectively examined women. Three of the 21 women carrying early twin pregnancies ultimately delivered twins, and of the two remaining multiple gestations, one triplet pregnancy resulted in normal twins, and a quadruplet pregnancy resulted in a normal singleton birth. One explanation for this phenomenon is that the nonviable gestation represented an anembryonic gestation, which is proposed to be the cause of 50% to 90% of early spontaneous abortions.[7] Histopathologic examination of these anembryonic gestations reveals autosomal trisomies (52%), triploidies (20%), and monosomy X (15%), among other disorders. Slowed gestational sac growth early on can suggest the diagnosis of an anembryonic gestation, because a normal sac grows at a rate of approximately 0.12 cm/day and a nonviable pregnancy at 0.025 cm/day. Later on, the nonviable gestational sac may begin to involute.

Sonographic criteria for this vanishing sac include a smaller gestational sac than expected for menstrual age, an irregular margin of the sac, and a crescent-shaped sac with an incomplete trophoblastic ring.[20] A small, echogenic focus may be seen even later, corresponding to a totally involuted gestational sac. In cases where an anembryonic gestation or vanishing sac is suspected, a transvaginal examination may be helpful in excluding the possibility of a viable or nonviable gestation, by noting a yolk sac or small fetal pole where none was seen on transabdominal scanning.

Individual gestations of multiple-gestation pregnancies have been seen to vanish even later in pregnancy, even after fetal poles have been identified. One prospective study of multiple-gestation pregnancies documented a group of cases in which twins were identified with fetal cardiac activity at first trimester ultrasound, but subsequent scans revealed only a singleton pregnancy.[33] They documented this to occur in approximately 21% of these prospectively imaged twins. This rate of spontaneous demise is actually similar to that of spontaneous singleton demise. In the situations in which one live twin has vanished, the remaining fetus appears to have a normal prognosis for survival.

A study by Benson and colleagues looked at first trimester twin pregnancies to determine criteria for predicting pregnancy outcome with regard to number of live born infants.[6] Of 137 patients evaluated, 110 (80.3%) had viable twins, 12 (8.8%) had 1 infant, and 15 (10.9%) had none. The criteria they found to be statistically significant included gestational age at the time of the ultrasound (the inference being that the earlier the gestation, the more time in which demise might occur), chorionicity of the pregnancy, and abnormal sonographic findings. Maternal age, type of conception (i.e., assisted fertility), and indication for the sonogram had no independent effect on outcome.

In fetal loss in the second or third trimester and in MZ twin gestation in which there is a fetal demise, the demise may develop into a fetus papyraceus (Fig. 23-6).[18] Instead of the usual complete decomposition and absorption of the fetus, the fetus papyraceus ("paper like") is preserved in a distorted form. In twins, a postulated cause of fetus papyraceus is transient polyhydramnios of one fetus in a monochorionic–diamniotic pregnancy exerting a lethal compressive effect on the other twin. Fetal papyraceus occurs in 1 of 12,000 live births, but is more common in the subgroup of twin gestations (1 in 184 twin births).[33]

TECHNICAL PITFALLS

Technical pitfalls exist in imaging multiple gestations. An important factor that should be borne in mind when determining if there is a multiple-gestation pregnancy is that crescentic areas of implantational hemorrhage or amniotic–chorionic separation may be mistaken for second pregnancies or nonviable pregnancies (Fig. 23-7). The distinction is usually obvious by the configuration of the fluid collections and the lack of a well-defined decidual rind in nongestational collections. A ghosting artifact[11] may be seen when scanning the pelvis in a transverse plane, where small anatomic areas such as early gestations are being investigated; this creates the illusion of two sacs when there is only

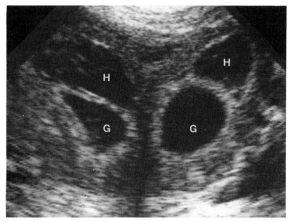

Figure 23-7. *Sector scan demonstrating two normal gestational sacs (G). Above each of the sacs is an implantational hemorrhage (H) with ill-defined margins and low-level echoes within.*

one (Fig. 23-8). The effect is most pronounced in muscular patients, although it can occur in any patient; the phenomenon is secondary to the rectus muscle acting as a lens, refracting the ultrasound beam. Examining the patient in the longitudinal plane makes this artifact disappear and prevents misdiagnosis. The same artifact may also duplicate ovarian follicles or the uterus, may cause overestimation of the crown–rump length, and may even mimic fetal omphalocele.

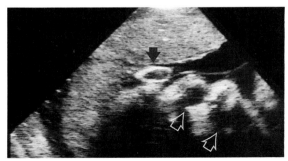

Figure 23-6. *Sector real-time image demonstrates a thin membrane (monochorionic) separating the small, distorted skull of a fetus papyraceus (black arrow) and the normal face of the surviving, large twin (open white arrows indicate orbits in transaxial scan with fetus looking upward and to the right in the image).*

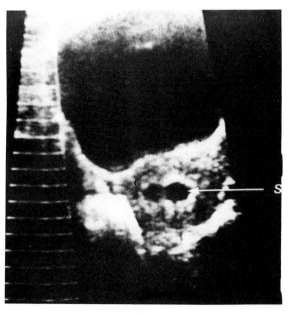

Figure 23-8. *Ghosting artifact creating the illusion of 2 sacs when only one was present. S, gestational sac. (Buttery B, Davison G. The ghost artifact. J Ultrasound Med. 1984; 3:49–52.)*

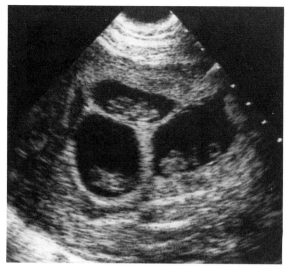

Figure 23-9. *Real-time scan of early triplet gestation demonstrates three separate gestational sacs with small fetal poles within.*

Although it seems intuitively unlikely, late in pregnancy a second fetus may be completely overlooked because the nondependent fetus obscures the underlying one. Sonographers should be alerted to this possibility if the visualized fetus is situated more anteriorly than would be expected and if there are more fetal parts in the image than seems appropriate. Later in pregnancy, owing to relative decreases in amniotic fluid with respect to the fetal volume, important areas of fetal anatomy may be hidden, and an effort must be made to evaluate obscured anatomy by scanning from multiple angles and with the mother in different positions.

Multiple Gestations Other Than Twins

SPONTANEOUS HIGHER-ORDER GESTATIONS

Although the average incidence of twins is 1 in 100 pregnancies, triplets occur in only approximately 1 in 7600 pregnancies (Fig. 23-9), and the spontaneous rates for quadruplet and quintuplet pregnancies are 1 in 729,000 and 1 in 65,610,000, respectively.[13] Interestingly, triplet pregnancies—and even quadruplet pregnancies—may be MZ. For example, 60% of triplet pregnancies are secondary to the fertilization of two ova (Fig. 23-10), 30% arise from the fertilization of three ova, and 10% arise from the fertilization of a single ovum.[25]

FERTILITY AUGMENTATION

Fertility drugs alter the rate of higher-order gestations. Three are currently used in fertility augmentation.[50] The first is clomiphine citrate; its use in ovulation induction results in an 8% to 13% rate of multiple gestation, most being twins. Although this drug has several mechanisms of action, the predominant one is thought to be the displacement of estrogen from hypothalamic receptors, which augments release of gonadotropin-releasing hormone, and ultimately causes follicular maturation and ovulation. The second agent, human menopausal gonadotropin (HMG), is a combination of follicle-stimulating hormone and lutenizing hormone. When ultrasound demonstrates follicles measuring 1.8 to 2.0 cm, HMG is administered to simulate the luteinizing hormone surge, resulting in ovulation. The rate of multiple gestations when this type of stimulation is used has approached 42% in some series; however, if estrogen levels are monitored closely, it is possible to decrease this to a more acceptable rate of 10%. Higher-order multiple gestations are more frequent with HMG than with clomiphine: triplets occur in as many as 5% to 6% of HMG-induced pregnancies. Bromocriptine, the third agent, acts directly on the pituitary, decreasing the production of prolactin in patients with hyperprolactinemia. This diminishes the inhibition of the release of hypothalamic gonadotropin-releasing hormone by prolactin, allowing the return

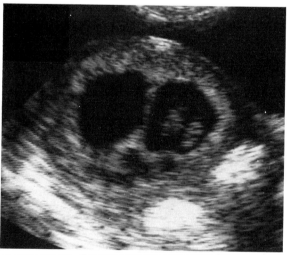

Figure 23-10. *Triplet pregnancy resulting from the fertilization of two ova, with one gestational sac on the left without the fetus in the field of view, and two monoamniotic twins in the gestational sac to the right with no dividing membrane.*

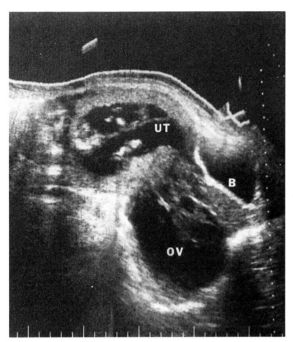

Figure 23-11. Longitudinal articulated arm scan in a patient who received human menopausal gonadotropin ovulation induction. A large, hyperstimulated ovary (OV) is identified in the cul-de-sac posterior to the uterus (UT). The maternal urinary bladder (B) is identified for reference.

area. Thoracopagus (joined at the thorax), omphalopagus (joined at the abdominal wall), or a combination of the two constitute approximately 70% of all conjoined twins (Figs. 23-12 and 23-13). Other varieties (Figs. 23-14 and 23-15) are craniopagus (joined at the head), pygopagus (joined at the buttocks), ischiopagus (joined at the ischia), and cephalothoracopagus.[25,36,52]

Developmentally, conjoined twins arise from monochorionic–monoamniotic gestations in which division of the embryo occurs after the 13th day of conception. They are always of the same sex, and 70% are female. Sonographic findings in conjoined twins include lack of visualization of a separating membrane between the twins, inability to separate the fetal bodies (Fig. 23-16) or heads despite changes in fetal position, more than three vessels in a single umbilical cord, and complex fetal structural anomalies.[32] Polyhydramnios is more common in conjoined twins, occurring in approximately 50% of cases (in contrast to 5% to 10% of normal twins).[51] It is important to make the diagnosis of conjoined twins, because approximately

of the hypothalamic–pituitary–gonadal axis to nearly normal function. Because this approximates the restoration of normal physiologic situation, the incidence of twinning is not much greater than normal. Approximately 1.2% to 1.8% of these pregnancies are multiple, mostly twins.

There are extrauterine complications of the ovulation induction technique, especially with HMG. Ovarian hyperstimulation syndrome may occur, in which multiple, large cysts cause the ovaries to attain huge proportions (Fig. 23-11). These changes may lead to ascites from cyst rupture, and ovarian torsion. Rarely in twin and higher-order gestations, ovarian hyperstimulation may occur spontaneously when no fertility drug was administered.

Abnormal Twinning

A variety of unusual abnormal twin types may occur. Conjoined twins occur in approximately 1 in 50,000 to 1 in 100,000 live births.[51] Conjoined twins are defined by the conjoined (shared) body

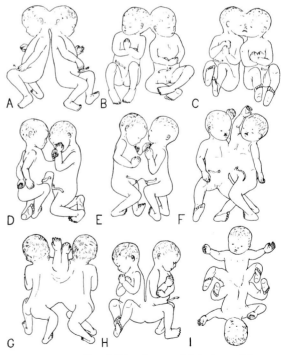

Figure 23-12. Possibilities for partial fusion of fetuses: (A–C) craniopagus; (D–G) thoracopagus; (H,I) pygopagus. (From Patten BM. Human Embryology. New York: McGraw Hill; 1968.)

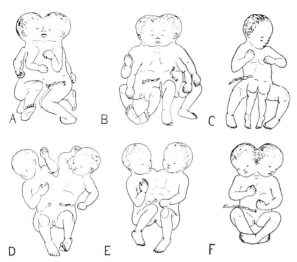

Figure 23-13. More complete forms of conjoined twinning. (From Patten BM. Human Embryology. New York: McGraw Hill; 1968.)

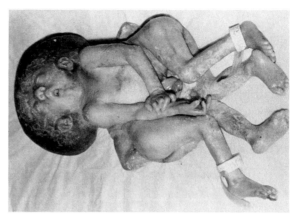

Figure 23-15. Photograph of fetus in Figure 23-14 after cesarean section delivery demonstrates fusion at the level of the heads, thoraces, and abdomens. Note the associated gastroschisis.

one third are stillborn and an additional one third die on day 1. Because the relation of the heart to each fetus is a critical determinant of survival, fetal echocardiography is essential for all conjoined twins. Conjoined twins can occur in higher-order gestations. In one series, without antenatal ultrasound to help plan for delivery, five of nine extra fetuses coexisting with conjoined twins died in the perinatal period.[31]

Another form of abnormal twinning is the parasitic twin found within the abdomen of its sibling. This is referred to as fetus in fetu[42] and should not be confused with a teratoma. Although the distinction between parasitic twin and teratoma may be difficult, it is an important point to establish, because teratomas have a definite malignant potential,

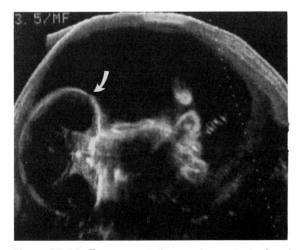

Figure 23-14. Transverse static scan demonstrates fused crania (*curved arrow*) in cephalothoracoomphalopagus (conjoined twins) with grossly abnormal intracranial contents.

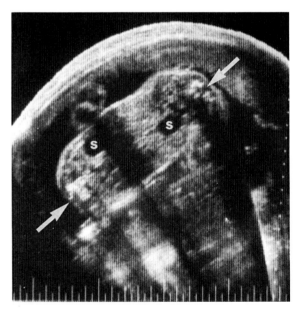

Figure 23-16. Image of thoracoomphalopagus demonstrates opposing spines (*arrows*) and fetal stomachs (s). In this case, the fetuses were obviously conjoined and could not be identified as separate fetuses despite multiple maneuvers.

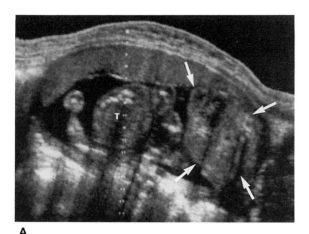
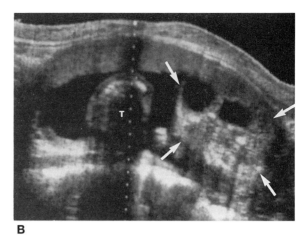

A   **B**

Figure 23-17. Two different longitudinal static scans demonstrate a normal twin (T) and a disorganized mass of tissue (*arrows*) in the lower uterine segment representing an amorphous, acardiac twin. On other images, an umbilical cord was identified entering the acardiac monster.

whereas the fetus in fetu is technically a hamartoma and entirely benign. Fetus in fetu occurs more commonly in the upper retroperitoneum, whereas teratomas usually arise in the lower abdomen, most commonly in the ovaries or the sacrococcygeal region. Also, there is usually radiographic or at least microscopic evidence of a vertebral column in fetus in fetu.

One type of parabiotic twinning, termed the *twin reversed arterial perfusion* (TRAP) syndrome,[19] leads to the development of a grossly malformed twin, referred to as an acardiac monster or acardiac anomaly (Fig. 23-17). The syndrome may arise whenever there is the potential for vascular communication between twins through the placenta (i.e., in monochorionic pregnancies) and results from one large arterial–arterial and one large venous–venous anastomosis between the twins. The acardiac twin, which possesses either no heart of its own or a grossly malformed heart, is completely perfused by the donor twin through the arterial–arterial communication. Because the blood perfusing the parasitic twin is not well oxygenated and enters through the abdominal aorta, preferential development of the lower extremities and body occurs, with frequent sacrifice of development of the fetus' upper thorax, head, and upper extremities. If this anomaly is detected, close monitoring should be considered during the third trimester, because there is a 20% mortality rate if the normal donor twin becomes hydropic due to high-output cardiac failure. Fortunately, this anomaly is rare,

occurring in 1 in 35,000 live births. This anomaly occurs exclusively in MZ twin gestations or triplets, and is most common with monochorionic–monoamniotic pregnancies. It carries with it no increased risk of recurrence.[15] In utero, ablation of arterial and venous communications marks a promising form of antenatal therapy, with selective termination of the anomalous twins.[28]

A normal twin may coexist with a complete hydatidiform mole (Fig. 23-18). This is a rare occurrence, with the more common presentation being a partial mole occurring in conjunction with a chromosomally abnormal (triploid) fetus (Figs.

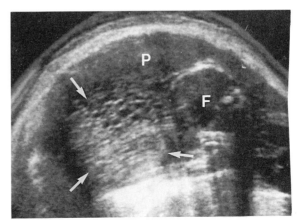

Figure 23-18. Transverse sonogram demonstrates a normal fetus (F) to the right, the placenta associated with the normal fetus (P), and an adjacent complete mole to the left (*arrows*).

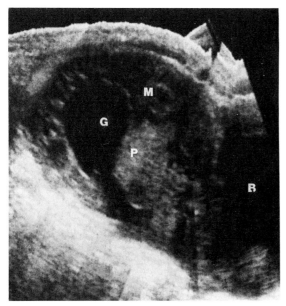

Figure 23-19. Longitudinal scan shows bladder (B) as reference, remnant portion of normal placenta (P), molar tissue (M), and the gestational sac (G). Note the small amount of shadowing in the dependent portion of the gestational sac from fetal parts.

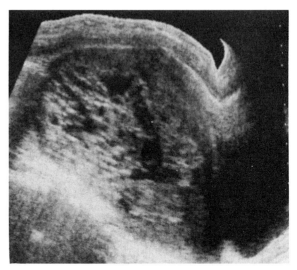

Figure 23-20. Longitudinal scan adjacent to Figure 23-19 more clearly demonstrates the abnormal, inhomogeneous molar placental tissue with sonolucent areas.

23-19 and 23-20).[53] See Chapter 25 for a complete discussion of molar pregnancies.

Heterotopic pregnancies may even be considered a type of twinning when single or multiple intrauterine pregnancies coexist with an ectopic pregnancy.[48] The incidence of this was once thought to be 1 in 30,000 pregnancies, but owing to the increase in ectopic pregnancies, it is now thought to be 1 in 6000 or lower.[24] Predisposing conditions include ovulation induction, a history of pelvic inflammatory disease or tubal surgery, endometriosis, and in vitro implantation of multiple embryos.[48] Heterotopic pregnancy or heterotopic twinning should not be confused with two pregnancies each within one of the horns of a bicornuate uterus or with an early singleton, unicornuate gestation within a bicornuate uterus and a pseudogestational sac in the contralateral horn (Fig. 23-21). The differentiation may be difficult to make using ultrasound.

Other twinning abnormalities include superfetation, in which there is fertilization of two separate ova months apart, (i.e., ovulation occurs after conception), and superfecundation, in which two ova are fertilized at different times by the sperm of two different fathers or by the same father at different times within the same cycle.[44,45]

Complications of Multigestational Pregnancies

MATERNAL COMPLICATIONS

Both maternal and fetal complications may occur in multiple gestations. Premature labor is the most common fetal and maternal complication. At least 52% of multiple fetuses are delivered before term, and 18% before 35 weeks.[13] Premature labor may ensue because the large fetoplacental mass causes

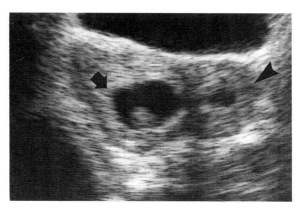

Figure 23-21. Transverse sector scan shows the two horns of a bicornuate uterus with a fetal pole in the gestational sac in the right horn (*arrow*), and the "pseudogestational sac" in the left horn (*arrowhead*) caused by vicarious stimulation of the endometrium in the left horn.

uterine overdistention and subsequent contractions, or because of premature rupture of the membranes resulting from increased intraamniotic pressure.[40] There is also an increased incidence of third trimester bleeding, possibly related to the increased prevalence of placenta previa, placental abruption, and velamentous insertion of the cord with placenta previa. Miscellaneous maternal complications that can occur with greater frequency in multiple gestations include hypertension of pregnancy, anemia, pyelonephritis, hepatic cholestasis, preeclampsia, and eclampsia.[27]

FETAL COMPLICATIONS

All fetuses in multiple gestations are at risk. Congenital anomalies occur approximately twice as often in twins and in even higher rates in triplets as in singleton fetuses. Malformation occurrence rates in twins have been reported to be as high as 2.71%, compared to 1.4% in single births. In triplets, congenital anomalies may occur in as many as 6.09%.[15] Fetal complications in multiple pregnancies are extensive, and because ultrasound can have a significant impact on reducing the high rate of mortality and morbidity due to these complications by early diagnosis, it should be used routinely to monitor these fetuses. Discordancy or intrauterine growth retardation (IUGR) in one of the fetuses in a multiple pregnancy is a major complication, second only to prematurity of all of the fetuses in the pregnancy due to early labor. The smaller fetus in the discordant pair is at risk for perinatal anoxia. Normal intrauterine growth of twins parallels that of singleton pregnancies until approximately 31 or 32 weeks.[23] After that point, the head and abdominal growth rates are thought by some authors to slow down while the femurs continue to grow normally.[23] Abnormal intrauterine growth or discordancy results in a weight difference greater than 15% to 20% between the twins,[4,10] with an overall weight differential of 500 g at birth.

To identify these fetuses at risk, several sonographic criteria have been used, including a difference in biparietal diameter of 5 mm or greater. The biparietal diameter alone, however, is a poor indicator of fetal growth and a poor standard for comparison in twin gestations, because there are inherent problems in accurately measuring normal fetal heads in unusual positions or when they are obscured by fetal superimposition. Second, the cal-

varia of normal fetuses not uncommonly become dolichocephalic secondary to uterine crowding or breech presentation.

A more sensitive measurement to identify discordant fetuses was found to be a discrepancy in the abdominal circumference measurement of greater than 20 mm.[4] This is a sensitive indicator because the fetal liver mass, as reflected in the abdominal circumference, is the first parameter to become abnormal in fetuses with asymmetric IUGR. It is important to realize, however, that the sensitivity and specificity for detecting IUGR in any one fetus, even using multiple criteria, is not 100%, and the sonographer is encouraged to be vigilant for other signs associated with IUGR, such as oligohydramnios (Fig. 23-22) or abnormal umbilical artery Doppler waveforms.

Discordancy of measurements may be secondary to either idiopathic IUGR of one fetus with the other fetus growing normally, or to the parabiotic syndrome, of which twin–twin transfusion and the previously mentioned acardiac anomaly are manifestations. To date, the twin–twin transfusion syndrome (TTS) has been found to occur only with monochorionic twins, whether they be diamniotic or monoamniotic, and has not been definitely demonstrated when there are separate placentas. Again, this underscores the importance of determining the amnioticity and chorionicity of a gestation.

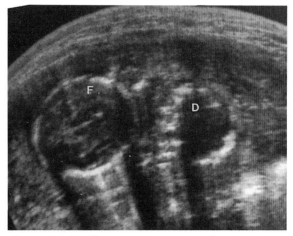

Figure 23-22. *Transverse sonogram demonstrates a normal-appearing fetal head (F), a somewhat distorted cranial vault in the adjacent nonviable twin (D), and oligohydramnios. Although both fetuses' growth was retarded, this demonstrates the ultimate form of discordancy—one live fetus and one nonviable fetus.*

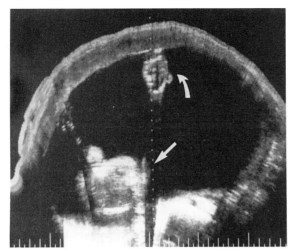

Figure 23-23. Curved arrow demonstrates a "stuck" twin in the nondependent portion of the uterine cavity due to oligohydramnios and a restrictive membrane. Gross polyhydramnios surrounds the more normal-looking fetus (*straight arrow*) in the dependent portion of the uterine cavity.

In TTS, the sharing of a common placenta allows abnormal anastomoses to develop between arterial and venous circulations, resulting in abnormal shunting of blood from one fetus to the other. Approximately 15% to 20% of all monochorionic twins have TTS to some extent.[9,43] In TTS, the twin on the arterial side of the communication, referred to as the donor twin, shunts blood to the other twin, the recipient. This results in the donor twin becoming hypovolemic, which may lead to severe growth retardation. Poor renal perfusion and anuria also occur, which often leads to severe oligohydramnios. When this occurs in diamniotic pregnancies, the donor twin may be held in a fixed position by the membrane. This is often referred to as a "stuck twin"[43] (Fig. 23-23). The finding of a stuck twin may be helpful in the diagnosis of TTS; however, the stuck twin appearance is not peculiar to this syndrome. Any cause of oligohydramnios, such as IUGR or a bilaterally obstructed renal system affecting one of the twins, may give the same appearance. A pregnancy with a stuck twin need not be monochorionic. It may occur with dichorionic–diamniotic twins.[31] The recipient twin becomes hypervolemic, which leads to increased urine production, often causing polyhydramnios. If the polyhydramnios becomes extreme, premature labor may occur. Hypervolemia of the recipient twin may also lead to congestive heart failure, hydrops, and fetal

death (Fig. 23-24). Unfortunately, TTS carries a very poor prognosis for both twins. The mortality rate approaches 70% to 80%.[5,43] Reversal of the oligohydramnios and hydrops present in TTS has been documented in cases in which a therapeutic amniocentesis to remove excess fluid from the polyhydramniotic sac is performed.[16,49] Identification of the communicating vessels within the placenta using color Doppler, and subsequent laser ablation of the vessels has also been reported to be sucessful in some cases.[28]

Whether the problem is TTS or discordancy secondary to IUGR of indeterminant cause, pulsed Doppler examination can evaluate hemodynamic changes in the fetoplacental unit and may be a useful tool for assessing fetal well-being. Doppler studies in TTS have shown a difference in systolic–diastolic ratios between twins of greater than 0.4.[43] Umbilical arterial pulsed Doppler studies in TTS have identified the fetus in which placental vascular resistance is greater, but neither the identification of hydrops nor abnormal Doppler waveforms can consistently differentiate donor from recipient fetuses or provide useful prognostic information for the pregnancy (Fig. 23-25).[29,41]

The biophysical profile has also established itself as an important way of estimating fetal well-being in complicated pregnancies[34] (see Chap. 22).

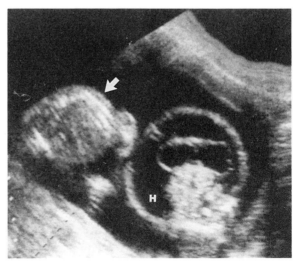

Figure 23-24. Obstetric static scan shows a normal (*arrow*) fetus adjacent to a grossly hydropic (H) fetus with a large amount of ascites. This appearance was secondary to twin–twin transfusion syndrome, and the relatively normal-looking fetus actually measured small for gestational age.

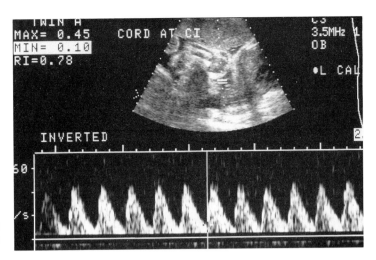

Figure 23-25. Umbilical artery waveform in a fetus with twin–twin transfusion syndrome demonstrates decreased diastolic flow.

Aside from discordancy and its deleterious effects, genetic and developmental abnormalities are also more common in twins. Genetically similar MZ twins are nearly 100% concordant for genetic defects (e.g., Down's syndrome). The most common discordant genetic defect in an MZ twin pair is a normal fetus paired with one that has Turner's syndrome. MZ twins are only 2% to 10% concordant for isolated developmental defects.[40] Because DZ twins are not genetically identical, they have a very low concordance for both genetic and developmental abnormalities.

Approximately 5% to 10% of twin pregnancies are complicated by polyhydramnios. When polyhydramnios does occur, it may be either chronic or acute. The chronic form usually develops over a period of weeks in the third trimester and is associated with an increased mortality rate (45%).[13] The even more ominous acute form usually develops over a period of days between 20 and 26 weeks, primarily among DZ twins, and carries with it a mortality rate of nearly 100%. This mortality figure is most likely secondary to prematurity because the polyhydramnios causes early labor.

The highest morbidity and mortality rates in multiple gestations are associated with monochorionic–monoamniotic twins. In addition to TTS, these pregnancies have associated cord accidents, including prolapse, entanglement, and nuchal cord, as well as an increased incidence of malpresentation and the interlocking twin phenomenon. The interlocking of fetal anatomy, in which one twin is breech and the second vertex, may prevent normal vaginal delivery. The possibility of these complications is so worrisome that in some centers all monochorionic–monoamniotic pregnancies are delivered by cesarean section.[13]

Invasive Fetal Evaluation

Amniocentesis and chorionic villus sampling in multiple gestations require special considerations that are described in Chapter 29.[12,14,39]

Selective Termination

Should serious complications occur or serious anomalies be detected in multiple gestations, selective termination may be offered to the parents as an option. In cases in which only one twin is affected with a serious chromosomal or congenital anomaly, or when decreasing the number of fetuses in a multifetal pregnancy might improve the perinatal result, selective termination of fetuses may be a reasonable alternative. This procedure usually involves the direct injection of air into the fetal heart or umbilical vein or fetal exsanguination by cardiac puncture. Selective termination should be performed only in dichorionic pregnancies (i.e., those in which the placentas are visualized in different locations, or where there appears to be one placenta [that is verified to be fused] but the dividing membrane is thick).

If selective termination is performed on a monochorionic pregnancy or if spontaneous fetal demise occurs in a monochorionic pregnancy, the potential exists for a thromboplastic substance to be released from the dead twin, passing into the surviving twin, and causing intrauterine disseminated intravascular coagulation with potential brain and multiorgan damage or death.[47] Because MZ twins are rarely discordant for genetic defects, selective termination in MZ pregnancies would involve cases of isolated congenital anomalies or would be performed to reduce the number of fetuses. The role of ultrasound in the procedure includes locating the appropriate fetus, guiding the needle for puncture, and monitoring the well-being of surviving fetuses. Hysterotomy may also be an option to correct certain defects instead of terminating the pregnancy.[35]

Conclusion

With the use of ultrasound, increased morbidity and mortality associated with multiple gestations can be dramatically reduced through early detection and through serial scanning, which identify associated abnormalities of structure or problems of growth.[17]

REFERENCES

1. American College of Obstetrics and Gynecology. Ultrasonography in Pregnancy. Technical bulletin #187. Washington, D.C.: ACOG; December 1993.
2. American College of Radiology. ACR standards for performance of antepartum obstetrical ultrasound. Reston, VA: ACR; 1990.
3. American Institute of Ultrasound in Medicine. American Institute of Ultrasound in Medicine guidelines for the performance of the antepartum obstetrical ultrasound examination. Rockville, MD: AIUM; 1991.
4. Barnea ER, Romero R, Scott D, et al. The value of biparietal diameter and abdominal perimeter in the diagnosis of growth retardation in twin gestation. Am J Perinatol. 1985; 2:221–222.
5. Benirschke K, Kim CK. Multiple pregnancy. N Engl J Med. 1973; 288:1276–1336.
6. Benson CB, Doubilet PM, David V. Prognosis of first trimester twin pregnancies: Polychotomous logistic regression analysis. Radiology. 1994; 192: 765–768.
7. Bernard KG, Cooperberg PL. Sonographic differentiation between blighted ovum and early viable pregnancy. AJR Am J Roentgenol. 1985; 144:597–602.
8. Brace RA, Wolf EJ. Normal amniotic fluid volume changes throughout pregnancy. Am J Obstet Gynecol. 1989; 382:161–165.
9. Brennan JN, Diwan RV, Rosen MG, et al. Fetal–

10. Brown CEL, Guzick DS, Levino KJ, et al. Prediction of discordant twins using ultrasound measurement of biparietal diameter and abdominal perimeter. Obstet Gynecol. 1987; 70:677–681.
11. Buttery B, Davison G. The ghost artifact. J Ultrasound Med. 1984; 3:49–52.
12. Cadikin AV, Ginsberg NA, Pergament E, et al. Chorionic villi sampling: A new technique for detection of genetic abnormalities in the first trimester. Radiology. 1984; 151:159–162.
13. Crane JP. Sonographic evaluation of multiple pregnancy. Semin Ultrasound CT MR. 1984; 5:144–156.
14. D'Alton ME, Alton ME, Dudley DKL. Ultrasound in the antenatal management of twin gestation. Semin Perinatol. 1986; 10:30–38.
15. Edwards MS, Ellings JM, Newman RB, et al. Predictive value of antepartum ultrasound examination for anomalies in twin gestations. Ultrasound in Obstetrics and Gynecology. 1995; 6:43–49.
16. Elliot JP, Urig MA, Clewell WH. Aggressive therapeutic amniocentesis for treatment of twin–twin transfusion syndrome. Obstet Gynecol. 1991; 77: 537–540.
17. Filly RA, Goldstein RB, Callen PW. Monochorionic twinning: Sonographic assessment. AJR Am J Roentgenol. 1990; 154:459–469.
18. Gericke GS. Genetic and teratological considerations in the analysis of concordant and discordant abnormalities in twins. S Afr Med J. 1986; 69:111–114.
19. Gibson JY, D'Cruz CA, Patel RB, et al. Acardiac anomaly: Review of the subject with case report and emphasis on practical sonography. J Clin Ultrasound. 1986; 14:541–545.
20. Gindoff PR, Yeh MN, Jewelewicz R. The vanishing sac syndrome: Ultrasound evidence of pregnancy failure in multiple gestations, induced and spontaneous. J Reprod Med. 1986; 31:322–325.
21. Goldstein RB, Filly RA. Sonographic estimation of amniotic fluid volume: Subjective assessment versus pocket measurement. J Ultrasound Med. 1988; 7:363–365.
22. Grennert L, Persson PH, Gennser G, et al. Ultrasound and human placental lactogen screening for early detection of twin pregnancies. Lancet 1976; 1:4–6.
23. Grumbach K, Coleman BG, Arger PH, et al. Twin and singleton growth patterns compared using ultrasound. Radiology. 1986; 158:237–241.
24. Hann LE, Bachman DM, McArdle CR. Coexistent intrauterine and ectopic pregnancy: A reevaluation. Radiology. 1984; 152:151–154.
25. Hartung RW, Yiu-Chiu V, Aschenbrener CA. Sono-

graphic diagnosis of cephalothoracopagus in a triplet pregnancy. J Ultrasound Med. 1984; 3:139–141.

26. Hashimoto B, Callen PW, Filly RA, et al. Ultrasound evaluation of polyhydramnios and twin pregnancy. Am J Obstet Gynecol. 1986; 154:1069–1072.

27. Hays PM, Smeltzer JS. Multiple gestation. Clin Obstet Gynecol. 1986; 29:264–285.

28. Hecher K, Ville Y, Nicolaides KH. Color Doppler ultrasonography in the identification of communicating vessels in twin–twin transfusion syndrome and acardiac twins. J Ultrasound Med. 1995; 14:37–40.

29. Hecher K, Ville Y, Nicolaides KH. Fetal arterial Doppler studies in twin–twin transfusion syndrome. J Ultrasound Med. 1995; 14:101–108.

30. Hertzberg BS, Kurtz AB, Choi HY, et al. Significance of membrane thickness in sonographic evaluation of twin gestations. AJR Am J Roentgenol. 1987; 148:151–153.

31. Hughey MJ, Olive DL. Routine ultrasound scanning for the detection and management of twin pregnancies. J Reprod Med. 1985; 30:427–430.

32. Koontz WL, Layman L, Adams A, et al. Antenatal sonographic diagnosis of conjoined twins in a triplet pregnancy. Am J Obstet Gynecol. 1985; 153:230–231.

33. Landy HJ, Weiner S, Corson SL, et al. The "vanishing twin": Ultrasonographic assessment of fetal disappearance in the first trimester. Am J Obstet Gynecol. 1986; 155:14–19.

34. Loderio JG, Vintzileos AM, Feinstein SJ, et al. Fetal biophysical profile in twin gestations. Obstet Gynecol. 1986; 67:824–827.

35. Longaker MT, Golbus MS, Filly RA, et al. Maternal outcome after open fetal surgery: A review of the first 17 human cases. JAMA. 1991; 265:737–741.

36. McLeod K, Tan PA, DeLange M, et al. Conjoined twins in a triplet pregnancy: Sonographic findings. JDMS. 1988; 4:9–12.

37. Mahony BS, Filly RA, Callen PW. Amnionicity and chorionicity in twin pregnancies: Prediction using ultrasound. Radiology. 1985; 155:205–209.

38. Moore TR, Cayle JE. The amniotic fluid index in normal human pregnancy. Am J Obstet Gynecol. 1990; 162:1168–1170.

39. Mulcahy MT, Roberman B, Reid SE. Chorion biopsy, cytogenetic diagnosis, and selected termination in a twin pregnancy at risk of haemophilia. Lancet. 1984; 2:866–867.

40. Newton ER. Antepartum care in multiple gestation. Semin Perinatol. 1986; 10:19–29.

41. Nimrod C, Davies D, Harder J, et al. Doppler ultrasound prediction of fetal outcome in twin pregnancies. Am J Obstet Gynecol. 1987; 156:402–406.

42. Nocera RM, Davis M, Hayden CK, et al. Fetus-infetu. AJR Am J Roentgenol. 1982; 138:762–764.

43. Pretorius DH, Manchester D, Barkin S, et al. Doppler ultrasound of twin transfusion syndrome. J Ultrasound Med. 1988; 7:117–124.

44. Pritchard JA. Multiple pregnancies. In: Pritchard JA, MacDonald PC, eds. Williams Obstetrics. 12th ed. New York: Appleton-Century-Crofts; 1961:687–688.

45. Pritchard JA. Multifetal pregnancy. In: Pritchard JA, MacDonald PC, eds. Williams Obstetrics. 16th ed. New York: Appleton-Century-Crofts; 1980:655–656.

46. Randel SB, Filly RA, Callen PW. Amniotic sheets. Radiology. 1988; 166:633–636.

47. Redwine FO, Hays PM. Selective birth. Semin Perinatol. 1986; 10:73–81.

48. Rowland DM, Geagan MB, Paul DA. Sonographic demonstration of combined quadruplet gestation, with viable ectopic and concomitant intrauterine triplet pregnancies. J Ultrasound Med. 1987; 6:89–91.

49. Saunders NJ, Snijders RJM, Nicholaides KH. Theraputic amniocentesis in twin–twin transfusion syndrome appearing in the second trimester of pregnancy. Am J Obstet Gynecol. 1992; 166:820–825.

50. Scialli AR. The reproductive toxicity of ovulation induction. Fertil Steril. 1986; 45:315–323.

51. Strauss S, Tamarkin M, Engleberg S, et al. Prenatal sonographic appearance of diprosopus. J Ultrasound Med. 1987; 6:93–95.

52. Wilson DA, Young GZ, Crumley CS. Antepartum ultrasonographic diagnosis of ischiopagus: A rare variety of conjoined twins. J Ultrasound Med. 1983; 2:281–282.

53. Woo JSK, Wong LC, Hsu C, et al. Sonographic appearances of the partial hydatidiform mole. J Ultrasound Med. 1983; 2:261–264.

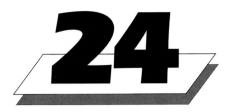

Intrauterine Growth Retardation (IUGR)

WAYNE PERSUTTE

According to the United States Bureau of Census, there were ~4,296,710 babies born in this country in 1995. While these births were usually joyous events, one in 100 families experienced a perinatal death. Why did more than 40,000 babies die? More than 75% of these perinatal deaths occur in babies that are born too early or are too small in size. Infants born too small for their gestational age are thought to be affected by *intrauterine growth retardation* (IUGR). Growth retarded infants are a significant concern for perinatal clinicians because of their high incidence of perinatal morbidity.[73] These infants account for ~7% of all deliveries, yet are responsible for 35% of all medical costs for children younger than 1 year of age.[87] Infants born with birth weights between 1000 and 2500 g, and without respiratory distress syndrome, are six times more costly than those of normal birth weight ($11,900 vs. $1900).[89] Additionally, 25% of these infants have long-term physical and intellectual deficits.[58] There is a higher incidence of karyotype abnormality among these infants. Reliable identification and treatment of these small infants before birth may greatly affect United States health care and its costs.

Presently, a fetus at risk for growth retardation and maladaptation is first identified by clinical and laboratory measures such as poor symphysis to fundal height growth, poor maternal weight gain, unexplained elevation in maternal serum alphafetoprotein (MSAFP), or underlying maternal complication(s) (Table 24-1).[7] Prenatal ultrasonography is then used to evaluate the existence of a potential discordancy between fetal size (as ascertained by ultrasonography) and gestational age

TABLE 24-1. MATERNAL RISK FACTORS ASSOCIATED WITH IUGR

Low socioeconomic status/poor maternal nutrition (prepregnancy weight <50 kg)

Coexisting maternal disease, infection, or genetic disorder, including:
  Collagen vascular disease
  Maternal renal/cardiovascular disease
  Rh sensitization
  Hypertension
  Diabetes
  Metabolic disease

Maternal drug use/teratogenic exposure
  Alcohol
  Narcotics
  Nicotine
  Dilantin
  Propranolol
  Steroids
  Irradiation
Prior child of unexplained low birth weight

High altitude

(as ascertained by the date of the last menstrual period or conception). Once this is established, ultrasonography is of great help in assessing interval growth and fetal well-being.

Definition of IUGR

The *estimate of fetal weight* (EFW) has served as the basis from which fetal size and growth are assessed. IUGR has been defined as an EFW below the 3rd, 5th, or 10th percentile for a population, 2 standard deviations below the mean for gestational age (≤97.5%) or a weight decline of at least 10% between two weight estimates as determined by ultrasonographic biometry.[64,101,118,133] It has also been defined using EFW combined with physiologic or clinical parameters, ponderal indices <10%, and most recently, failure to achieve growth potential.[132] In this chapter, the most widely accepted prenatal definition of IUGR will be used: an EFW of <10% and/or poor growth as evidenced by a significant decline in the predicted EFW percentile (for gestational age) over the course of two or more examinations.

Prevalence

The prevalence of IUGR in the general population is directly related to the definition used. That is, if we choose <10th percentile to define IUGR, 10% of infants in a low risk population will be affected; if one chooses percentile <3, 3% will be affected, and so on. However, in populations at risk, the prevalence increases. For example, in women with hypertension or in a woman with a previous growth retarded infant, the prevalence may be as high as 25% or more.[127,133] According to the Colorado Department of Health, 8.4% of live births in 1993 were born at <2500 g (5 lb 8 oz, which is considered low birth weight and is ~10% for 37 weeks of gestation and the 3% for 40 weeks).[40]

Adverse Effects

Many clinical problems occur more commonly in growth retarded individuals during their perinatal life, childhood, and adulthood than in the normal population (Table 24-2).

▰▰▰ **TABLE 24-2. PATHOLOGY ASSOCIATED WITH IUGR**
Perinatal
Intrapartum fetal distress
Hypoglycemia
Hypocalcemia
Meconium aspiration pneumonia
Hypothermia
Encephalopathy
Childhood
Hypertension
Poor neural outcome
Adult
Cardiovascular disease
Hypertension
Diabetes

EFFECTS AND ASSOCIATIONS DURING PERINATAL LIFE

The perinatal period is the interval between the onset of fetal survivability (~24–26 weeks) and the end of the neonatal period (~28 days after delivery). Such growth retarded infants are usually small with diminutive subcutaneous tissue resulting in wrinkled skin and a wizened look (Fig. 24-1). The fetus with poor intrauterine growth has a fivefold to tenfold increase in risk for perinatal mortality (≈0.5%–1% risk), compared with the normal size fetus (0.1%).[88,123] Twenty-percent of stillborn fetuses are small for gestational age.

EFFECTS DURING CHILDHOOD

Surviving children who were growth retarded bear a 50% risk of significant short- and long-term morbidity. Hospitalizations are often prolonged.[73] Physical, metabolic, and neurologic complications are frequently seen. However, only one study has been published that relates poor perinatal outcome with postnatal behavior in the same infants.[54] Fitzhardinge and Steven showed that ~25% of affected infants have long-term neurologic deficits and remain disabled for life.[58] Children with IUGR have been found to have higher blood pressure compared with controls.[73]

EFFECTS IN ADULTHOOD

Adults who had suffered from IUGR as fetuses are at a much higher risk for acquired heart disease, lipid abnormalities, and diabetes in later life.[14,74,102,134]

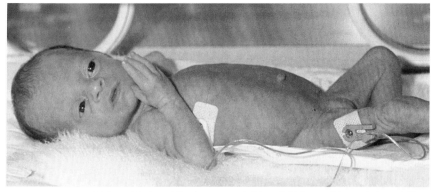

Figure 24-1. IUGR in a 12-day-old neonate weighing 1400 g at 36 weeks' gestation. Notice the wrinkling of the skin in the lower extremities and the right arm secondary to diminished subcutaneous tissue. Additionally, the infant has a wizened look, which was more prominent in the first days of life.

Etiology

Fetal growth abnormalities are thought to be idiopathic in half of the cases and multifactorial in the remainder. Some infants are constitutionally small because of genetic or racial influences.[14] The difficulty is in discerning this normal group from infants compromised because of malnourishment, uteroplacental insufficiency, or other hemodynamic malady. Recent advances in prenatal Doppler interrogation are reducing the number of idiopathic cases by identifying the underlying causes of disease. However these mechanisms, which cause the poor growth, are not well understood.

Poor intrauterine growth and subsequent low birth weight are common features of many chromosomal abnormalities and in other fetuses with structural abnormalities.[38,114,136] The incidence of chromosomal abnormality in an infant of low birth weight is ~10%.[81] Many of these fetuses have multisystem malformations and altered body proportionality. When no ultrasonographically identifiable malformation can be seen the incidence falls to 4% to 7%.[130] With severely impaired fetal growth, the risk of chromosomal abnormality is increased even more if there are abnormal amounts of amniotic fluid or there are abnormal placentofetal Doppler indices.[130]

Abnormal placental development is associated with poor placental function, and the chromosomally abnormal fetus has a chromosomally abnormal placenta. Therefore, the IUGR associated with the aneuploid (karyotypically abnormal) fetus may be caused by primary placental insufficiency due to placental maldevelopment.

Identification of IUGR

WEIGHT-BASED THEORIES

As stated, the sonographic prediction of estimated fetal weight forms the foundation for the identification of the small fetus and poor fetal growth. A list of birth weight percentiles from the 23rd to the 44th week of pregnancy is shown in Table 24-3. This table shows, for example, that low birth weight fetuses weigh less than ~2510 g and 2750 g at the 38th and 40th weeks of pregnancy, respectively. It should be noted that the birth weights listed in Table 24-3 are derived from pregnant women living at or near sea level. No tables have been published for populations at high altitude in the United States where infants are normally lighter in weight than those at sea level. The tables formulated at sea level may consequently be inaccurate for these infants.[15]

SYMMETRIC AND ASYMMETRIC IUGR

The traditional model for abnormal fetal growth defines two types of aberrant growth: symmetric and asymmetric IUGR. This model has lost favor in recent years because it does not appear to withstand scrutiny. Doubilet and Benson argued that the ratio of head circumference to abdominal circumference (HC/AC) measurement would have a bimodal distribution with a lower value for cases of symmetric

◢◣◢◣ TABLE 24-3. FETAL WEIGHT PERCENTILES THROUGHOUT PREGNANCY

Gestational Age (Menstrual Weeks)	Smoothed Percentiles				
	10	25	50	75	90
23	370	460	550	690	990
24	420	530	640	780	1080
25	490	630	740	890	1180
26	570	730	860	1020	1320
27	660	840	990	1160	1470
28	770	980	1150	1350	1660
29	890	1100	1310	1530	1890
30	1030	1260	1460	1710	2100
31	1180	1410	1630	1880	2290
32	1310	1570	1810	2090	2500
33	1480	1720	2010	2280	2690
34	1670	1910	2220	2510	2880
35	1870	2130	2430	2730	3090
36	2190	2470	2650	2950	3290
37	2310	2580	2870	3160	3470
38	2510	2770	3030	3320	3610
39	2680	2910	3170	3470	3750
40	2750	3010	3280	3590	3870
41	2800	3070	3360	3680	3980
42	2830	3110	3410	3740	4060
43	2840	3110	3420	3780	4100
44	2790	3050	3390	3770	4110

Adapted from Brenner WE, Edelman DA, Hendricks CH: A standard of fetal growth for the United States of America. Am J Obstet Gynecol. 1976, 126:555.

IUGR and a higher value for those with asymmetric IUGR if these two different types of IUGR truly exist.[47] The fact that the HC/AC ratio has a unimodal distribution in IUGR with a mean value higher than that for normal fetuses argues for their point.[18,37]

CALCULATING WEIGHT PERCENTILE

Doubilet and Benson described a *"straightforward"* approach to screen for IUGR by assessing for an EFW of <10%.[47] Calculating the weight percentile requires three steps[20]:

1. *A gestational age is assigned to the fetus.* The optimal gestational age estimate (OGA) should be determined at the time of the first ultrasound examination during a pregnancy. It may be based on the last menstrual period, the conception date, or fetal biometry obtained at the time of that examination. For every subsequent examination, the OGA should be calculated as the OGA plus the number of weeks since the first examination. Biometry obtained at all subsequent examinations should never be used to redate the pregnancy. The examiner should be mindful that the sonographic prediction of gestational age based on biometry is less exact with advancing gestation (±0.7 weeks in the first trimester to ±3 to 4 weeks in the last trimester).

2. *The fetal weight is estimated.* There have been more than 57 published articles that provide formulas or tables that use various body parts in the estimation of fetal weight.[19,84] Schemes using two, three, or more measurements have been offered, including those using the biparietal diameter, head circumference, abdominal circumference, femur length, as well as the humerus length (discussed in Chapter 19). A reasonable model for estimating the fetal weight would include measurement of the fetal head, abdomen, and femur.[60,67,143] The use of multiple parameters has been shown to decrease both interobserver and intraobserver error.

The accuracy of the predicted EFW will fall within 10% to 20% of the actual weight in 80% to 95% of cases.[4,18] The reliability of EFW predictions is not influenced by amniotic fluid amounts or maternal weight.[56,95]

Most of these formulas for EFW use the BPD, HC, AC, or FL measurements. Campbell et al, Ferrero et al, Hadlock et al, and Warsof et al formulas use the FL and AC; Shepard et al used BPD and FL; Hadlock et al, Hill et al, Woo et al, and Benson et al used FL, AC, and BPD; Roberts et al used FL, AC, BPD, and HC; and Sabbagha et al used HC, AC, and FL[4,21,35,55,67,68,72,117,121,125,146,151] (see Appendixes L, M, N). In this chapter we discuss the three most popular formulas:

Formula by Shepard and Coworkers[125]

This formula incorporates only BPD and AC. Its predictive error is high ($\pm$10% to 15%) and it is particularly accurate in small infants.[67] Although there have been more than 18 articles published that validate the efficacy of this formula, it has two limiting factors. First, BPD measurements can be altered by *"normal"* changes in head shape as pregnancy continues or because of normal variants in head shape such as dolichocephaly and brachycephaly. Second, it does not use the HC and FL, considered by some as important measurements in determining weight. Despite these problems, many recommend this technique for estimating the fetal weight.[84]

Formula by Hadlock and Coworkers[67]

This formula incorporates three basic measurements: HC, AC, and FL (Table 24-4).[67] With this approach the 2 SD variation in the prediction of birth weight has been reduced.[68] However, the authors have reported a wide error ($\pm$ 19.4%) in estimating the size of fetuses that weigh <1500 g. The formula has been found more accurate in fetuses >2500 g, and it does not consider the proportional contributions of HC and AC to birth weight. These

contributions are known to be in a dynamic state of change. In other words, the HC/AC ratio normally changes throughout pregnancy and with some pathologic states. The following examples illustrate the dynamic differences that exist in the HC/AC ratios: (1) Before the 36th pregnancy week the HC/AC ratio is >1.0. (2) Following the 36th pregnancy week the HC/AC ratio is <1.0. (3) In the macrosomic fetus the HC/AC ratio is <1.0.

Formulas by Sabbagha and Coworkers[121]

To account for the dynamically varying proportional contributions of the HC and the AC, these investigators derived three formulas, one from each of three fetal groups: large, appropriate, and small for gestational age; each of the three formulas is targeted to a specific group of fetuses. All three targeted formulas incorporate the following four parameters: gestational age in weeks, HC, AC (multiplied by 2), and FL. The accuracy of the assigned gestational age should be within $\pm$2 weeks, and preferably decided by one of the following criteria: (1) early CRL or BPD (measurements obtained before 13 and 26 weeks' gestation, respectively); (2) known ovulation dates or certain last menstrual period; (3) confirmation of menstrual dates by early CRL or BPD, as defined in criterion 1; (4) the average of different dates estimated by early CRL and/or BPD, and FL, if the estimates do not differ from each other by more than 1 week; and (5) the average of different dates provided by early CRL, and/or HC, or AC, and FL, again, if the estimates do not differ from each other by more than 1 week.

In estimating fetal weight by the targeted formulas, the percentile rank of the AC determines which of the three formulas should be employed. For example, if the AC is at least in the 90th percentile, the formula for the large-for-dates fetus is used. On the other hand, if the AC is average (between 10th and 90th percentile), the formula for the appropriate-for-dates fetus is used. Finally, if the AC is below the 5th percentile, the formula for the small-for-dates fetus is used.

 TABLE 24-4. FORMULA FOR ESTIMATION OF FETAL WEIGHT

$Log_{10}BW = 1.5662 - 0.0108(HC) + 0.0468(AC) + 0.171(FL) + 0.00034(HC)^2 - 0.003685(AC \times FL)$

From Hadlock FP, Harrist RB, Sharman RS, et al. Estimation of fetal weight with the use of head, body, and femur measurements: A prospective study. Am J Obstet Gynecol. 1985; 151:333–337.

In comparison to Hadlock's formula, the targeted formulas reduce the cumulative 2 SD variation by 8.4%. On the other hand, the cumulative absolute 2 SD variation of the targeted formulas is 12% versus 15.6% for Hadlock's formula, a reduction of 23%.[68] It should be emphasized that the advantage of reduction in the 2 SD variation achieved by the targeted formulas may be lost if gestational age cannot be determined within a range of ±2 weeks.

The format of deriving estimates of fetal weight by the sum of four variables allows the sonographer the choice of reading the estimated fetal weight directly from a concise chart or entering all three formulas into a computer for automatic calculation of the estimated fetal weight.

3. *The weight percentile is calculated from the estimated weight and the gestational age.* This is typically accomplished using a published table that reports normal weight for gestational age. Of particular importance is the determination about whether the fetus' weight falls below the 10%.

NON-WEIGHT BASED PARAMETERS

Several other biometric methods have been proposed to aid in the identification of IUGR. These include the brain's gyral patterns,[5] the transcerebellar diameter, evidence of decreased adipose deposits,[13] foot length, the imaging of the distal femoral epiphysis or proximal humeral epiphysis, ratios of the HC to the AC[33,41] or the AC to the FL,[66] amniotic fluid volumes (without PROM),[91] the presence of a Grade 3 placenta,[80] or echogenic bowel[47] (Table 24-5). For an independent technique to be clinically useful, it must have a high degree of sensitivity, specificity, and have high predictive values. Unfortunately, no single ultrasonographic parameter will allow for the confident diagnosis of IUGR. The most accurate diagnosis is achieved by using multiple biometric and structural parameters.[47]

CLINICAL PARAMETERS

Benson and Doubilet offered a quantitative method of assessing IUGR that uses clinical parameters to improve predictability.[18] This technique allows the diagnosis of IUGR if the EFW corresponding to

TABLE 24-5. CONVENTIONAL SONOGRAPHIC CRITERIA FOR IUGR: PERFORMANCE CHARACTERISTICS[25]

Criterion	Sensitivity (%)	Specificity (%)	Predictive Values	
			Positive (%)	Negative (%)
Advanced placental grade	62	64	16	94
Elevated FL/AC	34–49	78–83	18–20	92–93
Low total intrauterine volume	57–80	72–76	21–24	92–97
Small BPD	24–88	62–94	21–44	92–98
Small BPD and advanced placental grade	59	86	32	95
Slow rate of BPD growth	75	84	35	97
Low amniotic fluid volume	89	88	45	99
Low EFW	89	88	45	99
Decreased AVF	24	98	55	92
Elevated HC/AC	82	94	62	98

Sensitivity = the ratio of affected fetuses (true positive) identified per all affected fetuses (e.g., if 90 fetuses with IUGR are identified with ultrasound of 100 fetuses that actually have IUGR, the test is 90% sensitive for IUGR detection); specificity = the ratio of unaffected fetuses (true negative) identified per all unaffected fetuses (e.g., 990 fetuses with normal growth are identified with ultrasound among 1000 fetuses that actually have normal growth, the test is 99% specific for IUGR detection); positive predictive value = the ratio of affected fetuses (true positives) identified per all affected fetuses plus the number of unaffected fetuses that test positive (false positives). This measures the likelihood that a positive test will identify affected status and it incorporates the defined prevalence of the condition in the equation.

Modified from Doubilet PM, Benson CB. Sonographic evaluation of intrauterine growth retardation. Am J Roentgenol. 1995, 164:709–717.

the gestational age, amniotic fluid volume, and maternal blood pressure status (Table 24-6) falls below the designated values. An EFW between these two groups of values is indeterminate for IUGR, whereas an EFW that falls in a higher zone of values excludes or "rules out" IUGR (with a similar high degree of confidence). Both the diagnosis and the exclusion of IUGR are 85% predictive.

Fetal Growth Rate

The idea of monitoring interval growth in IUGR or at-risk fetuses is relatively new.[46] Whenever possible, measurements should be obtained at several points during pregnancy showing longitudinal changes in growth. Affected fetuses grow at a slower rate than unaffected fetuses. As a result their birth weights are lower. Growth assessment can either be direct (monitoring the growth rate) or indirect (deviations from the expected size). Indirect assessment implies that the normal range of growth over time is known. This would allow for a compu-

tation of the growth rate by dividing the growth by the time interval. The growth rates for the BPD, AC, and FL have been recently reported.[97]

Fetal Physiology

Fetal maladaptation syndrome (FMS) occurs when the fetus can no longer compensate physiologically in a stressful environment. One of the first sequelae of maladaptation is poor intrauterine fetal growth. Commonly this finding is followed by observations of decreased amniotic fluid amounts (from oliguria), abnormal fetal/umbilical arterial and venous Doppler assessment (reflecting declining cardiac output, increasing or decreasing vascular resistance in the fetus or placenta, or fetal hypoxia/acidemia with resultant arterial and venous cardiovascular adaptations), and pathologic fetal behavior (no movement or poor tone). Many fetuses with poor growth are found to have a primary disorder of uteroplacental or fetoplacental hemodynamics.

Changes in fetal size/growth, developmental

TABLE 24-6. CRITICAL VALUES FOR ESTIMATED FETAL WEIGHT FOR DIAGNOSING OR EXCLUDING IUGR USING THE IUGR SCORE[25]

| Gestational Age (weeks) | Status of Maternal Blood Pressure and Amniotic Fluid Volume | | | | | |
| | Normal Blood Pressure | | | Hypertension | | |
	Norm/Poly	M-M Oligo	Sev Oligo	Norm/Poly	M-M Oligo	Sev Oligo
26	516–660	646–826	743–950	610–780	7663–976	878–1123
27	597–791	745–949	855–1090	704–898	878–1119	1009–1285
28	693–877	859–1087	982–1244	813–1030	1008–1276	1153–1460
29	803–1008	988–1239	1124–1410	937–1176	1152–1446	1312–1646
30	931–1155	1132–1405	1281–1589	1078–1337	1311–1627	1483–1840
31	1075–1317	1293–1584	1452–1779	1234–1512	1484–1819	1667–2042
32	1235–1493	1468–1774	1635–1976	1404–1698	1670–2018	1860–2248
33	1411–1682	1656–1973	1830–2180	1590–1895	1865–2223	2061–2456
34	1600–1880	1853–2177	2031–2386	1785–2098	2067–2429	2266–2662
35	1798–2083	2055–2382	2236–2590	1987–2302	2272–2633	2471–2863
36	1997–2285	2257–2593	2437–2789	2189–2504	2474–2830	2671–3056
37	2192–2479	2452–2774	2631–2976	2383–2696	2666–3016	2861–3236
38	2371–2658	2631–2949	2807–3147	2563–2872	2843–3186	3034–3400
39	2526–2812	2785–3101	2961–3296	2717–3025	2996–3335	3185–3545
40	2645–2933	2906–3223	3083–3419	2838–3147	3118–3458	3307–3668
41	2717–3013	2985–3310	3166–3511	2915–3232	3202–3551	3396–3766
42	2736–3405	3016–3356	3205–3567	2942–3274	3243–3609	3447–3836

For each pair an EFW less than the lower value corresponds to an IUGR score of more than 60, allowing a confident diagnosis of IUGR (positive predictive value of 74%). An EFW value greater than the higher number corresponds with a score below 50, virtually excluding IUGR (negative predictive value of 97%). An EFW between the two values is equivocal (probability of IUGR is 13%).

Modified from Doubilet PM, Benson CB. Sonographic evaluation of intrauterine growth retardation. Am J Roentgenol. 1995, 164:709–717.

TABLE 24-7. PREDICTORS THAT HAVE BEEN USED IN THE PRENATAL IDENTIFICATION OF IUGR

Past obstetric history
Roll-over test, blood pressure
Angiotensin-II test
Fibronectin, atrial natriuretic factor, or calcium β-hCG
Plasma volume, hemoglobin, hematocrit
Uricemia, microalbuminuria
Platelet count
Umbilical artery Doppler
Uterine artery Doppler
Placental lateralization

anatomy, physiology, and behavior, have been observed to precede fetal compromise and eventual fetal death.[1] These changes can portend acute and chronic fetal deterioration. Several prenatal diagnostic techniques have been offered as predictors of poor growth (Table 24-7). In this discussion, we focus on the sonographic tools used in the diagnosis of IUGR.

Doppler Assessment in IUGR[9,11,16,25,63,70,94,104,119,139,141,142,145]

In the fetus with IUGR, there is a normal redistribution of blood within the fetus and placenta. Doppler technology has had a significant impact on our ability to assess the physiologic status of the fetus. It can help in identifying changes in the fetal circulation at a time when other tests are normal and in so doing identify the truly hypoxic fetus. Interval changes in Doppler values may be useful in determining the optimal time for delivery to reduce perinatal mortality and any subsequent complications.

During Doppler interrogation it is important to remember that fetal blood flow is influenced by cardiac contractility, the physical properties of the arterial walls and the blood viscosity within, the size of small blood vessels, and the outflow impedance from the arterial tree.[32,78,113,131,140] Most reports regarding the interrogation of the fetal circulation use the pulsatility index because it is Doppler angle independent.

While Doppler interrogation has not been universally accepted for screening low-risk populations, it has been proven to be effective in the evaluation

of high-risk pregnancies.[61,135] Several have shown that it is of value in identifying the physiologically compromised fetus. Most now agree that women at risk should have access to equipment with pulsed Doppler capabilities.[3]

UTERINE ARTERY DOPPLER

Normally, uterine vascular resistance decreases with advancing gestational age. During the first 10 weeks of pregnancy, a persistent diastolic component of the uterine artery Doppler (utD) waveform is observed and the systolic/diastolic (S/D) ratio is normally about 3.0, with an early diastolic notch.[113] At ~13 weeks, the S/D ratio decreases to 2.6.[113] After 26 weeks, the utD S/D ratio is ~2.0.[113] Higher ratios may suggest abnormality and increasing resistance to flow (Fig. 24-2). Uterine arterial Doppler assessment has been reported during four distinct periods of gestation:

Early Pregnancy (12–13 weeks)

The pulsatility index of a utD waveform was analyzed in women of advanced maternal age (>34 years) carrying fetuses between 12 and 13 weeks gestation. Women with abnormally high values had higher risks of developing hypertensive disorders

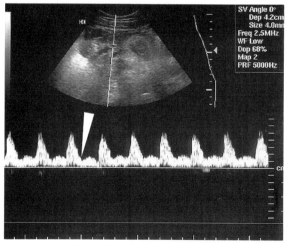

Figure 24-2. Pulsed Doppler waveform of the uterine artery showing a resistivity index of 0.76, a pulsatility index of 1.63, and a systolic to diastolic ratio of 4.25, and a *dichrotic notch* (*arrow*). This represents an abnormal uterine artery waveform at 34 weeks and 2 days of gestation because of the presence of the notching and diminutive diastolic flow.

(four times normal), Small for Gestational Age (SGA) (twice normal), preterm delivery (three times normal), and gestational diabetes (nine times normal). Pulsatility index values of <1.24 were considered overtly normal and >1.67 was abnormal.[34,59,136,138] In preeclampsia, a prominent diastolic notch is seen in ≈60% of cases.[126]

Early Second Trimester (16–20 weeks)

UtD interrogation during the midsecond trimester has been successfully used to predict outcome in cases at risk for pregnancy-induced hypertension, IUGR, preterm delivery, gestational diabetes, and fetal asphyxia.[22,28,30,31,53,100,116,138,148] However, the value of routine screening for predicting preeclampsia and IUGR has yet to be accepted by all authors.[27,100]

Bromley and colleagues investigated the relationship between utD and the presence of uterine artery notching in terms of perinatal outcome.[30] In a population of women with elevated MSAFP test values, they found an incidence in adverse outcome of 13% without notching and 47% with Grade II notching.

Mid-second Trimester (23–27 weeks)

Van den Elzen and colleagues found abnormal PI values (>1.24) with an 11-fold increased risk for preterm delivery when compared with normals (<1.09).[138]

Third Trimester (29–41 weeks)

IUGR neonates with abnormal prenatal utD resistivity index have placental ischemia and clinical difficulties (including preterm delivery, cesarean section for fetal distress, lower mean pH, higher carbon dioxide pressure, and lower oxygen pressure) in ≈92% of cases.[76,77,85,103,116]

UMBILICAL ARTERIAL DOPPLER

Assessment of blood flow through the umbilical cord, primarily the umbilical artery, has been widely reported.[12,48,99,135,152] Abnormal umbilical Doppler (umD) waveforms may show reduced, absent, or even reversed diastolic flow velocities. When this happens, the indices of resistance are increased. This is thought to result from increased placental vascular resistance. Absent end-diastolic flow is normal before 24 weeks. The diastolic component of the

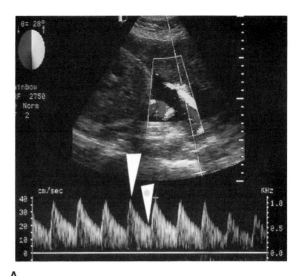

A

B

Figure 24-3. (**A**) B-mode sonography with pulsed Doppler of the umbilical artery in normal fetus at ~34 weeks and without IUGR shows an S/D ratio of 2.23 (*arrow, systole; dotted arrow, diastole*). (See also Color Plate 19.) (**B**) Conversely, in a compromised fetus of the same age, the diastolic component of the waveform will progressively diminish until absent (*arrow*), or in the most severe cases, reversed diastolic flow can be seen.

waveform gradually increases with advancing gestation. A persistent reduced diastolic component in the mid- to late third trimester is indicative of poor perinatal outcome. Further, abnormally reduced diastolic flow velocities are predictive in the identification of infants requiring early delivery and neonatal intensive care.[136]

The Doppler spectral finding that has received the most notoriety is *absent or reversed end-diastolic flow,* after 30 weeks' gestation (Fig. 24-3). This finding is indicative of impending fetal demise and it has been associated with perinatal mortality in 28% of cases (and in ~ 100% of cases if untreated) and in IUGR in ~ 100% of cases.[6,79] The observation of absent end-diastolic flow may occur nearly 8 days before pathologic cardiotocographic findings are present.[6] The appearance of reversed end-diastolic flow is evidence of (1) the lowest vascular resistance being in the fetal circulatory network rather than the placenta and (2) preplacental blood with low oxygen content from the descending aorta and pulmonary artery is being shifted toward the brain.[44] This is to be considered an alarming finding affecting obstetrical diagnosis and management.

While an association clearly exists, several investigators have tried to establish the applicability of umD (excepting absent diastolic flow) in the *prediction* of IUGR.[36,135] Fetuses with abnormal umD indices have only a twofold to fourfold risk of IUGR, compared with controls.[36] While there is an increased risk of cesarean section, preterm delivery, neonatal intensive care unit admissions, the need for assisted ventilation, and perinatal mortality, the low sensitivity of umD in the detection of IUGR makes it a poor screening tool in a low-risk population.[147]

MIDDLE CEREBRAL ARTERY DOPPLER

Prenatal interrogation of cerebral blood flow can be accomplished by assessing the common carotid artery, the internal carotid artery, or the anterior, middle, or cerebral arteries. The efficacy and utility of middle cerebral artery (MCA) Doppler have been proven useful in detecting hypoxia associated with IUGR.[99,141,150] The flow velocity in the middle cerebral artery is normally highly pulsatile and the frequency of detectable end-diastolic flow increases with advancing gestation (75% at 18 weeks and 100% at 34 weeks).[43,145] In fetuses with IUGR, pulsatility indices in all major intracranial arteries are significantly reduced.[44] It is thought that a hormonally mediated increase in fetal peripheral vascular resistance occurs so that cerebral, cardiac, and adrenal gland blood flow is conserved. These phenomena result in the *"brain sparing effect"*[8,23,44,65,106,116,145,149] and the *"cardiac sparing*

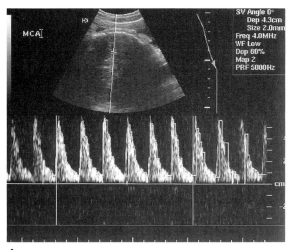
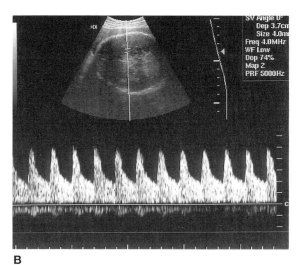

A   B

Figure 24-4. In hypoxia, the fetus will compensate by redistributing its cardiovascular load so that more blood is circulated to the fetal head (the *brain-sparing effect*), heart, and adrenal glands. Therefore, when compensating, the diastolic component of the middle cerebral artery (MCA) waveform will show increased flow. (**A**) Transverse ultrasonographic image of the fetal head in duplex mode (B-mode and pulsed Doppler) showing normal middle cerebral arterial flow at ~34 weeks. This fetus is uncompromised. (**B**) This transverse ultrasonographic image of the fetal head in duplex mode, also at ~34 weeks, shows an increased diastolic component, consistent with circulatory redistribution in a compromised fetus.

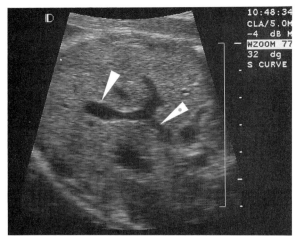

Figure 24-5. This transverse ultrasonographic image of the fetal abdomen at ~30 weeks of gestation, shows the (*arrow*) ductus venosus.

effect"[141] to preserve the function of these important structures (Fig. 24-4). In the brain it may prevent fetal hypoxia and is a sign of impending brain damage.[24,44,122,145]

The MCA and umD are the best individual predictors of adverse fetal outcome, respectively. However, better results have been obtained using the ratio of these two values. Compared with controls, infants with IUGR and umD/MCA values >95% were found to have a higher incidence of preterm delivery (33 vs. 36 weeks, p = 0.001), lower birth weight (1414 vs. 2104 g, p = 0.001), incidence of emergency cesarean section for fetal distress (58% vs. 8%, p = 0.001), prenatal/neonatal mortality (22% vs. 0%, p = 0.001), low 5-minute Apgar score (24% vs. 2%, p = 0.001), and admission to neonatal intensive care unit for asphyxia (27% vs. 0%, p = 0.001). Early in 1995, Harrington and coworkers reaffirmed these findings when they reported that abnormal umD/MCA ratios were found in pregnancies with adverse outcomes, but with normal umD values.[69] If growth retardation is suspected at >34 weeks, Harrington and coworkers stated that it is not sufficient to observe that the umD resistance is normal; fetal Doppler studies should include the umD/MCA ratio because fetal hemodynamic redistribution may exist in the presence of a normal umD index. Whereas an abnormal umD/MCA requires intensive fetal surveillance, a normal test value may be reassuring.

DUCTUS VENOSUS AND UMBILICAL VEIN DOPPLER

The ductus venosus (DV) is a regulator of oxygen to the fetus.[82] Half the oxygenated blood returning from the placenta is directed through the DV (Figs. 24-5, 24-6). This forms a preferential bloodstream through the foramen ovale to the left heart, into the aorta and to the cranial vessels.[16,29,49,51,82,83]

Between 17 and 39 weeks, growth retarded fetuses with normal chromosomes and no concomitant malformations have reduced DV flows seen during atrial contraction.[71,82] This serious finding has been linked to a raised utD PI, and reversed or absent end-diastolic UmD flow and umbilical vein pulsations. During hypoxia an increase in pressure in the umbilical vein occurs and more blood is shunted through the DV, when compared with the liver. In fetal compromise, as much as 70% of blood returning from the placenta is directed into the inferior vena cava through the DV.[50,105]

Increased pulsatility of the venous circulation reflects cardiac compromise from increased cardiac afterload. Umbilical vein (UV) pulsation is a common finding in the early, normal pregnancy and in association with fetal breathing. However, this phenomenon is associated with compromised fetal hemodynamics in later pregnancy.[82] Thirty percent

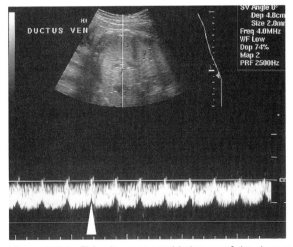

Figure 24-6. This ultrasonographic image of the ductus venosus shows an abnormal venous Doppler waveform. Note the marked notching (*arrow*) during diastole (considered abnormal if >50% of the systolic peak). This is a severely compromised fetus.

of cases with abnormal umD indices have umbilical vein pulsations (without breathing).[82]

Other Tools in the Antenatal Surveillance of the IUGR Fetus

In addition to maternal diabetes, hypertension, postdatism, and a history of unexplained stillbirth, IUGR is thought to place the fetus at significant risk for fetal death and thus warrants close antepartum surveillance. Furthermore, IUGR is often an indicator of chronic fetal compromise and it may precede acute fetal deterioration and fetal death. Therefore, enhanced antenatal surveillance is needed to identify that the fetus is deteriorating. In this way, the most suitable time for delivering the affected fetus can be better determined—the point in pregnancy when the fetus has attained maximum pulmonary maturity but has not yet developed central nervous system compromise. Once the diagnosis of poor growth is made the exact mode of surveillance used by different clinical departments will vary. Nonetheless, the usual modalities may include the biophysical profile (BPP), nonstress test (NST), or contraction stress test (CST). Importantly, when results of these tests are normal they accurately predict fetal well-being. On the other hand, abnormal test results do not have a high correlation with poor outcome or fetal hypoxia; in other words, the false-positive rate of these tests is high.

BIOPHYSICAL PROFILE (BPP)

The biophysical profile is presented in detail in Chapter 22. In this discussion the reader is reminded that the BPP score is based on the evaluation of five biophysical functions: fetal breathing movement (FBM), fetal motion (FM), fetal tone (FT), amniotic fluid volume (AFV), and NST. A score of 2 is assigned for each normal variable and a score of 0 when the biophysical function is absent. All observations are made within an interval of 30 minutes.

The reactivity of the biophysical variables is dependent on an intact central nervous system (CNS). The reason for this is thought to relate to the *"gradual hypoxia concept."*[57,144] This concept has been formulated on the premise that (1) the later a neuroanatomic center develops, the more sensitive it is to the manifestations of acute hypoxia (the area of the fetal brain that regulates FT develops at

7 to 9 weeks, FM at 9 weeks, FBM at 20 to 21 weeks, and NST at 26 weeks to term), (2) FBM, FM, FT, and NST are acute biophysical parameters that represent the acute fetal condition, and (3) the amniotic fluid volume is a predictor of the chronic fetal condition. The biophysical profile is a better predictor of normality than of abnormality (fetal hypoxia). First, the result is likely to be negative in 97.5% of tested fetuses, and the predictive value of a normal test is high.[90] It would be extremely unlikely for a preterm or term fetus to die within 7 days of a normal biophysical profile result (≥ 8) or for a postterm fetus to die within 3 days. The biophysical profile can be equivocal in 2% of fetuses. Under such circumstances it should be repeated or a CST performed, depending on the management protocol of the particular institution.

The biophysical profile is clearly abnormal in a very small number (1%) of tested fetuses (value of ≤ 4), but the subsequent management of such fetuses is not uniform.[90] In some centers delivery of the fetus may be performed, particularly if it is pulmonically mature. In other centers a CST may be performed first to confirm fetal hypoxia or continuous fetal biophysical survey may be observed for 2 to 3 hours before decisive action is taken. The rationale for the latter thinking is that absence of some biophysical functions may reflect normal periodicity rather than hypoxia. The absence of some biophysical functions for periods of 20 minutes to more than 2 hours can be normal. Absence of some biologic function may also be related to the time of testing or to medication used by the mother. FBMs follow a circadian rhythm (i.e., appear more frequently at specific times), are more common 2 hours after meals, and can be suppressed by medication used to sedate the mother or treat her hypertension. The accuracy of the BPP will be enhanced if the mother is tested 2 hours after meals and is not using medication known to depress the fetal CNS. Two important components of the BPP are discussed below. It is important to emphasize that different institutions may employ different protocols for assessment. For example, one institution may consider weekly BPP assessments to evaluate the IUGR fetus, while another may use NST and AFV assessment; still others may use Doppler assessment in their *"first-line"* of interrogation.

NONSTRESS TEST

Abnormal fetal heart rate patterns are thought to suggest heart failure and serve as an indirect measure of CNS integrity and function (Fig. 24-7).[112] These patterns are thought to precede the development of hypoxia. A major advantage of the NST is its ease of performance. A drawback of the NST is that it is sensitive (most "*abnormal*" fetuses have abnormal results), but not very specific (most "*abnormal*" test results occur in normal fetuses). Normal fetuses may have an abnormal test result because of gestational immaturity, sleep cycles, or maternal sedation.

Although NSTs are usually conducted by a nurse-specialist, knowledge of the method of interpreting the test is important for sonographers. The NST is frequently called a bioelectric test. It involves computation of the baseline fetal heart rate (FHR) and any changes that occur in response to fetal movement. A normal (or reactive) test depends on detection of at least two FHR accelerations above the baseline. Normally, in a 20-minute period the FHR should accelerate by 15 beats per minute (bpm) for at least 15 seconds.[86] Indicators of well-being also include a baseline FHR falling between 120 and 160 bpm and absence of any decelerations, that is, decreases in the FHR below baseline. A normal or reactive result implies good fetal CNS integrity; that is, absence of asphyxia for 7 days in the preterm and term fetus and for 3 days in the postterm fetus. A reactive test correctly predicts fetal well-being in 62% to 89% of cases.

An abnormal or nonreactive NST is defined by absence of fetal movements or by FHR accelerations <15 bpm. Additionally, the presence of spontaneous heart rate decelerations and/or loss of beat-to-beat heart rate variability (a characteristic of normal fetuses) may be associated with poor outcome. A nonreactive test correctly predicts fetal death (within 1 week of testing) in only 3% to 29% of cases. The reason may be partly related to the normal periodicity.

ASSESSMENT OF AMNIOTIC FLUID

Assessment of the amount of amniotic fluid is an important, albeit indeterminate, measure of the fetal condition. The amount of amniotic fluid is, at best, a weak predictor of perinatal morbidity and it needs to be used together with other biophysical parameters. While decreased amounts of amniotic fluid can be the result of premature rupture of the membranes or renal anomalies, it can also occur as the result of decreased urine production from poor renal perfusion. Amniotic fluid is derived from fetal

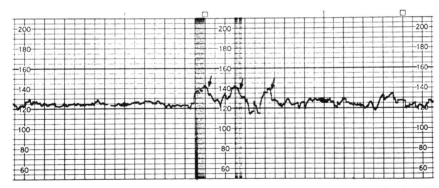

Figure 24-7. Bioelectric tracing shows a reactive nonstress test. The vertical line (y-axis) delineates the FHR per minute. The horizontal (x-axis) delineates time, ~10 seconds per small box (20 small boxes are placed between the vertical printed FHR numbers and are run through the NST machine at a rate of one box per 10 seconds or 20 boxes every 3.33 minutes, ~200 seconds). Note the following characteristics of a reactive test: (1) baseline in normal, ranging from 120 to 125 beats per minute, (2) beat-to-beat variability is clearly seen with the baseline heart rate having a jagged appearance, (3) no decelerations are recorded, and (4) three heart rate accelerations are recorded (*arrows*), each exceeding 15 bpm. A reactive test is normal.

and maternal sources. The exchange occurs in two directions within each of three compartments.[75]

Compartment 1, Mother and Amniotic Fluid

The bidirectional flow takes place across the decidua and fetal membranes; at term, the normal net hourly exchange is ~135 ml in the direction of amniotic fluid.

Compartment 2, Mother and Fetus

The bidirectional flow takes place across the intervillous space; at term, the normal net hourly exchange is ~50 to 90 ml in the direction of the fetus.

Compartment 3, Fetus and Amniotic Fluid

The flow mainly occurs through the respiratory, gastrointestinal, and urinary tracts. At term, the normal net hourly exchange is ~150 to 225 ml in the direction of the amniotic fluid compartment.

There are three methods of assessing the amounts of fluid in the amniotic cavity. First, quantitative methods were employed using the instillation of dye into the amniotic cavity and removal of the amniotic fluid. This was then titrated. The precise amount of amniotic fluid can then be determined. Second, semiquantitative methods were proposed such as the maximum sonographically detectable vertical pocket of amniotic fluid or using the *amniotic fluid index* (AFI, discussed in the following section). Last, subjective assessment using ultrasonography by an experienced observer is highly predictive of oligohydramnios and polyhydramnios.

The method that seems to have garnered a great deal of recent favor is the AFI. Phelan and coworkers developed this ultrasound method that allows quantification of normal amniotic fluid volume.[107] They divide the uterine cavity into four quadrants using two imaginary lines, one running transversely across the umbilicus and the other vertically using the linea nigra (Fig. 24-8). The vertical

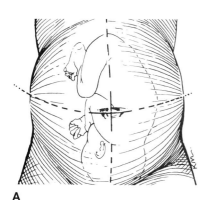

A

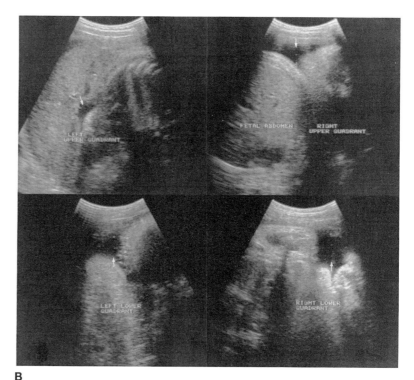

B

Figure 24-8. (**A**) Photograph shows division of the pregnant abdomen into four quadrants for obtaining the *amniotic fluid index* (AFI). (**B**) Sonograms depicting amniotic fluid volume (*arrows*) in the four quadrants. The AFI is ~5 (not cm because an index has no unit of measure) because there is no measurable fluid in the left upper quadrant. This AFI is diagnostic of oligohydramnios.

diameter of the largest pocket in each quadrant is measured and the sum of the four pockets is determined. This sum is called the AFI. The mean values (±2 SD) of the AFI throughout pregnancy are then determined (Fig. 24-9). In the third trimester of pregnancy, the 2 SD variation about the mean AFI is wide. Additionally, a progressive increase in the AFV is noted until the 28th to 30th week.

In the third trimester of pregnancy, oligohydramnios exists when (1) the diameter of the largest pocket of amniotic fluid is <2 to 3 cm (depending on the guidelines used),[42] (2) the AFI is <6,[120] or (3) the experienced sonographer subjectively observes an overall paucity in AFV.

Using the subjective method of assessing AFV in a large unselected population of pregnant women, Philipson and coworkers showed that the prevalence of oligohydramnios is 3.9%.[109] The predictive value of oligohydramnios in the diagnosis of IUGR was only 19% to 40%.[26,109] The sensitivity of the test (i.e., presence of oligohydramnios) is also low, 16%.[107] The fact that only 16% of all IUGR is associated with oligohydramnios may be related to the marked variation in AFV noted in different pregnancies. In other words, the AFV may be low in many normal pregnancies.

Phelan and colleagues showed that in postterm pregnancies with severe oligohydramnios (largest vertical AF pocket <1 cm) the incidence of abnormal fetal heart tracings requiring cesarean section was 16.7%.[108] By comparison in postterm pregnancies with normal AFV the incidence of abnormal fetal heart tracings requiring cesarean section was only 1.05%.[108] Thus, the presence of oligohydramnios in postterm pregnancy is an ominous finding and points to the need to deliver the fetus. Similarly, the presence of oligohydramnios in a fetus whose EFW is below the 10th percentile is predictive of poor outcome and is an indication for strict surveillance and of the fetus to decide the most appropriate time for delivery.

Some investigators argue that there is no need to spend a long time waiting to evaluate all the components of the biophysical profile and that the results of both the NST and AFV suffice. The rationale: (1) a reactive NST implies that fetal motion is indeed present and indirectly tests for this important function of fetal motion; (2) an NST should always be part of the antenatal testing schema because it may show variable decelerations, a finding that may be missed completely if one relies only on the other four functions of the biophysical profile; and (3) oligohydramnios may be a significant indicator of chronic hypoxia, particularly in the IUGR or postdate fetus, and should always be considered. Because specific management protocols are not universally accepted, the sonographer should follow the guidelines established by the institution.

OTHER METHODS OF ASSESSMENT

Two additional methods of assessment have also been used for fetal evaluation with controversial results. These are *fetal acoustic stimulation (FAS) during an NST or a BPP* and *contraction stress test (CST)*.

FAS is accomplished using an artificial larynx (EAL Bell Telephone) to generate an acoustic-vibratory stimulus lasting 2 to 5 seconds to stimulate a fetus to respond.[110,124,128,129] The average sound energy produced at 1 m of air equals 82 dB.[62,86] The frequency of the emitted sound is 80 Hz, with harmonics ranging from 20 to 9000 Hz.[128]

The CST is only rarely used in modern obstetrics. It was one of the first forms of fetal surveillance and is the only modality that uses the principle of induced stress to reveal marginal placental insuffi-

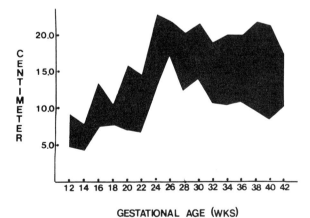

Figure 24-9. The black area of the graph depicts the mean values (± 2 SD variation) of the AFI, from the 12th to the 42nd weeks of pregnancy. Note that at 40 weeks' gestation an AFI of 8 falls at a critical 2 SD level below the mean. (Reprinted with permission from Phelan JP, Ahn MO, Smith CV, et al: Amniotic fluid index measurements during the pregnancy. Reprod Med 1987, 32:602.)

ciency. Several have reported that this test is poorly specific (only ~50%), it is time-consuming to perform, invasive, and expensive.

In the CST three uterine contractions are induced during a 10-minute interval, either by controlled intravenous pitocin drip or by nipple stimulation. A hypoxic or compromised fetus will not tolerate the low intervillous blood flow and oxygen level caused by the stress of the induced uterine contractions. As a result, fetal myocardial hypoxia is manifested as repetitive, uniform, and late heart rate decelerations (decelerations that occur at the end of a uterine contraction). The CST, like the NST, is much better at predicting the normal uncompromised fetus and its false-negative rate is low (30% to 60%).[39,60]

Protocol for Reporting Ultrasound Findings

The sonographer in possession of the background information discussed in this chapter is in a position to present the comprehensive data to the referring physician. The challenge is to present it in an effective and practical way. The referring physician would like to have specific information regarding the following areas:

1. The *optimal gestational age* and the method used to assign this age. An example of important comments would be as follows:
   a. Dates are established by concurrence between the early ultrasound (before 26 weeks' gestation) and the menstrual dates, or, menstrual dates are confirmed by known ovulation day.
   b. Dates are established by CRL.
2. The *estimated fetal weight* and the 2 SD variation of the formula used.
3. The *birth weight percentile,* as outlined in Table 24-3. For example, it should be stated that an EFW of 2120 g at 36 weeks' gestation falls below the 10th percentile rank. The sonographer should specify which table was used.
4. The *fetal growth pattern,* once the diagnosis of IUGR is suspected (by an EFW below the 10th percentile), other ultrasound data should be carefully examined and follow-up examinations are appropriate. The interval between these examinations should be agreed upon by the physician and the sonographer.

5. *Amniotic fluid volume.* The sonographer should enter one or more of the following diagnostic criteria for oligohydramnios:
   a. Diagnosis of oligohydramnios is based on the subjective evaluation of AFV.
   b. Diagnosis of oligohydramnios is based on the largest vertical pocket of AF at <2 to 3 cm (depending on the accepted threshold for oligohydramnios in the ultrasound department).
   c. Diagnosis of oligohydramnios is based on an amniotic fluid index <6.
6. *Placental grade.* A Grade 3 placenta may be associated with IUGR if it is noted before 36 weeks' gestation; this should be described.
7. *Biophysical profile score.* The biophysical profile score should be reported when requested. The results can be entered on one line, as in the following example: FBM = 0, FM = 2, FT = 2, AFV = 2, NST = 2; total score = 8.
8. *Doppler velocimetry.* Doppler assessment of the umbilical artery, MCA, and other vessels should be described in terms of the systolic/diastolic ratio, pulsatility index, or resistivity index (in accordance with your departmental policy) (see Chapter 20).

Treatment and Management

A variety of treatment regimens have been considered for IUGR. Maternal bedrest, nutrification, and prenatal treatment with 75 mg oral aspirin have been shown to improve the outcome of pregnancies with unexplained IUGR.[137]

One center has suggested that maternal hyperoxygenation should be considered as a treatment for poor growth.[2,98,101] Arduini and colleagues reported that no effect was observed on placental resistance indices, but cerebral arterial waveforms were altered by hyperoxygenation. This positive response is thought to be a good prognostic sign. Further, Molenidijk and coworkers showed that daily intravenous hypervolumic hemodilution (1500 ml), with hydroxyethylstarch and ringers solution is effective in positively altering fetal circulation, in otherwise compromised fetuses.[96] This is thought to enhance oxygenation of the fetus and it may be an easy and effective method to increase placental perfusion.

Several studies are currently underway to determine if low-dose aspirin (antiplatelet) therapy is useful in correcting the pathological increases in angiotensin II sensitivity that precede the clinical development of preeclampsia and IUGR.[45] Whether aspirin therapy will be useful in combating or preventing IUGR remains to be determined.[45]

Conclusions

The concern with any diagnostic test is that of encouraging inappropriate early or late deliveries. Failure to diagnose poor growth and associated IUGR bears considerable risk. Although the diagnosis of IUGR carries alarming concerns, the consequences

of the misdiagnosis can be similarly alarming (Fig. 24-10). Ringa and coworkers studied the rate preterm elective cesarean section in pregnancies thought to have an EFW <10%.[115] They reported in a series of almost 17,000 deliveries that 118 infants were falsely diagnosed as IUGR and 13% of these had a needless elective cesarean section. Their investigation illustrated the importance of supplemental tests to interrogate for fetal distress to avoid unnecessary interventions.[115]

When a fetus is identified to have poor interval growth, IUGR should be suspected and the fetus should be closely monitored for physiological compromise, and properly delivered at an appropriate time. A typical pattern of fetal deterioration in

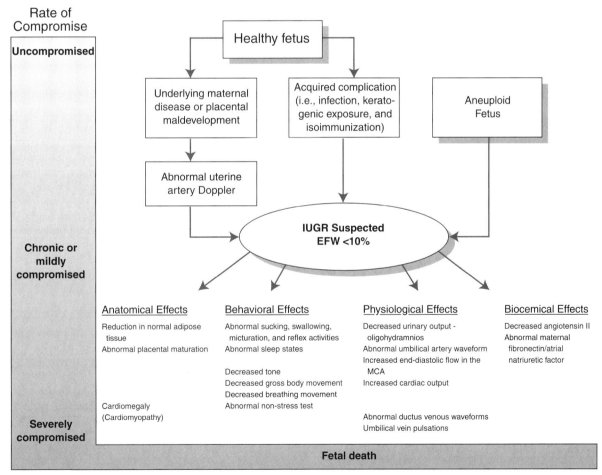

Figure 24-10. This algorithm shows the complexity of fetal deterioration. As the fetal condition evolves from health to death, many anatomic, behavioral, physiologic, and biochemical changes occur. The task of the prenatal diagnostician is to determine the risk and level of deterioration based on the sonographic variables.

IUGR is an early abnormal utD index (typical in women at risk for placental abnormality [i.e., elevated MSAFP] or pregnancy-induced hypertension), followed by abnormal fetal growth, abnormal umD and MCA Doppler values (or their ratio), abnormal UV pulsatility, and abnormal DV.

Any technique must be subjected to rigorous evaluation before its widespread acceptance. Several pharmacological agents are known to affect fetal cerebral blood flow. Diminished flow has been observed with agents such as ritodrine, magnesium, indomethacin, and nicotine.[32,52,92,93] Oxygen has been shown to positively affect cerebral circulation.[10] Administration of a 2% to 3% prepared gas mixture of carbon dioxide can cause a decrease in resistance in the fetal cerebral circulation.[17,111] While EFW, umD, and utD are now accepted and have been proven effective for routine clinical management, other Doppler applications are undergoing further evaluation. Because significant scientific advances are being achieved yearly, in the next decade clinicians should have a firm grasp on the physiologic processes underlying IUGR and preceding perinatal morbidity and mortality.

Postscript

The terms, intrauterine growth retardation (IUGR), intrauterine growth restriction, small-for-gestational-age (SGA), low birth weight, and intrauterine maladaptation, have all been used to describe the result of poor intrauterine fetal growth. The terminology concerning fetal size and growth is very confusing; no single term seems to define this entity adequately. The term IUGR bears the stigmata associated with "retardation." Many patients, after hearing that their fetus may be "growth retarded" panic because of the association with intellectual deficiency. While this may or may not be the case, it seems imprudent to suggest this during the prenatal period. As an alternative, the term intrauterine growth restriction was suggested (to minimize inherent concerns). Lastly, IUGR or "small for gestational age" is a neonatal diagnosis and cannot be definitively diagnosed prenatally. We can however identify infants at risk for IUGR in the prenatal period. Each of the aforementioned terms is inaccurate and fails to describe the process of deficient growth and fetal maladaptation that may result, so I suggest using the terms "poor fetal growth" and "fetal maladaptative sequence." The problem with traditional definitions using estimated fetal weight (EFW) alone is that they often do not account for the noncompromised infant who is constitutionally small, or the fetus of normal birth weight who is really physiologically compromised. It is important to emphasize that compromise may be acute or chronic, and when chronic, it may encompass poor fetal growth (exclusive of fetal aneuploidy and other genetic syndrome). The most widely accepted term to describe poor intrauterine growth is *intrauterine growth retardation*. For convention, we have used the term IUGR in this chapter.

REFERENCES

1. Akalin-sel T, Nicholaides KH, Peacock J, Campbell S. Doppler dynamics and their complex interrelation with fetal oxygen pressure, carbon dioxide pressure, and pH in growth-retarded fetuses. Obstet Gynecol. 1994; 84:439–444.

2. Alahuhta S, Rasanen J, Jouppila R, Jouppila P, Kangas-Saarela T, Hollman AI. Uteroplacental and fetal hemodynamics during extradural anaesthesia for caesarean section. Br J Anaesth. 1991; 66:319–323.

3. Alfirevic Z, Neilson JP. Doppler ultrasonography in high-risk pregnancies: Systematic review with meta-analysis. Am J Obstet Gynecol. 1995; 172:1379–1387.

4. Alfonso K, Portman E. Fetal weights and measurements as determined by postmortem examination and their correlation with ultrasound examination. Arch Pathol Lab Med. 1995; 119:179–180.

5. Amiel-Toson C, Petigrew AG. Adaptive changes in the developing brain during intrauterine stress. Brain Dev. 1991; 13:67–76.

6. Arabin B, Siebert M, Jimenez E, Saling E. Obstetrical characteristics of a loss in end-diastolic velocities in the fetal aorta and/or umbilical artery using Doppler ultrasound. Gynecol Obstet Invest. 1988; 25:173–180.

7. Arbeille P, Bose M, Valilant MC, Tranguant F. Nicotine-induced changes in the cerebral circulation in ovine fetuses. Am J Perinatol. 1992; 9:270–274.

8. Arbeille P, Roncin A, Berson M, et al. Exploration of the fetal cerebral blood flow by Doppler ultrasound in normal and pathological pregnancies. Ultrasound Med Biol. 1987; 13:329.

9. Arduini D, Rizzo G. Prediction of fetal outcome in small for gestational age fetuses: Comparison

of Doppler measurements obtained from different fetal vessels. J Perinat Med. 1992; 20:29–38.

10. Arduini D, Rizzo G, Romanini C, Mancuso S. Fetal haemodynamic response to acute maternal hyper-oxygenation as a predictor of fetal distress in intra-uterine growth retardation. Br J Med. 1989; 298:1561–1562.

11. Arduini D, Rizzo G, Romanini C, Mancuso S. Fetal blood flow velocity waveforms as predictors of growth retardation. Obstet Gynecol. 1987; 70:7–10.

12. Atkinson MW, Maher JE, Owen J, Hauth JC, Goldenberg RL, Copper RL. The predictive value of umbilical artery Doppler studies for preeclampsia or fetal growth retardation in a preeclampsia preventive trial. Obstet Gynecol. 1994; 83:609–612.

13. Balouet P, Hamel P, Domessent D, et al. The estimation of fetal weight by measurement of the adipose tissue of the extremities: Use in the diagnosis of hypotrophy. J Gynecol Obstet Biol Reprod. 1994; 23:64–68.

14. Barker DJP, Gluckman PD, Godrey KM, Harding JE, Owens JA, Robinson JS. Fetal nutrition and cardiovascular disease in adult life. Lancet. 1993; 341:938–941.

15. Battaglia FC, Lubchenco LO. A practical classification of newborn infants by weight and gestational age. J Pediatr. 1967; 71:159.

16. Behrman RE, Lees MH, Peterson EN, Mehannoy CW, Seeds AE. Distribution of the circulation in the normal and asphyxiated fetal primate. Am J Obstet Gynecol. 1970; 108:956.

17. Beille JC, Penry M. Effects of maternal administration of 3% carbon dioxide on umbilical and fetal renal and middle cerebral artery Doppler waveforms. Am J Obstet Gynecol. 1992; 167:1668–1671.

18. Benson CB, Doubilet PM. Head-sparing in fetuses with intrauterine growth retardation: Does it really occur? Radiology. 1986; 161:75.

19. Benson CB, Belville JS, Lentini JF, Saltzman DH, Doubilet PM. Intrauterine growth retardation: Diagnosis based on multiple parameters—prospective study. Radiology. 1990; 177:499–502.

20. Benson CB, Doubilet PM. Fetal measurements: Normal and abnormal growth. In: Rumack C, Charboneau W, Wilson S, eds. *Diagnostic Ultrasound*. St. Louis, Mosby-Year Book, 1992; pp 723–728.

21. Benson CB, Doubilet PM, Saltzman DH. Sonographic determination of fetal weights in diabetic pregnancies. Am J Obstet Gynecol. 1987; 156:441–444.

22. Berkowitz GS, Mehalek KE, Chitkara U, Rosen-berg J, Cogswell C, Berkowitz RL. Doppler umbilical velocimetry in the prediction of adverse outcome in pregnancies at risk for intrauterine growth retardation. Obstet Gynecol. 1988; 71:742–746.

23. Berman RE, Less MH, Peterson EN, DeLannoy CW. Distribution of the circulation in the normal and asphyxiated fetal primate. Am J Obstet Gynecol. 1970; 108:956–969.

24. Bilardo CM, Nicholaides KH, Campbell S. Doppler measurements of fetal and uteroplacental circulations: Relationship with umbilical venous blood gasses measured at cordocentesis. Am J Obstet Gynecol. 1990; 162:115–120.

25. Bilardo CM, Campbell S, Nicholaides KH. Mean blood velocities and flow impedance in the fetal descending thoracic aorta and common carotid artery in normal pregnancy. Early Hum Dev. 1988; 18:213–218.

26. Bottoms SF, Welch RA, Zador IE, et al. Limitations of using maximum vertical pocket and other sonographic evaluations of amniotic fluid volume to predict fetal growth: Technical or physiologic. Am J Obstet Gynecol. 1986; 155:154.

27. Bower S, Schuchter K, Campbell S. Doppler ultrasound screening as part of routine antenatal scanning: Prediction of pre-eclampsia and intrauterine growth retardation. Br J Obstet Gynaecol. 1993; 100:989–994.

28. Brar HS, Platt LD. Reverse end-diastolic flow velocity on umbilical artery velocimetry in high risk pregnancies: An ominous finding with adverse pregnancy outcome. Am J Obstet Gynecol. 1988; 159:559–561.

29. Bristow J, Rudolph AM, Itskovitz J, Barnes R. Hepatic oxygen and glucose metabolism in the fetal lamb. J Dev Physiol. 1983; 71:1047–1061.

30. Bromley B, Frigoletto FD, Harlow BL, Pauker S, Benacerraf B. The role of Doppler velocimetry in the structurally normal second-trimester fetus with elevated levels of maternal serum α-fetoprotein. Ultrasound Obstet Gynecol. 1994; 4:377–380.

31. Burke G, Stuart B, Crowley P, Scanaill SN, Drumm J. Is intrauterine growth retardation with normal umbilical artery blood flow a benign condition? Br J Med. 1990; 300:1044.

32. Cameron AS, Nicholson SF, Nimrod CA, Harder JR, Davies DM. Doppler waveforms in the fetal aorta and umbilical artery in patients with hypertension in pregnancy. Am J Obstet Gynecol. 1988; 158:339–345.

33. Campbell S, Thomas A. Ultrasound measurements of the fetal head to abdominal circumference ratio in the assessment of growth retardation. Br J Obstet Gynaecol. 1977; 84:165–174.

34. Campbell S, Diaz-Recasens J, Griffin DR, et al. New Doppler technique for assessing uteroplacental blood flow. Lancet. 1983; 1:675.

35. Campbell WA, Vintzileos AM, Neckkles E, et al. The use of the femur to estimate weight in premature infants: Preliminary results. J Ultrasound Med. 1985; 151:333–337.

36. Chang TC, Ronson SC, Spencer JAD, Gallivan S. Identification of fetal growth retardation: Comparison of Doppler waveform indices and serial ultrasound measurements of abdominal circumference and fetal weight. Obstet Gynecol. 1993; 82:230–236.

37. Chard T, Toong A, Macintosh M. The myth of growth retardation at term. Br J Obstet Gynecol. 1993; 100:1076–1081.

38. Chen ATL, Chan YK, Falek A. The effects of chromosomal abnormalities on birth weight in man. Hum Hered. 1972; 22:209–224.

39. Collea JV, Holls WM. The contraction stress test. Clin Obstet Gynecol. 1982; 4:707.

40. Colorado Department of Health, Health Statistics Section, WWW site. http://hsvrd@state.co.us

41. Crane JP, Kopta MM. Prediction of intrauterine growth retardation via ultrasonically measured head/abdominal circumference ratios. Obstet Gynecol. 1979; 54:597–601.

42. Crowley P, O'Herlihy C, Boylan P. The value of ultrasound measurement of amniotic fluid volume in the management of prolonged pregnancies. Br J Obstet Gynaecol. 1984; 91:444.

43. de. Mari S, Moise KJ, Deter RL, Carpenter RJ. Fetal heart rate influence in the pulsatility index in the middle cerebral artery. J Clin Ultrasound. 1991; 19:149–153.

44. Degani S, Paltieli Y, Gonen R, Sharf M. Fetal internal carotid artery pulsed Doppler flow velocity waveforms and maternal plasma glucose levels. Obstet Gynecol. 1991; 77:379.

45. Dekker GA, Sibai BM. Low-dose aspirin in the prevention of preeclampsia and fetal growth retardation: Rationale, mechanisms, and clinical trials. Am J Obstet Gynecol. 1993; 168:214–227.

46. Deter RL. Evaluation of intrauterine growth retardation in the fetus and neonate: Are simple-minded methods good enough? Ultrasound Obstet Gynecol. 1995; 6:161–163.

47. Doubilet PM, Benson CB. Sonographic evaluation of intrauterine growth retardation. Am J Roentgenol. 1995; 164:709–717.

48. Downing GJ, Yarlagadda AP, Maulik D. Comparison of pulsatility index and input impedance parameters in a model of altered hemodynamics. J Ultrasound Med. 1991; 155:317–321.

49. Edelstone DI, Rudolph AM, Heymann MA. Liver and ductus venosus blood flows in fetal lambs *in utero.* Circ Res. 1978; 42:426–433.

50. Edelstone DI, Rudolph AM, Heymann MA. Effect of hypoxia and decreasing umbilical flow on liver and ductus venosus blood flows in fetal lambs. Am J Physiol. 1980; 238:H656–H663.

51. Edelstone DI, Rudolph AM. Preferential streaming of the ductus venosus blood flow to the brain and heart in fetal lambs. Am J Physiol. 1979; 237:H724–H729.

52. Facchinetti F, Battaglia C, Benatti R, Borella P, Genazzani AR. Oral magnesium supplementation improves fetal circulation. Magnesium Res. 1992; 5:179–181.

53. Fairlie FM, Moretti M, Walker JJ, Sibai BM. Umbilical artery and uteroplacental velocimetry in pregnancies complicated by idiopathic low birth weight centile. Am J Perinatol. 1992; 9:250–253.

54. Fancourt R, Campbell S, Harvey D, Norman AP. Follow-up study of small-for-dates babies. Br Med J. 1976; 1:1435–1437.

55. Ferrero A, Maggi E, Giancotti A, Torcia F, Pachi A. Regression formula for estimation of fetal weight with use of abdominal circumference and femur length: A prospective study. J Ultrasound Med. 1994; 13:823–833.

56. Field NT, Piper JM, Langer O. The effect of maternal obesity on the accuracy of fetal weight estimation. Obstet Gynecol. 1995; 86:102–107.

57. Finberg HJ, Kurtz AB, Johnson RL, Wapner RJ. The biophysical profile: A literature review and reassessment of its usefulness in the evaluation of fetal well-being. J Ultrasound Med. 1990; 9:583–591.

58. Fitzhardinge PM, Steven EM. The small-for-dates infant II: Neurological and intellectual sequelae. Pediatrics. 1972; 50:50.

59. Fleischer A, Schulman H, Farmakides G, et al. Uterine artery Doppler velocity in pregnant women with hypertension. Am J Obstet Gynecol. 1986; 154:806.

60. Freeman RE, Anderson G, Dorcester W. A prospective multi-institutional study of antepartum fetal heart rate monitoring: I. Risk of perinatal mortality and morbidity according to antepartum fetal heart rate test results. Am J Obstet Gynecol. 1982; 143:771.

61. Gaziano EP. Antenatal ultrasound and fetal Doppler: Diagnosis and outcome in intrauterine growth retardation. Clin Perinatol. 1995; 22:111–140.

62. Goodlin RC. Possible deleterious effects of sound or vibratory fetal stimuli (letter to the editors). Am J Obstet Gynecol. 1988; 159:1016.

63. Grammelini D, Folli MC, Raboni S, Vadora E, Me-

rialdi A. Cerebral umbilical Doppler ratio as a predictor of adverse fetal outcome. Obstet Gynecol. 1992; 79:416–420.

64. Gruenwald P. Infants of low birth weight among 5000 deliveries. Pediatrics. 1964; 34:157.

65. Hackett GA, Campbell S, Gamsu H, et al. Doppler studies in the growth retarded fetus and prediction of neonatal necrotizing enterocolitis, hemorrhage, and neonatal morbidity. Br Med J. 1987; 294:13.

66. Hadlock FP, Deter RL, Harrist RB, Roecker E, Park SK. A date-independent predictor of intrauterine growth retardation: Femur length/abdominal circumference ratio. Am J Roentgenol. 1983; 141:979–984.

67. Hadlock FP, Harrist RB, Sharman RS, et al. Estimation of fetal weight with the use of head, body, and femur measurements: A prospective study. Am J Obstet Gynecol. 1985; 151:333–337.

68. Hadlock FP, Harrist RB, Carpenter RJ. Sonographic estimation of fetal weight: The value of femur length in addition to head and abdomen measurements. Radiology. 1984; 150:535–540.

69. Harrington K, Carpenter RG, Nguren M, Campbell S. Changes observed in Doppler studies of the fetal circulation in pregnancies complicated by preeclampsia or the delivery of a small-for-gestational-age baby: I. Cross sectional analysis. Ultrasound Obstet Gynecol. 1995; 6:19–28.

70. Hecher K, Spernol R, Stettner H, Szalay S. Potential for diagnosing imminent risk to appropriate and small-for-gestational-age fetuses by Doppler sonographic examination of umbilical and cerebral blood flow. Ultrasound Obstet Gynecol. 1992; 2:266–271.

71. Hecker K, Campbell S, Doyle P, Harrington K, Nicholaides K. Assessment of fetal compromise by Doppler ultrasound investigation of the fetal circulation: Arterial, intracardiac, and venous blood flow velocity studies. Circulation. 1995; 91:129–138.

72. Hill LM, Breckle R, Gehrking WC, et al. Use of femur length in the estimation of fetal weight. Am J Obstet Gynecol. 1985; 152:847–852.

73. Hinchcliffe SA, Lynch MRJ, Sargent PH, Howard CV, van Velzen D. The effect of intrauterine growth retardation on the development of renal nephrons. Br J Obstet Gynaecol. 1992; 99:296–301.

74. Hollard P. Placental insufficiency and its effect on the fetus and adult disease. Lancet. 1993; 341:827–828.

75. Hutchinson DL, Gray MJ, Plentl AA, et al. The role of the fetus in the water exchange of the amniotic fluid in normal and hydramniotic patients. J Clin Invest. 1959; 38:971.

76. Iwata M, Matsuzaki N, Shimizu I, Mitsuda A, Nakayama M, Suehara N. Prenatal detection of ischemic changes in the placenta of the growth-retarded fetus by Doppler flow velocimetry of the maternal uterine artery. Obstet Gynecol. 1993; 82:494–499.

77. Jackson MR, Walsh AJ, Morrow RJ, Mullen JBM, Lye SJ, Ritchie JWK. Reduced placental villous tree elaboration in small-for-gestational-age pregnancies: Relationship with umbilical artery Doppler waveforms. Am J Obstet Gynecol. 1995; 172:518–525.

78. Jouppila P, Kirkinen P. Noninvasive assessment of fetal aortic blood flow in normal and abnormal pregnancies. Clin Obstet Gynecol. 1989; 32:703–709.

79. Karsdorp VH, van Vugt, van Geijn HP, et al. Clinical significance of absent or reversed end-diastolic velocity waveforms in the umbilical artery. Lancet. 1994; 8938:1664–1668.

80. Kazzi GM, Gross TL, Sokol RJ, Kazzi NJ. Detection of intrauterine growth retardation: A new use of sonographic placental grading. Am J Obstet Gynecol. 1983; 145:733–737.

81. Khoury MJ, Erickson JD, Cordero JF, McCarthy BJ. Congenital malformations and intrauterine growth retardation: A population study. Pediatrics. 1988; 82:83–90.

82. Kiserud T, Eik-Nes SH, Blaas HG, Hellevik LR, Simensen B. Ductus venosus blood velocity and the umbilical circulation in the seriously growth-retarded fetus. Ultrasound Obstet Gynecol. 1994; 4:109–114.

83. Kiserud T, Eik-Nes SH, Blaas HG, Hellevik LR. Foramen ovale. An ultrasonographic study of its relation to the inferior vena cava, ductus venosus, and hepatic veins. Ultrasound Obstet Gynecol. 1992; 2:389–396.

84. Kurtz AB, Goldberg BB. Combined fetal head and body measurements. In: Kurtz AB, Goldberg BB, (eds): Obstetrical Measurements in Ultrasound: A Reference Manual. Chicago: Year Book Medical Publishers, 1988; p 147.

85. Laurini R, Laurin J, Marsal K. Placental histology and fetal blood flow in intrauterine growth retardation. Acta Obstet Gynecol Scand. 1994; 73:529–534.

86. Lavery PJ. Nonstress fetal heart rate testing. Clin Obstet Gynecol. 1982; 25:689.

87. Lewitt EM, Monheit AC. Expenditures on health care for children and women. Future of Children. 1992; 2:95–114.

88. Lockwood CJ, Weiner S. Assessment of fetal growth. Clin Perinatol. 1986; 13:3–35.

89. Long SH, Marquis MS, Harrison GR. The cost and financing of perinatal care in the United States. Am J Public Health. 1994; 84:1473–1478.

90. Manning FA, Morrison I, Lange MB, et al. Fetal assessment based on fetal biophysical profile scoring: Experience in 12,620 referred high-risk pregnancies. Perinatal mortality by frequency and etiology. Am J Obstet Gynecol. 1985; 151:343–350.

91. Manning FA, Hill LM, Platt LD. Quantitative amniotic fluid volume determination by ultrasound antepartum detection of intrauterine growth retardation. Am J Obstet Gynecol. 1981; 139:254–258.

92. Mari G, Moise K, Deter RL, et al. Doppler assessment of the pulsatility index of the middle cerebral artery during constriction of the ductus arteriosus after indomethacin therapy. Am J Obstet Gynecol. 1989; 161:1528–1531.

93. Mari G, Kirschon B, Moise K, Lee W, Cotten DB. Doppler assessment of the fetal and uteroplacental circulation during nifedipine therapy for preterm labor. Am J Obstet Gynecol. 1989; 161:1514–1518.

94. Mari G, Deter R. Middle cerebral artery flow velocity waveforms in normal and small for gestational age fetuses. Am J Obstet Gynecol. 1992; 166:1262–1270.

95. Meyer WJ, Font GE, Gauthier DW, Myles TD, Bieniarz A, Rodriguez A. Effect of amniotic fluid volume on ultrasonic fetal weight estimation. J Ultrasound Med. 1995; 14:193–197.

96. Molendijk L, Malburg I, Kopecky P. Doppler ultrasound studies in placental insufficiency as an indication of the effectiveness of hemodilution therapy. Z Geburtshife Perinatol. 1995; 199:18–22.

97. Nazarian LN, Halpern EJ, Kurtz AB, Hauck WW, Needleman L. Normal interval fetal growth rates based on obstetrical ultrasonographic measurements. J Ultrasound Med. 1995; 14:829–836.

98. Nicolaides KH, Campbell S, Bradley KJ, Bilardo CM, Soothill PW, Gibb D. Maternal oxygen therapy for intrauterine growth retardation. Lancet. 1987; 1:942–945.

99. Noordam MJ, Heydanus R, Hop WCJ, Hoekstra FME, Wladimiroff JW. Doppler colour flow imaging of the fetal intracerebral arteries and umbilical artery in the small-for-gestational-age fetus. Br J Obstet Gynaecol. 1994; 101:504–508.

100. North RA, Ferrier C, Long D, Townend K, Kincaid-Smith P. Uterine artery Doppler flow velocity waveforms in the second trimester for the prediction of preeclampsia and fetal growth retardation. Obstet Gynecol. 1994; 83:378–386.

101. Olofsson P, Laurini RN, Marsál K. A high uterine artery pulsatility index reflects a defective development of placental bed spiral arteries in pregnancies complicated by hypertension and fetal growth retardation. Eur J Obstet Gynecol Reprod Biol. 1993; 49:161–168.

102. Oslen SF. Further on the association between retarded foetal growth and adult cardiovascular disease: Could low intake or marine diets be a common cause? J Clin Epidemiol. 1994; 47:565–569.

103. Park YW, Cho JS, Kim HS, Kim JS, Song CH. The clinical implications of early diastolic notch in third trimester Doppler waveform analysis of the uterine artery. J Ultrasound Med. 1996; 15:47–51.

104. Paton JB, Fisher DE, Dehannoy CW, Behrman RE. Umbilical blood flow, cardiac output, and organ flow in immature baboon. Am J Obstet Gynecol. 1973; 117:560–569.

105. Paulick RP, Meyers RL, Rudolph CD, Rudolph MA. Venous responses to hypoxemia in the fetal lamb. J Dev Physiol. 1990; 15:81–88.

106. Peters LLH, Sheldon RE, Makowski EL, Neschin G. Blood flow to fetal organs as a function of arterial oxygen content. Am J Obstet Gynecol. 1979; 135:637–646.

107. Phelan JP, Ahn MO, Smith CV, et al. Amniotic fluid index measurements during pregnancy. J Reprod Med. 1987; 32:601.

108. Phelan JP, Platt LD, Yeh SY, et al. The role of ultrasound assessment of amniotic fluid volume in the management of the postdate pregnancy. Am J Obstet Gynecol. 1985; 151:304–308.

109. Philipson EH, Sokol RJ, Williams T. Oligohydramnios: Clinical associations and predictive value for intrauterine growth retardation. Am Obstet Gynecol. 1983; 146:271.

110. Polzin GB, Blakemore KJ, Petrie RH, Amon E. Fetal vibro-acoustic stimulation: Magnitude and duration of fetal heart rate accelerations as a marker of fetal health. Obstet Gynecol. 1988; 72:621–626.

111. Potts P, Connors G, Gillis S, Hunse C, Richardson B. The effects of carbon dioxide on Doppler flow velocity waveforms in human fetus. J Dev Physiol. 1992; 17:119–123.

112. Read JA, Miller FC. Fetal heart rate acceleration in response to acoustic stimulation as a measure of fetal well-being. Am J Obstet Gynecol. 1977; 129:512–519.

113. Reese EA, Homko CJ, Wiznitzer A. Doppler velocimetry and the assessment of fetal well-being in normal and diabetic pregnancies. Ultrasound Obstet Gynecol. 1994; 4:508–514.

114. Reisman IE. Chromosomal abnormalities and intrauterine growth retardation. Pediatr Clin North Am. 1970; 17:101–110.

115. Ringa V, Carrat F, Blondel B, Breast G. Consequences of misdiagnosis of intrauterine growth retardation for preterm elective cesarean section. Fetal Diagn Ther. 1993; 8:325–330.

116. Rizzo G, Pietropolli A, Capponi A, Cacciatore C, Arduini D, Romanini C. Evaluation of pulsatility index nomograms based on fetal biometry in small for gestational age fetuses. J Ultrasound Med. 1994; 13:267–274.

117. Roberts AV, Lee AJ, James AG. Ultrasonographic estimation of fetal weight: A new predictive model incorporating the femur length for the low-birth-weight fetus. J Clin Ultrasound. 1985; 13:555–559.

118. Rosenberg K, Grant J, Hepburn M. Antenatal detection of growth retardation: Actual practice in a large maternity hospital. Br J Obstet Gynaecol. 1982; 89:12.

119. Rudolph AM, Haemin MA. Circulatory changes during growth in the fetal lamb. Circ Res. 1970; 26:289–299.

120. Rutherford SE, Phelan JP, Smith CV, et al. The four-quadrant assessment of amniotic fluid volume: An adjunct to antepartum fetal heart rate testing. Obstet Gynecol. 1987; 70:353.

121. Sabbagha RE, Minogue J, Tamura RK, et al. Estimation of birth weight by the use of ultrasound formulas targeted to large, appropriate, and small-for-gestational age fetuses. Am J Obstet Gynecol. 1989; 160:854.

122. Scherjon SA, Smolders-Dehaas H, Kok J, Zondervan HA. The "brain-sparing" effect: Antenatal cerebral Doppler findings in relation to neurologic outcome in very preterm infants. Am J Obstet Gynecol. 1993; 169:169–175.

123. Seeds JW. Impaired fetal growth: Definition and clinical diagnosis. Obstet Gynecol. 1984; 64:303–310.

124. Serfini P, Lindsay MBJ, Nagay DA, Pupkin MJ, Tseng P, Crenshaw C. Antepartum fetal heart rate response to sound stimulation: The acoustic stimulation test. Am J Obstet Gynecol. 1984; 148:41–45.

125. Shepard MJ, Richards VA, Berkowitz RL, et al. An evaluation of two equations for predicting fetal weight by ultrasound. Am J Obstet Gynecol. 1982; 142:47.

126. Shulman H. The clinical implications of Doppler ultrasound examination of the uterine and umbilical arteries. Am J Obstet Gynecol. 1987; 136:889.

127. Simon NC, Surosky BA, Shearer DM, Levisky JS. Effect of the pretest probability of intrauterine growth retardation on the predictiveness of sonographic estimated fetal weight in detecting IUGR: A clinical application of Bayes' theorem. J Clin Ultrasound. 1990; 18:145–153.

128. Smith CV, Phelan JP, Paul RH, et al. Fetal acoustic stimulation testing: A retrospective experience with the fetal acoustic stimulation test. Am J Obstet Gynecol. 1985; 153:567.

129. Smith CV. Vibroacoustic stimulation. Clin Obstet Gynecol. 1995; 38:68–77.

130. Snijders RJM, Sherrod C, Gosden CM, Nicholaides KH. Fetal growth retardation: Associated malformations and chromosomal abnormalities. Am J Obstet Gynecol. 1993; 168:547–555.

131. Soothill PW, Nicholaides KH, Bilardo CN, Campbell S. Relation of fetal hypoxia growth retardation to mean blood velocity in the fetal aorta. Lancet. 1986; 2:118.

132. Stratton JF, Scanaill SN, Staurt B, Turner MJ. Are babies of normal birth weight who fail to reach their growth potential as diagnosed by ultrasound at increased risk? Ultrasound Obstet Gynecol. 1995; 5:114–118.

133. Tejani N, Mann LI, Weiss RR. Antenatal diagnosis and management of the small-for-gestational age fetus. Obstet Gynecol. 1976; 47:31.

134. Tejanis NA. Recurrence of intrauterine growth retardation. Obstet Gynecol. 1982; 59:329–331.

135. Todros T, Ferrazzi E, Arudini D, Bastonero S. Performance of Doppler ultrasonography as a screening test in low risk pregnancies: Result of a multicentric study. J Ultrasound Med. 1995; 14:343–348.

136. Trudinger BJ, Giles WB, Cook CM. Uteroplacental blood flow velocity-time waveforms in normal and complicated pregnancy. Br J Obstet Gynaecol. 1985; 151:502.

136a. Trudinger BJ, Cook CM, Giles WB, Fong E, Connelly A, Wilcox W. Fetal umbilical artery velocity waveforms and subsequent neonatal outcome. Br J Obstet Gynaecol. 1991; 98:378.

137. Uzan S, Beaufils M, Breast G, Bazin B, Capitant C, Paris J. Prevention of fetal growth retardation with low-dose aspirin: Findings of EPREDA trial. Lancet. 1991; 337:1427–1431.

138. van den Elzen HJ, Cohen-Overbeek TE, Grobbee DE, Quartero RWP, Wladimiroff JW. Early uterine artery Doppler velocimetry and outcome of pregnancy in women aged 35 years and older. Ultrasound Obstet Gynecol. 1995; 5:328–333.

139. Van den Wijngaard JAGW, Greenberg IAL, Wladimiroff JW, Hop WCJ. Cerebral Doppler ultrasound in the human fetus. Br J Obstet Gynaecol. 1989; 96:845–849.

140. VanEyck J, Wladimiroff JW, Van der Wijngaard JA, Noordam MJ, Prechtl HF. The blood flow velocity

waveform in the fetal internal carotid and umbilical artery: Its relation to fetal behavior in normal pregnancy at 37–38 weeks. Br J Obstet Gynaecol. 1987; 94:736.

141. Veille JC, Hanson R, Sivakoff M, Hoen H, Ben-Ami M. Fetal cardiac size in normal, intrauterine growth retarded, and diabetic pregnancies. Am J Perinatol. 1993; 10:275–279.

142. Veille JC, Hanson RA, Tatum K, Kelley K. Quantitative assessment of human fetal renal blood flow. Am J Obstet Gynecol. 1993; 169:1399–1402.

143. Vintzileos AM, Campbell WA, Rodis JF, et al. Fetal weight estimation formulas for head, abdomen, femur, and thigh circumference measurements. Am J Obstet Gynecol. 1987; 157:410–414.

144. Vintzileos AM, Campbell WA, Ingardia CJ, et al. The fetal biophysical profile and its predictive value. Obstet Gynecol. 1983; 62:271.

145. Vyas S, Nicolaides KH, Bower S, Campbell S. Middle cerebral artery waveforms in fetal hypoxemia. Br J Obstet Gynaecol. 1990; 97:797–803.

146. Warsof SL, Wolf P, Coulehan J, et al. Comparison of the fetal weight estimation formulas with and without head measurements. Obstet Gynecol. 1986; 67:569–573.

147. Whittle MJ, Hanretty KP, Primrose MH, Neilson JP. Screening for the compromised fetus: A randomized trial of umbilical artery velocimetry in unselected pregnancies. Am J Obstet Gynecol. 1994; 170:555–559.

148. Wladimiroff JW. A review of the etiology, diagnostic techniques, and management of IUGR, and clinical application of Doppler in the assessment of placental blood flow. J Perinatol Med. 1991; 19:11–13.

149. Wladimiroff JW, Tonge HM, Stewart PA. Doppler ultrasound assessment of cerebral blood flow in the human fetus. Br J Obstet Gyn. 1986; 93:471–475.

150. Wladimiroff JW, Wijngeerd JAGW, Delgani S, Noordam MJ, Van Eyck J, Tange HM. Cerebral and umbilical arterial blood flow velocity waveforms in normal and growth-retarded pregnancies. Obstet Gynecol. 1991; 31:705–709.

151. Woo JSK, Wan MCW. An evaluation of fetal weight prediction using a simple equation containing the fetal femur length. J Ultrasound Med. 1986; 5:453–457.

152. Yoon BH, Lee CM, Kim SW. An umbilical artery waveform: A strong and independent predictor of adverse pregnancy outcome in patients with preeclampsia. Am J Obstet Gynecol. 1994; 171:13–21.

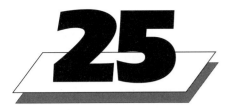

Gestational Trophoblastic Disease

MARIE DeLANGE, PHIL-ANN TAN-SINN, and GERALD L. GRUBE

Gestational trophoblastic diseases are rare but important conditions that constitute a range of benign and malignant processes, including hydatidiform mole, invasive mole, and choriocarcinoma. Sonography plays a crucial role in diagnosing hydatidiform mole, in evaluating its progression to invasive mole or choriocarcinoma, and in monitoring the efficacy of treatment. By correlating the sonographic findings with clinical and laboratory findings, obstetric and gynecologic conditions with similar sonographic appearances can be distinguished from gestational trophoblastic disease.

Gestational trophoblastic diseases are related to abnormalities of the trophoblast. The trophoblast, from which the chorion and amnion are derived, provides the attachment to the uterine wall, invading the wall and its vessels to supply nutrition to the embryo.[9] Gestational trophoblastic disease results from a combination of male and female gametes. Nongestational trophoblastic disease does not involve a gestational event and includes testicular and ovarian choriocarcinoma.[8]

Hydatidiform Mole

Hydatidiform mole is the most common neoplasm that arises from the trophoblast. Complete hydatidiform moles are masses that arise from fertilization of a defective ovum by a single sperm that duplicates, yielding a homozygous mole of 46,XX karyotype, or from fertilization of one ovum by two sperm, resulting in a heterozygous mole with a 46,XX or 46,XY karyotype.[11] A defective ovum fertilized by a single sperm with a Y sex chromosome would not be viable without some X-linked genetic material.[9]

Histologically, complete hydatidiform moles are characterized by hydropic degeneration and swelling of the chorionic villus stroma, absence of blood vessels in the swollen villi, proliferation of the trophoblastic epithelium in varying degrees, and absence of fetus and amnion (Fig. 25-1).[20]

A partial (incomplete) hydatidiform mole results from a normal egg with a 23,X haploid chro-

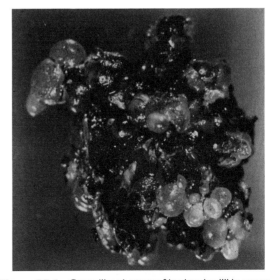

Figure 25-1. Grapelike clusters of hydropic villi in a specimen from a complete hydatidiform mole.

507

mosome set being fertilized by two sperm carrying either sex chromosome, giving a karyotype of 69,XXY, 69,XXX, or 69,XYY. A triploid karyotype of XXY can also result from fertilization of a normal egg by a sperm with a 46,XY diploid set.[11] A partial mole has focal and less advanced hydatidiform changes with slowly progressing swelling of some avascular villi, whereas vascular villi are spared. The hyperplasia of the trophoblast is focal rather than generalized.[20] There may be a coexistent fetus, fetal parts, or an amniotic sac. Approximately 5% of all hydatidiform moles are incomplete or partial.

Both complete and partial hydatidiform moles are regarded clinically as benign trophoblastic disease, although the complete moles, especially the rare heterozygous type, have a definite malignant potential. Partial moles have very little malignant potential.[9] A complete heterozygous mole is 1000 times more likely to develop into a choriocarcinoma than a complete homozygous mole.[6]

Ovarian theca lutein cysts are found in 20% to 35% of patients with hydatidiform mole and are caused by overstimulation of ovarian lutein elements by large amounts of human chorionic gonadotropin (hCG) secreted by the proliferating trophoblast.[20] They are bilateral, contain multiple cysts and septa, and are largest when hCG production is greatest (at 12 to 24 weeks' gestation; Fig. 25-2). Theca lutein cysts may twist and hemorrhage, causing areas of solid echogenicity seen within the cysts that correspond to contained areas of thrombus.

Sonography's role is to assess and determine whether there has been regression of the cysts after uterine evacuation of the molar pregnancy. Theca lutein cysts may persist for as long as 2 to 4 months after evacuation. This may cause confusion during serial follow-up studies for possible recurrence of a molar pregnancy.

INCIDENCE

Hydatidiform moles occur in 1 of every 1000 to 2000 pregnancies in the United States and Europe.[2,20] The highest national incidences occur in the Far Eastern countries, especially Taiwan, Japan, and Indonesia. The incidence in these countries is 10 times greater than that in the United States. An epidemiologic study of Asian women in the United States, however, did not find them to be at signifi-

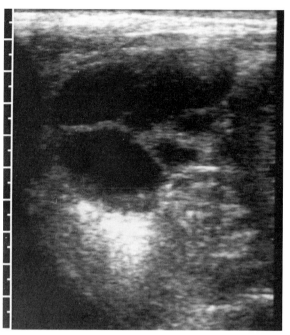

Figure 25-2. Transverse view of an enlarged ovary with theca lutein cysts.

cantly greater risk for molar pregnancy than women of other races living in the United States.[2] In Mexico, the prevalence is twice that of the United States.[9,20]

Women 46 years of age or older and 14 years of age or younger are at higher risk for a molar pregnancy.[2,11] Women between 20 and 29 years of age are at lowest risk. Although ovarian hydatidiform moles are rare, they have been reported; the estimated incidence is 1 in 50–80 million gestations.[21] Risk of recurrence of hydatidiform mole increases by 2% to 3% with each subsequent pregnancy.[2,9]

SYMPTOMS AND COMPLICATIONS

A woman who is considered to be pregnant may experience vaginal bleeding, which may follow a missed period. Spotting or bleeding of a brownish discharge has been described in 97% of women with a molar pregnancy. Some pass grapelike clusters of maternal blood and molar tissue.[9] Other common clinical symptoms are discrepant uterine height, hyperemesis, and preeclampsia.

On physical examination, the uterus in most cases is noted to be large for gestational age, which may be a result of rapid proliferation of the trophoblastic tissue; however, the uterine size also may be consistent with or small for the gestational age.[9]

Hyperemesis and preeclampsia occur in approximately 25% of cases and are thought to be caused by the increased levels of β-hCG in the bloodstream. Projectile vomiting and nausea are some of the clinical findings with hyperemesis gravidarum. With eclampsia or preeclampsia, varying degrees of proteinuria and hypertension are present. Preeclampsia occurs more frequently in cases of complete than partial molar pregnancies.[11]

With a nonmolar gestation, pregnancy-induced hypertension usually occurs after the 24th week of pregnancy. A molar pregnancy must, therefore, be considered when hypertension and elevated β-hCG are present before the 24th gestational week.

The following complications may develop as a result of a molar pregnancy:

1. Hemorrhage from an existing mole or local invasion
2. Anemia due to maternal blood loss
3. Rupture or hemorrhage of theca lutein cysts
4. Pulmonary embolization or pulmonary edema due to the migration of trophoblastic tissue through the uterine veins
5. Hyperthyroidism associated with 2% to 10% of cases due to elevated β-hCG levels, which stimulate thyroxine production
6. Progression to invasive mole or choriocarcinoma

LABORATORY FINDINGS

Hydatidiform moles usually show elevated serum β-hCG levels (>100,000 mIU/ml). This is especially significant if the levels are persistently high or continue to rise beyond 100 days after the last menstrual period, when normally there is a decline in the hCG level.[20]

Ultrasound-guided chorionic villus sampling has been performed with coexistent molar and normal gestations in separate sacs to determine the karyotype of the molar pregnancy because a triploid karyotype would have a low malignant potential and the pregnancy might be allowed to continue.[10]

SONOGRAPHIC APPEARANCE

Reported cases of first trimester molar pregnancy document that a variable appearance is possible. Some first trimester moles may have an appearance that simulates a blighted ovum, missed abortion, degenerating leiomyoma, or hydropic placenta (Fig. 25-3, Table 25-1). Others may demonstrate a small, echogenic mass filling the entire uterine cavity.[19] In any of these situations, careful clinical correlation is important in differentiating these possible causes (Table 25-2).

The more advanced hydatidiform mole, which contains numerous hydropic villi, can be well visualized by sonography. Owing to the hydropic villi, uterine enlargement greater than is appropriate for dates may be present. The hydatidiform mole appears as a large, soft tissue mass containing cystic spaces of varying sizes (Fig. 25-4). This appearance has previously been referred to as a "snowflake" or "lacy" pattern. No fetal parts are seen. When the tumor volume is small, the myometrium may be perceived as less echogenic soft tissue surrounding the echogenic mass that fills the uterus. These classic sonographic findings are specific only for a second trimester hydatidiform mole.[12] The identification of fetal parts within or adjacent to the molar tissue helps to classify an incomplete mole (Fig. 25-5). With a significant rise in the β-hCG level, bilateral, multicystic, multiseptated ovarian theca lutein cysts may be identified in the adnexa.

Invasive Mole (Chorioadenoma Destruens)

The invasive mole (chorioadenoma destruens) is classified clinically as malignant, nonmetastatic trophoblastic disease. These all result from malignant

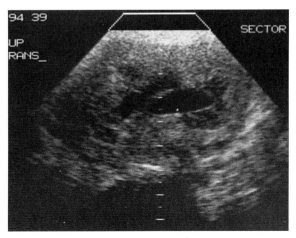

Figure 25-3. Missed abortion with an irregular gestational sac and placental degeneration. A molar pregnancy may have a similar appearance.

TABLE 25-1. SONOGRAPHIC APPEARANCE OF GESTATIONAL TROPHOBLASTIC DISEASE

Trophoblastic Process	Sonographic Appearance
Hydatidiform mole (first trimester)	May have appearance of a blighted ovum, threatened abortion, or variable echogenicity filling the entire uterus without the characteristic vesicular appearance[2]
Hydatidiform mole (after first trimester)	Large soft tissue mass of low- to moderate-amplitude echoes filling the uterine cavity and containing fluid-filled spaces
Incomplete or partial mole	May present as a gestational sac that is relatively large and intact surrounded by a thick rim of placenta-like echoes with well-defined sonolucent spaces within. It may be empty or contain a disproportionately small viable or nonviable fetus. Echogenic fetal parts may be visualized with or without normal placenta.[23]
Coexisting mole and fetus	Concurrent presence of normal-appearing placenta and fetus and a separate area of cystic vesicular appearance
Invasive mole	Enlarged uterus with foci of increased echogenicity and cystic spaces in the myometrium
Choriocarcinoma	Cystic to solid areas of necrosis, coagulated blood, or tumor tissue invading and extending as a mass outside the uterine wall with metastatic lesions located in the liver

progression of hydatidiform moles; approximately 15% to 18% manifest these changes. Histologically, the invasive mole is distinguished by excessive trophoblastic overgrowth and penetration by the trophoblastic elements, including whole villi, into the depths of the myometrium, sometimes penetrating through the uterine wall and involving the peritoneum, adjacent parametrium, or vaginal vault. Such moles show local invasion but not widespread metastasis.[20] The diagnosis of invasive mole is made primarily from the myometrial tissue if hysterectomy is performed.

Invasive trophoblastic disease is recognized sonographically by the presence of hemorrhagic necrosis within the myometrium, which appears as irregular anechoic and echogenic areas in the homogeneously hypoechoic myometrium secondary to extension of the intrauterine soft tissue mass or hydatidiform mole (Fig. 25-6). Placental site tumors are an extremely rare and aggressive solid or serpiginous cystic mass seen within the myometrium, and may be considered as a differential diagnosis along with invasive trophoblastic diseases.[1,12] The hCG levels for these tumors, however, would be much lower than in the trophoblastic disease. Sonography should not be considered a screening procedure for invasive trophoblastic disease because in some cases no recognizable textural abnormalities of the uterus can be demonstrated.[8]

Choriocarcinoma

Choriocarcinoma is classified clinically as malignant, metastatic gestational trophoblastic disease. Microscopically, choriocarcinoma is characterized by sheets of highly malignant trophoblast of both cytotrophoblast and syncytiotrophoblast elements, with no villous structures. Choriocarcinoma, the most malignant form of gestational trophoblastic disease, has an incidence of approximately 1 in 40,000 pregnancies in the United States.[4] Two to 5% of hydatidiform moles progress to choriocarcinoma. Approximately 50% of choriocarcinomas develop from a hydatidiform mole, and 50% evolve from a normal-term pregnancy, or spontaneous abortion.[9]

In general, this condition is first suspected clinically in a patient with a history of gestational trophoblastic disease who has undergone evacuation

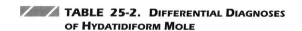 **TABLE 25-2. DIFFERENTIAL DIAGNOSES OF HYDATIDIFORM MOLE**

Missed abortion
Hydropic placenta
Degenerating leiomyoma
Endometrial carcinoma
Adenomyosis
Blighted Ovum

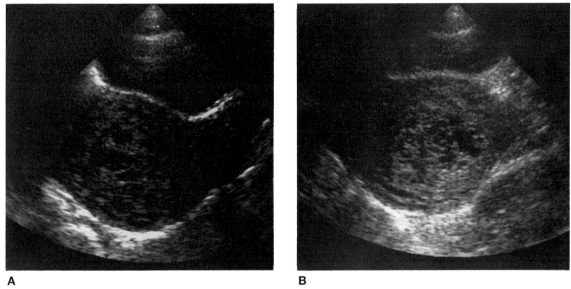

Figure 25-4. Longitudinal (**A**) and transverse (**B**) views of a complete mole filling the uterine cavity at 10 weeks after last menstrual period.

of the uterine contents but presents with continued vaginal bleeding, persistently elevated β-hCG levels, or persistent theca lutein cysts. Sonographically, choriocarcinoma may present with marked hemorrhagic necrosis in the myometrium. The factors involved in malignant transformation of the tropho-

blast are unknown. The tumor spreads rapidly through the uterus and disseminates either locally in the pelvis or by hematogenous spread to the lungs, lower gastrointestinal tract, central nervous system, liver, and urinary tract. The lungs and vagina are the most common sites of metastases.[20]

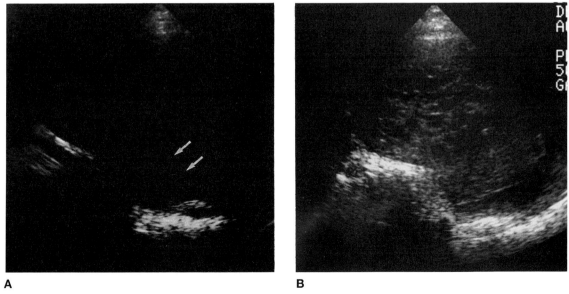

Figure 25-5. Longitudinal (**A**) and transverse (**B**) views of a partial molar pregnancy demonstrating a fetal pole (*arrows*) surrounded by a large multicystic mass.

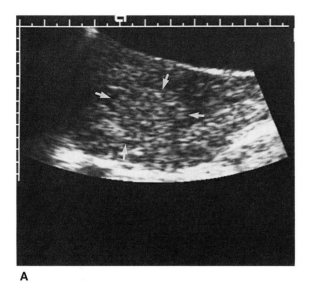

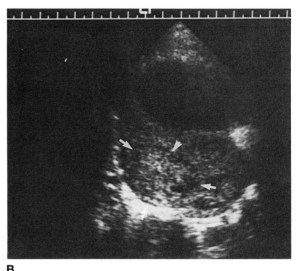

A   **B**

Figure 25-6. Longitudinal (**A**) and transverse (**B**) views of an invasive mole with an echogenic lesion surrounded by a hypoechoic rim, invading peripherally into the uterine wall (*arrows*).

Fetus and Coexisting Mole

Several reports in the literature have noted a molar pregnancy associated with a living fetus. Unfortunately, their statistics included patients whose placenta had undergone hydropic degeneration as well as those with a proliferating trophoblast in a classic hydatidiform mole.[3,7,21]

A coexisting complete mole and a normal fetus in a normal gestational sac arise from transformation of the trophoblast of one of two dizygotic twin placentas.[24] Ultrasound examination may suggest the diagnosis by demonstrating fetal echoes adjacent to a trophoblastic process (Fig. 25-7). However, the findings should ultimately be confirmed histologically because these lesions are considered to have the same malignant potential as the classic hydatidiform mole.

Sonographic Differentiation

Sonographic findings for a hydatidiform mole include an enlarged uterus containing complex echoes without evidence of a viable fetus. A leiomyoma could mimic a mole, but is most often homogeneous to complex, rounded, and well circumscribed. It does not transmit sound well and occupies only a portion of the uterus. A mole, on the other hand, occupies the entire uterus and has the appearance of placental tissue with anechoic areas. Detection of fetal parts or a viable fetus is very important in evaluating for coexisting or partial mole. When scanning the uterus for coexisting fetal parts, various gain settings and postprocessing techniques should be used to better resolve subtle echogenic areas that may represent fetal parts. Scans should also be performed of the liver to look for metastases. Patients who have undergone evacuation of a molar pregnancy can be followed sonographically to assess the uterine contents and the resolution of theca lutein cysts.

Doppler Examination

Duplex Doppler and color Doppler ultrasound are also helpful in distinguishing gestational trophoblastic disease from other, similar-looking conditions in the first trimester. Doppler waveform analysis of the uterine artery flow demonstrates a high impedance pattern with little diastolic flow in patients with hydropic degeneration of the placenta, degenerating fibroids, and incomplete abortion. A lower resistive index is found in a normal first trimester pregnancy and also in gestational trophoblastic disease. There is increased peak systolic velocity in the uterine arteries at 5 to 8 weeks in a normal gestation, indicating increased blood flow for the developing embryo.[13,14] The resistive index

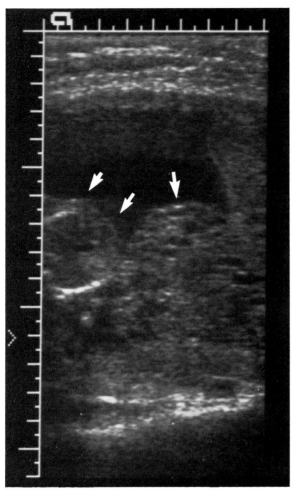

Figure 25-7. Transverse view of a fetal abdomen adjacent to apparently multicystic molar tissue in a coexisting mole (*arrows*).

in the uterine arteries decreases at 9 to 12 weeks' gestation because of trophoblastic destruction of the uterine vasculature and increase of the vascular bed causing a lower-impedance uteroplacental flow.[16] Gestational trophoblastic disease also exhibits increased peak systolic velocity and increased diastolic flow with a low resistive index due to extensive invasion and replacement of the smooth muscles in the spiral arteries. Enlargement of the spiral arteries results from arteriovenous shunting and pooling of blood within these lacunar spaces. The resistive index may range between 0.37 to 0.51, but this alone may not be specific for gestational trophoblastic processes.[15] When velocities are compared, intratumoral vessels demonstrate sig-

nificantly lower systolic velocities and increased diastolic velocities than do uterine arteries.[13] Color Doppler should demonstrate multiple, dilated, serpiginous vessels in the myometrium or some localized flow in the uterine mass with gestational trophoblastic disease.[5]

Doppler evaluation may also be useful in following the response of gestational trophoblastic disease to chemotherapy, which should result in increasing resistive indices and a decrease in the peak systolic velocity of the uterine arteries, compatible with a decreasing trophoblastic mass. A sudden decrease in the resistive index may indicate recurrent gestational trophoblastic disease and decreased response to chemotherapy.[13] However, destruction of the uterine vasculature by trophoblasts may be permanent, resulting in a low resistive index value despite complete remission.

Evaluation of uterine hemodynamics with Doppler ultrasound may also help in distinguishing the histopathologic type of gestational trophoblastic disease by the degree of uterine vascular alteration and destruction. A solid or compact lesion within the myometrium may exhibit central avascularity and a higher resistive index in the uterine artery, correlating histologically with choriocarcinoma. More cystic, tubular masses demonstrating a lower resistive index have been shown to correlate with invasive trophoblastic disease.[13,14] The vascular dynamics, however, should be correlated with the serum β-hCG levels in monitoring the gestational trophoblastic disease.

Treatment

After confirmation of the molar pregnancy by sonographic evaluation of the pelvis, most women undergo cervical dilation and suction and curettage of the trophoblastic contents from the uterine cavity.

The patient is placed on oral contraception for 1 year to prevent pregnancy-induced elevation of β-hCG. A quantitative β-hCG test is performed every 1 to 2 weeks after primary treatment until results of three consecutive tests are normal, then monthly for 6 months, and then every other month for 6 months. Regression should occur within 2 to 3 months. Recurrence is suspected if the β-hCG level reaches a plateau and remains there for 3 consecutive weeks or increases over 2 weeks.

Recurrent molar pregnancy confined to the

pelvic region is treated with single-agent chemotherapy such as methotrexate or actinomycin D. The risk of toxicity from these agents is high, but their use has been found to decrease the incidence of persistent gestational trophoblastic disease by 90%.[9,17] Multiple chemotherapeutic agents are used for widespread or persistent disease.

Surgical intervention, such as hysterectomy or hysterotomy, is performed only for control of local tumor symptoms and if fertility is not a concern. Older women in the high-risk category and women with invasive trophoblastic disease are the most likely candidates for surgery.

Women who have a clinical diagnosis other than a nonmetastatic, molar pregnancy are treated according to the malignant gestational trophoblastic disease group by pathologic presence and confirmation of choriocarcinoma or an invasive mole. The treatment of these women is further determined by whether they are in the nonmetastatic or low-risk group or the metastatic or high-risk group, which carries a poorer prognosis.[8,20]

Women with choriocarcinoma in the high-risk group have a urine level of β-hCG greater than 100,000 mIU/24 hours or serum levels of β-hCG greater than 40,000 mIU/ml. Liver or brain metastasis is present in the high-risk group. Single-agent chemotherapy will have failed and the duration of the disease will be greater than 4 months. Radiation therapy may be used in conjunction with chemotherapy for brain or liver metastases. If choriocarcinoma is associated with a term pregnancy, the woman is also considered to be at high risk.

Transvaginal ultrasonography is a sensitive modality when used in conjunction with β-hCG levels to monitor and assess changes in tumor size in patients during chemotherapy, and to determine further possible surgical intervention in patients with myometrial invasion.[18]

REFERENCES

1. Abulafia O, Sherer DM, Fultz PJ, Sternberg LB, Angel C. Unusual endovaginal ultrasonography and magnetic resonance imaging of placental site trophoblastic tumor. Am J Obstet Gynecol. 1993; 170:750–752.
2. Atrash HK, Hogne JR, Grimes DA. Epidemiology of hydatidiform mole during early gestation. Am J Obstet Gynecol. 1986; 154:906–909.
3. Bree RL, Silver TM, Wicks JD, et al. Trophoblastic disease with coexistent fetus: A sonographic and clinical spectrum. J Clin Ultrasound. 1978; 6:310–314.
4. Callen PW. Ultrasonography in evaluation of gestational trophoblastic disease. In: Callen PW, ed. Ultrasonography in Obstetrics and Gynecology. 2nd ed. Philadelphia: WB Saunders; 1988; 20:259–270.
5. Carter J, Fowler J, Carlson J, et al. Transvaginal color flow Doppler sonography in the assessment of gestational trophoblastic disease. J Ultrasound Med. 1993; 12:595–599.
6. Fisher RA, Sheppard DM, Lawler SD. Two patients with complete hydatidiform mole with 46,XY karyotype. Br J Obstet Gynaecol. 1984; 91:690–693.
7. Fleischer AC, James AE, Krause DA, et al. Sonographic patterns in trophoblastic diseases. Radiology. 1978; 126:215–220.
8. Fleischer AC, Jones HW III, James AE. Sonography of trophoblastic disease. In: Sanders RC, James AE, eds. The Principles and Practice of Ultrasonography in Obstetrics and Gynecology. 3rd ed. Norwalk, CT: Appleton-Century-Crofts; 1985.
9. Heath JM, Bu TH, Brereton WF. Hydatidiform moles. Am Fam Physician. 1985; 31:123–131.
10. Hertzberg BS, Kurtz AB, Wagner AB, et al. Gestational trophoblastic disease with coexistent normal fetus: Evaluation by ultrasound-guided chorionic villus sampling. J Ultrasound Med. 1986; 5:467–469.
11. Hiscock K. Ultrasound diagnosis of partial hydatidiform mole: A case report and review. Journal of Diagnostic and Medical Sonography. 1987; 3:91–94.
12. Hoffman JS, Silverman AD, Gelber J, Cartun R. Placental site trophoblastic tumor: A report of radiologic, surgical, and pathological methods of evaluating the extent of disease. Gynecol Oncol. 1993; 50:110–114.
13. Hsieh FJ, Wu CC, Chen CA, Chen TM, Hsieh CY, Chen HY. Correlation of uterine hemodynamics with chemotherapy response in gestational trophoblastic tumors. Obstet Gynecol. 1994; 83:1021–1025.
14. Hsieh FJ, Wu CC, Lee CN, et al. Vascular patterns of gestational trophoblastic tumors by color Doppler ultrasound. Cancer. 1994; 74:2361–2365.
15. Jaffe R. Investigation of abnormal first-trimester gestations by color Doppler imaging. J Clin Ultrasound. 1993; 21:521–526.
16. Jauniaux E, Jurkovic D, Campbell S, Hustin J. Doppler ultrasonographic features of the developing placental circulation: Correlation with anatomic findings. Am J Obstet Gynecol. 1992; 166:585–587.
17. Kim DS, Moon H, Kim KT. Effects of prophylactic chemotherapy for persistent trophoblastic disease in

patients with complete hydatidiform mole. Obstet Gynecol. 1986; 67:690–694.

18. Mangili G, Spagnolo D, Valsecchi L, Maggi R. Transvaginal ultrasonography in persistent trophoblastic tumor. Am J Obstet Gynecol. 1993; 169:1218–1223.

19. Munyer TP, Callen PW, Filly RA, et al. Further observations on the sonographic spectrum of gestational trophoblastic disease. J Clin Ultrasound. 1981; 9:349–358.

20. Pritchard JA, MacDonald PC, Gant NG. Abnormalities of the placenta and fetal membranes. In: Williams' Obstetrics. 17th ed. Norwalk, CT: Appleton-Century-Crofts; 1985; 104–107.

21. Sauerbrei EE, Salem S, Fayle B. Coexistent hydatidiform mole and live fetus in the second trimester. Radiology. 1980; 135:415–417.

22. Switzer JM, Weckstein ML, Campbell LF, et al. Ovarian hydatidiform mole. J Ultrasound Med. 1984; 3:471–473.

23. Szulman AE, Surti U. The syndromes of hydatidiform mole: I. Cytogenic and morphologic conditions. Am J Obstet Gynecol. 1978; 131:20–27.

24. Szulman AE, Surti U. The syndromes of hydatidiform mole: II. Morphologic evaluation of the complete and partial mole. Am J Obstet Gynecol. 1978; 132:20–27.

25. Taylor JW, Schwartz PE, Koharn EI. Gestational trophoblastic neoplasia: Diagnosis with Doppler ultrasound. Radiology. 1987; 165:445–448.

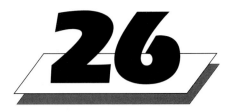

The Effect of Maternal Disease on Pregnancy

DUNSTAN ABRAHAM, WILLIAM M. GREENHUT,
and MORDECAI KOENIGSBERG

Maternal disease may have a wide spectrum of effects on pregnancy, ranging from destruction of the early zygote or embryo to major malformation and demise of the developing fetus. The mechanisms through which maternal disease can affect the fetus are varied; however, it has been clearly established that the placenta can play a crucial role in preventing or facilitating the transmission process.[3,63]

The major physiologic function of the placenta is to exchange gas, nutrients, and waste products between the maternal and fetal circulations. This is achieved by various methods, including diffusion, active transport, and pinocytosis. For example, blood gases move or diffuse speedily and easily across the placenta from maternal to fetal circulation, but larger molecules, such as carbohydrates, must be assisted or actively transported across the placental membranes. Some substances, usually those that have larger molecules, are unable to cross the placenta and are thus effectively barred from entering the fetal circulation by the "placental barrier." This barrier prevents the mixing of the maternal and fetal circulations. Nevertheless, a variety of substances and agents are able to move across this barrier and harm the developing fetus. Examples include infectious agents, drugs, and antibodies.

Some maternal diseases may directly injure the placenta, thereby harming the fetus indirectly. Maternal vascular disease, such as hypertension, decreases uteroplacental blood flow and compromises the placenta's function of providing nutrients for the fetus. Intrauterine growth retardation (IUGR) is not uncommonly encountered in these cases.

Sonography has a valuable role in evaluating pregnancies complicated by maternal disease. In general, a fetus at risk can be screened for gross malformations and IUGR. In addition, sonography can assess placental maturation and amniotic fluid volume and can date pregnancies to determine the best time for cesarean section. In diagnostic procedures such as amniocentesis and percutaneous umbilical blood sampling (PUBS) of the umbilical vein, ultrasound is used for needle guidance.[13,46]

Information about the fetoplacental circulatory unit has been obtained with Doppler ultrasound. Technically, this is performed by recording the flow velocity waveform of the umbilical artery and, less frequently, the uterine artery. From this waveform, a systolic-to-diastolic (S/D) ratio can be calculated, and abnormal values, indicating disease, can be detected.[15] Doppler velocity waveform monitoring of the umbilical artery has proven to be a useful indicator of fetal well-being. Normally, as pregnancy progresses, increased diastolic flow is observed, representing reduced resistance to flow. High resistance to flow has been found in complicated pregnancies such as premature rupture of membranes, toxemia, IUGR, sickle cell disease, and diabetes mellitus.[15,24,71]

In this chapter, we discuss some of the more commonly encountered maternal diseases and conditions that may adversely affect fetal outcome. These include infectious disease, endocrine and metabolic disorders, hematologic disorders, toxemia, drug addiction, and malnutrition. The specific role of sonography in these various situations is also discussed.

Infections

Fetal infection from maternal disease can occur at various times during gestation and can have a variety of clinical outcomes. Maternal infection even before conception may also have an adverse effect on future pregnancies.

The extent of damage to the fetus depends on several factors, including the virulence of the agent and the route of transmission. The gestational age at the time of infection is also of major importance, because in many cases this determines the susceptibility of the fetus to the agent. Because organogenesis occurs during the first trimester, the fetus is particularly susceptible during that time; but infection can occur before conception, before implantation, after implantation, and in the puerperium.[78]

Infection before conception has been studied in mouse systems by researchers using retroviruses. Results have demonstrated that these viruses can infect the embryo, integrate into the germ line, and cause disease in future generations.

Infection before implantation may result from local infection of the maternal reproductive tract. The most likely routes of transmission are through the genital tract and through the circulation. At this early stage, infection may destroy the zygote or embryo, although local barriers such as the zona pellucida prevent most agents from causing damage.

Infection after implantation, particularly during organogenesis, accounts for the largest number of adverse fetal effects. The disruption of normal development at this stage may lead to serious fetal abnormalities. Usually, after the infectious agent enters the mother, she contracts viremia, bacteremia, or parasitemia. The agent then reaches and infects the placenta by a hematogenous route. Organisms cross the placenta, enter the fetal circulation, and spread throughout the fetus' body. The fetus is harmed as these agents destroy parenchymal cells and blood vessels. They replicate in fetal tissue, changing growth patterns and eliciting autoimmune responses. Fetal damage may be less severe if the mother has been immunized through prior exposure to the agent.

VIRAL INFECTION

The human herpesviruses (cytomegalovirus [CMV], herpes hominis types I and II [herpes simplex viruses], varicella-zoster virus, and Epstein-Barr virus [EBV] infect most people at some time during life. The viruses usually remain latent in the body but may reactivate periodically and produce disease.

Gestational herpesvirus infections may reach the embryo or fetus through the placenta, or by ascending through the cervix or through fetal contact with the birth canal during vaginal delivery. CMV is the most common known cause of congenital infections in humans. Reports indicate that 6% to 19% of infants infected in utero contract the disease.[59] Features of CMV disease in neonates include hepatosplenomegaly, jaundice, thrombocytopenia, chorioretinitis, cerebral calcifications, and microcephaly (Fig. 26-1). Other reported associated congenital defects and findings include inguinal hernia, anomalies of the first branchial arch, and central nervous system anomalies. Antenatal findings may include ascites, splenomegaly, IUGR, hydrocephaly, and polyhydramnios.[17,50]

Herpes simplex virus infection occurs in 1 to 6 newborns per 10,000 deliveries per year.[39] Primary infection during the first half of pregnancy has been associated with an increased frequency of spontaneous abortions and stillbirths.[40] Associated congenital malformations include microcephaly, hydranencephaly, intracranial calcifications, microphthalmia, and hepatosplenomegaly. If the virus is present in the maternal genital tract at the time of delivery, there is a 50% chance that the infant will be infected as it passes through the birth canal, so cesarean section is indicated in such cases.

Serologic evidence of past varicella-zoster (chickenpox) infection is found in 95% of women of childbearing age in the United States. Three outcomes have been described in pregnancies infected

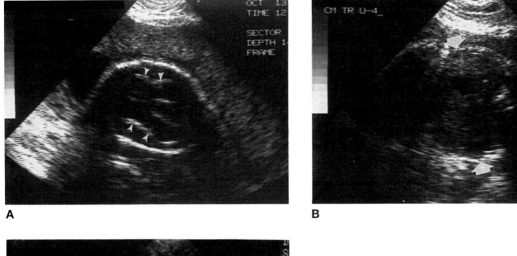

A   B

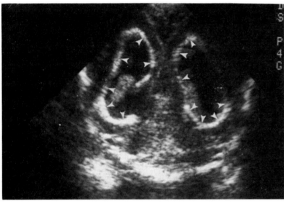

C

Figure 26-1. Fetal cytomegalovirus infection. (**A**) Cephalic sonogram of a fetus that appeared smaller on clinical examination than was expected by maternal dates. On a sonogram 8 weeks before this examination, a fetal biparietal diameter of 44 mm was measured, consistent with 18.5 weeks' gestation on average. Femoral length was 33 mm, consistent with 20.5 weeks on average. On this axial sonogram there is evidence of microcephaly. A biparietal diameter of 62 mm is obtained, consistent with 24 weeks on average. A head circumference of 225 mm was calculated, consistent with 24.5 weeks' gestation on average. In comparison, a femoral length of 55 mm was measured at this time, consistent with 29 weeks' gestation on average. Hydrocephaly is also evident, with a ventricular–hemispheric ratio of 0.52. Note the thick echogenic margin of the ventricular wall (*arrowheads*), due to diffuse periventricular calcification. (**B**) Transverse abdominal sonogram using the same image scale as in **A.** Abdominal diameter from side to side (*arrows*) measures 81 mm. The circumference is calculated at 250 mm, consistent with 30.5 weeks' gestation on average. (**C**) Postnatal coronal neurosonogram confirmed the presence of hydrocephaly and periventricular calcification (*arrowheads*). The cerebral tissue in the periphery shows a paucity of echogenic sulci because of failure of normal migration of fetal ventricular lining cells to the periphery as a result of the periventriculitis. Cytomegalovirus was cultured from the neonatal nasopharynx and urine, and markedly elevated viral antibody titers were measured in the serum of mother and infant.

with the varicella virus: congenital abnormalities, postnatal newborn disease ranging from benign to fatal, and zoster (shingles), which may appear months or years after birth.[59] Congenital abnormalities, identified as early as 1947, include IUGR,

limb aplasia, microphthalmia, and brain calcifications.[78] These abnormalities are observed when the virus is transmitted to the fetus during weeks 8 to 20 of pregnancy.

Although EBV infection is very common during childhood, primary EBV infection in pregnancy is not. In one study, only 3 of more than 12,000 pregnant women tested positive.[22] EBV infection, which causes mononucleosis, has been linked to spontaneous abortions, stillbirths, low–birth-weight infants, as well as congenital heart anomalies and microphthalmia.[21,31] But questions have been raised about the validity of these associations, and further research is required to determine the extent of the correlation between EBV and fetal congenital abnormalities.

Up to 20% of reproductive age women are thought to be susceptible to rubella.[23] Infection during pregnancy may result in spontaneous abortion, stillbirth, or congenital defects. Reported congenital defects include microcephaly, hydrocephaly, cephalocele (Fig. 26-2), and cardiac anomalies.

The evidence linking influenza virus to adverse pregnancy outcome has been inconsistent. Early reports of congenital malformation of the heart and central nervous system[59] have not been confirmed by later studies.

Most cases of human immunodeficiency virus (HIV) (the agent of acquired immunodeficiency syndrome) infection in children are a consequence of transmission of infection from mother to infant, most of which is estimated to occur near the time of birth. Factors affecting this transmission include the total number of maternal HIV particles, the effectiveness of the maternal and fetal immune response, and the integrity of the placental barrier.[11] In utero, effects of HIV on the fetus may lead to prematurity, IUGR, hepatomegaly, and lymphadenopathy.[69,78]

BACTERIAL INFECTION

Infections with syphilis early in pregnancy may result in spontaneous abortion. At a later stage, the fetus may be stillborn or may die in the neonatal period from congenital disease. If infection occurs very late in pregnancy, the clinical signs of congenital syphilis may not be apparent for 2 to 4 weeks.[59] Syphilis in neonates is characterized by hepatosplenomegaly, hyperbilirubinemia, evidence of hemolysis, and generalized lymphadenopathy. Gonorrhea has been reported by Handsfield and colleagues[29] to be implicated in an increased incidence of prematurity, prolonged rupture of fetal membranes, chorioamnionitis, sepsis, and IUGR. Gonococcal infections in neonates can result in meningitis and arthritis. Syphilis and gonorrhea can be treated successfully with penicillin, or with other antibiotics in those patients who are allergic to penicillin.[67]

Lyme disease, transmitted by ticks borne by deer, has become a cause for increasing concern in the northeast United States. There has also been heightened awareness of the risk of contracting this infection elsewhere in this country and in Europe. One large investigation has neither ruled out nor been able to discover specific abnormalities associated with the infection if it is left untreated.

Urinary tract infections (UTIs) represent one of the most common medical complications of pregnancy. If not managed properly, they may cause considerable adverse effects to both mother and fetus. UTIs include asymptomatic bacteriuria, acute cystitis, and acute pyelonephritis. Asymptomatic bacterial infection has been implicated as a cause in premature delivery and low birth weight, although some studies do not support this finding.[68] Pyelonephritis in pregnancy has been associated with low birth weight, increased perinatal mortality, anemia, toxemia, and premature rupture of membranes.[64] Mental and motor development of children of pyelonephrotic mothers has been found to be impaired. Patients with UTIs during pregnancy should be treated with antibiotics and monitored by frequent urine cultures.

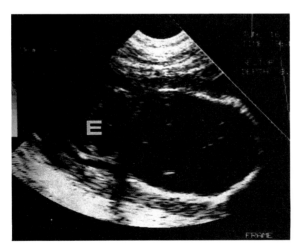

Figure 26-2. Cephalocele in 22-week fetus with rubella. Axial sonogram of the fetal head demonstrates a large occipital encephalocele (E) containing fluid and echogenic brain tissue.

PARASITIC INFECTION

Parasitic infection during pregnancy may not always pose a risk to the fetus or mother. The clinical manifestations of parasitic disease are determined by several factors: the life cycle in the human host, the quantity and location of the parasite, and the host–parasite interaction.[34] Parasites that penetrate and invade the host's viscera are a threat to the fetus. These organisms may directly penetrate and infect the uterus and placenta or may infect the fetus through the blood. Moreover, they are clearly a threat to both mother and fetus if they multiply within the human host. Toxoplasmosis and malaria are two of the more common parasitic diseases of humans. In the United States, the incidence of congenital toxoplasmosis is approximately 1 per 1000 live births. Toxoplasmosis occurring early in pregnancy is less frequently transmitted to the fetus than is infection acquired during the last trimester. In early pregnancy the small placenta usually protects the fetus from parasites. In late pregnancy this barrier is not as effective, owing to the expanded maternoplacental interface and the aging placenta. Fetal effects are usually devastating. These include severe IUGR, hydrocephaly, microcephaly, cerebral calcifications, hepatosplenomegaly, and fetal demise.

The incidence of congenital malaria in immune mothers residing in areas with a high incidence of the disease is 0.3%. Maternal malaria promotes placental insufficiency, which causes IUGR, low birth weight, abortion, and stillbirth.[34] Antiparasitic drug therapy has been used successfully to treat toxoplasmosis and malaria infections during pregnancy, but some effective medications are potential teratogens.

Ultrasound has a useful role in evaluating fetuses exposed to infectious diseases. For example, fetal echocardiography should be performed to exclude cardiac abnormalities in patients exposed to CMV and rubella. IUGR, seen in some bacterial infections, can be diagnosed by serial scans and measurements of the fetal growth parameters. Fetuses who require delivery by cesarean section because of infections such as herpes or syphilis can be accurately dated by sonography.

Endocrine and Metabolic Disorders

DIABETES MELLITUS

Diabetes mellitus is perhaps the most common maternal disorder the obstetric sonographer encounters. It has been estimated that it occurs in 1 of every 324 to 350 pregnancies in the United States.[3] The condition is a disorder of carbohydrate metabolism related to insulin deficiency and characterized by hyperglycemia.

Diabetes mellitus is classified as type I (insulin dependent; formerly known as juvenile-onset diabetes), type II (noninsulin dependent; formerly known as adult-onset diabetes), and other, or secondary, diabetes. Causes of secondary diabetes include pancreatic disease or pancreatectomy, hormones, drugs, or chemicals, and certain genetic syndromes. Additional classes of diabetes mellitus are impaired glucose tolerance and gestational diabetes, a condition manifested only during pregnancy.[41]

The association between diabetes mellitus and fetal congenital anomalies was recognized as early as 1885. Today, the frequency of anomalies among offspring of diabetic mothers is estimated at 3% to 6%.[53] The pathogenesis of these anomalies is ascribed to the hyperglycemia of diabetes, which disrupts organogenesis. Early diabetes control has been found to reduce the incidence of congenital malformations.[47]

Congenital anomalies in infants of diabetic mothers include skeletal, central nervous system (Fig. 26-3), cardiac, renal, and gastrointestinal types.[26] In addition, a single umbilical artery (SUA) has been found in about 6.4% of diabetic mothers' pregnancies. An SUA has been associated with various malformations, including cardiac and great vessel anomalies, pulmonary hypoplasia, genitourinary tract anomalies, vertebral anomalies, talipes equinovarus (clubfoot), inguinal hernias, and polydactyly.[53] The finding of an SUA, therefore, warrants a thorough examination of the fetus to exclude these malformations. In addition to malformations, fetuses of diabetic mothers may also experience growth disturbance problems such as IUGR or macrosomia (increased body tissues and fat). Growth retardation of a fetus of a mother with severe diabetes is attributed to uteroplacental vascular insufficiency, which results in less nutrients being transferred to the fetus. Fetal hyperinsulinemia is thought to be responsible for the development of macrosomia, as continuous maternal hyperglycemia gains access to the fetal circulatory system. Macrosomia is described as fetal weight in excess of 4000 g or a birth weight above the 90th percentile for gestational age, which predisposes the fetus to complications such as stillbirth and intrapartum

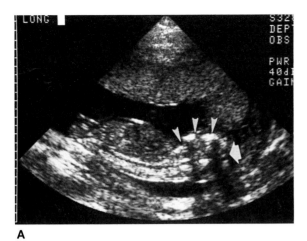
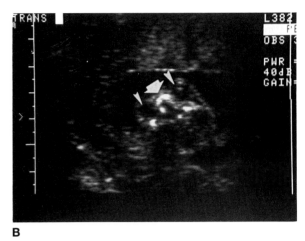

A   **B**

Figure 26-3. Anencephaly in the fetus of a diabetic mother. (**A**) Longitudinal sonogram demonstrates the fetal trunk and the facial structures (*small arrowheads*). No cranial vault is discerned (*large arrowhead*). The fetus was 15 weeks' size by femoral length. (**B**) Sonographic section of the fetal orbits in a semiaxial plane. Note the nasal bridge (*large arrowhead*) separating the echopenic globes of the eyes (*small arrowheads*). A lens is seen anterolaterally in the globe on the right side of the image.

trauma.[76] In addition, both maternal and perinatal morbidity and mortality increase in relation to increasing fetal birth weight.[26,78]

Several growth parameters can be examined with ultrasound to monitor the diabetic mother's pregnancy. These include the biparietal diameter, the abdominal circumference, and the estimated fetal weight. Less commonly used parameters are chest size determination and the assessment of fetal breathing movements.[6,27,30,43,55]

In the sonographic evaluation of the diabetic mother's pregnancy, it is recommended that an initial first trimester examination be done to establish dates, followed by an examination between 18 and 22 weeks to screen for neural tube defects, caudal regression syndrome (with variable agenesis of the lower spinal segments, variable fusion of the lower extremities, and variable absence of the long bones), and cardiac defects, and to exclude other gross malformations.[53] Follow-up examinations should then be done every 4 to 6 weeks for fetal growth and estimated weight. Attention should be paid to placental size because chronic hyperglycemia can cause placental enlargement (Fig. 26-4). Macrosomic and growth-retarded fetuses should be examined more frequently (Fig. 26-5). Umbilical artery flow tracings, specifically high-resistance Doppler velocity patterns, have also proven significant.[71]

Gestational diabetes—diabetes that occurs only during pregnancy—affects about 25 of 1000 pregnant women. Historical risk factors for this condition include a previous stillbirth, a baby with congenital anomalies, a previous macrosomic infant, or a family history of diabetes.[44] Gestational diabetes can affect the fetus in the same way that pregestational diabetes can, but the later the onset in pregnancy the less likely the fetus will have been affected during periods of major organogenesis. Because the onset of clinical symptoms may lag behind

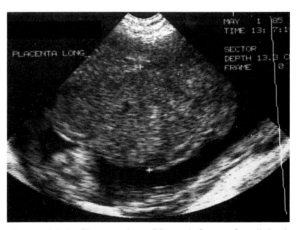

Figure 26-4. Placenta in a 29-week fetus of a diabetic mother. The placenta measures 7 cm in maximal thickness (between markers).

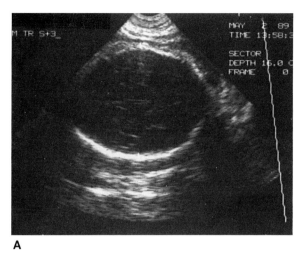
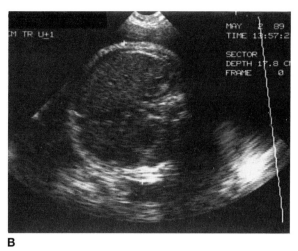

A   **B**

Figure 26-5. Macrosomia in the fetus of an insulin-dependent diabetic mother. (**A**) Axial cephalic sonogram demonstrates a biparietal diameter of 87 mm, consistent with 34 weeks' gestation on average. A head circumference (HC) of 320 mm is calculated. (**B**) Transverse abdominal sonogram using a depth scale greater than that in **A** shows a larger fetal abdomen. An abdominal circumference (AC) of 356 mm is calculated. HC-to-AC ratio equals 0.90, which is markedly small for a 34-week fetus. The fetal abdominal integument is thickened to 1 cm.

maternal metabolic changes, there is no certainty that the fetus has gone through organogenesis unaffected, no matter how late in pregnancy the clinical diagnosis is established. A common-sense approach, such as examining all fetuses whose mothers manifested symptoms before 24 weeks' gestation, is best.

HYPERTHYROIDISM

Hyperthyroidism, also known as thyrotoxicosis, occurs in approximately 2 of every 1000 pregnancies.[5] The additional thyroid stimulation produces thyroxine, which disrupts normal cell development, causing a significant increase in the incidence of low–birth-weight infants and a slight increase in the neonatal mortality rate.

The most common cause of clinical hyperthyroidism is Graves' disease (toxic diffuse goiter). Plummer's disease (toxic nodular goiter), trophoblastic tumors, and hydatidiform mole may also cause hyperthyroidism.[5]

HYPOTHYROIDISM

The incidence of hypothyroidism is very low in pregnant women, because the absence of normal hormone stimulation makes it unlikely that the woman will conceive. When pregnancy does occur, incidence of stillbirth is high.[5] The most common causes of hypothyroidism are thyroidectomy and radioactive iodine therapy.[12]

HYPERPARATHYROIDISM

The incidence of hyperparathyroidism in pregnancy is very low. The most common cause is parathyroid adenoma. An increase in prematurity, spontaneous abortions, fetal demise in late pregnancy, and hypocalcemia and tetany in newborns can be seen.[12]

PHENYLKETONURIA

Phenylketonuria is a genetic disorder that exposes the developing fetus of an affected mother, who is not following a low-phenylalanine, low-protein diet, to potentially toxic levels of otherwise important metabolic products. The risks of spontaneous abortion, microcephaly, mental retardation, and congenital heart disease are increased.[35] Dietary restriction of phenylalanine should be started before conception to maximize the chances of producing a normal fetus. Maternal dietary adjustments reinstated after inception of pregnancy have been unsuccessful in preventing abnormalities.

Hematologic Disorders

Rh ISOIMMUNIZATION

Rh isoimmunization refers to the development of maternal antibodies to the surface antigens on fetal red blood cells. The maternal antibodies perceive these fetal antigens as foreign invaders, and they attack and destroy them. Erythroblastosis fetalis, a condition characterized by rapid destruction of fetal red blood cells and hepatosplenomegaly, may occur when an Rh-positive fetus is carried by an Rh-negative mother who has been sensitized to Rh antigen in a previous pregnancy.[32] In its most severe form, a fluid overload condition known as hydrops fetalis results (Fig. 26-6). With the introduction of preventive maternal immunologic blocking treatment, clinical Rh isoimmunization to the Rh factor is much less common. However, isoimmunization due to major blood type (ABO) maternofetal incompatibility occasionally occurs.

Amniocentesis is an important procedure for monitoring the bilirubin concentration in amniotic fluid; the severity of hemolytic disease is related to the bilirubin level. Ultrasound is not only helpful in detecting changes in extrafetal and intrafetal fluid and noting growth rate disturbances, but in establishing accurate dates for timing amniocentesis and delivery and for guidance in needle placement for amniocentesis, particularly when serial procedures may be indicated. Ultrasound-guided PUBS now allows direct sampling of fetal blood from which antibody titers can be determined and a prompt diagnosis rendered. In recent years, isoimmunized pregnancies have been treated successfully by transfusing blood into the umbilical vein, through the cord near its insertion into the placenta, or into the fetal peritoneal cavity under ultrasound guidance.[4,60]

Doppler ultrasound is also helpful in assessing the well-being of potentially affected fetuses. A correlation between increasing velocity of blood flow to the fetus in compensation for decreasing hemoglobin carried in the blood implies that periodic Doppler examinations may be of value in timing intervention.[25,73,74]

Hydrops can be caused by factors other than isoimmunization. This nonimmunologic hydrops may be caused by over 40 conditions.[18,48] Most commonly, nonimmunologic hydrops may result from fetal problems such as cardiovascular conditions (hypoplastic left heart, dysrhythmias), infections (toxoplasmosis, herpes simplex), obstructive vascular problems (umbilical vein thrombosis), pulmonary diseases (cystic adenomatoid malformation), neoplasms (neuroblastoma, teratoma), chro-

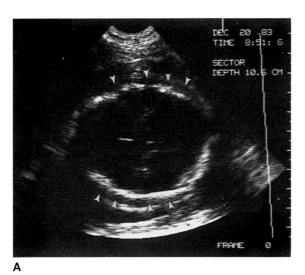
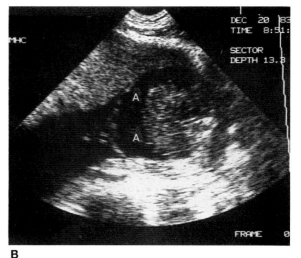

A   **B**

Figure 26-6. Hydrops fetalis in 24-week fetus of a mother with Rh sensitization. (**A**) Cephalic sonogram in axial view shows scalp edema (*arrowheads*) measuring 7 to 8 mm in thickness. (**B**) Transverse abdominal sonogram demonstrates fetal ascites (A). There is also polyhydramnios, especially prominent if one estimates what the true abdominal circumference would be in the absence of the fetal ascites.

mosomal anomalies (trisomy 18 or 21), and congenital nephrosis. Maternal causes include diabetes mellitus and toxemia.[51]

The ultrasound findings associated with hydrops include polyhydramnios, fetal ascites, pleural and pericardial effusions, fetal anasarca (subcutaneous edema with skin thickness greater than 5 mm), abnormally thickened placenta (greater than 6 cm), fetal hepatosplenomegaly and cardiomegaly, and umbilical vein dilatation.[19,20,47,71] The sonographically detectable structural anomalies associated with fetal hydrops are numerous and varied (Table 26-1).

SICKLE CELL ANEMIA

Sickle cell anemia is an inherited disorder that affects the black population predominantly. Normally round, the red blood cells are instead sickle shaped. This leads to abnormally high red cell destruction

and occlusion of arterioles. Incidences of spontaneous abortion, prematurity, and stillbirth are increased. Perinatal morbidity and mortality have also been reported.[61] Short femurs may be present and low birth weight may occur.[56]

Fetuses should be followed sonographically for growth retardation and increased placental resistance to umbilical artery and uterine artery flow. The S/D velocity ratio can be monitored using Doppler techniques. An S/D ratio of 3.0 or higher after 30 weeks' gestation has been reported as predictive of fetal distress when detected in both umbilical and uterine arteries. The same study recorded abnormal flow in at least one of these arteries, with abnormal flow in 88% of pregnant women with sickle cell disease, as opposed to 4% to 7% of normal pregnant women.[1]

Management of sickle cell patients during pregnancy includes dietary supplementation of iron and folic acid.[14,36] Prophylactic transfusions have been

TABLE 26-1. STRUCTURAL ANOMALIES ASSOCIATED WITH HYDROPS FETALIS THAT MAY HAVE SONOGRAPHIC MANIFESTATION

Structure	Sonographic Finding	Abnormality
Head	Intracranial mass, associated with congestive heart failure and microcephaly	Arteriovenous malformation, vein of Galen aneurysm, cytomegalovirus or toxoplasmosis infection
Neck	Cystic neck masses	Lymphatic dysplasias
Thorax	Poorly contracting heart	Congestive heart failure
	Pericardial effusion, tachycardia	Cardiac anomaly
	Asystole	Demise
	Mediastinal mass	Tumor
	Chest mass	Cystic adenomatoid malformation
	Small thorax	Dwarfism
	Cystic masses crossing diaphragm	Diaphragmatic hernias
Abdomen	Tubular sonolucent structures	Gastrointestinal obstruction, atresia, or volvulus
	Abdominal masses	Tumors, neurofibromatosis
Retroperitoneum	Retroperitoneal mass	Neurogenic mass
	Hydronephrotic kidney	Hydronephrosis, posterior urethral valves
Extremities	Short arms, legs	Dwarfism
	Contractures	Arthrogryposis
	Fractures	Osteogenesis imperfecta
Placenta	Thick placenta	Infection, extramedullary hematopoiesis, anemia
	Mass	Chorioangioma
Amniotic cavity	Number of fetuses, relative size, amniotic membrane	Twin–twin transfusion
	Umbilical cord anomalies	Single umbilical artery, umbilical cord torsion

(Adapted from Fleischer AC, Killam AP, Boehm FH, et al. Hydrops fetalis: Sonographic evaluation and clinical implications. 1981; 141:163–168.)

reported to improve both maternal and fetal morbidity and mortality, although this procedure carries the risk of blood-borne infection and the formation of alloantibodies that may affect future transfusions.[38]

THALASSEMIA

Thalassemia has been cited as the most common maternal genetic abnormality associated with pregnancy worldwide.[75] This form of red blood cell production presents in multiple variations, the most common of which is referred to as Cooley's anemia or thalassemia major. Thalassemia often shortens the life span of an affected person because of the iron overload that develops from the necessary multiple transfusions. Most women with thalassemia major die before reaching reproductive age. In cases of successful pregnancy, effects on the fetus range from hydrops and death to no effect at all.[28,30]

Toxemia and Hypertension

Toxemia of pregnancy is a disease occurring in the third trimester characterized by maternal edema, hypertension, proteinuria, and central nervous system irritability. The disease has been classified into two stages, preeclampsia and eclampsia. The preeclamptic stage is marked by development of hypertension with proteinuria or edema, or both. In the eclamptic stage one or more convulsions occur, significantly increasing the risk of maternal and fetal mortality.[19] Preeclampsia affects less than 1.5% of all pregnancies, but, when it develops before 36 weeks' gestation, a prenatal mortality rate as high as 20% has been reported. The disorder has been found to occur most commonly in young primigravidas and in older multiparas. Although the etiology of preeclampsia remains unclear, immunologic, hormonal, and nutritional factors are thought to be responsible. It has been postulated that the reduction in prostaglandin synthesis seen in preeclamptic patients promotes placental vascular disease and decreased uteroplacental blood flow. Low birth weight, fetal distress, and placental abruption are all associated with toxemia.[19] Treatment of this condition depends on the severity of the disease. Antihypertensive drugs can be used to control blood pressure, and in severe disease anticonvulsant medication is prescribed for seizures. Immediate delivery of the fetus is indicated in most cases of toxemia.

Hypertension during pregnancy may also occur without the development of toxemia. Hypertension preceding or persisting after pregnancy is diagnosed as essential hypertension, whereas hypertension that occurs during pregnancy and disappears after parturition is considered to be pregnancy-induced hypertension. Hypertension during pregnancy, regardless of the type, always poses a risk to both mother and fetus. In a prospective study of 14,833 women, Page and Christianson[45] reported that a mean arterial pressure of 90 mm Hg or more during the middle trimester of pregnancy significantly increased the risk of stillbirth, preeclampsia, and IUGR. Other reports have concluded that the maternal risk of mild chronic hypertension is small unless preeclampsia develops.[62]

Sonography can reliably monitor preeclamptic pregnancies and detect abnormalities early. A spectrum of ultrasound findings has been described in these patients: IUGR, oligohydramnios, decreased placental volume, accelerated placental maturation, and fetal demise.[7] In addition, S/D ratios can be followed serially by Doppler to detect the development of increased placental vascular resistance.

A protocol for evaluating patients with hypertension has been described by Zuspan.[79] He advises that at least three ultrasound examinations be done. The first examination should be performed at 10 to 14 weeks, to date the pregnancy; the second, at 20 to 26 weeks; and the third, at 32 weeks' gestational age. The later examinations should focus on detecting early evidence of IUGR and on documenting the amount of amniotic fluid, because this is a good index of fetal well-being.

A complaint of abdominal pain in a woman with chronic hypertension should raise the clinical suspicion of placental abruption. These patients should be carefully monitored by ultrasound and clinical observation.

Systemic Lupus Erythematosus

Systemic lupus erythematosus is a multisystem autoimmune disease that is not uncommon in women, particularly in the childbearing years. Fetal effects may be caused by the transfer of autoantibodies across the placenta, or indirectly as a result of the lack of maternal well-being. Pregnancy disorders that have been reported with this disease include fetal death, recurrent abortion, growth retardation, and toxemia.[52] Best fetal outcomes are obtained when pregnancies are planned for time periods when disease activity has been well controlled by small doses of steroids and aspirin.

Drug Use and Nutritional Disorders

Drug use during pregnancy may affect its outcome by promoting fetal addiction, teratogenesis, altered uteroplacental blood flow, or IUGR.[54] It is estimated that drug exposure accounts for approximately 2% to 3% of birth defects in humans.[42] This teratogenic effect depends on several factors, including the drug, its dosage, time of exposure, host susceptibility, genetic differences in the host, and interactions with other agents in the environment.[42] In general, in the early period of gestation teratogens affect organs that develop first, such as the heart.

Although many drugs and chemicals have been sporadically associated with various fetal malformations, only a few are proven teratogens (Table 26-2). Some, unfortunately, are important medications, such as Coumadin (warfarin), whose use during pregnancy must be restricted.

Drugs used abusively include alcohol, amphetamines, barbiturates, and narcotics (heroin, methadone, and cocaine). These agents have reportedly been associated with a variety of effects in the fetus, ranging from mild to severe, but in other than proven teratogens, the main effect appears to be IUGR as a result of poor nutrition associated with drug use (Fig. 26-7). Excessive consumption of al-

TABLE 26-2. PROVEN TERATOGENS AND THEIR FETAL EFFECTS

Teratogen	Fetal Effects
Aminopterin	Meningoencephalocele, hydrocephalus, clubfoot, hypoplasia of fibula
Antithyroid drugs	Polydactyly, goiter
Azathioprine	Pulmonary valvular stenosis
Carbon monoxide	Cerebral atrophy, hydrocephalus, cleft lip
Coumadin	Encephalocele, anencephaly, spina bifida, congenital heart disease, skeletal deformities, growth retardation
Cyclophosphamide	Tetralogy of Fallot, syndactyly, missing digits
Daunorubicin	Anencephaly, cardiac defects
Ethanol	Microcephaly, cardiac defects, growth retardation
Heparin	Absence of thumbs
Methotrexate	Oxycephaly, absence of frontal bone, dextrocardia, growth retardation
Methyl mercury	Microcephaly, head asymmetry
Phenytoin	Microcephaly, cardiac malformations, hypertelorism, cleft palate or lip, growth retardation
Polychlorinated biphenyl	Growth retardation
Procarbazine	Cerebral hemorrhage
Retinoic acid	Hydrocephalus, microcephaly, congenital heart defects, malformation of cranium, face, and ribs, limb deformities
Thalidomide	Congenital heart malformations, spine malformations, limb reduction, duodenal stenosis or atresia, pyloric stenosis, microtia
Trimethadione	Microcephaly, cardiac defects, club foot, esophageal atresia, growth deficiency
Valproic acid	Meningomyelocele, microcephaly, growth deficiency, tetralogy of Fallot, oral cleft

(Adapted from Koren A, Edwards MB, Miskin M. Antenatal sonography of fetal malformation associated with drugs and chemicals: A guide. Am J Obstet Gynecol. 1987; 156:79–85.)

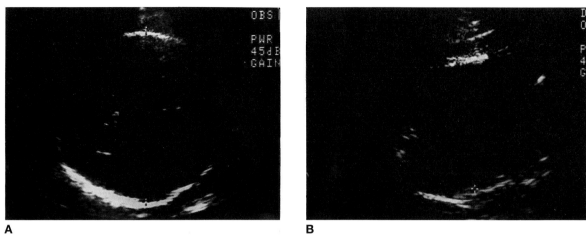

A   **B**

Figure 26-7. Severe intrauterine growth retardation in the fetus of a drug abuser. (**A**) Axial cephalic sonogram demonstrates a biparietal diameter (BPD) of 74 mm. Head circumference (HC) was calculated at 245 mm. BPD and HC are both 4 to 5 weeks less than expected for this fetus, which should be at 32 weeks, based on a sonogram at 17 weeks' gestation. (**B**) Transverse abdominal sonogram using the same scale as in **A** shows a much smaller fetal abdomen. The abdominal contour is not optimal owing to compression by the uterine wall as a result of severe oligohydramnios. Abdominal circumference (AC) is estimated at 190 mm. HC/AC ratio is 1.29, markedly increased for a 32-week fetus.

cohol, a known teratogen, during pregnancy can result in the fetal alcohol syndrome (FAS). This syndrome includes features of gross physical retardation, central nervous system dysfunction, and facial dysmorphology, including microcephaly and microphthalmia. Additional effects of alcohol include cardiac anomalies (such as ventricular septal defect), increased risk of infections, placental abruption, and spontaneous abortion.[54,57,65] It is estimated that 11% of pregnant women are problem drinkers and about 5% to 10% of their offspring demonstrate full-blown FAS. FAS occurs at a rate of 1 in 1500 to 2000 live births.[54]

The role of street drugs (amphetamines, barbiturates, narcotics) in the development of congenital anomalies has been difficult to define because of complicating factors such as drug potency and purity, multiple drug use, and the high incidence of perinatal infection and malnutrition among drug abusers.[2] Amphetamines have been implicated as a cause of cleft palate and IUGR. Barbiturate use has been reported to carry an increased risk for cardiac anomalies as well as cleft lip and palate.[54,77] The major effects of narcotics are drug dependency in both mother and fetus, and IUGR. In addition, cocaine use has been associated with an increased risk of abruptio placentae, genitourinary malforma-

tions, limb reduction anomalies, and cardiac defects.[8–10,54,72] Nicotine and caffeine have also been associated with adverse fetal outcome. Nicotine use has been linked to an increased risk of spontaneous abortion, perinatal mortality, and low birth weight. Light smoking (<1 pack per day) was found to increase this risk by 20%; heavy smoking (>1 pack per day) by 35%.[16,37] Excessive caffeine consumption (150 mg/day) has been associated with an increased rate of spontaneous abortion.[66]

Closely associated with drug abuse is the problem of malnutrition. Drug abuse not uncommonly leads to neglect of personal care, including nutrition. Mild degrees of maternal malnutrition have been associated with prematurity, low birth weight, and IUGR.[33] Maternal starvation in early gestation has been reported to be associated with central nervous system abnormalities (spina bifida and hydrocephalus). In later gestation, it can result in IUGR.

The most common nutritional disorder in developed countries is obesity. This is defined as weight 20% above standard for height at the onset of pregnancy.[70,72] Three major antenatal complications of moderate obesity are hypertension, preeclampsia, and gestational diabetes.[58,69] Massive obesity is a major technical problem when cesarean section is indicated.

Sonography has an important role in evaluating fetuses of drug-addicted, malnourished, and obese mothers. A considerable number of fetal structural anomalies can be detected in fetuses exposed to teratogenic agents. Careful sonography with high-resolution equipment can rule out malformations such as hydrocephalus, limb reduction defects, and cardiac anomalies, as early as 17 to 18 weeks of gestation. Serial scans should be performed to follow growth patterns and to detect IUGR or macrosomia. Pregnancies of malnourished or obese patients who require cesarean section can be dated accurately with sonography for correct planning of this procedure.

TABLE 26-3. SONOGRAPHIC FINDINGS IN FETUSES OF MOTHERS WITH DISEASE

Maternal Disease	Sonographic and Associated Findings
Viral Infection	
Cytomegalovirus	Microcephaly, hydrocephaly, cardiac abnormality, IUGR, splenomegaly, ascites, polyhydramnios, hydrops
Herpes simplex	Microcephaly, hydranencephaly, intracranial calcifications, microphthalmia, hepatosplenomegaly, hydrops
Varicella-zoster	IUGR, limb aplasia, microphthalmia, intracranial calcifications
Epstein-Barr	Cardiac, IUGR, microphthalmia
Rubella	Microcephaly, cardiac anomaly, hydrocephaly, cephalocele, agenesis of the corpus callosum
Influenza	Cardiac anomalies
Human immunodeficiency virus	IUGR, hepatomegaly
Bacterial Infection	
Syphilis	Hydrocephaly, iniencephaly, thick placenta, hydrops, osteitis, fetal demise
Gonorrhea	IUGR, oligohydramnios
Urinary tract infection	IUGR, oligohydramnios
Parasitic Infection	
Toxoplasmosis	IUGR, hydrocephaly, microcephaly, cerebral calcification, agenesis of the corpus callosum, hepatosplenomegaly, hydrops
Malaria	IUGR
Endocrine and Metabolic	
Diabetes mellitus	Thickened placenta
Hyperthyroidism	IUGR
Hypothyroidism	Fetal demise, goiter
Hyperparathyroidism	Fetal demise, goiter
Phenylketonuria	Microcephaly, cardiac disease
Hematologic	
Isoimmunization	Pleural and pericardial effusion, ascites, skin thickening, polyhydramnios
Sickle cell anemia	Short femurs, IUGR
Thalassemia	Hydrops
Toxemia	IUGR, oligohydramnios, abruptio placentae, decreased placental volume, early placental maturation, fetal demise
Malnutrition	IUGR, oligohydramnios, decreased placental volume

IUGR, intrauterine growth retardation.

Other Maternal Disorders

Women with cyanotic congenital heart disease have pregnancies with a higher incidence of premature births, IUGR, and abortions.[49] The incidence of congenital heart disease in these infants is also somewhat higher than that in the normal population.

Summary

Pregnancies complicated by maternal disease represent a difficult and challenging problem for the obstetrician. Diagnostic sonography offers a safe and reliable modality for evaluating fetuses at risk for growth retardation and malformations produced by maternal disease (Table 26-3). Technologic advancements, such as Doppler ultrasound, have enhanced our ability to obtain more information about the fetus and to make better diagnoses. Moreover, as invasive obstetric procedures such as PUBS are performed more frequently, sonography is assuming a broader and more significant role in fetal surveillance.

REFERENCES

1. Anyaegbunam A, Langer O, Brustman L, et al. The application of uterine and umbilical artery velocimetry to the antenatal supervision of pregnancies complicated by maternal disease. Am J Obstet Gynecol. 1988; 159:544–547.
2. Beckman DA, Brent RL. Mechanism of known environmental teratogens: Drugs and chemicals. Clin Perinatol. 1986; 13:649–687.
3. Benson RC. Handbook of Obstetrics and Gynecology. 8th ed. Los Altos, CA: Lange Medical Publications; 1983:365.
4. Berkowitz RL, Chitkara U, Goldberg JD, et al. Intravascular transfusion in utero: The percutaneous approach. Am J Obstet Gynecol. 1986; 154:622–623.
5. Burrow GN. Thyroid diseases. In: Burrow GN, Ferris TF, eds. Medical Complications During Pregnancy. 3rd ed. Philadelphia, WB Saunders; 1988.
6. Campbell S, Wilkin D. Ultrasonic measurement of fetal abdomen circumference in the estimation of fetal weight. Br J Obstet Gynaecol. 1975; 82:689.
7. Carroll B. Ultrasound features of preeclampsia. J Clin Ultrasound. 1980; 8:483–488.
8. Chasnoff IJ, Burns WJ, Schnolls, H, et al. Cocaine use in pregnancy. N Engl J Med. 1985; 313:666.
9. Chavez GF, Mulinare J, Cordero JF. Maternal cocaine use and the risk for genitourinary tract defects: An epidemiologic approach. Am J Hum Genet. 1988; 43(Suppl):A43.
10. Cherukuri R, Minkoff H, Feldman J, et al. A cohort study of alkaloidal cocaine ("crack") in pregnancy. Obstet Gynecol. 1988; 72:147–151.
11. Connor EM, McSherry G. Immune-based interventions in perinatal human immunodeficiency virus infection. Pediatr Infect Dis J. 1994; 13:440–448.
12. Creasy RK, Resnick R. Maternal–Fetal Medicine: Principles and Practice. Philadelphia: WB Saunders; 1984:926.
13. Daffos F, Capella-Pavlovsky M, Forestier F. A new procedure for fetal blood sampling in utero: Preliminary results of fifty-three cases. Am J Obstet Gynecol. 1985; 146:985–987.
14. Desforges JF, Warth J. The management of sickle cell disease in pregnancy. Clin Perinatol. 1974; 1:385–394.
15. De Vore GR, Brar HS, Platt LD. Doppler ultrasound in the fetus: A review of current applications. J Clin Ultrasound. 1987; 15:687–703.
16. Di Franza JR, Lew RA. Effect of maternal cigarette smoking on pregnancy complications and sudden infant death syndrome. J Fam Pract. 1995; 40:385–394.
17. Eliezer S, Ester F, Ehud W, et al. Fetal splenomegaly: Ultrasound diagnosis of cytomegalovirus infection: A case report. J Clin Ultrasound. 1984; 12:520–521.
18. Etches PC, Lemons JA. Nonimmune hydrops fetalis: Report of 22 cases including three siblings. Pediatrics. 1979; 64:326–332.
19. Ferris TF. Toxemia and hypertension. In: Burrow GM, Ferris TF, eds. Medical Complications During Pregnancy. 3rd ed. Philadelphia: WB Saunders; 1988.
20. Fleischer AC, Killam AP, Boehm FH, et al. Hydrops fetalis: Sonographic evaluation and clinical implications. Radiology. 1981; 141:163–168.
21. Fleischer G, Bolognese R. EBV infection in pregnancy: A prospective study. J Pediatr. 1984; 104:374.
22. Freij BJ, Sever JL. Herpesvirus infection in pregnancy: Risks to embryo, fetus and neonate. Clin Perinatol. 1988; 15:203–231.
23. Freij BJ, South M, Sever JL. Maternal rubella and the congenital rubella syndrome. Clin Perinatol. 1988; 15:247–257.
24. Friedman DM, Rutkowski M, Synder JR, et al. Doppler blood velocity waveforms in the umbilical artery as an indicator of fetal well-being. J Clin Ultrasound. 1985; 13:161–165.
25. Gill RW. Doppler assessment in obstetrics and fetal

physiology. Clin Diagn Ultrasound. 1984; 13:131–147.

26. Golditch IM, Kirkman K. The large fetus: Management and outcome. Obstet Gynecol. 1978; 52:26–30.

27. Grandjean SH, Saraman MF, DeMouzo J, et al. Detection of gestational diabetes by means of excessive fetal growth. Am J Obstet Gynecol. 1980; 138:790–792.

28. Guy G, Coady DJ, Jansen V, et al. Alpha-thalassemia hydrops fetalis: Clinical and ultrasonographic considerations. Am J Obstet Gynecol. 1985; 153:500–504.

29. Handsfield HH, Hodson WA, Holmes KK. Neonatal gonococcal infections: 1. Orogastric contamination with *Neisseria gonorrhoeae*. JAMA. 1973; 225:697.

30. Houchang D, Modanlou ND, Komatsu G, et al. Large-for-gestational-age neonates: Anthropometric reasons for shoulder dystocia. Obstet Gynecol. 1982; 60:417–423.

31. Icarf J, Didier J, Dalens M, et al. Prospective study of EBV infection during pregnancy. Biomedicine. 1981; 34:160.

32. Kelton JG, Cruickshauk M. Hematologic disorders of pregnancy. In: Burrows GN, Ferris TF, eds. Medical Complications During Pregnancy. 3rd ed. Philadelphia: WB Saunders; 1988.

33. Landon MB, Gabbe SG, Mullen JL. Total parenteral nutrition during pregnancy. Clin Perinatol. 1986; 13:57–72.

34. Lee RV. Parasites and pregnancy: The problems of malaria and toxoplasmosis. Clin Perinatol. 1988; 15:351–363.

35. Lenke RR, Levy HC. Maternal pheylketonuria and hyperphenylalaninemia: An international survey of the outcome of untreated and treated pregnancies. N Engl J Med. 1980; 303:1202.

36. Lindenbaum J, Klipstein FA. Folic acid deficiency in sickle cell anemia. N Engl J Med. 1963; 269:875.

37. Meyer MB, Tonascia JA. Maternal smoking, pregnancy complications and perinatal mortality. Am J Obstet Gynecol. 1977; 128:494–502.

38. Morrison JC, Blake PG, Reed CD. Therapy for the pregnant patient with sickle hemoglobinopathies: A national focus. Am J Obstet Gynecol. 1982; 144:268–269.

39. Nahmias AJ, Josey WE, Naib WE, et al. Perinatal risk associated with maternal genital herpes simplex virus infection. Am J Obstet Gynecol. 1971; 110:825–837.

40. Naib ZM, Nahmias AJ, Josey WE, et al. Association of maternal herpetic infection with spontaneous abortion. Obstet Gynecol. 1970; 35:260–263.

41. National Diabetes Data Group. Classification and diagnosis of diabetes mellitus and other categories of glucose intolerance. Diabetes. 1979; 28:1039.

42. Niebyl JR. Genetics and teratology, drug use in pregnancy. In: Pitkin R, Zlatnik F, eds. 1984 Year Book of Obstetrics and Gynecology. Chicago: Year Book Medical Publishers; 1984.

43. Ogata ES, Sabbagha R, Metzger BE, et al. Serial ultrasonography to assess evolving fetal macrosomia. JAMA. 1980; 243:2405.

44. Olson C. Diagnosis and Management of Diabetes Mellitus. 2nd ed. New York: Raven Press; 1985:181.

45. Page EW, Christianson R. The impact of mean arterial pressure in the middle trimester upon the outcome of pregnancy. Am J Obstet Gynecol. 1976; 125:740–746.

46. Pearce JM, Chamberlain GV. Ultrasonically guided percutaneous umbilical blood sampling in the management of intrauterine growth retardation. Br J Obstet Gynaecol. 1987; 94:318–321.

47. Pedersen J, Molsted-Pedersen L, Andersen B. Assessors of fetal perinatal mortality in diabetic pregnancy: Analysis of 1,332 pregnancies in the Copenhagen series 1946–1972. Diabetes. 1974; 23:302.

48. Perlin BM, Pomerance JJ, Schifrin BS. Nonimmunologic hydrops fetalis. Obstet Gynecol. 1981; 57:584–588.

49. Presbitero P, Somerville J, Stone S, et al. Pregnancy in cyanotic congenital heart disease: Outcome of mother and fetus. Circulation. 1994; 89:2673–2676.

50. Price JM, Fisch AE, Jacobson J. Ultrasound findings in fetal cytomegalovirus infection. J Clin Ultrasound. 1978; 6:268.

51. Queenan JT, O'Brien GD. Diagnostic ultrasound in erythroblastosis fetalis. In: Sanders RC, James AE Jr, eds. Ultrasonography in Obstetrics and Gynecology. 3rd ed. Norwalk, CT: Appleton-Century-Crofts; 1985.

52. Ramsey-Goldman R, Kutzer LH, Guziick D, et al. Previous pregnancy outcome is an important determinant of subsequent pregnancy outcome in women with systemic lupus erythematosis. Am J Reprod Immunol. 1992; 28:195–198.

53. Reece AE, Hobbins JC. Ultrasonography and diabetes mellitus in pregnancy. In: Sanders RC, James AE Jr, eds. Ultrasonography in Obstetrics and Gynecology. 3rd ed. Norwalk, CT: Appleton-Century-Crofts; 1985.

54. Rodgers BD, Lee RV. Drug abuse. In: Burrow GN, Ferris TF, eds. Medical Complications During Pregnancy. 3rd ed. Philadelphia: WB Saunders; 1988.

55. Romero R, Chervenak FA, Berkowitz RL, et al. Intrauterine fetal tachypnea. Am J Obstet Gynecol. 1982; 144:356–357.

56. Roopnarinesingh S, Ramsewaks S. Decreased birth weight and femur length in fetuses of patients with the sickle-cell trait. Obstet Gynecol. 1986; 68:46–48.

57. Rosett HL, Weinger L. Alcohol and the Fetus: A Clinical Perspective. New York: Oxford University Press; 1984.

58. Ruges S, Anderson T. Obstetric risks in obesity: An analysis of the literature. Obstet Gynecol Surv. 1985; 40:57.

59. Saltzman RL, Jordan MC. Viral infections. In: Burrow GN, Ferris TF, eds. Medical Complication During Pregnancy. 3rd ed. Philadelphia: WB Saunders; 1988.

60. Seeds JW, Watson AB. Ultrasound-guided fetal intravascular transfusion in severe rhesus immunization. Am J Obstet Gynecol. 1986; 154:1105–1107.

61. Serjeant GR. Sickle haemoglobin and pregnancy. Br Med J. 1983; 287:628.

62. Sibai BM, Abdella TM, Anderson DG. Pregnancy outcome in 211 patients with mild chronic hypertension. Obstet Gynecol. 1983; 61:571–576.

63. Simmons MA, Battaglia FC, Quilligan EJ. The fetus and newborn. In: Romney SL, Gray JM, Little AB, et al, eds. Gynecology and Obstetrics: The Health Care of Women. New York: McGraw-Hill; 1975: 315.

64. Simpson ML, Graziano EP, Lupo VR, et al. Bacterial infections during pregnancy. In: Burrow GN, Ferris TF, eds. Medical Complications During Pregnancy. 3rd ed. Philadelphia: WB Saunders; 1988.

65. Sokol RJ, Miller SI. Identifying the alcohol abusing obstetric/gynecologic patient: A practical approach. Alcohol Health Res World. 1980; 4:3.

66. Srisuphan W, Braken MB. Caffeine consumption during pregnancy and association with late spontaneous abortion. Am J Obstet Gynecol. 1986; 154:14–20.

67. Strobino BA, Williams CL, et al. Lyme disease and pregnancy outcome: A prospective study of two thousand prenatal patients. Am J Obstet Gynecol. 1993; 69:367–374.

68. Sweet RL. Bacteriuria and pyelonephritis during pregnancy. Semin Perinatol. 1977; 1:25.

69. Temmerman M, Chomba EN, et al. Maternal immunodeficiency virus-1 infection and pregnancy outcome. Obstet Gynecol. 1994; 83:495–501.

70. Treharne L. Obesity in pregnancy. Progress in Obstetrics and Gynecology. 1984; 4:127–138.

71. Trudinger BJ. The umbilical circulation. Semin Perinatol. 1987; 11:311–321.

72. Wall RE. Nutritional problems during pregnancy. In: Abrams RS, Waxler P eds. Medical Care of the Pregnant Patient. Boston: Little, Brown; 1983.

73. Warren PS, Gill RW, Fisher CC. Doppler flow studies in rhesus isoimmunization. Semin Perinatol. 1987; 11:375.

74. Weiner S, Bolognese RJ, Librizzi, DO. Ultrasound in the evaluation and management of the isoimmunized pregnancy. J Clin Ultrasound. 1981; 9:315–323.

75. White JM, Richards B, Byrne M, et al. Thalassemia trait and pregnancy. J Clin Pathol. 1985; 38:810.

76. Wladimiroff JW, Bloemsma CA, Wallenburg HCS. Ultrasonic diagnosis of the large-for-dates infant. Obstet Gynecol. 1978; 52:285–288.

77. Wladimiroff JW, Stewart PA, Reuss A, et al. The role of ultrasound in the early diagnosis of fetal structural defects following maternal anticonvulsant therapy. Ultrasound Med Biol. 1988; 14:657–660.

78. Zeichner SL, Plotkin SA. Mechanisms and pathways of congenital infections. Clin Perinatol. 1988; 15:163–188.

79. Zuspan FP. Hypertensive disorders of pregnancy. In: Pauerstein CJ, ed. Clinical Obstetrics. New York: John Wiley and Sons; 1987:645.

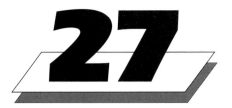

Sonography of the Postpartum Uterus

DIANE M. KAWAMURA

The puerperium is the postpartum period (after parturition), commencing with the expulsion of the placenta and extending to the time when the maternal physiology and anatomy are restored to their approximate prepregnant states.[32] A sonographic examination during the puerperium may be indicated to (1) examine the uterine cavity for the cause of postpartum hemorrhage; (2) evaluate complications such as puerperal infection; (3) determine the extent of postpartum ovarian vein thrombophlebitis; and (4) survey cesarean section incision sites of the uterine and abdominal wall for complications such as hematomas and abscesses.

Normal Postpartum Anatomy and Physiology

The postpartum period lasts 6 to 8 weeks and involves both biochemical and physiologic changes.[40] These changes are a consequence of the withdrawal of luteal and placental estrogen and progesterone, which reverses the morphologic and functional changes of pregnancy, resulting in involution of the uterus.[40] Lactation begins at this time, and when it is discontinued the normal reproductive organ functions, such as ovulation and menstruation, resume.[25,40]

Immediately after delivery the uterus is heavy, and retrodisplacement occurs when the patient lies supine.[43] As involution or contraction progresses, the uterus assumes its normal prepregnant shape and position unless supportive pelvic structures have undergone extensive stretching and tearing due to big infants, difficult forceps delivery, or lacerations.[40,43] The fundus descends from its subxyphoid location to a level just above the umbilicus, assuming a slightly dextroverted position referred to as "physiologic right torsion of the uterus."[32,40] Within 1 week after delivery, rapid uterine involution results in a change in uterine weight from approximately 1100 to 500 g.[32,40] This event also restores the uterus to a position between the symphysis pubis and umbilicus.[32,40]

Under normal conditions, uterine involution is assessed by clinical examination, consisting of external or bimanual palpation.[32,40] In obese patients, patients who are in pain, or patients who have recently undergone surgery (e.g., cesarean section, cholecystectomy), sonography provides a complementary, noninvasive way to follow uterine involution.

Scanning Technique

Selecting the transducer should be based on the sonographer's ability to maintain adequate skin contact with a minimal amount of external pressure and to visualize the pelvic structure interfaces, which are nonperpendicular to the abdominal wall. In the early postpartum period, the uterus is extremely pliable and the normal scanning pressure from routine transabdominal examination can lead to a reduction in the anteroposterior diameter, an increase in the transverse measurement, and diminished visualization of myometrial vessels.[42] As the postpartum period progresses, the degree of uterine distortion from scanning pressure decreases as the spongy consistency diminishes with normal uterine involution.[40]

The preferred transducer is one that is of high enough frequency to provide the best resolution and yet low enough for adequate penetration. The frequency ranges usually selected for transabdominal scanning are 3.5 to 5 MHz, and for endovaginal scanning are 5 to 8 MHz. Improved spatial detail is obtained with an electronically focused sector (phased) transducer.[18] Distention of the urinary bladder is necessary for transabdominal examination of the ovoid puerperal uterus and the pelvic cavity.[32] The time gain compensation or slope should be adjusted to compensate for enhanced sound transmission through the urine-filled bladder.[8]

Visualization and measurement of the entire puerperal uterus require examination of the pelvis in both transverse and sagittal planes transabdominally or in transverse and coronal planes endovaginally.[17] For accurate measurements, it may be necessary to angle the transducer in both transabdominal or endovaginal examinations to obtain a true longitudinal and transverse plane through the uterus when there is the aforementioned physiologic right torsion of the uterus.[17,29,32]

The transperineal scanning technique can be used to augment or complete an examination of a symptomatic patient recovering from a cesarean surgery. If transabdominal scanning is limited because of pain caused by scanning pressure on the incision site or when there is bleeding or oozing of the incisional site, transperineal scanning can provide an image, although with a limited field of view, of the lower uterine segment. This technique does not allow adequate imaging of the body and fundus of the enlarged postpartum uterus. Ultrasonic gel is placed on a 2.25- to 3.5-MHz transducer. A commercial plastic wrap is placed over the transducer and more gel is applied. The patient position is the same as for an endovaginal examination, but the transducer is positioned on the perineum between

the labia majora[21] and is adjusted best to demonstrate images of the vagina, cervix, and lower uterine segment as well as subfascial tissue.[20] The transperineal approach does not require a full bladder technique, but a moderate amount of fluid in the urinary bladder allows differentiation of the region anterior to the uterine incision from soft tissue located anterior to the bladder.[20]

Sonographic Appearance of Normal Postpartum Anatomy

UTERUS

Bimanual examination alone may not be sufficient precisely to determine postpartum uterine size.[39] Sonography not only permits reliable measurement of uterine dimensions but provides a noninvasive method that allows multiple follow-up studies to establish physiologic and pathologic changes.[13,34,39]

Uterine involution has been assessed with sonography by several investigators.[13,23,25,27,34,39] The postpartum uterus can assume varying shapes, from long and narrow to short and wide, and can produce a wide range of measurements in each dimension. The endometrial cavity shape, however, remains the same, eventually appearing as an inverted triangle in all patients.[34] On day 1, the internal os may be open and ill defined compared to its appearance on subsequent days.[34]

In the anteroposterior dimension, the uterine myometrium is homogeneous in echogenicity and is 3 to 6.5 cm in thickness.[27] The range for total uterine thickness is 7 to 10 cm.[27] Prominent myometrial vessels can be sonographically visualized within the normal uterine wall.[25] The endometrial cavity appears as a central linear echogenicity with an anteroposterior thickness measurement as great as 5 to 13 mm initially, but involuting to 0.3 to 0.6 mm within 10 postpartum days.[27,40] An anechoic separation of the internal endometrial walls (because of residual blood or serous fluid[17]) can normally be seen measuring up to 1.3 cm.[32] Focal areas of greater separation are considered abnormal.[32]

Uterine length after delivery ranges from 14.5 to 25 cm, decreasing as the puerperium advances.[25,27,34,39] In the early postpartum period, when uterine size is still relatively large and the organ arches over the sacrum, uterine length can be determined by summing segmental measurements to determine the true length.[42] The uterine width is measured at right angles to the sagittal measurement at the widest uterine segment. The maximum width measurement of the uterus has been reported as 7 to 14 cm[25,27,34,39] (Fig. 27-1). Errors in uterine measurements are associated with: (1) the degree of bladder filling, which influences the cavity distance between the fundus and the internal os[34]; (2) external scanning pressure from a hand-held transabdominal transducer[42]; (3) location of the points of measurement; and (4) uterine contractions.[34,42]

In a study conducted by Wachsberg and colleagues,[42] normal measurements in the first postpartum month were slightly larger with increasing maternal parity. Several studies have noted that there is no difference in regression size between breast-feeding and bottle-feeding mothers,[25,26,32,39,42] or in relationship to infant birth weight.[42] Table 27-1 provides the normal range of postpartum sonographic measurements presented in the literature.[13,23,25,34,39,42]

ADNEXA

The eight ligaments supporting the uterus are flaccid after delivery but assume normal prepregnancy firmness within a few weeks.[40] Of these, only the

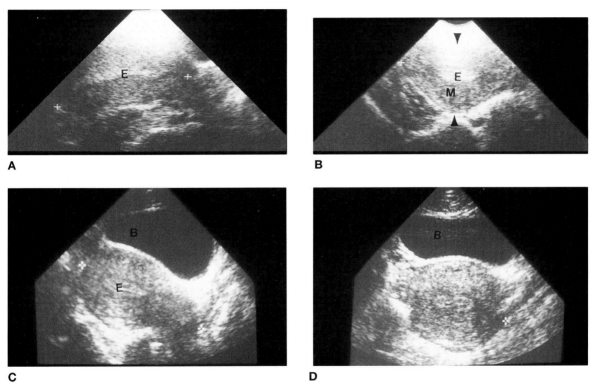

Figure 27-1. (**A** and **B**) A normal uterus is imaged on a 2-day postpartum patient. (**A**) The sagittal section demonstrates an endometrial cavity distance of 12.5 cm (between cursors). In this early postpartum stage, the uterus arches over the sacrum. The most accurate method of determining the true length is to sum two or more segmental measurements of the arched endometrium, which appears as a central linear echogenicity (E, endometrium). (**B**) The transverse section demonstrates the widest measurement of 10.7 cm (between cursors; E, endometrium; M, myometrium). The black arrowheads indicate the location for an anteroposterior measurement. (**A** and **B** courtesy of Tamara Salsgiver, RDMS, Hill Air Force Base, Ogden, UT.) (**C** and **D**) A normal uterus is imaged on a 3 weeks' postpartum patient. Moderate global uterine enlargement is identified on both the sagittal and transverse sections. (**C**) Uterine length measures 10.9 cm (cursors) on the sagittal section (E, endometrium). (**D**) The transverse section measured 7.1 cm (cursors; B, urinary bladder). (**C** and **D** courtesy of Catherine Carr-Hoefer, RT(R), RDMS, RDCS, Good Samaritan Hospital, Corvallis, OR.)

▨▨▨ **TABLE 27-1. RANGES OF NORMAL SONOGRAPHIC POSTPARTUM MEASUREMENTS**[13,23,25,34,39,42]

Structure	Dimensions (cm)
Anteroposterior thickness	
Endometrium	0.4–1.3
Myometrium	3.0–6.5
Uterus	7.0–10.0
Length (sagittal measurement)	14.5–25.0
Width (transverse measurement)	7.0–14.0

broad ligaments and their components can occasionally be visualized sonographically in the puerperal patient. To avoid any confusion with a pathologic abnormality, it is important to recognize the broad ligaments and their components when they are imaged.[32] As the uterus regresses, the adnexa become more readily identifiable.[25]

The ovaries can be demonstrated approximately 50% of the time on routine scanning.[25] During the first trimester, ovaries frequently present with cysts. After the first trimester, the ovaries regress in volume as the cysts disappear, and do not undergo any significant size or contour change during the remainder of the pregnancy.[24]

Postpartum Pathology

POSTPARTUM HEMORRHAGE

Postpartum hemorrhage is defined as blood loss exceeding 500 ml.[40] It occurs after less than 5% of all deliveries but is potentially the most lethal complication of the puerperium, accounting for 35% of maternal deaths.[32,41,43] Death can be prevented with immediate blood replacement.[43] Acute postpartum hemorrhage occurs within the first 24 hours; delayed postpartum hemorrhage occurs between days 2 and 31 of the puerperium.[40]

Predisposing Factors

Uterine muscles must contract rapidly and firmly after delivery to occlude the uterine vessels at the point of placental separation. Factors that delay contraction and interfere with the normal mechanisms that control bleeding are listed in Table 27-2.

Etiology

The most common causes of acute hemorrhage are uterine atony and soft tissue injury. Delayed hemorrhage is most commonly caused by retained secundines (i.e., products of conception such as the placenta, umbilical cord, and fetal membranes) or subinvolution (local endometritis) at the former placental site.

Acute Hemorrhage

After the placenta separates from the maternal decidua spongiosa, uterine bleeding is initially controlled by uterine contraction and compression of blood vessels at the site of separation. The healing process produces lochia, a copious (dark red-brown) exudate, which is discharged through the vagina. Uterine atony is the failure of the uterus to contract after delivery. Treatments for acute postpartum hemorrhage due to uterine atony include keeping the patient in a supine position, manual uterine massage, and intravenous oxytocin.[40]

Sonographically, there is no significant difference between the size or shape of the uterus of patients with uterine atony and of those with a normal postpartum uterus.[27,32] Therefore, if the sonographic appearance is that of a normal postpartum uterus and no retained products of conception are identified, uterine atony must be considered the most likely cause for the hemorrhage.[32] Acute postpartum hemorrhage can also result from torn blood vessels in soft tissue lacerations of the cervix, vagina, or perineum or from hematomas located in the uterus or adnexa.[43,46] If bleeding continues after treatment, sonography can be used to investigate the cause of this prolonged hemorrhage.

Delayed Hemorrhage

Retention of secundines and subinvolution are the leading causes of delayed postpartum hemorrhage. Uterine subinvolution is a localized form of endometritis that contributes to continued delay in the normal regression of the uterus. The sonographic appearance is the same as that of uterine atony, and so is the treatment.

With retained secundines, the uterine cavity remains distended and bleeding continues at the previous placental attachment site. Retained products of conception produce variable sonographic appearances, depending on the type of tissue retained

▨◢ TABLE 27-2. PREDISPOSING FACTORS TO POSTPARTUM PATHOLOGIES

Complication	Predisposing Factors
Postpartum hemorrhage	Delayed contraction if the uterus: 1. emptied very rapidly; 2. has been overdistended (large infant, multiple gestation, or hydramnios), causing muscle fibers to be stretched excessively; 3. does not contract normally because the patient received deep inhalation anesthesia; 4. was manipulated or massaged in an attempt to expel the placenta before it was completely separated; 5. retains a large fragment or a succenturiate lobe of the placenta; and when there is a history of postpartum bleeding of unknown cause in a multipara.[43]
Postpartum infection	1. Poor nutrition and hygiene; 2. prepartum and postpartum anemia; 3. vaginitis or cervicitis; 4. coitus late in pregnancy; 5. toxemia; 6. prolonged labor; 7. prolonged rupture or membranes; 8. frequent internal examination during labor; 9. use of invasive (intrapartum) fetal and maternal monitoring devices; 10. lacerations resulting from spontaneous or operative vaginal delivery; 11. manual removal of the placenta; 12. cesarian section; and 13. retention of secundines.[31,40,43]
Postpartum ovarian vein thrombophlebitis	1. Endometritis; 2. increasing age and parity; 3. obesity; 4. previous history of thromboembolism; 5. administration of high estrogen doses to suppress lactation; 6. heart disease; and 7. anemia.[30,39]
Cesarean section	1. Protracted operation time; 2. amniotic fluid bacterial contamination before surgery or other preexisting infection; 3. duration of labor; 4. number of vaginal examinations; 5. length of internal fetal monitoring; 6. estimated blood loss; 7. obesity; and 8. surgery as a result of labor dystocia (difficult labor associated with either a large fetus or too small a maternal pelvis[38]).[14]

and its degree of necrosis at the time of the examination.[27] Two separate studies[19,22] concluded that an intrauterine space-occupying collection should be judged as retained products of conception. In symptomatic patients evaluated after a first trimester spontaneous abortion, pathologically proven retained products of conception were associated with the sonographic findings of an intrauterine gestational sac-like structure or a space-occupying collection within the endometrial cavity.[14] Products of conception were found in 14% of the cases with an endometrial stripe measurement less than 2 mm in the anteroposterior dimension, in 43% of the cases with an endometrial stripe measurement between 2 and 5 mm in the anteroposterior dimension, and in 100% of the cases with an endometrial stripe measurement greater than 5 mm in the anteroposterior dimension[22] (Fig. 27-2). There were no

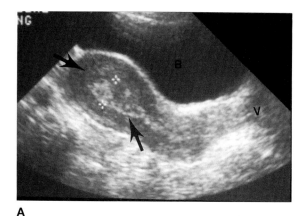

A

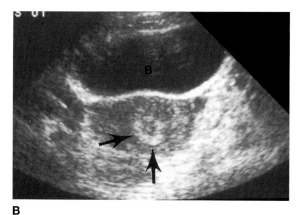

B

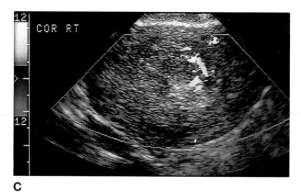

C

Figure 27-2. This patient was referred after a dilation and curettage procedure to terminate an 18-week anencephalic pregnancy. Two passes obtained large amounts of clot. The sonograms demonstrate a complex, primarily hyperechoic mass in the endometrial canal. This appearance could represent blood or infection, but the color flow Doppler scan is highly suspect for residual trophoblast. (**A**) A transabdominal sagittal midline section showing a 1.6-cm (cursors), primarily hyperechoic ovoid collection in the endometrium (*arrows*; B, urinary bladder). (**B**) The ovoid collection is clearly identified in a transabdominal transverse section (*arrows*; B, urinary bladder). (**C**) A color flow Doppler coronal endovaginal section demonstrates the nature of blood flow in the collection. (See also Color Plate 20.) (**A–C** courtesy of Stephanie Ellingson, BA, RT(R), RDMS, The University of Iowa Hospital and Clinics, Iowa City, IA.)

pathologically proven retained products of conception in symptomatic patients evaluated after a second or third trimester delivery who either had a normal linear pattern of endometrial echoes or had endometrial fluid; however, 90% of the cases with an echogenic mass had pathologically proven retained products of conception.[19] In a transvaginal duplex Doppler study on postpartum and postabortion patients with excessive hemorrhage suspected of having residual trophoblast,[1] the resistance index (RI) in the myometrial vessels was significantly higher in patients without residual trophoblast (RI > 0.35) than in patients with confirmed residual trophoblast (RI < 0.35)[1] (Fig. 27-3). With further research, duplex Doppler may prove to aid in the differentiation between retained products of conception and intrauterine blood clots with decidual debris.

Echogenic foci present within the endometrial cavity after such instrumentations as dilation and curettage or dilation and evacuation may be due to the introduction of air by the instrumentation instead of being evidence of retained placenta. Echogenic foci may obscure an existing intrauterine mass or the foci may be mistaken for either echogenic fragments of retained placenta or air produced by gas-forming organisms.[19]

In cases of postpartum hemorrhage, sonography provides valuable information for narrowing the differential diagnostic possibilities of the cause. Even though sonographic appearances are not tissue specific, the sonographic examination can delineate normal and abnormal structures and determine the presence of a mass, its organ of origin, and its internal consistency. The sonographic appearances of lesions that can cause hemorrhage are listed in Table 27-3.

PUERPERAL INFECTION

Puerperal infection occurs in 6 to 8 mothers per 100,000 and accounts for approximately 20% of maternal deaths.[41] It should be suspected when the postpar-

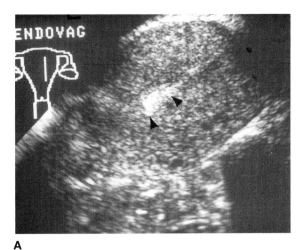

A

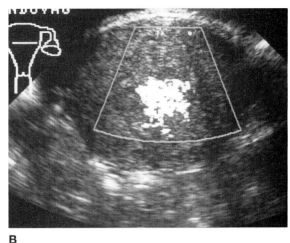

B

Figure 27-3. This patient presented 3 weeks postpartum with bleeding. The enlarged uterus demonstrates heterogenous endometrial echoes. (**A**) Endovaginal sagittal section through the left endometrium demonstrates an intrauterine space occupying collection with echogenic foci (*arrowheads*). (**B**) On a transverse section, the collection measures 7.6 cm and the color flow Doppler scan through the heterogenous collection demonstrates increased flow. (**C**) On duplex Doppler, the heterogenous collection is highly suspect for being residual trophoblast with a low-impedance flow resulting in a low resistance index (0.29). (**A–C** courtesy of Catherine Carr-Hoefer, RT(R), RDMS, RDCS, Good Samaritan Hospital, Corvallis, OR.)

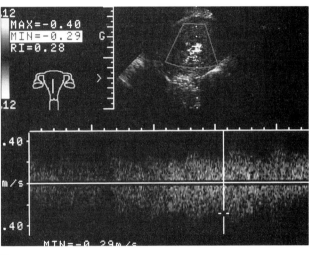

C

tum patient experiences elevated body temperatures of 38°C (100.4°F) or greater on any 2 of the first 10 postpartum days (not including the first day of fever).[41] Certain factors increase the risk of infection, but they do so inconsistently[43] (see Table 27-2).

Etiology

The vagina is the most common route of infection into the uterine cavity. The normal acidity of the vagina prevents many pathogens from proliferating within the uterus, but after the rupture of membranes and parturition, the amniotic fluid, blood, and lochia have a neutralizing effect and the vagina becomes alkaline, providing an environment conducive to the growth of bacteria and other microor-

ganisms.[41] Vaginal bacteria and microorganisms can readily enter the uterine cavity. Seventy percent of puerperal infections are caused by anaerobic bacteria, and the remaining 30% are caused by aerobic microorganisms. The devitalized intrauterine tissues, especially the thrombosed uteroplacental vessels, provide a congenial culture site that can allow the spread of infection outside the uterus and result in parametritis, septic pelvic thrombophlebitis, femoral thrombophlebitis, peritonitis, and pulmonary infarct or abscess (septic embolus).[41]

In most cases, puerperal infections are treated with antibiotics. Clinically, it is difficult to distinguish between urinary tract infections and endometritis[32] because both may present with either nega-

TABLE 27-3. SONOGRAPHIC APPEARANCE OF POSTPARTUM PATHOLOGY

Complication	Sonographic Appearance
Hemorrhage due to:	
Retained products	Endometrial cavity echogenic and expanded with round, oval, or lobulated intracavitary tissues; stippled echo pattern; may have hyperechoic foci, with or without associated acoustic shadowing or ring-down; may have fluid within the uterine cavity
Local endometritis	Normal postpartum appearance except for size; uterus fails to return to normal postpartum size owing to imperfect involution
Uterine atony	Appearance of normal postpartum uterus with expanded and echogenic endometrial cavity
Endometritis	In advanced stages, separation of uterine cavity walls by anechoic space with smooth or irregular margins; may have echogenic shadows due to gas formation
Puerperal ovarian vein thrombophlebitis	Anechoic to hypoechoic round to oval mass in mid- to upper retroperitoneum; Doppler shows limited blood flow
Bladder flap hematoma	Complex mass, poorly defined borders, primarily anechoic with internal septations or debris located at junction of uterus and bladder measuring 2.5 to 15 cm
Cesarean section hematoma	Anechoic to hypoechoic, smooth or irregular masses in the incision site area
Cesarean section abscess	Echogenic, smooth or irregular masses; may have hyperechoic areas with shadowing, indicating gas formation

tive blood cultures or with elevated white blood cell count. In the event of worsening patient condition resulting from the puerperal infection, a curettage procedure may be performed if retention of secundines is suspected. If no improvement is observed with curettage and antibiotic therapy, the findings suggest infectious myometrial necrosis (gangrene), and a hysterectomy may be performed.[41]

Endometritis

After delivery, endometritis develops in 3% to 4% of all women and in 13% to 27% of those who are delivered by cesarean section.[41] Endometritis results from retention of secundines or from vaginal microorganisms contaminating the uterine cavity, usually with a mixed flora of both anaerobic and aerobic pathogens.[32,41]

The sonographic appearances of retained secundines and endometritis can overlap.[32] In mild to moderate intrauterine infections, endometritis is not detectable sonographically. In advanced stages, sonographic examination should demonstrate widening of the uterine cavity because of inflammation and contained exudate.[28] The endometrial cavity may be imaged as an anechoic space that has either smooth or irregular margins[4] (Fig. 27-4A,B). The normal postpartum uterus can also present with an anechoic separation representing blood or serous fluid in the endometrial cavity, supporting the need to correlate sonographic appearance and clinical evidence of endometritis[4] (see Fig. 27-4C–E). With pyometra, pus fills the endometrial canal. The contained endometrial fluid may or may not be echogenic. Pyometra is rare, with a reported incidence of 0.5% in all gynecologic patients, including patients presenting with postpartum endometritis.[11] When presented with an image of endometrial separation, the sonographer can make a substantial contribution to the diagnostic process by knowing that the normal range of postpartum endometrial cavity measurements is 0.4 to 1.3 cm[13,23,25,34,39,42] (see Table 27-1).

Before any surgical manipulations, the presence of gas in the endometrial cavity of a patient suspected of puerperal infection is most commonly caused by gas-forming microorganisms. The sonographic examination to rule out endometritis should be performed before curettage because air can be introduced into the uterine cavity during surgical manipulation.[32] Air produces echogenic streaks and ring-down on ultrasound (see Table 27-3).

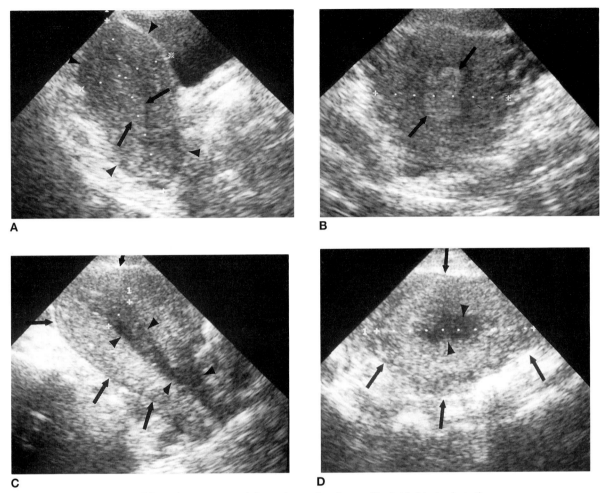

Figure 27-4. (A and **B)** This patient presented 6 weeks postpartum with right-sided adnexal and hypogastric pain. Because the patient was anovulatory (6 weeks postpartum), the small amounts of free fluid in the pelvis seen on other images were considered abnormal. Sonographically, this fluid cannot be differentiated as serous, inflammatory, or hemorrhagic, but should be correlated with the patient's clinical presentation. The ovaries, vasculature, and abdominal organs were all normal. **(A)** The sagittal midline section shows the anteverted postpartum uterus (*arrowheads*) to be well within normal measurements (8.9 cm sagittal × 6.8 cm transverse × 4.8 cm anteroposterior). The normal myometrial echoes are homogeneous, symmetrically surrounding a thickened (1.2 cm) endometrium (*arrows*). Although this appearance is consistent with the secretory menstrual phase, the patient is not pregnant, has a negative serum β-human chorionic gonadotropin, and is anovulatory. **(B)** Noted on the transverse section is the thickened endometrium. When correlated with the patient's history, the sonographic appearance could represent either blood or pus. **(C–E)** This postcesarean section patient presented with fever, chills, and severe pelvic pain with tenderness directly over the uterus. The patient was treated with antibiotics. The uterine cavity was dilated, fluid-filled, and contained amorphous echoes that may represent retained products of conception or blood clots. Because of the patient's history, associated endometritis was considered in the differential diagnosis. **(C)** The uterus (*arrows*) in the sagittal section measures 13.5 cm in length and 7.4 cm anteroposteriorly. The endometrial cavity is dilated to 1.9 cm anteroposterior diameter (*arrowheads*) and contains amorphous echoes. **(D)** In the transverse section, the uterus (*arrows*) measures 9.6 cm. The fluid-filled cavity (*arrowheads*) containing amorphous echoes can be identified. (*continued on next page*)

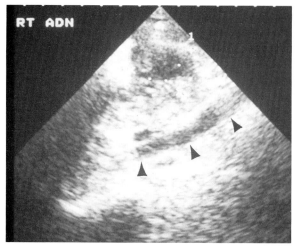

E

Figure 27-4. (CONTINUED) (**E**) In the right adnexa, an ill-defined mass is seen measuring approximately 4.5 × 2.7 × 2.8 cm (cursors) that was thought to represent the right ovary or a mass. A somewhat tubular-shaped, anechoic structure was identified posteriorly. Differential diagnoses included an infected cyst, hydrosalpinx, pyosalpinx, or a pelvic abscess. (**A–E** courtesy of Barbara Abney, RDMS, Carol Benoit, Sandra Bringhurst, RDMS, LDJ Hospital, Salt Lake City, UT.)

OVARIAN VEIN THROMBOPHLEBITIS

Thrombophlebitis is inflammation of a vein secondary to the formation of a contained thrombus. Postpartum ovarian vein thrombophlebitis (POVT) is an uncommon complication of the puerperium. The prevalence is 1 in 2000 to 1 in 600 (0.05% to 0.18%) pregnancies,[2,12] and 1% to 2% after cesarean section.[9,35] Thromboembolic disease remains a major cause of maternal mortality.[31]

Etiology and Predisposing Factors

The pathogenesis of POVT is related to Virchow's triad: (1) the natural hypercoagulability of blood during pregnancy and the puerperium, (2) venous stasis of blood, and (3) alterations in the vein walls.[32,33,37,40] The incidence among patients delivered by cesarean section is probably increased because they are immobilized longer and the risk of thrombus is thus greater.[40] POVT is a significant, life-threatening postpartum sequela to metritis.[9,33,35,38,40,43,44] In most cases, uterine infection and anaerobic streptococci are present or are suspected before the onset of POVT symptoms.[32,33,40,43]

Thrombus formation can be secondary to injury during delivery or to the effect of bacterial inflammation and toxins on the endothelium of the blood vessels of the pelvis, vagina, perineum, and superficial muscle of the legs. Other predisposing factors are listed in Table 27-2.

The ovarian veins are predominantly involved in puerperal pelvic thrombophlebitis, but the disease process can extend into or be isolated to the pelvic and femoral veins.[3] POVT has a 90% right-sided preponderance.[12,16] The right ovarian vein is involved more often than the left, probably because of compression from normal uterine dextrorotation during pregnancy and early postpartum,[9,33,37] and its greater length than the left ovarian vein. The ovarian veins contain multiple incompetent valves that may be sites of venous stasis, providing a nidus for thrombus development.[16]

Symptoms

The POVT syndrome is difficult to diagnose clinically because consistent findings are noted in only about half of the affected patients.[9,33] The most remarkable and dependable physical finding is a palpable lower abdominal mass. Unilateral lower abdominal pain, tenderness, fever, and an elevated pulse rate related to the fever are the most frequent symptoms.[33,43] Nausea, vomiting, and bowel ileus are noted less commonly.[33] These symptoms are usually experienced within the first few days after delivery. The pain can radiate to the groin, flank, or the costophrenic angle.[43]

Diagnosis

Sectional imaging contributes significantly to the diagnosis of POVT. Before the availability of sonography, computed tomography (CT), and magnetic resonance imaging (MRI), POVT was diagnosed indirectly by intravenous pyelography or venography.

Sonography, CT, and MRI have been shown to be reliable and accurate methods of detecting POVT and for monitoring patients with proven POVT.[16] CT remains the method of choice because of its sensitivity and specificity for the diagnosis.[35,37,38] Sonography can be used to make the diagnosis, but its role is secondary because of its inability directly to image the full length of the right ovarian vein because of overlying bowel gas or ileus.[16] At present, MRI is used as an adjunct to sonography

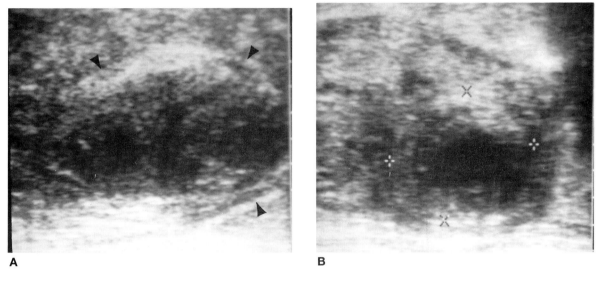

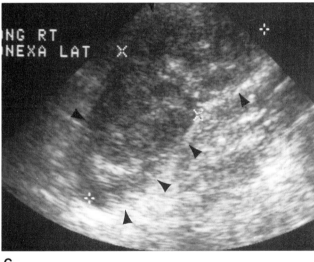

Figure 27-5. (**A** and **B**) A 29-year-old presented with nausea, vomiting, right flank pain, and a 20,000 white blood cell count 4 days after delivering triplets at 35 weeks' gestation. The transverse (**A**) and sagittal (**B**) sections made in the right lower quadrant demonstrated a complex, mostly hypoechoic mass in the right adnexal region measuring 3.0 × 2.3 × 0.3 cm. On the transverse image, the structure has a laminated appearance with surrounding echogenic fat (*arrowheads* on **A**). The typical sonographic appearance of an inflamed appendix was not visualized. An exploratory laparotomy procedure provided the diagnosis of ovarian vein thrombosis. (**C**) This is a 32-year-old woman, G5P3, 8 days postpartum with right lower quadrant pain, fever, and a palpable mass. The sonographic examination demonstrated increased ovarian size with an adnexal mass most consistent with ovarian vein thrombosis. The mass measured 3.4 × 8.5 cm (*arrowheads*). An exploratory laparotomy one day after sonographic examination provided the diagnosis of an edematous right ovary, a fallopian tube three times normal size, and an 8 × 10 cm mass in the right broad ligament containing thrombosed vessels by biopsy. (**A–C** courtesy of Stephanie Ellingson, BA, RT(R), RDMS, The University of Iowa Hospital and Clinics, Iowa City, IA.)

or CT. Coronal MRI scans can demonstrate the full extent of ovarian vein involvement.[37]

With current and future equipment improvements, sonographic evaluation has great potential for becoming the imaging modality of choice.[33] Sonographically, a thrombosed ovarian vein has the appearance of an anechoic to hypoechoic, round to oval mass in the middle to upper retroperitoneum[2,37] (see Table 27-3; Fig. 27-5). In scanning, the sonographer must make every effort to demonstrate the phlebitic vein from the adnexal area to the suprarenal inferior vena cava.[35,37]

Doppler evaluation of deep abdominal vessels documents vascular flow and can be used adjunctively to diagnosis POVT and to follow flow restoration after treatment.[37] In the acute stage of POVT, duplex Doppler imaging may demonstrate absence of flow in these veins.[7]

The leading sonographic pitfall in scanning symptomatic patients is that POVT can sonographically (and clinically) mimic appendicitis.[2,16] The ultrasonographic differential diagnoses includes appendicitis, ovarian torsion, tuboovarian abscess, pelvic abscess, broad ligament hematoma, and volvulus of the bowel.[32,35,37,38,44]

Treatment

A conservative approach is used in the treatment of POVT. The patient is given antibiotics and anticoagulation therapy. Surgical intervention is associated with significant mortality and is indicated in some cases only after failure of conservative therapy.[44] Septic pulmonary emboli may develop in as many as one third of patients with POVT.[9]

Cesarean Section Complications

In many high-risk centers in the United States, 15% to 20% of deliveries are by cesarean section.[6,30] In an effort to reduce this number and allow patients to deliver vaginally in the future, a transverse incision of the lower uterine segment is commonly used.[5,30] The sonographic appearance of the incision is variable and is related to local tissue reaction and to the type of suture material used.[6,10,32] Interposed between the lower uterine segment and the posterior urinary bladder wall, it is normal for it to be seen as (1) a symmetric region of distinct echogenicity generated by the suture material; (2) a region of medium-intensity echoes, relative to the myometrium, surrounding the suture material; (3) an anechoic area anterior to the wound between the uterus and bladder; or (4) anechoic areas both at the wound site and anterior to it.[4,6,32]

HEMATOMAS

During a cesarean section, the surgeon incises the vesicouterine reflection of the peritoneum to obtain access to the lower uterine segment. This creates a potential space between the bladder and uterus, commonly known as the bladder flap[45] (Fig. 27-6). If hemostasis is not obtained after closure of the uterine incision, a hematoma forms between the lower uterine segment and the urinary bladder (bladder flap)[5] or anywhere the surgical scalpel made an incision (e.g., abdominal wall, muscle).[26]

A patient with a hematoma can present with an elevated temperature, a mass, or dropping hematocrit. An infected hematoma can manifest itself with the same symptoms, but the patient can also have leukocytosis and more pain. The elevated temperature can be caused by the infected hematoma alone or by postsurgical complications such as endometritis, septic thrombophlebitis, abscess, hematoma, or wound infection.[45]

The incidence of bladder flap hematoma is un-

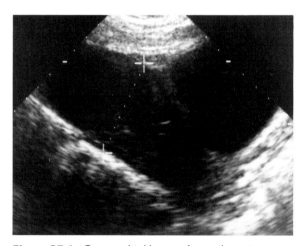

Figure 27-6. *On a sagittal image, 1-month postcesarean section of a normal uterus (U) measuring 11.5 cm in length and 5.6 cm anteroposteriorly, echogenic densities in the myometrium (arrowheads) represent suture material. The contour of the uterus is broken at the incision site (arrow), the potential area for a bladder flap hematoma (B, urinary bladder). (Courtesy of Helen Johnson, RDMS, Cottonwood Hospital, Murray, UT.)*

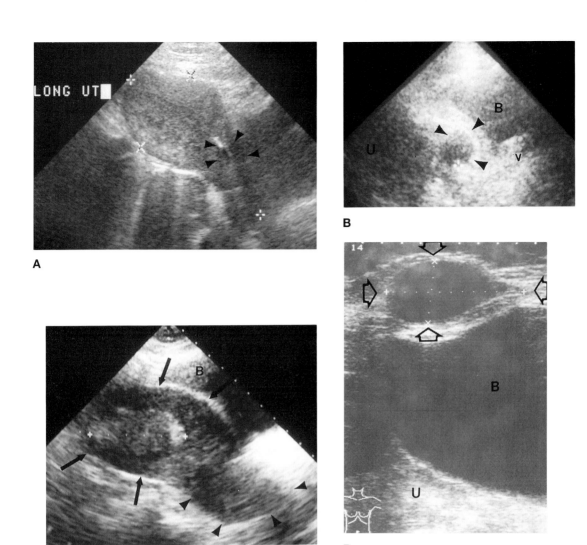

A

B

C

D

Figure 27-7. (**A**) This sagittal section is of a 6-week postcesarean section patient with a persistently large uterus (10.6 cm in length, 4.9 cm anteroposteriorly, and 7.8 cm transverse) and heavy bleeding. The homogeneous prominent uterus (cursors) appears empty and the endometrial cavity line is thin (0.6 cm) down to the level of the lower uterine segment, posterior to the region of the cesarean incision. The lower uterine segment is enlarged with internal echogenic and anechoic areas measuring approximately 1.6 cm in length and 0.8 cm in width (*arrowheads*). The echogenic appearance could represent calcified retained products of conception or calcified hematoma. The hypoechoic area may represent a bladder flap hematoma. (Courtesy of JoDee Pundt, BS, RDMS, LDS Hospital, Salt Lake City, UT.) (**B**) On this patient's images, between the uterus (U) and the urinary bladder (B), an anechoic mass (*arrowheads*) could represent a bladder flap hematoma or a local abscess. An abscess correlates with leukocytosis, whereas a hematoma correlates with dropping hematocrit. Without the patient's laboratory values, either an abscess or a hematoma is included in the differential diagnosis (v, vagina). (**C**) This patient presented with low pelvic tenderness postcesarean section. A prominent uterus (*arrows*) measures 10.8 cm in length, 4.6 cm anteroposteriorly and 5.8 cm transverse. The endometrial cavity is markedly hyperechoic and expanded, and contains a lobulated mass (cursors) representing endometritis, infected or noninfected hematomas, or retained secundines. A small amount of fluid in the pelvis surrounds the uterus. A large solid mass is seen posterior on a sagittal section made to the right of midline that is consistent with an intrapelvic hematoma (*arrowheads*) or an infected hematoma (B, urinary bladder). Correlating these findings to the patient's laboratory values aids in the differential of a hematoma (dropping hematocrit) or an infected hematoma (dropping hematocrit with leukocytosis). (**B** and **C** courtesy of Susan Olson, LDS Hospital, Salt Lake City, UT.) (**D**) A subfascial hematoma (*arrowheads*) measuring 7.2 cm transverse by 3.2 cm anteroposteriorly is seen on a postcesarean delivery patient. The uterine measurements were normal.

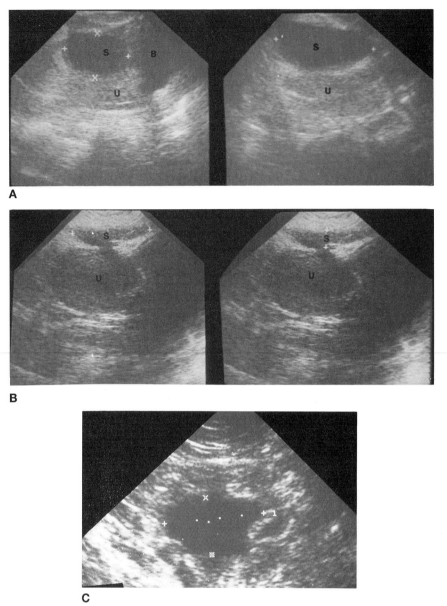

A

B

C

Figure 27-8. (**A**) The sagittal (*left*) and transverse (*right*) sections on a 21-year-old, postcesarean patient with a clinical history of fever and anemia demonstrates an anechoic mass representing a bladder flap seroma (S) measuring 5.6 cm in length, 3.9 cm in thickness, and 8.7 cm in width. An aspiration was performed on both the seroma and on a subfascial (abdominal wall) wound abscess (U, uterus; B, bladder). (**B**) The sonographic findings on the same patient on an 18-day follow-up demonstrates the seroma (S) is a more heterogenous collection and measures 6.6 cm in length (*left*) and 1.5 cm in thickness (*right;* U, uterus). (**A** and **B** courtesy of sonographers, Kings County Hospital, Brooklyn, NY.) (**C**) This 30-year-old patient presented with severe lower abdominal pain and fever 11 days postcesarean section and hysterectomy. This transverse image demonstrates a primarily cystic mass measuring 4.4 cm transverse by 2.4 cm anteroposteriorly (cursors). The mass was located more in the right adnexal region than near midline. Based on sonographic appearance alone, the contents cannot be distinguished as blood or pus.

known and the sonographic appearances described in the literature vary significantly, and include a mass as great as $15 \times 12 \times 9$ cm (length $\times$ width $\times$ height).[5,45] Most bladder flap hematomas are complex masses with poorly defined borders that are primarily anechoic with contained internal septations or debris[45] (see Table 27-3; Fig. 27-7A).

Because it is not possible to differentiate sonographically between a hematoma, an infected hematoma, and an abscess, the patient's clinical presentation is important.[5,32,45] A symptomatic patient with a clinical history of leukocytosis suggests an abscess; a dropping hematocrit, a hematoma; and a dropping hematocrit with leukocytosis, an infected hematoma. Figure 27-7B and C demonstrates the importance of obtaining laboratory values and of having the patient's clinical history.

If there is a hematoma suspected near the incisional site of the abdominal wall, a high frequency and a standoff pad may be required to examine the superficial area. This area may be more difficult to examine because of incisional pain and tenderness. To distinguish between a superficial wound versus a subfascial hematoma, the rectus muscle must be identified. Superficial hematomas are located anterior to the rectus muscle and a subfascial hematoma is located posterior to it.[36] The typical location for a subfascial hematoma is in the prevesicular space, ventral to the bladder[15,20,36] (see Fig. 27-7D). Based on sonographic appearance, a superficial hematoma or a subfascial hematoma may appear the same as an abscess or an infected hematoma.[24]

INFECTIONS

A wound infection develops in approximately 5% of patients after cesarean section.[14] Factors that contribute to wound infection are included in Table 27-2.

Hypoechoic masses in the area of the incision in afebrile patients probably represent small seromas or hematomas that develop as a normal surgical complication[32] (Fig. 27-8A,B). In febrile patients, fluid collections may represent abscess, especially if strong echoes with associated acoustic shadowing are seen, indicative of an abscess with gas formation[32] (see Table 27-3).

Wound infection can develop in the uterine incision and in the abdominal wall incision from the same vaginal microorganisms that cause infected endometritis.[14] Abdominal wall disorders can be difficult to detect clinically because of tenderness and induration due to edema.[32] At various stages, seromas, hematomas, and abscesses can have similar sonographic appearances.

In addition to incision wound infections, abscess formations can also occur deep in the pelvis, in the broad ligament, or in the cul-de-sac. These cesarean section complications can appear anechoic, primarily cystic with internal echoes, without a wall or margin (abscess), or with a wall or margin of varying degrees of thickness (phlegmon)[24] (see Fig. 27-8C). Sonographically, there may be no distinction between an abscess formation, an infected hematoma, or a sterile hematoma. CT may provide a more global view of the abdominopelvic contents.

Conclusion

There maybe several indications for a noninvasive ultrasound examination to be performed in the postpartum period. Even though the sonographic findings are not tissue specific, correlating these findings with the patient's clinical history and laboratory values can greatly assist in the diagnostic process and make a substantive contribution to the management of postpartum complications.

REFERENCES

1. Achiron R, Goldenberg M, Lipitz S, et al. Transvaginal duplex Doppler ultrasonography in bleeding patients suspected of having residual trophoblastic tissue. Obstet Gynecol. 1993; 81:507–511.
2. Adkins J, Wilson S. Unusual course of the gonadal vein: A case report of postpartum ovarian vein thrombosis mimicking acute appendicitis clinically and sonographically. J Ultrasound Med. 1996; 15:409–412.
3. Allan TR, Miller GC, Wabrek AJ, et al. Postpartum and postabortal ovarian vein thrombophlebitis. Obstet Gynecol. 1976; 47:525–528.
4. Athey PA. Uterus: Abnormalities of the endometrial cavity. In: Athey PA, Hadlock FP, eds. Ultrasound in Obstetrics and Gynecology. 2nd ed. St. Louis: CV Mosby; 1985:194–205.
5. Baker ME, Bowie JD, Killam AP. Sonography of post-cesarean-section bladder-flap hematoma. Am J Roentgenol. 1985; 144:757–759.
6. Baker ME, Kay H, Mahony BS, et al. Sonography of the low transverse incision, cesarean section: A

prospective study. J Ultrasound Med. 1988; 7:389–393.

7. Baran GW, Frisch KM. Duplex Doppler evaluation of puerperal ovarian vein thrombosis. Am J Roentgenol. 1987; 149:757–759.

8. Bowie JD. Sonography of the uterus. In: Sabbagha RD, ed. Diagnostic Ultrasound: Applied to Obstetrics and Gynecology. 2nd ed. Philadelphia: JB Lippincott; 1987:474–496.

9. Brown TK, Munsick RA. Puerperal ovarian vein thrombophlebitis: A syndrome. Am J Obstet Gynecol. 1971; 109:263–273.

10. Burger NF, Darazs B, Boes EGM. An echographic evaluation during the early puerperium of the uterine wound after cesarean section. J Clin Ultrasound. 1982; 10:271–274.

11. Deutchman ME, Hartman KJ. Postpartum pyometra: A case report. J Fam Pract. 1993; 36:449–452.

12. Dunnihoo DR, Gallaspy W, Wise RB, et al. Postpartum ovarian vein thrombophlebitis: A review. Obstet Gynecol Surg. 1991; 46:415–427.

13. Defoort P, Benijts G, Thiery M, et al. Ultrasound assessment of puerperal uterine involution. Eur J Obstet Gynecol Reprod Biol. 1978; 8:95–97.

14. Emmons SL, Krohn M, Jackson M, et al. Development of wound infections among women undergoing cesarean section. Obstet Gynecol. 1988; 72:559–564.

15. Fleischer AC, Cullinan JA, Goncalves L, et al. Obstetrical sonography. In: Fleischer AC, Kepple DM, eds. Diagnostic Sonography: Principles and Clinical Applications. 2nd ed. Philadelphia: WB Saunders; 1995:36–243.

16. Grant TH, Schoettle BW, Buchsbaru MS. Postpartum ovarian vein thrombosis: Diagnosis by clot protrusion into the inferior vena cava at sonography. Am J Roentgenol. 1993; 160:551–552.

17. Hall DA, Yoder IC. Ultrasound evaluation of the uterus. In: Callen PW, ed. Ultrasonography in Obstetrics and Gynecology. 3rd ed. Philadelphia: WB Saunders; 1994:586–614.

18. Hedrick WR, Hykes DL, Starchman DE. Ultrasound Physics and Instrumentation. 3rd ed. St. Louis: Mosby; 1995.

19. Hertzberg BS, Bowie JD. Ultrasound of the postpartum uterus. J Ultrasound Med. 1991; 10:451–456.

20. Herzberg BS, Bowie JD, Kliewer MA. Complications of cesarean section: Role of transperineal US. Radiology. 1993; 188:533–536.

21. Herzberg BS, Bowie JD, Weber TM, et al. Sonography of the cervix during the third trimester of pregnancy: Value of the transperineal approach. Am J Roentgenol. 1991; 157:73–76.

22. Kurtz AB, Shlansky-Goldberg RD, Choi HY, et al. Detection of retained products of conception following spontaneous abortion in the first trimester. J Ultrasound Med. 1991; 10:387–395.

23. Land JA, Stoot JE, Evers JL. Puerperal ultrasonic hysterography. Gynecol Obstet Invest. 1984; 18:165–168.

24. Lavery JP, Gadwood KA. Postpartum ultrasound. In: Fleischer AC, Manning FA, Jeanty P, et al, eds. Sonography in Obstetrics and Gynecology: Principles and Practice. 5th ed. Norwalk, CT: Appleton & Lange; 1995:739–754.

25. Lavery JP, Shaw LA. Sonography of the puerperal uterus. J Ultrasound Med. 1989; 8:481–486.

26. Lavery JP, Shaw LA. Postpartum ultrasonography. In: Chervenak FA, Isaacson GC, Campbell S, eds. Ultrasound in Obstetrics and Gynecology. Vol 2. Boston: Little, Brown; 1993:1589–1597.

27. Lee CY, Madrazo B, Drukker BH. Ultrasound evaluation of the postpartum uterus in the management of postpartum bleeding. Obstet Gynecol. 1981; 58:227–232.

28. Lee CY, Madrazo BL, Parks S, et al. Ultrasonic evaluation in the management of postpartum infection. Henry Ford Hospital Medical Journal. 1987; 35:58–62.

29. Leopold GR. Pelvic ultrasonography. In: Sarti DA, ed. Diagnostic Ultrasound: Text and Cases. 2nd ed. Chicago: Year Book Medical Publishers; 1987:684–696.

30. Lonky NM, Worthen N, Ross MG. Prediction of cesarean section scars with ultrasound imaging during pregnancy. J Ultrasound Med. 1989; 8:15–19.

31. Macklon NS, Barry J, Greer IA. Duplex ultrasound screening for deep venous thrombosis in the puerperium. Br J Obstet Gynaecol. 1995; 102:255–256.

32. Madrazo B. Postpartum sonography. In: Saunders RC, James AE, eds. The Principles and Practice of Ultrasonography in Obstetrics and Gynecology. 3rd ed. Norwalk, CT: Appleton-Century-Crofts; 1985:449–456.

33. Munsick RA, Gillanders LA. A review of the syndrome of puerperal ovarian vein thrombophlebitis. Obstet Gynecol Surv. 1981; 36:57–66.

34. Rodeck CH, Newton JR. Study of the uterine cavity by ultrasound in the early puerperium. Br J Obstet Gynaecol. 1976; 83:795–801.

35. Rudoff JM, Astrauskas LJ, Rudoff JC, et al. Ultrasonographic diagnosis of septic pelvic thrombophlebitis. J Ultrasound Med. 1988; 7:287–291.

36. Salem S. The uterus and adnexa. In: Rumack C, Wilson S, Charboneau J, eds. Diagnostic Ultrasound (Vol. 1). St. Louis: Mosby Year Book; 1991:383–412.

37. Savader SJ, Otero PR, Savader BL. Puerperal ovarian

vein thrombosis: Evaluation with CT, US, and MR imaging. Radiology. 1988; 167:637–639.

38. Shaffer PB, Johnson JC, Bryan D, et al. Diagnosis of ovarian vein thrombophlebitis of the ovarian vein. J Comput Assist Tomogr. 1981; 4:436–439.

39. VanRees D, Bernstine RL, Crawford W. Involution of the postpartum uterus: An ultrasonic study. J Clin Ultrasound. 1981; 9:55–57.

40. Vorherr H. Puerperium: Maternal involutional changes—management of puerperal problems and complications. In: Sciarra JJ, ed. Gynecology and Obstetrics. Philadelphia: Harper and Row; 1982:1–44.

41. Vorherr H. Puerperium: Puerperal genitourinary infection. In: Sciarra JJ, ed. Gynecology and Obstetrics. Philadelphia: Harper and Row; 1982:1–31.

42. Wachsberg RH, Kurtz AB, Levine CD, et al. Real-time ultrasonographic analysis of the normal postpartum uterus: Technique, variability, and measurements. J Ultrasound Med. 1994; 13:215–221.

43. Willson JR, Carrington ER. Obstetrics and Gynecology. 7th ed. St. Louis: CV Mobsy; 1983.

44. Wilson PC, Lerner RM. Diagnosis of ovarian vein thrombophlebitis by ultrasonography. J Ultrasound Med. 1983; 2:187–190.

45. Winsett MZ, Fagan CJ, Bedi DG. Sonographic demonstration of bladder-flap hematoma. J Ultrasound Med. 1986; 5:483–487.

46. Yamashita Y, Torashima M, Harada M. Postpartum extraperitoneal pelvic hematoma: Imaging findings. Am J Roentgenol. 1993; 161:805–808.

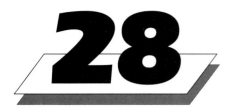

Role of Sonography in Infertility Management and in Contraception

FRANCES R. BATZER

Infertility is defined as the failure to conceive a child after a year of unprotected intercourse. One in six couples in the United States is considered infertile, with 2 to 4 million American couples affected.[113] When analyzed by the female partner's age group, one in seven couples are infertile at age 30 to 34, 1 in 5 at age 35 to 39, and 1 in 4 at age 40 to 44 years. The increased incidence of sexually transmitted disease, the age delay of childbearing by women, the scope and use of infertility treatments, both medical and surgical, all combine to increase the need for medical intervention.

The process of conception is such an intricate one that even the most fertile couple has only one chance in four of conceiving in a given month. For conception to occur, many events must be coordinated. Adequate sperm must be deposited at the cervix at the appropriate mid-cycle moment when the cervical mucus is thin, permitting passage into the uterus (Fig. 28-1). The oocyte (egg) is swept from the surface of the ovary by the fimbria (or distal end) of the tube. Fertilization occurs in the ampullary (enlarged) end of the fallopian tube. The resulting zygote continues to divide into a morula and then a blastocyst, which move down the tube, arriving in the uterus after 4 to 5 days. Implantation

may occur at this point if the endometrium lining is capable of supporting it. A growing chorionic sac can be visualized by ultrasound as early as 18 days after fertilization (see Chap. 12).

The scope of infertility treatment has changed dramatically over the last 20 years, due in great part to the birth of Louis Brown in 1978, the first child conceived with the use of in vitro fertilization (IVF).[115] Today IVF is only one of several forms of assisted reproductive technologies (ART) available, but it was the first major technological breakthrough and provided the impetus for the development of transvaginal imaging techniques.[33] Although originally designed for women with damaged or absent tubes, IVF can also provide the ultimate treatment for male infertility.[81,126] Pregnancies can now be achieved by direct injection of a single sperm into an oocyte, a procedure known as intracytoplasmic sperm injection.[89] It was as a result of these procedures that transvaginal ultrasound techniques developed from the initial placement of an abdominal probe within the vagina for better visualization of follicular development, to the use of a specifically designed vaginal probe as the preferred manner of oocyte retrieval. Although success rates of 12% to 24% per attempt for ART procedures

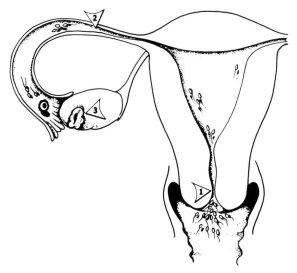

Figure 28-1. Diagram of cervix, uterus, fallopian tubes, and ovary, indicating the path of sperm and oocyte to their intersection: sperm are deposited at the cervix (1) and swim through the uterus into the ampullary portion of the tube (2). The dominant follicle on the ovary grows and ruptures with ovulation of an oocyte, which is picked up by the fimbria of the tube and swept into the ampullary portion of the tube to meet with sperm (3).

may seem low,[2] the monthly fecundity of a fertile couple is only 15% to 20%.

Ultrasound, in particular transvaginal sonography, is an invaluable tool in assessing this complex process. First, ultrasound is used for diagnosing disease or structural barriers in either partner that may hinder fertilization. Second, ultrasound may be used in conjunction with therapy for patients in whom ovulation must be hormonally induced. Third, ultrasound is indispensible for ART procedures, not only for monitoring ovulation changes but as a method of oocyte collection from the ovaries. Fourth, it allows documentation of anatomic changes coincident with ovulation and identification of the hormonal response from the uterus and the cervix. Fifth, ultrasound is used to confirm and follow a pregnancy through implantation and its early growth.

Etiology

Etiologies of infertility are usually divided into 40% due to the female partner, 40% due to the male, 5% to 10% related to both partners, and 5% to 10% unknown etiologies. Female factor infertility in-cludes ovulatory dysfunction (40%), tubal, including adhesions, and endometriosis (30% to 50%), uterine (5% to 10%), cervical (5% to 10%), immunologic (5%), and unknown (5%)[61,113] (Table 28-1). Male factor infertility is idiopathic in 25% or more of cases. The presence of a varicocele accounts for 40% of cases, testicular failure 10%, tubular obstruction 5% to 10%, cryptorchidism 5% to 10%, and other semen disorders 10%.

Diagnosis

Many factors can contribute to female infertility (see Table 28-1). Anatomic abnormalities can be congenital, infectious, or unknown in etiology (Table 28-2). Most of these are considered at length in other chapters. The typical sonographic appearance for each is noted for reference.

OVULATION MONITORING

Ovulatory dysfunction exists in 30% to 40% of patients undergoing an evaluation for infertility.[113] In the normal menstrual cycle, folliculogenesis begins in the late part of the preceding cycle and ends with the mid-cycle gonadotropin surge (Fig. 28-2). The ovary, endometrium, and cervix undergo characteristic changes in response to the hormonal milieu that result in ovulation. But the only definitive proof of ovulation is the identification of an oocyte

▨▨▨ TABLE 28-1. CAUSES OF MALE AND FEMALE INFERTILITY

FEMALE INFERTILITY DISORDERS	
Ovulatory dysfunction	40%
Mechanical factors (including tubal, adhesions, endometriosis)	30%–50%
Cervical factors	5%–10%
Unexplained	5%–10%
MALE INFERTILITY DISORDERS	
Varicocele	40%
Cryptorchidism	6%
Obstruction	6%
Testicular failure	10%
Semen disorders	10%
Idiopathic	25%–30%

(Modified from Speroff L, Glass RH, Kase NG, eds. Clinical Gynecologic Endocrinology and Infertility. 4th ed. Chaps. 17 and 19. Baltimore: Williams & Wilkins; 1989.)

▰▰▰▰ **TABLE 28-2. ANATOMIC CAUSES OF FEMALE INFERTILITY: SONOGRAPHIC IMAGES**

Lesions	Pathology	Etiology	Sonographic Image
UTERUS			
Myoma	Subserosal, intramural, submucosal	Unknown	Varies with location: hyperechoic/hypoechoic with shadowing
Congenital anomaly	Bicornuate, septate, unicollate, single or double cervix/vagina	Congenital	Varies with abnormality; smooth vs. indented fundal surface, single vs. double endometrial stripe; check for associated kidney anomaly
Endometrial lesion	Polyp, retained secundines	Overgrowth of endometrium, pregnancy loss	Hyperechoic/hypoechoic irregularities within the endometrial stripe
Asherman's	Uterine scarring	Unknown, almost always follows pregnancy loss	Absence or discontinuation of endometrial stripe
TUBES			
Hydrosalpinx	Blocked or scarred tubes	Infection, prior surgery	Varies: echogenic tube-shaped structure often surrounding the ovary
Paratubal cyst	Cystic structure	Congenital	Cyst of Morgagni or paratubal cyst, echogenic structure distinct from ovary
Adhesions	Scarring around tubes/ovaries	Infection, prior surgery	Varies: fixed, echogenic fluid areas surrounding ovary, tubes
OVARY			
Endometriosis	Implants, loculations of old blood	Unknown; ectopic growth of endometrial tissue	Classic "snowstorm" pattern of cystic area within ovary
Cyst	Cystic teratomas, serous/mucinous cyst adenomas, simple cyst, corpus luteum, solid tumors	Unknown	Classic irregular hypoechoic areas within a fluid-filled structure; cystic teratoma: various images dependent on kind of tissue present; corpus luteum "great pretender"

under the microscope outside the ovary, or the early detection of pregnancy.

The tests commonly used to evaluate ovulation include measurement of the basal body temperature, serum progesterone levels, and an endometrial biopsy from the lining of the uterus. These tests are indirect and assess only the biochemical result of progesterone secretion. The actual event of ovulation, which is extrusion of the oocyte cumulus complex from the ovary, cannot be assessed by such indirect methods. Since Hackeloer and colleagues[56] first described the ultrasonographic monitoring of follicular development throughout the menstrual cycle, ultrasound has become an important and reliable method of assessing follicular maturation and ovulation (Fig. 28-3).

An ovarian follicle destined to ovulate is derived from a cohort of growing follicles that in turn are derived from the pool of primordial follicles present since birth. By days 5 to 7 of the menstrual cycle (cycle day 1 is the beginning of the menses), as the volume of follicular fluid increases, these small developing follicles become visible ultrasonographically (>5 mm). In the following days, the dominant follicle is differentiated from the cohort as its size and rate of growth exceed the others.[69] Because subordinate follicles that go on to become atretic rarely grow larger than 14 mm, visualization of a large follicle suggests that it is likely to ovulate.[100] Follicles appear as echo-free structures within ovarian tissue. Follicular measurement involves taking three measurements, two in the sagittal plane and one in the coronal plane. A mean diameter is calculated ($L + H + W/3$ = mean follicular diameter [mm]) (Fig. 28-4). A vol-

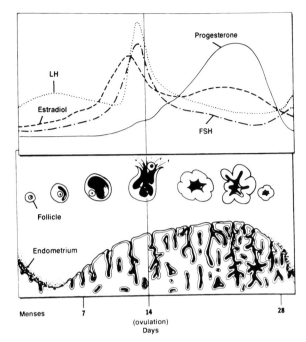

Figure 28-2. Physiology of a normal menstrual cycle. *Upper portion:* hormonal changes (estradiol and progesterone rise) in response to pituitary signals (luteinizing hormone [LH] and follicle-stimulating hormone [FSH]), centered on the LH surge, with ovulation occurring 24 hours later. *Lower portion:* Growth of the endometrium with subsequent breakdown and bleeding (menses). Note the change in thickness of the endometrium that occurs throughout the cycle.

umetric calculation can also be made, but it is more cumbersome for serial scanning of multiple follicles. In the 4 to 5 days preceding ovulation, the dominant follicle grows approximately 1 to 2 mm daily.[100] The growth in diameter of this single dominant follicle is directly proportionate to the rise in serum estradiol[56] (see Fig. 28-3). At the time of ovulation, the mean diameter of the lead follicle measures approximately 20 to 24 mm, although the range has been reported to be from 18 to 28 mm (Fig. 28-5). This disparity in follicle size precludes the use of ultrasound as the only index for the prediction of the exact time of ovulation.[13,87,95] However, other preovulatory sonographic features that reflect the hormonally induced morphologic changes in the follicle have been described.[5] With the luteinizing hormone (LH) surge, the theca, the outer cellular layer of the follicle, becomes edematous and begins to separate from the granulosa layer. This can be appreciated sonographically by noting a line of decreasing reflectivity around the follicle.[93] The granulosa layer inside the theca

begins to fold. Sonographically, this appears as a crenated pattern in the lining of the follicle. The cumulus–corona–oocyte complex can occasionally be detected as a small, echogenic area projecting into the follicle, a finding present in approximately 20% of follicles greater than 18 mm in diameter.[69]

Characteristic ultrasonographic findings[27,82,86,95] have been noted to occur at the time of ovulation (Table 28-3). At the time of ovulation, follicular rupture occurs, seen as a rapid reduction in follicle size with collapse of the follicular wall.[27,86,95] Follicular emptying requires between 1 to 45 minutes to complete. Within an hour, the follicle partially refills and appears as a cyst, usually smaller, containing numerous echoes, which likely represent hemorrhage (Fig. 28-6). In addition to the changes in the appearance of the follicle, fluid can often be detected in the cul-de-sac.[27,82] The now corpus luteum can be differentiated from the preovulatory follicle by its irregular shape, internal echoes, and thickened walls, the latter of which is a result of luteinization.[55,58] It is usually gone with the onset of the next menses.

Because the ultrasound findings of normal ovulation are well documented, ultrasound can be used to detect ovulatory dysfunction. Polan and colleagues[94] noted that in some cycles, despite the fact

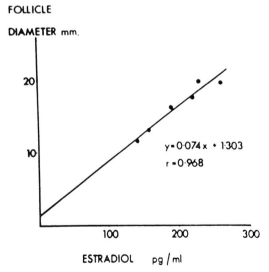

Figure 28-3. Linear correlation between mean values for follicular diameter and mean levels of estradiol on days −5 to 0. (Hackeloer BJ, Fleming R, Robinson HP, Adam AH, Coutts JRT. Correlation of ultrasonic and endocrinologic assessment of human follicular development. Am J Obstet Gynecol. 1979; 135:122.)

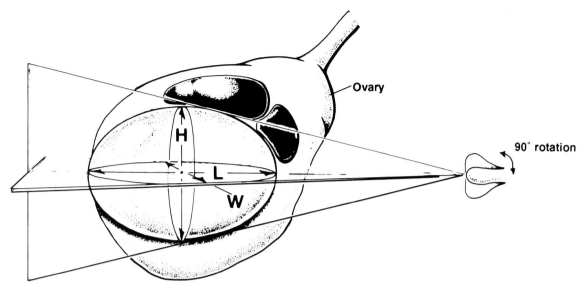

Figure 28-4. Diagram illustrating the manner in which follicular measurements are made: length plus height plus width (L + H + W/3) = mean follicular diameter.

that the basal body temperature chart appears biphasic, suggesting ovulation, there is asynchrony between the estradiol peak, the LH surge, and the growth and rupture of ovarian follicles. In such cases, the follicle is usually less than 14 mm in diameter and either ruptures prematurely or ceases to grow, becoming atretic, a process that can be detected only with ultrasonographic monitoring.

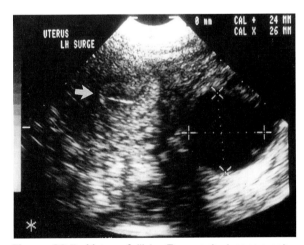

Figure 28-5. Mature follicle. Transvaginal sonography showing the uterus and ovary at the time of the luteinizing hormone surge. An echo-free area is identified on the ovary measuring about 24 mm, compatible with a mature follicle. The endometrium (*arrow*) shows a triple-layered texture with a thickness greater than 8 mm, compatible with a well developed periovulatory endometrium.

Another type of ovulatory dysfunction, detected best by ultrasound, is ovum entrapment in an unruptured follicle. The phenomenon has been termed luteinized unruptured follicle syndrome and has been reported to occur in 6% to 79% of cycles as assessed at laparoscopy.[75] Using ultrasound for diagnosis, it has been reported to occur in 9% to 29% of patients with unexplained infertility.[24,79] The persistence or growth of a dominant follicle with an echo-free cystic appearance more than 38 hours after the LH peak, with no sign of collapse despite biochemical changes consistent with ovulation, is evidence of failure of oocyte extrusion.[100]

ENDOMETRIAL INDICATORS

Endometrial abnormalities and luteal phase defects, inappropriate delayed hormonal changes in the endometrium, account for 5% to 10% of all infertil-

TABLE 28-3. DOCUMENTATION OF OVULATION: ULTRASONOGRAPHIC CRITERIA FOR CHANGE IN THE DOMINANT FOLLICLE

Disappearance of the dominant follicle
Presence of internal echoes within the follicle
Collapse of the dominant follicle with crenation of the edges
Free cul-de-sac fluid

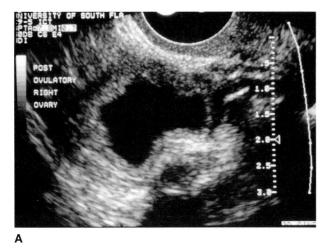

A

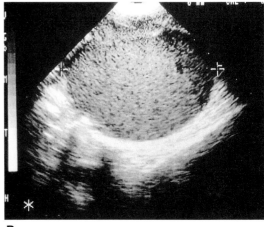

B

Figure 28-6. Transvaginal sonography of a corpus luteum (**A**) and an endometrioma (**B**). A "snowstorm" pattern, homogeneous in nature, is seen in the endometrioma. The corpus luteum shows an irregular border with some internal echogenicity throughout. Follow-up ultrasound at the beginning of a new cycle demonstrated resolution of the corpus luteum with the ongoing presence of the endometrioma. (**A** courtesy of Charlene Croyt, ATL, Bothell, Washington.)

ity.[113] An endometrial biopsy is usually required to make such a diagnosis, although several investigators rely on serum progesterone levels. The endometrium, as a hormone-dependent tissue, demonstrates marked changes throughout the menstrual cycle. The ultrasonographic characteristics of these changes noted during the menstrual cycle appear to relate to fecundity and pregnancy outcome. Studies have indicated that thickness measurements of less than 6 mm correlate with a poor chance of pregnancy,[31,66,110] whereas 11 mm or greater connotes a good prognosis for pregnancy, with any measurement of at least 8 mm being reasonable.[30] The texture of the endometrium has also been correlated with fecundity and pregnancy outcome.[46,108,117] The presence of specific lesions (e.g., polyps, submucosal fibroids) is thought to play a role in infertility. Sonographic recognition of these abnormalities is discussed in other chapters.

The endometrium undergoes cyclic changes during the normal menstrual cycle that are related to hormonal stimulation. Noting the characteristic sonographic images consistent with the phases of the menstrual cycle is a necessary part of assessing normal ovulatory function. Several imaging characteristics of the endometrium have been presented as important in terms of denoting normality or underlining pathology (Fig. 28-7): (1) thickness; (2) texture (hyperechoic, isoechoic, or hypoechoic with respect to the myometrium; (3) homogeneous or

irregular echogenicity signifying potential intracavitary lesions; and (4) presence or absence of intracavitary fluid.

The increased resolution available with transvaginal ultrasound has provided information that suggests a possible role of the endometrium at the mid-cycle. Abramowicz and colleagues[1] found that increased peristaltic endometrial and myometrial movements appear to occur in women around mid-

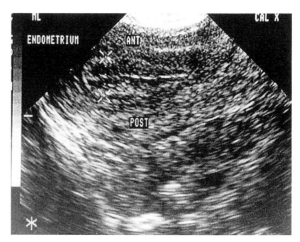

Figure 28-7. Transvaginal ultrasound of the preovulatory uterus and endometrium. Measurement of the endometrium includes two thicknesses, from one myometrial interface to the opposite interface (between markers); texture grading suggests a triple-stripe preovulatory pattern.

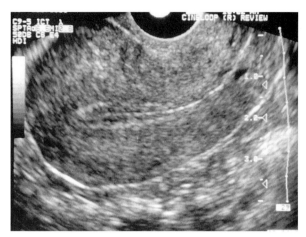

Figure 28-8. Transvaginal ultrasound of the uterus and endometrium. The endometrium is thin and hypoechoic in relation to the myometrium, compatible with proliferative change. A measurement of 6 mm was obtained.

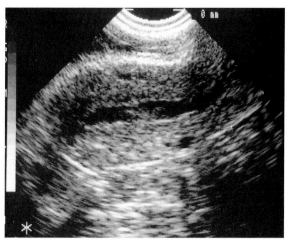

Figure 28-9. Transvaginal ultrasound of the uterus and endometrium with evidence of fluid (blood) in the cavity and an irregular, thin endometrium, compatible with menstrual sloughing of the endometrium.

cycle. They postulated that these movements, which are decreased in patients on oral contraceptives, probably enhance sperm propulsion toward the tubal ostia. Further investigation in this area is required.

Thickness

Thickness depends on the hormonal status of the patient (Fig. 28-8). During the reproductive years, an increase in endometrial thickness as well as uterine volume parallels follicular development.[78] The endometrium consists of two layers, a basal and a functional layer.[3,104] It is primarily the functional layer that changes with hormonal fluctuation. Normal endometrial thickness can be seen to vary from 3 to 14 mm within the menstrual cycle (see Chap. 4).[2]

Texture

Circulating estrogen and progesterone as well as the presence or absence of anatomic abnormalities account for textural changes. The menstrual endometrium is a thin, echogenic interface with the myometrium[41] (Fig. 28-9). During the proliferative phase it thickens, becoming isoechoic with regard to the myometrium[41] (see Fig. 28-8). The variable echogenicity that is seen just before ovulation is thought to reflect the growth of endometrial glands with their secretions.[53] The multilayered (the "triple line") appearance of the endometrium in this periovulatory period seems to be predictive of

a positive pregnancy outcome[40,53,70,123] (see Fig. 28-7). Echogenicity and thickness continue to increase during the secretory phase of the cycle, with the endometrium becoming hyperechoic compared to the myometrium (Fig. 28-10).

Intracavitary Lesions

Transvaginal sonography has demonstrated accuracy in identifying the presence of intracavitary abnormalities. Sonohysterography can be used for further char-

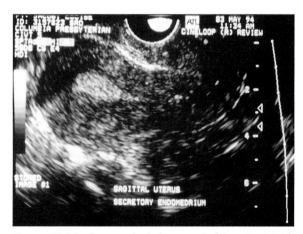

Figure 28-10. Transvaginal ultrasound of the uterus and endometrium. The endometrium is thickened and hyperechoic with respect to the myometrium, compatible with a luteal-phase endometrium. (Courtesy of Charlene Croyt, ATL, Bothell, Washington.)

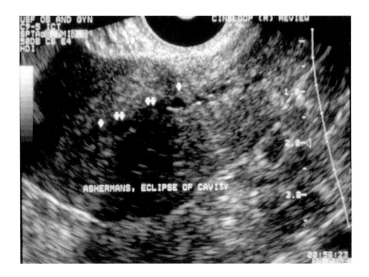

Figure 28-11. *Transvaginal ultrasound of the uterus with no identifiable endometrial stripe, compatible with Asherman's syndrome. (Courtesy of Charlene Croyt, Bothell, Washington.)*

acterization of endometrial abnormalities, as shown by Parsons and Lense.[90] Saline infusion by a catheter system passed through the cervix under direct sonographic guidance was able to permit correct identification of polyps, myomas, synechiae, retained secundines, endometrial hyperplasia, and carcinoma in 39 women with surgical confirmation. Others have corroborated the use of sonohysteroscopy.[43,57,65,72,91]

Transvaginal sonography can verify the extension of particularly submucosal lesions into or through the myometrium, even to the serosa. Especially when future fertility and uterine integrity are of concern, the exact location of leiomyomata is important to planning a surgical approach.[35]

Intrauterine adhesions, which are often the result of a postpartum or postabortal curettage, have been reported in 5% to 39% of women,[54] usually with the concomitant symptom of hypomenorrhea or amenorrhea. Sonographically, they appear as sonolucent defects within the bright, thickened endometrium during the secretory phase, or as obliteration of the normal endometrium[18,109] (Fig. 28-11). Sonohysterography has been demonstrated successfully to identify intrauterine adhesions or Asherman's syndrome,[90] although hysteroscopy has been the traditional technique and a better diagnostic tool.

Intracavitary Fluid

The presence of intracavity mucus may accompany the periovulatory endometrial change. Intracavitary fluid in the form of blood can be seen perimenstrually (see Fig. 28-9).

Following the endometrial line from the fundus in the longitudinal plane while withdrawing or angling the transducer facilitates visualization of the cervix and endocervical canal. Normal cervical findings include inclusion cysts (Nabothian cysts) of various sizes, not to be confused with ovarian follicular development or early pregnancy.[81] They are usually fluid-filled cystic areas with distal acoustic enhancement noted because the fluid is mucinous in type. Hormonal status can be inferred by noting the presence or absence of cervical mucus.[81] At midcycle, the cervical canal is most prominent because of the presence of mucus produced in response to the elevated estradiol level coincident with impending ovulation (Fig. 28-12).

DOPPLER ULTRASOUND

Characteristic changes in blood flow dynamics occur during the menstrual cycle. Doppler ultrasound is a noninvasive technique that can be applied to measure blood flow and note physiologic changes involving the uterine and ovarian arteries. Goswamy and colleagues[48] suggested that poor uterine perfusion may be a cause of infertility. Through hormonal manipulation, they were able to effect changes in uterine perfusion that resulted in a normalization of the pregnancy rate in patients with evidence of poor uterine perfusion in comparison to other patients undergoing ART. Consistent studies in this area are difficult. In general, the rising estradiol (E2) levels of the follicular phase result in a vasodilatory effect.[39,48] Decreased E2 levels result

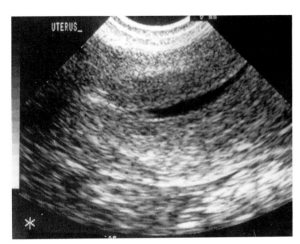

Figure 28-12. Transvaginal sonography of the cervix showing an echo-free area within the cervical canal, compatible with watery, thin cervical mucus of a mid-cycle nature.

in decreased perfusion. The presence of E2 and progesterone in the luteal phase results in continued increased uterine perfusion. These changes are measured as a decrease in resistance index or pulsatility index during the late follicular phase, persisting throughout the luteal phase. The ovarian artery shows similar changes, with marked neovascularization of the dominant follicle, now the corpus luteum, occurring after ovulation.

UTERINE FACTORS

Anatomic uterine abnormalities, which include congenital abnormalities, leiomyomata, and adenomyosis, account for approximately 5% of cases of infertility.[21] These abnormalities act by interfering with normal implantation. Evaluation of the uterine cavity is an important part of the infertility workup. Although it is usually performed using hysterosalpingography, sonohysterography yields comparable results.

Müllerian duct abnormalities occur in 1% to 5% of women, 25% of whom experience infertility and pregnancy loss.[17] Because the treatments of the various kinds of uterine malformation differ, it is of paramount importance to establish the correct diagnosis before undertaking any intervention[37,98] (see Chap. 5). Normality and presence of both kidneys must also be evaluated when a congenital uterine anomaly is identified.

Leiomyomata can also play a role in pregnancy loss and, to a lesser degree, infertility. They can act in several ways: distorting the shape of the uterine cavity, interfering with uterine/endometrial blood flow, occluding the tubal ostia, or as a kind of intrauterine device (IUD), preventing implantation (see Chap. 7).

Adenomyosis describes the presence of endometrial glands and stroma within the myometrium below the endomyometrial junction. Prevalence data are poor because diagnosis before hysterectomy is difficult. Symptoms include dysmenorrhea, pelvic pain, menomenorrhagia, and infertility. Adenomyosis coexists with other pathology two thirds of the time, including leiomyoma (19% to 56%), endometriosis (6% to 28%), and endometrial hyperplasia.[111] It can present in a diffuse or focal form.[36,84] Fedele and colleagues[36] showed a sensitivity of 87% and a specificity of 98% using transvaginal ultrasound for the diagnosis. Results seem to be somewhat operator dependent. Magnetic resonance imaging has proven increasingly useful in the diagnosis.[83,102] Varied patterns to adenomyoma have been imaged, including multiple cysts within distinct lesions[7] (Fig. 28-13).

TUBAL PERITONEAL FACTORS

Tubal/peritoneal disease is believed to play a role in 30% to 50% of cases of female infertility.[113] Typically, hysterosalpingography has been the procedure of choice to evaluate tubal patency. Alternative methods using ultrasound to evaluate tubal patency, called sonohysterography or hysterosonography,[90] which eliminate the risks of ionizing radiation, are being explored[92,96,99] (Fig. 28-14). Randolph and colleagues[96] evaluated tubal patency in 56 patients by observing the pelvis with transabdominal ultrasound during the instillation of saline into the uterus. Free fluid in the cul-de-sac was considered diagnostic of tubal patency. Ultrasound was found to have a sensitivity of 100% and a specificity of 91%. Unfortunately, it was difficult to discern the side of tubal patency. More recently, color Doppler was applied to this technique with encouraging results.[92] The fallopian tubes, without instillation techniques, are almost impossible to visualize unless the tube is diseased and obstructed, as in the case of hydrosalpinx or in the presence of significant ascites (Fig. 28-15; see Chap. 10).

Transcervical fallopian tube catheterization as described by Jansen and Anderson[63] for diagnosis and treatment of proximal tube disease can be performed through the vagina under transvaginal sonographic

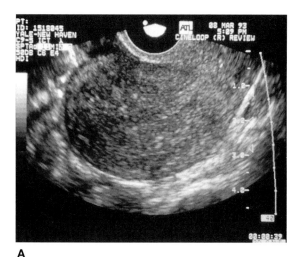
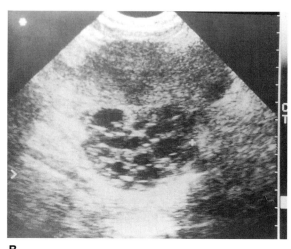

A   **B**

Figure 28-13. (**A**) Transvaginal ultrasound of the uterus demonstrating adenomyosis. Note the irregular echogenicity within the myometrium at the uterus. (Courtesy of Charlene Croyt, ATL, Bothell, Washington.) (**B**) Transvaginal ultrasound of an adenomyoma. It is a cystic mass extending from the posterior aspect of the cervix and consisting of multiple, small cystic areas measuring up to 1.5 cm in diameter with relatively thick walls and intervening stroma, encompassing the entire length of the cervix from the internal to the external os, and measuring 6.7 × 5.4 × 7.2 cm.

guidance. The technique involves sonographically guided placement of an initial stiff, distally curved, flexible Teflon catheter through the cervix up toward the tubal ostia with a metal obturator (Fig. 28-16). On removing the obturator, a thinner, tapered cathe-

ter is then passed through the cannula and into the isthmus of the tube. When treating cornual obstruction, passage of a metal wire is first attempted, followed over by the tapered catheter. There are much data on fluoroscopically guided tubal cannulization procedures[22,122] and abdominal sonographically guided procedures,[12,26,60,107] but there is little re-

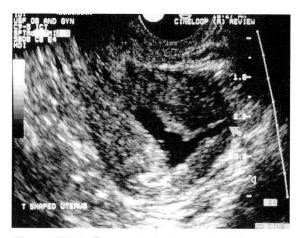

Figure 28-14. Transvaginal ultrasound of the uterus after saline injection (sonohysterography). Uterine distention is noted, along with a T-shaped uterus (arrow) compatible with maternal diethylstilbestrol ingestion. The lack of flow through the interstitial tubal portions indicate probable cornual tubal obstruction. (Courtesy of Charlene Croyt, ATL, Bothell, Washington.)

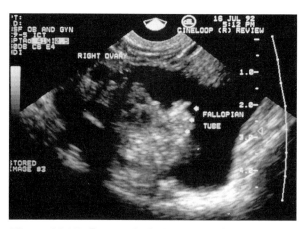

Figure 28-15. Transvaginal ultrasound of the uterus in the presence of ascites. The patient was experiencing symptoms of moderate to severe hyperstimulation with fluid loss into the third space, the peritoneal cavity. A normal fallopian tube is shown floating in the serous fluid. (Courtesy of Charlene Croyt, ATL, Bothell, Washington.)

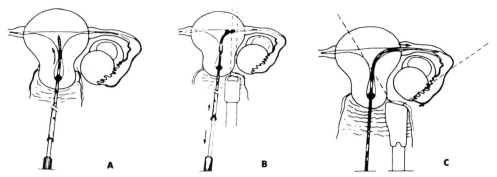

Figure 28-16. System for catheterization of the fallopian tubes. (**A**) A metal obturator is used to guide the cannula through the curve of the cervix into the uterus. (**B**) As the obturator is withdrawn, the cannula regains its lateral curve and is advanced to the uterotubal junction. (**C**) The catheter is then passed down the cannula and through the isthmus of the fallopian tube. (Jansen RPS, Anderson JC. Catheterisation of the fallopian tubes from the vagina. Lancet. 1987; 2:309.)

ported experience with transvaginally guided techniques.[121] The technique is similar to that discussed later in the section on ART (sonographically guided gamete intrafallopian transfer and tubal embryo transfer). Patients must be closely counseled about the risk of ectopic pregnancy after the procedure regardless of how it is performed, because the isthmic portion, the smallest-diameter point of the tube, has been potentially traumatized with instrumentation or was abnormal.

Endoluminal ultrasound with a small, high-frequency transducer has been used to visualize and evaluate the fallopian tubes.[44] Initial results have been encouraging, although more investigation and development are required.

Included in the category of peritoneal factor infertility is endometriosis, which has typically been diagnosed at the time of laparoscopy. Although transvaginal sonography cannot usually detect peritoneal implants, it can detect an endometrioma within the ovary. In general, an endometrioma is characterized by uniform low-level echoes that reflect the hemorrhagic content of the cyst, giving a uniform, typical "ground glass" appearance (see Chap. 10). Although an endometrioma can be mistaken for a corpus luteum, follow-up scan in the follicular phase of the subsequent cycle helps make the distinction because the endometrioma persists and perhaps even grows, while the functional cyst disappears (see Fig. 28-6).

CERVICAL FACTORS

Cervical factor infertility, in which the sperm are prevented from ascending into the uterus, presents in 5% to 10% of patients with infertility. Cervical

mucus can be seen within the periovulatory cervical canal (see Fig. 28-11). In one study, it was observed in only 5% of cases.[59] Others report its identification approximately 40% to 50% of the time.[5,18] Surgical trauma, diethylstilbestrol-related abnormalities, ovulatory dysfunction, or medications such as clomiphene citrate can be responsible for the absence of cervical mucus.

Treatment

OVULATION INDUCTION

If ovulatory dysfunction is established during the infertility evaluation, ovulation induction is instituted, usually using clomiphene citrate, an oral medication, or human menopausal gonadotropins, an injectable medication containing the gonadotropins follicle-stimulating hormone or LH. In addition, ovulation induction, particularly with human menopausal gonadotropins (hMG), is used empirically in patients with long-standing infertility and ART. The goal of therapy is to induce satisfactory ovulation of one or more follicles and to avoid excessive follicular development, ovarian hyperstimulation, and multiple-gestation pregnancies.[5,100] The use of ultrasound monitoring for ovulation induction has improved outcome by determining the timely injection of human chorionic gonadotropin (hCG) to trigger ovulation by mimicking the normal LH surge (see Fig. 28-2). Similarly, the morbidity associated with hyperstimulation and the risk of a multiple-gestation pregnancy are reduced with the use of ultrasound. Ovulation induction is also

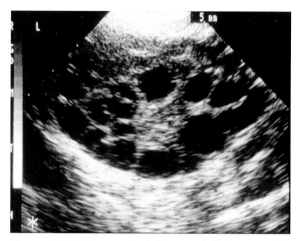

Figure 28-17. Transvaginal ultrasound of the ovary with sonographic evidence of polycystic ovarian disease: multiple, small subcortical echogenic areas (less than 5 mm), the "necklace" appearance, within an ovary of upper-normal size.

used in ART to increase the number of oocytes recovered, and hence embryos generated, to improve pregnancy rates.

The usefulness of a baseline ultrasound performed transabdominally with transvaginal follow-up at the onset of the menses before the initiation of drug therapy is to be emphasized. Any persistent abnormalities can be identified at this time because all normal follicular development should be gone or minimal in size. Frequently it is necessary to wait between stimulated cycles to allow the ovaries to return to their normal, unstimulated state. Polycystic ovaries (PCO) have a unique sonographic appearance that must be noted at this time because stimulatory therapy should be altered to prevent problems of hyperstimulation that are especially prevalent with PCO (Fig. 28-17). The sonographic picture of PCO is one of multiple, small cystic follicles (measuring less than 10 mm) along the periphery of the frequently top normal-sized or enlarged

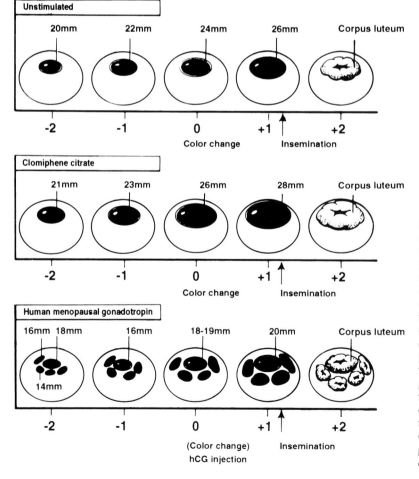

Figure 28-18. Follicular size in unstimulated and stimulated cycles (clomiphene citrate and human menopausal gonadotropins). Based on urinary luteinizing hormone testing (color change) or timing of human chorionic gonadotropin (hCG) injection, patients in unstimulated cycles ovulate at a smaller dominant follicle diameter than do patients in a clomiphene citrate-stimulated cycle. Patients stimulated with human menopausal gonadotropin with multiple follicular development are ready to ovulate at smaller follicular diameters. (Modified from Yee B, Rosen GF, Cassidenti DL. Transvaginal Sonography in Infertility. Philadelphia: Lippincott–Raven; 1995:89.)

ovary.[100] Although the etiology is unknown, the disorder affects 3% to 5% of women.

The rate of follicular growth as followed by transvaginal sonography is the same in both stimulated and unstimulated cycles (i.e., approximately 1- to 2-mm increase in mean follicular diameter daily). Follicular size at which ovulation occurs is bigger, 26 to 28 mm, in clomiphene citrate-stimulated ovulation induction cycles[18,100] compared to spontaneous or hMG-stimulated cycles (Fig. 28-18). Multiple follicular development apparently is seen in 35% to 60% of clomiphene citrate-stimulated cycles.[100] hMG stimulation, because it bypasses the central hypothalamic–pituitary axis, is quite different. Recruitment of many follicles at different stages of development often occurs because patients with endogenous estrogen activity often harbor antral follicles (less than 5 mm) at various stages of growth. Multiple follicular development is seen in up to 80% of hMG-stimulated cycles (Fig. 28-19). Assessment of follicular mean diameter along with serum estradiol levels is used to time hCG administration, usually when the lead follicles have a mean diameter of at least 16 to 18 mm[100] (see Fig. 28-18).

Complications

OVARIAN HYPERSTIMULATION SYNDROME. Ovarian hyperstimulation syndrome is a serious potential complication of ovulation induction, and ultrasound plays an important role in decreasing its likelihood. Hyperstimulation occurs to some degree in most patients undergoing ovulation induction, and ranges from mild abdominal discomfort to, in its most severe form, circulatory compromise and electrolyte imbalance (Table 28-4). In severe ovarian hyperstimulation syndrome, the ovaries are markedly enlarged (greater than 10 cm) and edematous. Ascites (see Fig. 28-19) and pleural effusions are present, with concomitant hemoconcentration and oliguria. There is increased risk of ovarian cyst rupture or torsion. In the absence of pregnancy, the syndrome spontaneously resolves within a few days. The syndrome, however, is most commonly seen with pregnancy, and resolution occurs more slowly, over 6 to 8 weeks. Hospitalization and abdominal paracentesis with an indwelling catheter placed under ultrasound guidance are often required.

Severe hyperstimulation occurs in cycles with enlarged ovaries, high estradiol levels, and many small or intermediate, rather than large, follicles.[10] This situation can often be avoided by withholding hCG, and thus not triggering ovulation and canceling cycles with these characteristics. Hyperstimulation occurs infrequently in ART programs, probably as a result of damage to the follicles at the time of follicular aspiration and retrieval.

MULTIPLE GESTATIONS. The use of ovulation-inducing drugs has dramatically increased the incidence of

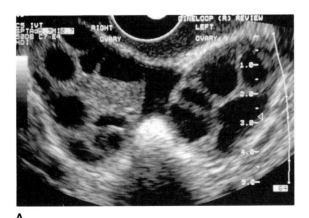
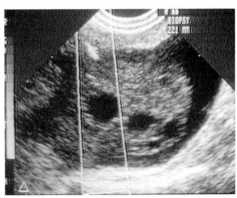

A
B

Figure 28-19. (**A**) Transvaginal ultrasound of a human menopausal gonadotropin-stimulated ovary. Multiple echogenic areas compatible with multiple follicular development are evident. (Courtesy of Charlene Croyt, ATL, Bothell, Washington.) (**B**) Transvaginal ultrasound of a human menopausal gonadotropin-stimulated ovary at the time of oocyte retrieval. The aspirating needle is visualized within the biopsy guidelines. Follicular aspiration for in vitro fertilization is being performed. Within the ovary, the echogenic needle tip is approaching a follicle. Bleeding around the ovary permits exact delineation of the ovarian capsule.

TABLE 28-4. CLASSIFICATION OF OVARIAN HYPERSTIMULATION SYNDROME

Parameter	Mild	Moderate	Severe
Incidence	10%–30%	1%–3%	<2%
Ovarian enlargement	≤5 cm	5–12 cm	>12 cm
Weight gain	≤5 lb	5–10 lb	>10 lb
Abdominal symptoms	Bloating	Slight distention	Moderate distention
Nausea/vomiting	Absent	Present	Present
Other symptoms	—	—	Ascites/pleural effusions
			Hemoconcentration/ electrolyte imbalance
			Possible rupture of ovarian cysts
			Possible ovarian torsion

(Modified from Yee B, Rosen GF, Cassidenti DL. Transvaginal Sonography in Infertility. Philadelphia: Lippincott–Raven; 1995:89.)

multiple gestation,[105] but ultrasound monitoring during gonadotropin therapy has helped to control the rate of high-order multiple gestations.[97] The increased incidence of multiple gestations has had an impact on maternal health, fetal outcome, and associated costs.[16] Transvaginal ultrasound is essential not only for early monitoring of fetal viability, but for assessing fetal number. The "vanishing twin" phenomenon,[73] by which one or more of the initial gestational sacs or fetuses disappears, seemingly absorbed without affecting the ongoing gestation, appears to occur more frequently than initially reported[29] (see Chap. 23). Spontaneous fetal reduction may occur at up to at least 12 weeks' gestation.[11] Therefore, multifetal reduction should not be electively performed before at least 10 weeks' gestation.[120] When necessary, the technique involves either transabdominal[6] or transvaginal[45] sonographic guidance for needle puncture into the chorionic sac, with potassium chloride instillation or amniotic fluid aspiration. Although there can be complications, elective reduction appears to be a safe, viable option to the delivery of a high-order multiple gestation.

ASSISTED REPRODUCTIVE TECHNOLOGIES

Assisted reproductive technologies, which began officially with the birth of Louise Brown in 1978, refers to all the multiple forms of applied technology whereby matured gametes—oocytes and sperm—are brought into direct contact (Table 28-5). ART is the result of the interaction of reproductive endocrinol-

ogy, cellular biology, ultrasound, and endoscopy. ART uses ovarian stimulation to allow retrieval of multiple oocytes with subsequent replacement of multiple embryos to improve the per-attempt pregnancy rate. As a result, ART relies extensively on ultrasound for surveillance of the induction of ovulation and also for oocyte retrieval. Follicle assessment for ART is similar to that for hMG-stimulated cycles. With the added use of gonadotropin-releasing hormone analogs, which suppress the pituitary–ovarian axis as part of the stimulation protocol, a premature LH surge possibly triggering ovulation is unlikely to occur. Given this, hCG administration is deferred until the larger follicles achieve a mean diameter of at least 16 to 18 mm.

In Vitro Fertilization

In IVF, fertilization occurs outside of the body. Although IVF was originally described as a laparoscopic oocyte retrieval procedure,[116] it was readily apparent that oocyte retrieval could be performed

TABLE 28-5. THE "ALPHABET SOUP" OF MODERN REPRODUCTIVE TECHNOLOGY

Acronym	Procedure Described
ART	Assisted reproductive technologies
IVF	In vitro fertilization
GIFT	Gamete intrafallopian transfer
ZIFT	Zygote intrafallopian transfer
TET	Tubal embryo transfer
ICSI	Intracytoplasmic sperm injection

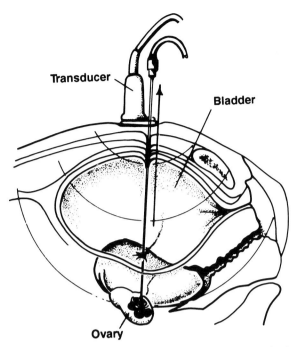

Figure 28-20. Diagram illustrating transabdominal, transvesicular (through the bladder) follicular aspiration. Note the necessity for a full bladder and the long traverse of the needle.

without laparoscopy, using sonographic guidance. Initially, transabdominally guided ultrasound oocyte retrieval was used[77] (Fig. 28-20). Transurethral and transvaginal oocyte retrieval methods followed, both using transabdominal sonographic guidance.[28] With the development of the transvaginal probe, most oocyte retrieval today is accomplished by the vaginal route[38] (Figs. 28-21 and 28-22). There is a low complication rate despite the nonantiseptic preparation of the vagina (normal saline wash only). The use of antiseptic solutions such as povidone iodine (10%) is contraindicated because of oocyte toxicity.

Occasionally, transuterine puncture is necessary to access an ovary. This can be performed with successful return of oocytes, although the patient may experience some increased discomfort.

Transvaginal Puncture Technique

Although IVF was the initial impetus for the development of transvaginally guided puncture technology, this technique has many uses in addition to treatment of infertility (Table 28-6). In the normal pelvis, any transvaginal puncture technique requires transversing minimal tissue depth to reach the site of interest. Normal or abnormal ovarian enlargement often distends the ovary

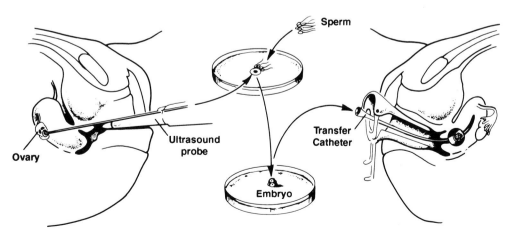

Figure 28-21. Diagram illustrating the in vitro fertilization procedure. The ovary is stimulated to produce multiple mature follicles. Transvaginal ultrasound-guided follicular aspiration is performed. Oocytes are placed in a Petri dish and inseminated with pretreated sperm. Fertilization is observed at 24 hours. Division indicating ongoing development of the oocyte into first a zygote and then an embryo is observed at 48 hours. Embryos are placed into the uterus through the cervix, using a small catheter.

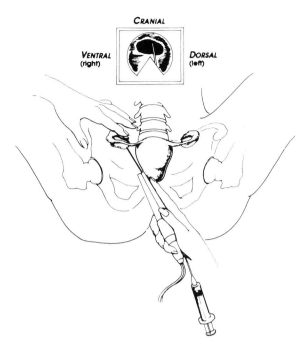

Figure 28-22. Diagram of the pelvis with transvaginal transducer in place and attached needle and biopsy guide, showing a bimanual approach to transvaginal ultrasound-guided evaluation and aspiration.

against the vaginal wall and into the potential space of the cul-de-sac, facilitating and shortening the needle path. Measurements from the vagina to the ovary or area of interest should be made if there is any question about access through a transvaginal route.

The technique is simply applied and well tolerated even without any more analgesia than a local anesthetic injected through the advancing needle. Most transvaginal probes are manufactured with compatible biopsy guides that can be sterilized and fixed to the probe (Fig. 28-23). A visual biopsy guide is reflected onto the monitor by the software program of the machine (see Figs. 28-19B and 28-26). Needles of an appropriate gauge (no larger than 16-gauge) are passed through the guide along or between a superimposed biopsy guideline on the monitor. The biopsy guideline is usually marked by centimeter lines to indicate depth and allow for an estimate of penetration. Aspirating needles have sonographically marked tips to help with visualization (Fig. 28-24). The needle is connected directly to a pump device by intravenous fluid tubing for

oocyte retrieval, or to a syringe for fluid collection and flushing. The needle is placed through the needle guide, fastened directly to the transducer probe (see Fig. 28-24). The position of the entire length of the needle is thus kept within the scanning plane, under direct visualization.

The needle can be moved manually or by an automated needle puncture system. With the first method, the needle is placed within the needle guide and manually advanced into the area of interest along the monitor's superimposed biopsy lines. The target is kept centralized as much as possible between the biopsy needle guides (see Fig. 28-19). An automated spring-loaded needle puncture device fixed to the shaft of the vaginal probe also has been developed (Fig. 28-25). Precise depth of penetration can be programmed using the same linear biopsy monitor guide. The advantage with this technique is that because of the force with which the needle is directed into the target, a thinner needle can be used, minimizing tissue trauma and pain. The disadvantage is that separate vaginal punctures must be made at each target. The manual technique allows for a single vaginal entry, with change in angulation in the probe and needle about that point facilitating targeting and aspiration of multiple areas, as is essential for oocyte retrieval.

Transvaginal ultrasound guidance can be used for transcervical embryo transfer or transmyometrial embryo transfer,[67,76] and is particularly helpful in the presence of severe cervical stenosis or distortion. The technique is similar to that of other transvaginally guided punctures.

TABLE 28-6. SONOGRAPHICALLY GUIDED OPERATIVE AND PUNCTURE PROCEDURES

PUNCTURE PROCEDURES
Oocyte retrieval
Ovum/pelvic cyst aspiration
Transmyometrial embryo transfer
Selective fetal reduction
Chorionic villus sampling/early amniocentesis
Ectopic pregnancy treatment
Culdocentesis
Pelvic fluid/abscess drainage

OPERATIVE PROCEDURES
Tubal embryo transfer
Tubal cannulization
Intrauterine device retrieval

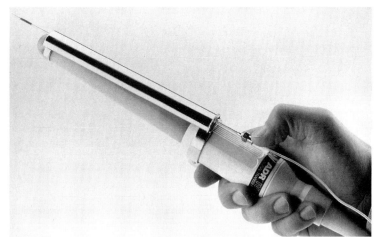

Figure 28-23. Transvaginal ultrasound probe (mechanical sector) with biopsy guide and needle aspirator in place. (Courtesy of ATL, Bothell, Washington.)

Aspiration of Abnormal Adnexal Lesions

Cyst aspiration in the early follicular phase before the initiation of an IVF cycle has been advocated by some to facilitate better follicular development and enhance pregnancy outcome.[101,124] Relief of pelvic pain by cyst aspiration is also easily accomplished, although there is a high recurrence rate. Endometriomas, although they can be aspirated under ultrasonic guidance, must ultimately be treated surgically.

Ovarian or pelvic cyst aspiration, although easily performed (Fig. 28-26), should be carefully contemplated before being carried out. The potential risk of malignancy and the consequences of performing vaginal aspiration in such an instance are unclear. Risk assessment by scoring systems related to the sonographic picture,[50,103] application of color flow Doppler analysis,[71] and documentation of serum CA 125 levels before aspiration are essential before transvaginal cyst aspiration should be performed. Analysis of cyst fluid content,[49,51] although diagnostic of a benign lesion in most instances (i.e., elevated estradiol and progesterone levels), can be indeterminate in others.[9] Analysis of cyst fluid CA 125 content does not aid diagnosis, nor does cytology. The controversy stems from the potential change in status and prognosis in a patent when spillage of malignant cells occurs within the peritoneal cavity and the potentially inconclusive evidence provided by cyst fluid analysis. Further discussion of this issue can be found in several publications,[9,51] and the arguments against it do not differ greatly from those against laparoscopic aspiration.

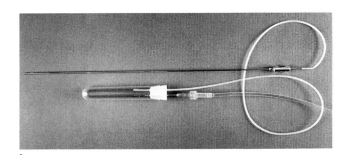

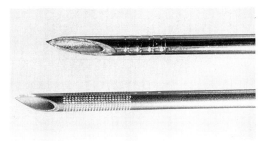

A **B**

Figure 28-24. (**A**) Swemed needle system attached for transvaginally guided aspiration for in vitro fertilization (Swemed Lab, V. Frolunda, Sweden). (**B**) Two types of etched needle systems available.

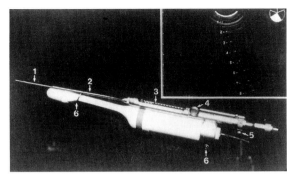

Figure 28-25. The spring-loaded, automated puncture device attached to the transvaginal ultrasound probe. 1, Needle; 2, needle guide; 3, depth setting; 4, trigger; 5, safety screw; 6, attachment brackets. *Inset:* On the screen, software-generated biopsy guide and depth markers. (Courtesy of Ilan E. Timor-Tritsch, MD, The Presbyterian Hospital in the City of New York, NY.)

Selective Fallopian Tube Cannulization

The technique of selective fallopian tube cannulization under sonographic guidance can be used to transfer embryos, zygotes, sperm, or oocytes into the ampullary portion of the tube by way of the cervix, as well as relieve cornual obstruction[15,63,106] (see Fig. 28-16). There is a potential for mucosal damage within the isthmic portion of the fallopian tube, which may be of concern because it will be the transport route for embryos shortly thereafter into the uterus. The initial experience showed a slight increase in ectopic pregnancies.[4,34] The technique does offer an alternative to laparoscopically guided gamete intrafallopian transfer (Fig. 28-27), but there has been little mention of it in the current literature.

Male Factor Infertility

Forty percent of all infertility is thought to be male in origin.[113] Adequate semen parameters (i.e., sperm density, motility, morphology) must be present for conception to occur. Etiologies for poor semen quality are varied and include testicular failure, vasoepididymal obstruction of congenital or infectious origin, as well as varicocele, systemic disease, or idiopathic causes.[114] Of these, varicoceles are the most common abnormality associated with male factor infertility (25% to 37%). Varicoceles are

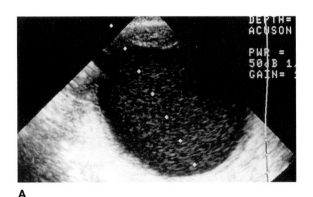

A

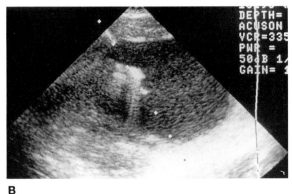

B

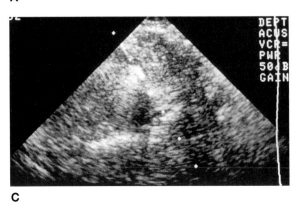

C

Figure 28-26. Puncturing a cyst that has an "endometrioma appearance." (**A**) The center of the cyst is targeted using the 2.5-cm depth. (**B**) The needle is in place; its tip is exactly 2.5 cm deep in the center of the cyst (ring-down artifacts are created by the needle itself). (**C**) The scan at the completion of the aspiration.

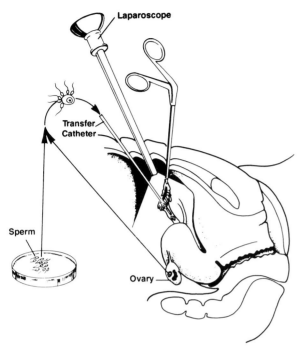

Figure 28-27. Diagram illustrating laparoscopic gamete intrafallopian transfer procedure. The ovary is stimulated to produce multiple mature follicles. Laparoscopic guidance with an aspirating needle placed transabdominally in the lower pelvis is used for oocyte retrieval. Mature gametes (oocytes and sperm) are placed in a catheter, threaded into the ampullary portion of the tube from the peritoneal cavity, and deposited there. Fertilization and subsequent passage of the embryos into the uterus for implantation occur in the normal fashion and time frame.

evidenced by dilatation and tortuosity of the veins of the pampiniform plexus surrounding the spermatic cord. Left-side varicoceles are more common because of the insertion of the left spermatic vein into the left renal vein. The right spermatic vein enters the inferior vena cava directly. Varicoceles are present in a significantly higher percentage of men with secondary infertility (81%) compared to primary (35%) infertility, according to Gorelick and Goldstein.[47] This suggests that varicoceles promote a progressive decline in infertility. A World Health Organization study of 9034 men found that the incidence of varicocele in men with abnormal semen was more than twice that in men with normal semen, and that varicoceles may be accompanied by decreases in testicular volume.[125]

Semen parameters are often abnormal in the presence of varicocele, with decreases in sperm density and motility and changes in morphology.[20]

Which of several proposed etiologies for this is most significant is unclear. Perhaps the effects of scrotal temperature, hormonal abnormalities, and biochemical and immunologic factors combine to provide a bilateral disease entity with the eventual symptom of infertility.[20]

Although the diagnosis of a varicocele can be made on the basis of a physical examination alone, smaller, subclinical varicoceles are diagnosed by Doppler sonography (Fig. 28-28) or venography. Treatment includes surgical interruption of the internal spermatic vein. An embolism technique to occlude the vein is also available. The pregnancy rate after therapy as well as the identification of which men might benefit most from surgery are controversial.[20]

Fertility Control

Fertility control includes hormonal, barrier and chemical agents, the IUD and surgical methods including elective abortion. While sonography can be applied in the evaluation of pain, bleeding, or pelvic masses, in the context of hormonal, barrier, or surgical contraceptive methods, it plays a critical role in only two of these areas: IUD localization and elective abortion.

INTRAUTERINE CONTRACEPTIVE DEVICES

Although IUD use has decreased from its all-time high in the 1960s and 1970s, it remains one of the most effective coitus-independent forms of contra-

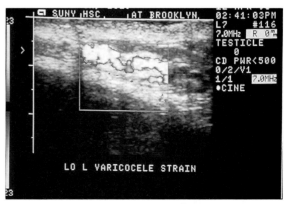

Figure 28-28. Varicocele with color flow on straining. Longitudinal image superior to testicle showed tubular areas that filled with color (seen as white on this black-and-white slide) on straining. Straining as imaging in standing position can make subclinical varicoceles more readily imaged.

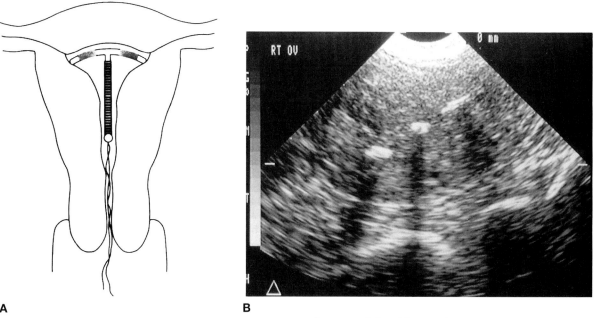

A   **B**

Figure 28-29. (**A**) Diagram of ParaGard intrauterine device. (Courtesy of GynoPharma, Inc., Somerville, New Jersey.) (**B**) Transvaginal ultrasound of intrauterine device (Lippes loop) in an appropriate intrauterine position. Note the drop-out of sound around the plastic device.

ception available.[14] Currently, only two types of IUDs are marketed in the United States: the Para-Gard T380A (Copper T) (GynoPharma, Inc., Somerville, NJ) and Progestasert (ALZA Pharmaceutical, Palo Alto, CA). Both have similar shapes (Fig. 28-29), but IUDs have had many shapes and forms[127] (Fig. 28-30). The contraceptive action of the IUD is not totally understood, but all devices act as a foreign body within the uterus. The bioactive devices, such as those with copper or progesterone, have added properties. The copper is released continuously, affecting the receptivity of the endometrium. The steady release of microdoses of progesterone within the uterus from the Progestasert device creates an endometrium that is hostile to implantation and cervical mucus that is too thick to permit sperm entry into the uterus. Regardless of which type of IUD is used, excellent contraceptive efficacy is obtained as long as the patient is a suitable candidate and proper placement within the uterus has been achieved. Efficacy rates for the copper device are 2.2 pregnancies for 100 women per year.[14]

Although IUDs are usually easily located by the string attached to the tailpiece and extending through the cervix,[14] the string may retract into the uterus or break at the time of an attempted removal.

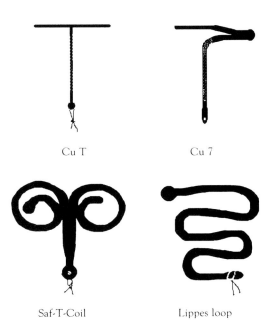

Cu T   Cu 7

Saf-T-Coil   Lippes loop

Figure 28-30. IUD: Diagram of the most common intrauterine devices. The ParaGard and the Progestasert look like the Copper T.

Ultrasound has replaced the standard radiograph in such cases, permitting easy identification of the IUD's location as long as it is within the uterus. Evidence of perforation, malpositioning within the uterine cavity, embedding in the myometrium, or incomplete removal can also be assessed by ultrasound, replacing hysterosalpingogram contrast injection. Difficult removals due to shifts in IUD positioning in the uterus or its embedding can be anticipated and removal guided with ultrasound.

Expulsion or partial expulsion of the IUD from the uterine cavity with resultant embedding of a portion of the IUD device, especially the stem, can occur without the user being aware. Absence of the string or strong cramping are indications for ultrasound evaluation. Uterine perforation, although usually occurring at the time of insertion, is rarely identified until later.[127] If the device is no longer within the uterus, ultrasound is rarely of use in localization. A flat plate for copper devices or magnetic resonance imaging for plastic devices are most useful.[127,128] Immediate removal is necessary to prevent further complications, including bowel perforation.

Pregnancy and Intrauterine Devices

Pregnancy in the presence of an IUD poses many serious problems. The risk of spontaneous abortion in the presence of an IUD is about 50%.[14] Removal is recommended if it can be accomplished without significant uterine manipulation. Complications of allowing the IUD to remain in the uterus include spontaneous abortion, sepsis, premature delivery, and maternal death.[19,62,64] Removal early in pregnancy decreases the miscarriage rate to 15% to 25%.[42,106] No gestational abnormalities have been associated with the presence of an IUD within the uterus throughout gestation. The device usually remains extraembryonic in location.[119] Ultrasound is essential in locating the device in relation to the ongoing gestation. According to one report, ultrasound guidance has been used successfully in removing an occult IUD and maintaining the ongoing gestation in all but one of eight cases.[119]

Although the incidence of ectopic pregnancy is not increased with IUD use, a high percentage of pregnancies that occur in patients with an IUD are ectopic in location.[112] Vaginal bleeding in the presence of an IUD and a suspected pregnancy must be aggressively evaluated by ultrasound and pregnancy testing.

Questions with regard to associated pelvic infection with the IUD have been the major deterrent to its more widespread use. Although many believe the risk and instance of pelvic inflammatory disease are increased with IUD use,[32] evidence is confounded by the general increase in the incidence of pelvic inflammatory disease and differences in occurrence rates with different devices (e.g., Dalkon Shield)[74] and within different relationships (e.g., monogamous as opposed to multiple partners).[52,88] Again, transvaginal as well as transabdominal ultrasound may be of use in the diagnosis. Immediate removal of the IUD is recommended when pelvic infection is suspected. In general, use of IUDs is suggested for primarily parous women.

HYSTEROSCOPIC STERILIZATION WITH SILICONE PLUGS

The insertion of hysteroscopically placed tubal plugs as potentially reversible or permanent forms of contraception was attempted in the 1970s and 1980s.[23] Placement of most of the devices was performed under direct visualization of the uterine cavity through the cervix.

Hysteroscopic sterilization has never moved out of the experimental phase and into general use because the silicone plugs proved to be irreversible, expensive, sophisticated equipment was required for their placement, and there was an increased rate of failure both at the time of placement and in the following 3 months after placement. However, patients are still seen who have had silicone plugs placed. Sonographically, they appear hyperechoic, with shadowing similar to the plastic of an IUD. Their shape is irregular. Their presence illustrates well the extent of the interstitial portion of the tube (Fig. 28-31), and they should be easily recognized when seen sonographically. They may contribute to irregular bleeding by acting as a kind of IUD.

ELECTIVE ABORTION

When a patient has made a decision to undergo an elective abortion, ultrasound can be useful in clinical management before, during, and after the procedure.

Preoperative Evaluation

Although there are no data to support the routine use of ultrasound for pregnancy dating in first trimester abortions, most practitioners believe it is

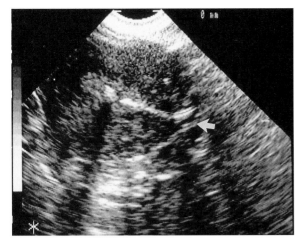

Figure 28-31. *Transvaginal ultrasound of the fundus of the uterus. The interstitial portion of the tube is visualized because it is filled with a silicone rubber plug (arrow), a portion of a hysteroscopically formed-in-place tubal plug. The patient was experiencing dysfunctional uterine bleeding because the plug had slipped into the uterine cavity, acting like an intrauterine device and irritating the uterine cavity.*

than expected dates could indicate the presence of a leiomyoma, congenital anomalies of the uterus, adnexal cysts, multiple gestation, hydatidiform mole, or just a date discrepancy, or possibly no pregnancy at all. When necessary, simultaneous quantitative β-hCG pregnancy testing and ultrasound should be performed to help define the true clinical situation.[8]

Intraoperative Ultrasound Guidance

Ultrasound guidance is indicated in cases of congenital anomaly of the uterus, cervical abnormalities—either diethylstilbestrol- or surgically induced, or in the presence of fibroids. Placement of the suction cannula with ultrasound direction permits the operator to be certain of reaching the chorionic sac while avoiding injury or perforation. Guidance should be applied when there is any concern on the part of the operator that the procedure was not complete (e.g., absence of villi in the curettings suggestive of an incomplete procedure, congenital anomaly of the uterus, or ectopic pregnancy).[68]

indicated in pregnancies judged to be 15 weeks or greater.[68,118] Ultrasound should be used in establishing gestational age before an abortion procedure when there is any concern regarding a discrepancy between menstrual dates (from last menstrual period) and physical examination. A uterus larger

Postoperative Ultrasound

When, after dilatation and evaluation, a patient has complaints of immediate or delayed severe pain or bleeding (Fig. 28-32), ultrasound can be particularly useful in identifying retained products of conception. This finding may indicate a need to repeat

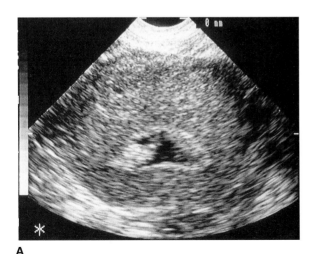

A

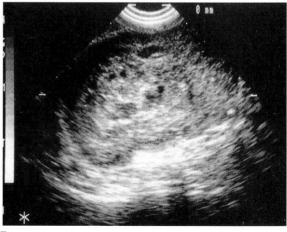

B

Figure 28-32. **(A)** *Transvaginal ultrasound of the uterus. Irregularity of the endometrium and fluid (blood) within the cavity are visualized. Retained secundines were confirmed at hysteroscopy.* **(B)** *Transvaginal ultrasound of the uterus. Irregular cystic tissue filling the uterine cavity was confirmed as retained secundines at the time of a repeat dilatation and curettage procedure.*

the surgical procedure.[68] Particularly in later mid-trimester abortions, retained osseous tissue within the uterine cavity may be present. Fetal endochondral ossification occurs after 12 weeks of gestation.[85] The presence of highly echogenic structures within the endometrial cavity with the history of a recent miscarriage or therapeutic abortion should raise this concern.[25]

Conclusion

Many of the development and clinical applications of ultrasound, particularly transvaginal sonography, have been borne of the demands of clinicians who treat infertility and the patients who suffer from it. Diagnostic ultrasound is an essential component of infertility management, from diagnosis to treatment and therapeutic intervention.

REFERENCES

1. Abramowicz JS, Archer DF. Uterine endometrial peristalsis: A transvaginal ultrasound study. Fertil Steril. 1990; 54:451–454.
2. The American Fertility Society, Society for Assisted Reproductive Technology. Assisted reproductive technology in the United States and Canada: 1992 results generated from the American Fertility Society/Society for Assisted Reproductive Technology Registry. Fertil Steril. 1994; 62:1121–1128.
3. Bakos O, Lundkvist O, Bergh T. Transvaginal sonographic evaluation of endometrial growth and texture in spontaneous ovulatory cycles: A descriptive study. Hum Reprod. 1993; 8:799–806.
4. Balmaceda JP, Alam V, Borini A. Fallopian tube catheterization. Infertility and Reproductive Medicine Clinics of North America. 1991; 2:783–787.
5. Batzer FR. Ultrasonic indices of ovulation. J Reprod Med. 1986; 31:764–769.
6. Batzer FR, Gocial B, Corson SL, Weiner S, Wapner RJ. Multiple pregnancies with GIFT: Complications of a new technique. Journal of In Vitro Fertilization and Embryo Transfer. 1988; 5:35–37.
7. Batzer FR, Hansen L. Bizarre sonographic appearance of an adenomyoma and its presentation. J Ultrasound Med. 1996; 15:599–602.
8. Batzer FR, Hasty LA, Corson SL, et al. Redefining the landmarks of early pregnancy utilizing transvaginosonography. Am J Gyn Health. 1993; 7:71–75.
9. Batzer FR, Roitman S, Becker N, et al. Benign versus malignant disease: Correlation of ovarian cyst fluid parameters with transvaginal sonographic appearance. In: Fleischer AC, Jones HW, eds. Early

10. Detection of Ovarian Carcinoma With Transvaginal Sonography: Potentials and Limitations. Part II. New York: Raven Press; 1993:75–81.
10. Blankstein J, Shalev J, Saadon T, Kukio EE. Ovarian hyperstimulation syndrome: Prediction by number and size of preovulatory ovarian follicles. Fertil Steril. 1987; 47:597–602.
11. Blumenfeld Z, Dirnfeld M, Abramovici H, Amit A, Bronshtein M, Brandes JM. Spontaneous fetal reduction in multiple gestations assessed by transvaginal ultrasound. Br J Obstet Gynaecol. 1992; 99:333–337.
12. Breckenridge JW, Schinfeld JS. Technique for US-guided fallopian tube catheterization. Radiology. 1991; 180:569–570.
13. Bryce RL, Shuter B, Sinosich MJ, Stiel JN. The value of ultrasound, gonadotropin, and estradiol measurements for precise ovulation prediction. Fertil Steril. 1982; 37:42–45.
14. Burnhill MS. Intrauterine contraception. In: Corson SL, Derman RJ, Tyrer LB, eds. Fertility Control. Boston: Little, Brown; 1984:271–285.
15. Bustillo M, Murabi AK, Schulman JD. Pregnancy after nonsurgical ultrasound-guided gamete intrafallopian transfer. N Engl J Med. 1988; 319:313.
16. Callahan TL, Hall JE, Ettner SL, Christiansen CL, Greene MF, Crowley WF Jr. The economic impact of multiple-gestation pregnancies and the contribution of assisted-reproduction techniques to their incidence. N Engl J Med. 1994; 331:244–249.
17. Carrington BM, Hricak H, Nuruddin RH, Secaf E. Müllerian duct anomalies: MR imaging evaluation. Radiology 1990; 176:715–720.
18. Cassidenti DL, Yee B. Ultrasound in the evaluation and management of the infertile woman. Ultrasound Quarterly. 1993; 11:169–175.
19. Cates W, Ory HW, Rochat RW, Tyler CW. The intrauterine device and deaths from spontaneous abortion. N Engl J Med. 1976; 295:1155–1159.
20. Chehval MJ, Purcell MH. Deterioration of semen parameters over time in men with untreated varicocele: Evidence of progressive testicular damage. Fertil Steril. 1992; 57:174–177.
21. Clark RL, Keefe B. Infertility: Imaging of the female. Urol Radiol. 1989; 11:233–237.
22. Confino E, Friberg J, Gleicher N. Transcervical balloon tuboplasty. Fertil Steril. 1986; 46:963–966.
23. Cooper JM. Hysteroscopic sterilization. In: Corson SL, Derman RJ, Tyrer LB, eds. Fertility Control. Boston: Little, Brown; 1984:119–131.
24. Daly DC, Soto-Albors C, Walters C, Ying YK, Riddick DH. Ultrasonographic assessment of luteinized unruptured follicle syndrome in unexplained infertility. Fertil Steril. 1985; 43:62–65.
25. Dawood YM, Jarrertt JC III. Prolonged intrauter-

ine retention of fetal bones after abortion causing infertility. Am J Obstet Gynecol. 1982; 143:715–717.

26. Deaton JL, Gibson M, Riddick DH, Brumsted JR. Diagnosis and treatment of cornual obstruction using a flexible guide wire. Fertil Steril. 1990; 53:232–236.

27. de Crespigny LCh, O'Herlihy C, Robinson HP. Ultrasonic observation of the mechanism of human ovulation. Am J Obstet Gynecol. 1981; 139:177–183.

28. Dellenbach P, Njsand I, Moreau L, Feger B, Plumere C, Gerlinger P. Transvaginal sonographically controlled ovarian follicle puncture for egg retrieval. Lancet 1984; 1:1467.

29. Dickey RP, Olar YY, Curole DN, Taylor SN, Rye PH, Matulich EM. The probability of multiple births when multiple gestational sacs or viable embryos are diagnosed at first trimester ultrasound. Hum Reprod. 1990; 5:880–882.

30. Dickey RP, Olar TT, Taylor SN, Curole DN, Harrigill K. Relationship of biochemical pregnancy to pre-ovulatory endometrial thickness and pattern in patients undergoing ovulation induction. Hum Reprod. 1993; 8:327–330.

31. Dickey RP, Olar TT, Taylor SN, Curole DN, Matulich EM. Relationship of endometrial thickness and pattern to fecundity in ovulation induction cycles: Effect of clomiphene citrate alone and with human menopausal gonadotropin. Fertil Steril. 1993; 59:756–760.

32. Edelman DA, Berger GS, Keith L. The use of IUDs and their relationship to pelvic inflammatory disease: A review of epidemiologic and clinical studies. Current Problems in Obstetrics and Gynecology. 1982; 6:5.

33. Edwards RG, Steptoe PC, Purdy JM. Establishing full-term pregnancies using cleaving embryos grown in vitro. Br J Obstet Gynaecol. 1980; 87:737–756.

34. Lucena E, Ruiz JA, Mendoza JC, Ortiz JA. Vaginal intratubal insemination (VITI) and vaginal GIFT endosonographic technique: Early experience. Hum Reprod. 1989; 4:658–662.

35. Fedele L, Bianchi S, Dorta M, Brieschi D. Transvaginal ultrasonography versus hysteroscopy in the diagnosis of uterine submucous myomas. Obstet Gynecol. 1991; 77:745–748.

36. Fedele L, Bianchi S, Dorta M, Zanotti F, Brioschi D, Carinelli S. Transvaginal ultrasonography in the differential diagnosis of adenomyoma versus leiomyoma. Am J Obstet Gynecol. 1992; 167:603–606.

37. Fedele L, Ferrazzi E, Dorta M, Vercellini P, Candiani GB. Ultrasonography in the differential diagnosis of "double" uteri. Fertil Steril. 1988; 50:361–364.

38. Feichtinger W, Kemeter P. Transvaginal sector scan sonography for needle guided transvaginal follicle aspiration and other applications in gynecologic routine and research. Fertil Steril. 1986; 45:722–725.

39. Fleischer AC. Ultrasound imaging—2000: Assessment of utero-ovarian blood flow with transvaginal color Doppler sonography: Potential clinical applications in infertility. Fertil Steril. 1991; 55:684–691.

40. Fleischer AC, Herbert Cm, Hill GA, Kepple DM, Worrell JA. Transvaginal sonography of the endometrium during induced cycles. J Ultrasound Med. 1991; 10:93–95.

41. Fleischer AC, Kalemeris GC, Entmann SS. Sonographic depiction of the endometrium during normal cycles. Ultrasound Med Biol. 1986; 12:271–277.

42. Foremann H, Bruce SV, Schlesselman S. Intrauterine device usage and fetal loss. Obstet Gynecol. 1981; 58:669–677.

43. Foy PM, Blumenfeld ML, Fleming CM. Secondary dysmenorrhea associated with residual calcified chorionic villi. J Diagn Med Sonogr. 1993; 9:79–81.

44. Goldberg BB, Liu JB, Kuhlman K, Merton DA, Kurtz AB. Endoluminal gynecologic ultrasound: Preliminary results. J Ultrasound Med. 1991; 10:583–590.

45. Gonen Y, Blankier J, Casper RAF. Transvaginal ultrasound in selective embryo reduction for multiple pregnancy. Obstet Gynecol. 1990; 75:720–722.

46. Gonen Y, Casper RF. Prediction of implantation by the sonographic appearances of the endometrium during controlled ovarian stimulation for in vitro fertilization (IVF). J In Vitro Fert Embryo Trans. 1990; 7–146.

47. Gorelick JI, Goldstein M. Loss of fertility in men with varicocele. Fertil Steril. 1993; 59:613–616.

48. Goswamy RK, Williams G, Steptoe PC. Decreased uterine perfusion: A cause of infertility. Hum Reprod. 1988; 3:955–959.

49. Granberg S, Crona N, Enk L, Hammarberg K, Wikland M. Ultrasound-guided puncture of cystic tumors in the lower pelvis of young women. J Clin Ultrasound. 1989; 17:107–111.

50. Granberg S, Norstrom A, Wikland M. Tumors in the lower pelvis as imaged by vaginal sonography. Gynecol Oncol. 1990; 37:224–229.

51. Granberg S, Norstrom A, Wikland M. Comparison of endovaginal ultrasound and cytological evaluation of cystic ovarian tumors. J Ultrasound Med. 1991; 10:9–14.

52. Grimes DA. The intrauterine device, pelvic inflammatory disease, and infertility: The confusion between hypothesis and knowledge. Fertil Steril. 1992; 58:670–673.

53. Grunfeld L, Walker B, Bergh PA, Sandler B, Hofmann G, Havot D. High-resolution endovaginal ultrasonography of the endometrium: A noninvasive test for endometrial adequacy. Obstet Gynecol. 1991; 78:200–204.

54. Gutmann JN. Imaging in the evaluation of female infertility. J Reprod Med. 1992; 37:54–61.

55. Hackeloer BJ. The role of ultrasound in female infertility management. Ultrasound Med Biol. 1984; 10:35–50.

56. Hackeloer BJ, Fleming R, Robinson HP, Adam AH, Coutts JRT. Correlation of ultrasonic and endocrinologic assessment of human follicular development. Am J Obstet Gynecol. 1979; 135:122.

57. Haddad S, Ruach M, Ohel G. Sonographic demonstration of endometrial fluid collection following termination of pregnancy. Obstet Gynecol. 1992; 79:703–704.

58. Hecht BR, Hoffman DI. The use of ultrasound in infertility. Clin Obstet Gynecol. 1989; 32:541–549.

59. Hill LM, Coulam CB, Kislak SL, et al. Sonographic evaluation of the cervix during ovulation induction. Am J Obstet Gynecol. 1987; 157:1170–1174.

60. Hughes EG, Shekelton P, Leonie M, Leeton J. Ultrasound guided fallopian tube catheterization per vaginum: A feasibility study with the use of laparoscopic control. Fertil Steril. 1988; 50:986–989.

61. Hull MGR, Glazener CMA, Kelly NJ, Conway DI. Population study of causes, treatment, and outcome of infertility. Br Med J. 1985; 291:1693.

62. Hurt WG. Septic pregnancy associated with Dalkon Shield device. Obstet Gynecol. 1974; 44:491–495.

63. Jansen RPS, Anderson JC. Catheterisation of the fallopian tubes from the vagina. Lancet. 1987; 2:309–310.

64. Kahn HS, Tyler CW. An association between the Dalkon Shield and complicated pregnancies among women hospitalized for intrauterine contraceptive device-related disorders. Am J Obstet Gynecol. 1976; 125:83–86.

65. Karlsson B, Norstrom A, Wikland M, Granberg S, Anderson H. The use of endovaginal ultrasound to diagnose invasion of endometrial carcinoma. Ultrasound Obstet Gynecol. 1992; 2:35–39.

66. Karlstrom PO, Bakos O, Bergh T, Lundkvist O. Hormone and ultrasound parameters in ovarian stimulation cycles for direct intraperitoneal insemination. Hum Reprod. 1992; 7:813–820.

67. Kato O, Takatsuka R, Asch RH. Transvaginal–transmyometrial embryo transfer: The Towako method. Experiences of 104 cases. Fertil Steril. 1993; 59:51–53.

68. Kaunitz AM, Grimes DA. First-trimester abortion technology. In: Corson SL, Derman RJ, Tyrer LB, eds. Fertility Control. Boston: Little, Brown; 1984:63–76.

69. Kerin JF, Edmonds DK, Warnes GM, et al. Morphological and functional relationships of graafian follicle growth to ovulation in women using ultrasonic, laparoscopic and biochemical measurements. Br J Obstet Gynaecol. 1981; 88:81–90.

70. Khalifa E, Brzyski RG, Oehninger S, Acosta AA, Muasher SJ. Sonographic appearance of the endometrium: The predictive value for the outcome of in-vitro fertilization in stimulated cycles. Hum Reprod. 1992; 7:677–680.

71. Kurjak A, Zalud I, Alfirevic Z. Evaluation of adnexal masses with transvaginal color ultrasound. J Ultrasound Med. 1991; 1:295–297.

72. Kurtz AB, Shlansky-Goldberg RD, Cho HY, Needleman L, Wapner RJ, Goldberg BB. Detection of retained products of conception following spontaneous abortion in the first trimester. J Ultrasound Med. 1991; 10:387–395.

73. Landy HJ, Weiner S, Corson SL, Batzer FR, Bolognese RJ. The vanishing twin: Ultrasonographic assessment of fetal disappearance in the first trimester. Am J Obstet Gynecol. 1986; 155:14–19.

74. Lee NC, Rubin GL, Ory HW, Burkman, RT. Type of intrauterine device and the risk of pelvic inflammatory disease. Obstet Gynecol. 1983; 62:1–6.

75. Leerentveld RA, Van Gent I, van der Stoep M, Wladimiroff JW. Ultrasonographic assessment of Graafian follicle growth under monofollicular and multifollicular conditions in clomiphene citrate-stimulated cycles. Fertil Steril. 1985; 43:565–569.

76. Lenz S, Leeton J, Rogers P, Trounson A. Transfundal transfer of embryos using ultrasound. Journal of In Vitro Fertilization and Embryo Transfer. 1987; 4:13–17.

77. Lenz S, Lauritzen JG, Kjellow M. Collection of human oocytes for in vitro fertilization by ultrasonically guided follicular puncture. Lancet. 1981; 1:1163–1164.

78. Lewit N, Thaler I, Rottem S. The uterus: A new look with transvaginal sonography. J Clin Ultrasound. 1990; 18:331–336.

79. Liukkonen S, Koskimies AL, Tenhunen A, Ylostalo P. Diagnosis of luteinized unruptured follicle (LUF) syndrome by ultrasound. Fertil Steril. 1984; 41:26–30.

80. Mahadevan MM, Trounson AO. The influence of

seminal characteristics on the success rate of human in vitro fertilization. Fertil Steril. 1984; 42:400–405.

81. Mahony BS. Translabial and transvaginal ultrasound of the cervix. Nyberg DA, Hill LM, Bohm-Velez M, Mendelson EB, eds. Transvaginal Ultrasound. St. Louis: Mosby Year Book; 1992:169–186.

82. Marinho AO, Sallam HN, Goessens LKV, Collins WP. Real time pelvic ultrasonography during the periovulatory period of patients attending an artificial insemination clinic. Fertil Steril. 1982; 37:633.

83. Mark AS, Hricak H, Heinrichs LW, Hendrickson MR. Adenomyosis and leiomyoma: Differential diagnosis with MR imaging. Radiology. 1987; 163:527–529.

84. Marshak RH, Eliasoph J. The roentgen findings in adenomyosis. Radiology. 1955; 64:846–852.

85. Melius FA, Julian TM, Nagel TC. Prolonged retention of intrauterine bones. Obstet Gynecol. 1991; 78:919–921.

86. Nitschke-Dabelstein S, Hackeloer BJ, Sturm G. Ovulation and corpus luteum formation observed by ultrasonography. Ultrasound Med Biol. 1981; 7:33–39.

87. O'Herlihy C, de Crespigny LJCh, Robinson HP. Monitoring ovarian follicular development with real-time ultrasound. Br J Obstet Gynaecol. 1980; 87:613–618.

88. Ory HW. A review of the association between intrauterine devices and acute pelvic inflammatory disease. J Reprod Med. 1978; 20:200–204.

89. Palermo G, Horis H, Devroey P, Van Steirteghem AC. Pregnancies after intracytoplasmic injection of a single spermatozoon into an oocyte. Lancet. 1992; 340:17–18.

90. Parsons SK, Lense JJ. Sonohysterography for endometrial abnormalities: Preliminary results. J Clin Ultrasound. 1993; 21:87–95.

91. Patten RM. The fallopian tube and pelvic inflammatory disease. In: Nyberg DA, Lill LM, Bohm-Velez M, Mendelson EB, eds. Transvaginal Ultrasound. St. Louis: Mosby Year Book; 1992:209–221.

92. Peters AJ, Coulam CB. Hysterosalpingography with color Doppler ultrasonography. Am J Obstet Gynecol. 1991; 164:1530–1532.

93. Picker RH, Smith DH, Tucker MH, Saunders DM. Ultrasonic signs of imminent ovulation. J Clin Ultrasound. 1983; 11:1–2.

94. Polan ML, Totora M, Caldwell BV, Decherney AH. Abnormal ovarian cycles as diagnosed by ultrasound and serum estradiol levels. Fertil Steril. 1982; 37:342–347.

95. Queenan JT, O'Brien GD, Bains LM, Simpson J. Ultrasound scanning of ovaries to detect ovulation in women. Fertil Steril. 1980; 34:99–105.

96. Randolph JR Jr, Ying YK, Maier DB, Schmidt CL. Comparison of real-time ultrasonography, hysterosalpingography, and laparoscopy/hysteroscopy in the evaluation of uterine abnormalities and tubal patency. Fertil Steril. 1986; 46:828–832.

97. Rein MS, Barbieri RL, Greene MF. The causes of high-order multiple gestation. Int J Fertil. 1990; 35:154–156.

98. Reuter KL, Daly DC, Cohen SM. Septate versus bicornuate uteri: Errors in imaging diagnosis. Radiology. 1989; 173:749–752.

99. Richman T, Viscomi GN, DeCherney A, et al. Fallopian tube patency assessed by ultrasound following fluid injection. Radiology. 1984; 152:507.

100. Ritchie WG. Ultrasound in the evaluation of normal and induced ovulation. Fertil Steril. 1985; 43:167–181.

101. Rizk B, Tan SL, Kingsland C, Steer C, Mason BA, Campbell S. Ovarian cyst aspiration and the outcome of in vitro fertilization. Fertil Steril. 1990; 54:661–664.

102. Rogashi K, Ozasa I, Konishi I, et al. Enlarged uterus: Differentiation between adenomyosis and leiomyoma with MR imaging. Radiology 1989; 171:531–534.

103. Sassone M, Timor-Tritsch IE, Artner A, Westhoff C, Warren WB. Transvaginal sonographic characterization of ovarian pathology: Evaluation of new scoring system to predict ovarian malignancy. Obstet Gynecol. 1991; 78:70–76.

104. Saxton DW, Farquhar CM, Rae T, Beard RW. Accuracy of ultrasound measurements of female pelvic organs. Br J Obstet Gynaecol. 1990; 97:695–699.

105. Schenker J, Yarkoni S, Granat M. Multiple pregnancies following induction of ovulation. Fertil Steril. 1981; 35:105–123.

106. Schultes MCW, Roozenburg BFG, Alderba AT, Zeilmaker GH. Transcervical intrafallopian transfer of zygotes. Fertil Steril. 1990; 54:283–286.

107. Segars JH, Herbert CM, Moore DE, Hill GA. Selective fallopian tube cannulation: Initial experience in an infertile population. Fertil Steril. 1990; 53:357–359.

108. Shapiro H, Cowell C, Casper RF. The use of vaginal ultrasound for monitoring endometrial preparation in a donor oocyte program. Fertil Steril. 1993; 59:1055–1058.

109. Shapiro BS, DeCherney AH. Ultrasound and infertility. J Reprod Med. 1989; 34:151–155.

110. Shoham Z, Di Carlo C, Patel A, Conway GS, Jacobs HS. Is it possible to run a successful ovulation induction program based solely on ultrasound

monitoring? The importance of endometrial measurements. Fertil Steril. 1991; 56:836–841.

111. Siedler D, Laing FC, Jeffrey RB Jr, Wing VW. Uterine adenomyosis: A difficult sonographic diagnosis. J Ultrasound Med 1987; 6:345–349.

112. Sivin I. IUDs and ectopic pregnancy. Stud Fam Plann. 1983; 14:57–63.

113. Speroff L, Glass RH, Kase NG, eds. Clinical Gynecologic Endocrinology and Infertility. 4th ed. Chap. 17. Baltimore: Williams & Wilkins; 1989: 513–546.

114. Speroff L, Glass RH, Kase NG, eds. Clinical Gynecologic Endocrinology and Infertility. 4th ed. Chap. 19. Baltimore: Williams & Wilkins; 1989: 565–582.

115. Steptoe PC, Edwards RG. Birth after the reimplantation of a human embryo. Lancet. 1978; 2:366.

116. Steptoe PC, Edwards RG. Laparoscopic recovery of preovulatory human oocytes after priming of ovaries with gonadotropins. Lancet. 1970; 1:683–689.

117. Sterzik K, Grab D, Rosenbusch B, Hamers S, Dallenbach-Hellweg G. Receptivity of the endometrium: Comparison of ultrasound and histologic findings after hormonal stimulation. Gerburtshilfe Frauenheilkd. 1991; 51:554–558.

118. Stubblefield PG. Induced abortion in the midtrimester. Corson SL, Derman RJ, Tyrer LB, eds. Fertility Control. Boston: Little, Brown; 1984: 77–87.

119. Sviggum O, Skjeldestad FE, Tuveng JM. Ultrasonically guided retrieval of occult IUD in early pregnancy. Acta Obstet Gynaecol Scand. 1991; 70: 355–357.

120. Tabsh KM. A report of 131 cases of multifetal pregnancy reduction. Obstet Gyneol. 1993; 82:57–60.

121. Thurmond AS, Patton PE, Hector DM, Jones MK. US-guided fallopian tube catheterization. Radiology. 1991; 180:571–572.

122. Thurmond A, Rosch J. Nonsurgical fallopian tube recanalization for treatment of infertility. Radiology. 1990; 174:371–374.

123. Ueno J, Oehninger S, Bryzyski RG, Acosta AA, Philput CB, Muasher SJ. Ultrasonographic appearance of the endometrium in natural and stimulated in-vitro fertilization cycles and its correlation with outcome. Hum Reprod. 1991; 6:901–904.

124. Waegemaekers CT, Berg-Helder A, Blankart A, Naaktgeboren N. Transvaginal ovarian cyst puncture in the early follicular phase of an IVF cycle: Indications and results. Hum Reprod. 1988; 3(suppl):80.

125. World Health Organization. The influence of varicocele on parameters of fertility in a large group of men presenting to infertility clinics. Fertil Steril. 1992; 57:1289–1293.

126. Yovich JL, Stanger JD. The limitations of in vitro fertilization from males with severe oligospermia and abnormal sperm morphology. Journal of In Vitro Fertilization and Embryo Transfer. 1984; 1:172–179.

127. Zakin D, Stern W, Rosenblatt R. Complete and partial uterine perforation and embedding following insertion of intrauterine devices, I: Classification, complications, mechanism, incidence and missing string. Obstet Gynecol Surv. 1981; 36:335–353.

128. Zakin D, Stern W, Rosenblatt R. Complete and partial uterine perforation and embedding following insertion of intrauterine devices, II: Diagnostic methods, prevention and management. Obstet Gynecol Surv. 1981; 36:401–417.

29

Amniocentesis and Chorionic Villus Sampling

GEORGE I. SOLISH and LUIS A. BRACERO

Amniocentesis and chorionic villus sampling (CVS), the two most common clinical techniques for obtaining living fetal cells or fetal cell products from the pregnant uterus for prenatal diagnosis, are heavily dependent on the use of ultrasound for their performance. Percutaneous umbilical blood sampling (PUBS), also known as cordocentesis,[15] is another technique requiring the use of ultrasound to obtain fetal cells, but this technique carries a much higher procedure-related risk than either amniocentesis or CVS. PUBS is performed by carefully inserting a long, fine-gauged needle under ultrasound guidance through the skin of the mother's abdomen, through the subcutaneous tissues, peritoneum, uterus, amniotic sac, and tapping one of the fetal umbilical vessels directly for microliter amounts of fetal whole blood to analyze. It is associated with a higher risk for complications and is therefore reserved for special indications and special analyses when, for example, fetal whole blood samples are needed for chemical assays or rapid blood cell cultures for chromosome studies in patients who are too far advanced in pregnancy for amniocentesis or CVS.

The ever-increasing number of genetic disorders that can now be diagnosed prenatally, particularly with the advent of DNA technology, has brought amniocentesis and CVS into the realm of everyday medical practice. These are invasive procedures carrying defined complication rates of which the patient must be made aware, along with these procedures' benefits and limitations. Genetic counseling sessions provide the opportunity to impart this information to patients and their families.

Genetic counseling has been described as a communication process by which the occurrence and the risk of recurrence of a genetic disorder within a family is discussed.[44] In fact, it is more than this, for the genetic counselor also has the obligation and the responsibility of providing the patient or the family with the most recent relevant facts concerning a genetic disorder, including the risks involved in diagnosis, and the available treatment options.[44,45]

Manipulations of the pregnant uterus and the developing fetus within are highly charged emotional issues with moral and ethical overtones that must also be addressed with each patient. To meet current standards of care in prenatal diagnosis, just as in all of today's general medical care, all relevant questions must be thoroughly discussed and appropriately answered. A team approach is therefore found to be useful, usually involving not only the obstetrician but a genetic counselor, a sonographer, and appropriate surgical and medical specialists.

Amniocentesis

"Amniocentesis," derived from the Greek, means "puncture of the amniotic sac." The amnion and the chorion, the two major membranous structures surrounding and protecting the developing fetus within the uterus throughout pregnancy, develop from the same fertilized ovum as does the fetus. They serve their function during pregnancy, and are then discarded with expulsion of the placenta after the birth of the child.

HISTORY

The technique of amniocentesis was first described in the last century by Lambl (1881)[31] and by Schatz (1882)[43] as a method for relieving intrauterine pressure resulting from abnormal accumulation of amniotic fluid. Parvey (1933),[38] who was one of the first in this country to report successful management of acute hydramnios with abdominal puncture, credits Bumm[9] as the first to have attempted this procedure, as early as 1900. The same theoretic objections to the blind insertion of a needle into the pregnant uterus were voiced by prominent physicians of that day as have been raised by critics of today. Objections included possible injury to the fetus, damage to the placenta, uterine hemorrhage, infection, and interruption of the pregnancy. These objections were apparently sufficient to discourage further progress until Bevis (1950)[4] showed that certain characteristics of amniotic fluid had diagnostic and prognostic value for hemolytic disease of the newborn. Walker (1957)[51] and later Liley (1961)[33] were able to demonstrate the relative safety of the procedure by performing serial amniocenteses on one patient without incident. Today, the amniocentesis needle is no longer inserted blindly into the abdomen, but rather under sonographic guidance. This has eliminated many of the previously encountered complications of the procedure, although some inherent risks still remain. Originally, prenatal diagnostic amniocentesis was recommended for patients who were at risk for congenital malformations because of advanced maternal age or because of a history in a previous pregnancy of a child with a specific birth defect. However, the President's Commission for Study of Ethical Problems in Medicine and Biomedical and Behavioral Science, which was convened in 1983,[40] recommended that the criteria for eligibility for genetic amniocentesis be reexamined so that women of all ages might benefit from this procedure, if they chose.

The increasing diagnostic accuracy, the decreasing risk of complications, and publicity in television and other mass media have increased the acceptability of amniocentesis among most populations of the world. The risk of complications has been variously reported to be of the order of 0.5%, and in many centers where this procedure is performed regularly and by well trained personnel, the actual procedure-related complication rate is less than 3 per 1000 procedures.[18]

The number of requests for amniocentesis and for CVS has escalated significantly in the past few years, with the advent of newer DNA technology and the identification of an increasing number of genetic disorders detectable by molecular genetic methods.

INDICATIONS FOR GENETIC AMNIOCENTESIS

The most frequent requests for genetic amniocentesis come from women aged 35 years or older, because of the maternal age-related increased chance of chromosome abnormalities. This category accounts for 65%[14] to 80%[21] of requests for prenatal diagnosis. Women whose serum α-fetoprotein (AFP) screening results are either elevated[7,8] or decreased below the median values for the general population[34] comprise the next largest group of requests, accounting for 10% to 15% of the total. The association between abnormally high levels of this protein and neural tube defects was first described by Leek and colleagues in 1972,[32] whereas maternal serum AFP (MSAFP) values below the mean levels for a given gestational age have been associated with an increased risk for fetal chromosomal trisomy.[34]

α-Fetoprotein is a serum protein found normally in the fetal circulatory system and produced by the fetal liver. If the circulation of amniotic fluid is obstructed, the protein accumulates in the amniotic fluid, backs up, and subsequently appears in the mother's serum in increasing amounts. Other conditions associated with MSAFP elevations include multiple pregnancy, fetal demise, and a number of other fetal abnormalities.[35] MSAFP levels as well as AFP levels in amniotic fluid differ at different weeks of gestation. The AFP level must therefore be evaluated in relation to the normal level for that specific gestational age. An MSAFP value in excess of 2.5 times the mean for that gestational age is suspect. The currently accepted protocol for screening recommends an ultrasound examination to confirm gestational age, and to determine the presence or absence of multiple pregnancies or the presence of other ultrasound-detectable abnormalities. Failure to determine correctly the gestational age may

lead to incorrect interpretation of the MSAFP results. Careful ultrasound examination discloses neural tube defects as the cause for MSAFP elevation in almost all cases (Figs. 29-1 and 29-2).

A varying but steadily growing number of well-informed patients who are in no specific risk category but are overly concerned about the possibility of an abnormal pregnancy outcome are asking to be tested. Maternal anxiety has therefore become a recognized indication for prenatal genetic diagnosis regardless of maternal age.

Amniocentesis is also recommended for women who have borne children with chromosomal defects or metabolic disorders in the past. More than a 100 metabolic disorders and an escalating number of

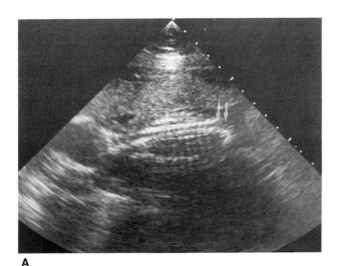

A

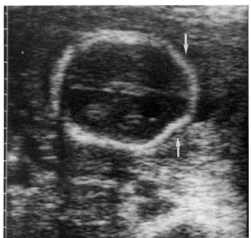

B

Figure 29-1. A pregnant 36-year-old woman had a routine amniocentesis for prenatal diagnosis because of advanced maternal age. A markedly elevated level of α-fetoprotein in the amniotic fluid led to reexamination of the fetus in utero, which disclosed (**A**) splaying of the distal sacral vertebral column (*arrows*) and (**B**) a positive "lemon" sign of the fetal skull (*arrows*). (**C**) These findings were the basis for the termination of this pregnancy. Spina bifida was seen after abortion.

C

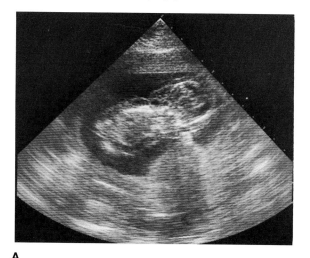
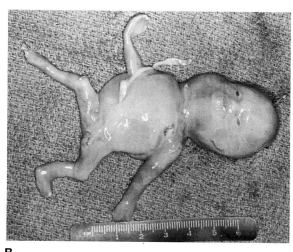

A   **B**

Figure 29-2. A cystic hygroma identified on sonographic examination (**A**) before amniocentesis and confirmed after abortion (**B**). The chromosomes and α-fetoprotein value were normal.

DNA fetal defects are now detectable biochemically in the prenatal period. The recurrence risks of genetic conditions depend on the mode of inheritance. The chances for recurrence range from less than 1% in the case of a previous child with a chromosomal defect not found in the parents, to 25% in the case of an autosomal recessive biochemical defect such as Tay-Sachs disease or cystic fibrosis, to 50% (for male children) in X-linked muscular dystrophy.

TIMING OF AMNIOCENTESIS

Amniocentesis is optimally performed between the 14th and 20th gestational weeks. The fluid volume is adequate at this time for obtaining useful samples with minimal threat to the fetus, and sufficient numbers of viable amniocytes are present to obtain a timely result. Furthermore, the fetal anatomy is better defined sonographically at this gestational age, permitting easier detection of abnormalities.

Prenatal diagnosis attempts to obtain results as early in pregnancy as possible, but performing amniocentesis earlier than 14 weeks has been shown significantly to increase the risk for pregnancy loss.[36] Technically, amniocentesis can be safely performed at any time in the second and third trimesters; the deadline is related more closely to individual state legal restrictions for pregnancy termination than to any other factor. Amniocentesis for determining fetal maturity by the ratio of lecithin to sphingomyelin (L/S ratio) and severity of erythroblastosis (by optical density measurements of the amniotic fluid) can be and is commonly performed with safety much later in pregnancy. However, because of increasing cell culture difficulties as the gestational age increases beyond 20 weeks, amniocentesis for prenatal diagnosis is likely to be unsuccessful when performed in the late second or third trimesters, and therefore is not recommended.

The legal limit for elective termination of pregnancy in New York State is 24 weeks; in many other states it is 20 weeks. The timing of genetic amniocentesis must therefore allow for completion of all laboratory testing to permit the option of legal pregnancy termination to those who might choose this alternative. The average waiting period for results (i.e., detecting abnormalities in chromosome number such as trisomy 21 [Down's syndrome], chromosome monosomy such as Turner's syndrome, or chromosome structural rearrangements, translocations, deletions, insertions, and so forth) is 7 to 10 days. Up to 3 weeks, in some cases, may be required to grow a sufficient number of cells to obtain a final result. Biochemical (enzyme) defects such as galactosemia, Gaucher's disease, Niemann-Pick disease, phenylketonuria, and Tay-Sachs disease, to name but a few, are usually diagnosed sooner than chromosome culture analyses can be completed. With the advent of molecular probes for detecting DNA defects, however, many biochemical defects such as those mentioned previously, as well as diseases like cystic fibrosis, Duchenne's muscular dystrophy, Prader-Willi syndrome, and the hemoglobinopathies can be diagnosed within hours after collection of the specimen.

To deal with problems of terminating pregnancies that have gone beyond the legal limit, particularly when a severely malformed fetus is at issue, many institutions have appointed ethics committees to evaluate each situation individually. The committee is composed of laymen, clergy, and nonmedical and medical professionals. They hear the evidence, evaluate the case, and make recommendations regarding these critical issues. Anencephalic fetuses have been legally aborted after 28 weeks of pregnancy in some cases.[12]

PROCEDURE FOR ULTRASOUND-GUIDED AMNIOCENTESIS

After genetic counseling and completion of the informed consent process, ideally done days or weeks before the performance of the procedure, an appointment is made for simultaneous ultrasound and amniocentesis. Amniocentesis is an outpatient procedure and is performed in the ultrasound laboratory in accordance with the guidelines of the American Institute of Ultrasound in Medicine.[1]

At our institution, the following information was found useful and is therefore routinely obtained by the sonographer before amniocentesis.

1. Number of fetuses, fetal position, and viability are determined.
2. Amniotic fluid volume is estimated as normal, decreased, or increased.
3. Placental location is recorded.
4. Gestational age is determined using the following measurements: biparietal diameter, femur length, abdominal circumference, head circumference, and binocular (interorbital) distance.
5. The following anatomic structures are identified and assessed: the cerebral ventricles, fetal heart (four-chamber view), stomach, urinary bladder, umbilical cord insertion, number of cord vessels, kidneys, spinal column, and limbs.
6. The optimal fluid pocket for amniocentesis is located.
7. Fetal heart rate is determined and noted before and after the procedure.

The operative site is draped with sterile towels. Strict sterile precautions are observed (Figs. 29-3 and 29-4) because complications after amniocentesis have been related to infection. The ultrasound transducer is coated with regular transmission gel and held by an assistant as the physician covers the transducer with a sterile plastic bag.[16] The plastic bag over the functional surface of the transducer is, in turn, coated with sterile gel. Under sonographic visualization, a 3.5-inch long, 20-gauge, sterile, disposable spinal needle with a stylet is used to enter the amniotic sac (see Fig. 29-3). Progress of the

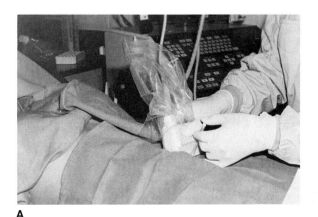
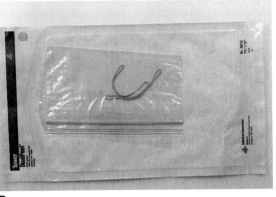

A   **B**

Figure 29-3. **(A)** Insertion of amniocentesis needle under direct ultrasonic visualization. The abdomen has been prepared and draped with sterile towels. The ultrasound transducer is encased in a sterile plastic bag. **(B)** Plastic bag is gas sterilized along with rubber bands for covering ultrasound scanner for amniocentesis.

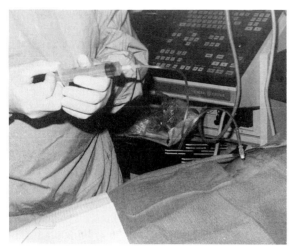

Figure 29-4. *The amniotic fluid specimen is withdrawn under sterile conditions by means of a sterile plastic catheter attached at one end to the amniocentesis needle and to a 20-ml syringe at the other.*

needle through the tissue layers is easily followed on the ultrasound screen. The beveled tip of the needle is seen as a bright spot on the ultrasound screen, described as a "flare" by Simpson and Elias (Fig. 29-5).[47] The amniocentesis site is thus documented on film. During the insertion procedure, extra caution must be exercised in directing the needle tip into the amniotic sac. It must be remembered that the ultrasound image of the needle position can be grossly distorted when viewed penetrating through liquid versus solid tissue interfaces.[47] Ultrasound monitoring and amniocentesis can be performed simultaneously by the same operator.

The stylet is removed and the first few drops of fluid are discarded, to avoid contaminating the specimen with maternal cells.[2,3] A 20-inch length of sterile, flexible extension tubing is attached to the Luer-lok needle hub. A sterile 20-ml syringe is attached to the other end of the tubing. The extension tubing provides greater ease and stability for amniotic fluid aspiration (see Fig. 29-4); alternatively, the syringe can be directly attached to the needle hub without the use of tubing. Approximately 20 to 30 ml of amniotic fluid is withdrawn and transferred to sterile, properly labeled, conical tubes for transport to the laboratory. After aspiration of the fluid sample, the needle is withdrawn. Although needle injuries to the fetus have been

reported, using the technique described here, none has been noted in our experience of 20 years. A final check of the fetal heart is made before the patient is discharged.

The amniocytes are separated in the laboratory from the amniotic fluid by centrifugation. The fluid is assayed for AFP or other biochemical substances, as indicated, and the cells are cultured for karyotyping.

MULTIPLE GESTATION

Ultrasound is used to determine gestational age, to verify viability, and to note the number and location of fetuses and placentas and to identify the presence of a membrane separating fetal compartments. In the event of diamniotic twins, each sac is identified sonographically and labeled A or B, according to its position in the mother's abdomen. In most instances the amniotic membrane separating the diamniotic twin sacs can be easily recognized. This is helpful in planning strategy for tapping each sac separately. Each fetus is scanned, measured, and treated as if it were a singleton.

After removing the amniotic fluid from the first sac (twin A), 1 to 2 ml of indigo carmine dye is instilled into sac A. A second amniocentesis is performed on twin B. Blue-stained fluid withdrawn from the second sac indicates that either a communication exists between the sacs, such as occurs with monoamniotic twins, or that the first sac was reentered. Direct simultaneous visualization of the in-

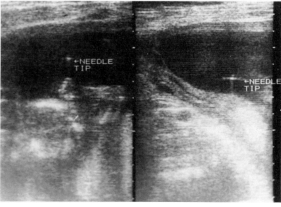

Figure 29-5. *The beveled tip of the needle is easily identified in the amniotic sac as a "flare."*

serted needle's progress with ultrasound helps to avoid reentry. Sampling of both fetal sacs is successful in approximately 88% of twin pregnancies. If triplets are encountered, the "blue dye procedure" is repeated once more after successful tapping of the second sac.

Chorionic Villus Sampling

HISTORY

Chorionic villus sampling (CVS) is one of the more recently developed techniques for effectively and safely obtaining living trophoblastic tissue for genetic diagnosis in the first trimester of pregnancy. The tissue obtained can be tested for a rapidly increasing number of biochemical and molecular disorders of the fetus, as well as for fetal chromosomal abnormalities. The trophoblast, the tissue actually sampled, is one of the extraembryonic structures that develop from the fertilized egg, becoming the placenta as the pregnancy progresses.

Working in the pre-ultrasound era, the earliest investigators[23,30] passed a rigid endoscope called a hysteroscope through the uterine cervix to obtain trophoblastic tissue for analysis. Chinese physicians used a metal cannula with no ultrasound guidance to aspirate tissue for sex determination.[24] Kazy and colleagues[29] were the first to use ultrasound to guide a flexible biopsy forceps into the uterus to obtain tissue under direct vision. An Italian group[5,46] deserves most of the credit for defining the risks and benefits of the procedure and for demonstrating the value of CVS in biochemical fetal tissue diagnoses. Their results served to popularize the method and to stimulate further investigation into this procedure.

ADVANTAGES AND DISADVANTAGES

The desire for earlier diagnosis of fetal genetic disorders and inherited metabolic derangements in pregnancy as well as the accuracy of the procedure used was, and continues to be, the impetus for further development of CVS.[39] The earlier diagnosis, and shorter waiting period for results (24 to 48 hours rather than the 7 to 10 days for amniocentesis) are especially appealing to patients. A diagnosis can therefore be forthcoming before outward physical changes associated with pregnancy are apparent

to others and deeper psychological attachment of the patient to the growing fetus is established. CVS can be performed between the 9th and 12th weeks after the last menstrual period rather than waiting to 14 or more gestational weeks for amniocentesis. Preliminary laboratory results are obtainable within 48 hours by the short-term culture method.[25] These results are confirmed by the long-term culture method, which provides results in 4 to 7 days.

TRANSVERSE LIMB DEFECTS

The possibility of a diagnosis of a severely affected fetus before the 40th day of pregnancy would have made termination, if desired, a more acceptable option to some orthodox Jewish religious groups.[17] However, the reports by Firth and colleagues[19] in 1991 and others since then[10,20,26,37] have discouraged this by raising the issue of the association of CVS, both transcervical and transabdominal, with transverse limb deficiencies. CVS was found to carry an increased risk for transverse limb deformities at 10 weeks' gestation (70 to 76 days), either solely or as part of the oromandibular–limb hypogenesis syndrome, which is about three times the background population rate of 0.3 per 1000 for similar defects.[13] The limb defect was found to decrease in frequency and severity as gestational age increases. Although the risk may be higher at later gestational ages than the general population rate in non-CVS patients, it is thought to be very small, not as well defined, and much smaller than the risk of the procedure itself. The recommendation is, therefore, that patients be counseled regarding the increased risk for transverse limb defects at least up to 76 postmenstrual days[12,13] (10 weeks).

Until recently, the fetal loss rate after CVS was reported to be 4%, compared to the 0.3% to 1.0% loss rate after amniocentesis.[18] More recent information from a compilation of the CVS registry data[27] indicate a significant reduction in fetal loss in centers with the largest experience, making the risk for this procedure comparable to that for amniocentesis.[39,41]

The problem of discordance in the chromosome results among cells obtained from the chorion, from amniotic fluid, and from the newborn has yet to be resolved. A recent report by Callen and coworkers,[11] for example, noted a discordance in 22 karyotypes of 1312 diagnostic CVS procedures, an incidence 20-fold higher than that reported for amniocentesis. Chorionic cells may therefore not always be a true representation of the fetus.

PROCEDURE FOR ULTRASOUND-GUIDED SAMPLING

In all methods of prenatal fetal evaluation, ultrasound visualization has become a *sine qua non* whether the prenatal procedure is for diagnostic or operative guidance purposes. More important than the equipment used is the training and experience of the sonographer, who must be able to work in coordination with the operator obtaining the tissue sample. For CVS, the type of real-time equipment used is secondary.[42] Scanning and sampling can be performed simultaneously by the same person, or one person can scan while the other obtains the tissue. A third alternative is for the obstetrician to scan while manipulating the cannula and then to hand the transducer to the sonographer, leaving both of the obstetrician's hands free to obtain the specimen.

Transcervical Technique

Like amniocentesis, CVS is considered to be an outpatient procedure, performed in an ultrasound laboratory. The aim is to obtain a small sample of viable chorionic tissue uncontaminated with maternal cells and without injuring the pregnancy. The patient at risk for a genetic problem must be identified early in pregnancy, properly counseled, and scheduled for the procedure between the 10th and 11th gestational weeks.

A careful obstetric and gynecologic history should be taken before scheduling the patient for testing. Among the contraindications to CVS are active infection of the vagina or any part of the genital tract, the presence of an intrauterine device, and stenosis of the cervical os. The patient's bladder may be full or empty, depending on which affords a better view of the pelvic organs. A distended bladder at times can cause undesirable distortion of the uterine contents. In the face of an abnormal appearance of the gestational sac on sonography or absence of fetal heart tones, the patient must be so informed before proceeding.

Ultrasound examination before CVS is essential, not only to confirm pregnancy and the presence of a viable fetus in the uterus but to evaluate the gestational age and location of the placenta. Vaginal and cervical smears are usually taken for culture to rule out *Neisseria gonorrheae* and other pathogens before preparing the vagina and cervix with povidone iodine solution. A vaginal speculum is inserted; the cervix is visualized and carefully grasped with a tenaculum. A uterine sound may be used to confirm the patency and the location of the internal os on the ultrasound screen (Fig. 29-6).

A variety of rigid instruments and an equal number of flexible catheters or cannulas are used by different operators. Whichever is used, its course into the uterus through the cervix is guided by ultrasound visualization. The thickest part of the trophoblast, the chorion frondosum where the umbilical cord is attached, is the target area for obtaining samples (Figs. 29-7 and 29-8). The yolk sac is used as the landmark and target area by many. The crown–rump length is measured; the shape of the uterus is noted, and the direction of the uterine axis determined. If a flexible catheter is used, its shape is adjusted to the shape of the uterus, using the obturator, to match the direction it must traverse to reach the proposed biopsy site.

When the catheter tip has reached the proper site, the malleable aluminum obturator is removed. A 20-ml syringe, previously prepared and containing 3 to 5 ml of sterile culture medium and a

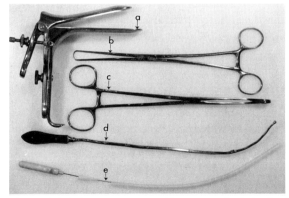

Figure 29-6. Instruments used in transvaginal chorionic villus sampling: (a) vaginal speculum, (b) tenaculum, (c) ring forceps, (d) uterine sound, (e) plastic catheter enclosed in plastic sleeve with the malleable obturator withdrawn slightly from the catheter.

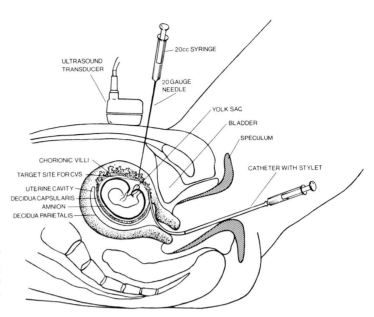

Figure 29-7. Diagram of the target area for chorionic villus sampling (CVS). The vaginal approach uses a pliable plastic catheter. The abdominal approach uses a spinal needle introduced transabdominally.

small amount of heparin, is attached to the outer end of the catheter, and the specimen is obtained by aspiration. Negative pressure is generated by sharply withdrawing the barrel of the syringe either once or repeatedly as the catheter is slowly withdrawn. This is done under constant ultrasound visualization.

An average of 20 to 30 mg of tissue is obtained

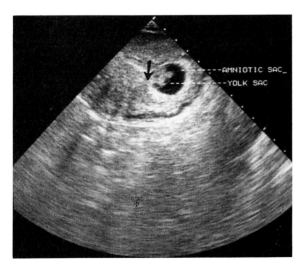

Figure 29-8 A vaginal ultrasound scan of the target area for chorionic villus sampling.

and transferred to a sterile Petri dish containing culture medium. The specimen is then washed with sterile culture media or saline solution and examined under a low-power dissecting microscope to verify the presence of chorionic villi. The specimen is separated from possible maternal cell contamination with a dissecting needle under the dissecting microscope. The washed chorionic tissue specimen is then taken to the tissue culture laboratory for processing.

After collection of the specimen, the instruments are removed and the patient is reexamined sonographically before being released. The examiner looks for evidence of hematoma formation or other complications that may have occurred as a result of the procedure. Follow-up ultrasound examinations are often scheduled at intervals, a few days to a week later.

Transabdominal Technique

The transabdominal approach differs from the transcervical only in the anatomic access route and the instrument used to obtain the specimen. The preparation of the patient, the treatment place, and the goals are the same in both approaches. In the transabdominal approach the patient is in the supine rather than the lithotomy position. The placenta is identified and its thickness measured. The abdomen, at the elected site, is cleansed with providone iodine solution. A 20-gauge, 3.5-inch spinal needle with a stylet, like that used in amniocentesis, is introduced into the the placenta (Fig. 29-9) and held by the sonographer, while the physician–operator removes the stylet, holding the needle steady in place, attaches a 20-ml Luer-lok syringe containing 3 ml of Hanks culture medium mixed with a few drops of heparin, and collects the specimen. By intermittent, vigorous withdrawal of the barrel of the syringe, negative pressure is created as the needle tip is slowly moved up and down until a specimen of about 30 mg of tissue is obtained. The needle is then withdrawn and the patient is treated as described previously for amniocentesis and transcervical CVS. In both transcervical and transabdominal CVS, the patient is informed before the procedure that amniocentesis may be necessary if the results are equivocal.

Transcervical Versus Transabdominal Technique

Until recently, the more accepted method of CVS was the transcervical technique introduced by Brambati and coworkers.[6] This method uses a flexible plastic catheter with a malleable inner obturator

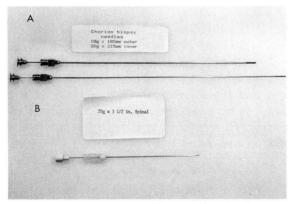

Figure 29-9. (A) Double-needle set with stylets for transabdominal chorionic villus sampling (CVS). The larger-bore needle is inserted first through the abdominal wall to just proximal to the target site. The stylet is withdrawn and the second, smaller (20-gauge) needle is inserted through the first one to the site of sampling, and the specimen obtained as described in the text. (B) Spinal needle with stylet partially withdrawn. This needle can be used for both amniocentesis and for transabdominal CVS.

that is inserted into the cervix *per vaginum,* guided by an abdominally placed transducer (see Fig. 29-7). On the other hand, the transabdominal method first introduced by Smidt-Jensen and Hahnemann in 1984[48] has gained wide acceptance because of the reported decreased chance of infection and the greater success rate in obtaining specimens. The transabdominal approach is successful in situations in which the transcervical method has failed, as, for example, in the case of the anteriorly implanted placenta. Figure 29-6 shows the instruments used for transcervical CVS; Figure 29-9 shows two different types of needles used in the transabdominal method.

There have been a few large, prospective, randomized studies comparing transabdominal and transcervical CVS done worldwide. In the United States, Jackson and colleagues[28] report on a study population in which 1944 women were randomized to a transcervical group and 1929 to a transabdominal group. They found that the sampling success after the first attempt was 94% when using the abdominal route versus 90% when using the cervical route. Maternal complications such as fluid leakage and vaginal spotting and bleeding were statistically significantly higher in the group that underwent transcervical CVS. They also found that the rate of spontaneous miscarriage was 2.3% in the transabdominal group and 2.5% in the transcervical group. The authors conclude, however, that both methods are equally safe. Smidt-Jensen and colleagues[49] in a Danish study compared the two approaches in 2882 women. They reported the sampling success for the first attempt to be 98.1% in the transabdominal group and 96% in the transcervical group. They found that the rate of unintentional pregnancy loss was significantly higher in the transcervical group (7.7%) compared to the transabdominal group (3.7%). Contamination with blood and maternal cells was greater with transcervically obtained specimens. These investigators have abandoned transcervical CVS because of the associated high pregnancy loss rate.

The data from these and other randomized trials[6] lead us to conclude that transabdominal CVS is the better procedure because of the higher sampling success, fewer minor complications, and fewer pregnancy losses.

Amniocentesis Versus Chorionic Villus Sampling

Rhoads and colleagues[41] compared the safety and efficacy of transcervical CVS in 2278 women to amniocentesis in 671 women. They obtained cytogenetic diagnoses in 97.8% of cases in which CVS was performed and 99.4% of cases in which amniocentesis was performed. In the CVS group, if inadequate amounts of tissue were obtained on the first try, the procedure was repeated up to four times. The overall pregnancy loss rate was 7.2% in the CVS group and 5.7% in the amniocentesis group. This included spontaneous and missed abortions, termination of abnormal pregnancies, stillbirths, and neonatal deaths. There was a greater number of minor complications in the CVS group, including cramping, spotting, bleeding, and leakage of amniotic fluid. Seventeen patients underwent amniocentesis after CVS because the diagnosis was ambiguous. Smidt-Jensen and coworkers[49] compared transabdominal and transcervical CVS to amniocentesis. They found that the transcervical CVS group had the highest postprocedure fetal loss rate (7.63%), followed by the transabdominal CVS group (2.34%), and finally by the amniocentesis group (1.16%).

Studies suggest that amniocentesis is the safest and most accurate of the three procedures. CVS, by whichever route chosen, carries a higher risk of repeated procedures, maternal cell contamination, sampling failures, and multiple insertions because of inadequate amounts of tissue, and a higher incidence of false-positive and false-negative results.

Early Amniocentesis Versus Transabdominal Chorionic Villus Sampling

There has been an attempt by researchers to perform amniocentesis earlier than the traditional 15 weeks. Nicolaides and associates[36] performed a prospective study of women with pregnancies at 10 to 13 weeks who requested fetal karyotyping. There were 731 women who underwent early amniocentesis, of whom 238 were randomized to this group, and 570 who underwent transabdominal CVS, of whom 250 were randomized to this group. They reported that the successful sampling rate was the same for both groups (97.5%). The rate of fetal loss was significantly higher in the early amniocentesis group (5.3%) than in the CVS group (2.3%). In the subgroups of randomized women, the fetal loss rate for early amniocentesis was 5.9%, and for transabdominal CVS, 1.2%. There were more culture failures after early amniocentesis (2.3%) versus CVS (0.53%). Vandenbussche and colleagues,[50] in a letter to the editor, confirm the results of Nicolaides and associates, reporting that in 120 early amniocenteses there were 8 fetal losses compared to none in the 64 women who underwent transabdominal CVS.

The main advantages of early amniocentesis are the decreased rate of mosaicism, decreased need for repeat testing, and the ability to do direct AFP determinations. The principal disadvantages are the increases in the rates of fetal loss and culture failure when the procedure is done before the 13th week. It is therefore recommended that early amniocentesis not be attempted before 14 weeks of gestation. Transabdominal CVS appears to be superior to early amniocentesis based on the information obtained from the studies mentioned here.

Conclusion

The rapid development that has marked the progress of these methods of prenatal diagnosis is noteworthy. In many countries, both amniocentesis and CVS have become standard medical practice. The success of these prenatal diagnostic methods is the result in no small measure of the availability of high-resolution ultrasound. The machinery that has been developed for viewing the fetus in utero is the essential element that has made all of this possible. Furthermore, ultrasound techniques have demonstrated a potentially greater utility for intrauterine fetal manipulation and treatment of developmental and genetic defects of the fetus, promising to be even more valuable in the future. It is becoming abundantly clear that any center offering prenatal genetic testing will need to be able to provide all of the aforementioned accepted techniques so that individual situations can be accommodated.

REFERENCES

1. American Institute of Ultrasound. Guidelines for Second and Third-Trimester Sonography. American Institute of Ultrasound, Laurel, MD; 1994:1–8.

2. Benn PA, Hsu LYF. Maternal cell contamination of amniotic fluid cell cultures. Results of a U.S. nationwide survey. Am J Med Genet. 1983; 15:297–305.

3. Benn PA, Schonhaut AG, Hsu LYF. A high incidence of maternal cell contamination of amniotic fluid cell cultures. Am J Med Genet. 1983; 14:361–365.

4. Bevis DCA. Composition of liquor amnii in haemolytic disease of newborn. Lancet. 1950; 2:443.

5. Brambati B, Simoni G. Fetal diagnosis of trisomy 21 in the first trimester of pregnancy. Lancet. 1983; 1:586.

6. Brambati B, Terzian E, Tognoni G. Randomized trials of transabdominal vs transvaginal chorionic villus sampling methods. Prenat Diagn. 1991; 11:285–292.

7. Brock DJH, Sutcliffe R. Alpha-fetoprotein in the diagnosis of anencephaly and spina bifida. Lancet. 1972; 2:197–199.

8. Brock DJH, Baron L, Duncan P, Scrimgeour JB, Watt M. Significance of elevated mid-trimester maternal plasma alpha-fetoprotein values. Lancet. 1979; 1:1281–1282.

9. Bumm E. Cited by Wormser E. Uber Punktion des Uterus bei Hydramnion. Zentralbl Gynakol. 1920; 44:137–140.

10. Burton BK, Schulz CJ, Burd LI. Limb anomalies associated with chorionic villus sampling. Obstet Gynecol. 1992; 79:726–730.

11. Callen DF, Korban G, Dawson G, et al. Extraembryonic/fetal karyotypic discordance during chorionic villus sampling. Prenat Diagn. 1988; 8:453–460.

12. Chervenak FA, Farley MA, Walter L, Hobbins JC, Mahoney MJ. When is termination of pregnancy during third trimester morally justifiable? N Engl J Med. 1984; 310:501–504.

13. Centers for Disease Control and Prevention. Chorionic villus sampling and amniocentesis: Recommendations for prenatal counseling. MMWR 1995; 44(No. RR-9):1–12.

14. Dacus JV, Wilroy RS, Summitt RL, et al. Genetic amniocentesis: A twelve years' experience. Am J Med Genet. 1985; 20:443–452.

15. Daffos F, Capella-Pavlosky M, Forestier F. A new procedure for fetal blood sampling in utero: Preliminary results of 53 cases. Am J Obstet Gynecol. 1983; 146:985–987.

16. Duff P, Brady WK, Robertson AW. An important medical use for the baggie. N Engl J Med. 1986; 315:1681.

17. Edelman C, Heimler A, Stamberg J. Acceptability of chorionic villus sampling in view of the Orthodox Jewish views on abortion. L. I. Jewish Hospital, New York, NY; unpublished manuscript, 1988.

18. Elias S, Simpson JL. Amniocentesis. In: Milunsky A, ed. Genetic Disorders and Fetus: Diagnosis, Prevention and Treatment. 3rd. ed. Baltimore, MD: The Johns Hopkins University Press; 1992:33–57.

19. Firth HV, Boyd PA, Chamberlain P, Mackenzie IZ, Lindenbaum RH, Huson SM. Severe limb abnormalities after chorionic villus sampling at 56–66 days gestation. Lancet. 1991; 337:762–763.

20. Firth HV, Boyd PA, Chamberlain PF, MacKenzie IZ, Morriss-Kay GM, Huson SM. Analysis of limb reduction defects in babies exposed to chorionic villus sampling. Lancet 1994; 343:1069–1071.

21. Golbus MS, Loughman WD, Epstein CJ, Halbasch G, Stephens JD, Hall BD. Prenatal diagnosis in 3000 amniocenteses. N Engl J Med. 1979; 300:157–163.

22. Gruber B, Burton BK. Oromandibular–limb hypogenesis syndrome following chorionic villus sampling. Int J Pediatr Otorhinolaryngol. 1994; 29:59–63.

23. Hahnemann N. Early prenatal diagnosis: A study of biopsy techniques and cell culturing from extraembryonic membranes. Clin Genet. 1974; 6:294–306.

24. Han A, Zhou B, Wang H. Long-term follow-up results after aspiration of chorionic villi during early pregnancy. In: Fraccaro M, Simoni G, Brambati B, eds. First-Trimester Fetal Diagnosis. Berlin: Springer-Verlag; 1985:1–6.

25. Heaton DE, Czepulkowski BH. Chorionic villi and direct chromosome preparation. In: Liu DTY, Symonds EM, Golbus MS, eds. Chorionic Villus Sampling. Chicago: Year Book Medical Publishers; 1987:273–286.

26. Hsieh F, Shyo M, Sheu B, Lin S, Chen C, Huang F. Limb defects after chorionic villus sampling. Obstet Gynecol. 1995; 85:84–88.

27. Jackson LG. CVS Newsletter No. 26. Philadelphia: Jefferson Medical College; 1988.

28. Jackson LG, Zachary JM, Fowler SE, et al. A randomized comparison of transcervical and transabdominal chorionic villus sampling. N Engl J Med. 1992; 327:594–598.

29. Kazy Z, Rozovsky IS, Bakharev VA. Chorion biopsy in early pregnancy: A method of early prenatal diagnosis for inherited disorders. Prenat Diagn. 1982; 2:39–45.

30. Kullander S, Sandahl B. Fetal chromosome analysis after transcervical placental biopsies during pregnancy. Acta Obstet Gynecol Scand. 1973; 52:355–359.

31. Lambl D. Ein seltener Fall von Hydramnios. Zentralbl Gynakol. 1881; 5:329–334.

32. Leek AF. Raised alpha-fetoprotein maternal serum with anencephalic pregnancy. Lancet. 1972; 2:385.

33. Liley AW. Liquor amnii analysis in the management of the pregnancy complicated by rhesus sensitizaton. Am J Obstet Gynecol. 1961; 82:1359–1370.

34. Merkatz IR, Nitowsky HM, Macri JN, Johnson WE. An association between maternal serum alpha-fetoprotein and fetal chromosome abnormalities. Am J Obstet Gynecol. 1984; 148:1331–1334.

35. Milunsky A. Maternal serum screening for neural tube and other defects. In: Milunsky A, ed. Genetic Disorders and the Fetus: Diagnosis, Prevention and Treatment. 3rd ed. The Johns Hopkins University Press. Baltimore, MD; 1992:507–563.

36. Nicolaides K, Brizot ML, Patel F, Snijders R. Comparison of chorionic villus sampling and amniocentesis for fetal karyotyping at 10–13 weeks' gestation. Lancet. 1994; 344:435–439.

37. Olney RS, Khoury MJ, Botto LD. Limb defects and gestational age at chorionic villus sampling. Lancet. 1994; 344:476.

38. Parvey B. Report of a case of acute hydramnion treated by abdominal puncture. N Engl J Med. 1933; 208:683–685.

39. Pergament E, Verlinsky Y, Ginsberg NA, Cadkin A, Brandt T. Assessment of the safety and accuracy of chorionic villus sampling in first trimester fetal diagnosis. In: Fraccaro M, Simoni G, Brambati B, eds. First Trimester Fetal Diagnosis. Berlin: Springer-Verlag; 1985:314–320.

40. President's Commission for the Study of Ethical Problems in Medicine and Biomedical and Behavioral Science. Screening and Counseling for Genetic Conditions. Washington, DC: U.S. Government Printing Office; 1983.

41. Rhoads GG, Jackson LG, Schlesseiman SE, et al. The safety and efficacy of chorionic villus sampling for early diagnostic abnormalities. N Engl J Med. 1989; 320:609–617.

42. Richardson RE, Liu DTY. Ultrasound for transcervical chorionic villus sampling. In: Liu DTY, Symonds EM, Golbus MS, eds. Chorionic Villus Sampling Chicago: Year Book Medical Publishers; 1987:107–125.

43. Schatz F. Eine besondere Art von ein seitiger Poly bei Zwillingen. Arch Gynackol. 1882; 19:329–369.

44. Shaw MW. Genetic counseling. Science. 1974; 184:751.

45. Shaw MW. Review of published studies of genetic counseling: A critique. In: Lubs HA, de la Cruz F, eds. Genetic Counseling. A Monograph of the National Institute of Child Health and Human Development. New York: Raven Press; 1977:252–259.

46. Simoni G, Brambati B, Danesino C, et al. Diagnostic application of first-trimester trophoblast sampling in 100 pregnancies. Hum Genet. 1984; 66:252–259.

47. Simpson JL, Elias E. Genetic amniocentesis. In: Sabbagha RE, ed. Diagnostic Ultrasound Applied to Obstetrics and Gynecology. 2nd ed. Philadelphia: JB Lippincott; 1987:64–82.

48. Smidt-Jensen S, Hahnemann N. Transabdominal fine-needle biopsy from chorionic villi in the first trimester. Prenat Diagn. 1984; 4:163–169.

49. Smidt-Jensen S, Permin M, Philip J, et al. Randomized comparison of amniocentesis and transabdominal and transcervical chorionic villus sampling. Lancet. 1992; 340:1237–1244.

50. Vandenbussche FPHA, Kanhai HHH, Keirse MJNC. Safety of early amniocentesis. Lancet 1994; 344:1032.

51. Walker AHC. Liquor amnii studies in the prediction of haemolytic disease of the newborn. Br Med J. 1957; 2:376–378.

PART III

Psychosocial, Professional, and Technical Topics

30

Artifacts in Obstetric and Gynecologic Ultrasound

LINDA W. GRAVES, MARIA SYKORA, SUSAN E. NEALER,
and BEVERLY A. SPIRT

Artifacts are an integral part of ultrasound that can both clarify and confuse the diagnostic picture. Sonographers must have a basic understanding of the physics of ultrasound to obtain optimal examinations, and to recognize the various artifacts. The reader is referred to one of the many basic texts on ultrasound physics for a more detailed discussion of physical principles.

The design of ultrasound instrumentation is based on four primary assumptions[8,9]:

1. Transducer acoustic beams travel in a straight line
2. The returning pulse is received before the next pulse is sent
3. The round-trip time of the pulse is proportional to the distance it travels
4. Objects viewed are located in the central portion of the sound beam

These assumptions are not true in every case, and artifacts are a manifestation of that fact.

This chapter describes and explains the artifacts most often encountered in obstetric and gynecologic scanning, including artifacts that are specific to Doppler ultrasound.

Artifacts in gray-scale ultrasound can be divided into four basic categories of physical principles: 1) reflection and refraction, 2) reverberation, 3) attenuation, and 4) side lobe and slice thickness, plus a fifth category, operator-dependent artifacts.

Reflection and Refraction

Sound does not always travel in a straight line. When a sound beam travels from one medium to another, it may be transmitted, refracted, and/or reflected, depending on the velocity of sound in the two media, the angle of transmission, and the angle of incidence (Fig. 30-1). This occurs according to Snell's law:

$$\frac{\text{sin angle of transmission}}{\text{sin angle of incidence}} = \frac{\text{velocity of medium 2}}{\text{velocity of medium 1}}$$

Refraction refers to the change in direction of the acoustic beam as it travels from one medium to another. When a sound beam crosses an interface between a low-velocity medium and a high-velocity medium, it is refracted away from the vertical. In the reverse, a beam traveling from a high-velocity to a low-velocity medium is bent toward the vertical. *Reflection* occurs when the sound beam bounces off

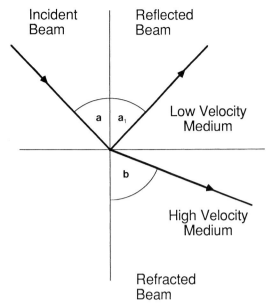

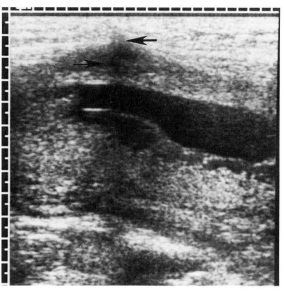

Figure 30-1. Reflection and refraction. With oblique incidence, the angle of incidence (a) equals the angle of
reflection (a₁). The angle of transmission (b) depends on
the incident angle and the velocities of the media.

Figure 30-2. Reflection. Obstetric sonogram demonstrates total reflection (*arrows*) of the sound beam caused
by the transducer–air interface at the umbilicus.

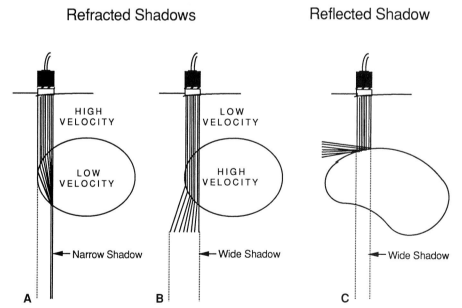

Figure 30-3. Curved edge refraction and reflection. (**A**) High to low velocity. (**B**) Low
to high velocity. (**C**) Critical angle shadowing.

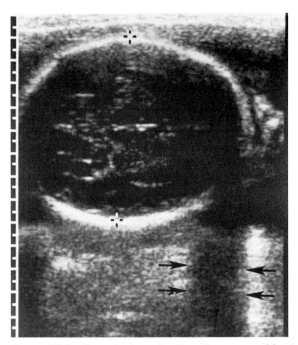

Figure 30-4. Curved edge refraction. Sonogram of fetal skull demonstrates wide edge shadowing (*arrows*) as a result of the sound beam traveling from a low-velocity medium such as amniotic fluid to a high-velocity medium such as bone.

the interface without entering the second medium (Fig. 30-2).[8,19]

The impact of a beam on a curved specular reflector results in *curved-edge refraction*, which may be of two types. A wide shadow results from the sound beam traveling from a low-velocity to a high-velocity medium when it intersects a curved surface; a narrow shadow results if the beam goes from high-velocity to low-velocity tissue (Fig. 30-3). Multiple examples of curved-edge refraction are found in obstetric and gynecologic scanning (Fig. 30-4).

A third type of curved-edge shadowing is *reflective shadowing*, also referred to as *critical angle shadowing*. This is a wide acoustic shadow that is produced when the angle of the incident beam is such that the angle of transmission equals 90°. At this critical angle, the sound beam is completely reflected (see Fig. 30-3).[10,19,21] This artifact is often a source of difficulty in pelvic scanning. When the sound beam intersects the bladder wall at a certain angle, it is reflected completely (Fig. 30-5A). This lack of sound transmission should not be misinterpreted as an acoustic shadow caused by calcification, as in a myoma or mass. The artifact may be eliminated by changing the angle of the transducer or incident beam (see Fig. 30-5B).

A striking example of refraction is the *split-*

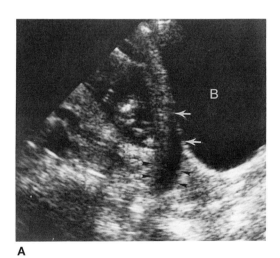

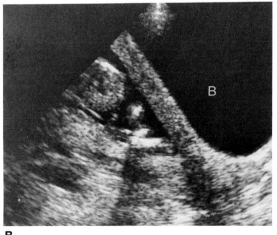

A   **B**

Figure 30-5. Critical angle shadowing. (**A**) Sagittal sector scan of the lower uterine segment demonstrates complete reflection of the sound beam (*arrowheads*) at the bladder wall (*arrows*; B, bladder). (**B**) By changing the transducer angle and further filling the bladder, this artifact is eliminated.

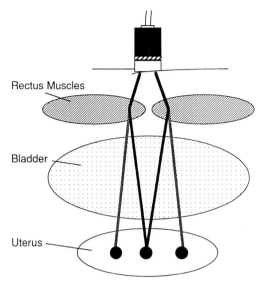

Figure 30-6. Double-image artifact. Line representation of acoustic path as it passes through rectus muscles and bladder. The solid line represents the actual sound path and the dotted lines the computer-calculated direction that causes the double image.

image or *double-image* artifact. In the pelvis, the sound beam passes through fat and the rectus muscles before reaching the bladder. The beam is refracted away from the perpendicular at the fat–muscle interface and toward the perpendicular

when it leaves the muscle. The equipment does not perceive that the beam has been refracted and that the sound is no longer traveling in a straight line. It places the structure in accordance with the time elapsed for the returned signal, causing an extra image to appear. If a structure is located at a particular depth, the image will be totally duplicated (Fig. 30-6).[2,16,21] If the depth is not optimal, partial duplication results. This artifact frequently produces a false double gestational sac, which could be misinterpreted as twins (Fig. 30-7). It may also cause the appearance of a double intrauterine device, an increased crown–rump length, enlargement of a uterine mass, or a bicornuate uterus. To avoid the split-image artifact, the sonographer should scan to the right or left of the midline or have the patient void partially. It has been demonstrated that this artifact appears less frequently when a linear-array transducer is used.[22]

Reverberation

Reverberation is defined as multiple reflections of sound. It occurs when the sound wave strikes an interface with a high degree of acoustic mismatch, such as soft tissue and gas, and most of the sound is reflected back to the transducer. The returning sound is reflected again off the transducer surface,

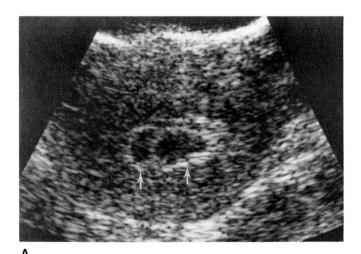

A

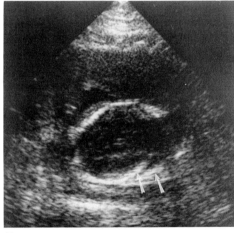

B

Figure 30-7. Split image. (**A**) Transverse sonogram of an early gestation demonstrates artifactual partial duplication of the gestational sac (*arrows*) due to refraction of the sound beam at the muscle–fat interface. (**B**) Artifactual double edge of fetal skull (*arrows*) should not be confused with overlapping of fetal skull bones.

reenters the body, and thus produces more than one reflection from the same surface. Returning echoes are then registered on the monitor at both incorrect and correct locations, equidistant from each other, with decreasing amplitude. The greater the acoustic mismatch, the greater the number of reverberant echoes produced.

The *pseudomass* is a dramatic example of this phenomenon, wherein a mass effect is created by a combination of reflection and reverberation. This occurs when a highly reflective surface creates strong reverberation echoes that, when mapped into an anechoic or hypoechoic region by the instrument, create the false appearance of a mass (Fig. 30-8).[10,21] Pseudomasses are common artifacts and should be identified promptly by the sonographer. In a thin patient, it should be obvious that a mass of the size visualized cannot possibly exist within the patient and that the image must represent artifactual echoes beyond the body cavity. Reducing the gain or changing the direction of the transducer

may cause the mass to disappear. If there is doubt, it may help to have the patient void to rearrange the pattern of reflected echoes. If the mass changes or disappears completely, further imaging studies are not necessary. Correlation with physical examination is useful to confirm the presence or absence of a mass.

Multipath reflection or reverberation is a similar artifact. It is caused by the beam striking a curved specular surface, intersecting other curved interfaces, and reflecting in an indirect path back to the transducer. Additional signals are received by the transducer that may be interpreted as part of the primary beam pattern.[8-10] In the pelvis, this artifact can duplicate the bladder posteriorly, owing to the increased time required for the reflected beam to return (see Figs. 30-8 and 30-9). It may be avoided by having the patient void or by repositioning the scanning angle.

Two artifacts that are similar in appearance but are caused by two disparate mechanisms are the

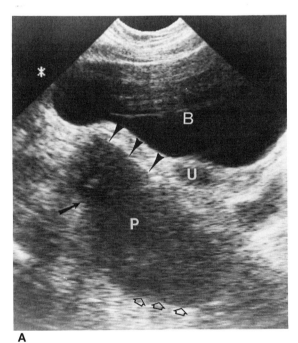

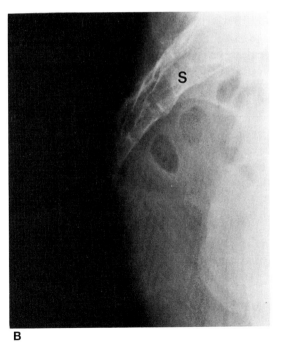

A **B**

Figure 30-8. Pseudomass. **(A)** Longitudinal sonogram of the pelvis demonstrates a pseudomass (P) posterior to the uterus (U). The back wall of the superior aspect of this pseudomass (*arrow*) is created by a reverberation from the highly reflective sacrum (*arrowheads*) in this thin patient. The inferior portion of this pseudomass (*open arrows*) is a duplicated bladder effect secondary to multiple-path reflection (see Fig. 30-9). (B, urinary bladder.) **(B)** Lateral radiograph confirms the absence of any mass anterior to the sacrum (S).

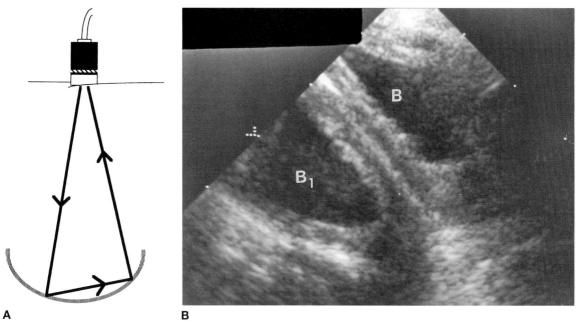

Figure 30-9. Multiple-path reflection: mirror image artifact. (**A**) The sound beam undergoes multiple reflections as it intersects a curved specular surface. (**B**) Longitudinal sonogram of the pelvis demonstrates posterior duplication (B₁) of the bladder (B).

comet-tail and the *ring-down* artifacts. In the first, internal reverberations that occur in dense, highly reflective objects such as metal are intense enough and close enough together to produce a distinct and characteristic pattern that appears to merge into a comet-tail configuration (Fig. 30-10).[26,29] Reverberations from intrauterine devices, shotgun pellets, and metal surgical clips produce comet tail artifacts.

Ring-down is caused by a unique mechanism that is a function of resonance. It is associated with gas collections. It is included here because of its similar sonographic appearance to the comet tail. Ring-down appears as a solid line or a series of parallel bands emanating from below a gas pocket. Experiments have shown that it originates from a "fluid bugle," which occurs in the center of a layer of bubbles or a bubble tetrahedron.[1] The fluid bugle acts as an oscillator of the sound beam and causes the liquid in it to vibrate, sending a continuous signal of decreasing amplitude back to the transducer (Fig. 30-11). The fluid bugle resonates at a frequency determined by its individual size and shape. The frequencies received by the transducer are thus independent of the original frequency.

Reverberations in the fetal head may lead to misinterpretation of brain anatomy. These reverberations may originate from the highly reflective fetal skull, from the transducer–skin interface, or from maternal tissue layers, particularly in an obese patient. This results in obscuration of the near field, causing a false impression of a unilateral abnormality in a bilateral condition (Fig. 30-12). An arc-shaped structure may appear in the posterior portion of the fetal head. This is referred to as the *pseudoepidural artifact* because of its similarity to epidural collections on computed tomographic scans of the brain. The reverberation echo that produces this artifact originates from the anterior surface of the fetal skull and is placed at twice its depth (Fig. 30-13).[24] With real-time imaging, this artifact may be circumvented by adjusting the angle of the probe while scanning.

Attenuation

When a sound wave travels through a medium, its amplitude and intensity decrease. This phenomenon is referred to as *attenuation*. An ex-

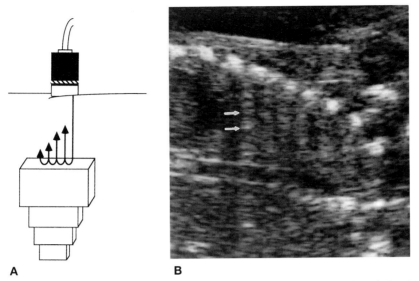

Figure 30-10. Comet tail. (**A**) This artifact is characterized by a series of closely spaced reverberations that taper. (**B**) Coronal section through fetal thorax demonstrates intense comet-tail reverberations (*arrows*) from fetal ribs.

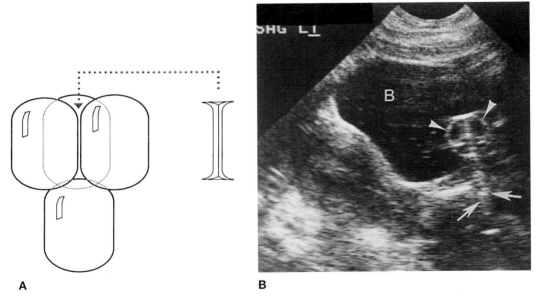

Figure 30-11. Ring-down. (**A**) Diagram of bubble-tetrahedron with "fluid bugle" (*arrow*) within. (**B**) Sagittal scan of pelvis shows ring-down artifact (*arrows*) from gas in Foley catheter balloon (*arrowheads;* B, bladder).

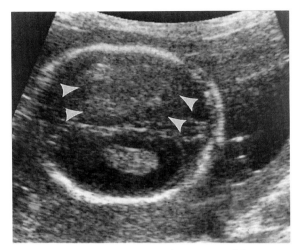

Figure 30-12. Reverberations. Sonogram of fetal skull shows multiple reverberations in the near-field portion (*arrows*) that completely obscure the brain anatomy.

tremely dense medium such as bone attenuates the sound beam to such an extent that an acoustic shadow is produced. This phenomenon is useful in diagnostic ultrasound, because an acoustic shadow behind an echogenic focus in an ovarian mass or in the fetal brain or abdomen indicates the presence of calcification (Fig. 30-14*A*). The degree of shadowing in fetal long bones also provides useful information, because bone absorbs approximately 20 times more sound than soft tissue.[10,28] If the normal degree of shadowing is not seen, an underlying problem of bone mineralization such as osteogenesis imperfecta (see Fig. 30-14*B*) should be considered.[9]

The opposite of shadowing is *enhancement*, an increase in amplitude from reflectors that lie posterior to a weakly attenuating material such as fluid. There is increased transmission of the sound beam through the fluid ("through transmission"), so that echoes from structures deep to the fluid are of greater amplitude than echoes from tissue adjacent to those structures (Fig. 30-15). The presence of posterior enhancement is the key to determining whether a mass contains a low attenuating medium such as fluid, hematoma, or abscess (Fig. 30-16). An anechoic mass without posterior enhancement does not represent a simple cyst but rather a complex collection.

Slice-Thickness and Side-Lobe Artifacts

Slice-thickness and *side-lobe* artifacts result from the fact that two of the basic assumptions of ultrasound instrumentation cited earlier are not always true: 1) the round-trip time of the pulse is proportional to the distance it travels, and 2) objects viewed are located in the central portion of the sound beam. Both slice-thickness and side-lobe artifacts may cause a cyst to appear complex.

Side-lobe artifacts result from multiple side beams of lower intensity that emanate from the transducer, surrounding the main beam.[11,21] These lower-intensity lobes radiate to the periphery of the main sound beam, scattering it against specular reflectors such as the bladder or diffuse reflectors like bowel gas. This artifact is frequently seen in the urinary bladder as a debris level or as a line anterior to its floor (Fig. 30-17). Side-lobe artifacts depend on transducer angle and beam intensity but are independent of gravity. They may be eliminated by changing the angle of the transducer and decreasing the gain.

Slice-thickness artifact refutes the assumption that all objects viewed are in a central, finite plane. In fact, a sound beam has width and diverges beyond the focal zone. Despite their true origin, all returning echoes

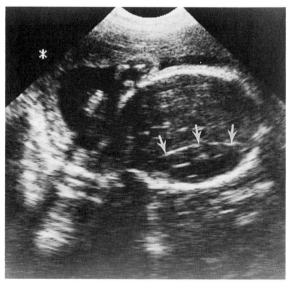

Figure 30-13. Pseudoepidural artifact. An arc-shaped reverberation (*arrows*) is seen in the posterior aspect of the fetal skull. This should not be confused with an epidural fluid collection.

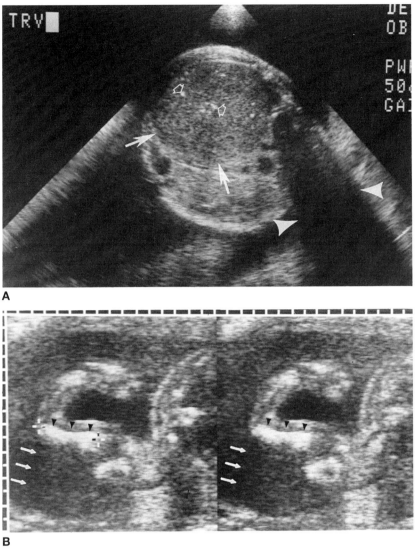

Figure 30-14. Acoustic shadow. (**A**) Transverse scan of fetal abdomen shows prominent acoustic shadow from fetal spine (*arrowheads*). Note acoustic shadows from calcifications (*open arrows*) in abdominal mass (*arrows*), which aided in the diagnosis of fetal neuroblastoma. (Courtesy of Dr. Michael Oliphant, Syracuse, NY.) (**B**) Note the decreased degree of shadowing (*arrows*) posterior to the humerus (*arrowheads*) of a 17-week fetus with osteogenesis imperfecta.

are placed by the equipment on a narrow axis. This produces a "partial volume" effect.[3,5,6,8] For example, if a beam is "off axis" to a cyst, an averaging effect of the cyst and surrounding tissue occurs, causing the cyst to fill in with echoes from adjacent structures (Fig. 30-18). To minimize this artifact, a narrowly focused beam should be used and the structure should be scanned along its central axis. As with side lobes, the slice-thickness artifact depends on equipment output and disappears when the gain setting is lowered.

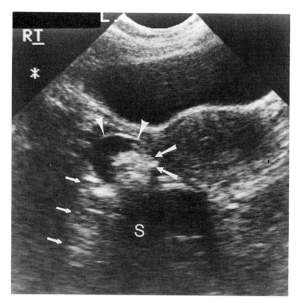

A

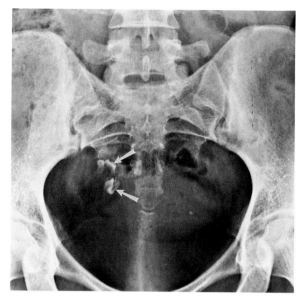

B

Figure 30-15. Posterior enhancement. Transverse sonogram (**A**) and corresponding radiograph (**B**) of the pelvis in a young woman with dermoid cyst (*arrowheads*) of the right ovary. Both posterior enhancement (*small arrows*) and acoustic shadowing (S) are present on the sonogram. Calcification (*large arrows*) within the dermoid is confirmed on the radiograph.

Operator-Dependent Artifacts

Of all the imaging modalities, ultrasound is the most operator dependent. In ultrasound scanning, three variables exist: the sonographer, the instrumentation, and the patient. The unknown variable is the patient. With proper technical and didactic foundation, and appropriate use of equipment, the

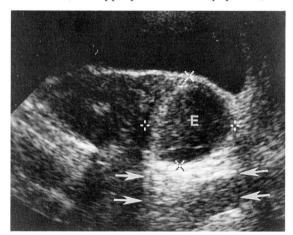

Figure 30-16. Posterior enhancement. Transverse sonogram of endometrioma (E) in the left adnexa. Posterior enhancement (*arrows*) is present owing to the weakly attenuating material within the mass.

experienced sonographer can produce anatomically and technically accurate images. The sonographer must select the proper transducer and focal zone and determine machine output and optimal gain curves. Inappropriate transducer and focal zone selection may result in overlooking vital diagnostic information (Fig. 30-19). Improper time gain compensation and output adjustments lead to a nonuniform display of echoes (Fig. 30-20).

In addition to an understanding of the physical principles involved in sonography, a thorough knowledge of the pertinent anatomy is necessary to perform an optimal examination. Artifacts may be produced by inappropriate scan planes that can confuse the appearance of normal anatomy. An example of this is the "bifid sacrum artifact," which is produced by a steeply angled scan plane causing a skewed appearance of normal ossification centers (Fig. 30-21).[7]

Artifacts Specific to Doppler Ultrasound

Doppler ultrasound is used to detect the presence or absence of flow, and flow direction, velocity, and pulsatility. Color Doppler is also used to profile

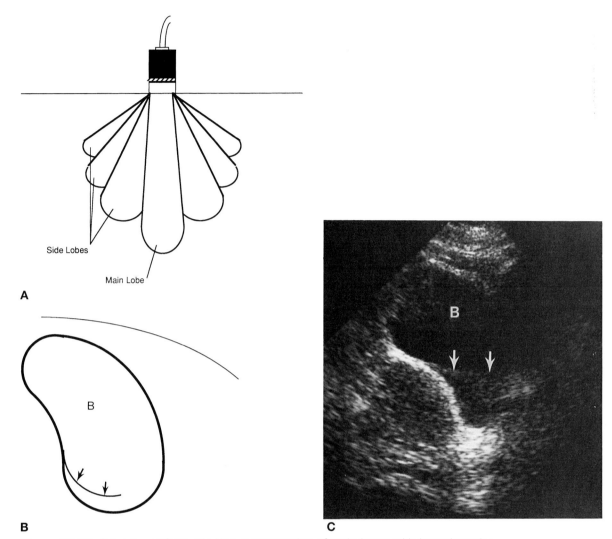

Figure 30-17. Side-lobe artifacts. (**A**) Line representation of main beam with lower-intensity side lobes. (**B**) Transducer side-lobe artifact (*arrows*) located in posterior portion of bladder (B). (**C**) Sagittal sector scan of pelvis shows low-level echoes (*arrows*) in the dependent portion of the bladder (B) caused by side lobes.

areas of turbulence. Artifacts occur with both spectral and color Doppler; these are often a source of confusion, and may lead to misinterpretation of the flow information. As with conventional ultrasound, a thorough understanding of the equipment and of Doppler physics is necessary to recognize and avoid various artifacts.[4]

Inappropriate gain settings are a common source of Doppler artifact.[15,17] A gain setting that is too low may inaccurately suggest a lack of flow and therefore thrombosis of a patent vessel. Conversely, an inappropriately high gain setting can mimic spectral broadening. Loss of the sharp "velocity envelope," when it fills in with noise, incorrectly suggests poststenotic turbulence.

Proper gain adjustment is of the utmost importance in the performance of a color Doppler examination. With color Doppler, a high gain setting

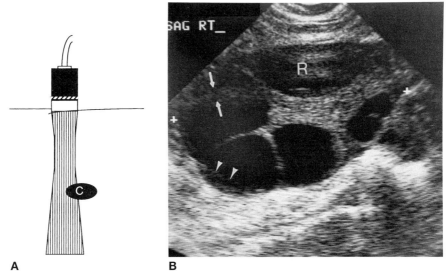

A   **B**

Figure 30-18. Slice thickness artifact. (**A**) Sound beam partially intersects tissue adjacent to cyst (C). Echoes from the tissue are misplaced by the equipment into the cyst. (**B**) Sagittal scan of right ovary in patient with ovarian hyperstimulation syndrome shows spurious band of echoes (*arrows*) emanating from adjacent soft tissue. Note also reverberations (R) and side-lobe artifact (*arrowheads*).

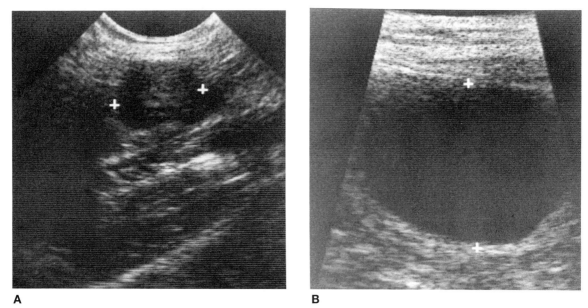

A   **B**

Figure 30-19. Operator-dependent artifacts: transducer selection. (**A**) Superficial ovarian cyst (cursors) imaged with 5-MHz sector transducer demonstrates no posterior enhancement. Multiple echoes are noted within. (**B**) the same cyst imaged with 10-MHz transducer shows posterior enhancement and no internal echoes. (**C**) Transabdominal transverse scan through pelvis of obese patient shows uterus (U) and solid-looking right adnexal mass (*arrows;* B, bladder). (**D**) Transvaginal scan shows that the right adnexal mass actually represents a cyst.

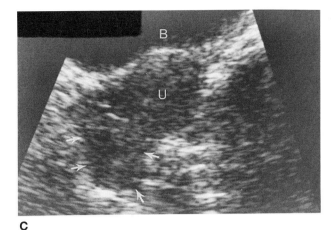

C

D

Figure 30-19. (CONTINUED)

causes the image to become "cluttered" with color noise, making it difficult to identify structures. Decreased gain settings may produce the incorrect impression of diminished or absent flow. The highest gain setting with the lowest threshold that does not

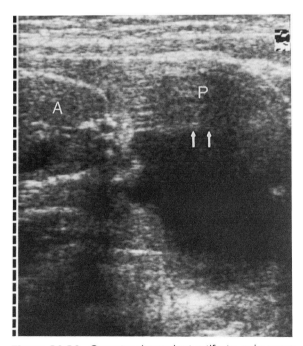

Figure 30-20. Operator-dependent artifacts: gain curve selection. Sagittal fetal sonogram shows an apparent anterior placenta (P), which is actually an artifact caused by improper gain curve selection. Note the absence of a chorionic plate (*arrows; A, fetal abdomen*).

cause noise in the image must be used. Motion in fluid-filled, nonvascular structures such as a full bladder or amniotic fluid causes flashes of color (Fig. 30-22). This color noise is a random mixture of red and blue that does not change with cardiac or respiratory cycles. Spectral analysis is useful to confirm vascular flow in a questionable area of color. This works because the Doppler spectrum is obtained differently than the color Doppler image, and is not changed by the signal process. Color Doppler noise is removed by reducing the color gain.[15,17]

Transmitted pulsations can produce a similar problem, but the color varies with the cardiac cycle and cannot be corrected even with proper gain settings[12] (Fig. 30-23). In setting technique, care should be taken that such factors as motion from vessel walls, organs moving during respiratory motion, and transmitted pulsations are unable to produce color signal. However, by preventing the assignment of color signals to these structures, signals from actual moving objects may be suppressed.[25]

Aliasing is an important Doppler artifact that depends on the pulse repetition frequency (PRF). It is akin to the appearance of reversed motion in old movies, wherein a frame rate that was too slow would cause a wheel that was actually turning forward to look as though it were going backward. The PRF must be equal to at least twice a particular frequency (the Nyquist frequency) to sample that frequency.[25] The Nyquist frequency thus sets a limit on the maximum flow velocity that Doppler can

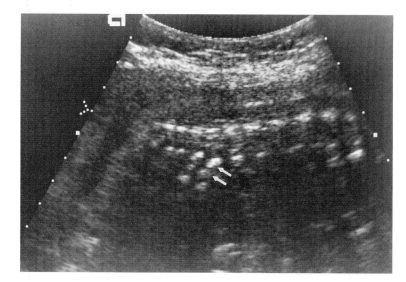

Figure 30-21. Operator-dependent artifacts: the bifid sacrum artifact. The appearance of the "bifid sacrum" (*arrows*) is produced by a steeply angled scan plane, approximately 20° to 30° off the coronal plane, causing the normal ossification centers of the sacral ala to appear in the same plane as the lumbosacral spine. This artifact may be seen after 25 weeks.

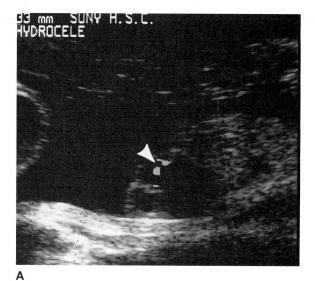

A

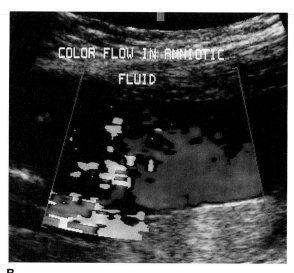

B

Figure 30-22. Color noise. (**A**) Color noise occurred in this fetal hydrocele (*arrowhead*) because of fluid motion. (**B**) Fetal movement caused this color flash in the amniotic fluid. (See also Color Plates 21 and 22.)

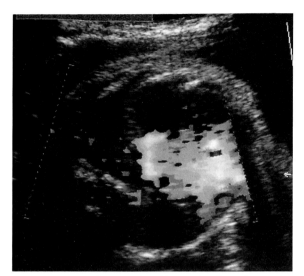

Figure 30-23. *Color noise. Transmitted cardiac pulsations caused this color noise in the fetal heart. (See also Color Plate 23.)*

measure at a given PRF. The Nyquist limit is equal to one half the PRF. If this limit is exceeded, aliasing occurs in both spectral and color Doppler, with "wrap-around" of the Doppler display (Fig. 30-24). With color Doppler, this is recognized by the fact that there is no black stripe from the low-velocity filter between the two reversed colors. Most commercially available ultrasound equipment does not allow the operator direct control of the PRF; instead, the PRF is automatically set as high as possible for depth interrogation. The PRF function is closely related to the velocity scale and frequency shift, and varies as the image depth is changed. The following methods may be used to correct aliasing: the Doppler angle can be increased, which decreases the Doppler shift; the velocity scale may be increased, which increases the PRF; the baseline may be changed; or a lower frequency transducer may be used.[14,20] Despite these methods, it may be impossible to prevent aliasing in a vessel that has a high velocity and is located deep in the body.[25]

Mirror-image artifact caused by multipath reflection or reverberation occurs with Doppler ultrasound, just as it does in B-mode sonography.[17,23] With color Doppler, instead of duplicating an organ such as the bladder, duplication of a vessel may occur with evidence of flow in both the true vessel

and the created vessel (Fig. 30-25).[13,18] With spectral Doppler, the waveform appears both above and below the zero baseline. Changing the direction of the ultrasound beam or the scanning angle and reduction of the overall gain should eliminate this artifact.[14]

Directional ambiguity occurs when the ultrasound beam is perpendicular to the object that is being interrogated. With spectral analysis, a tracing above and below the baseline is displayed and direction of flow is uncertain. This may be corrected by changing the angle of insonation. Directional ambiguity occurs with color Doppler imaging when both colors are adjacent, with the flow appearing to divide in the middle of the image. Angling the transducer or steering the color box to the right or to the left clarifies the direction of flow.[17]

The wall filter setting is critical for the proper evaluation of flow. A wall filter setting that is too high causes a loss of information in low flow states, whereas an inappropriately low setting obscures the presence of flow.[17,27]

As with conventional ultrasound, the Doppler

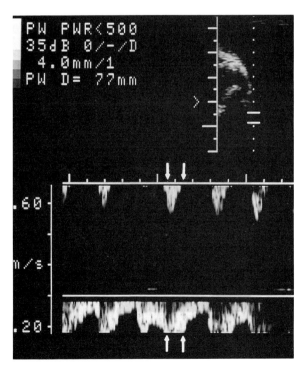

Figure 30-24. *Aliasing. Improper baseline and gain settings cause wrap-around of the Doppler signal (arrows).*

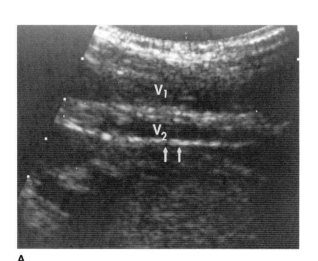

A

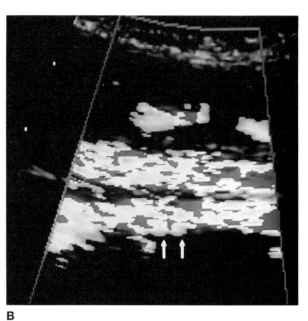

B

Figure 30-25. Mirror-image artifact. (**A**) Gray-scale image shows apparent duplication (*arrows;* V_2) of iliac vessel (V_1) caused by multipath reflection. (**B**) Color Doppler image shows color in both the true vessel (*arrowheads*) and the "ghost" vessel (*arrows*). (See also Color Plate 24.)

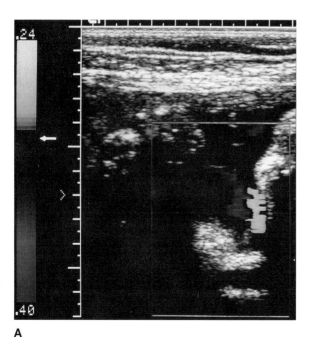

A

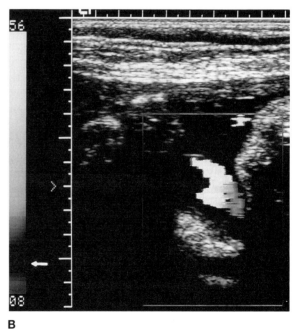

B

Figure 30-26. Operator-dependent artifact: incorrect baseline setting. (**A, B**) Color Doppler images of the umbilical vessels emphasize the fact that incorrect baseline settings can depict a false direction of flow. As the baseline (*arrow*) is changed, the direction of flow appears to reverse. (See also Color Plates 25 and 26.)

examination is extremely operator dependent. Inappropriate equipment settings may exaggerate or conceal diagnostic information (Fig. 30-26); a complete understanding of the operation of the equipment and of the physical principles involved is necessary to obtain an optimal diagnostic examination.

REFERENCES

1. Avruch L, Cooperberg PL. The ring-down artifact. J Ultrasound Med. 1985; 4:21.
2. Buttery B, Davison G. The ghost artifact. J Ultrasound Med. 1984; 3:49.
3. Fiske CE, Filly RA. Pseudo-sludge. Radiology. 1982; 144:631.
4. Foley WD, Erickson SJ. Color Doppler flow imaging. Am J Roentgenol. 1991; 156:3–13.
5. Goldstein A, Madrazzo BI. Slice-thickness artifacts in gray-scale ultrasound. J Clin Ultrasound. 1989; 9:365.
6. Jaffe CC, Rosenfield AT, Sommer G, et al. Technical factors influencing the imaging of small anechoic cysts by B-scan ultrasound. Radiology. 1980; 135:429.
7. Kliewer MA, Hertzberg BS, George P, et al. Fetal bifid sacrum artifact: Normal developmental anatomy simulating malformation. Radiology. 1995; 195:673–676.
8. Kremkau FW. Diagnostic Ultrasound Principles, Instrumentation, and Exercises. 2nd ed. Orlando, FL: Grune & Stratton; 1984.
9. Kremkau FW, Taylor KJW. Artifacts in ultrasound imaging. J Ultrasound Med. 1985; 5:227–237.
10. Laing FC. Commonly encountered artifacts in clinical ultrasound. Semin Ultrasound. 1983; 4:27.
11. Laing FC, Kurtz AB. The importance of side-lobe artifacts. Radiology. 1982; 145:763.
12. Middleton WD, Erickson SJ, Melson GL. Perivascular color artifact: Pathological significance and appearance on color Doppler US images. Radiology. 1989; 171:647–652.
13. Middleton WD, Melson GL. The carotid ghost: A color Doppler ultrasound mirror image artifact. J Ultrasound Med. 1990; 9:487–493.
14. Mitchell DG. Color Doppler imaging: Principles, limitations, and artifacts. Radiology. 1990; 177:1–10.
15. Mitchell DG, Burns P, Needleman L. Color Doppler artifact in anechoic regions. J Ultrasound Med. 1990; 9:255–260.
16. Muller N, Cooperberg PL, Rowley VA, et al. Ultrasonic refraction by the rectus abdominis muscles: The double image artifact. J Ultrasound Med. 1984; 3:515.
17. Pozniak MA, Zagzebski JA, Scanlan KA. Spectral and color Doppler artifacts. Radiographics. 1992; 12:35–44.
18. Reading CC, Charbonneau JW, Allison JW, Cooperberg PL. Color and spectral Doppler mirror-image artifact of the subclavian artery. Radiology. 1990; 174:41–42.
19. Robinson DE, Wilson LS, Kossoff G. Shadowing and enhancement in ultrasonic echograms by reflection and refraction. J Clin Ultrasound. 1981; 9:181.
20. Rubin JM. AAPM tutorial: Spectral Doppler US. Radiographics. 1994; 12:139–150.
21. Sarti DA. Diagnostic ultrasound: Text and cases. Chicago: Year Book Medical Publishers; 1987:54–67.
22. Sauerbrie EE. The split-image artifact in pelvic sonography: The anatomy and the physics. J Ultrasound Med. 1985; 4:29.
23. Scanlan KA. Sonographic artifacts and their origins. Am J Roentgenol. 1991; 156:1267–1272.
24. Stanley JH, Harrell B, Horger EO. Pseudoepidural reverberation artifact: A common ultrasound artifact in the fetal cranium. J Clin Ultrasound. 1986; 14:251–254.
25. Taylor KJW, Holland S. Doppler US: I. Basic principles, instrumentation, and pitfalls. Radiology. 1990; 174:297–300.
26. Thickman DI, Ziskin MC, Goldenberg NJ, et al. Clinical manifestations of the comet tail artifact. J Ultrasound Med. 1983; 2:225.
27. Winkler P, Helmke K, Mahl M. Major pitfalls in Doppler investigations. Pediatr Radiol. 1990; 20:304–310.
28. Ziskin MC. Basic principles. In: Goldberg BB, Kotler MN, Ziskin MC, et al, eds. Diagnostic Uses of Ultrasound. New York: Grune & Stratton; 1975:1–30.
29. Ziskin MC, Thickman DI, Goldenberg NJ, et al. Clinical manifestations of the comet tail artifact. J Ultrasound Med. 1982; 1:1.

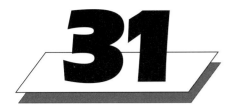

Controversies in Obstetric and Gynecologic Ultrasound

MARVEEN CRAIG

Technologic advances are often achieved much faster than technical, legal, and ethical protocols are developed to guide them. This chapter explores some of the major areas of controversy involving the use of diagnostic ultrasound in the practice of obstetrics and gynecology, and their impact on patients, fetuses, sonologists and sonographers.

Obstetric Ultrasound

The unparalleled information obtained from diagnostic ultrasound studies of the gravid patient, especially during the critical stages of fetal development, have earned widespread acceptance for obstetric ultrasound. The additional bonuses of safety and low cost have made it the preferred tool for many obstetric applications. But obstetric ultrasound has implications beyond diagnosis; those who would unravel the mysteries of life in utero have an obligation to maintain the dignity of that life.

Routine Versus Selective Scanning

For discussion, it is helpful to define the differences between the use of ultrasound in routine scanning or as a screening device. Routine scanning consists of regular scans of an unvarying nature, applied to each and every pregnancy. Screening refers to systematic searches that use special techniques or measurements and are conducted to separate specific pregnancy abnormalities from normally progressing pregnancies.

The standard of care in many countries calls for routine ultrasound examinations in the second trimester, yet the United States, although unofficially adopting this concept, continues to debate the issue, citing questions of safety, cost, lack of established standards or protocols, and the inconsistent quality of operators, interpreters, and equipment.[16]

Most proponents of routine scanning are members of the medical community who recognize the fetus as a patient, albeit one inaccessible to the traditional forms of clinical investigations such as palpation and inspection.[51] Among the opponents of this concept are some physicians, policy makers, insurance carriers, and their lobbyists who decry even the notion of such a practice.[40,51,79]

The difficult task of judging a technology that has been widely embraced by both physicians and their patients is further compounded now that concerns for safety have lessened. Studies addressing the issues of safety have shown no convincing proof of damage and have not allowed any firm conclusions to be drawn.[48] Even while the debate about routine versus selective scanning continues, there is an increasing demand from physicians and their patients for ultrasound scans. The previous stumbling blocks—primitive technology, lack of skilled operators, and the need to prove the clinical value of the technique—have been overcome to such a degree that a form of routine scanning may actually be taking place, as progressively more and more pregnancy patients are being scanned.

BENEFITS OF ROUTINE SCANNING

The benefit of routine obstetric ultrasound is its ability to answer basic questions about the embryo or fetus: Is it alive? Is it growing normally or is it malformed? What is its current age? Recognizing preterm delivery as a major cause of perinatal mortality and that postmaturity syndromes are associated with fetal distress and long-term developmental disorders, it is easy to see what a boon to obstetrics ultrasound can be.[48,51]

The earliest detection of fetal growth disorders is critical if appropriate changes in obstetric management are to be made to avoid further fetal compromise. Early documentation of unsuspected multiple gestation (with its high-risk implications) is also advantageous because of its potential to improve both fetal and maternal outcomes. Although the incidence of placenta previa is only a few in every thousand pregnancies, it is an obstetric problem with serious consequences. The most crucial case favoring routine obstetric scanning, however, centers on early detection of congenital malformations, which affect approximately 2% to 4% of all newborns.[51] Advance knowledge is of critical importance in terms of mortality and because of the emotional and economic stresses that morbidity places on the family and society. Such information is vital to patients who must decide whether to continue or terminate such pregnancies.[46,47]

EFFICACY

Routine obstetric ultrasound has become standard practice in other countries because, by their criteria, it has improved patient care and fetal outcome. In 1988, the published results of a large-scale study in Sweden concluded that significant benefits could be obtained from even a single routine obstetric sonogram at approximately 15 weeks' gestation.[81]

POTENTIAL DISADVANTAGES TO ROUTINE SCANNING

Before American medicine adopts ultrasound as a routine or screening test in pregnancy, the following considerations must be explored: its rate of sensitivity and specificity (efficacy), its potential risks (safety), its cost, patient acceptance, and quality control. Sensitivity is the probability that a test demonstrates an abnormality or disease when it is in fact present. Specificity is the probability that test results will be negative when indeed a patient has no disease. (See Chap. 34 for further discussion of these concepts.)

COST FACTORS

Why does American medicine resist officially sanctioning the practice of routine scanning? Could the answer lie in the differences between European and American health care delivery systems? The cost of diagnostic ultrasound is vastly different in America from that in equally developed countries such as England, Germany, and France, where routine scanning is widely practiced. European scanning costs are well under $50. In America, examination time, cost of equipment, personnel, and miscellaneous institutional and insurance costs can boost the price of a single ultrasound scan to a range of $100 to $450. The major deterrent to routine obstetric scanning is, and will continue to be, *cost*. The current shift in focus from patient-focused care to cost-effective and preventive care in the United States may eventually favor routine pregnancy screening if it is proven to be cost effective.[24,51,75]

A desperate need exists for a comprehensive and well designed cost–benefit analysis of routine ultrasound screening of pregnancy. Previous attempts have not represented the entire spectrum of patients, or were studies in which only one or two conditions were correlated with limited variables (i.e., length of hospital stay, improved quality of life, increased life span).[51] A thorough cost–benefit analysis must also address more complicated issues than the purely financial ones—issues that involve ethical and philosophic factors.

SAFETY FACTORS

Although no adverse effects have been reported in patient populations scanned in the early 1960s and 1970s, and despite the fact that more than 10 million newborns have been scanned worldwide without evidence of ill effects due to ultrasound exposure, we in the United States are reluctant to surrender our concerns for safety.[51] Opponents to routine scanning are quick to point out that follow-up of infants exposed to ultrasound in utero has been insufficient to test for delayed effects. The bitter lessons learned from thyroid and thymus irradiation and from diethystilbestrol exposure exert a powerful influence. Thus, the lingering concerns that ultrasound exposure may produce subtle effects in subsequent generations is the underlying force behind today's policy of using diagnostic ultrasound very prudently or only when it is clinically indicated.

NATIONAL INSTITUTES OF HEALTH CONSENSUS PANEL FINDINGS

A 1984 National Institutes of Health (NIH) task force addressing the issue of routine obstetric ultrasound found it to be of diagnostic value where clinical questions existed, but that it offered no demonstrable improvement in perinatal outcome. Their decision was based on: 1) the lack of well controlled studies demonstrating improved pregnancy outcome resulting from routine obstetric scanning; 2) the lack of consensus among professionals that ultrasound should be used to examine all pregnant women; and 3) the inconclusive evidence about long-term effects.[79] The Food and Drug Administration, as one of the panel members, reaffirmed its policy that, until risks are better defined, only prudent and judicious use of ultrasound should occur and exposure, duration, and ultrasound intensity should be limited to what is needed to produce the necessary diagnostic information.[40]

RADIUS

The Routine Antenatal Diagnostic Imaging with Ultrasound trial (RADIUS) was a practice-based, multicenter study of pregnant women at low risk for adverse pregnancy outcomes. The 5-year-long, highly publicized study was designed to test the hypothesis that routine screening with standardized ultrasound would reduce the primary outcome variables of perinatal morbidity and mortality. A select, asymptomatic, low-risk population (53,367 women) was examined in 28 tertiary and nontertiary care centers. Only 16.6% of major congenital

anomalies were detected before 24 weeks' gestation, with the rate of detection greater in tertiary care centers (35%) than in the nontertiary care centers (13%). Based on these data, the authors concluded that routine ultrasound did not improve perinatal outcome compared with its selective use on the basis of clinician judgment. It became obvious that cost was the issue that compelled the RADIUS study when the authors concluded that adopting the practice of routine obstetric ultrasound in the United States would considerably raise the cost of pregnancy care without demonstrated improvement.

This study, like its NIH predecessor, was slanted toward patient therapy and management protocols rather than ultrasound protocols, and attempted to tie the usefulness of diagnostic ultrasound testing solely to pregnancy outcome.[34] The study patients selected were not truly representative of most American pregnant women; furthermore, no distinction was made between the diagnostic accuracy of casual ultrasound practitioners versus those with formal training and extensive experience. For these, and other reasons, many experts in the ultrasound community felt that the findings of both the NIH and RADIUS studies were incomplete at best, and at worst, that the RADIUS study design and analysis, in particular, were flawed.[34,78]

Now, some 2 years poststudy, predictions that the RADIUS findings would have little impact on the regular use of ultrasound in low-risk pregnancy have been borne out. Because most routine scanning takes place in obstetric office practices, the current trend can be expected to continue; it is difficult to convince any pregnant woman not to have a sonogram once she understands that even in low-risk situations there is always the possibility of some degree of abnormality.

Maternal Versus Fetal Rights

THE FETUS AS A PATIENT

The modern concept of the fetus as a patient owes much of its status directly to the use of diagnostic ultrasound in pregnancy. Although the first direct view of ovulation occurred in 1930, followed in 1944 by the microscopic observation of fertilization, it was not until the 1960s that accurate and specific fetal diagnosis and therapy became a reality.

That one instance was the treatment of Rh isoimmunization disease with serial amniocentesis and intrauterine fetal transfusions. At about the same time, diagnostic ultrasound was being hailed as a promising tool for evaluating fetal response to this maternal condition.[46,47] Since then, many ultrasound milestones have been passed:

1. Identification of the fetus during embryonic development
2. Demonstration of fetal physiology and fetal disease
3. Detection of the need for fetal therapy, including therapy guidance or monitoring, and follow-up monitoring of fetal tolerance and response to treatment

Prenatal ultrasound testing can actually produce a paradoxic effect. On the one hand, its use in developing new tests and therapies for common disorders is very positive; on the other, its use to justify pregnancy termination can create moral dilemmas when we consider that the protection of life is medicine's highest calling.

Some oppose fetal diagnosis and therapy, seeing it as a means of carrying out search-and-destroy missions, a method for selective breeding and possible genocide (e.g., screening for Down syndrome, Tay-Sachs, thallasemia). To those who embrace the concept, the goal is to provide deeper understanding of a wide range of fetal illnesses and to be able to offer brighter prospects than the present alternatives of neonatal death, abnormality, or abortion.[47]

FETAL THERAPY

Specific therapies exist to improve fetal life in utero, and are categorized as indirect, specific, invasive, and surgical. Indirect fetal therapy involves the use of drugs to manipulate the fetus' physiologic status. Sonography's role in indirect and specific therapy is obviously detection and follow-up of therapeutic response.

Invasive therapies involve entering the uterus, amniotic cavity, or fetus to administer agents such as hormones or red blood cells. In these instances, sonography plays an additional role: mapping the area of interest, monitoring the procedure, and in some cases guiding it.

Surgical intervention, clearly a more potentially dangerous form of fetal therapy, involves the de-

compression of cysts, shunt placement in fetal hydronephrosis or hydrocephaly, and draining abnormal fluid collections. The fact that all of these procedures are greatly improved with the aid of diagnostic ultrasound has contributed to its increasing use.

Perhaps the most daring feat of all is intrauterine fetal surgery, in which the gravid uterus is exposed through a midline incision, a hysterotomy is performed, and the appropriate fetal part is exteriorized and subjected to corrective surgery. Experience has proven that open fetal surgery with continuation of pregnancy or delivery near term is feasible. This knowledge has increased hope for both parents and health care providers.[47,72] The work accomplished in this area relies heavily on diagnostic ultrasound. Proponents point to these procedures as leading to a greater understanding of fetal problems and alternative solutions, acknowledging, however, that it will be many years before the benefits of these activities can be fully evaluated (Hobbins, JC, personal communications).

The primary reason for performing fetal surgery is to free the fetus from a life of physical suffering and to ease any potential economic burdens. Opposition to intrauterine surgery is based chiefly on its high cost and the uncertainty of long-term effects. Fletcher estimates the cost of congenital defects to be $1.5 billion, with an additional $1.4 billion in lost earnings from parents and children who will never work.[39] Although it is obvious that costs would soar if every fetus was treated in utero, selective fetal surgery represents only a fraction of that cost and also results in a contributing member of society.

FETAL TISSUE RESEARCH

Would sonography play a role in evaluating the living fetus before a selection process? Would its use extend to recipients as a means of detecting and demonstrating their abnormality? And once fetal tissue transplantation was completed, would it be used in follow-up studies to determine the positive or negative effects?

Although fetal tissue can be obtained from miscarriages and stillbirths, the major available source of fetal tissue for research would be from elective abortions. This factor poses the most difficult ethical dilemma. Religious groups in particular are concerned that the routine use of fetal organs could result in a morally unacceptable collaboration with the "abortion industry." Would researchers be tempted to declare fetuses dead prematurely or to encourage more abortions? Would such practices result in one generation living off another by using fetuses as spare parts for a senescent population? Unless genetic engineering is perfected to the extent that fetal organs can be "grown" in the laboratory, the source of fetal tissue will continue to be primarily abortions.

Fetal tissue research holds important potential benefits for victims of major disease, such as diabetes, Parkinson's disease, and other brain disorders, and also for medical research. Implanted fetal tissue grows rapidly and is less likely than adult tissue to be rejected by the recipient's immune system. Transplantation of fetal tissues involved in the formation of blood and immune cells, to be used as a powerful tool against acquired immunodeficiency syndrome and other immune-mediated diseases, is being investigated.[55,72]

The magnificent medical advances of recent decades have also produced monstrous ethical problems related to maternal and fetal rights and resource allocation. Fetal tissue research fell victim to politics when it was seriously curtailed during the Reagan and Bush administrations. In 1988, the United States National Organ Transplant Act was amended to ban the sale of "fetal organs or subparts," and the NIH banned research involving the transplantation of fetal tissue from elective abortions. The Reagan–Bush moratorium was finally overturned early in the course of the Clinton administration.[72,80]

Fetal tissue transplantation raises the ethical fear of fetal exploitation, and voices have already been raised demanding that this particular aspect of medical research be safeguarded from any possible commercial enterprise.[55] An NIH study panel determined that fetal tissue research should continue to receive federal funding, and it proposed adoption of the following procedural guidelines: 1) no mention of tissue donation should be made until after a patient elected to have an abortion; 2) the donor should not know the recipient; 3) the tissue should not be donated expressly for a particular person; and 4) no money should be exchanged for any fetal material, nor should there be any financial incentive

for obstetricians or staff members to encourage patients to make donations.[31,53,72]

European legislation permits routine organ procurement, and in Britain a Medical Research Council Intermediate Tissue Bank has been established as an intermediary between those performing abortions and those using fetal tissue. A special "conscience" clause allows dissenting medical personnel to be released from involvement.[30,72]

MATERNAL RIGHTS

There are numerous reasons why a woman might decide not to undergo procedures such as fetal therapy or fetal surgery. Often a patient has personal and family responsibilities that place her in conflict with her physician's advice. Religious beliefs and personal values such as bodily integrity are also powerful factors in this issue. In extreme circumstances, physicians have resorted to court-ordered intrauterine transfusions, cesarean sections, and hospital detention in the interest of the fetus, even though such actions would seriously impair patient–doctor communication and mutual trust.[16] Murray suggests that "the fetus becomes a patient when its welfare becomes the physician's concern." Should obligations to the fetus equal or exceed our obligations to a born child?[59] Should a mother be legally obligated to undergo invasive surgery for the sake of her fetus?

PREGNANCY TERMINATION

It is unlikely that there is a more divisive aspect of obstetric sonography than its use in pregnancy termination. A growing number of sonographers find themselves in direct conflict with their moral principles and the demands of their profession. As the bitter drama of pro-life versus pro-choice continues to unfold around them, sonographers are not likely to escape the crossfire.

The best advice seems to be that sonographers should take a personal inventory of their feelings and beliefs regarding abortion and medical intervention procedures. Those unable to accept the current abortion laws and medical practices regarding them should express their convictions and request to be relieved of the duty of working with patients destined to undergo such procedures. Depending on an institution's patient population and activities, this may not be easily arranged. Nonetheless, sonographers should never be forced through fear of professional or economic reprisal to perform ultrasound procedures that conflict with their personal beliefs; and a sonographer who once accepts responsibility toward a patient must never refuse to carry out or complete a procedure.

The common practice of permitting patients to view the display screen during ultrasound studies and sonographers' willingness to point out fetal structures during routine scanning can create potential problems. Should women who are contemplating abortion watch their fetuses? Should sonographers freely answer questions that such patients may be prompted to ask as a result of seeing their fetus? Shouldn't such patients be clearly identified as potential or certain elective abortion candidates before arriving in the ultrasound facility?

The failure of referring physicians to inform the ultrasound center that the patient being scheduled for sonography is *also* scheduled for an abortion forces sonographers into compromising situations. Such problems could be eased if 1) clinicians fully explained the ultrasound procedure to patients before scheduling and communicated their combined wishes regarding patient viewing of the study, and 2) sonographers offered patients the option of viewing the screen during a study instead of assuming that all patients wish to do so. They could then adjust the position of the display screen and restrict their comments during the examination. It is not the province of diagnostic ultrasound and its purveyors to attempt to dissuade, encourage, or punish patients.

FETAL REDUCTION

That multiple gestation can produce complications in pregnancy is well known. Studies have shown that the risk of stillbirth and infant deaths is greater when a woman is carrying three or more fetuses. This problem surfaces most often in women who have undergone ovulation induction or in vitro fertilization. To increase the chances of viable infants in such situations, reducing the number of fetuses may be suggested. This can be achieved by cardiac puncture, injection of formaldehyde into the fetal heart, or injection of filtered air into an umbilical vessel in fetuses targeted for selective feticide or abortion.[73]

Because diagnostic ultrasound plays a pivotal role in the performance of such selective reduction therapies, sonographers may be confronted with a personal moral dilemma; sonographers who view abortion as unacceptable under any circumstances would decline to be involved in such procedures. Even those who think that abortion might be appropriate under special circumstances would be forced to wrestle with the concept of sacrificing some fetuses so that others might survive.

FETAL RIGHTS

What began as a physician dilemma of choosing to sacrifice the life of a fetus to save the life of its mother (e.g., third trimester abortions) has widened to take in additional fundamental moral questions: Does the fetus have a right to life? What are the mother's rights with respect to her fetus? What is the state's interest in a fetus?

The concept of the fetus as a patient in need of consideration, care, and sometimes corrective protection has been widely accepted. Thus far, however, all parties concerned have been unable to achieve emotional satisfaction and political clarity regarding the sanctity of life in this particular context. In light of the prevailing legal, ethical, and moral climate surrounding the issues, sonographers, sonologists, and their institutions must be aware of the assertion of fetal rights—aware that they are legally responsible for their actions and diagnosis until the fetal patient reaches the majority at 21 years of age. This responsibility demands that they produce well documented records of all studies involving pregnancy and fetuses and keep them for longer periods (two decades) than other types of patient studies are traditionally kept.

The Obstetric and Gynecologic Sonographer's Role

Beside the moral issues that confront sonographers, there are many ethical considerations to resolve. One leading area of controversy surrounds the role of sonographers in dispensing information to patients and to referring or interpreting physicians. Another is the proper degree of involvement of the patient's family and loved ones during sonography.

SONOGRAPHER–PATIENT INTERACTION

Sonographers must consider carefully not only *what* they say to patients but *how* they deliver the information. Considering the apprehension and concerns that patients bring to the scanning experience, one of our goals should be to prepare them psychologically by explaining the procedure and establishing realistic expectations.[19,20,54]

FAMILY-CENTERED SONOGRAPHY

Pregnancy differs from other medical situations because it springs from a partnership that creates a family as well as a fetus. This is a compelling reason to admit the mother's loved ones into the examination room. The institution of childbirth classes, birthing rooms, rooming in, and similar innovations has transformed pregnancy into more of a social event than ever before. It is not surprising that today's pregnant women want to share the first views of their unborn child with family and friends, especially because close family members can experience bonding as a direct result of viewing fetal images on an ultrasound display. But whatever the reason, the positive results of allowing family and friends into the examining room during obstetric scanning far outweigh the risk that any problems or abnormalities will be encountered.

There are two practical reasons for turning a diagnostic study into a family event: 1) diagnostic ultrasound poses no harm to bystanders, and 2) pregnancy is a family affair that produces anxiety as well as joy.[19] There are also two arguments against such a practice. Many sonographers fear discovering an unexpected anomaly and do not want to be placed in the position of handling the distress of the patient, let alone that of her support group. Others complain that the presence of family members is distracting and is likely to interfere with the complete concentration necessary to produce a diagnostic study, regardless of whether abnormalities are discovered.

If an institution wishes to encourage or permit family involvement, participation guidelines should be established to prevent compromising the diagnostic quality of the study:

1. Admit only one or two people at a time.
2. Require guests be seated.
3. Admit no small children.
4. Reserve for the sonographer the option of first performing the study in private and then admitting guests for a review of selected highlights of the fetal examination.[19]

A brief explanation of departmental policies and of the actual ultrasound procedure should establish a professional tone and allow the sonographer to control the situation.

If an abnormality is discovered, it is necessary to extend scanning time to provide complete documentation of the problem. The interpreting physician should be contacted immediately and consulted on the further handling of the case. Ideally, the sonologist should become personally involved, because most patients can sense when something is wrong and expect to be informed of the result of the examination. In such settings, the physician acts as the sonographer's "supporter," and the patient's loved ones are there to support her at a time when she needs them most.

It is extremely important that an ultrasound facility's internal policies and procedures be developed in such a way that the sonographer's role is clearly defined. All parties involved in the delivery of diagnostic ultrasound should provide input to any policy-making session, so that a set of guidelines is developed that allows sonographers to discharge their duties without evading their responsibilities or breaking the patient's trust. The following list offers a practical approach to developing obstetric ultrasound scanning policies:

1. Review the patients' rights document adopted by your institution.
2. Establish what information (e.g., gender identification, viability) sonographers are permitted to deliver and what they should withhold.
3. Establish the number of family members permitted to view an examination and rules for their conduct.
4. Explain to the patient and family members how you plan to conduct the examination.
5. Inform the patient before commencing the examination that the privilege of delivering medical results belongs solely to the physician.
6. Treat family members with the same respect you accord the patient.
7. Describe the routine portions of the examination in a basic way without referring to specific fetal or maternal abnormalities or results.
8. If an abnormality is discovered, contact the physician in charge as soon as possible and seek further instructions.

The concept of family-centered care is actively promoted by consumer groups, physicians, midwives, nurses, and administrators, and is changing attitudes toward the services provided by others in related fields. Sonographers must realize and accept the fact that obstetric patients no longer submit passively to procedures but are becoming increasingly aware of the options available to them.[19]

SONOGRAPHER REPORTS

A sonographer's desire to generate preliminary impressions or reports that contribute to the patient's diagnosis must be weighed against medicolegal implications and self-doubt. In the course of their daily practice, sonographers are consulted by some people and threatened by others, and must constantly avoid being manipulated. Although they are fully aware that rendering a diagnosis is not included in their professional or job descriptions, they are nevertheless frequently urged to "share their thoughts" about a case. This request may be made by the interpreting or referring physician, patients, or family members.[49,50]

Initially, when ultrasound was still a new entity—not yet included in physician training—sonographers were *required* to contribute written or verbal findings to their supervising physician. This concept developed either because the trained physician was not able to be present for the patient study or because the interpreting physician had less training and experience than the sonographer. Today, the increased number of physicians with ultrasound training and experience has limited such reliance on preliminary impressions.

Every health care worker knows the value, and sometimes urgent need, for an instant report. Because of economic pressures, some sonographers are required to work in unsupervised settings, where they are frequently pressured by referring physicians to interpret a study.[49] Every ultrasound facility should draw up policies to guide sonographers in these situations, and when they are established, should circulate a letter to all house staff and referring physicians stating the valid reasons for adopting such policies.

The basic problem with sonographers rendering their impressions seems to stem from misunderstanding on the part of referring physicians: sonographers' impressions must be recognized not as diagnoses but as technical interpretations, and the final diagnosis must be rendered by the interpreting physician. When properly used, sonographers' impressions promote an open environment and offer them an opportunity for their intellectual growth.[19]

VIDEOTAPING PRACTICES

Today's patients are definitely more aware and want (at times demand) filmed or taped documentation of the time they spend in the ultrasound laboratory. Some bring blank videotapes for copying the images of their fetus and some even seek permission to bring home video cameras into the scanning environment to record the entire event.[22]

As in any controversial issue, there are pros and cons to these practices; some of the pros include:

Satisfies patient/obstetrician request
Encourages family-centered sonography
Enhances family bonding
Enhances attractiveness of diagnostic ultrasound

The following, however, are adduced against the practice of videotaping:

Should not be provided for nonmedical or unofficial use
Distracts sonographer's concentration
Extends scanning time and patient exposure
Negative sequelae occur when poorly trained sonographers or sonologists perform the study, when patients misunderstand the information they are given, or when unsuspected fetal anomalies surface, either during taping or afterward, at delivery

If videotaping for the patient is offered, a specific time should be set aside for carrying out this service. Physicians should be aware of the examination results before any videotape is made for the patient. Nothing that was not visualized on the diagnostic recording should appear on the patient's copy.[22]

In obstetric office practices, Polaroid films are given to patients, and most, if not all, pregnant patients are scanned. Although families now press for tangible mementos of the examination, even in office practices these should not be given until a complete diagnostic study has been performed and reviewed.

Historically, obstetric ultrasound examinations have happy endings. The rewards of parental bonding, patient education and cooperation, and an improved public image for diagnostic ultrasound and the sponsoring institution are strong incentives to share information with the patient.[54] Along with being one of the most interesting and rewarding ultrasound experiences, however, obstetric sonography is an area in which real, written, and sonographic statements may return to haunt a person.

Every department, clinic, or office practice must address this issue independently because there are no national standards. Common sense and experience would indicate the following considerations:

1. A written policy should be established for providing patients with hard-copy images of their ultrasound study.
2. Nothing should appear on a patient's hard-copy that was not seen on the diagnostic study or survey.
3. The physician in charge of the imaging facility should view the tape or images before they are released to the patient and should retain the right to deny the tape or photos for patient use if an abnormality is found or suspected.

The legal representatives of some ultrasound facilities have indicated that providing a tape of the patient's ultrasound examination does not increase their liability, but that to allow these practices without physician approval or preview might. Any existing department protocols should be viewed by the institution's or the physician's legal representative. All personnel involved should remember that, in the event of litigation, national, not local, standards, will apply.[33]

COMMERCIAL FETAL IMAGING

A new facet of fetal videotaping has begun attracting the attention of the public and the ultrasound community as a result of local and national newspaper articles reporting on the work of prenatal portrait studios.[32] Many of these businesses are sonographer-owned, and operated for the express purpose of providing expectant mothers with keepsake videotapes of their fetuses. But of greatest concern are those enterprises operated by nonmedical personnel who have taken weekend "training courses" and are operating with suboptimal imaging equipment. The American Institute of Ultrasound in Medicine (AIUM), the Society of Diagnostic Medical Sonographers, and The American Registry of Diagnostic Medical Sonographers (ARDMS) have each issued position statements expressing the view that diagnostic ultrasound should not be used for casual entertainment and exploitation.[2]

Alerted by the degree of publicity, the Food and Drug Administration, which disapproves of ultrasound for nonmedical uses, has investigated many of these businesses, and in some instances, in cooperation with state health agencies, has been instrumental in their closing.[23,36] Despite this fact, because of the wide variation in state laws and the fact that some of the entrepreneurial videographers have structured their business plans to require physician referrals and "readings," quite a few are still operating. Their existence not only mirrors the lack of established standards in the field of sonography, but will undoubtedly fuel controversy for a long time to come.

EDUCATION AND COMPETENCY

Who should perform diagnostic ultrasound studies? Who should interpret them? Sadly, the lack of rules governing these aspects of diagnostic ultrasound has opened wide the potential for abuse of this profession. A sonologist must not only be skilled in interpreting images but must be sure that images are obtained with optimal examination technique and equipment. Expert performance of ultrasound examinations is an art that cannot be learned from books alone but requires consistent practice and the use of intelligence, medical knowledge, and experience.[10,37,64,68] Even the RADIUS study pointed out the need to improve the quality of obstetric ultrasound (particularly in nontertiary centers) through more extensive training for sonologists and sonographers.

Unfortunately, the deceptively simple appearance of the scanning technique is enhanced by the fact that anyone can purchase diagnostic ultrasound equipment and offer scanning services. This has attracted some practitioners of questionable competency. The crux of the problem, once again, is that there are no national standards. As sonography advances in both years and experience, it might be thought that the number of incompetent or poorly trained practitioners would decline. There are two main reasons this has not happened: enthusiastic patient acceptance has increased demands for the technique, and the manufacture and sale of less expensive "basic" models to private offices has spawned a casual approach to using ultrasound. In such settings, many people are asked to learn to perform ultrasound studies on their own and are entirely unaware of the educational demands on and resources available to professional sonographers. This situation contributed to the adoption of two levels of ultrasound examination in obstetrics today.

In a level 1 study, ultrasound is used as an everyday clinical tool, by physicians with little skill, to make immediate—albeit crude—decisions. In a level 2 study, ultrasound is used to look at intricate intraabdominal or fetal anatomy and pathology to make much more subtle decisions. To those whose focus is primarily imaging, there is little tolerance for the concept of two levels of performance. In their view, every study should be expertly performed by personnel as knowledgeable about imaging as they are about clinical medicine.[37,64]

Filly has pointed out that for all intents and purposes, level 1 sonography is the standard second or third trimester obstetric examination as described in the AIUM and American College of Radiology guidelines, and although the specific purpose of the examination is not to detect fetal anomalies, there is a reasonable probability that, during the course of the data acquisition, many anomalies will be recognized and that a prudent effort should be made toward this end. He expresses concern that the term "level 1" might be used as a shield for incompetency and notes that patients have a right to expect that the person performing and interpreting their examination has the appropriate knowledge to do so. He has lobbied tirelessly for the elimination of level 1 and level 2 examinations, stressing that there should be only one level of ultrasound that is optimal. His concern is that too often the term "level 1 scan" is used as an excuse for lack of knowledge and for shoddy performance, or as a shield for incompetence.[37] Most legal suits involving ultrasound have been shown to relate primarily to obstetric scanning or interpretation by relatively inexperienced individuals.[68]

The training criteria for all specialties that use diagnostic ultrasound are just beginning to be defined. Only small segments of the radiology, obstetric, and cardiology boards are devoted to diagnostic ultrasound, and there are no universal mandates or requirements regarding the length of practical ultrasound training or the minimum number of examinations required for proficiency.[58,68]

In 1993, AIUM, in collaboration with the American College of Obstetrics and Gynecology (ACOG), published recommended training guidelines for physicians who perform or interpret ultrasound examinations. These guidelines recommend that physicians be able to show evidence of training and competence in interpretation, and those who perform ultrasound studies should have completed at least 3 months of physician-supervised training (including involvement in at least 500 diagnostic ultrasound examinations) or provide evidence of 100 hours of AMA Category 1 continuing medical education activity dedicated to diagnostic ultrasound and evidence of involvement with the evaluation and interpretation of at least 500 diagnostic examinations within a 3-year period. Through the efforts of the Commission on Ultrasound of the American College of Radiology, ACOG, and AIUM, development of guidelines for residency training programs is now under way.[76]

Since 1975, ARDMS has conducted voluntary registry examinations for sonographers. For more than a decade their test was the only available yardstick for measuring minimum levels of competency of the people who perform a variety of diagnostic ultrasound studies. In 20 years of offering examinations, a total of 30,000 sonographers have been registered. Among them are a small, but growing number of physicians who have seen the value of establishing their own competency. ARDMS' greatest contribution, however, may well be their insistence on mandatory continuing education (evidence of 30 continuing medical education units over a 3-year period) to maintain a registered status.

IMPACT OF HEALTH CARE REFORM

In the early days of the Clinton administration, great emphasis was placed on reforming the health care system through federal legislative actions. Although the federal initiative was unsuccessful, interest in reform remains and has spurred considerable action at the state level. Fiscal reform is another area of great activity, and has produced directives relating to vascular and obstetric ultrasound requiring sonographers who perform studies in these specialties to be certified. Concerns about health care reform have made deep inroads on ultrasound laboratories by limiting scanning time, increasing patient loads, and restricting insurance reimbursement.[23]

CROSS-TRAINING AND MULTISKILLING

Evidence of the impact of health care reform on sonography can be seen in the growing number of sonographers who have been laid off or whose jobs have been eliminated by administrative decisions to cut back and downsize. Those still employed work under increasing pressure to operate within tighter budgets. Wages are frozen, existing employees are expected to assume the work of those who have been let go, some are required to take mandatory call, and many are forced to assume nonimaging duties through cross-training rather than formal training. They are then required to cross-train hospital employees without imaging backgrounds to perform ultrasound examinations, if they wish to retain their jobs.[4,25–27]

These practices, especially in the area of cross-training, have dealt a body blow to the ongoing efforts of sonographers to reach professional status. They have also created many questions and few answers: Who will train sonographers to perform nursing procedures? Will they and the people they are cross-training receive any formal training? If so, how long will they go to "school?" Where will they get adequate clinical experience? How will they maintain state-of-the-art knowledge? Will educators have to revamp sonography programs so that students can extend their studies to become certified in other related fields (e.g., medical assisting) as well as sonography? Will cross-trained personnel be expected to become credentialed to meet the reimbursement demands of insurance companies? These questions point out the difference between being multiskilled, multicompetent, and being multicredentialed.

LIMITED ULTRASOUND EXAMINATIONS

The Association of Women's Health, Obstetric, Gynecologic, and Neonatal Nurses (AWHONN, formerly NAACOG) has published a document entitled "Nursing Practice Competencies for Limited Ultrasound Examinations." In it, following the definitions of limited ultrasonography as set forth by ACOG, they define the minimum competencies and training necessary for nurses to perform limited ultrasound studies:

- Evaluation of early first trimester pregnancies
- Evaluation of fetal number
- Confirmation of fetal life and presentation
- Localization of the placenta
- Assessment of amniotic fluid volume, biophysical profile, ultrasound-guided amniocentesis, and external version

They have further mandated that nurses have 12 hours of didactic education and "sufficient supervised clinical hands-on training to obtain competency."[9] This statement has roused the ire of sonographers who are required to demonstrate from 1 to 4 years of formal or on-the-job training to be considered competent to take the registry exams.[9] According to the AWHONN document, nurses have the responsibility of both performing and interpreting limited ultrasound examinations. They consider performing limited ultrasound studies and providing interpretations of those studies one of the many competencies that nurses are authorized to do by virtue of the fact that the sonographic activities they have outlined are part of nursing practice.[9,41–43]

The Society of Diagnostic Medical Sonographers does not endorse the performance of limited obstetric examinations that do not meet current guidelines established by the AIUM, ACOG, and American College of Radiology. Nor do they endorse individuals whose scope of practice in sonography does not conform to the certification standards for obstetrics and gynecology of the ARDMS.[70]

Only time will tell whether acceptance of the AWHONN document will prove to be a professional and educational defeat or a boon by serving as a precedent for autonomy, professional interpretation, and billing rights. Sonographers who favor creating an advanced practice tier on the sonographer career ladder will follow the outcome closely.[62]

LEGAL CONSIDERATIONS

The continuing 1980s trend toward medical malpractice litigation strikes most deeply in the area of obstetric ultrasound. In fact, ultrasound appears to have created new medicolegal corridors. Some areas that can potentially lead to legal difficulties (those marked with an asterisk relate specifically to sonographers) are:

> Failure to conform to a standard of care in performing or not performing an ultrasound examination
>
> Performing an incomplete study and "missing" a lesion
>
> Improper interpretation of the sonogram
>
> Failures and misdiagnoses due to instrumentation
>
> Complications from invasive ultrasound procedures
>
> Failure to adequately inform the referring physician
>
> *Professional misconduct
>
> *Misinterpreting and reporting a diagnosis
>
> *Failure to provide for patient safety during the ultrasound examination[66,67]

In each diagnostic ultrasound study, there are four important variables to consider: the knowledge and skill of the sonographer, the knowledge and skill of the sonologist, the quality of the ultrasound instrument, and the patient's unique sonographic characteristics.

Obviously, high standards offer the best protection against obstetric sonography claims. One critical component is the need for detailed documentation of all studies. Most ultrasound-related malpractice suits in the United States are the result of missed diagnosis.[50,66,67] The obvious causes of such misadventures are poor-quality images, poor documentation, and poor technical performance of the study. These factors frequently result from failure to use state-of-the-art equipment and transducers. Sometimes they result from failure of the sonography service to communicate the limitations of ultrasound to the referring doctor and patient, or from inappropriate use of ultrasound during a specific stage of pregnancy.

At the root of malpractice is the lack of quality-control guidelines for obstetric sonography. Although the AIUM published guidelines for the use of ultrasound in obstetrics, there is still concern that they will not be widely circulated and adopted.[44,45] Predictions that reimbursement will require performance of studies only by certified or registered health care professionals has prompted many orga-

nizations like the AIUM to begin designing and implementing voluntary diagnostic ultrasound laboratory accreditation processes.[7,8]

SONOGRAPHY AS A PROFESSION

Some believe sonography does not currently enjoy professional status and it is unlikely ever to achieve professional status until it earns recognition of authenticity and endorsement from the professional branches of medicine.

In a visionary article, Persutte concluded that there are two tiers of clinical sonographers practicing in the United States: those with standard skills and those with advanced skills in a particular specialty.[62] His words are a comfort for every sonographer who has felt frustrated by occupational and clinical advancement limits. Some sonographers, after years of study and supervised experience, are able and willing to use their independent judgment and discretion in their daily clinical activities. Having met and exceeded all of the educational requirements to be sonographers, they long to take the next step and become practitioners. If denied those opportunities, there is heightened concern that many valuable sonographers will leave the field to pursue advanced opportunities in nonultrasound professions.

The innovative concept of advanced practice sonography would be very popular with health care reformists who wish to improve primary care and at the same time contain costs. Sonographers performing low-risk obstetric ultrasound studies would relieve physicians and allow them to concentrate on high-risk patients, provide care at lower costs, and provide service to patients who could otherwise not afford care.[29,62]

Conclusion

Sonography is vulnerable to political and economic pressures and to the encroachment of other medical professions. It is also vulnerable to both apathy and unrealistic expectations. Now, more than ever before, it is the duty of all sonographers to become familiar with the issues and to remain current with the medical, professional, legal, and economic solutions regarding them as they attempt to explore the contours of an unknown horizon.

The issues of what constitutes a sonographer's

professional relationship with patients and physicians is complex and still evolving. While we go about the task of recognizing the obligations, duties, benefits, and liabilities of being sonographers, we must not diminish the potential for good that diagnostic ultrasound can provide.

REFERENCES

1. American Registry of Diagnostic Medical Sonographers Directory and Informational Booklet—1994. Rockville, MD: American Registry of Diagnostic Medical Sonographers; 1994.
2. Anderhub B. Letter from the president. [SDMS] NewsWave. 1994; 15:2.
3. Anderhub B. Letter from the President. [SDMS] NewsWave. 1993; 14:6.
4. Anderhub B. Letter from the President. [SDMS] NewsWave. 1995; 16:1.
5. Anderhub B. Letter from the President. [SDMS] NewsWave. 1994; 15:3.
6. Anderhub B. Letter from the President. [SDMS] NewsWave. 1995; 16:3.
7. Arger PH. President's letter. AIUM Reporter. 1995; 11:7.
8. Arger PH. President's letter. AIUM Reporter. 1995; 11:8.
9. Association of Women's Health, Obstetric, Gynecologic, and Neonatal Nursing. Nursing Practice Competencies and Educational Guidelines for Limited Ultrasound Examinations in Obstetric and Gynecologic/Infertility Settings. Chicago, IL: AWHONN; 1993.
10. Benacerraf BR. Editorial: Who should be performing fetal ultrasound? Ultrasound in Obstetrics and Gynecology. 1993; 3:1–2.
11. Berman MC. Mandatory licensure for sonographers. J Diagn Med Sonogr. 1989; 4:191.
12. Callen PW. The obstetric ultrasound examination. In: Ultrasonography in Obstetrics and Gynecology. 3rd ed. Philadelphia: WB Saunders; 1994:1–14.
13. Chervenak FA, McCullough LB. The fetus as patient: Implications for directive vs. nondirective counseling for fetal benefits. Fetal Diagn Ther. 1991; 6:93–100.
14. Chervenak FA, McCullough LB. Clinical guides to preventing ethical conflicts between pregnant women and their physicians. Obstet Gynecol. 1990; 162:303–307.
15. Chervenak FA, McCullough LB. Ethical issues in obstetric sonography. In: Berman MC, Craig MC, Kawamura DM, eds. Diagnostic Medical Sonography: A Guide to Clinical Practice. Vol. I. Philadelphia: JB Lippincott; 1991:609–613.
16. Chervenak FA, McCullough LB. Perinatal ethics: A practical method of analysis of obligations to mother and fetus. Obstet Gynecol. 1985; 66:442–446.
17. Concalves LF, Romero R. A critical appraisal of the RADIUS study. The Fetus. 1993; 3:6.
18. Craig M. The challenge of patient interaction. J Diagn Med Sonogr. 1987; 3:147–150.
19. Craig M. Family centered sonography. J Diagn Med Sonogr. 1986; 2:96–103.
20. Craig M. Treating patients with patience. J Diagn Med Sonogr. 1989; 1:16–18.
21. Craig M. The eternal controversy: Sonographer's reports. J Diagn Med Sonogr. 1987; 3:244–248.
22. Craig M. Baby videos: A boon or liability? J Diagn Med Sonogr. 1988; 4:19–22.
23. Craig M. The ripple effect: Final chapter on fetal imaging services. J Diagn Med Sonogr. 1995; 4:210–212.
24. Craig M. Impact of healthcare reform on sonography. J Diagn Med Sonogr. 1994; 10:175–179.
25. Craig M. Cross-training: A double-edged sword? J Diagn Med Sonogr. 1987; 3:99–100.
26. Craig M. Cross-training: Palliative, panacea, or professional suicide? J Diagn Med Sonogr. 1995; 6:329–331.
27. Craig M. Mandatory call. J Diagn Med Sonogr. 1994; 10:339–343.
28. Craig M. Inventing the future. J Diagn Med Sonogr. 1994; 10:41–45.
29. Demarais H. Government health policy and the non-physician practitioner: A closer look. In: Clawson D, Osterweis M, eds. The Role of Physician Assistants and the Nurse Practitioners in Primary Care. Washington, DC: Association of Academic Health Centers; 1993.
30. Easton SS, Lamb D. Transplanting fetal tissue. Nursing Times. 1991; 87:39–40.
31. Elsom MK. Fetal tissue transplants. Canadian Nurse. 1992; 88:30–31.
32. Evans H. Womb with a view: Unborn babies star in fetal film fests. Wall Street Journal. November 30, 1993.
33. Everett SL. Ultrasound: Legal issues. Presented at the meeting of the Redwood Society of Sonographers, Santa Rosa, California, May 7, 1987.
34. Ewigman BG, Crane JP, Frigoletto FD, LeFevre ML, Bain RP, McNellis D, and the RADIUS Study Group. Effect of prenatal ultrasound screening on perinatal outcome. N Engl J Med. 1993; 328:821–827.
35. Falke DS, Weisfeld N, Tochen C. Perspectives on Health Occupational Credentialing. Washington, DC: U.S. Government Publications Office; 1980.
36. FDA investigates fetal sonogram video businesses. [SDMS] NewsWave. 1994; 4:1.

37. Filly RA. Level 1, level 2, level 3 obstetric sonography: I'll see your level and raise you one. Radiology. 1989; 172:312.

38. Finberg HJ. Routine ultrasound screening in pregnancy: Tough questions. Radiology Today. 1993; 10:3–7.

39. Fletcher JC. Ethical considerations in and beyond experimental fetal therapy. Semin Perinatol. 1985; 9:130–135.

40. Frigoletto FD. Obstetrical ultrasound: Selective use. In: McGahan JP, ed. Controversies in Ultrasound. New York: Churchill Livingstone; 1987:123–127.

41. Gegor CL, Paine LL, Johnson TRB. Antepartum fetal assessment: A nurse midwifery perspective. J Nurse Midwifery. 1991; 36:153–167.

42. Gegor CL. Antepartum fetal assessment techniques: An update for today's perinatal nurse. Journal of Perinatal and Neonatal Nursing. 1992; 5:1–8.

43. Gegor CL. Obstetric ultrasound: Who should perform sonograms. Birth. 1992; 19:92–99.

44. Guidelines for performance of the antepartum obstetrical ultrasound examination. J Ultrasound Med. 1991; 10:577.

45. Guidelines for the Performance of Antepartum Obstetrical Ultrasound Examination. Laurel, MD: American Institute of Ultrasound in Medicine; 1994.

46. Harrison MR, Adzick NS, Flake AW. Prenatal management of the fetus with a correctable defect. In: Callen PW, ed. Ultrasonography in Obstetrics and Gynecology. 3rd ed. Philadelphia: WB Saunders; 1994:536–547.

47. Harrison MR, Golbus MS, Filly RA, eds. The Unborn Patient: Prenatal Diagnosis and Treatment. 2nd ed. Philadelphia: WB Saunders; 1984.

48. Hughey MJ. Routine vs. indicated scans. In: Sabbagha RE, ed. Diagnostic Ultasound Applied to Obstetrics and Gynecology. 2nd ed. Philadelphia: JB Lippincott; 1987.

49. James AE, Fleischer AC, Thieme G, et al. Diagnostic ultrasonography: Certain legal considerations. J Ultrasound Med. 1985; 4:427–431.

50. James AE, Bundy A, Fleischer AC, et al. Legal aspects of diagnostic medical sonography. Semin Ultrasound CT MRI. 1985; 5:207–216.

51. Jeanty P, Romero R, Hobbins JC. Obstetrical ultrasound: Routine use. In: McGahan JP, ed. Controversies in Ultrasound. New York: Churchill Livingstone; 1987:113–122.

52. Joint Task Group on Training for Diagnosis in Obstetrical and Gynecologic Ultrasound, American Institute of Ultrasound in Medicine. Guidelines for minimum post residency training in obstetrical and gynecologic ultrasound. J Ultrasound Med. 1982; 1:R40.

53. Kassirer JP, Angell M. The use of fetal tissue from elective abortions in transplantation research? N Engl J Med. 1992; 327:1592–1595.

54. Lea JH. Psychosocial progression through normal pregnancy. A model for sonographer–patient interaction. J Diagn Med Ultrasound. 1985; 1:55–58.

55. Leary WE. U.S. panel backs research use of fetal tissue from abortions. New York Times. September 17, 1988.

56. LeFevre ML, Bain RP, Ewigman BG, et al. A randomized trial of prenatal ultrasonographic screening: Impact on maternal management and outcome. Am J Obstet Gynecol. 1993; 169:483.

57. Leopold G. Antepartum obstetrical ultrasound examination guidelines. J Ultrasound Med. 1986; 5:241–242.

58. Miller EI. Specialty certification in diagnostic ultrasound: disadvantages. In: McGahan JP, ed. Controversies in Ultrasound. New York: Churchill Livingstone; 1987:47–51.

59. Murray TH. Moral obligations to the not-yet-born: The fetus as a patient. Clin Perinatol. 1987; 14:329–342.

60. Nelson LJ, Milliken N. Compelled medical treatment of pregnant women: Life, liberty, and law in conflict. JAMA. 1988; 259:1060–1066.

61. Persutte WH. Professional credibility for the sonographer: How to get there from here. Sociopolitical Symposium. J Diagn Med Sonogr. 1990; 6:336–342.

62. Persutte WH. Advanced practice sonography in obstetrics and gynecology. J Diagn Med Sonogr. 1995; 3:147–152.

63. Platt LD. Assessment of gestational age. In: Queenan JT, Hobbins JC, eds. Protocols for High Risk Pregnancies. Oradell, NJ: Medical Economics Books; 1982:23–27.

64. Platt LD. Editorial: Leveling out. Ultrasound in Obstetrics and Gynecology. 1991; 1:83–85.

65. Romero. Editorial: Routine obstetric ultrasound. Ultrasound Obstet Gynecol 1993; 3:303.

66. Sanders RC. The effect of the malpractice crisis on obstetrical and gynecological ultrasound. In: Chervenak F, et al, eds. Textbook of Obstetrical and Gynecological Ultrasound. Boston: Little, Brown & Co; 1993.

67. Sanders RC. Malpractice ultrasound. In: Sanders RC, Hill MC, eds. Ultrasound Annual—1986. New York: Raven Press; 1986.

68. Sanders RC. Specialty certification in diagnostic ultrasound: Advantages. In: McGahan JP, ed. Controversies in Ultrasound. New York: Churchill-Livingstone; 1987.

69. Saari-Kemppainen A, Karjalainen O, Ylostalo P, et

al. Ultrasound screening and perinatal mortality: Controlled trial of systematic one-stage screening in pregnancy. The Helsinki Ultrasound Trial. Lancet. 1990; 336:387.

70. Scope of Practice for the Diagnostic Sonographer. Dallas, TX: Society of Diagnostic Medical Sonographers; 1993.

71. SDMS position on non-diagnostic use of ultrasound. [SDMS] NewsWave. 1994; 2:1.

72. Sills L. Fetal tissue research and prenatal fetal therapy: Ethical dilemmas. J Diagn Med Sonogr. 1994; 10:208–212.

73. Simpson JL, Sherman E. Genetic amniocentesis. In: Sabbagha RE, ed. Diagnostic Ultrasound Applied to Obstetrics and Gynecology. 2nd ed. Philadelphia: JB Lippincott; 1987:64–82.

74. Spitz JL. Sonographer support of maternal–fetal bonding. In: Berman MC, Craig MC, Kawamura DM, eds. Diagnostic Medical Sonography: A Guide to Clinical Practice. Vol 1. Philadelphia: JB Lippincott; 1991:565–571.

75. Spitz JL. Editorial. J Diagn Med Sonogr. 1994; 3:135–136.

76. Tenner MS. Letter from the president. AIUM Reporter. May, 1993.

77. Tenner MS. Letter from the president. AIUM Reporter. November, 1993.

78. Tenner MS. Letter from the president. AIUM Reporter. 1995; 2:1–4.

79. U. S. Department of Health and Human Services, Public Health Service, National Institutes of Health. Diagnostic Ultrasound Imaging in Pregnancy. NIH Publication No. 84-667. Washington, DC: U. S. Government Printing Office; 1984.

80. Vawter DE, Caplan A. Strange brew: The politics and ethics of fetal tissue transplant research in the United States. J Lab Clin Med. 1992; 120:30–34.

81. Waldenstrom U, Axelsson O, Nilsson S, et al. Effects of routine one-stage ultrasound screening in pregnancy: A randomized controlled trial. Lancet. 1988; 11:585–588.

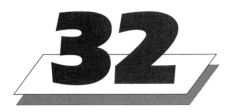

Sonographer Support of Parental–Fetal Bonding

JEAN LEA SPITZ

Attachment and bonding are interactions between parents and infant that reinforce their relationship; they are vital for the survival and normal development of the infant. Extensive research on bonding during the postnatal period has shown that bonding is an ongoing process that is apparent immediately after birth and throughout infancy and childhood.[19] Recognition of the prenatal origins of maternal attachment and the importance of a relationship between a mother and fetus has changed obstetric management. Fostering the development of bonding has become a central issue for modern obstetric practice and has led to a humanizing of the obstetric process.[23]

The importance of a strong parental–child bond cannot be overemphasized. According to Klaus and Kennell, the bond that is formed between mother and baby is the "well-spring for all the infant's subsequent attachments and is the formative relationship in the course of which the child develops a sense of himself. Throughout his lifetime, the strength and character of this attachment will influence the quality of all future bonds to other individuals."[19] A weak or dysfunctional bond may be associated with emotional and physical child abuse, neglect, and abandonment, all of which are major problems in our society. It has been postulated that prenatal bonding may promote prenatal care and the mother's adherence to health regimens beneficial to the pregnancy.[30]

For many years, the lack of reliable measures of prenatal attachment hindered research during pregnancy. Cranley[7] defined maternal–fetal attachment as the extent to which a woman differentiates self from the fetus, attributes characteristics and intentions to the fetus, interacts with the fetus, gives of herself, and assumes a maternal role. This definition led to the development of a maternal-fetal attachment scale (MFA), whose validity and reliability has been documented.[7] The Cranley MFA has been used to quantify factors that may facilitate prenatal bonding.

With the advent of ultrasound imaging in pregnancy, reactions of the mother to prenatal visualization of the baby have been described.[10,14,20,26,28,30] Although visualization is essentially a reaction in the mother, and not an interaction between the mother and fetus, many observers of ultrasound examinations have speculated that the visualization process facilitates earlier and stronger bonding with the child by increasing the mother's recognition of and attachment to the baby before birth.

Obstetric ultrasound imaging has potential societal and individual psychosocial impacts that have been discussed not only in the medical literature, but in the sociologic, legal, and ethical literature as well. Ultrasound imaging in pregnancy has become

629

a cultural ritual[32] with expected components and results. There are profound and controversial effects of ultrasound imaging on society and individuals,[27,32] including not only bonding, but, among many others, gender identification, individualization and separation of the image of the fetus from the mother, and expansion of pregnancy from a private into a public format.[27,32] As the public mediators of this technology, sonographers need to maximize the examination potential for the individual patient's good. In obstetric examinations, it is important for sonographers to encourage prenatal bonding and promote protocols that positively influence bonding.

A Review of the Literature Related to Maternal–Fetal Bonding

Early studies and anecdotal information suggest that the ultrasound examination in normal pregnancies at least transiently affects the mother's perception of the fetus. In a small sample of patients, Holland found that the mother was less likely to characterize her baby as smaller or weaker than other babies and rated her baby as more active in postscan questionnaires than in prescan questionnaires.[14] Geisler found that 71% of the women in her survey indicated that being able to see the baby on the screen made them feel "closer to the baby or more maternal."[10] Milne and Rich observed mothers during an examination and studied the process of recognizing the baby and the excitement of the mothers. The same researchers observed anecdotally that several women continued mentally to visualize their babies as they had been observed on the ultrasound instrument screen weeks after the examination.[26] Kohn and colleagues observed a greater sense of attachment to the fetus among patients who received ultrasound examinations that included a good deal of feedback from the sonographer.[20] Reading and Cox assessed maternal attitudes toward pregnancy by adjective analysis. They found prescan and postscan differences and more positive attitudes in the group who received the greatest feedback from the sonographers.[28] Hyde, in a study involving postscan interviews, reported that ultrasound allayed anxiety associated with pregnancy in most women, but that not all women found it reassuring.[16]

Later studies have shown equivocal results,

and many have found ultrasound not to be significantly related to maternal–fetal attachment.[4,9,13,18,24,33] In a later study, Reading and Cox could not confirm a relationship between ultrasound feedback conditions and attitudes toward the pregnancy or the baby.[29] A study of women in the third trimester[18] failed to demonstrate any attachment effect from ultrasound. The authors suggested ultrasound might accelerate attachment early in pregnancy, but make no difference in later pregnancy or postnatally when multiple other factors have contributed. This hypothesis is supported by reports[11,12] that indicate that maternal bonding activities during the first 5 days after birth show no relationship to the number or timing of ultrasound scans during pregnancy. Quickening is a major factor in prenatal attachment scores, with mothers who have experienced movement demonstrating higher scores. In a study of maternal–fetal attachment[23] during the second trimester, maternal age and the physical symptoms of pregnancy were not related to attachment, but the experience of quickening as well as the degree and frequency of fetal movement were strongly correlated. Economic status, ultrasound, and the planning of the pregnancy were also significant factors, but to a lesser degree than quickening. Another study found that high levels of social support seem to be consistent with high levels of attachment.[9] These results confirm that for the mother, internal body sensations of pregnancy and personal satisfaction are much more powerful attachment stimuli than is external visualization of the fetus. The role of ultrasound in hastening early attachment may be secondary. Women who have not associated mild physical sensations with fetal movement may do so when they see the fetus move on the screen at the same time they feel the sensation. By helping women identify the early sensations of fetal movement, ultrasound may accelerate quickening. The earlier sensation of quickening may be the primary factor related to attachment, with ultrasound imaging a secondary, facilitating event.

Women having an amniocentesis show lower attachment scores until after the amniocentesis results are obtained. This probably demonstrates a hesitancy to bond with the fetus until a definite choice related to the pregnancy has been made. In a study[13] comparing three groups of women, one group scheduled to have amniocentesis and ultrasound, one scheduled to have ultrasound to determine fetal age, and one group scheduled to have neither, Heidrich and Cranley measured prenatal attachment at 16 and at 20 weeks. They found that the group scheduled for amniocentesis showed lower attachment scores at 16 weeks, but by 20 weeks after the amniocentesis results were known, these scores were not significantly different from those of the other women. Maternal–fetal attachment scores increased in all the women between 16 and 20 weeks. Women who reported quickening earlier had higher attachment scores at both tests. Ultrasound did not demonstrate a significant effect in this study. When women who have chorionic villus sampling are compared to women who have genetic amniocentesis,[2] it is found that attachment begins earlier in the chorionic villus sampling group, presumably because of earlier verification of chromosomal normality.

Maternal anxiety has been measured before and after an ultrasound examination by several authors. Reading and Cox demonstrated anxiety in obstetric patients before an ultrasound scan and found that it was not significantly changed afterwards.[28] Others have demonstrated anxiety and have speculated that it is due to fear of finding an anomaly[28] or fear of having to exercise a "choice" in the pregnancy if an anomaly is found.[27] One study[34] found that anxiety is actually increased in women during ultrasound examinations, but that this increase in anxiety can be alleviated in most patients by the sonographer if she provides a high level of feedback to the patient. In low-feedback conditions, the anxiety is less likely to be dissipated. Sonographers who do not provide high levels of feedback can cause women to feel excluded from their own pregnancy.[6,16] A fear that strangers may know more about their baby than they do may contribute to an increasing number of women requesting that they be informed of fetal gender.[31]

In another study of pregnant women, Reading and Cox documented better adherence to health-related regimens, particularly the advice to stop smoking, when the advice is associated with an ultrasound examination.[30] A group of Swedish researchers found that women who had sonograms delivered larger babies, on average, and that the weight differences were most pronounced among women who at their first visit reported being smok-

ers.[34] The inference is that the sonography enhanced adherence to smoking advice, which resulted in larger babies. This study is cited as evidence of a beneficial effect for routine scanning in all pregnancies.

The Impact of Ultrasound Imaging in Pregnancy on Fathers

The greatest impact of ultrasound imaging on parental–fetal attachment may be in the attachment of the fathers.[31] Before ultrasound imaging, the mother controlled access of the father to the fetus, and the father could experience the fetus only through maternal descriptions or by feeling movements on the mother's abdomen. The external imaging of the fetus by ultrasound is a more direct experience for fathers, and anecdotal interviews[31] cite its impact. To accompany his partner to the physician's office to view the ultrasound examination is a culturally supported reason for a man to miss work. It may be one of the few pregnancy-related activities in which he is involved. Ultrasound enhances the pregnancy experience for men by allowing them to see what the women may feel and describe. For women, the ultrasound examination is a time to share the fetus with her partner. The only drawback to the involvement of the father in the ultrasound experience is that the mother may feel excluded in a situation where the sonographer talks primarily to the father, or may feel that her own personal sensations of the pregnancy are trivialized by the importance placed on the visualization by the father.[31]

Psychological Responses of Pregnant Patients

Studies and discussions of parental bonding recommend high-feedback scanning in which the sonographer provides information and descriptions of the ultrasound image seen. Obstetric sonographers need to develop an advanced professional level of communication skills. Knowledge of the normal psychological progression of pregnancy is not only interesting but very important to the development of communication strategies for sonographers. The optimal strategy may be one that serves to reduce patient anxiety and enhance attachment to the fetus. Because the major anxieties of pregnancy change during its course, it follows that appropriate and supportive interaction strategies may vary throughout the mother's pregnancy. Sonographers' ability to discern that stage and to adapt their communication to individual needs—or to the particular concerns of that pregnancy—may be heightened by attention to the psychological process of pregnancy.

In a previous review article, a graphic model (Fig. 32-1) characterizing the psychological process of pregnancy was presented.[22] The base of the model represents conditions with which the mother enters pregnancy, variables such as age, parity, socioeconomic status, culture, previous mothering experience, and family support systems, all of which affect her adaptation to pregnancy. Major sources of anxiety during pregnancy are also listed. Activi-

ties typical of each trimester of pregnancy are shown within the triangular sections of the model. The activities express the paths for resolving the underlying anxieties of pregnancy. It is hypothesized that through supportive activities, the anxieties of pregnancy are reduced and attachment to the fetus can grow. In the model, anxieties, activities, and attachment typical of each trimester are listed.

FIRST TRIMESTER

During the first trimester of pregnancy, anxiety is related to acceptance of the reality of pregnancy and normal ambiguity toward the pregnancy. Teenagers have difficulty accepting the reality of pregnancy

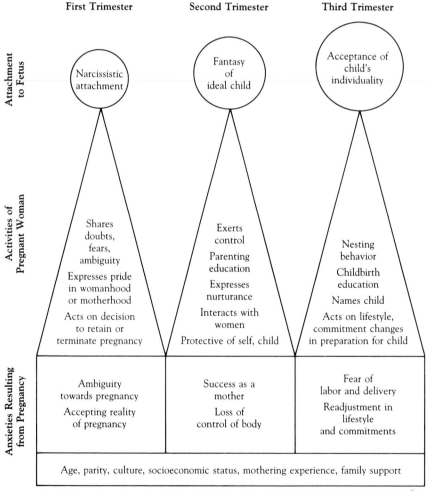

Figure 32-1. A model of the psychological process of pregnancy. Variables that may affect adaptation to pregnancy are presented at the base of the model. Anxieties common to pregnancy (squares) may be resolved by activities (triangles). Through such resolution, maternal–fetal bonding processes (circles) are enhanced.

because they have not fully accepted their womanhood. Teenagers often perceive themselves more as children than as adults, and so have difficulty acknowledging a pregnancy. Older patients generally are capable of accepting the reality of pregnancy, but may deny ambiguous feelings toward it. Even under optimal conditions, when the pregnancy was planned and actively sought, women can expect to feel some ambiguity. Pregnancy entails a major commitment and life change for women and is therefore greeted with both positive and negative expectations. Psychologically healthy women accept, express, and share doubts and fears related to the pregnancy with support people. Such women resolve their ambiguity by making a decision either to retain or terminate the pregnancy and then act on that decision.

Remarks that express disbelief, excitement, disappointment, and worry are typical during the first trimester. Sonographers working with these patients may encourage them to accept the reality of the pregnancy and openly explore their own feelings about the fetus. The ultrasound image, when it is seen by the patient, is powerful evidence of the reality of pregnancy. Connecting the image to the patient's body by verbally pointing out the area within which the fetus lies further emphasizes this reality. The sonographer may be a supportive and nonjudgmental listener to positive or negative expressions concerning the pregnancy. Ambiguity is normal, and the more openly it is expressed, the more quickly it can be resolved.

Women initially attach to the fetus because it is part of themselves. They do not perceive it as a separate person. The recognition of the fetus as a separate individual begins at quickening, when the mother first perceives fetal motion. The internal sensations of movement are strongly associated with attachment. Ultrasound imaging may accelerate the recognition of fetal movement and have a positive impact on bonding during this stage of pregnancy.

SECOND TRIMESTER

Along with the perception of the fetus as a separate person, anxiety related to the woman's ability to mother arises. Sonographers are often asked by patients about their own children or their own parenting experiences. This is a natural expression of the need to explore mothering alternatives. Parenting classes are often helpful at this stage. Along with concern about her mothering ability, a strong protectiveness toward herself and toward the fetus develops in most women. This may be expressed to the sonographer as concern about the safety of the ultrasound procedure or concern about adequate visualization of all parts of the fetus. The continuing growth of the fetus creates in the woman a sense of a loss of control over her own body. Anxiety related to this loss of control may lead to activities that express the desire to control the environment, herself, or others. Rearranging furniture, changing diets, or beginning exercise programs are examples of external efforts to control.

Second trimester is the ideal time to talk with patients about changes in diets or habits that may benefit the fetus. The desire to control and the increasing sense of protection toward the fetus lead many women to incorporate advice regarding changes in diet or smoking habits. If a sonographer is uncomfortable providing this type of patient education, a poster in the ultrasound laboratory about healthy eating or other habits might be effective. Such posters are available from many sources, including March of Dimes, the American Lung Association, and the American Dietetics Association.

Attachment to the fetus may grow rapidly during the second trimester. The mother is generally feeling well, the sickness of early pregnancy has subsided, and the heaviness of later pregnancy has not yet begun. The mother perceives the fetus as a separate individual, and often an individual endowed with characteristics of the mother's ideal child.

THIRD TRIMESTER

During the third trimester, anxiety is related to fear of labor and delivery. The need to readjust lifestyles or relationships with others to create more time for the new baby may cause anxiety as well. "Nesting," or nursery preparation, is undertaken, and professional commitments may be reduced. Childbirth education classes taken at this time may alleviate some of the anxiety related to labor and delivery. It is helpful for obstetric sonographers to have some knowledge of labor alternatives to answer patients' questions.

Attachment to the fetus continues to grow, but less rapidly than in the second trimester. The "ideal child" is by now kicking quite hard, making the mother feel heavy and uncomfortable, and often interrupting her sleep. The mother's perceptions of the fetus contain positive and negative elements, and the child is increasingly perceived as a separate individual with unique personal characteristics. Mothers who did not want to know the sex of the child earlier may change their minds during the third trimester. Many mothers settle on a name or names at this point in pregnancy, and if the sex is known may refer to the baby by name. The perception of separateness and fetal individuality that develops at this stage promotes the development of an optimal mother–child relationship after the birth.

Sonographer–Patient Interactions

It is apparent from the studies cited earlier that ultrasound scanning may have a positive effect on pregnancy and that this effect may be influenced by the communication style of the sonographer during the examination. It is also apparent that interactions that minimize anxiety and enhance attachment may vary somewhat from trimester to trimester. Communication may also differ depending on the specific needs of that pregnancy or the results of the examination.

Sonographers have been leaders in developing strategies to make the ultrasound examination a positive experience for expectant mothers. In the literature and at national meetings, anecdotal and researched communication strategies to lessen maternal anxiety before the examination and improve maternal understanding of the examination have been shared. There remains widespread controversy and confusion about what feedback is appropriate for obstetric patients. Sonographers are caught between institutional needs to schedule more patients, marketers' demands to cater to patients' requests and produce videotapes and images for them to take home, and lawyers' warnings to be realistic and not overly reassuring. It is no wonder that in the midst of this complexity there is confusion.

The goal of interactions between the sonographer and the patient is to reduce the patient's anxiety and promote fetal attachment. It can be assumed that pointing out fetal anatomy and allowing the mother to watch the fetus move enhance attachment. Connecting the image to the patient's body by pointing out where the fetus is enhances bonding to the fetus as part of oneself. Spending additional time to visualize the face and holding the transducer in one place to watch the fetus yawn, suck, or shift positions may be a very memorable experience for the mother. Linda Carter-Jessop has suggested teaching mothers in late pregnancy to rub their baby's back, talk to it, and otherwise interact with it when it is active.[3] This is a strategy that sonographers could adopt as well.

The careless use of terminology (i.e., *breech,* the placenta is not *right,* checking for intrauterine growth *retardation*) may increase anxiety.[1] Similarly, other interactions that alarm or anger the mother may interfere with the attachment process during the examination. Lumley refers to feedback that includes inappropriate comments, incorrect or indefinite diagnoses, and language that is unfamiliar or alarming to the parents as the "diagnostic toxicity" of ultrasound.[25] If only a small percentage of women experience this type of communication, the large numbers of women receiving ultrasound means that the numbers of women subject to "diagnostic toxicity" may be a major problem. It is essential that anxiety-provoking comments be carefully avoided during obstetric examinations.

COMMUNICATION BASICS

It is generally agreed that the approach of the sonographer working with obstetric patients at any stage of pregnancy should include but not necessarily be limited to the following:

- Prior maternal knowledge of and consent to the presence of nonessential personnel, whose number is kept to a minimum

- An intent to share with parents, either during an examination or shortly thereafter, the information derived

- An offer of choice about viewing the fetus

- An offer of choice about learning the sex of the fetus if such information becomes available.[5]

Additional guidelines first suggested in *Medical Ultrasound*[21] and subsequently modified are listed in Display 32-1. The International Childbirth Education Association, in a position paper on diagnostic ultrasound, discusses "family-centered aspects" of ultrasound examinations and includes several suggestions for sonographer communication with the patient.[17]

Display 32-1 Communication Guidelines for Obstetric Ultrasonography

Dos

Do try to maintain an easy flow of conversation throughout the examination.

Do encourage the patient to talk.

Do ask for the patient's version of the referral reason. This will give them the security of knowing that you are addressing their perceived need.

Do point out normal anatomy when asked.

Do discuss or clarify information that the patient has already been given by the physician.

Do be firm about information you will and will not discuss.

Do know laboratory guidelines relative to revealing obvious diagnoses.

Do be supportive and honest about invasive procedures.

Do strive to maintain a positive attitude. Since we do not know for certain the outcome during any examination, we should strive to think positively in order not to alarm the patient.

Don'ts

Don't be falsely reassuring.

Don't compare physicians or recommend other procedures.

Don't discuss the diagnosis of the current examination.

Don't play dumb.

Don't express negative feelings about your ability, your job, or your day.

Don't talk about other patients or other staff members.

Don't be afraid to touch the patient.

In an article on legal malpractice risks in radiology,[8] Dr. Edward Bartlett, president of a consulting firm that specializes in finding communications solutions to the problem of malpractice risk, contends that most malpractice suits can be attributed to lack of communication, and are thus preventable. "We have to look at that 79% of cases filed that were the result of temporary, emotional and minor injuries and ask why people go to the bother of filing that claim when the chances are they won't recover a penny through the litigation process." Anger resulting from misconceptions about what the procedure will yield or what it entails may prompt many malpractice claims, Bartlett suggests. Similarly, if a patient is frustrated with one aspect of care and there is a negative outcome, the patient may blame the outcome on those who frustrated her.

Communication important to legally safeguarding sonographers is communication that facilitates the following ends:

- The patient leaves feeling that she has been treated in a competent, professional, and empathetic manner.

- The patient is not surprised by any aspect of the ultrasound procedures, the sonographer's care, or the possible outcomes.

- Pertinent patient communications shared with the sonographer are in turn shared with those on the medical team responsible for acting on that information.

ABNORMAL PREGNANCIES, ADOPTIONS, AND TERMINATIONS

Specific guidelines for communication during examinations involving abnormal fetuses have not been developed. The guidelines discussed earlier relate to these examinations as well, however, and during the initial examination it is important for the sonographer to be firm about information that can and cannot be discussed without "playing dumb" or sowing doubts about his or her skill or the care the patient is receiving. A child who spends a lot of time in the hospital, who is handicapped, or who has special needs is a child at greater risk for neglect and abuse than are more typical children.[15] Once the mother has been informed of the diagnosis, bonding activities during the examination may be more important than usual. In follow-up examinations, as in all examinations, it is important to ask the mother whether she wants to see the screen and to follow the mother's lead in determining how much information she is ready to accept. In general, parents preparing for the birth of an abnormal child need every opportunity to acknowledge and accept that child. Unless the abnormality is unequivocally lethal, the sonographer should not hesitate to point out portions of the baby if the mother seems interested and has been given basic information about the diagnosis. Allowing the mother to observe any normal activities of the baby may help her attach and better prepare her for the challenges she and the family will face after the birth.

Sonographers should ask each pregnant patient whether she wishes to see the screen before beginning the ultrasound examination. This is particularly important in situations in which the mother is giving up the child for adoption, a termination is planned, or a lethal anomaly is present. If the mother indicates that she wants to see the screen, the sonographer should allow her to do so and should answer any questions that arise during the examination and that fall within these guidelines. Spending time on bonding activities, unless this is specifically requested by the mother, is inappropriate.

The evidence of prenatal bonding mandates continued development by sonographers of appropriate, realistic, and efficient communication during all obstetric examinations. Sonographers' interactions with pregnant patients are as varied as the individuals involved, and often challenge the best instincts. Studying and optimizing the value of their communication and creating additional guidelines for patients who face adoptions, terminations, or abnormalities is an important role for obstetric sonographers.

Future Research

There is no evidence that the transient impact on the mother of the obstetric ultrasound examination relates to long-term beneficial effects. There may be negative psychological effects of ultrasound imaging in abnormal pregnancies or in mothers before termination of pregnancy. The present state of knowledge in these and other areas is largely speculative or anecdotal. Sonographers are in an optimal position to study prenatal bonding. Some of the questions that need to be answered are presented in the NIH Consensus Conference monograph[5]:

- Are there incidences of deleterious effects of ultrasound imagery on maternal perception of the fetus?

- Can ultrasound imaging produce a positive effect on patients who are highly anxious prenatally?

- Would a positive effect on anxiety have clinical significance as measured by pregnancy outcome and child development?

- How many women are receiving prenatal gender information through ultrasound imagery?

- Does prenatal knowledge of fetal gender affect prenatal attachment or anxiety?

- What is the appropriate role of sonography personnel in relation to patients' image perceptions?

- Is attachment of the mother to the fetus enhanced by ultrasound imagery?

- If enhancement occurs, should it be encouraged in special situations such as high-risk pregnancies, terminations, or adoption?

The answers to these questions and others may be learned by careful observation and inquiry by sonographers.

Sonographers and consumers have long been aware that ultrasound imaging is not just another diagnostic tool used in pregnancy. The social and psychological ramifications of ultrasound imaging are enormous. The potential for its therapeutic use in stimulating bonding is largely unexplored. The possibility that sonographers may be able to use instruments not only to diagnose but to help mothers with a poor bonding history, teenagers who deny the reality of pregnancy, and others, carries with it an awesome responsibility to observe, to study, and to learn more about these complex interactions.

REFERENCES

1. Boyce K. Patients' reactions to medical terminology. Student research paper. University of Oklahoma, Department of Radiologic Technology, Norman, Oklahoma; 1983.

2. Caccia N, Johnson JM, Robinson GE, Barna T. Impact of prenatal testing on maternal–fetal bonding:

Chorionic villus sampling versus amniocentesis. Am J Obstet Gynecol. 1991; 165:1122–1125.

3. Carter-Jessop L. Promoting maternal attachment through prenatal intervention. Maternal Child Nurs J. 1981; 6:107–112.

4. Clark ME. The relationship between ultrasonic imaging and maternal–fetal attachment. Unpublished masters thesis. The University of Oklahoma Health Sciences Center Graduate College, Norman, Oklahoma; 1990.

5. Consensus Development Conference. The Use of Diagnostic Ultrasound Imaging in Pregnancy. NIH Publication No. 84-667. Washington, DC: U.S. Government Printing Office; 1984; 173–174.

6. Cox DN, Witman BK, Hess M, Ross AG, Lindah S. The psychological impact of diagnostic ultrasound. Obstet Gynecol. 1987; 70:673–676.

7. Cranley M. Development of a tool for the measurement of maternal attachment during pregnancy. Nurs Res. 1985; 30:281–284.

8. Dakins D. Radiologists at greater legal risk as role in patient care expands. Diagnostic Imaging. 1987; 9:8.75–83.

9. Gaffney KF. Prenatal maternal attachment. Image. 1988; 20:106–109.

10. Geisler D. The effects of ultrasound examinations on maternal–infant bonding. Student research paper. State University of New York Health Science Center at Brooklyn, Department of Radiologic Sciences and Technology, Brooklyn, New York; 1987.

11. Grace JT. Does a mother's knowledge of fetal gender affect attachment? Maternal Child Nurs J. 1985; 9:42–45.

12. Grace JT. Prenatal ultrasound examinations and mother–infant bonding [letter]. N Engl J Med. 1983; 309:561.

13. Heidrich SM, Cranley MS. Effect of fetal movement, ultrasound scans, and amniocentesis on maternal–fetal attachment. Nurs Res. 1989; 38:81–84.

14. Holland M. Evidence of bonding between a mother and fetus during an ultrasound examination. Student research paper. University of Oklahoma, Department of Radiologic Technology, Norman, Oklahoma; 1988.

15. Hunner R. Child abuse and the special-needs child. Presented at the 7th National Conference on Child Abuse and Neglect, Chicago, Illinois; December 1985.

16. Hyde B. An interview study of pregnant women's attitudes to ultrasound scanning. Soc Sci Med. 1986; 22:S587–S592.

17. International Childbirth Education Association. Position Paper: Diagnostic Ultrasound in Obstetrics. ICEA News. 1983; 22:2.

18. Kemp VH, Page CK. Maternal prenatal attachment in normal and high-risk pregnancies. J Obstet Gynecol Neonatal Nurs. 1987; 116:179–184.

19. Klaus MH, Kennell JH. Maternal–Infant Bonding. St. Louis: CV Mosby; 1976; 3.

20. Kohn CL, Nelson A, Weiner S. Gravidas responses to real time ultrasound fetal image. JOGN Nursing. 1980; 9:77–80.

21. Lea JH. Educationally speaking: The value of role playing in sonography education. Medical Ultrasound. 1983; 7:81–82.

22. Lea JH. Psychosocial progression through normal pregnancy: A model for sonographer–patient interaction. J Diagn Med Sonogr. 1985; 1:2.

23. Lerum CW, LoBiondo-Wood G. The relationship of maternal age, quickening, and the physical symptoms of pregnancy to the development of maternal–fetal attachment. Birth. 1989; 16:13–17.

24. LoBiondo-Wood G. The progression of pregnancy symptoms in pregnancy and the development of maternal–fetal attachment. Dissertation Abstracts International, 46, 2625-B. New York: New York University; 1985.

25. Lumley J. Through a glass darkly: Ultrasound and prenatal bonding. Birth. 1990; 17:214–217.

26. Milne LS, Rich OJ. Cognitive and affective aspects of the responses of pregnant women to sonography. Maternal Child Nurs J. 1981; 10:15–39.

27. Rapp R. Real-time is prime time: The role of the sonographer in the age of mechanical reproduction. Presented at the American Anthropological Association Annual Meeting, Washington, DC, November 17–21, 1993.

28. Reading AE, Cox DN. The effects of ultrasound examination on maternal anxiety levels. J Behav Med. 1982; 5:237–247.

29. Reading AE, Cox DN. Psychological changes over the course of pregnancy: A study of attitudes toward the fetus/neonate. Health Psychol. 1984; 3:211–221.

30. Reading AE, Cambell S, Cox D, et al. Health beliefs and health care behavior in pregnancy. Psychol Med. 1982; 12:379–383.

31. Sandelowski M. Separate but less unequal: Fetal ultrasonography and the transformation of expectant mother/fatherhood." Gender and Society. 1994; 8:230–245.

32. Taylor JS. The public fetus and the family car: From abortion politics to a Volvo advertisement. Public Culture. 1992; 4(2):67–80.

33. Vito KO. The development of maternal–fetal attachment and the association of selected variables. Dissertation Abstracts International, 47, 998-B. Washington, DC: The Catholic University of America; 1986.

34. Waldenstrom U, Axelsson O, Nilsson S, et al. Effects of routine one-stage ultrasound screening in pregnancy: A randomized controlled trial. Lancet. 1988; 2:585–588.

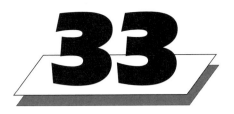

Statistical Methods in Obstetric Ultrasound

HARRY J. KHAMIS and ROGER W. WARNER

The methods of applied statistics can be used effectively and clearly to formulate and solve important problems in obstetric ultrasonography. Specifically, statistical principles are used to formulate proper experimental designs and sampling techniques and to analyze and interpret the resulting data. This chapter discusses basic statistical concepts and terminology as well as many of the common techniques used in obstetric ultrasonography.

The need for statistical techniques in analyzing ultrasonographic data (or, for that matter, any other kind of data) arises from the basic inherent variability in the data; specifically, variation among the individuals being measured. For instance, if an investigator using real-time sonography takes fetal abdominal circumference measurements on several fetuses, it is unlikely that all of the measurements will be identical. The variation observed in such measurements results from the natural differences among the fetuses. If more than one investigator takes the measurements, then additional variation will be observed in the data (interobserver variability[12]). It is the purpose of applied statistics to take this variation into account or to assess the reliability of the measurements, to facilitate description, analysis, and interpretation of the data.

A measure or test that is consistent from one use to the next is said to have high *reliability*. So,

if a method to measure head circumference is applied to the same infant repeatedly, the method is reliable (although not necessarily accurate) if the same, or nearly the same, value is observed each time. The *validity* of a measure or test refers to its ability to measure accurately what is intended. For example, an instrument that is not adjusted properly provides invalid data. Therefore, measures that have high reliability are free of random error, whereas measures that have high validity are free of systematic error. Finally, *integrity* of the measurements concerns the accuracy with which the measurements are recorded and used in analyses. When measurements are incorrectly coded or entered, the integrity of those measurements is undermined.

In statistical terms, the set of measurements (from a group of subjects) that characterizes a phenomenon under study is called a *population,* and a *sample* is some subset of the population. It is of paramount importance in ultrasound studies to define the population of interest, the sample that is obtained, the method of data collection, and the kinds of statistical analyses used to make inferences from the sample to the population. A sample should represent the population that is to be studied. If the sample consists of randomly selected measurements from the population of interest (random sampling), then the sample is said to be *representative* of the population; otherwise the sample is *biased*. For instance, if the study population is the set of all second trimester femur lengths (FLs) of fetuses measured in the last 2 years at Hospital X, a random sample (using a random number table or a random number generator on a computer) of case records containing such measurements obtained from Hospital X would be considered to be representative of the study population. If the study population is the set of all second trimester FLs of fetuses measured in the last 2 years at all hospitals in the country, then the sample from Hospital X would not be considered representative of the study population unless Hospital X does not differ substantively from other hospitals in the country with regard to any parameters that influence FL.

In addition to defining the sample and how it was obtained, the investigator must describe the measurement procedure fully. There is great potential in any study for the validity, reliability, and integrity of the measurements to be compromised. Such compromise can be caused by an error on the part of the investigator or inexperience of the investigator with the measuring instrument, or by a measuring instrument that is not adjusted properly. A high degree of quality control must be maintained with regard to the measurements that are recorded, because the entire quantitative approach is based on these measurements (garbage in, garbage out!).

In general, two different kinds of measurements can be observed, those that are *discrete* and those that are *continuous*. Discrete measurements correspond to values that are finite in number or that can be counted. Examples of discrete measurements are sex of the fetus (M, F), disease state (mild, intermediate, severe), and number of fetuses (1, 2, 3, 4, . . .). Such data are referred to as discrete data. Continuous measurements correspond to values that come from a continuum on the real number line. Examples of continuous measurements are fetal blood flow velocity in centimeters per second, biparietal diameter of a fetal head in centimeters, and age of the fetus in weeks. These kinds of data are referred to as continuous data. Different statistical techniques are used to describe and analyze data generated by these two different kinds of measurements.

Typically, the first thing that an investigator

wishes to do on obtaining the sample data is to summarize the findings in an efficient and useful manner. Second, the investigator may wish to make inferences about the study population based on the sample, such as prediction, estimation, and answering research questions about population characteristics. *Descriptive statistics* is that branch of statistics that deals with the description and summarization of data. Some techniques in descriptive statistics applied to ultrasonographic data are given in the next section of this chapter. *Inferential statistics* is the area of statistics that deals with making an inference or generalization about the study population based on information contained in a sample.

Descriptive Statistical Techniques in Medical Sonography

In general, there are two different but related ways in which data can be summarized and described effectively. One is to use *graphic techniques* for data description; the other is to use *numeric measures* of important characteristics of the data. The use of graphic techniques for describing data is particularly effective: it provides a visual presentation of important characteristics of the data, and typically the techniques are very simple.

BAR GRAPH

Suppose a set of discrete data is to be summarized graphically. A bar graph is constructed as follows: list the values of the discrete measurement on a horizontal axis, and for each of these values draw a rectangle whose height is equal to the frequency with which that value is observed in the data set. An example should clarify the technique.

> *Example 1.* A sample of 85 pregnant women is taken, 15 of whom are younger than 20 years of age, 50 are between 20 and 30 years of age, and 20 are older than 30 years of age. The bar graph of this discretized age variable is in Figure 33-1.

Note that in the use of the bar graph, the vertical axis can designate the relative frequency, or percentage of the sample, that corresponds to each value on the horizontal axis (e.g., in Example 1, 17.7% of the women in the sample are younger than 20 years of age, 58.8% are between 20 and 30

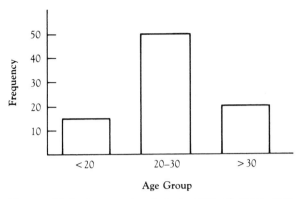

Figure 33-1. Bar graph of frequency of three age groups.

years of age, and 23.5% are older than 30 years of age.

PLOTTING DATA

To investigate the relationship between two continuous variables, it is useful to plot the paired observations on the x-y coordinate axis system. Consider the following example:

> *Example 2.* A longitudinal study was made of the ascending aortic cross-sectional area (A_{A_0}) in 31 healthy infants from birth through the first year of life using M-mode echocardiography. The data, which appear in an article by Alverson and coworkers,[1] are plotted in Figure 33-2.

From this plot, it is easy to see that the average A_{A_0} increases with age in a nearly linear fashion, because the points fall approximately along a straight line. Such a relationship is referred to as a simple linear regression (see later).

Many other graphic techniques are used to summarize and describe data, including pie charts, box-plots, and histograms (see, for example, the text by McClave and Dietrich[9]).

In addition to depicting graphically important features of the data, certain key characteristics can be determined through numeric measures. Two particularly important characteristics of any set of numerical data are its *central tendency* and its *variability*.

MEASURES OF CENTRAL TENDENCY

The central tendency of a set of measurements is the value around which the measurements tend to cluster or tend to be centered. The most common

measure of central tendency is the mean. The *mean* of the sample, denoted by $\bar{x}$, is defined as the sum of the measurements divided by the number of measurements. Notationally, we write $\bar{x} = \Sigma x/n$, where n represents the sample size, and Σx represents the sum of the measurements in the sample.

> *Example 3.* Consider the following set of measurements: 8, 12, 7, 10, 8, 6, 10, 8, 5, 9. The mean of this sample is computed as follows: $\Sigma x = 8 + 12 + 7 + 10 + 8 + 6 + 10 + 8 + 5 + 9 = 83$, and $n = 10$; so $\bar{x} = \Sigma x/n = 83/10 = 8.3$.

Another measure of central tendency is the median. The *median* of a sample of size n is obtained by first listing the measurements from smallest to largest. If n is an odd number, the median is defined as the middle measurement from this ordered list of measurements. If n is an even number, then the median is defined as the midpoint (or average) of the middle two measurements from the list.

> *Example 4.* For the sample given in Example 3, the ordered list of measurements is: 5, 6, 7, 8, 8, 8, 9, 10, 10, 12. Because $n = 10$, the median of this sample is the average of the middle two measurements: median $= (^1/_2) (8 + 8) = 8$.

MEASURES OF VARIABILITY

The *variability* of a set of measurements refers to how closely the measurements cluster about the central location, or, alternatively, how spread out the measurements are. One very simple measure of variability is the range. The *range* of a sample is defined as the difference between the largest measurement and the smallest measurement.

> *Example 5.* Consider the following sample: 3, 4, 2, 5, 1, 2. The range of this sample is $5 - 1 = 4$. One might also say that these data range from 1 to 5.

Intuitively, the range is a reasonable measure of variability: the more spread out the measurements in a sample are, the larger the range will be. However, two very different data sets can give rise to the same range. For instance, the following two samples have the same range (49): sample 1: 1, 1, 1, 1, 50; sample 2: 1, 10, 25, 35, 50.

A measure of variability that is sensitive to distinctions of this kind is the *variance*. The variance of a sample, denoted by S^2, measures the average squared distance between the measurements and $\bar{x}$.

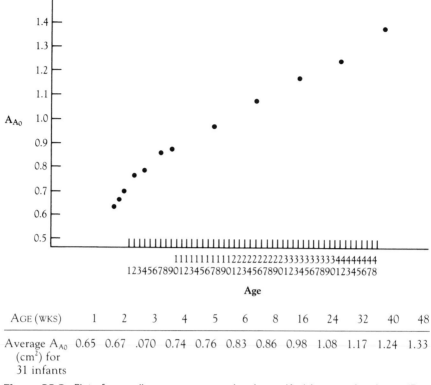

AGE (WKS)	1	2	3	4	5	6	8	16	24	32	40	48
Average A_{A_0} (cm²) for 31 infants	0.65	0.67	.070	0.74	0.76	0.83	0.86	0.98	1.08	1.17	1.24	1.33

Figure 33-2. Plot of ascending aorta cross-sectional area (A_{A_0}) by gestational age. (Data from Alverson, DC, Aldrich M, Angelus P, et al. Longitudinal trends in left ventricular cardiac output in healthy infants in the first year of life. J Ultrasound Med. 1987; 6:519–524.)

The formula for S^2 is: $S^2 = [n\Sigma x^2 - (\Sigma x)^2]/n(n-1)$, where n is the sample size, Σx the sum of the measurements in the sample, and Σx^2 the sum of the squares of the measurements. For sample 1 earlier, $S^2 = 480.2$, and for sample 2, $S^2 = 380.7$; so the variance of sample 1 is greater (the measurements are more dispersed) than the variance of sample 2.

Example 6. For the sample of Example 5, $n = 6$, $\Sigma x = 3 + 4 + 2 + 5 + 1 + 2 = 17$ and $\Sigma x^2 = 9 + 16 + 4 + 25 + 1 + 4 = 59$. So, $S^2 = [6 \cdot 59 - (17)^2]/6 \cdot 5 = (354 - 289)/30 = 2.167$.

Although the variance is more complicated to compute than the range, it is the most common measure of variability used in data description. Note, however, that the variance is expressed in terms of squared units. For instance, if the units of measurement are centimeters, then S^2 is expressed in square centimeters. To have a measure of variability that is in the same units as the original measurements, the *standard deviation* (SD) is used.

The standard deviation of a sample is denoted by S and is defined as the positive square root of S^2; $S = \sqrt{S^2}$. For the data given in Example 5, the SD is $S = \sqrt{2.167} = 1.472$.

Example 7. Sonographic studies were performed on a random sample of 50 normal pregnant women whose fetuses' gestational ages ranged from 30 to 40 weeks. For each fetus the transverse cerebellar diameter was obtained. Suppose the diameters (in millimeters) are as follows: 44.4, 41.7, 41.4, 47.4, 42.0, 41.5, 39.5, 42.6, 36.8, 40.7, 36.8, 39.4, 41.2, 40.3, 45.1, 37.5, 43.4, 44.8, 38.5, 41.9, 43.2, 45.6, 35.4, 41.4, 42.4, 39.7, 37.3, 39.0, 40.3, 42.5, 40.2, 39.8, 36.4, 43.3, 39.4, 45.7, 38.7, 34.3, 38.8, 40.5, 38.2, 37.4, 38.4, 39.4, 44.5, 46.1, 40.5, 40.4, 42.3, 43.1.

For these data, we have $n = 50$, $\Sigma x = 2,041.2$, and $\Sigma x^2 = 83,746.84$. Then, $\bar{x} = \Sigma x/n = 40.824$. From the ordered data values, it is easy to count up to the 25th and 26th measurements (the middle two measurements); they are 40.5 and 40.5. The median is the average of these two values, 40.5. The variance is $S^2 = [50 \cdot (83,746.84) - (2,041.2)2]/50 \cdot 49$

= 8.508, and the SD is $S = 2.917$. The range is $47.4 - 34.3 = 13.1$.

INTERPRETATION OF THE STANDARD DEVIATION

A set of data is said to have a *bell-shaped* or *normal* distribution if the mean is approximately the same as the median (so that the measurements are symmetric about the mean) and the measurements tend to cluster around the mean while becoming less and less frequent farther from the mean. The distribution of many measurements used in sonographic studies is bell shaped. In fact, many different kinds of data sets from all disciplines take on bell-shaped distributions; that is, most of the measurements tend to be close to the mean (95% within 2 SDs of the mean), with few that are distant from the mean (only 5% that are more than 2 SDs away). This is why a laboratory test result is often classified as normal when it falls within 2 SDs of the mean and abnormal when it falls outside this range. Note here that we measure distance in terms of SD units.

It will be shown that the data in Example 7 are bell shaped. The mean and SD have been computed to be $\bar{x} = 40.824$ and $S = 2.917$, respectively (note that the mean is very close to the median, 40.5). Therefore, $(\bar{x} - S, \bar{x} + S) = (37.91, 43.74)$, $\bar{x} - 2S, \bar{x} + 2S) = (34.99, 46.66)$, and $(\bar{x} - 3S, \bar{x} + 3S) = (32.07, 49.58)$. Now, referring to the data in Example 7, we can determine that 34 of the 50 measurements, or 68%, fall between $\bar{x} - S$ and $\bar{x} + S$; 48 of the 50 measurements, or 96%, fall between $\bar{x} - 2S$ and $\bar{x} + 2S$; and all 50 of the measurements, or 100%, fall between $\bar{x} - 3S$ and $\bar{x} + 3S$.

These conclusions illustrate criteria for interpreting a standard deviation for bell-shaped data. For such data sets, the *empirical rule* provides criteria for interpreting the standard deviation, *S:*

1. About 68% of the measurements fall between $\bar{x} - S$ and $\bar{x} + S$
2. About 95% of the measurements fall between $\bar{x} - 2S$ and $\bar{x} + 2S$
3. Almost 100% of the measurements fall between $\bar{x} - 3S$ and $\bar{x} + 3S$

Note that the data set in Example 7 follows the empirical rule very closely, the 1-, 2-, and 3-SD percentages being 68%, 96%, and 100%, respectively.

It is usually desirable to have a small SD for a given set of data because then the interval from $\bar{x} - 2S$ to $\bar{x} + 2S$, where about 95% of the measurements are located (by the empirical rule), is small. Consequently, most of the measurements would be very close to the mean, $\bar{x}$. In this sense, such measurements would be considered to be of *low variability;* that is, the measurements would be considered to be *reliable*.

MEASURES OF RELATIVE STANDING

The researcher is often interested in where a particular measurement falls in a given data set in relation to the other measurements. Is it the largest measurement? Is it the smallest measurement? Is it close to the largest or close to the smallest? One way to measure the *relative standing* of a measurement is to count the number of measurements in the data set that are smaller than that measurement. That number of measurements, expressed as a percentage of the total number of measurements in the data set, is referred to as the *percentile ranking* of the measurement of interest. For instance, in the data set presented in Example 7, the 10th percentile is 37.3 because 5 of the 50 measurements, or 10% of the measurements, are smaller than 37.3. The measurement 46.1 is the 96th percentile because 48 of the 50 measurements, or 96% of the measurements, are smaller than 46.1. Percentile rankings are of practical value only for large data sets. Note that the median is, by definition, the 50th percentile, because half, or 50%, of the measurements are smaller than the median. When using charts, one of the considerations sonographers should keep in mind is the percentile in which the fetus' measurement falls; this is especially true of fetal weight.

Another measure of relative standing is the z score: the z score for a measurement x is $z = (x - \bar{x})/\text{SD}$. That is, z measures the distance that x lies from the mean in terms of SD units. For the data in Example 7, the z score for 40.3 is $z = (40.3 - 40.824)/2.917 = -0.18$; so, 40.3 lies 0.18 SDs below the mean.

SLOPE AND CORRELATION

There are two numeric measures, the slope and the correlation coefficient, that are useful in helping to describe the linear relationship between two continuous variables, say x and y. To provide the formulas for these measures, some notation must be established that will make the formulas easier to write.

Let $S_{xx} = \Sigma x^2 - \frac{1}{n} (\Sigma x)^2$, $S_{yy} = \Sigma y^2 - \frac{1}{n} (\Sigma y)^2$, and $S_{xy} = \Sigma xy - \frac{1}{n} (\Sigma x)(\Sigma y)$, where Σxy represents the sum of the products of the x measurements and the y measurements.

> *Example 8.* Consider the following sample of (x,y) values: $(1, 2)$, $(1, 1)$, $(3, 2)$, $(2, 2)$, $(2, 4)$.
>
> Then, with $n = 5$, we have $S_{xx} = 19 - (9)^2/5 = 2.8$, $S_{yy} = 29 - (11)^2/5 = 4.8$, and $S_{xy} = 21 - (9)(11)/5 = 1.2$. The *slope* for a sample of (x,y) measurements represents the change in the y measurement that corresponds to a 1-unit increase in the x measurement. The *slope* is denoted by b, $b = S_{xy}/S_{xx}$. If b is negative, then y decreases as x increases; if b is positive, then y increases as x increases. If b is 0, then y remains constant for all values of x. For the sample in Example 8, $b = 1.2/2.8 = 0.429$. This means that, on average, for every unit increase in x, y *increases* by 0.429.

The *correlation coefficient* is a measure of the strength of the linear relationship between the x measurements and the y measurements. The correlation coefficient is denoted by r, and $r = S_{xy}/S_{xx} \cdot S_{yy}$. It can be proven that r always lies between -1 and $+1$. If r is positive, then the y measurements tend to increase as the x measurements increase; if r is negative, the y measurements tend to decrease as the x measurements increase. If r is 0, then the x measurements and y measurements are not linearly related. For the data given in Example 8, $r = 1.2/(2.8)(4.8) = 0.327$, indicating that y increases as x increases in this sample. Because $r = 0.327$ is not very close to -1 or $+1$, this correlation is not considered to be strong.

In Example 2, the correlation coefficient $r = 0.982$ indicates a very strong, positive linear relationship between age and ascending aortic cross-sectional area (A_{A_0}). The plot in Figure 33-2 confirms these conclusions: the dots tend to increase at the rate of 0.0142 cm² per week $(b = 0.0142)$, and the dots fall very nearly along a straight line rising from left to right $(r = 0.982)$.

It is important to emphasize that no causal relationships can be inferred from the value of b or r. So, although a value of r close to 1 or close to -1 establishes a linear relationship between x and y, it provides no information about the reason for that linear relationship, in particular, whether it is causal

or not. For instance, it may be that x and y are highly correlated but that both are influenced by a third intervening variable.

Consider as an example the high positive correlation between blood pressure and cholesterol in a random sample of men ranging in age from 18 to 72 years. It would be incorrect to conclude that high blood pressure causes cholesterol (or vice versa) based on this correlation because both blood pressure and cholesterol increase with age. So, in this case age is the intervening variable that is correlated with both of the study variables.

SUMMARY TABLES

When presenting the descriptive statistics of a study, it is important to include all pertinent information in an effective format. For a discrete measurement, a bar graph is useful for visual purposes, and the frequencies and relative frequencies, or percentages, should be given for each level of the measurement (frequency table). For continuous measurements, sample means are usually recorded. Some investigators display $\bar{x} \pm 2S$, because this interval contains about 95% of all of the measurements in the sample, and so represents the interval within which "normal" values fall.

When the mean and median for a given set of data are about equal, then the distribution for those data is said to be *symmetric*. For instance, in the data of Example 7, $\bar{x} = 40.824$ and median $= 40.5$. However, for data having an *asymmetric* distribution, these measures of central tendency differ. In these cases, it is important that both the mean and the median be presented. The more asymmetric the distribution is, the farther apart the mean and median will be.

Finally, when discussing the linear relationship between two continuous variables, plots of the type given in Figure 33-2 are useful, as well as the slope (b) and the correlation coefficient (r).

Testing in Medical Sonography

In addition to summarizing and describing experimental data in ultrasound studies, the researcher typically wishes to make inferences about the study population based on information contained in a random sample from the population. Such inferences can be made by testing research hypotheses.

TESTING

Very often in a research paper, especially one involving the collection and analysis of data, a certain amount of statistical jargon and notation arises with respect to testing research hypotheses, and a familiarity with statistical concepts is helpful for fully understanding the research being presented. For instance, phrases such as the following are very often encountered: "significantly higher," "velocity did not change significantly," "a linear increase in the blood flow amount," "did not reach statistical significance at 0.05," and "$0.05 < P < 0.1$." This section provides an intuitive understanding of the concept of significance testing and how it is used in research articles.

Certain elements occur in every statistical testing problem. They constitute a *five-step procedure for a test of hypothesis.*

1. The researcher begins by setting up two hypotheses, the *null* and the *alternative* hypotheses, keeping in mind that the data will be analyzed to determine how strongly they contradict the null hypothesis. Typically, the null hypothesis is the hypothesis of no change or status quo and the alternative hypothesis is the hypothesis of change. For instance, a researcher may be interested in knowing whether the average umbilical vein blood flow velocity is the same for women in the 33rd week of pregnancy as for women in the 39th week of pregnancy. The null hypothesis would be that the average blood flow velocity is the same for both groups of women; the alternative hypothesis would state that the average blood flow velocity differs between the two groups of women. Then the data would be collected and analyzed to determine how strongly they contradict the null hypothesis and support the alternative hypothesis.

2. The investigator must decide how strongly the data should contradict the null hypothesis before he or she concludes that the null hypothesis is indeed false. This decision is made by choosing a *level of significance* for the test, namely, the probability that the null hypothesis will be rejected erroneously. The level of significance most commonly used in ultrasonographic studies is 0.05. So with a 0.05 level of significance in the test for deciding whether the null hypothesis is false, there will be only a 5% chance of rejecting a true null hypothesis.

To decide whether the null hypothesis is false, a measure called the P value is compared to the level of significance. The P value is calculated from the data and is a measure of how strongly the data contradict the null hypothesis (or, equivalently, how strongly the data support the alternative hypothesis); the smaller the P value, the more the data contradict the null hypothesis. So, the null hypothesis is rejected when the P value is small; otherwise, the null hypothesis is not rejected. Specifically, the null hypothesis is rejected when the P value is smaller than the chosen level of significance (e.g., 0.05).

3. The data are collected. Again, the sample must be representative of the population being studied.

4. The P value that corresponds to the data is calculated. Computation of the P value is based on mathematical properties of the measurement representing the characteristic being studied and the kind of statistical test being conducted. In general, the z test is used to make inferences about proportions, the t test is used to make inferences about means, and the chi-squared test is used to make inferences involving discrete variables. Most statistical software programs provide the P value automatically.

5. Compare the P value to 0.05 (or whatever level of significance was chosen in step 2); if it is smaller, reject the null hypothesis, and if it is larger, do not reject the null hypothesis.

This five-step procedure can be generalized to handle an enormous variety of statistical testing problems, and for each one the P *value is the measure of the extent to which the null hypothesis is contradicted by the data.* A few of the more common test hypotheses are presented in the following sections.

Proportion

In the 1986 Society of Diagnostic Medical Sonographers Professional Profile Survey, Khamis and Warner[8] report that 377 of the 2479 respondents had a bachelor's degree or higher education. Assuming that the 2479 respondents form a representative sample of all U.S. sonographers, suppose we are interested in knowing if more than, say, 13% of all U.S. sonographers have a bachelor's degree or higher education (this may represent a goal of the professional society, for example). To address this question, set up the null hypothesis as the claim that 13% or less of all U.S. sonographers have a bachelor's degree or higher education, and the alternative hypothesis as the claim that over 13% of U.S. sonographers have a bachelor's degree or higher education. Then, the *P* value corresponding to the sample proportion observed above, 377/ 2479 = 15.2%, is *P* = 0.0011 (this value is obtained from a table or a computer software program). The test used to obtain this *P* value is the *z* test. More specifically, it is called an *upper-tail z* test because the alternative hypothesis specifies that the proportion under study exceeds 13%.

Because the computed *P* value is smaller than 0.05, our level of significance, we would reject the null hypothesis and conclude that over 13% of all U.S. sonographers have a bachelor's degree or higher education. That is, the extent to which the sample proportion, 15.2%, exceeds the hypothesized proportion, 13%, is more than can be attributed to chance alone.

Mean

It is often of interest to test hypotheses concerning the mean of a population. Suppose we hypothesize that the mean velocity of umbilical venous blood flow for pregnant women in their 33rd week is 15 cm/sec, and a random sample of 30 normal pregnant women rendered a sample mean velocity of 13.9 cm/sec, as reported by Chen's group.[2]

In this problem, the null hypothesis is that the mean velocity of umbilical venous blood flow for pregnant women in their 33rd week is 15 cm/sec. The alternative hypothesis is that it is different from 15 cm/sec. Suppose the level of significance is set at 0.05. Does the sample value of 13.9 cm/sec differ from 15 cm/sec enough to enable us to reject the null hypothesis? Based on the so-called *t* test, the *P* value corresponding to 13.9 cm/sec turns out to be *P* = 0.603. This test is referred to as a *two-tailed t* test, because the alternative hypothesis specifies that the true mean velocity is either larger or smaller than the hypothesized value of 15 cm/sec.

Because the *P* value exceeds 0.05, we conclude that the null hypothesis cannot be rejected. The reason that the null hypothesis cannot be rejected is that 13.9 cm/sec is not unusually far from 15

cm/sec, certainly not far enough away for us to doubt the null hypothesis.

Two Means

It is sometimes useful to compare two different means. For instance, suppose we wish to test the null hypothesis that the average umbilical venous blood flow velocity is the same for women in the 33rd week of pregnancy as for women in the 39th week. Suppose that a sample of 30 women in their 33rd week have an average velocity of 13.9 cm/sec and a sample of 26 women in their 39th week of pregnancy have an average velocity of 13.4 cm/ sec.[2] Do these two sample means differ enough to enable us to reject the null hypothesis? The *P* value associated with the difference between these two sample means is 0.772 (*two-sample* t *test*). This value far exceeds the 0.05 level of significance, so we fail to reject the null hypothesis and conclude that the average umbilical venous blood flow velocity does not differ significantly between the two groups of women.

These examples should help focus the logic behind the decision-making process involving a given parameter. Khamis[7] provides an easy-to-follow procedure for determining the most appropriate statistical method to use in analyzing the most common types of data structures.

Diagnostic Test Evaluation in Medical Sonography

An important consideration among investigators in ultrasound is the ability to assess the comparative usefulness of diagnostic techniques such as sonography, computed tomography, and magnetic resonance imaging. The following discussion focuses on how to determine the diagnostic and predictive value of tests that are designed to make such assessments.

Consider a new test designed to discriminate between people with a particular disease (or condition) and people who are disease free. Two traditional measures of the diagnostic value of such a test are the *sensitivity* and the *specificity*. The *sensitivity* of a test, or *true-positive ratio,* is defined to be the proportion of those having the disease whose test result is positive for it (i.e., for whom the test indicates presence of the disease). Hence, it is a

TABLE 33-1. A 2 × 2 TABLE OF THE GOLD STANDARD VERSUS THE ULTRASOUND EXAMINATION RESULT

Ultrasound Examination Result	Gold Standard		Total
	Diseased	**Disease Free**	
Positive	*a*	*b*	*a + b*
Negative	*c*	*d*	*c + d*
Total	*a + c*	*b + d*	*a + b + c + d*

a = Number of patients who are diseased and test positive, *b* = number of patients who are disease free and test positive, *c* = number of patients who are diseased and test negative, and *d* = number of patients who are disease free and test negative.

measure of how sensitive the test is in detecting the disease. Analogously, the *specificity* of a test, or *true-negative ratio,* is the proportion of people who do not have the disease whose test result is negative.

To quantify these two measures, suppose that it is possible to distinguish accurately between those who have the disease and those who do not have the disease (e.g., through surgery or autopsy). Call this the *gold standard.* Then a 2 × 2 table can be set up, as in Table 33-1.

Based on this table, simple formulas can be given for the sensitivity and specificity of the test:

$$\text{Sensitivity} = a/(a + c);$$

$$\text{Specificity} = d/(b + d)$$

The *prevalence rate* of the disease is defined as the proportion of people who have the disease:

$$\text{Prevalence rate} = (a + c)/(a + b + c + d)$$

Note that *a* and *d* correspond to the patients whose test result is correct, and that *b* and *c* correspond to those whose test result is incorrect. More specifically, positive results for people who are disease free (*b*) are called *false positives,* and negative results

for people who are diseased (*c*) are called *false negatives.* Note that an overall measure of the accuracy of the test is the proportion of correct results: $(a + d)/(a + b + c + d)$.

Consider Table 33-2. According to the previous formulas, we have:

$$\text{Sensitivity} = 600/750 = 80\%$$

$$\text{Specificity} = 675/750 = 90\%$$

$$\text{Prevalence rate} = 750/1500 = 50\%$$

$$\text{False positives} = 75$$

$$\text{False negatives} = 150$$

Interpretation

Eighty percent of diseased patients test positive and 90% of disease-free patients test negative. The prevalence rate of the disease is 50%. There are 225 people for whom the test is inaccurate: 75 false positives and 150 false negatives. A major advantage of sensitivity and specificity as measures of the diagnostic value of a test is that they are independent of the prevalence rate of the disease, so they can be

 TABLE 33-2. A 2 × 2 TABLE FOR A DISEASE WITH A 50% PREVALENCE RATE

Ultrasound Examination Result	Gold Standard		Total
	Diseased	**Disease Free**	
Positive	600	75	675
Negative	150	675	825
Total	750	750	1500

TABLE 33-3. A 2 × 2 TABLE FOR A DISEASE WITH 10% PREVALENCE RATE

Ultrasound Examination Result	Gold Standard		Total
	Diseased	Disease Free	
Positive	120	135	255
Negative	30	1215	1245
Total	150	1350	1500

used in cases involving a rare disease, that is, one that has a very low prevalence rate.

Now, suppose it is of interest to predict a person's disease status, given the test result. The two measures of particular interest to clinicians that are used for this purpose are the *positive predictive value (PPV)* of a test and the *negative predictive value (NPV)* of a test. The PPV is defined to be the proportion of those with a positive test result who are diseased, as determined by the gold standard. The NPV is defined to be the proportion of those with a negative test result who are disease free, as determined by the gold standard. From Table 33-1, we have:

$$PPV = a/(a + b); \quad NPV = d/(c + d)$$

Plugging in the values from Table 33-2, we have:

$$PPV = 600/675 = 88.9\%; \text{ and}$$
$$NPV = 675/825 = 81.8\%$$

Interpretation

A person whose test result is positive has an 88.9% chance of being diseased; a person whose test result is negative has an 81.8% chance of being disease free.

One drawback of these two predictive measures is that they are a function of the prevalence rate. So, if the prevalence rate in the previous example is 10% instead of 50% (perhaps a more realistic situation),

then the predictive values may be very different from the values found above. As an illustration, consider Table 33-3.

The data in Table 33-3 indicate that the sensitivity of the examination is 80% and the specificity 90%, exactly as in Table 33-2; however, the PPV is 47.1% and the NPV is 97.6%. Note that for a test with equal sensitivity and specificity, the reduction in the prevalence rate has the effect of reducing the PPV and increasing the NPV. That is, if fewer diseased people are tested, fewer diseased people will have a positive test result, so the PPV is lower. Likewise, if more disease-free people are tested, more disease-free people will have a negative result, so the NPV is higher.

Whereas the sensitivity and specificity are important indicators of the effectiveness of a diagnostic test, it is the PPV and NPV that are of primary interest to those in clinical obstetrics. They want to know what a given test result means for the patient.

Example 9. In a 1988 article, Townsend and colleagues[11] report on a retrospective review of initial sonograms performed on 65 twin gestations to evaluate the ability of sonography to distinguish monochorionic from dichorionic gestations based on the thickness of the membrane separating the fetuses. The results are shown in Table 33-4.

For this examination, the indicators of diagnostic accuracy are:

TABLE 33-4. DATA FOR EXAMPLE 9

Ultrasound Examination Result	Gold Standard		Total
	Two Chorions	One Chorion	
Thick membrane	39	8	47
Thin membrane	3	15	18
Total	42	23	65

$$\text{Sensitivity} = 39/42 = 93\%;$$

$$\text{Specificity} = 15/23 = 65\%$$

The predictive values are:

$$\text{PPV} = 39/47 = 83\%; \quad \text{NPV} = 15/18 = 83.3\%$$

The prevalence rate of two chorions is 42/65, or 64.6%. Hence, a thick membrane detected dichorio-

nic gestation with a sensitivity of 93%, and a thin membrane detected monochorionic gestation with a specificity of 65%. The PPV of a thick membrane for two chorions is 83%, and the NPV of a thin membrane for one chorion is 83.3%.

The association of two chorions with a thick membrane and of one chorion to a thin membrane was correct in 54 patients, for an accuracy of 54/

TABLE 33-5. GLOSSARY OF STATISTICAL TERMS

Term	Meaning
Alternative hypothesis	Also called research hypothesis: a claim indicating a change or difference, denoted by H_1 or H_A
Bar chart	A graphic way to depict frequency distributions of discrete variables
Bell-shaped data	Continuous measurements that cluster symmetrically about the mean and become less frequent as they become more distant from the mean
Continuous variable	A measure that assumes values from a continuum on the real number line
Correlation coefficient	A measure of the strength of the linear relationship between the x measurements and y measurements; falls between -1 and $+1$
Discrete variable	A measure whose levels are finite or can be counted
Frequency distribution	A tally of the frequency with which each measurement occurs in a set of measurements
Hypothesis test	A test procedure used to determine the exent to which data support a claim or hypothesis
Level of significance	The probability of rejecting a true null hypothesis in the hypothesis testing procedure; denoted by α
Mean	Central location of a set of numeric data; sometimes called the average
Median	That value in a data set for which half the measurements are higher and half are lower
Negative predictive value	The rate of true-negative results; calculated as the proportion of true-negative test results over all negative (true-negative and false-negative) test results
Normal values	Values that fall within two standard deviations of the mean
Null hypothesis	A claim, the accuracy of which is to be tested; typically involves a statement of "no change" or "status quo"; denoted by H_0
pth Percentile	That measurement for which p% of the measurements in the data set are smaller, where $0 \le p \le 100$
Population	The set of measurements obtained from all of the people or things that are under study; sometimes called the universe
Positive predictive value	The rate of true positive results; calculated as the proportion of true-positive test results over all positive (true-positive and false-positive) test results
P value	A measure of the extent to which the data in a hypothesis testing procedure contradict the null hypothesis; a small value of *P* (e.g., less than 0.05) leads to rejection of H_0
Range	The largest measurement minus the smallest measurement
Sample	A subset of a population
Scatterplot	A pattern of points that results from plotting two variables on the x-y coordinate axis system; each point represents one subject or unit of analysis
Sensitivity	Proportion of proven diseased individuals for whom the diagnostic test is positive
Slope	The change in the y measurement corresponding to a unit increase in the x measurement
Specificity	Proportion of proven disease-free individuals for whom the diagnostic test is negative
Standard deviation	The square root of the variance (see *Variance*)
Variance	A measure of the variability in a set of data; its formula is the sum of squared deviations between the measurements and the mean divided by one less than the sample size

65, or 83%. The conclusion of the article is that the appearance of the membrane can be useful in sonographic evaluation of chorionicity and amnionicity in twin gestations.

Further information on diagnostic test evaluation can be found in articles by Stempel[10] and Khamis.[4,6]

Conclusion

Often when data analyses are conducted, certain of the assumptions necessary for the testing procedures discussed previously are invalid. For instance, the sample size may be small ($n < 30$) or the sample mean may not be distributed normally. In these instances, so-called *nonparametric procedures* must be used to make inferences based on the sample data (see, for example, McClave and Dietrich,[9] Chapter 10).

One of the important considerations in planning any experiment involving statistical analysis of data is the sample size. The appropriate sample size for a given experiment depends on the hypotheses being tested, the kind of statistical test being applied, and the degree of accuracy required by the researcher, among other factors. In general, it is not appropriate to make an intuitive guess as to what the appropriate sample size should be. Further reading on sample size choice is available in Khamis.[5] For a more detailed presentation of statistical methods in obstetric sonography, see the text by Deter and colleagues.[3] Table 33-5 is a statistics glossary.

If researchers are uncertain about the statistical aspect of their study, they should consult a professional statistician.

REFERENCES

1. Alverson DC, Aldrich M, Angelus P, et al. Longitudinal trends in left ventricular cardiac output in healthy infants in the first year of life. J Ultrasound Med. 1987; 6:519–524.
2. Chen H-Y, Lu C-C, Cheng Y-T, et al. Antenatal measurement of fetal umbilical venous flow by pulsed Doppler and B-mode ultrasonography. J Ultrasound Med. 1986; 5:319–321.
3. Deter RL, Harrist RB, Birnholz JC, et al. Quantitative Obstetrical Ultrasonography. New York: John Wiley & Sons; 1986.
4. Khamis HJ. A statistics refresher: Tests of hypothesis and diagnostic test evaluation. J Diagn Med Sonogr. 1987; 3:123–129.
5. Khamis HJ. Statistics refresher: II. Choice of sample size. J Diagn Med Sonogr. 1988; 4:176–183.
6. Khamis HJ. An application of Bayes' Rule to diagnostic test evaluation. J Diagn Med Sonogr. 1990; 6:212–218.
7. Khamis HJ. Deciding on the correct statistical technique. J Diagn Med Sonogr. 1992; 193–198.
8. Khamis HJ, Warner RW. A discussion of the 1986 Society of Diagnostic Medical Sonographers professional profile survey: Part II. J Diagn Med Sonogr. 1986; 2:328–333.
9. McClave JT, Dietrich FH II. Statistics. 3rd ed. San Francisco: Dellen Publishing Company; 1985.
10. Stempel LE. Einie, meenie, minie, mo . . . What do the data really show? Am J Obstet Gynecol. 1982; 144:745–752.
11. Townsend RR, Simpson GF, Filly RA. Membrane thickness in ultrasound prediction of chorionicity of twin gestations. J Ultrasound Med. 1988; 7:327–332.
12. Zador IE, Sokol RJ, Chik L. Interobserver variability, a source of error in obstetric ultrasound. J Ultrasound Med. 1988; 7:245–249.

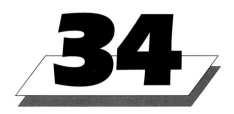

Ethical Issues in Obstetric Sonography

FRANK A. CHERVENAK and LAURENCE B. McCULLOUGH

Ethical issues frequently arise in the relationships of sonographers with their patients and with physicians who supervise them.[5] After a discussion of ethics in general, medical ethics, and obstetric ethics, this chapter examines four ethical issues in obstetric ultrasound examinations with special reference to the sonographer's role: competence to perform obstetric ultrasound and referral to specialists; routine screening; disclosure of results; and confidentiality.

The authors understand sonographers to be members of a not fully autonomous profession. There is no science of sonography independent of medical science. Therefore, sonographers have no method independent of medicine and physicians for establishing reliable diagnostic categories and nomenclature. Sonographers apply but do not originate the science of ultrasound imaging. This contrasts sharply with, for example, social workers, who have developed more autonomous diagnostic categories (e.g., the troubled family or the parent at risk for child abuse). As a consequence of its less-than-full autonomy, the ethics of sonography are most usefully analyzed in terms of the sonographer's role as member of the health care team.

Ethics

Ethics is the disciplined study of morality. Morality concerns right and wrong conduct (what we ought or ought not do) and good and bad character (the kinds of people we should aspire to be and the virtues we should cultivate). Both are of importance for the ethics of sonographers.

There are many sources of moral beliefs and behavior in our society, including personal experience; the traditions and experiences of families, communities, ethnic and racial groups, and geographic regions; the variety of world religions; and national identity and history, including the laws of the states and of the federal government. These sources of moral beliefs are frequently in conflict. Morality should not be confused with ethics, which seeks to articulate clear, consistent, coherent, and applicable accounts of moral conduct and character.

Historically, two academic disciplines have contributed to ethics. The first, theologic or religious ethics, is based on particular or general religious commitments. There are several problems with this approach. First, religions disagree both intramurally and extramurally about conduct and

This chapter is modified from an earlier version that appeared in Chervenak FA, McCullough LB. Ethics in obstetric ultrasound. J Ultrasound Med. 1989; 8:493–497.

character. Second, people of no religious persuasion are excluded from the dialogue. Finally, medical ethics, at least in countries such as the United States, must confront the fact that the health care professions are secular and that the society they serve is morally pluralistic.[5] Religious ethics provides an inadequate foundation for secular professional ethics in a diverse society such as the United States.[7]

The second academic discipline involved in ethics is philosophy. To be applicable in a medical context, ethics must transcend moral pluralism by offering an approach with minimal—ideally, non-existent—ties to any substantive prior commitment about moral conduct and character. This is what philosophic ethics attempts to do. It requires only a commitment to the results of rational discourse, in which all substantive commitments about what morality ought to be are open to question. Every such substantive claim requires intellectual justification in the form of a rigorous ethical analysis and argument. Philosophic ethics, therefore, properly serves as the foundation for medical ethics, especially in an international context.[10]

Medical Ethics

Perhaps the most useful beginning point for a discussion of ethics in sonography is an analysis of the ethical obligation that serves as the foundation of the patient–sonographer relationship: the sonographer's obligation to protect and promote the interests of the patient. This commitment creates the health care professional's moral authority (i.e., ethical justification for the professional's power), which takes the forms of clinical judgment, recommendations, and technical interventions. This relationship derives from the patient–physician relationship, because the sonographer's moral authority to care for patients derives from the physician's moral authority as the patient's principal caregiver.

From its recorded beginnings in ancient Greece in about the fifth century B.C.E., Western medicine has made a distinctive claim to know what is in the interests of the patient. One expression of this claim is "*Primum non nocere,*" which means "First, do no harm." In ethics, this is known as the *principle of nonmaleficence.*[1] This principle only partially explains what is in the patient's interests, however,

because medicine, and therefore sonography, seeks to benefit patients, not simply avoid harming them. The use of obstetric ultrasound, like other medical interventions, must be justified by the goal of seeking the greater balance of "goods" over "harms,"[1] not simply avoiding harm to the patient at all cost. This ethical principle is called *beneficence,* and is a more adequate basis for ethics in sonography than is nonmaleficence.[1,2]

The principle of beneficence obligates the sonographer to seek the greater balance of goods over harms in the care of patients. Goods and harms are to be defined and balanced from a rigorous clinical perspective.[11] The goods that sonography should seek for patients are preventing early or premature death (not preventing death itself); preventing and managing disease, injury, and handicapping conditions; and alleviating unnecessary pain and suffering.[2] Pain and suffering are unnecessary and therefore represent harms to be avoided when they do not contribute to seeking the goods of the beneficence-based clinical judgment. Pain is a physiologic phenomenon involving central nervous system processing of tissue damage. Suffering is a psychological phenomenon involving blocked intentions, plans, and projects. Pain usually causes suffering, although a person can suffer without being in pain.

In the 20th century, first in the United States and more recently in other Western democracies, it has been recognized that patients have their own perspective on their interests that should be respected as being equal to the clinician's perspective on the patient's interests. A patient's perspective on her interests is shaped by wide-ranging and sometimes idiosyncratic values and beliefs.[2] *Autonomy* refers to a person's capacity to formulate, express, and carry out value-based preferences. The ethical principle of respect for autonomy obligates the sonographer to acknowledge the integrity of a patient's values and beliefs and of her value-based preferences; to avoid interfering with the expression or implementation of these preferences; and, when necessary, to assist in their expression and implementation. This principle generates the autonomy-based obligations of the sonographer.[11] Unlike beneficence-based clinical judgment, no specific goods and harms can be defined because these definitions are left to each individual patient. These range widely and include biopsychosocial dimensions of health as well as spiritual, religious, aesthetic, and other personal concerns.

Obstetric Ethics

Protecting and promoting the interests of the pregnant woman and the interests of the fetal patient in a pregnancy going to term are the basic goals or purposes of obstetric care.[4,11] Sonographic examination helps to implement these goals.

Maternal interests are protected and promoted by both autonomy-based and beneficence-based obligations of the sonographer to the pregnant woman. Fetuses are incapable of having their own perspective on their interests, because the immaturity of their central nervous system renders them incapable of having the necessary values or beliefs. So, there are no autonomy-based obligations to the fetus.[4,11] Fetal interests in sonography are understood exclusively in terms of beneficence. This principle explains the moral—as distinct from legal—status of the fetus as a patient, and generates the serious ethical obligations owed to it.[4,11] In the technical language of beneficence, the sonographer has beneficence-based obligations to the fetal patient in a pregnancy going to term, to protect and promote its interests and those of the child it will become, as these are understood from a rigorous clinical perspective.[4,11] The goods to be sought for the fetal patient include prevention of premature death, disease, and handicapping conditions and of unnecessary pain and suffering. It is appropriate, therefore, to refer to fetuses as patients, with the exception of previable fetuses that are to be aborted.[4,11]

The pregnant woman also has beneficence-based obligations to the fetal patient, because she is its moral fiduciary when the pregnancy will be taken to term. She is expected to protect and promote the fetal patient's interests and those of the child it will become.[4,11] When a pregnant woman elects to have an abortion, however, these fiduciary obligations do not exist. A sonographer with moral objections to abortion should keep two things in mind: First, the moral judgment of the pregnant woman should not be criticized or commented on in any way; her autonomy demands respect in the form of the sonographer and physician being neu-

tral to her judgment and decision. Second, the sonographer is free to follow his or her conscience and to withdraw from further involvement with patients who elect abortion. Physicians should as a matter of office policy respect this important matter of individual conscience on the part of the sonographer.[11]

Ethical Issues in Obstetric Ultrasound

COMPETENCE AND REFERRAL

The ethical obligation to provide competent obstetric ultrasound examinations is based on both beneficence and respect for autonomy. Either principle alone, and certainly both in combination, require sonographers and physicians to provide patients with accurate and reliable information. To meet this ethical obligation, the clinician must address the following ethical considerations.

First, ensuring an appropriate level of competence imposes a rigorous standard of training and continuing education. Two problems result when sonographers do not maintain this baseline level of competence in the techniques and interpretation of ultrasound imaging. First, they may cause unnecessary harm to the pregnant woman or fetal patient, thus violating beneficence-based obligations. Second, incomplete or inaccurate reporting of results by the sonographer to the physician and, therefore, by the physician to the pregnant woman undermines the informed consent process regarding the management of pregnancy, thus violating autonomy-based obligations of the sonographer to the pregnant woman. Because physicians rely heavily on them, the general competence of sonographers is essential to avoid these ethically unacceptable consequences for the exercise of the pregnant woman's autonomy.

Second, these obligations have important implications for physicians who employ a sonographer. Such physicians are ethically obligated to supervise adequately the sonographer's work. To do this, the physician must know substantially more than the sonographer, especially about the application of sonographic findings to the diagnosis of anomalies. This more advanced fund of knowledge is essential for the physician to fulfill the additional obligation regularly to review the sonographer's work. In addition, physicians should provide the opportunity for continuing education.

In medical care, patients properly rely for their protection on the personal and professional integrity of their clinicians. An important facet of that integrity on the part of physicians is willingness to refer to specialists when the limits of their own knowledge are being approached. Integrity should also be one of the fundamental virtues of sonographers, and, thus, a standard for judging professional character. Like other virtues, such as self-sacrifice and compassion, integrity directs sonographers to focus primarily on the patient's interests, as a way to blunt mere self-interest.[11] As sonography continues to develop as a profession, it will need to identify and address incentives to mere self-interest on the part of sonographers, especially concerning compensation packages and productivity.

Sonographers who work with specialists who receive patients on referral confront two principal ethical concerns. Like all sonographers, they have an ethical obligation to ensure that they maintain their standards of general competence. Sonographers as a group have beneficence-based obligations to the patient population. The patient population relies on sonographers' self-regulation as the means to guarantee that these beneficence-based obligations are fulfilled. This ethical concern becomes even more important in the clinically complex and demanding setting of a specialty referral practice.

The second concern for sonographers involves discovering avoidable errors that a colleague has made. The specialist may sometimes face the obligation to present findings to a pregnant woman that the referring physician should have been competent to detect but did not, possibly because of faulty technique or interpretation. In such an instance, the sonographer's integrity is an essential safeguard of the patient's autonomy against the self-interest of the specialist, who may wish to avoid potential loss of income that might result from a conflict with the referring physician. The sonographer should not fail to bring to the attention of the referral specialist (not the patient directly) his or her concern about the inadequacies of the referring physician's sonographic technique. If necessary, the sonographer should become an advocate, even a vigorous advocate, for disclosure of such informa-

tion to the pregnant woman. Failure to make such a disclosure undermines professional integrity and therefore the moral authority of health care professionals.

ROUTINE SCREENING

In many countries, such as Germany, Great Britain, and those of Scandinavia, routine obstetric ultrasound examination at about 18 weeks' gestation has become the standard of care. In others, including the United States, this is not the case. Debate in the United States about routine ultrasound examination has been conducted almost exclusively in terms of the principle of beneficence applied to both the fetus and the pregnant woman. The Routine Antenatal Diagnostic Imaging with Ultrasound Study (RADIUS), for example, used exclusively beneficence-based outcomes of perinatal morbidity and mortality.[8] Its findings that routine obstetric ultrasound had no effect on these outcomes and, therefore, would involve unjustified costs, have been strongly challenged.[12] The result of this ongoing debate is residual uncertainty about how to balance the goods and harms of routine obstetric ultrasound examinations.[6]

The ethical issues concern the physician's responsibilities under informed consent, an autonomy-based concern. The authors believe that this debate should therefore be expanded to include reference to the health care professional's autonomy-based obligations regarding the informed consent process. This process includes disclosure of and discussion about what ultrasound examinations can and cannot detect, the level of sophistication of the ultrasound techniques used, and the incomplete and sometimes uncertain interpretation of ultrasound images.

In the face of medical uncertainty about the goods and harms of routine ultrasound, it is obligatory to inform patients about that uncertainty and to give them the opportunity to make their own choices about how that uncertainty should be managed. We have argued that prenatal informed consent for sonogram (PICS) should be an indication for the routine use of obstetric ultrasound,[6] despite the contested claim that routine ultrasound has no effect on perinatal morbidity and mortality.[8]

The timing of routine ultrasound should be

governed in large part by the principle of respect for autonomy, because the information obtained is relevant to the woman's decision about whether she will seek an abortion. In pregnancies that will be taken to term, routine ultrasound during the second trimester can enhance a pregnant woman's autonomy. If anomalies are detected, she may begin to prepare herself for the decisions that she will confront later about the management of those anomalies in the intrapartum and postpartum periods. Providing this information early in pregnancy permits a pregnant woman ample time to deal with its psychological and other sequelae before she must confront such decisions.

DISCLOSURE

A number of ethical issues arise about the disclosure of results of ultrasound examinations. First, there must be an adequate informed consent process, as mentioned previously. In routine examinations, it may also be important to inform women of the possibility of confronting an anomaly that will force them to decide whether to terminate the pregnancy or take it to term.[9] Sonographers are justified to disclose findings of normal anatomy directly to the pregnant woman. Disclosure of, and discussion about, abnormal findings—if these are to respect and to enhance maternal autonomy and avoid unnecessary psychological harm to the pregnant woman—are the responsibilities of the physician. This is because such discussion should occur in the context of the alternatives available to manage a pregnancy complicated by abnormal ultrasound findings. Sonographers, neither by trainig nor experience, can claim the competence to engage in such discussions; physicians can and therefore should.

The second ethical issue arises in connection with the phenomenon of apparent bonding of pregnant women to their fetuses as a result of the pregnant woman seeing the ultrasound images.[3] Such bonding may benefit pregnancies that will be taken to term, but could also complicate decisions to terminate a pregnancy. It is recommended that these matters, like abnormal findings, be discussed with the pregnant woman.

A third issue is a matter of ongoing debate: the disclosure of the fetus's gender.[11,13] The authors propose that respect for maternal autonomy dictates responding frankly to requests from the pregnant woman for information about the fetus's gender. The pregnant woman should be made aware of the uncertainties of ultrasound gender identification as part of the disclosure process. The sonographer can use his or her own experience to help the pregnant woman understand those uncertainties.

A final issue is that of videotaping or the Polaroid photography of "baby pictures." There is nothing intrinsically wrong with the practice if it is a side product of a legitimate ultrasound examination. In fact, it may help the bonding of the prospective parents to the fetal patient. However, when videotaping or Polaroid photography is performed to generate revenues, this practice trivializes the ultrasound examination and may result in harm because problems that could be diagnosed would be missed.

CONFIDENTIALITY

The principles of beneficence and respect for autonomy govern the sonographer's ethical obligations to his or her *patient*. The pregnant woman is indisputably the patient of the sonographer and the physician. Others, including the pregnant woman's spouse, sex partner, and family, should be understood as third parties to the patient–sonographer relationship. Diagnostic information about a woman's pregnancy is confidential. It can be justifiably disclosed to third parties only with the pregnant woman's explicit permission. This is because a potentially acceptable condition for releasing confidential information, avoiding grave harm to others, does not apply in this context.[1,11] To avoid awkward situations, sonographers and their supervising physicians should establish policies and procedures that reflect this analysis of the ethics of confidentiality.

Conclusion

Sonographers are in an ethically significant relationship with patients and thus are significant members of the health care team. Sonographers have ethical obligations generated by the principes of beneficence and respect for autonomy. It is important to distinguish, however, limits on those obligations, and therefore limits on the freedom of sonographers that derive from the patient–physician relationship. Where these limits should be drawn is the fundamental agenda for the future of ethical issues in obstetric sonography. Because sonography is a new and still-evolving profession, this distinction is not always easy to make in practice. However, this distinction is crucial for an understanding of the proper role of the sonographer in the health care team.

REFERENCES

1. Beauchamp TL, Childress JF. Principles of Biomedical Ethics. 3rd ed. New York: Oxford University Press; 1989.
2. Beauchamp TL, McCullough LB. Medical Ethics: The Moral Responsibilities of Physicians. Englewood Cliffs, NJ: Prentice-Hall; 1984.
3. Campbell S, Reading AE, Cox DN, et al. Ultrasound scanning in pregnancy: The short-term psychological effects of early real time scans. J Psychosom Obstet Gynaecol. 1986; 1:57–61.
4. Chervenak FA, McCullough LB. Perinatal ethics: A practical analysis of obligations to mother and fetus. Obstet Gynecol. 1985; 66:442–446.
5. Chervenak FA, McCullough L. Ethics in obstetric ultrasound. J Ultrasound Med. 1989; 8:493–497.
6. Chervenak FA, McCullough LB, Chervenak JL. Prenatal informed consent for sonogram (PICS): An indication for obstetrical ultrasound. Am J Obstet Gynecol. 1989; 161:857–860.
7. Engelhardt HT Jr. The Foundations of Bioethics. New York: Oxford University Press; 1986.
8. Ewigman BG, Crane JP, Frigoletto FP, LeFevre ML, Bain RP, McNellis D. Effect of prenatal ultrasound screening on perinatal outcome. N Engl J Med. 1993; 329:483–489.
9. Faden RR, Becker C, Lewis C, Freeman J, Faden AI. Disclosure of information to patients in medical care. Med Care. 1981; 19:718–733.
10. McCullough LB. Methodological concerns in bioethics. J Med Philos. 1986; 11:17–37.
11. McCullough LB, Chervenak FA. Ethics in Obstetrics and Gynecology. New York: Oxford University Press; 1994.
12. Skupski DW, Chervenak FA, McCullough LB. Is routine ultrasound screening for all patients? Clin Perinatol. 1994; 21:707–721.
13. Warren MA. Gendercide: The Implications of Sex Selection. Totowa, NJ: Rowman and Littlefield; 1985.

Appendixes

Mean Predicted Gestational Sac (mm)	Gestational Age (weeks)	Mean Predicted Gestational Sac (mm)	Gestational Age (weeks)
10.0	5.0		
11.0	5.2	36.0	8.8
12.0	5.3	37.0	8.9
13.0	5.5	38.0	9.0
14.0	5.6	39.0	9.2
15.0	5.8	40.0	9.3
16.0	5.9	41.0	9.5
17.0	6.0	42.0	9.6
18.0	6.2	43.0	9.7
19.0	6.3	44.0	9.9
20.0	6.5	45.0	10.0
21.0	6.6	46.0	10.2
22.0	6.8	47.0	10.3
23.0	6.9	48.0	10.5
24.0	7.0	49.0	10.6
25.0	7.2	50.0	10.7
26.0	7.3	51.0	10.9
27.0	7.5	52.0	11.0
28.0	7.6	53.0	11.2
29.0	7.8	54.0	11.3
30.0	7.9	55.0	11.5
31.0	8.0	56.0	11.6
32.0	8.2	57.0	11.7
33.0	8.3	58.0	11.9
34.0	8.5	59.0	12.0
35.0	8.6	60.0	12.2

Equation*: $\text{Gestational age (wks)} = \dfrac{\text{Gestational sac (mm)} + 25.43}{7.02}$

* This formula was expressed in centimeters in its original form.
 (From Hellman LM, Kobayashi M, Fillisti L, et al. Growth and development of the human fetus prior to the 20th week of gestation. Am J Obstet Gynecol. 1969;103:784–800.)

APPENDIX B. **MEAN DIAMETER OF GESTATIONAL SAC
AND CORRESPONDING ESTIMATES OF GESTATIONAL AGE***
ASSESSED WITH TRANSVAGINAL SCANNING

Mean Sac Diameter (mm)	Mean Gestational Age (weeks)	Gestational Age (days)	
		Mean	95% Confidence Interval
2	5.0	34.9	34.3–35.5
3	5.1	35.8	35.2–36.3
4	5.2	36.6	36.1–37.2
5	5.4	37.5	37.0–38.0
6	5.5	38.4	37.9–38.9
7	5.6	39.3	38.9–39.7
8	5.7	40.2	39.8–40.6
9	5.9	41.1	40.7–41.4
10	6.0	41.9	41.6–42.3
11	6.1	42.8	42.5–43.2
12	6.2	43.7	43.4–44.0
13	6.4	44.6	44.3–44.9
14	6.5	45.5	45.2–45.8
15	6.6	46.3	46.0–46.6
16	6.7	47.2	46.9–47.5
17	6.9	48.1	47.8–48.4
18	7.0	49.0	48.6–49.4
19	7.1	49.9	49.5–50.3
20	7.3	50.8	50.3–51.2
21	7.4	51.6	51.2–52.1
22	7.5	52.5	52.0–53.0
23	7.6	53.4	52.9–53.9
24	7.8	54.3	53.7–54.8
25	7.9	55.2	54.6–55.7
26	8.0	56.0	55.4–56.7
27	8.1	56.9	56.3–57.6
28	8.3	57.8	57.1–58.5
29	8.4	58.7	58.0–59.4
30	8.5	59.6	58.8–60.4

* The mean gestational age was calculated from a regression equation.
(From Table 2. Daya S, Woods S, Ward S, et al. Early pregnancy assessment with transvaginal ultrasound scanning. Can Med Assoc J. 1991;441–445.)

APPENDIX C. PREDICTED MENSTRUAL AGE (WEEKS) FROM CRL MEASUREMENTS (MM) FROM 5.7 TO 12 WEEKS

CRL (mm)	MA (wk)	CRL (cm)	MA (wk)	CRL (cm)	MA (wk)
2	5.7	22	8.9	42	11.1
3	5.9	23	9.0	43	11.2
4	6.1	24	9.1	44	11.2
5	6.2	25	9.2	45	11.3
6	6.4	26	9.4	46	11.4
7	6.6	27	9.5	47	11.5
8	6.7	28	9.6	48	11.6
9	6.9	29	9.7	49	11.7
10	7.1	30	9.9	50	11.7
11	7.2	31	10.0	51	11.8
12	7.4	32	10.1	52	11.9
13	7.5	33	10.2	53	12.0
14	7.7	34	10.3	54	12.0
15	7.9	35	10.4		
16	8.0	36	10.5		
17	8.1	37	10.6		
18	8.3	38	10.7		
19	8.4	39	10.8		
20	8.6	40	10.9		
21	8.7	41	11.0		

MA = menstrual age. The 95% confidence interval is ±8% of the predicted age.

(From Table 3; only 5.7 to 12.0 weeks are reported. Hadlock FP, Shah YP, Kanon DJ, et al. Fetal crown-rump length: Reevaluation of relation to menstrual age (5–18 weeks) with high-resolution real-time ultrasound. Radiology. 1992;182:501–505.)

APPENDIX D. Estimation of Gestational Age by Biparietal Diameter

Biparietal Diameter (mm)	Gestational Age (weeks) Mean*	Gestational Age (weeks) 90% Variation†	Biparietal Diameter (mm)	Gestational Age (weeks) Mean*	Gestational Age (weeks) 90% Variation†
20	12.0	12.0	60	23.8	22.3–25.5
21	12.0	12.0	61	24.2	22.6–25.8
22	12.7	12.2–13.2	62	24.6	23.1–26.1
23	13.0	12.4–13.6	63	24.9	23.4–26.4
24	13.2	12.6–13.8	64	25.3	23.8–26.8
25	13.5	12.9–14.1	65	25.6	24.1–27.1
26	13.7	13.1–14.3	66	26.0	24.5–27.5
27	14.0	13.4–14.6	67	26.4	25.0–27.8
28	14.3	13.6–15.0	68	26.7	25.3–28.1
29	14.5	13.9–15.2	69	27.1	25.8–28.4
30	14.8	14.1–15.5	70	27.5	26.3–28.7
31	15.1	14.3–15.9	71	27.9	26.7–29.1
32	15.3	14.5–16.1	72	28.3	27.2–29.4
33	15.6	14.7–16.5	73	28.7	27.6–29.8
34	15.9	15.0–16.8	74	29.1	28.1–30.1
35	16.2	15.2–17.2	75	29.5	28.5–30.5
36	16.4	15.4–17.4	76	30.0	29.0–31.0
37	16.7	15.6–17.8	77	30.3	29.2–31.4
38	17.0	15.9–18.1	78	30.8	29.6–32.0
39	17.3	16.1–18.5	79	31.1	29.9–32.5
40	17.6	16.4–18.8	80	31.6	30.2–33.0
41	17.9	16.5–19.3	81	32.1	30.7–33.5
42	18.1	16.6–19.8	82	32.6	31.2–34.0
43	18.4	16.8–20.2	83	33.0	31.5–34.5
44	18.8	16.9–20.7	84	33.4	31.9–35.1
45	19.1	17.0–21.2	85	34.0	32.3–35.7
46	19.4	17.4–21.4	86	34.3	32.8–36.2
47	19.7	17.8–21.6	87	35.0	33.4–36.6
48	20.0	18.2–21.8	88	35.4	33.9–37.1
49	20.3	18.6–22.0	89	36.1	34.6–37.6
50	20.6	19.0–22.2	90	36.6	35.1–38.1
51	20.9	19.3–22.5	91	37.2	35.9–38.5
52	21.2	19.5–22.9	92	37.8	36.7–38.9
53	21.5	19.8–23.2	93	38.8	37.3–39.3
54	21.9	20.1–23.7	94	39.0	37.9–40.1
55	22.2	20.4–24.0	95	39.7	38.5–40.9
56	22.5	20.7–24.3	96	40.6	39.1–41.5
57	22.8	21.1–24.5	97	41.0	39.9–42.1
58	23.2	21.5–24.9	98	41.8	40.5–43.1
59	23.5	21.9–25.1			

* From weighted least mean square fit equation: $Y = 3.45701 + 0.50157\chi - 0.00441\chi^2$.
† For each biparietal diameter, 90% of gestational age data points fell within this range.
(From Kurtz AB, et al. Analysis of biparietal diameter as an accurate indicator of gestational age. J Clin Ultrasound. 1980;8:319–326.)

▰▰▰ **APPENDIX E.** **CORRECTED BIPARIETAL DIAMETER (BPD)**

$$BPDa = \sqrt{(BPD \times FOD)/1.265}$$

BPDa = area-corrected BPD.
(From Doubilet PM, Greenes RA. Improved prediction of gestational age from fetal head measurements. Am J Roentgenol. 1984; 142:797–800.)

▰▰▰ **APPENDIX F.** **ESTIMATION OF GESTATIONAL AGE BY HEAD CIRCUMFERENCE MEASUREMENT**

Head Circumference (mm)	Gestational Age (weeks)		Head Circumference (mm)	Gestational Age (weeks)	
	Predicted Mean Values	95% Confidence Limits		Predicted Mean Values	95% Confidence Limits
80	13.4	12.1–14.7	220	23.9	22.3–25.5
85	13.7	12.4–15.0	225	24.4	22.1–26.7
90	14.0	12.7–15.3	230	24.9	22.6–27.2
95	14.3	13.0–15.6	235	25.4	23.1–27.7
100	14.6	13.3–15.9	240	25.9	23.6–28.2
105	15.0	13.7–16.3	245	26.4	24.1–28.7
110	15.3	14.0–16.6	250	26.9	24.6–29.2
115	15.6	14.3–16.9	255	27.5	25.2–29.8
120	15.9	14.6–17.2	260	28.0	25.7–30.3
125	16.3	15.0–17.6	265	28.1	25.8–30.4
130	16.6	15.3–17.9	270	29.2	26.9–31.5
135	17.0	15.7–18.3	275	29.8	27.5–32.1
140	17.3	16.0–18.6	280	30.3	27.6–33.0
145	17.7	16.4–19.0	285	31.0	28.3–33.7
150	18.1	16.5–19.7	290	31.6	28.9–34.3
155	18.4	16.8–20.0	295	32.2	29.5–34.8
160	18.8	17.2–20.4	300	32.8	30.1–35.5
165	19.2	17.6–20.8	305	33.5	30.7–36.2
170	19.6	18.0–21.2	310	34.2	31.5–36.9
175	20.0	18.4–21.6	315	34.9	32.2–37.6
180	20.4	18.8–22.0	320	35.5	32.8–38.2
185	20.8	19.2–22.4	325	36.3	32.9–39.7
190	21.2	19.8–22.8	330	37.0	33.6–40.4
195	21.6	20.0–23.2	335	37.7	34.3–41.1
200	22.1	20.5–23.7	340	38.5	35.1–41.9
205	22.5	20.9–24.1	345	39.2	35.8–42.6
210	23.0	21.4–24.6	350	40.0	36.6–43.4
215	23.4	21.8–25.0	355	40.8	37.4–44.2
			360	41.6	38.2–45.0

(Data from Tables 3 and 4 in Hadlock FP, Deter RL, Harrist RB, et al. Fetal head circumference: Relation to menstrual age. Am J Roentgenol. 1982; 138:649–653.)

APPENDIX G. ESTIMATION OF GESTATIONAL AGE BY ABDOMINAL CIRCUMFERENCE MEASUREMENT

Abdominal Circumference (mm)	Gestational Age (weeks) Predicted Mean	95% Confidence Limits	Abdominal Circumference (mm)	Gestational Age (weeks) Predicted Mean	95% Confidence Limits
100	15.6	13.7–17.5	235	27.7	25.5–29.9
105	16.1	14.2–18.0	240	28.2	26.0–30.4
110	16.5	14.6–18.4	245	28.7	26.5–30.9
115	16.9	15.0–18.8	250	29.2	27.0–31.4
120	17.3	15.4–19.2	255	29.7	27.5–31.9
125	17.8	15.9–19.7	260	30.1	27.1–33.1
130	18.2	16.2–20.2	265	30.6	27.6–33.6
135	18.6	16.6–20.6	270	31.1	28.1–34.1
140	19.1	17.1–21.1	275	31.6	28.6–34.6
145	19.5	17.5–21.5	280	32.1	29.1–35.1
150	20.0	18.0–22.0	285	32.6	29.6–35.6
155	20.4	18.4–22.4	290	33.1	30.1–36.1
160	20.8	18.8–22.8	295	33.6	30.6–36.6
165	21.3	19.3–23.3	300	34.1	31.1–37.1
170	21.7	19.7–23.7	305	34.6	31.6–37.6
175	22.2	20.2–24.2	310	35.1	32.1–38.1
180	22.6	20.6–24.6	315	35.6	32.6–38.6
185	23.1	21.1–25.1	320	36.1	33.6–38.6
190	23.6	21.6–25.6	325	36.6	34.1–39.1
195	24.0	21.8–26.2	330	37.1	34.6–39.6
200	24.5	22.3–26.7	335	37.6	35.1–40.1
205	24.9	22.7–27.1	340	38.1	35.6–40.6
210	25.4	23.2–27.6	345	38.7	36.2–41.2
215	25.9	23.7–28.1	350	39.2	36.7–41.7
220	26.3	24.1–28.5	355	39.7	37.2–42.2
225	26.8	24.6–29.0	360	40.2	37.7–42.7
230	27.3	25.1–29.5	365	40.8	38.3–43.3

(Data from Tables 3 and 4 in Hadlock FP, Deter RL, Harrist RB, et al. Fetal abdominal circumference as a predictor of menstrual age. Am J Roentgenol. 1982;139:367–370.)

APPENDIX H. ESTIMATION OF GESTATIONAL AGE BY FETAL THORACIC CIRCUMFERENCE (IN CENTIMETERS)

Gestational Age (weeks)	Sample Size No.	Predictive Percentiles								
		2.5	5	10	25	50	75	90	95	97.5
16	6	5.9	6.4	7.0	8.0	9.1	10.3	11.3	11.9	12.4
17	22	6.8	7.3	7.9	8.9	10.0	11.2	12.2	12.8	13.3
18	31	7.7	8.2	8.8	9.8	11.0	12.1	13.1	13.7	14.2
19	21	8.6	9.1	9.7	10.7	11.9	13.0	14.0	14.6	15.1
20	20	9.5	10.0	10.6	11.7	12.8	13.9	15.0	15.5	16.0
21	30	10.4	11.0	11.6	12.6	13.7	14.8	15.8	16.4	16.9
22	18	11.3	11.9	12.5	13.5	14.6	15.7	16.7	17.3	17.8
23	21	12.2	12.8	13.4	14.4	15.5	16.6	17.6	18.2	18.8
24	27	13.2	13.7	14.3	15.3	16.4	17.5	18.5	19.1	19.7
25	20	14.1	14.6	15.2	16.2	17.3	18.4	19.4	20.0	20.6
26	25	15.0	15.5	16.1	17.1	18.2	19.3	20.3	21.0	21.5
27	24	15.9	16.4	17.0	18.0	19.1	20.2	21.3	21.9	22.4
28	24	16.8	17.3	17.9	18.9	20.0	21.2	22.2	22.8	23.3
29	24	17.7	18.2	18.8	19.8	21.0	22.1	23.1	23.7	24.2
30	27	18.6	19.1	19.7	20.7	21.9	23.0	24.0	24.6	25.1
31	24	19.5	20.0	20.6	21.6	22.8	23.9	24.9	25.5	26.0
32	28	20.4	20.9	21.5	22.6	23.7	24.8	25.8	26.4	26.9
33	27	21.3	21.8	22.5	23.5	24.6	25.7	26.7	27.3	27.8
34	25	22.2	22.8	23.4	24.4	25.5	26.6	27.6	28.2	28.7
35	20	23.1	23.7	24.3	25.3	26.4	27.5	28.5	29.1	29.6
36	23	24.0	24.6	25.2	26.2	27.3	28.4	29.4	30.0	30.6
37	22	24.9	25.5	26.1	27.1	28.2	29.3	30.3	30.9	31.5
38	21	25.9	26.4	27.0	28.0	29.1	30.2	31.2	31.9	32.4
39	7	26.8	27.3	27.9	28.9	30.0	31.1	32.2	32.8	33.3
40	6	27.7	28.2	28.8	29.8	30.9	32.1	33.1	33.7	34.2

(From Chitkara U, Rosenberg J, Chervenak FA, et al. Prenatal sonographic assessment of the fetal thorax: Normal values. Am J Obstet Gynecol. 1987;156:1071.)

APPENDIX I. ESTIMATION OF GESTATIONAL AGE BY FEMUR AND HUMERUS MEASUREMENT

| Bone Length (mm) | Gestational Age (weeks) | | | |
| | Femur | | Humerus | |
	Predicted Mean	5th–95th Percentiles	Predicted Mean	5th–95th Percentiles
10	12.6	10.4–14.9	12.6	9.9–15.3
11	12.9	10.7–15.1	12.9	10.1–15.6
12	13.3	11.1–15.6	13.1	10.4–15.9
13	13.6	11.4–15.9	13.6	10.9–16.1
14	13.9	11.7–16.1	13.9	11.1–16.6
15	14.1	12.0–16.4	14.1	11.4–16.9
16	14.6	12.4–16.9	14.6	11.9–17.3
17	14.9	12.7–17.1	14.9	12.1–17.6
18	15.1	13.0–17.4	15.1	12.6–18.0
19	15.6	13.4–17.9	15.6	12.9–18.3
20	15.9	13.7–18.1	15.9	13.1–18.7
21	16.3	14.1–18.6	16.3	13.6–19.1
22	16.6	14.4–18.9	16.7	13.9–19.4
23	16.9	14.7–19.1	17.1	14.3–19.9
24	17.3	15.1–19.6	17.4	14.7–20.1
25	17.6	15.4–19.9	17.9	15.1–20.6
26	18.0	15.9–20.1	18.1	15.6–21.0
27	18.3	16.1–20.6	18.6	15.9–21.4
28	18.7	16.6–20.9	19.0	16.3–21.9
29	19.0	16.9–21.1	19.4	16.7–22.1
30	19.4	17.1–21.6	19.9	17.1–22.6
31	19.9	17.6–22.0	20.3	17.6–23.0
32	20.1	17.9–22.3	20.7	18.0–23.6
33	20.6	18.3–22.7	21.1	18.4–23.9
34	20.9	18.7–23.1	21.6	18.9–24.3
35	21.1	19.0–23.4	22.0	19.3–24.9
36	21.6	19.4–23.9	22.6	19.7–25.1
37	22.0	19.9–24.1	22.9	20.1–25.7
38	22.4	20.1–24.6	23.4	20.6–26.1
39	22.7	20.6–24.9	23.9	21.1–26.6
40	23.1	20.9–25.3	24.3	21.6–27.1
41	23.6	21.3–25.7	24.9	22.0–27.6
42	23.9	21.7–26.1	25.3	22.6–28.0
43	24.3	22.1–26.6	25.7	23.0–28.6
44	24.7	22.6–26.9	26.1	23.6–29.0
45	25.0	22.9–27.1	26.7	24.0–29.6
46	25.4	23.1–27.6	27.1	24.6–30.0
47	25.9	23.6–28.0	27.7	25.0–30.6
48	26.1	24.0–28.4	28.1	25.6–31.0
49	26.6	24.4–28.9	28.9	26.0–31.6

(continued)

APPENDIX I. (Continued)

Bone Length (mm)	Gestational Age (weeks)			
	Femur		Humerus	
	Predicted Mean	5th–95th Percentiles	Predicted Mean	5th–95th Percentiles
50	27.0	24.9–29.1	29.3	26.6–32.0
51	27.4	25.1–29.6	29.9	27.1–32.6
52	27.9	25.6–30.0	30.3	27.6–33.1
53	28.1	26.0–30.4	30.9	28.1–33.6
54	28.6	26.4–30.9	31.4	28.7–34.1
55	29.1	26.9–31.3	32.0	29.1–34.7
56	29.6	27.2–31.7	32.6	29.9–35.3
57	29.9	27.7–32.1	33.1	30.3–35.9
58	30.3	28.1–32.6	33.6	30.9–36.4
59	30.7	28.6–32.9	34.1	31.4–36.9
60	31.1	28.9–33.3	34.9	32.0–37.6
61	31.6	29.4–33.9	35.3	32.6–38.1
62	32.0	29.9–34.1	35.9	33.1–38.7
63	32.4	30.1–34.6	36.6	33.9–39.3
64	32.9	30.7–35.1	37.1	34.4–39.9
65	33.4	31.1–35.6	37.7	35.0–40.6
66	33.7	31.6–35.9	38.3	35.6–41.1
67	34.1	32.0–36.4	38.9	36.1–41.7
68	34.6	32.4–36.9	39.6	36.9–42.3
69	35.0	32.6–37.1	40.1	37.4–42.9
70	35.6	33.3–37.7		
71	35.9	33.7–38.1		
72	36.4	34.1–38.6		
73	36.9	34.6–39.0		
74	37.3	35.1–39.6		
75	37.7	35.6–39.9		
76	38.1	36.0–40.4		
77	38.6	36.4–40.9		
78	39.1	36.9–41.3		
79	39.6	37.3–41.7		
80	40.0	37.9–42.1		

(From Jeanty P, Rodesch F, Delbeke D, et al. Estimation of gestational age from measurements of fetal long bones. J Ultrasound Med. 1984; 3:75–79.)

APPENDIX J. Estimation of Gestational Age by Tibia Measurement

Tibia Length (mm)	Gestational Age (weeks)		Tibia Length (mm)	Gestational Age (weeks)	
	Predicted Mean	5th–95th Percentiles		Predicted Mean	5th–95th Percentiles
10	13.4	10.6–16.3	40	25.3	22.4–28.1
11	13.7	10.9–16.6	41	25.7	22.9–28.6
12	14.1	11.1–17.0	42	26.1	23.3–29.1
13	14.4	11.6–17.3	43	26.6	23.7–29.6
14	14.9	11.9–17.7	44	27.1	24.1–30.0
15	15.1	12.1–18.0	45	27.6	24.6–30.6
16	15.6	12.6–18.4	46	28.0	25.1–30.9
17	15.9	13.0–18.9	47	28.4	25.6–31.4
18	16.1	13.3–19.1	48	29.0	26.1–31.6
19	16.6	13.7–19.6	49	29.4	26.6–32.3
20	17.0	14.1–19.9	50	29.9	27.0–32.9
21	17.4	14.6–20.3	51	30.4	27.6–33.3
22	17.9	14.9–20.7	52	30.9	28.0–33.9
23	18.1	15.1–21.1	53	31.4	28.6–34.3
24	18.6	15.6–21.4	54	31.9	29.0–34.9
25	18.9	16.0–21.9	55	32.4	29.6–35.3
26	19.3	16.4–22.1	56	32.9	30.0–35.9
27	19.7	16.9–22.6	57	33.4	30.6–36.3
28	20.1	17.1–23.0	58	33.9	31.0–36.9
29	20.6	17.6–23.6	59	34.4	31.6–37.3
30	21.0	18.1–23.9	60	34.9	32.0–37.9
31	21.4	18.6–24.3	61	35.4	32.6–38.3
32	21.9	18.9–24.7	62	35.9	33.0–39.4
33	22.1	19.3–25.1	63	36.6	33.6–39.4
34	22.6	19.7–25.6	64	37.0	34.1–39.9
35	23.1	20.1–26.0	65	37.6	34.6–40.5
36	23.6	20.6–26.4	66	38.0	35.1–41.0
37	23.9	21.0–26.9	67	38.6	35.7–41.6
38	24.4	21.6–27.3	68	39.1	36.1–42.0
39	24.9	21.9–27.7	69	39.7	36.9–42.6

(From Jeanty P, Rodesch F, Delbeke D, et al. Estimation of gestational age from measurements of fetal long bones. J Ultrasound Med. 1984;3:75–79.)

APPENDIX K. ESTIMATION OF GESTATIONAL AGE BY ULNA MEASUREMENT

Ulna Length (mm)	Gestational Age (weeks) Predicted Mean	5th–95th Percentiles	Ulna Length (mm)	Gestational Age (weeks) Predicted Mean	5th–95th Percentiles
10	13.1	10.1–16.1	38	25.1	22.1–28.1
11	13.6	10.6–16.4	39	25.6	22.6–28.7
12	13.9	10.9–16.9			
13	14.1	11.1–17.3	40	26.1	23.1–29.1
14	14.6	11.6–17.7	41	26.7	23.6–29.7
15	15.0	11.9–18.0	42	27.1	24.1–30.3
16	15.4	12.3–18.4	43	27.7	24.7–30.9
17	15.7	12.7–18.9	44	28.3	25.1–31.3
18	16.1	13.1–19.1	45	28.9	25.9–31.9
19	16.6	13.6–19.6	46	29.4	26.3–32.4
			47	29.9	26.9–33.0
20	16.9	13.9–20.0	48	30.6	27.4–33.6
21	17.3	14.3–20.6	49	31.1	28.0–34.1
22	17.7	14.7–20.9			
23	18.1	15.1–21.1	50	31.6	28.6–34.7
24	18.6	15.6–21.6	51	32.1	29.1–35.3
25	19.0	16.0–22.1	52	32.9	29.7–35.9
26	19.4	16.4–22.6	53	33.4	30.3–36.4
27	19.9	16.9–22.9	54	34.0	30.9–37.0
28	20.3	17.3–23.4	55	34.6	31.6–37.7
29	20.9	17.7–23.9	56	35.1	32.1–38.3
			57	35.9	32.9–38.9
30	21.1	18.1–24.3	58	36.4	33.4–39.6
31	21.7	18.6–24.9	59	37.1	34.0–40.1
32	22.1	19.1–25.1			
33	22.7	19.6–25.7	60	37.7	34.6–40.9
34	23.1	20.1–26.1	61	38.3	35.3–41.4
35	23.6	20.6–26.7	62	39.0	35.9–42.0
36	24.1	21.1–27.1	63	39.6	36.6–42.7
37	24.6	21.4–27.7	64	40.3	37.1–43.3

(From Jeanty P, Rodesch F, Delbeke D, et al. Estimation of gestational age from measurements of fetal long bones. J Ultrasound Med. 1984;3:75–79.)

▰▰▰ APPENDIX L. ABBREVIATED FETAL WEIGHT ESTIMATION TABLE

BPD + AD (mm)	EFW (g)	AD + FEM SUM (mm)	EFW (g)
100	490	90	500
110	590	100	620
120	720	110	760
130	870	120	930
140	1050	130	1140
150	1280	140	1400
160	1550	150	1720
170	1880	160	2120
180	2280	170	2600
190	2770	180	3190
200	3350	190	3920
210	4070	200	4810
220	4940		

To use this table, obtain the BPD and/or FEM and two abdominal diameter measurements using standard sonographic methods. Compute the mean (average) AD in millimeters and add to BPD or FEM in millimeters. Look up the estimated fetal weight in the appropriate column.

BPD, biparietal diameter; FEM, femur diaphysis (shaft) length; AD, mean abdominal diameter, i.e., (AD1 + AD2)/2.

(Adapted from Rose BI. Abbreviated tables for estimating fetal weight with ultrasound. J Reprod Med. 1988;33:298–300.)

APPENDIX M. ESTIMATION OF FETAL WEIGHT (IN GRAMS) BY BIPARIETAL DIAMETER (BPD) AND ABDOMINAL CIRCUMFERENCE (AC)*

BPD (mm)	AC (mm)												
	155	160	165	170	175	180	185	190	195	200	205	210	215
31	224	234	244	255	267	279	291	304	318	332	346	362	378
32	231	241	251	263	274	286	299	312	326	340	355	371	388
33	237	248	259	270	282	294	307	321	335	349	365	381	397
34	244	255	266	278	290	302	316	329	344	359	374	391	408
35	251	262	274	285	298	311	324	338	353	368	384	401	418
36	259	270	281	294	306	319	333	347	362	378	394	411	429
37	266	278	290	302	315	328	342	357	372	388	404	422	440
38	274	286	298	310	324	337	352	366	382	398	415	432	451
39	282	294	306	319	333	347	361	376	392	409	426	444	462
40	290	303	315	328	342	356	371	386	403	419	437	455	474
41	299	311	324	338	352	366	381	397	413	430	448	467	486
42	308	320	333	347	361	376	392	408	424	442	460	479	498
43	317	330	343	357	371	387	402	419	436	453	472	491	511
44	326	339	353	367	382	397	413	430	447	465	484	504	524
45	335	349	363	377	393	408	425	442	459	478	497	517	538
46	345	359	373	386	404	420	436	454	472	490	510	530	551
47	355	369	384	399	415	431	448	466	484	503	524	544	565
48	366	380	395	410	426	443	460	478	497	517	537	558	580
49	376	391	406	422	438	455	473	491	510	530	551	572	594
50	387	402	418	434	451	468	486	505	524	544	565	587	610
51	399	414	430	446	463	481	499	518	538	559	580	602	625
52	410	426	442	459	476	494	513	532	552	573	595	618	641
53	422	438	455	472	489	508	527	547	567	589	611	634	657
54	435	451	468	485	503	522	541	561	582	604	627	650	674
55	447	464	481	499	517	536	556	577	598	620	643	667	691
56	461	477	495	513	532	551	571	592	614	636	660	684	709
57	474	491	509	527	547	566	587	608	630	653	677	701	727
58	488	505	524	542	562	582	603	625	647	670	695	719	745
59	502	520	539	558	578	598	619	642	664	688	713	738	764
60	517	535	554	573	594	615	636	659	682	706	731	757	784
61	532	550	570	590	610	632	654	677	700	725	750	777	804
62	547	566	586	606	627	649	672	695	719	744	770	797	824
63	563	583	603	624	645	667	690	714	738	764	790	817	845
64	580	600	620	641	663	686	709	733	758	784	811	838	867
65	597	617	638	659	682	705	728	753	778	805	832	860	889

▰▰▰ **APPENDIX M. (Continued)**

BPD (mm)	AC (mm)												
	155	160	165	170	175	180	185	190	195	200	205	210	215
66	614	635	656	678	701	724	748	773	799	826	853	882	911
67	632	653	675	697	720	744	769	794	820	848	876	905	935
68	651	672	694	717	740	765	790	816	842	870	898	928	958
69	670	691	714	737	761	786	811	838	865	893	922	952	983
70	689	711	734	758	782	807	833	860	888	916	946	976	1,008
71	709	732	755	779	804	830	856	883	912	941	971	1,002	1,033
72	730	763	777	801	827	853	880	907	936	965	996	1,027	1,060
73	751	775	799	824	850	876	904	932	961	991	1,022	1,054	1,087
74	773	797	822	847	874	901	928	957	987	1,017	1,049	1,081	1,114
75	796	820	845	871	898	925	954	983	1,013	1,044	1,076	1,109	1,143
76	819	844	870	896	923	951	980	1,009	1,040	1,072	1,104	1,137	1,172
77	843	868	894	921	949	977	1,007	1,037	1,068	1,100	1,133	1,167	1,202
78	868	894	920	947	975	1,004	1,034	1,065	1,096	1,129	1,162	1,197	1,232
79	893	919	946	974	1,003	1,032	1,062	1,094	1,126	1,159	1,193	1,228	1,264
80	919	946	973	1,002	1,031	1,061	1,091	1,123	1,156	1,189	1,224	1,259	1,296
81	946	973	1,001	1,030	1,060	1,090	1,121	1,153	1,187	1,221	1,256	1,292	1,329
82	974	1,001	1,030	1,059	1,089	1,120	1,152	1,185	1,218	1,253	1,288	1,325	1,363
83	1,002	1,030	1,059	1,089	1,120	1,151	1,183	1,217	1,251	1,286	1,322	1,359	1,397
84	1,032	1,060	1,090	1,120	1,151	1,183	1,216	1,249	1,284	1,320	1,356	1,394	1,433
85	1,062	1,091	1,121	1,151	1,183	1,216	1,249	1,283	1,318	1,355	1,392	1,430	1,469
86	1,093	1,122	1,153	1,184	1,216	1,249	1,283	1,318	1,354	1,390	1,428	1,467	1,507
87	1,125	1,155	1,186	1,218	1,250	1,284	1,318	1,353	1,390	1,427	1,465	1,505	1,545
88	1,157	1,188	1,220	1,252	1,285	1,319	1,354	1,390	1,427	1,465	1,504	1,543	1,584
89	1,191	1,222	1,254	1,287	1,321	1,356	1,391	1,428	1,465	1,503	1,543	1,583	1,625
90	1,226	1,258	1,290	1,324	1,358	1,393	1,429	1,456	1,504	1,543	1,583	1,624	1,666
91	1,262	1,294	1,327	1,361	1,396	1,432	1,468	1,506	1,544	1,584	1,624	1,666	1,708
92	1,299	1,332	1,365	1,400	1,435	1,471	1,508	1,546	1,586	1,626	1,667	1,709	1,752
93	1,337	1,370	1,404	1,439	1,475	1,512	1,550	1,588	1,628	1,668	1,710	1,753	1,796
94	1,376	1,410	1,444	1,480	1,516	1,554	1,592	1,631	1,671	1,712	1,755	1,798	1,842
95	1,416	1,450	1,486	1,522	1,559	1,597	1,635	1,675	1,716	1,758	1,800	1,844	1,889
96	1,457	1,492	1,528	1,565	1,602	1,641	1,680	1,720	1,762	1,804	1,847	1,892	1,937
97	1,500	1,535	1,572	1,609	1,547	1,686	1,726	1,767	1,809	1,852	1,895	1,940	1,986
98	1,544	1,580	1,617	1,654	1,693	1,733	1,773	1,815	1,857	1,900	1,945	1,990	2,037
99	1,589	1,625	1,663	1,701	1,740	1,781	1,822	1,864	1,907	1,951	1,996	2,042	2,089
100	1,635	1,672	1,710	1,749	1,789	1,830	1,871	1,914	1,958	2,002	2,048	2,094	2,142

(continued)

APPENDIX M. (Continued)

BPD (mm)	AC (mm) 220	225	230	235	240	245	250	255	260	265	270	275	280
31	395	412	431	450	470	491	513	536	559	584	610	638	666
32	405	423	441	461	481	502	525	548	572	597	624	651	680
33	415	433	452	472	493	514	537	560	585	611	638	666	693
34	425	444	463	483	504	526	549	573	598	624	652	680	710
35	436	455	475	495	517	539	562	587	612	638	666	695	725
36	447	466	486	507	529	552	575	600	626	653	681	710	740
37	458	478	498	519	542	565	589	614	640	667	696	725	756
38	470	490	510	532	554	578	602	628	654	682	711	741	772
39	482	502	523	545	568	592	616	642	669	697	727	757	789
40	494	514	536	558	581	606	631	657	684	713	743	773	806
41	506	527	549	572	595	620	645	672	700	729	759	790	828
42	519	540	562	585	609	634	660	688	716	745	776	807	841
43	532	554	576	600	624	649	676	703	732	762	793	825	859
44	545	567	590	614	639	665	692	719	749	779	810	843	877
45	559	581	605	629	654	680	708	736	765	796	828	861	896
46	573	596	620	644	670	696	724	753	783	814	846	880	915
47	588	611	635	660	686	713	741	770	801	832	865	899	934
48	602	626	650	676	702	730	758	788	819	851	884	919	954
49	617	641	666	692	719	747	776	806	837	870	903	938	975
50	633	657	683	709	736	765	794	824	856	889	923	959	996
51	649	674	699	726	754	783	812	843	876	909	944	980	1,017
52	665	690	717	744	772	801	831	863	895	929	964	1,001	1,039
53	682	708	734	762	790	820	851	883	916	950	986	1,023	1,061
54	699	725	752	780	809	839	870	903	936	971	1,007	1,045	1,084
55	717	743	771	799	828	859	891	924	958	993	1,030	1,068	1,107
56	735	762	789	818	848	879	911	945	979	1,015	1,052	1,091	1,131
57	753	780	809	838	869	900	933	966	1,001	1,038	1,075	1,114	1,155
58	772	800	829	858	889	921	954	989	1,024	1,061	1,099	1,139	1,180
59	792	820	849	879	911	943	977	1,011	1,047	1,085	1,123	1,163	1,205
60	811	840	870	900	932	965	999	1,035	1,071	1,109	1,148	1,189	1,231
61	832	861	891	922	955	988	1,023	1,058	1,095	1,134	1,173	1,214	1,257
62	853	882	913	945	977	1,011	1,046	1,083	1,120	1,159	1,199	1,241	1,284
63	874	904	935	967	1,001	1,035	1,071	1,107	1,145	1,185	1,226	1,268	1,311
64	896	927	958	991	1,025	1,059	1,096	1,133	1,171	1,211	1,253	1,295	1,339
65	919	950	982	1,015	1,049	1,084	1,121	1,159	1,198	1,238	1,280	1,323	1,368

APPENDIX M. (Continued)

BPD (mm)	AC (mm)												
	220	225	230	235	240	245	250	255	260	265	270	275	280
66	942	973	1,006	1,039	1,074	1,110	1,147	1,185	1,225	1,266	1,308	1,352	1,397
67	965	997	1,030	1,065	1,100	1,136	1,174	1,213	1,253	1,294	1,337	1,381	1,427
68	990	1,022	1,056	1,090	1,126	1,163	1,201	1,241	1,281	1,323	1,367	1,411	1,458
69	1,015	1,048	1,082	1,117	1,153	1,190	1,229	1,269	1,310	1,353	1,397	1,442	1,489
70	1,040	1,074	1,108	1,144	1,181	1,219	1,258	1,298	1,340	1,383	1,427	1,473	1,521
71	1,066	1,100	1,135	1,171	1,209	1,247	1,287	1,328	1,370	1,414	1,459	1,505	1,553
72	1,093	1,128	1,163	1,200	1,238	1,277	1,317	1,358	1,401	1,445	1,491	1,538	1,586
73	1,121	1,156	1,192	1,229	1,267	1,307	1,348	1,390	1,433	1,478	1,524	1,571	1,620
74	1,149	1,184	1,221	1,259	1,297	1,338	1,379	1,421	1,465	1,511	1,557	1,605	1,655
75	1,178	1,214	1,251	1,289	1,328	1,369	1,411	1,454	1,499	1,544	1,592	1,640	1,690
76	1,207	1,244	1,281	1,320	1,360	1,401	1,444	1,487	1,533	1,579	1,627	1,676	1,727
77	1,238	1,275	1,313	1,352	1,393	1,434	1,477	1,522	1,567	1,614	1,663	1,712	1,764
78	1,269	1,306	1,345	1,385	1,426	1,468	1,512	1,557	1,603	1,650	1,699	1,749	1,801
79	1,301	1,339	1,378	1,418	1,460	1,503	1,547	1,592	1,639	1,687	1,737	1,787	1,840
80	1,333	1,372	1,412	1,453	1,495	1,538	1,583	1,629	1,676	1,725	1,775	1,826	1,879
81	1,367	1,406	1,446	1,488	1,531	1,575	1,620	1,666	1,714	1,763	1,814	1,866	1,919
82	1,401	1,441	1,482	1,524	1,567	1,612	1,657	1,704	1,753	1,803	1,854	1,906	1,960
83	1,436	1,477	1,518	1,561	1,605	1,650	1,696	1,744	1,793	1,843	1,895	1,948	2,002
84	1,473	1,513	1,555	1,599	1,643	1,689	1,735	1,784	1,833	1,884	1,936	1,990	2,045
85	1,510	1,551	1,594	1,637	1,682	1,728	1,776	1,825	1,875	1,926	1,979	2,033	2,089
86	1,548	1,589	1,633	1,677	1,722	1,769	1,817	1,866	1,917	1,969	2,022	2,077	2,134
87	1,586	1,629	1,673	1,717	1,764	1,811	1,859	1,909	1,960	2,013	2,067	2,122	2,179
88	1,626	1,669	1,714	1,759	1,806	1,854	1,903	1,953	2,005	2,058	2,113	2,169	2,226
89	1,667	1,711	1,756	1,802	1,849	1,897	1,947	1,998	2,050	2,104	2,159	2,216	2,274
90	1,709	1,753	1,799	1,845	1,893	1,942	1,992	2,044	2,097	2,151	2,207	2,264	2,322
91	1,752	1,797	1,843	1,890	1,938	1,988	2,039	2,091	2,144	2,199	2,255	2,313	2,372
92	1,796	1,841	1,888	1,936	1,984	2,035	2,086	2,139	2,193	2,248	2,305	2,363	2,423
93	1,841	1,887	1,934	1,982	2,032	2,083	2,135	2,188	2,242	2,298	2,356	2,414	2,475
94	1,887	1,934	1,982	2,030	2,080	2,132	2,184	2,238	2,293	2,350	2,407	2,467	2,527
95	1,935	1,982	2,030	2,080	2,130	2,182	2,235	2,289	2,345	2,402	2,460	2,520	2,582
96	1,984	2,031	2,080	2,130	2,181	2,233	2,287	2,342	2,398	2,456	2,515	2,575	2,637
97	2,033	2,082	2,131	2,181	2,233	2,286	2,340	2,396	2,452	2,510	2,570	2,631	2,693
98	2,085	2,133	2,183	2,234	2,286	2,340	2,395	2,451	2,508	2,567	2,627	2,688	2,751
99	2,137	2,186	2,237	2,288	2,341	2,395	2,450	2,507	2,565	2,624	2,684	2,746	2,810
100	2,191	2,241	2,292	2,344	2,397	2,452	2,507	2,564	2,623	2,682	2,743	2,806	2,870

(continued)

APPENDIX M. (Continued)

BPD (mm)	AC (mm)												
	285	290	295	300	305	310	315	320	325	330	335	340	345
31	696	726	759	793	828	865	903	943	985	1,029	1,075	1,123	1,173
32	710	742	774	809	844	882	921	961	1,004	1,048	1,094	1,143	1,193
33	725	757	790	825	861	899	938	979	1,022	1,067	1,114	1,163	1,214
34	740	773	806	841	878	916	956	998	1,041	1,087	1,134	1,183	1,235
35	756	789	823	858	896	934	975	1,017	1,061	1,107	1,154	1,204	1,256
36	772	805	840	876	913	953	993	1,036	1,080	1,127	1,175	1,226	1,278
37	788	822	857	893	931	971	1,012	1,056	1,101	1,147	1,196	1,247	1,300
38	805	839	874	911	950	990	1,032	1,076	1,121	1,168	1,218	1,269	1,323
39	822	856	892	930	969	1,009	1,052	1,096	1,142	1,190	1,240	1,292	1,346
40	839	874	911	949	988	1,029	1,072	1,117	1,163	1,212	1,262	1,315	1,369
41	857	892	929	968	1,008	1,049	1,093	1,138	1,185	1,234	1,285	1,338	1,393
42	875	911	948	987	1,028	1,070	1,114	1,159	1,207	1,256	1,308	1,361	1,417
43	893	930	968	1,007	1,048	1,091	1,135	1,181	1,229	1,279	1,331	1,385	1,442
44	912	949	987	1,027	1,069	1,112	1,157	1,204	1,252	1,303	1,355	1,410	1,467
45	932	969	1,008	1,048	1,090	1,134	1,179	1,226	1,275	1,326	1,380	1,435	1,492
46	951	989	1,028	1,069	1,112	1,156	1,202	1,249	1,299	1,351	1,404	1,406	1,518
47	971	1,010	1,049	1,091	1,134	1,178	1,225	1,273	1,323	1,375	1,430	1,486	1,545
48	992	1,031	1,071	1,113	1,156	1,201	1,248	1,297	1,348	1,401	1,455	1,512	1,571
49	1,013	1,052	1,093	1,135	1,179	1,225	1,272	1,322	1,373	1,426	1,482	1,539	1,599
50	1,034	1,074	1,115	1,158	1,203	1,249	1,297	1,347	1,399	1,452	1,508	1,566	1,626
51	1,056	1,096	1,138	1,181	1,226	1,273	1,322	1,372	1,425	1,479	1,535	1,594	1,655
52	1,078	1,119	1,161	1,205	1,251	1,298	1,347	1,398	1,451	1,506	1,563	1,622	1,683
53	1,101	1,142	1,185	1,229	1,276	1,323	1,373	1,425	1,478	1,533	1,591	1,651	1,713
54	1,124	1,166	1,209	1,254	1,301	1,349	1,399	1,452	1,506	1,562	1,620	1,680	1,742
55	1,148	1,190	1,234	1,279	1,327	1,376	1,426	1,497	1,534	1,590	1,649	1,710	1,773
56	1,172	1,215	1,259	1,305	1,353	1,402	1,454	1,507	1,562	1,619	1,678	1,740	1,803
57	1,197	1,240	1,285	1,332	1,380	1,430	1,482	1,535	1,591	1,649	1,709	1,770	1,835
58	1,222	1,266	1,311	1,358	1,407	1,458	1,510	1,564	1,621	1,679	1,739	1,802	1,866
59	1,248	1,292	1,338	1,386	1,435	1,486	1,539	1,594	1,651	1,710	1,770	1,834	1,899
60	1,274	1,319	1,366	1,414	1,464	1,515	1,569	1,624	1,682	1,741	1,802	1,866	1,932
61	1,301	1,346	1,393	1,442	1,493	1,545	1,599	1,655	1,713	1,773	1,835	1,899	1,965
62	1,328	1,374	1,422	1,471	1,522	1,575	1,630	1,686	1,745	1,805	1,868	1,932	1,999
63	1,356	1,403	1,451	1,501	1,552	1,606	1,661	1,718	1,777	1,838	1,901	1,967	2,034
64	1,385	1,432	1,481	1,531	1,583	1,837	1,693	1,751	1,810	1,872	1,935	2,001	2,069

APPENDIX M. (Continued)

BPD (mm)	AC (mm)												
	285	290	295	300	305	310	315	320	325	330	335	340	345
66	1,444	1,492	1,542	1,594	1,647	1,702	1,759	1,817	1,878	1,941	2,006	2,073	2,142
67	1,474	1,523	1,574	1,626	1,679	1,735	1,792	1,852	1,913	1,976	2,042	2,109	2,179
68	1,505	1,555	1,606	1,658	1,713	1,769	1,827	1,887	1,949	2,012	2,078	2,147	2,217
69	1,537	1,587	1,639	1,692	1,747	1,803	1,862	1,922	1,985	2,049	2,116	2,184	2,255
70	1,570	1,620	1,672	1,726	1,781	1,839	1,898	1,959	2,022	2,087	2,154	2,223	2,295
71	1,603	1,654	1,706	1,761	1,817	1,875	1,934	1,996	2,059	2,125	2,193	2,262	2,334
72	1,636	1,688	1,741	1,796	1,853	1,911	1,971	2,044	2,098	2,164	2,232	2,302	2,375
73	1,671	1,723	1,777	1,832	1,890	1,948	2,009	2,072	2,137	2,203	2,272	2,343	2,416
74	1,706	1,759	1,813	1,869	1,927	1,987	2,048	2,111	2,176	2,244	2,313	2,384	2,458
75	1,742	1,795	1,850	1,907	1,965	2,025	2,087	2,151	2,217	2,265	2,354	2,426	2,501
76	1,779	1,833	1,888	1,945	2,004	2,065	2,127	2,192	2,258	2,326	2,397	2,469	2,544
77	1,816	1,871	1,927	1,985	2,044	2,105	2,168	2,233	2,300	2,369	2,440	2,513	2,588
78	1,855	1,910	1,966	2,025	2,085	2,146	2,210	2,275	2,343	2,412	2,484	2,557	2,633
79	1,894	1,949	2,006	2,065	2,126	2,188	2,252	2,318	2,386	2,456	2,528	2,603	2,679
80	1,934	1,990	2,048	2,107	2,168	2,231	2,296	2,362	2,431	2,501	2,574	2,649	2,725
81	1,975	2,031	2,089	2,149	2,211	2,275	2,340	2,407	2,476	2,547	2,620	2,695	2,773
82	2,016	2,073	2,132	2,193	2,255	2,319	2,385	2,462	2,522	2,594	2,667	2,743	2,821
83	2,059	2,116	2,176	2,237	2,300	2,364	2,431	2,499	2,569	2,641	2,715	2,791	2,870
84	2,102	2,160	2,220	2,282	2,345	2,410	2,477	2,546	2,617	2,689	2,764	2,841	2,920
85	2,146	2,205	2,266	2,328	2,392	2,457	2,525	2,594	2,665	2,739	2,814	2,891	2,970
86	2,192	2,251	2,312	2,375	2,439	2,505	2,573	2,643	2,715	2,789	2,864	2,942	3,022
87	2,238	2,298	2,359	2,423	2,488	2,554	2,623	2,693	2,765	2,840	2,916	2,994	3,074
88	2,285	2,346	2,408	2,472	2,537	2,604	2,673	2,744	2,817	2,892	2,968	3,047	3,128
89	2,333	2,394	2,457	2,521	2,587	2,655	2,725	2,796	2,869	2,944	3,021	3,101	3,182
90	2,382	2,444	2,507	2,572	2,639	2,707	2,777	2,849	2,923	2,998	3,076	3,155	3,237
91	2,433	2,495	2,559	2,624	2,691	2,760	2,830	2,903	2,977	3,053	3,131	3,211	3,293
92	2,484	2,547	2,611	2,677	2,744	2,814	2,885	2,958	3,032	3,109	3,187	3,268	3,350
93	2,536	2,599	2,664	2,731	2,799	2,869	2,940	3,014	3,089	3,166	3,245	3,326	3,409
94	2,590	2,653	2,719	2,786	2,854	2,925	2,997	3,070	3,146	3,224	3,303	3,384	3,468
95	2,644	2,709	2,774	2,842	2,911	2,982	3,054	3,129	3,205	3,283	3,362	3,444	3,528
96	2,700	2,765	2,831	2,899	2,969	3,040	3,113	3,188	3,264	3,343	3,423	3,505	3,589
97	2,757	2,822	2,889	2,958	3,028	3,099	3,173	3,248	3,325	3,404	3,484	3,567	3,651
98	2,815	2,881	2,948	3,017	3,088	3,160	3,234	3,309	3,387	3,466	3,547	3,630	3,715
99	2,874	2,941	3,009	3,078	3,149	3,222	3,296	3,372	3,450	3,529	3,600	3,694	3,779
100	2,935	3,002	3,070	3,140	3,211	3,285	3,359	3,436	3,514	3,594	3,676	3,759	3,845

(continued)

APPENDIX M. (Continued)

BPD (mm)	AC (mm) 350	355	360	365	370	375	380	385	390	395	400
31	1,225	1,279	1,336	1,396	1,458	1,523	1,591	1,661	1,735	1,812	1,893
32	1,246	1,301	1,258	1,418	1,481	1,546	1,615	1,686	1,761	1,838	1,920
33	1,267	1,323	1,381	1,441	1,504	1,570	1,639	1,711	1,786	1,865	1,946
34	1,289	1,345	1,403	1,464	1,528	1,595	1,664	1,737	1,812	1,891	1,973
35	1,311	1,367	1,426	1,488	1,552	1,619	1,689	1,762	1,839	1,918	2,001
36	1,333	1,390	1,450	1,512	1,577	1,645	1,715	1,789	1,865	1,945	2,029
37	1,356	1,413	1,474	1,536	1,602	1,670	1,741	1,815	1,893	1,973	2,057
38	1,379	1,437	1,498	1,561	1,627	1,696	1,768	1,842	1,920	2,001	2,086
39	1,402	1,461	1,523	1,586	1,653	1,722	1,794	1,870	1,948	2,030	2,115
40	1,426	1,486	1,548	1,612	1,679	1,749	1,822	1,898	1,977	2,059	2,145
41	1,451	1,511	1,573	1,638	1,706	1,776	1,849	1,926	2,005	2,088	2,174
42	1,475	1,536	1,599	1,664	1,733	1,804	1,878	1,954	2,035	2,118	2,205
43	1,500	1,562	1,625	1,691	1,760	1,832	1,906	1,984	2,064	2,148	2,236
44	1,526	1,588	1,652	1,718	1,788	1,860	1,935	2,013	2,094	2,179	2,267
45	1,552	1,614	1,679	1,746	1,816	1,889	1,964	2,043	2,125	2,210	2,298
46	1,579	1,641	1,706	1,774	1,845	1,918	1,994	2,073	2,156	2,241	2,330
47	1,605	1,669	1,734	1,803	1,874	1,948	2,024	2,104	2,187	2,273	2,363
48	1,633	1,697	1,763	1,832	1,904	1,976	2,055	2,136	2,219	2,306	2,396
49	1,661	1,725	1,792	1,861	1,934	2,009	2,086	2,167	2,251	2,339	2,429
50	1,689	1,754	1,821	1,891	1,964	2,040	2,118	2,200	2,284	2,372	2,463
51	1,718	1,783	1,851	1,922	1,995	2,071	2,150	2,232	2,317	2,406	2,498
52	1,747	1,813	1,882	1,953	2,027	2,103	2,183	2,266	2,351	2,440	2,532
53	1,777	1,843	1,913	1,984	2,059	2,136	2,216	2,299	2,386	2,475	2,568
54	1,807	1,874	1,944	2,016	2,091	2,169	2,250	2,333	2,420	2,510	2,604
55	1,838	1,906	1,976	2,049	2,124	2,203	2,284	2,368	2,456	2,546	2,640
56	1,869	1,938	2,008	2,082	2,158	2,237	2,319	2,403	2,491	2,582	2,677
57	1,901	1,970	2,041	2,115	2,192	2,272	2,354	2,439	2,528	2,619	2,714
58	1,934	2,003	2,075	2,150	2,227	2,307	2,390	2,475	2,564	2,657	2,752
59	1,966	2,037	2,109	2,184	2,262	2,342	2,426	2,512	2,602	2,694	2,790
60	2,000	2,071	2,144	2,219	2,298	2,379	2,463	2,550	2,640	2,733	2,829
61	2,034	2,105	2,179	2,255	2,334	2,416	2,500	2,588	2,678	2,772	2,869
62	2,069	2,140	2,215	2,291	2,371	2,453	2,538	2,626	2,717	2,811	2,909
63	2,104	2,176	2,251	2,328	2,408	2,491	2,577	2,665	2,757	2,851	2,949
64	2,140	2,213	2,288	2,366	2,446	2,530	2,616	2,705	2,797	2,892	2,991
65	2,176	2,250	2,326	2,404	2,485	2,569	2,656	2,745	2,838	2,933	3,032

(continued)

APPENDIX M. (Continued)

BPD (mm)	AC (mm)										
	350	355	360	365	370	375	380	385	390	395	400
66	2,213	2,287	2,364	2,443	2,524	2,609	2,696	2,786	2,879	2,975	3,075
67	2,251	2,326	2,403	2,482	2,564	2,649	2,737	2,827	2,921	3,018	3,117
68	2,290	2,365	2,442	2,522	2,605	2,690	2,778	2,869	2,964	3,061	3,161
69	2,329	2,404	2,482	2,563	2,646	2,732	2,821	2,912	3,007	3,104	3,205
70	2,368	2,444	2,523	2,604	2,688	2,774	2,863	2,955	3,050	3,149	3,250
71	2,409	2,485	2,564	2,646	2,730	2,817	2,907	2,999	3,095	3,193	3,295
72	2,450	2,527	2,607	2,689	2,773	2,861	2,951	3,044	3,140	3,239	3,341
73	2,491	2,569	2,649	2,732	2,817	2,905	2,996	3,089	3,186	3,285	3,386
74	2,534	2,612	2,693	2,776	2,862	2,950	3,041	3,135	3,232	3,332	3,435
75	2,577	2,656	2,737	2,821	2,907	2,996	3,088	3,182	3,279	3,380	3,483
76	2,621	2,700	2,782	2,866	2,953	3,042	3,134	3,299	3,327	3,428	3,531
77	2,666	2,746	2,828	2,912	3,000	3,090	3,128	3,277	3,376	3,477	3,581
78	2,711	2,792	2,874	2,959	3,047	3,137	3,230	3,326	3,425	3,526	3,631
79	2,757	2,838	2,921	3,007	3,095	3,186	3,279	3,376	3,475	3,576	3,681
80	2,804	2,886	2,969	3,056	3,144	3,235	3,329	3,426	3,525	3,627	3,733
81	2,852	2,934	3,018	3,105	3,194	3,286	3,380	3,477	3,577	3,679	3,785
82	2,901	2,983	3,068	3,155	3,244	3,336	3,431	3,529	3,629	3,732	3,838
83	2,950	3,033	3,118	3,206	3,296	3,388	3,483	3,581	3,682	3,785	3,891
84	3,001	3,084	3,169	3,257	3,348	3,441	3,536	3,634	3,735	3,839	3,945
85	3,052	3,135	3,221	3,310	3,401	3,494	3,590	3,688	3,790	3,894	4,000
86	3,104	3,188	3,274	3,363	3,454	3,548	3,644	3,743	3,845	3,949	4,056
87	3,157	3,241	3,328	3,417	3,509	3,603	3,700	3,799	3,901	4,005	4,113
88	3,210	3,295	3,383	3,472	3,565	3,659	3,756	3,855	3,958	4,063	4,170
89	3,265	3,351	3,438	3,528	3,621	3,716	3,813	3,913	4,015	4,120	4,228
90	3,321	3,407	3,495	3,585	3,678	3,773	3,871	3,971	4,074	4,179	4,287
91	3,377	3,464	3,552	3,643	3,736	3,832	3,930	4,030	4,133	4,239	4,347
92	3,435	3,522	3,611	3,702	3,795	3,891	3,989	4,090	4,193	4,299	4,408
93	3,494	3,581	3,670	3,761	3,855	3,951	4,050	4,151	4,254	4,361	4,469
94	3,553	3,641	3,738	3,822	3,916	4,013	4,111	4,213	4,316	4,423	4,532
95	3,614	3,701	3,791	3,884	3,978	4,075	4,174	4,275	4,379	4,486	4,595
96	3,675	3,763	3,854	3,946	4,041	4,138	4,237	4,339	4,443	4,550	4,659
97	3,738	3,826	3,917	4,010	4,105	4,202	4,302	4,404	4,508	4,615	4,724
98	3,802	3,890	3,981	4,074	4,170	4,267	4,367	4,469	4,573	4,680	4,790
99	3,866	3,956	4,047	4,140	4,236	4,333	4,433	4,536	4,640	4,747	4,857
100	3,932	4,022	4,113	4,207	4,303	4,400	4,501	4,603	4,708	4,815	4,924

* Estimated fetal weights: Log (birth weight) = −1.7492 + 0.166 (BPD) + 0.046 (AC) − 2.646 (AC + BPD)/1,000.
(From Shepard MJ, Richards VA, Berkowitz RL, et al. An evaluation of two equations for predicting fetal weight by ultrasound. Am J Obstet Gynecol. 1982;147:47–54. Used by permission.)

APPENDIX N. ESTIMATION OF FETAL WEIGHT (IN GRAMS) BY ABDOMINAL CIRCUMFERENCE (AC) AND FEMUR LENGTH (FL)*

FL (mm)	AC (mm)									
	200	205	210	215	220	225	230	235	240	245
40	663	691	720	751	783	816	851	887	925	964
41	680	709	738	769	802	836	871	907	946	986
42	697	726	757	788	821	855	891	928	967	1,007
43	715	745	776	808	841	875	912	949	988	1,029
44	734	764	795	827	861	896	933	971	1,010	1,051
45	753	783	815	847	882	917	954	993	1,033	1,074
46	772	803	835	868	903	939	976	1,015	1,056	1,098
47	792	823	856	889	924	961	999	1,038	1,079	1,122
48	812	844	877	911	947	984	1,022	1,062	1,103	1,146
49	833	865	899	933	969	1,007	1,046	1,086	1,128	1,171
50	855	887	921	956	993	1,031	1,070	1,111	1,153	1,197
51	877	910	944	980	1,016	1,055	1,095	1,136	1,179	1,223
52	899	933	967	1,004	1,041	1,080	1,120	1,162	1,205	1,250
53	922	956	992	1,028	1,066	1,105	1,146	1,188	1,232	1,277
54	946	981	1,016	1,053	1,091	1,131	1,172	1,215	1,259	1,305
55	971	1,005	1,041	1,079	1,118	1,158	1,199	1,242	1,287	1,333
56	995	1,031	1,067	1,105	1,144	1,185	1,227	1,271	1,316	1,362
57	1,021	1,057	1,094	1,132	1,172	1,213	1,255	1,299	1,345	1,392
58	1,047	1,084	1,121	1,160	1,200	1,242	1,285	1,329	1,375	1,422
59	1,074	1,111	1,149	1,188	1,229	1,271	1,314	1,359	1,406	1,454
60	1,102	1,139	1,178	1,217	1,258	1,301	1,345	1,409	1,437	1,485
61	1,130	1,168	1,207	1,247	1,289	1,331	1,376	1,421	1,469	1,518
62	1,160	1,198	1,237	1,278	1,319	1,363	1,408	1,454	1,501	1,551
63	1,189	1,228	1,268	1,309	1,351	1,395	1,440	1,487	1,535	1,585
64	1,220	1,259	1,299	1,341	1,384	1,428	1,473	1,520	1,569	1,619
65	1,251	1,291	1,332	1,373	1,417	1,461	1,507	1,555	1,604	1,655
66	1,284	1,324	1,365	1,407	1,451	1,496	1,542	1,590	1,640	1,691
67	1,317	1,357	1,399	1,441	1,486	1,531	1,578	1,626	1,676	1,728
68	1,351	1,391	1,433	1,477	1,521	1,567	1,615	1,663	1,713	1,765
69	1,385	1,427	1,469	1,513	1,558	1,604	1,652	1,701	1,752	1,804
70	1,421	1,463	1,506	1,550	1,595	1,642	1,690	1,740	1,791	1,843
71	1,458	1,500	1,543	1,588	1,633	1,681	1,729	1,779	1,830	1,883
72	1,495	1,538	1,581	1,626	1,673	1,720	1,769	1,819	1,871	1,924
73	1,534	1,577	1,621	1,666	1,713	1,761	1,810	1,861	1,913	1,966
74	1,573	1,616	1,661	1,707	1,754	1,802	1,852	1,903	1,955	2,009
75	1,614	1,657	1,702	1,749	1,796	1,845	1,895	1,946	1,999	2,053
76	1,655	1,699	1,745	1,791	1,839	1,888	1,939	1,990	2,043	2,098
77	1,698	1,742	1,788	1,835	1,883	1,933	1,983	2,035	2,089	2,144
78	1,741	1,786	1,833	1,880	1,928	1,978	2,029	2,082	2,135	2,191
79	1,786	1,832	1,878	1,926	1,975	2,025	2,076	2,129	2,183	2,238
80	1,832	1,878	1,925	1,973	2,022	2,073	2,124	2,177	2,232	2,287
81	1,879	1,926	1,973	2,021	2,071	2,121	2,173	2,227	2,281	2,337
82	1,928	1,974	2,022	2,070	2,120	2,171	2,224	2,277	2,332	2,388
83	1,978	2,024	2,072	2,121	2,171	2,223	2,275	2,329	2,384	2,440

(continued)

APPENDIX N. (Continued)

AC (mm)										
250	**255**	**260**	**265**	**270**	**275**	**280**	**285**	**290**	**295**	**300**
1,006	1,048	1,093	1,139	1,188	1,239	1,291	1,346	1,403	1,463	1,525
1,027	1,070	1,115	1,162	1,211	1,262	1,315	1,371	1,429	1,489	1,551
1,049	1,093	1,138	1,186	1,235	1,287	1,340	1,396	1,454	1,515	1,578
1,071	1,116	1,162	1,209	1,259	1,311	1,365	1,422	1,480	1,541	1,605
1,094	1,139	1,185	1,234	1,284	1,336	1,391	1,448	1,507	1,568	1,632
1,118	1,163	1,210	1,259	1,309	1,362	1,417	1,474	1,534	1,596	1,660
1,142	1,187	1,235	1,284	1,335	1,388	1,444	1,501	1,561	1,623	1,688
1,166	1,212	1,260	1,310	1,316	1,415	1,471	1,529	1,589	1,652	1,717
1,191	1,237	1,286	1,336	1,388	1,442	1,498	1,557	1,618	1,681	1,746
1,216	1,263	1,312	1,363	1,415	1,470	1,527	1,585	1,647	1,710	1,776
1,243	1,290	1,339	1,390	1,443	1,498	1,555	1,615	1,676	1,740	1,806
1,269	1,317	1,367	1,418	1,471	1,527	1,584	1,644	1,706	1,770	1,837
1,296	1,344	1,395	1,447	1,500	1,556	1,614	1,647	1,737	1,801	1,868
1,324	1,373	1,423	1,476	1,530	1,586	1,645	1,705	1,768	1,833	1,900
1,352	1,401	1,452	1,505	1,560	1,617	1,675	1,736	1,799	1,865	1,933
1,418	1,431	1,482	1,535	1,591	1,648	1,707	1,768	1,832	1,897	1,966
1,411	1,461	1,513	1,566	1,622	1,679	1,739	1,801	1,864	1,931	1,999
1,441	1,491	1,544	1,598	1,654	1,712	1,772	1,834	1,898	1,964	2,033
1,472	1,523	1,575	1,630	1,686	1,744	1,805	1,867	1,932	1,999	2,068
1,503	1,555	1,608	1,663	1,719	1,778	1,839	1,902	1,966	2,034	2,103
1,535	1,587	1,641	1,696	1,753	1,812	1,873	1,936	2,002	2,069	2,139
1,568	1,620	1,674	1,730	1,788	1,847	1,908	1,972	2,038	2,105	2,175
1,602	1,654	1,709	1,765	1,823	1,882	1,944	2,008	2,074	2,142	2,212
1,636	1,689	1,744	1,800	1,858	1,919	1,981	2,045	2,111	2,180	2,250
1,671	1,724	1,779	1,836	1,895	1,956	2,018	2,082	2,149	2,218	2,289
1,707	1,760	1,816	1,873	1,932	1,993	2,056	2,121	2,188	2,256	2,328
1,743	1,797	1,853	1,911	1,970	2,031	2,094	2,160	2,227	2,296	2,367
1,780	1,835	1,891	1,949	2,009	2,070	2,134	2,199	2,267	2,336	2,408
1,819	1,873	1,930	1,988	2,048	2,110	2,174	2,240	2,307	2,377	2,449
1,857	1,913	1,970	2,028	2,089	2,151	2,215	2,281	2,348	2,418	2,490
1,897	1,953	2,010	2,069	2,130	2,192	2,256	2,322	2,391	2,461	2,533
1,938	1,994	2,051	2,110	2,171	2,234	2,299	2,365	2,433	2,504	2,576
1,979	2,035	2,093	2,153	2,214	2,277	2,342	2,408	2,477	2,547	2,620
2,021	2,078	2,136	2,196	2,196	2,321	2,386	2,453	2,521	2,592	2,665
2,065	2,122	2,180	2,240	2,302	2,365	2,431	2,498	2,566	2,637	2,710
2,109	2,166	2,225	2,285	2,347	2,411	2,476	2,543	2,612	2,683	2,756
2,154	2,211	2,270	2,331	2,393	2,457	2,523	2,590	2,659	2,730	2,803
2,200	2,258	2,317	2,378	2,440	2,504	2,570	2,638	2,707	2,778	2,851
2,247	2,305	2,365	2,426	2,488	2,553	2,618	2,686	2,755	2,827	2,899
2,295	2,353	2,413	2,474	2,537	2,602	2,668	2,735	2,805	2,876	2,949
2,344	2,403	2,463	2,524	2,587	2,652	2,718	2,785	2,855	2,926	2,999
2,394	2,453	2,513	2,575	2,638	2,702	2,769	2,837	2,906	2,977	3,050
2,446	2,504	2,565	2,626	2,690	2,754	2,821	2,889	2,958	3,029	3,102
2,498	2,557	2,617	2,679	2,743	2,807	2,874	2,942	3,011	3,082	3,155

(continued)

APPENDIX N. (Continued)

FL (mm)	AC (mm)									
	305	310	315	320	325	330	335	340	345	350
40	1,590	1,658	1,729	1,802	1,879	1,959	2,042	2,129	2,220	2,314
41	1,617	1,685	1,756	1,830	1,907	1,987	2,071	2,158	2,249	2,344
42	1,644	1,712	1,783	1,858	1,935	2,016	2,100	2,187	2,279	2,373
43	1,671	1,740	1,812	1,886	1,964	2,054	2,129	2,217	2,308	2,404
44	1,699	1,768	1,840	1,915	1,993	2,075	2,159	2,247	2,339	2,434
45	1,727	1,797	1,869	1,944	2,023	2,105	2,189	2,278	2,370	2,465
46	1,756	1,826	1,898	1,974	2,053	2,135	2,220	2,309	2,401	2,497
47	1,785	1,855	1,928	2,004	2,084	2,166	2,251	2,340	2,432	2,528
48	1,814	1,885	1,959	2,035	2,115	2,197	2,283	2,372	2,464	2,560
49	1,845	1,916	1,990	2,066	2,146	2,229	2,315	2,404	2,497	2,593
50	1,875	1,947	2,021	2,098	2,178	2,261	2,347	2,437	2,530	2,626
51	1,906	1,978	2,053	2,130	2,210	2,294	2,380	2,470	2,563	2,659
52	1,938	2,010	2,085	2,163	2,243	2,327	2,413	2,503	2,597	2,693
53	1,970	2,043	2,118	2,196	2,277	2,360	2,447	2,537	2,631	2,728
54	2,003	2,076	2,151	2,229	2,311	2,395	2,482	2,572	2,665	2,762
55	2,036	2,109	2,185	2,264	2,345	2,429	2,516	2,607	2,700	2,797
56	2,070	2,143	2,220	2,298	2,380	2,464	2,552	2,642	2,736	2,833
57	2,104	2,178	2,254	2,333	2,415	2,500	2,587	2,678	2,772	2,869
58	2,139	2,213	2,290	2,369	2,451	2,536	2,624	2,714	2,808	2,905
59	2,175	2,249	2,326	2,405	2,488	2,573	2,660	2,751	2,845	2,942
60	2,211	2,286	2,363	2,442	2,525	2,610	2,698	2,789	2,883	2,980
61	2,248	2,323	2,400	2,480	2,562	2,647	2,736	2,837	2,921	3,018
62	2,285	2,360	2,438	2,518	2,600	2,686	2,774	2,865	2,959	3,056
63	2,323	2,398	2,476	2,556	2,639	2,725	2,813	2,904	2,998	3,095
64	2,362	2,437	2,515	2,595	2,678	2,764	2,852	2,943	3,037	3,134
65	3,401	2,477	2,555	2,635	2,718	2,804	2,892	2,983	3,077	3,174
66	2,441	2,517	2,595	2,675	2,759	2,844	2,933	3,024	3,118	3,215
67	2,481	2,557	2,636	2,716	2,800	2,885	2,974	3,065	3,159	3,256
68	2,523	2,599	2,677	2,758	2,841	2,927	3,016	3,107	3,200	3,297
69	2,564	2,641	2,719	2,800	2,884	2,969	3,058	3,149	3,242	3,339
70	2,607	2,683	2,762	2,843	2,927	3,012	3,101	3,192	3,285	3,381
71	2,650	2,727	2,806	2,887	2,970	3,056	3,144	3,235	3,328	3,424
72	2,694	2,771	2,850	2,931	3,014	3,100	3,188	3,279	3,372	3,468
73	2,739	2,816	2,895	2,976	3,059	3,145	3,233	3,323	3,416	3,512
74	2,785	2,861	2,940	3,021	3,105	3,190	3,278	3,369	3,461	3,557
75	2,831	2,908	2,987	3,068	3,151	3,236	3,324	3,414	3,507	3,602
76	2,878	2,955	3,034	3,115	3,198	3,283	3,371	3,461	3,553	3,648
77	2,926	3,003	3,081	3,162	3,245	3,331	3,418	3,508	3,600	3,694
78	2,974	3,051	3,130	3,211	3,294	3,379	3,466	3,555	3,647	3,741
79	3,024	3,100	3,179	3,260	3,343	3,427	3,514	3,604	3,695	3,789
80	3,074	3,151	3,229	3,310	3,392	3,477	3,564	3,653	3,744	3,837
81	3,125	3,202	3,280	3,360	3,443	3,527	3,614	3,702	3,793	3,886
82	3,177	3,253	3,332	3,412	3,494	3,578	3,664	3,752	3,843	3,935
83	3,230	3,306	3,384	3,464	3,546	3,630	3,716	3,803	3,893	3,985

(continued)

◤◤◤◤ **APPENDIX N.** (Continued)

AC (mm)									
355	**360**	**365**	**370**	**375**	**380**	**385**	**390**	**395**	**400**
2,413	2,515	2,622	2,734	2,850	2,972	3,098	3,230	3,367	3,511
2,442	2,545	2,652	2,764	2,880	3,002	3,128	3,260	3,397	3,540
2,472	2,575	2,683	2,794	2,911	3,032	3,159	3,290	3,427	3,570
2,503	2,606	2,713	2,825	2,942	3,063	3,189	3,321	3,458	3,600
2,533	2,637	2,744	2,856	2,973	3,094	3,220	3,352	3,488	3,630
2,565	2,668	2,776	2,888	3,004	3,125	3,251	3,383	3,519	3,661
2,596	2,700	2,807	2,919	3,036	3,157	3,283	3,414	3,550	3,692
2,628	2,732	2,840	2,952	3,068	3,189	3,315	3,446	3,582	3,723
2,660	2,764	2,872	2,984	3,100	3,221	3,347	3,478	3,613	3,754
2,693	2,797	2,905	3,017	3,133	3,254	3,380	3,510	3,645	3,786
2,726	2,830	2,938	3,050	3,166	3,287	3,412	3,542	3,677	3,818
2,760	2,864	2,972	3,084	3,200	3,320	3,445	3,575	3,710	3,850
2,794	2,898	3,006	3,117	3,234	3,354	3,479	3,608	3,743	3,882
2,828	2,932	3,040	3,152	3,268	3,388	3,513	3,642	3,776	3,915
2,863	2,967	3,075	3,186	3,302	3,422	3,547	3,676	3,809	3,948
2,898	3,002	3,110	3,221	3,337	3,457	3,581	3,710	3,843	3,981
2,933	3,038	3,145	3,257	3,372	3,492	3,616	3,744	3,877	4,015
2,970	3,074	3,181	3,293	3,408	3,572	3,651	3,779	3,911	4,048
3,006	3,110	3,218	3,329	3,444	3,563	3,686	3,814	3,946	4,082
3,043	3,147	3,254	3,366	3,480	3,599	3,722	3,849	3,981	4,117
3,080	3,184	3,292	3,403	3,517	3,636	3,758	3,885	4,016	4,151
3,118	3,222	3,329	3,440	3,554	3,673	3,795	3,921	4,052	4,186
3,157	3,260	3,367	3,478	3,592	3,710	3,832	3,957	4,087	4,222
3,195	3,299	3,406	3,516	3,630	3,747	3,869	3,994	4,124	4,257
3,235	3,338	3,445	3,555	3,668	3,785	3,906	4,031	4,160	4,293
3,274	3,378	3,484	3,594	3,707	3,824	3,944	4,069	4,197	4,329
3,315	3,418	3,524	3,633	3,746	3,863	3,983	4,106	4,234	4,366
3,355	3,458	3,564	3,673	3,786	3,902	4,021	4,144	4,271	4,402
3,397	3,499	3,605	3,714	3,862	3,941	4,060	4,183	4,309	4,439
3,438	3,541	3,646	3,754	3,866	3,981	4,100	4,222	4,347	4,477
3,481	3,583	3,688	3,796	3,907	4,022	4,140	4,261	4,386	4,514
3,523	3,625	3,730	3,838	3,948	4,062	4,180	4,300	4,425	4,552
3,567	3,668	3,772	3,880	3,990	4,104	4,220	4,340	4,464	4,591
3,610	3,712	3,816	3,922	4,032	4,145	4,261	4,381	4,503	4,629
3,655	3,756	3,859	3,966	4,075	4,187	4,303	4,421	4,543	4,668
3,700	3,800	3,903	4,009	4,118	4,230	4,344	4,462	4,583	4,708
3,745	3,845	3,948	4,053	4,161	4,272	4,387	4,504	4,624	4,747
3,791	3,891	3,993	4,098	4,205	4,316	4,429	4,545	4,665	4,787
3,838	3,937	4,039	4,143	4,250	4,360	4,472	4,588	4,706	4,827
3,885	3,984	4,085	4,188	4,295	4,404	4,515	4,630	4,748	4,868
3,933	4,031	4,131	4,234	4,340	4,448	4,559	4,673	4,790	4,909
3,981	4,079	4,179	4,281	4,386	4,493	4,604	4,716	4,832	4,950
4,030	4,127	4,226	4,328	4,432	4,539	4,648	4,760	4,875	4,992
4,080	4,176	4,275	4,376	4,479	4,585	4,693	4,804	4,918	5,034

* Based on regression model: $\log_{10}$ body weight = 1.3598 + 0.051 (AC) + 0.1844 (FL) − 0.0037 (AC × FL).
  (From Hadlock FP, Harrist RB, Carpenter RJ, et al. Sonographic estimation of fetal weight: The value of femur length
in addition to head and abdomen measurements. Radiology. 1984;150:535–540. Used by permission.)

APPENDIX O. MEAN RENAL LENGTHS FOR VARIOUS GESTATIONAL AGES

Gestational Age (weeks)	Mean Length (mm)	95% CI Confidence Limit (mm)
18	22	16–28
19	23	15–31
20	26	18–34
21	27	21–32
22	27	20–34
23	30	22–37
24	31	19–44
25	33	25–42
26	34	24–44
27	35	27–44
28	34	26–42
29	36	23–48
30	38	29–46
31	37	28–46
32	41	31–51
33	40	31–47
34	42	33–50
35	42	32–52
36	42	33–50
37	42	33–51
38	44	32–56
39	42	35–48
40	43	32–53
41	45	39–51

(From Cohen HL, Cooper J, Eisenberg P, et al. Normal length of fetal kidneys: Sonographic study in 397 obstetric patients. Am J Roentgenol. 1991;157:545–548.)

APPENDIX P. FETAL CARDIAC MEASUREMENT TABLE

| | Linear Increase (mm) From 17 to 40 Weeks | | |
	17 Weeks	40 Weeks	Range From 5th to 95th Percentile
Left ventricle*	4	16	±1.7
Right ventricle*	4	19	±1.8
Left atrium†	4	16	±1.9
Right atrium†	6	16	±1.5
Aortic root	2.4	10	±1.3

* Measurements taken in end-diastole at the tips of the atrioventricular valves just prior to closure in a plane perpendicular to the interventricular septum.

† Measurements obtained in end-systole just after atrioventricular valve closure using widest visible internal diameter in a plane perpendicular to the interatrial septum.

(From Shime J, Gresser RN, Rakowski H. Quantitative two-dimensional echocardiographic assessment of fetal cardiac growth. Am J Obstet Gynecol. 1986;154:294–300.)

APPENDIX Q. REFERENCE VALUES FOR A/B RATIO IN THE UMBILICAL ARTERY

A/B Ratio (Gestation)	10%	50%	90%
16	3.01	4.25	6.07
20	3.16	4.04	5.24
24	2.7	3.5	4.75
28	2.41	3.02	3.97
30	2.43	3.04	3.8
32	2.27	2.73	3.57
34	2.08	2.52	3.41
36	1.96	2.35	3.15
38	1.89	2.24	3.1
40	1.88	2.22	2.68
41	1.93	2.21	2.55
42	1.91	2.51	3.21

(From Fogarty P, Beattie B, Harper A, et al. Continuous wave Doppler flow velocity waveforms from the umbilical artery in normal pregnancy. J Perinat Med. 1990;18:51–54.)

▰▰▰ APPENDIX R. AMNIOTIC FLUID INDEX (AFI) VALUES IN NORMAL PREGNANCY (IN CENTIMETERS)

Week	AFI Percentile Values		
	5th	50th	95
16	7.9	12.1	18.5
17	8.3	12.7	19.4
18	8.7	13.3	20.2
19	9.0	13.7	20.7
20	9.3	14.1	21.2
21	9.5	14.3	21.4
22	9.7	14.5	21.6
23	9.8	14.6	21.8
24	9.8	14.7	21.9
36	7.7	13.8	24.9
37	7.5	13.5	24.4
38	7.3	13.2	23.9
39	7.2	12.7	22.6
40	7.1	12.3	21.4
41	7.0	11.6	19.4
42	6.9	11.0	17.5

Note: The clinical validity of this table in the detection of oligohydramnios and polyhydramnios has not been fully established. Therefore, while an AFI can be stated, the ultrasound diagnosis of normal, increased, or decreased fluid should rest with the observer's subjective analysis.

(From Moore TR, Cayle JE. The amniotic fluid index in normal human pregnancy. Am J Obstet Gynecol. 1990;162:1168–1173).

Index

685